W9-CCK-553

# ■ MOLECULAR BASIS OF CARDIOVASCULAR DISEASE

## Second Edition

■ ■ ■ A Companion to Braunwald's Heart Disease

**KENNETH R. CHIEN, MD, PhD**

Director, Institute of Molecular Medicine

Professor, UCSD Department of Medicine and the Salk Institute (Adjunct)

American Heart Association Endowed Chair

La Jolla, California 92093

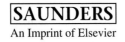

**SAUNDERS**

An Imprint of Elsevier

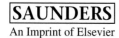

An Imprint of Elsevier

170 S Independence Mall W 300 E
Philadelphia, PA 19106-3399

Molecular Basis of Cardiovascular Disease:
A Companion to Braunwald's Heart Disease

ISBN 0-7216-9428-4

---

**NOTICE**

Medicine is an ever-changing field. Standard safety precautions must be followed, but as new research
and clinical experience broaden our knowledge, changes in treatment and drug therapy may become
necessary or appropriate. Readers are advised to check the most current product information provided
by the manufacturer of each drug to be administered to verify the recommended dose, the method and
duration of administration, and contraindications. It is the responsibility of the treating physician,
relying on experience and knowledge of the patient, to determine dosages and the best treatment for
each individual patient. Neither the publisher nor the editor assumes any liability for any injury and/or
damage to persons or property arising from this publication.

The Publisher

---

Previous edition copyrighted 1999

**Library of Congress Cataloging-in-Publication Data**

Molecular basis of cardiovascular disease: a companion to Braunwald's heart disease /
[edited by] Kenneth R. Chien - 2nd ed.
p. ; cm.
Includes bibliographical references and index.
ISBN 0-7216-9428-4
1. Heart–Diseases–Molecular aspects. I. Chien, Kenneth R. II. Heart disease.
[DNLM: 1. Cardiovascular Diseases–genetics. 2. Molecular Biology. WG 120 M7173 2004]
RC682.9.M64 2004
616.1'07–dc21                                            2003054301

*Editor:* Anne Lenehan
*Editorial Assistant:* Vera Ginsburgs
*Production Manager:* Mary Stermel

Printed in the United States of America

Last digit is the print number:   9   8   7   6   5   4   3   2   1

To my family: Pat, Marisa, and Elena.

The very substantial advances in the diagnosis and management of patients with cardiovascular diseases represent one of the medical triumphs of the last half century. These great strides have been based on solid foundations of cardiovascular physiology and pharmacology, and on the clinical applications of bioengineering. Notable examples include the development of a variety of accurate invasive and non-invasive diagnostic techniques, several classes of drugs that have profoundly beneficial effects on patients with cardiovascular disease, as well as open heart surgery, percutaneous catheter-based coronary revascularization, artificial cardiac valves, cardiac pacemakers, and internal cardioverter-defibrillators. These have prolonged and improved the quality of the lives of millions of persons world-wide.

However, despite these impressive advances, cardiovascular diseases still remain the most common fatal and disabling disorders in industrialized nations and are projected soon to be so on a world-wide basis. Clearly, bold new approaches to solving the problems posed by these conditions are still needed. There is a growing consensus that just as the first wave of advances was based largely on the applications of physiology, pharmacology, and bioengineering, the next wave is exploring the new biologic sciences—molecular biology, genetics and cell biology. Because most cardiovascular disorders now appear to have a molecular basis, it is clear that appropriate preventive or therapeutic strategies will require an understanding of the molecular pathology.

Kenneth Chien has enlisted a team of distinguished experts to produce the second edition of *Molecular Basis of Heart Disease,* a superb book that provides an up-to-date picture of the impact that the new biology will have on cardiovascular disease. In the first section they provide the background in genetics as well as molecular and cell biology required to apply these sciences to the study of a variety of cardiovascular disorders. They then go on to demonstrate how the new molecular techniques can be applied to understanding disorders of cardiovascular structure such as congenital heart disease, ventricular hypertrophy, heart failure, and arrhythmias. The molecular bases of atherogenesis, thrombosis, and angiogenesis are carefully considered.

This second edition of *Molecular Basis of Heart Disease* is totally revised and expanded and is even better than the first edition. Many of the authors and chapters are new to this edition. It is filled with important new concepts and explanations which are clearly presented. This book should serve as an especially important resource, not only to scientists and trainees in this rapidly growing field, but also to clinical cardiologists who wish to understand the biologic principles underlying cardiovascular disease. It is a most fitting companion to *Heart Disease: A Textbook of Cardiovascular Medicine.*

Eugene Braunwald, MD
Boston, MA

## A DECADE FULL OF DREAMS

*"There's a man who's been out sailing*
*In a decade full of dreams..."*
—Joni Mitchell (from "Cactus Tree")

For all of us in the field of molecular cardiology, this has indeed been a decade full of dreams. Over the past 10 years, cardiovascular medicine has fully embraced the tools of modern molecular biology, in effect creating a bridge between the traditional physiological and clinical discipline of cardiology and genetics, genomics, and biotechnology. Since the previous edition of MCVD, there has been a widespread appreciation of the power of new advances in genetically engineered animal models and novel strategies for rapidly identifying mutations in candidate human genes for diverse cardiovascular diseases, both of which have led to an exponential increase in our understanding of the molecular mechanisms that drive disease progression. In addition, a handful of new therapies have been approved that represent the direct fruits of biotechnology and rational drug design, including second generation thrombolytic agents, novel platelet antagonists, new anti-thrombins, and brain natriuretic factor therapy for acute, decompensated heart failure. A host of new prognostic and diagnostic markers for cardiovascular disease have also been developed, including BNP for heart failure and CRP as a powerful independent risk factor for acute coronary events. Finally, the first example of hybrid therapy at the interface of device technology and biotechnology has been provided by the approval of rapamycin coated stents, an outcome of earlier experimental studies that documented the utility of rapamycin to inhibit intimal proliferation in the setting of coronary restenosis. In short, the promise of molecular biology is starting to be realized by practicing cardiologists and their patients. The hope is that this new edition of MCVD captures the excitement in the field of molecular cardiology and is of value to the growing syncytium of physicians, molecular biologists, physiologists, geneticists, engineers, and biotech professionals during this exciting new era of scientific discovery in cardiovascular medicine.

In this regard, this new edition includes a number of new chapters, which highlight new technology that will probably have an impact on cardiovascular medicine within this decade. The genome databases of all creatures great and small are breaking down the barriers between fields, an opportunity created by the wonderful tools and model organisms that connect genes with biological function. New advances in cardiovascular signaling, stem cell biology, gene therapy, genome technology, model organisms, and human genetics are highlighted by several leaders in the field. In each chapter, direct examples of the potential of these technologies for cardiovascular medicine are provided. In addition, all of the chapters have been updated with comprehensive references, color figures, and new tables. Finally, many of the chapters contain an "Editor's Choice" section in the references, which lists recent papers of interest to readers with specialized interests in the particular subject area.

In many ways, the production of a text of this scope in a rapidly changing field is akin to "sailing" through the perfect storm. If it not were for the steadfast support of an experienced crew, this edition of MCVD would not have been possible. In particular, Anne Lenahan provided invaluable assistance as the Managing Editor of MCVD at Elsevier. We are especially grateful to Vera Ginsburgs at Elsevier and to Virginia McIlwain, who served as the Editorial Assistant at UCSD, who routinely kept the boat afloat when it often appeared that it was about to capsize. As ever, Gene Braunwald provided the necessary long-range vision, inspiration, and guidance to ensure that

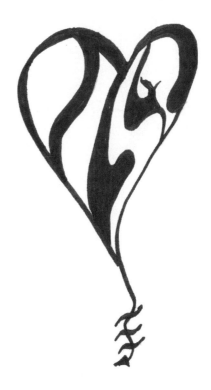

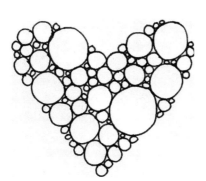

MCVD would stay on a course that would allow integration with his seminal text, "Heart Disease". Finally, I am indebted to my family, Pat, Marisa, and Elena, for their support and understanding during the long course of preparation of this text, and also for their artwork.

As we enter this "decade full of dreams," perhaps it is time to reflect on the future of molecular cardiology as a field. Although there may be some who view the molecular biology of the cardiovascular system as a separate field of cardiovascular science and medicine, my personal viewpoint is that it will rapidly become fully integrated with clinical cardiology in this decade. In the coming years, much of the work that is outlined in the current edition of MCVD may simply be viewed as part of the mainstream of cardiology itself as it becomes an essential part of the practice of cardiovascular medicine. Ironically, the value of MCVD may ultimately be to accelerate the integration of the principles, technology, and therapeutic potential of molecular cardiology into the mainstream texts of clinical cardiology, leading to a less compelling need for future editions of this and other specialized texts of molecular cardiology. In short, we are entering a new era in cardiovascular medicine, where biologically targeted therapy is positioned to replace the halfway technology that forms the cornerstone of most of our current clinical practice. Perhaps Lewis Thomas, the leader of an earlier generation of physician scientists, stated this concept most eloquently in this excerpt, which reflects on the merits of developing an artificial heart:

*"Halfway technology represents the kinds of things that must be done after the fact, in efforts to compensate for the incapacitating effects of certain diseases whose course one is unable to do very much about. By its nature, it is at the same time highly sophisticated and profoundly primitive... It is characteristic of this kind of technology that it costs an enormous amount of money and requires a continuing expansion of hospital facilities... It is when physicians are bogged down by their incomplete technologies, by the innumerable things they are obliged to do in medicine, when they lack a clear understanding of disease mechanisms, that the deficiencies of the health-care system are most conspicuous... The only thing that can move medicine away from this level of technology is new information, and the only imaginable source of this information is research. The real high technology of medicine comes as the result of a genuine understanding of disease mechanisms and when it becomes available, it is relatively inexpensive, relatively simple, and relatively easy to deliver...*

*I conclude that the greatest potential value of the successful artificial heart is, or ought to be, its power to convince the government as well as the citizenry at large that the nation simply must invest more money in basic biomedical research. We do not really understand the underlying mechanism of cardiomyopathies at all, and we are not much better off at comprehending the biochemical events that disable the heart muscle or its valves in other more common illnesses. But there are clues enough to raise the spirits of people in a good many basic science disciplines, and any number of engrossing questions are at hand awaiting answers."*

—Lewis Thomas (From *Lives of a Cell*)

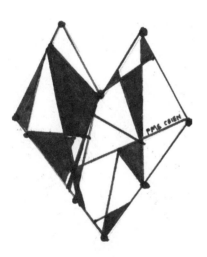

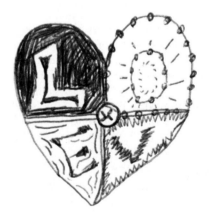

**Michael J. Ackerman, MD, PhD**
Assistant Professor of Medicine, Pediatrics, and Molecular Pharmacology; Director, Long QT Syndrome Clinic and Sudden Death Genomics Laboratory; Department of Medicine and Pediatrics, Mayo Clinic/ Mayo Foundation, Rochester, Minnesota
*Excitability and Conduction*

**Hiroshi Ashikaga, MD**
Institute of Molecular Medicine, University of California— San Diego, La Jolla, California; Division of Cardiology, UCSD Medical Center, San Diego, California
*Biotechnology and Cardiovascular Medicine: Recombinant Protein Therapy; Coronary Restenosis; Blood Coagulation and Atherothrombosis*

**Antonio Baldini, MD**
Associate Professor, Department of Pediatrics (Cardiology), Baylor College of Medicine, Associate, Department of Cardiology, Texas Children's Hospital, Houston, Texas
*Pharyngeal Apparatus and Cardiac Neural Crest Defects*

**Craig T. Basson, MD, PhD**
Associate Professor, Department of Medicine; Director, Molecular Cardiology Laboratory, Cell and Developmental Biology, Weill Medical College of Cornell University; Associate Attending Physician, Department of Medicine, The New York Presbyterian Hospital, New York, New York
*Genetic Approaches to Cardiovascular Disease*

**Ori Ben-Yehuda, MD, FACC**
Assistant Professor of Medicine, Department of Medicine, University of California—San Diego, La Jolla, California; Director, Coronary Care Unit, Division of Cardiology, UCSD Medical Center, San Diego, California
*Biotechnology and Cardiovascular Medicine: Recombinant Protein Therapy; Coronary Restenosis; Platelets and Antiplatelet Therapy in Cardiovascular Disease: Molecular Mechanisms*

**Joan Heller Brown, PhD**
Professor and Interim Chair, Department of Pharmacology, University of California—San Diego, La Jolla, California
*Cardiovascular Signaling Pathways*

**Roger W. Brown, MA, BM, BCh, MRCP, PhD**
Senior Lecturer in Medicine, Molecular Medicine Centre, School of Molecular and Clinical Medicine, Western General Hospital, University of Edinburgh; Honorary Consultant Physician, Metabolic Unit, Department of Medicine, Western General Hospital, Edinburgh, Scotland, United Kingdom
*Mechanisms and Molecular Pathways in Hypertension*

**Kevin P. Campbell, PhD**
Professor and Chair, Department of Physiology and Biophysics, University of Iowa; Investigator, Howard Hughes Medical Institute, Iowa City, Iowa
*Molecular Pathways for Dilated Cardiomyopathy*

**Ju Chen, PhD**
Assistant Professor, Department of Medicine, Institute of Molecular Medicine, University of California—San Diego, La Jolla, California
*Mouse Models of Human Cardiovascular Disease*

**Kenneth R. Chien, MD, PhD**
Director, Institute of Molecular Medicine; Professor, UCSD Department of Medicine and the Salk Institute (Adjunct); American Heart Association Endowed Chair, La Jolla, California
*Biotechnology and Cardiovascular Medicine: Recombinant Protein Therapy; Generation and Cloning of Genetically Modified Animals; Mouse Models of Human Cardiovascular Disease; Toward Stem Cell Therapy; Development of Cardiac Pacemaking and Conduction System Lineages; Cardiac Laterality and Congenital Heart Disease; Molecular Pathways for Cardiac Hypertrophy and Heart Failure Progression; Coronary Restenosis; Blood Coagulation and Atherothrombosis*

**Geir Christensen, MD, PhD**
Director of Molecular Cardiology, Institute for Experimental Medical Research, Ullevål University Hospital, Oslo, Norway
*Mouse Models of Human Cardiovascular Disease*

**David E. Clapham, MD, PhD**
Aldo R. Castaneda Professor of Cardiovascular Research, Department of Cardiology, Children's Hospital; Department of Neurobiology, Harvard Medical School, Howard Hughes Medical Institute/Children's Hospital of Boston, Boston, Massachusetts
*Excitability and Conduction*

**Ronald D. Cohn, MD**
Johns Hopkins Hospital Children's Center; McKusick-Nathans Institute of Genetic Medicine, Baltimore, Maryland
*Molecular Pathways for Dilated Cardiomyopathy*

**Leon J. De Windt, PhD**
Assistant Professor, Hubrecht Laboratory and Interuniversity Cardiology Institute Netherlands, Royal Netherlands Academy of Arts and Sciences, Utrecht, The Netherlands
*Generation and Cloning of Genetically Modified Animals*

**Pieter A. Doevendans, MD, PhD**
Associate Professor, Department of Cardiology, Utrecht University; Cardiologist, Department of Cardiology, Heart Lung Center Utrecht; Interuniversity Cardiology Institute of the Netherlands, Utrecht, The Netherlands
*Generation and Cloning of Genetically Modified Animals; Toward Stem Cell Therapy*

**Hervé Duplain, MD**
Postdoctoral Fellow, Department of Medicine, Division of Cardiology, University of California—San Diego, La Jolla, California
*Viral Infections of the Heart*

**Victor J. Dzau, MD**
Hersey Professor of the Theory and Practice of Physic, Harvard Medical School; Chairman, Department of Medicine, Brigham and Women's Hospital, Boston, Massachusetts
*Human Genome Project and Cardiovascular Disease Genes*

**Mark C. Fishman, MD**
Chief Executive Officer, Novartis Institutes for Biomedical Research, Cambridge, Massachusetts
*Model Organisms for Cardiac Disease Gene Discovery*

**Judah Folkman, MD**
Andrus Professor of Pediatric Surgery, Professor of Cell Biology, Department of Surgery, Harvard Medical School; Director, Surgical Research Laboratory, Department of Surgery, Children's Hospital, Boston, Massachusetts
*Angiogenesis in Cardiovascular Disease*

**Christopher K. Glass, MD, PhD**
Professor of Cellular and Molecular Medicine, Professor of Medicine, Department of Cellular and Molecular Medicine, School of Medicine, University of California—San Diego, La Jolla, California
*Lipoprotein Oxidation, Macrophages, Immunity, and Atherogenesis*

**Steve A. N. Goldstein, MA, MD, PhD**
Professor of Pediatrics and Cellular and Molecular Physiology; Chief, Section of Developmental Biology and Biophysics; Member, Boyer Center for Molecular Medicine, Department of Pediatrics, Yale University School of Medicine, Yale-New Haven Hospital, New Haven, Connecticut
*Cardiac Arrhythmias: Inherited Molecular Mechanisms*

**Robert G. Gourdie, PhD**
Associate Professor, Department of Cell Biology and Anatomy, Medical University of South Carolina, Charleston, South Carolina
*Development of Cardiac Pacemaking and Conduction System Lineages*

**Robert M. Graham, FAA, MD**
Professor and Executive Director, Victor Chang Cardiac Research Institute, Sydney, New South Wales, Australia
*Molecular Targets of Antihypertensive Drug Therapy*

**Göran K. Hansson, MD, PhD**
Professor, Center for Molecular Medicine, Department of Medicine, Karolinska Institute, Stockholm, Sweden
*Inflammation and Immunity in Atherogenesis*

**Stephen Heinemann, PhD**
Salk Institute Council Professor in Genetics, Molecular Neurobiology Laboratory, The Salk Institute La Jolla, California
*Molecular Basis for the Potential Use of NMDA Receptor Open-Channel Blockers in the Treatment of Cerebral Ischemia and Other Brain Insults*

**Patrick Hildbrand, MD**
Research Associate, Cardiac Transplant Research Laboratory; Cardiology Fellow, Swiss Cardiovascular Center Bern, Cardiology; University Hospital Bern, Bern, Switzerland
*Molecular Biology of Transplantation and Xenotransplantation*

**Masahiko Hoshijima, MD, PhD**
Assistant Project Scientist, Institute of Molecular Medicine, Department of Medicine, University of California—San Diego, La Jolla, California
*Molecular Pathways for Cardiac Hypertrophy and Heart Failure Progression*

**Ahsan Husain, PhD**
Professor and Deputy Director, Victor Chang Cardiac Research Institute, Sydney, New South Wales, Australia
*Molecular Targets of Antihypertensive Drug Therapy*

**Juan Carlos Izpisua-Belmonte, PhD**
Adjunct Professor, University of California—San Diego; Professor, Gene Expression Laboratory, The Salk Institute for Biological Studies, La Jolla, California
*Cardiac Laterality and Congenital Heart Disease*

**Michael Karin, PhD**
Professor of Pharmacology, American Cancer Society Research Professor, Department of Pharmacology, University of California—San Diego, La Jolla, California
*Cardiovascular Signaling Pathways*

**Mark T. Keating, MD**
Professor, Department of Cell Biology, Harvard Medical School; Senior Associate, Department of Cardiology, Children's Hospital; Investigator, Howard Hughes Medical Institute, Boston, Massachusetts
*Cardiac Arrhythmias: Inherited Molecular Mechanisms*

**Kirk U. Knowlton, MD**
Associate Professor of Medicine, Department of Medicine, Division of Cardiology, University of California—San Diego, La Jolla, California
*Viral Infections of the Heart*

**Steven W. Kubalak, PhD**
Associate Professor, Department of Cell Biology and Anatomy, Cardiovascular Developmental Biology Center, Medical University of South Carolina, Charleston, South Carolina
*Development of Cardiac Pacemaking and Conduction System Lineages*

**Peter Libby, MD**
Mallinckrodt Professor of Medicine, Harvard Medical School; Chief, Cardiovascular Medicine, Department of Medicine, Brigham and Women's Hospital, Boston, Massachusetts
*Inflammation and Immunity in Atherogenesis*

**Choong-Chin Liew, PhD**
Visiting Professor of Medicine, Harvard Medical School; Director, Cardiovascular Genome Unit, Brigham and Women's Hospital, Boston, Massachusetts; Professor of Clinical Biochemistry and Medicine, Laboratory Medicine and Pathobiology, University of Toronto, Toronto, Ontario, Canada.
*Human Genome Project and Cardiovascular Disease Genes*

**Roger Lijnen, PhD**
Professor, Department of Molecular and Cardiovascular Research, University of Leuven, Leuven, Belgium
*Thrombosis and Thrombolytic Therapy*

**Stuart A. Lipton, MD, PhD**
Professor and Scientific Director, Center for Neuroscience and Aging, The Burnham Institute; Professor Neurosciences, Department of Neurology and Neuroscience, Department of Psychiatry, University of California—San Diego; Adjunct Professor, Department of Molecular Neurobiology, The Salk Institute for Biological Studies; Adjunct Professor, Department of Neuropharmacology, Department of Molecular Medicine, The Scripps Research Institute, La Jolla, California
*Molecular Basis for the Potential Use of NMDA Receptor Open-Channel Blockers in the Treatment of Cerebral Ischemia and Other Brain Insults*

**Calum A. MacRae, MB, ChB**
Instructor, Department of Medicine, Harvard Medical School; Assistant in Medicine, Cardiology Division and Cardiovascular Research Center, Massachusetts General Hospital, Boston, Massachusetts
*Model Organisms for Cardiac Disease Gene Discovery*

**Takashi Mikawa, PhD**
Joseph C. Hinsey Professor, Department of Cell and Developmental Biology, Cornell University Medical College, New York, New York
*Development of Cardiac Pacemaking and Conduction System Lineages*

**Susumu Minamisawa, MD**
Assistant Professor, Department of Physiology, Yokohama City University, Yokohama, Japan
*Molecular Pathways for Cardiac Hypertrophy and Heart Failure Progression*

**Vincent Mooser, MD**
Director, Medical Genetics (Cardiovascular), Department of Genetic Research, GlaxoSmithKline, King of Prussia, Pennsylvania
*Molecular Biology of Lipoproteins and Dyslipidemias*

**Karen S. Moulton, MD**
Instructor, Department of Medicine, Harvard Medical School; Associate Physician, Cardiovascular Division, Brigham and Women's Hospital; Research Associate, Department of Surgery, Children's Hospital, Boston, Massachusetts
*Angiogenesis in Cardiovascular Disease*

**John Mullins, BSc., PhD**
Professor, Wellcome Trust Principal Research Fellow, Department of Medical and Radiological Science, University of Edinburgh, Edinburgh, Scotland, United Kingdom
*Mechanisms and Molecular Pathways in Hypertension*

**Christine L. Mummery, PhD**
Senior Staff Scientist/Group Leader, Hubrecht Laboratory, Netherlands Institute of Developmental Biology; ICIN Professor of Developmental Biology of the Heart, Interuniversity Cardiology Institute of The Netherlands, Utrecht, The Netherlands
*Toward Stem Cell Therapy*

**Elizabeth G. Nabel, MD**
Scientific Director, Clinical Research, National Heart, Lung, and Blood Institute, National Institutes of Health, Bethesda, Maryland
*Gene Transfer Approaches for Cardiovascular Disease*

**Terrence X. O'Brien, MD, FACC**
Associate Professor of Medicine, Department of Medicine and Cardiology; Director of Cardiovascular Clinical Research, Medical University of South Carolina; Director of Echocardiography, Department of Medicine and Cardiology, Veterans Affairs Medical Center, Charleston, South Carolina
*Development of Cardiac Pacemaking and Conduction System Lineages*

**Eric N. Olson, PhD**
Professor and Chairman, Department of Molecular Biology, University of Texas Southwestern Medical Center, Dallas, Texas
*Cardiac Development and Congenital Heart Disease*

**Hans Pannekoek, PhD**
Professor, Department of Biochemistry, Academic Medical Center, University of Amsterdam, Amsterdam, The Netherlands
*Thrombosis and Thrombolytic Therapy*

**Jordan S. Pober, MD, PhD**
Professor, Department of Pathology, Immunobiology, and Dermatology; Director, Interdepartmental Program in Vascular Biology and Transplantation, Yale University School of Medicine, New Haven, Connecticut
*Inflammation and Immunity in Atherogenesis*

**Ángel Raya, MD, PhD**
Research Associate, Gene Expression Laboratory, The Salk Institute for Biological Studies, La Jolla, California
*Cardiac Laterality and Congenital Heart Disease*

**John Ross Jr., MD**
Research Professor of Medicine, School of Medicine, Department of Medicine, Institute of Molecular Medicine, University of California—San Diego, La Jolla, California
*Mouse Models of Human Cardiovascular Disease*

**Pilar Ruiz-Lozano, PhD**
Assistant Project Scientist, Institute of Molecular Medicine, University of California—San Diego, La Jolla, California
*Cardiac Laterality and Congenital Heart Disease*

**Daniel R. Salomon, MD**
Associate Professor, Department of Molecular and Experimental Medicine, The Scripps Research Institute; Director, Center for Organ and Cell Transplantation, Department of Surgery, Scripps Health, Green Hospital, La Jolla, California
*Molecular Biology of Transplantation and Xenotransplantation*

**Michael C. Sanguinetti, PhD**
Professor, Department of Physiology, University of Utah, Salt Lake City, Utah
*Cardiac Arrhythmias: Inherited Molecular Mechanisms*

**Joachim P. Schmitt, MD**
Research Associate Department of Genetics, Harvard Medical School, Boston, Massachusetts
*Monogenic Causes of Congenital Heart Disease*

**Christine E. Seidman, MD**
Professor of Medicine and Genetics, Department of Genetics, Harvard Medical School; Director, Cardiovascular Genetics Center, Department of Medicine, Cardiovascular Division; Investigator, Howard Hughes Medical Institute, Boston, Massachusetts
*Monogenic Causes of Congenital Heart Disease; Molecular Genetics of Inherited Cardiomyopathies*

**Jonathan Seidman, PhD**
Henrietta and Frederick Bugher Professor of Cardiovascular Genetics, Department of Genetics, Harvard Medical School; Investigator, Howard Hughes Medical Institute, Boston, Massachusetts
*Molecular Genetics of Inherited Cardiomyopathies*

**Christopher Semsarian, MB, BS, PhD, FRACP**
Head, Molecular Cardiology Laboratory, Centenary Institute, University of Sydney; Cardiologist, Department of Cardiology, Royal Prince Alfred Hospital, Sydney, New South Wales, Australia
*Molecular Genetics of Inherited Cardiomyopathies*

**Deepak Srivastava, MD**
Associate Professor, Joel B. Steinberg Chair in Pediatrics, Departments of Pediatrics and Molecular Biology, University of Texas Southwestern Medical Center; Staff Pediatric Cardiologist, Department of Pediatrics, Children's Medical Center of Dallas, Dallas, Texas
*Cardiac Development and Congenital Heart Disease*

**Daniel Steinberg, MD, PhD**
Research Professor, Department of Medicine, University of California—San Diego, La Jolla, California
*Lipoprotein Oxidation, Macrophages, Immunity, and Atherogenesis*

**Susan F. Steinberg, MD**
Associate Professor, Department of Pharmacology and Medicine, Columbia University, New York, New York
*Cardiovascular Signaling Pathways*

**Ira Tabas, MD, PhD**
Professor, Department of Medicine, Department of Cell Biology, Columbia University, New York, New York
*Cellular Cholesterol Metabolism in Health and Disease*

**Sotirios Tsimikas, MD, FACC, FAHA**
Director, Vascular Medicine; Associate Professor of Medicine, Department of Medicine, University of California—San Diego, La Jolla, California
*Molecular Biology of Lipoproteins and Dyslipidemias; Lipoprotein Oxidation, Macrophages, Immunity, and Atherogenesis*

**Carl J. Vaughan, MD**
David S. Blumenthal Assistant Professor of Medicine, Department of Medicine, Weill Medical College of Cornell University; Assistant Attending Physician, Department of Medicine, The New York Presbyterian Hospital, New York, New York
*Genetic Approaches to Cardiovascular Disease*

**Jos Vermylen, MD, PhD**
Professor of Medicine, Center for Molecular and Vascular Biology, University of Leuven; Department Head, Department of Bleeding and Vascular Disorders, University Hospital Gasthuisberg, Leuven, Belgium
*Thrombosis and Thrombolytic Therapy*

**David Webb, MD, DSc, FRCP**
Professor of Clinical Pharmacology, Clinical Research Centre, Western General Hospital, University of Edinburgh, Edinburgh, Scotland, United Kingdom
*Mechanisms and Molecular Pathways in Hypertension*

**Ed Willems, PhD**
Professor, Victor Chang Cardiac Research Institute, Sydney, New South Wales, Australia
*Molecular Targets of Antihypertensive Drug Therapy*

**Joseph L. Witztum, MD**
Professor of Medicine; Director, SCOR in Molecular Medicine and Atherosclerosis, University of California—San Diego, La Jolla, California
*Lipoprotein Oxidation, Macrophages, Immunity, and Atherogenesis*

**Hideo Yasukawa, MD, PhD**
Assistant Professor, Cardiovascular Research Institute and the Third Department of Medicine, Kurume University, Kurume, Fukuoka, Japan
*Molecular Pathways for Cardiac Hypertrophy and Heart Failure Progression*

# CONTENTS

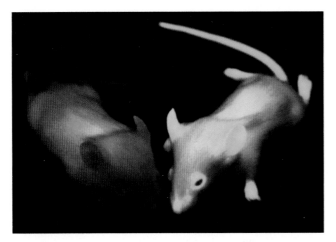

**FIGURE 4-1.** Green Fluorescent Protein (GFP) transgenic mice. GFP is responsible for the green bioluminescence of the jellyfish *Aequoria Victoria*. Transgenic mice were generated with an enhanced GFP cDNA under the control of a chicken beta-actin promoter and cytomegalovirus enhancer. All of the tissue from these eGFP transgenic mice, except for the hair and erythrocytes, were green under excitation light. The fluorescent nature of these cells from these eGFP transgenic mice would facilitate their use in many kinds of transplantation experiments. Also see the web site of these mice (http://kumikae01. gen-info.osaka-u.ac.jp/greenmouse.cfm).

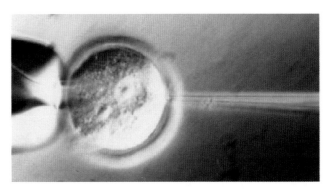

**FIGURE 4-3.** Microinjection of a fertilized mouse egg. The oocyte is held under suspension, free of underlying support, with a holding pipette, and the DNA suspension is injected into the male pronucleus with a microneedle.

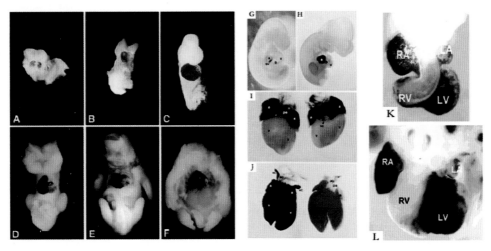

**FIGURE 4-4.** *(Left panel)* Whole mount staining of representative HF-1 LacZ transgenic embryos, using part of the MLC2v promoter driving LacZ expression. E 7-7.5. Late headfold stage/early foregut pocket; *A*, E 8-8.5; *B*, E 9-9.5; *C*, E 10-10.5; *D*, E 12-12.5; and *E*, E 14-14.5. In each case transgene expression was restricted to the heart with an anterior/posterior gradient similar to MLC2v (250 bp) LacZ transgenics. *(Middle panel)* Cardiac chamber-specific expression of an α-MyHC promoter-driven transgene. Whole-mount preparations of embryos *(G and H)* and postnatal hearts *(I and J)* are shown. *G*, Embryo at 9.5 days post coitum (dpc) shows *lacZ* expression in the primitive atrium (a) as it emerges from the sinus venosus (sv). *H*, By 10.5 dpc, *lacZ* staining is strong in the common atrium. *I*, Anterior *(left)* and posterior *(right)* views of the newborn animal's heart are shown. At birth, transgene expression is limited to the atria, the right superior vena cava (vc) as it enters the right atrium, and the pulmonary veins (out of the plane of focus). No expression is seen in the ventricles (v). *J*, Anterior view of *lacZ* expression in hearts from transgenic *(left)* and nontransgenic *(right)* littermates at 2 weeks of age. In the transgenic hearts, both atria and ventricles are intensely stained, as are the right and left superior vena cava and the pulmonary veins (not shown). ao, aorta; b, bulbus cordis; pa, pulmonary artery. *(Right panel)* Chamber specific nLacZ expression using the MLC3f transgene. Expression in E10.5 embryos *(K)* and in E14.5 embryos *(L)*, showing confinement of expression to the right atrium and left ventricle. *(Left panel modified from Ross et al. An HF-1a/HF-1b/MEF-2 combinatorial element confers cardiac ventricular specificity and establishes and anterior-posterior gradient of expression. Development 1996;122:1799-1809. Middle panel modified from Palermo, Gulick J, Colbert M, et al: Transgenic remodeling of the contractile apparatus in the mammalian heart. Circ Res 1996;78:504-509. Right panel modified from Franco et al: MLC3F transgene expression in iv mutant mice reveals the importance of left-right signaling pathways for the acquisition of left and right atrial but not ventricular compartment identity. Dev Dyn 2001;221:206-215.)*

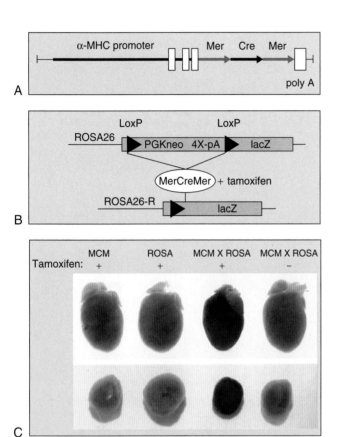

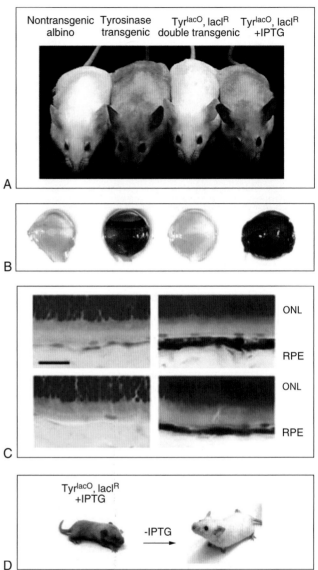

**FIGURE 4-8.** MerCreMer × ROSA lacZ transgenic mice. *A,* A cDNA encoding the mutant estrogen receptor ligand-binding domain (Mer) flanking the Cre recombinase was placed downstream of the 5.5 kb α-*MyHC* promoter to drive expression in the adult heart. *B,* Mice containing a single allele of the Cre recombinase-dependent lacZ gene knocked into the ROSA 26 locus were crossed with transgenic mice containing the MerCreMer transgene, permitting tamoxifen-inducible recombination within the heart. *C,* Assessment of tamoxifen-regulated Cre-mediated recombination in the heart of 6-week-old mice. Wholemount LacZ staining of the entire heart or a transverse section. The indicated experimental and control mice were treated with four injections of tamoxifen for 5 days or left untreated. *(Modified from Sobal DS, Nghiem M, Crackower, et al: Temporally regulated and tissuespecific manipulations in the adult and embryonic heart using a tamoxifen-inducible Cre protein. Circ Res 2001;89:20–25.)*

**FIGURE 4-9.** *Tyr*^lacO^*-SynLacI*^R^ transgenic mouse. IPTG controls *LacI*^R^ repression of the *Tyr*^LacO^ target gene in the mouse. Mice *(A),* dissected eyes *(B),* and cross-sections through eyes *(C).* Note the lack of pigmentation in the nontransgenic albino and the *Tyr*^LacO^, *LacI*^R^ double transgenic mice, whereas the tyrosinase transgenic and the *Tyr*^LacO^, *LacI*^R^ double transgenic mouse treated with IPTG are pigmented. ONL, outer nuclear layer; RPE, retinal pigment epithelium. *D,* Control of the *Tyr*^LacO^ target gene is reversible even after birth. Tyrosinase expression can be silenced after a period of derepression. Left and right panels show the same *Tyr*^LacO^, *LacI*^R^ double transgenic animal, on the left as an infant (day 8) and on the right as an adult. IPTG was discontinued at day 9, causing reversion to an albino phenotype in the adult. If the animal was left treated with IPTG, a fully pigmented adult animal would have been generated. *(Modified from Cronin CA, Gluba W, Scrable H, et al: The lac operator-repressor system is functional in the mouse. Genes Dev 2001;15:1506–1517.)*

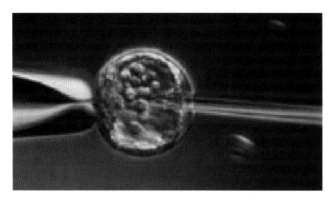

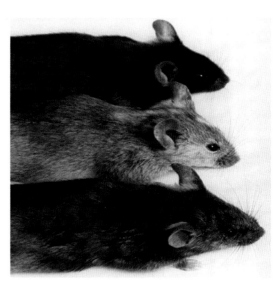

**FIGURE 4-10.** Microinjection of ES cells into the cavity of a mouse blastocyst. The blastocyst is held firmly with a holding pipette and the cavity of the blastocyst is punctured with a microneedle. In this photograph many ES cells have been deposited into the cavity and are resting on the inner cell mass of the blastocyst.

**FIGURE 4-11.** Chimeric mice. A chimeric mouse is created by mixing cells from a host embryo with ES cells and coat colors are used for the detection of chimerism. In this case, R1 ES cells were derived from 129/Sv-CP mice, which are agouti. The cells will give agouti coat color and dark eyes to the chimeras. When R1 cells are injected into C57BL/6 host blastocysts, the resulting chimera will be bicolored: black derived from the wild-type blastocyst and agouti derived from the R1 ES cells. In this picture, the top animal is not chimeric, the middle animal is 100% penetrant chimeric, and the bottom animal is partially chimeric.

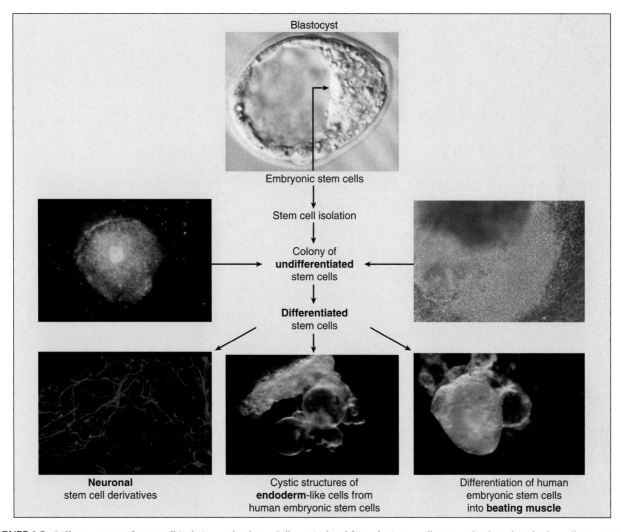

**FIGURE 6-2.** Different stages of stem cell isolation and culture. Cells are isolated from the inner cell mass and cultured on feeder cells to maintain the undifferentiated phenotype. Different differentiation pathways can then be followed by the stem cells, resulting in cells with different morphologies and phenotypes representative of all three embryonic germ layers.

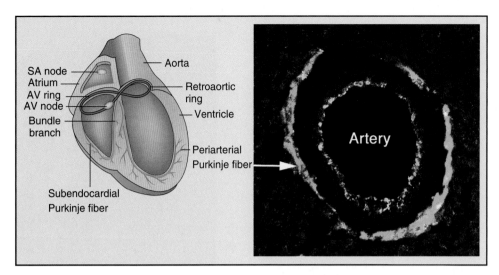

**FIGURE 11-1.** Basic structural and functional organization of the embryonic pacemaking and conduction system (PCS). The heartbeat is set by the ***sinuatrial (SA) node***. From this focus of pacemaking activity, propagating action potential spreads through atrial muscle, eventually focusing into the ***atrioventricular (AV) node*** where it is delayed briefly before ventricular activation. Following exit from the node, the propagating action potential accelerates along the His bundle and ***bundle branches,*** finally activating working ventricular muscle via a network of ***Purkinje fiber*** conduction cells. The model shown in the right hand panel is based on the embryonic chick heart. In the chick, the terminalmost component of the conduction system penetrates into the ventricular muscle in intimate association with coronary arteries. The ***periarterial Purkinje fiber*** shown in the left hand panel has been simultaneously labeled for three markers of conduction lineage: a gap junction protein Cx40 (yellow), a myosin heavy chain (green), and Nkx2.5 (red), a transcription factor. The endothelial cells lining the artery also contain Cx40 gap junctions. See the following references for further reading on the discovery of structure and function of the developing and mature PCS, including classics by Purkinje,[1] His,[2] Tawara,[3] Wenckebach,[4] Hering,[5] and Keith and Flack.[6] Also see references 1 to 16.

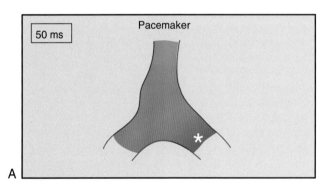

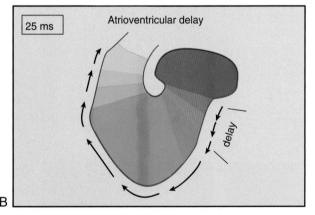

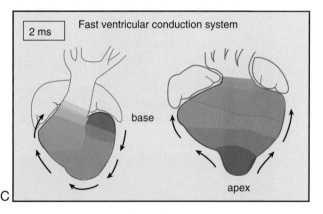

**FIGURE 11-2.** Functional emergence of the three major components of the PCS in the chick. *A,* A ***dominant pacemaker*** (i.e., SA nodelike) emerges initially in the left inflow region (star) of the tube heart (Hamburger and Hamilton (HH) developmental stage 10 to 11). *B,* AV impulse delay (i.e., an ***AV nodelike function***) develops first at the junction of the atria and ventricles in the looped tube heart (e.g., ~HH 15 to 17). *C,* A shift in the sequence of activation spread as observed from the ventricular epicardium marks differentiation of a ***His-Purkinje-like function*** of fast ventricular conduction. The righthand HH 28 heart retains the more primitive sequence, initiating activation from the left-ventricular base. Later in the HH 31 heart, activation spreads first from the apex of the ventricle. Note that the entire tubular heart (e.g., in A) is approximately 0.5 mm in length—less than one tenth of the ventricular base-apex distance of the HH 31 heart. The arrows indicate course of activation spread. Isochrones are in milliseconds in the right-hand corner of each box. *(B and C from Reckova M, Rosengarten C, deAlmeida A, et al: Hemodynamics is a key epigenetic factor in development of the cardiac conduction system. Circ Res 2003;93:77-85.)*

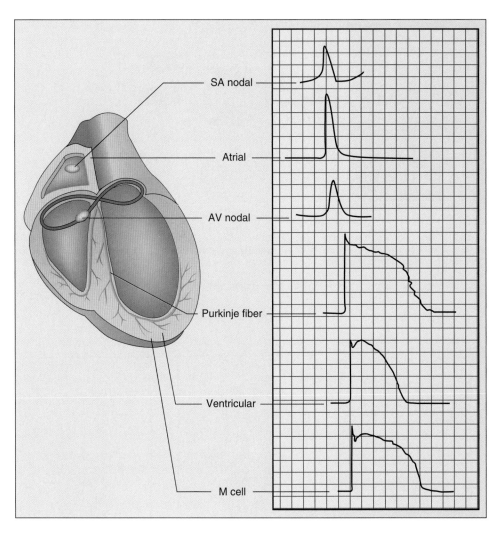

**FIGURE 11-3.** Cardiomyocyte electrophysiologic phenotypes. Each of the six APs shown are representative of different cardiomyocyte types present in the sinu-ventricular conduction pathway. All APs are drawn to the same scale. Horizontal lines on Aps (X-axis) show 0 potential level. Each of these lines is ~400 ms in duration. Position of the cellular AP along the X-axis indicates approximate order of the activation sequence. The maximum diastolic potential (Y-axis) of the SA node AP is ~50 millivolts.

SA nodal

Atrial

AV nodal

Purkinje fiber

Ventricular

M cell

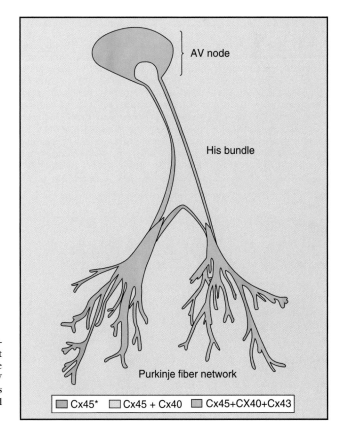

AV node

His bundle

Purkinje fiber network

Cx45*  Cx45 + Cx40  Cx45+CX40+Cx43

**FIGURE 11-4.** Connexin distribution patterns in the mouse AV conduction system (see references 37 and 39). Connexins define distinct compartments of cardiomyocytes along the axis of AV conduction. Note that the domain of Cx45 expressing tissue encompasses the entire AV conduction system and is always slightly broader than those domains coexpressing other connexins. Cx40 expression occurs within a coaxial core of cells found mainly in the His-Purkinje system.

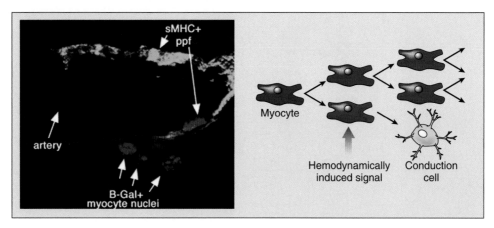

**FIGURE 11-6.** Induction of periarterial Purkinje fiber conduction cells. The right hand panel shows a cluster of red nuclei delineating a clone of LacZ expressing cells infected with a defective retrovirus. The clone contains both working myocytes and an sMHC+ (green) Purkinje fiber—a pattern consistent with the occurrence of localized recruitment of a multipotent progenitor cell to specialized myocardial lineages in the avian heart (e.g., Fig. 11-5). The left hand panel shows a model in which hemodynamically sensitive factors (e.g., the endothelin-1 signaling pathway) from arterial tissues locally mediate this divergence into either working myocytes or Purkinje fiber conduction cells within a cardiomyogenic lineage.

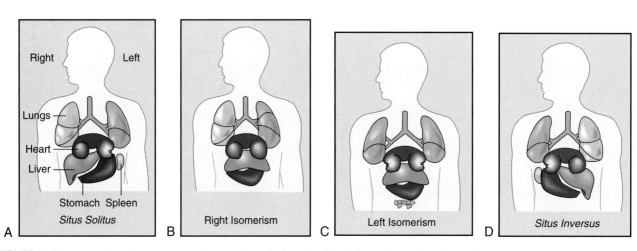

**FIGURE 12-1.** In normal conditions *(situs solitus, A)*, the right lung has three lobes, whereas the left lung has two. In addition, the apex of the heart points to the left side, the liver is on the right side, and the stomach and spleen are on the left side. Although not shown in the figure, the gut coils counterclockwise in the abdominal cavity. In the condition known as right isomerism *(B)*, also called asplenia syndrome, the heart and lungs are double-right (as indicated by the structure of the heart chambers and by both lungs having three lobes), as is the liver, which is generally found in a midline position. The stomach may be located on either side or in the midline, and the spleen is absent. In left isomerism *(C)*, also called polysplenia syndrome, the heart and lungs are double-left; the liver may be double-left, located in a midline position, or normal; and the stomach is usually found in a midline position. There is always more than one spleen (termed splenules), although multilobulated single spleens may also occur. *Situs inversus* refers to the complete mirror-image reversal of organ asymmetry *(D)*. Because laterality defects are highly variable, the figure depicts simplified cases, and is not intended to portray accurately the whole range of possible defects. The terms *situs inversus* and right or left isomerism can also be used to describe laterality defects in individual organs, even if they are not included in specific syndromes. *(Modified from Izpisua Belmonte JC: How the body tells left from right. Sci Am 1999;280[6]:46-51.)*

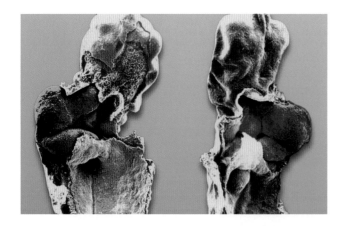

**FIGURE 12-2.** Developing heart (in red) in chick embryos shows the importance of retinoic acid on the correct heart asymmetry. Exposure to normal retinoic acid concentrations results in a heart that loops properly *(left image)*. After exposure to elevated levels of retinoic acid, however, the heart loops in the opposite direction *(right image)*. *(Modified from Izpisua Belmonte JC: How the body tells left from right. Sci Am 1999;280[6]:46-51.)*

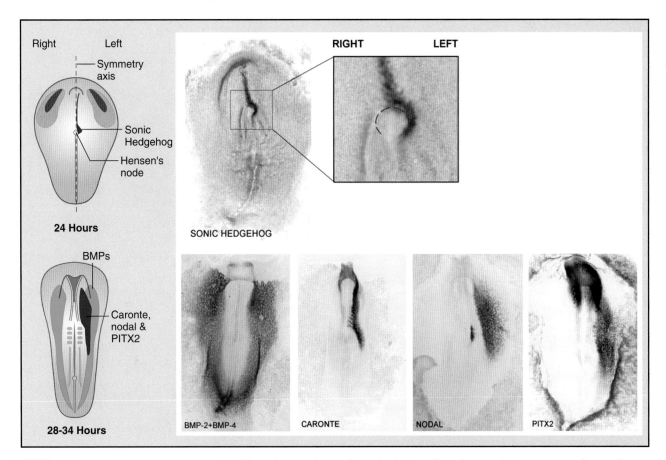

**FIGURE 12-5.** Genes that are active on one side of the embryo, such as in this early chick, establish the normal L-R asymmetry of internal organs. The gene encoding Sonic Hedgehog (dark blue in top images) is one of the first to become active, on the left side of the embryo above the Hensen's node. Ten hours later, Sonic Hedgehog is no longer active, and its activity has been replaced by that of *Nodal* and *Pitx2* (dark blue in the lower images). The transfer of asymmetric information is carried out by the protein Caronte (in dark blue in middle images), whose left-sided expression is induced by Sonic Hedgehog. Caronte allows the expression of Nodal on the left side of the embryo, by inhibiting BMPs activity (in green in middle images), which, in turn, represses Nodal expression on the right side. *(Modified from Izpisua Belmonte JC: How the body tells left from right. Sci Am 1999;280[6]:46-51.)*

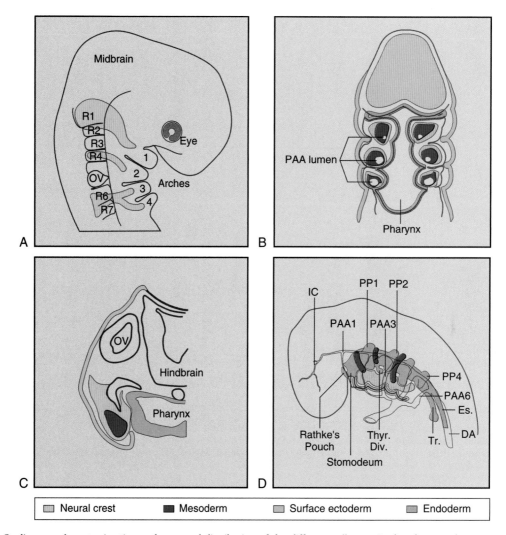

**FIGURE 13-1.** Cardiac neural crest migration pathways and distribution of the different cell types in the pharyngeal apparatus. *A,* Lateral view showing the three major streams directed to arches 1, 2, and 3-4. *B,* Coronal section showing the segmental organization of the embryonic pharynx. *C,* Transverse section at the level of the otic vesicle (OV) through the second pharyngeal arch. *D,* Pharyngeal endoderm-lined pouches and how they relate to vessels. DAo, dorsal aorta; Es, esophagus; PAA, pharyngeal arch arteries; PP, pharyngeal pouch; TD, thyroid diverticulum; Tr, trachea. *(A–C modified from Graham A, Smith A: Patterning the pharyngeal arches. Bioessays 2001;23:54-61. D, modified from Carlson BM: Patten's Foundations of Embryology. New York, McGraw-Hill, 1996.)*

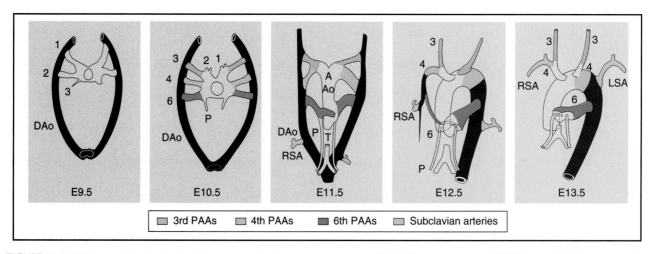

**FIGURE 13-2.** PAA remodeling during development, stages refers to mouse embryonic day. The arrangement at E13.5 is essentially the same as that in embryos at term. *Arrow* on E11.5 panel indicates the origin of the aorticopulmonary septum. DAo, dorsal aorta; LSA, left subclavian artery; P, pulmonary artery; RSA, right subclavian artery; T, trachea. Numbers refer to PAAs. *(Modified from Kaufman MH: The Atlas of Mouse Development. San Diego, Academic Press, 1992.)*

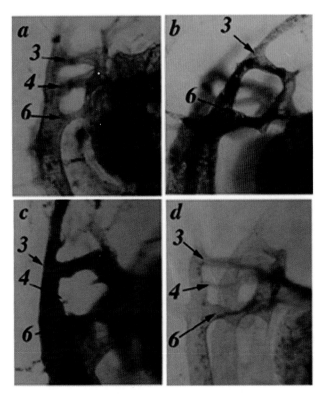

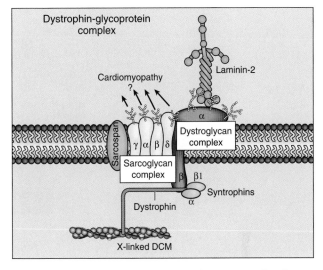

**FIGURE 13-4.** Diagnosis of fourth PAA abnormalities using intracardiac India ink injection. Lateral view of cleared E10.5 mouse embryos. *A,* Wild-type embryo showing the normal pattern, third, fourth, and sixth PAAs are clearly visible. *B, C,* and *D,* Show the same test on *Df1/+* embryos, which are heterozygously deleted for a chromosomal region homologous to the DGS deleted region on 22q11.2. *B,* The left fourth PAA is missing, whereas the right fourth PAA (visible in the background) is normal. *C,* The fourth PAA is greatly reduced in size and partially nonpatent to ink. *D,* The fourth PAA is present but very reduced in size. *(From Lindsay EA, Baldini A: Recovery from arterial growth delay reduces penetrance of cardiovascular defects in mice deleted for the DiGeorge syndrome region. Hum Mol Genet 2001;10: 997–1002.)*

**FIGURE 17-1.** The DGC and cardiomyopathies associated with mutations within the DGC.

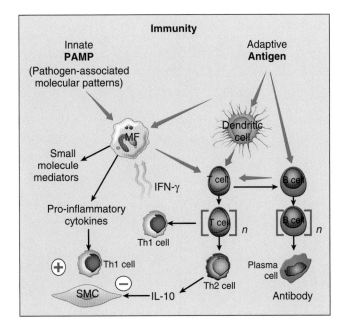

**FIGURE 20-2.** Interplay between adaptive and innate immunity during atherogenesis. The principal effector cell of innate immunity, the macrophage (MF), elaborates cytokines that critically regulate many functions of atheroma-associated cells involved with disease initiation, progression, and complication as well as thrombosis. IFN-γ, a product of the activated T cell, activates a number of these functions of the macrophage. In turn, the activated macrophage expresses high levels of MHC class II antigens, needed for antigen-dependent activation of T cells. *(From Hansson GK, Libby P, Schonbeck U, et al: Innate and adaptive immunity in the pathogenesis of atherosclerosis Circ Res 2002;91:281–291.)*

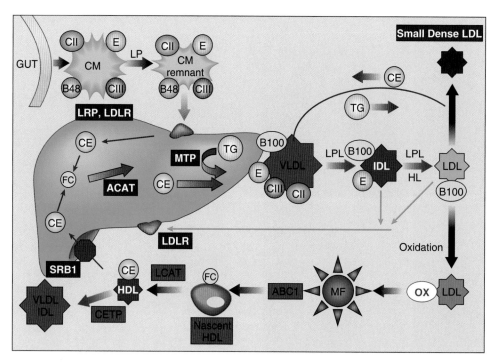

**FIGURE 21-1.** General overview of lipoprotein metabolism. CE, cholesteryl ester; FC, free cholesterol; HL, hepatic lipase; LPL, lipoprotein lipase; MΦ, macrophage; OxLDL, oxidized LDL; TG, triglycerides.

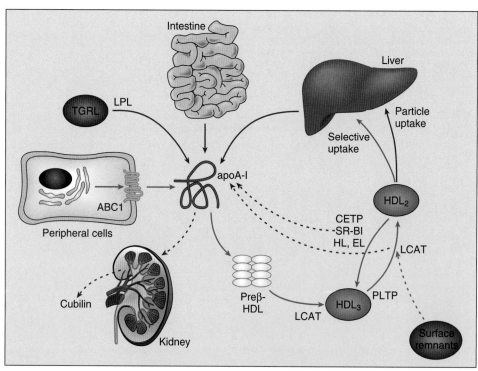

**FIGURE 21-2.** HDL lipoprotein metabolism. *(Reproduced with permission from von Eckardstein A, Nofer JR, Assmann G: High density lipoproteins and artereosclerosis: Role of cholesterol efflux and reverse cholesterol transport. Arterioscler Thromb Vasc Biol 2001;21:13–27.)*

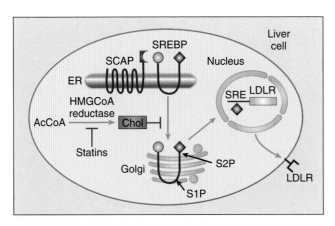

**FIGURE 21-3.** Regulation of cellular cholesterol metabolism by SREBPs. *(Reproduced with permission from Rader DJ: A new feature on the cholesterol-lowering landscape. Nat Med 2001;7:1282–1284.)*

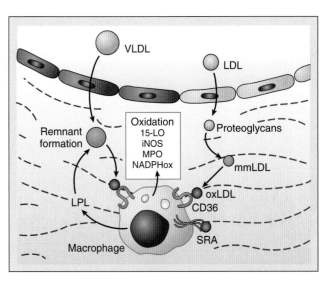

**FIGURE 22-3.** Mechanisms contributing to foam-cell formation. LDL penetrates into the artery wall where it is trapped after adhering to proteoglycans. It is then highly susceptible to oxidation by enzymes such as LOs, MPO, and iNOS. VLDL particles are subject to modification by LPL. The resulting remnant particles are also subject to trapping by proteoglycans, oxidative modification, and uptake by macrophages. mmLDL, minimally modified LDL; SR-A, scavenger receptor class A. *(Reproduced with permission from Li AC, Glass CK: The macrophage foam cell as a target for therapeutic intervention. Nat Med 2002;8: 1235–1242.)*

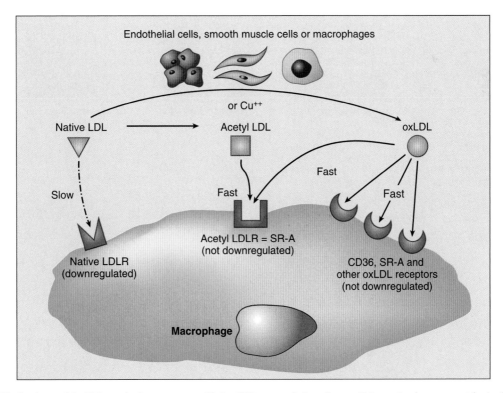

**FIGURE 22-2.** Mechanisms of OxLDL uptake by monocytes. Native LDL cannot induce foam cell formation because uptake is slow and because the LDL receptor downregulates. Either acetyl LDL or OxLDL can induce cholesterol accumulation in macrophages resulting in foam cell formation because uptake is rapid and the scavenger receptors do not downregulate in response to an increase in cellular cholesterol. *(Reproduced with permission from Steinberg D: Atherogenesis in perspective: Hypercholesterolemia and inflammation as partners in crime. Nat Med 2002;8:1211–1217.)*

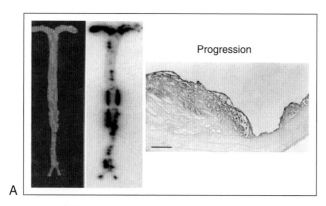

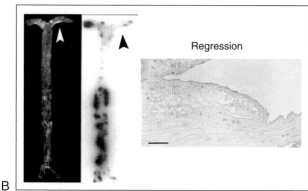

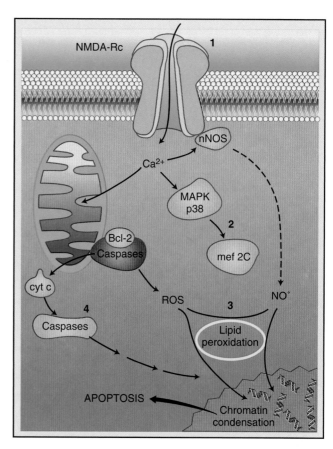

**FIGURE 22-4.** *In vivo* uptake of [125]I-MDA2, a prototype oxidation-specific antibody that was intravenously injected in LDLR-/- mice with preexisting atherosclerotic lesions. These mice were subsequently placed on either a dietary atherosclerosis progression diet *(A)* or a regression diet *(B)*. The aorta (left panels of each figure) represents the presence of plaque accentuated by Sudan IV staining and the aorta in the middle panels represents the corresponding autoradiograph. In the progression aorta, there is nearly 100% concordance of Sudan staining and *in vivo* distribution and plaque uptake of [125]I-MDA2. Immuno-staining for OxLDL (far right panel) shows strong staining pattern. In contrast in a regression mouse *(B)*, the arrowheads depict an area in the aortic arch where a Sudan-stained lesion does not take up [125]I-MDA2. Immunostaining of this segment, which is similar in size to the area in the progression mouse, shows essentially absent OxLDL staining following a regression antioxidant diet.[169] *(Reproduced with permission from Tsimikas S, Shortal BP, Witztum JL, Palinski W: In vivo uptake of radiolabeled MDA2, an oxidation-specific monoclonal antibody, provides an accurate measure of atherosclerotic lesions rich in oxidized LDL and is highly sensitive to their regression. Arterioscler Thromb Vasc Biol 2000;20:689–697.)*

**FIGURE 26-1.** Schematic model of the link of excessive NMDA receptor activity to apoptotic pathways. Steps to cell death include: (1) NMDA receptor (NMDA-Rc) hyperactivation; (2) activation of the p38 MAPK—MEF2C (transcription factor) pathway. MEF2 is subsequently cleaved by caspases to form an endogenous dominant-interfering form that contributes to neuronal cell death; (3) toxic effects of free radicals such as NO and reactive oxygen species (ROS); and (4) activation of apoptosis-inducing enzymes including caspases. Cyt c, cytochrome c; nNOS, nitric oxide synthase. *(From Okamoto S-i, Li Z, Ju C, Schölzke MN, et al: Dominant-interfering forms of MEF2 generated by caspase cleavage contribute to NMDA-induced neuronal apoptosis. Proc Natl Acad Sci USA 2002;99:3974–3979.)*

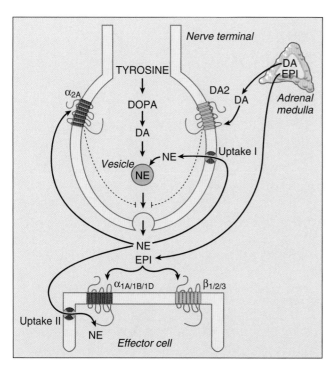

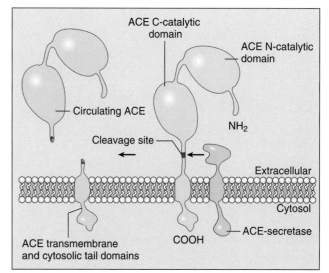

**FIGURE 30-1.** Sympathetic prejunctional and postjunctional neuroeffector events. Cytoplasmic enzymes mediating catecholamine biosynthesis (detailed in Fig. 30-2) catalyze the conversion of tyrosine to DOPA and dopamine (DA) and finally to the sympathetic neurotransmitter norepinephrine (NE), which is stored in vesicles. Arrival of an action potential at the sympathetic nerve terminal triggers fusion of the vesicle with the plasma membrane, resulting in exocytosis of NE (and other cotransmitters such as ATP and NPY; not shown). Most of the released NE, however, is taken back up into the prejunctional nerve terminal (via Uptake I) and either catabolized by MAO or restored in vesicles. Released NE activates postjunctional $\alpha_{1A/1B/1D}$- or $\beta_{1/2/3}$-adrenergic receptors on effector cells and prejunctional $\alpha_{2A}$-adrenergic receptors that negatively regulate exocytotic NE release *(dashed line)*. Some NE is taken up by the postjunctional effector cell (via Uptake II) and is rapidly metabolized by COMT to normetanephrine (not shown). Epinephrine (EPI) and dopamine released from the adrenal medulla activate postjunctional $\alpha_{1A/1B/1D}$-/$\beta_{1/2/3}$-adrenergic receptors at effector cells and prejunctional DA2 receptors, respectively; the latter inhibits the release of NE *(dashed line)*.

**FIGURE 30-4.** Schematic showing the cleavage of the somatic form of ACE by ACE-secretase. Both ACE-secretase and its substrate ACE are embedded in the same lipid bilayer. ACE-secretase cleaves ACE in its membrane-proximal stalk region, generating the soluble, circulating form of ACE.

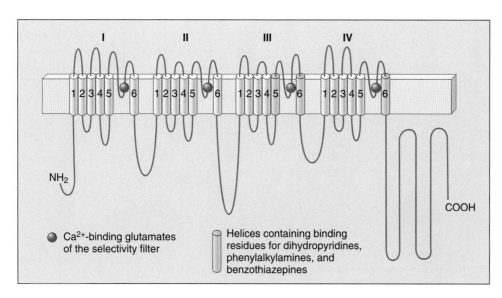

**FIGURE 30-5.** Structure of L-type $Ca^{2+}$ channel $\alpha^1$-subunits. *(Adapted from Striessnig J, Grabner M, Mitterdorfer J, et al: Structural basis of drug binding to L $Ca^{2+}$ channels. Trends Pharmacol Sci 1998;19: 108–115.)*

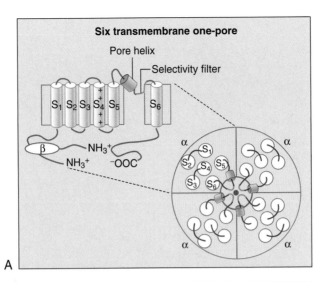

**Six transmembrane one-pore**

Pore helix

Selectivity filter

$S_1$ $S_2$ $S_3$ $S_4$ $S_5$ $S_6$

β

$NH_3^+$

$NH_3^+$

$^-OOC$

α α

$S_1$
$S_2$ $S_4$ $S_5$
$S_3$ $S_6$

α α

**A**

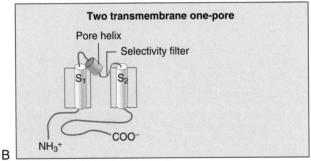

**Two transmembrane one-pore**

Pore helix

Selectivity filter

$S_1$ $S_2$

$NH_3^+$

$COO^-$

**B**

**FIGURE 30-6.** Schematic representation of six-TM (A) or two-TM (B) one-pore $K^+$ channel α subunits, which cluster to form the $K^+$ ion conducting pore. *A,* The six-TM, one-pore subunit. The voltage-gated $K^+$ channels are composed of four segments each containing six TM segments (S1 to S6) and a pore helix between S5 and S6 with a voltage sensor (positively charged amino acids) located at S4. Some of the voltage-gated $K^+$ channels include an auxiliary β subunit that binds to the N-terminus of the α subunit. The inset shows the general assembly of $K^+$ channel α subunits to form the channel's conducting pore *B,* A two-TM, one-pore subunit. The inwardly rectifying $K^+$ channels are members of this family, which are formed by the clustering of four subunits each containing two TM segments (S1 and S2) with a pore helix and selectivity filter in between. *(Adapted from Shieh CC, Coghlan M, Sullivan JP, Gopalakrishnan M: Potassium channels: Molecular defects, diseases, and therapeutic opportunities. Pharmacol Rev 2000;52:557-594.)*

■ ■ ■ chapter **1**

# Biotechnology and Cardiovascular Medicine: Recombinant Protein Therapy

*Hiroshi Ashikaga*
*Ori Ben-Yehuda*
*Kenneth R. Chien*

Recombinant deoxyribonucleic acid (DNA) technology has proven to be a powerful tool to elucidate fundamental biologic processes, disease pathways, and therapeutic targets and has had a major clinical impact in every facet of cardiovascular medicine over the past decade. On a clinical level, recombinant DNA technology has become a cornerstone of biologically targeted cardiovascular therapies, including the creation of new agents to treat acute coronary syndromes, sepsis, anemia, granulocytopenia, and heart failure. The first report of successful molecular cloning was reported in the mid-1970s, which was soon followed by the successful expression of human somatostatin, a 14-amino-acid peptide neurotransmitter, from recombinant DNA cloned into a plasmid in *Escherichia coli*.[1] Before long, human insulin came onto the market as the first commercialized recombinant protein. Recombinant DNA technology has thus evolved into biotechnology, which created an entirely new industry devoted to the cloning and production of recombinant proteins for therapy and diagnosis of human disease.[2] The intersection of biotechnology and clinical medicine has accelerated the development of large-scale production of recombinant proteins for human use, and its clinical applications have produced dozens of recombinant protein drugs for a diverse group of diseases (Table 1-1). Recent advances in protein design and engineering has led to the development of second generation therapeutic proteins that have been engineered to have improved pharmacokinetics, specificity, and side effect profiles. One of the most impressive advances in recent years has been the advent of humanized monoclonal antibodies in clinical practice, which can be administered with minimal or no immune response. Recombinant protein therapeutics has permeated almost every discipline of medical science: hematology, oncology, nephrology, gastroenterology, rheumatology, endocrinology, infectious disease, genetic disease, and cardiovascular disease. As we enter the era of molecular medicine, the recombinant protein technology will continue to shape the practice of medicine.

## RECOMBINANT PROTEIN PRODUCTION: EXPRESSION SYSTEMS

The production of recombinant proteins is based on the introduction of a cloned complementary DNA (cDNA), which encodes the particular protein of interest into a host cell and essentially provides the molecular machinery for protein synthesis (for a review, see reference 2). A wide variety of expression systems are currently available: bacteria, yeast, insect, mammalian cells, and transgenic animals. Each expression system has inherent advantages and disadvantages, and the choice of the expression system depends on many factors, including intrinsic structural features of the protein of interest, the stability of the protein, and the projected dose of protein per patient[3] (Table 1-2).

Bacterial cells, most commonly *E. coli*, are the most cost-effective among all expression systems and can be used to produce a large amount of proteins in a relatively short period. On the other hand, the bacterial cell machinery lacks the capability to complete critical aspects of posttranslational protein modifications that can be critical for therapeutic efficacy. In addition, foreign proteins expressed in bacteria are often insoluble, thus forming dense aggregates called inclusion bodies, necessitating a cumbersome denaturation/renaturation process to recover active protein.

Yeast cells maintain economic advantages comparable to those of bacteria and are capable of performing most of the eukaryotic posttranslational modifications, including phosphorylation, glycosylation, disulfide bond formation, and proteolytic cleavage of inactive precursors. Because of the sophisticated protein processing of yeast cells, recombinant proteins that are insoluble when expressed in bacteria may be soluble if the yeast system is used. Yeast cells can also be induced to secrete recombinant proteins into the growth medium for harvesting. The quantity of recombinant proteins expressed in yeast cells, however, is often limited by active proteases present in yeast cells that degrade foreign proteins. This problem may be circumvented by construction of yeast strains lacking the protease genes. Other disadvantages

■ ■ ■

## TABLE 1-1   RECOMBINANT PROTEIN DRUGS

| Product | Category | First Indication | First FDA approval |
|---|---|---|---|
| *Recombinant Protein* | | | |
| Humulin | Insulin | Diabetes | 1982 |
| Protropin (somatrem) | Growth hormone | Growth hormone deficiency in pediatrics | 1985 |
| Roferon-A | Interferon α2a | Hairy cell leukemia | 1986 |
| Intron A | Interferon α2b | Hairy cell leukemia | 1986 |
| Recombivax HB | Hepatitis B vaccine | Hepatitis B prophylaxis | 1986 |
| Activase (alteplase) | t-PA | Acute myocardial infarction | 1987 |
| Epogen | Erythropoietin (EPO) | Renal anemia | 1989 |
| Alferon N | Interferon αn3 | Genital warts | 1989 |
| Actimmune | Interferon γ1b | Chronic granulomatosis | 1990 |
| Neupogen | G-CSF | Chemotherapy-induced neutropenia | 1991 |
| Leukine | GM-CSF | Autologous bone marrow transplantation | 1991 |
| Proleukin | IL-2 | Renal cell carcinoma | 1992 |
| Recombinate | Factor VIII | Hemophilia A | 1992 |
| KoGENate | Factor VIII | Hemophilia A | 1993 |
| Betaseron | Interferon β1b | Multiple sclerosis | 1993 |
| Pulmozyme (dornase alfa) | Deoxyribonuclease I | Cystic fibrosis | 1993 |
| Nutropin (somatropin) | Growth hormone | Growth failure in pediatrics due to renal failure | 1994 |
| Cerezyme (ceredase) | Glucocerebrosidase | Gaucher's disease | 1994 |
| Nutropin AQ | Growth hormone; liquid | Growth failure in pediatrics due to renal failure | 1995 |
| Humalog | Insulin analog | Diabetes | 1996 |
| Avonex | Interferon β 1a | Multiple myeloma | 1996 |
| Retavase (reteplase) | Mutant t-PA | Acute myocardial infarction | 1996 |
| BeneFIX | Factor IX | Hemophilia B | 1997 |
| Infergen | Mutant interferon α1 | Hepatitis C | 1997 |
| Neumega | IL-11 | Chemotherapy-induced thrombocytopenia | 1997 |
| Regranex Gel | Platelet-derived growth factor-β | Diabetic neuropathic ulcers | 1997 |
| Enbrel (etanercept) | TNF receptor with human IgG₁ Fc | Rheumatoid arthritis | 1998 |
| GlucaGen | Glucagon | Hypoglycemia | 1998 |
| NovoSeven | Factor VIIa | Bleeding episodes in hemophilia A/B | 1999 |
| Nutropin Depot | Growth hormone; long-acting | Growth failure in pediatrics due to renal failure | 1999 |
| Refacto | Factor VIII SC; albumin-free | Hemophilia A | 2000 |
| TNKase (tenecteplase) | Mutant t-PA | Acute myocardial infarction | 2000 |
| Aranesp (darbepoietin alfa) | 2nd generation EPO | Renal anemia | 2001 |
| Kineret (anakinra) | IL-1 receptor antagonist | Rheumatoid arthritis | 2001 |
| Natrecor (nesiritide) | B-type natriuretic peptide | Congestive heart failure | 2001 |
| Xigris (drotrecogin alfa) | Activated protein C | Severe sepsis | 2001 |
| Peg-Intron (peginterferon alfa2b) | Interferon α2b modified with polyethylene glycol (PEG) | Chronic hepatitis C | 2001 |
| *Recombinant Monoclonal Antibody (mAb)* | | | |
| Orthoclone OKT3 (muromonab) | Anti-CD3 mouse mAb | Reversal of acute kidney transplant rejection | 1986 |
| ReoPro (abciximab) | Anti-GPIIb/IIIa chimeric mAb | Refractory UA when PTCA is planned | 1994 |
| Rituxan (rituximab) | Anti-CD20 chimeric mAb | B-cell non-Hodgkin's lymphoma | 1997 |
| Zenapax (daclizumab) | Anti-Tac humanized mAb | Prevention of acute kidney transplant rejection | 1997 |
| Simulect (brasiliximab) | Anti-CD25 chimeric mAb | Prevention of acute kidney transplant rejection | 1998 |
| Herceptin (trastuzumab) | Anti-HER2 humanized mAb | Metastatic breast cancer | 1998 |
| Remicade (infliximab) | Anti-TNFα chimeric mAb | Crohn's disease | 1998 |
| Synagis (palivizumab) | Anti-RSV humanized mAb | Prophylaxis of RSV infection in pediatrics | 1998 |
| Mylotarg (gemtuzumab ozogamicin) | Anti-CD33 humanized mAb with calicheamicin | Acute myeloid leukemia | 2000 |
| Campath (alemtuzumab) | Anti-CD52 humanized mAb | B-cell chronic lymphocytic leukemia | 2001 |

G-CSF, granulocyte colony-stimulating factor; GM-CSF, granulocyte-macrophage colony-stimulating factor; IL, interleukin; PTCA, percutaneous transluminal coronary angioplasty; RSV, respiratory syncytial virus; SC, subcutaneous; TNF, tumor necrosis factor; t-PA, tissue plasminogen activator; UA, unstable angina.

of the yeast system include overglycosylation of glycoproteins, which may alter the activity of the expressed proteins, vector instability, and entrapment of secreted proteins in the periplasmic space.

The baculovirus system uses viral vectors that infect and multiply in cultured insect cells to express foreign proteins. Baculovirus expression of foreign genes in insect cells permits protein folding, posttranslational modification, and oligomerization seen in mammalian cells. Recombinant proteins can be produced in large quantities either within the cells or secreted into the cul-

ture medium. One of the major disadvantages of the baculovirus system is that foreign proteins are expressed during acute lytic infection of insect cells, resulting in short production period and cell death.[4] In addition, generation and transfection of baculovirus vectors in insect cells may be difficult, and some proteins may not undergo proper modifications. Insect cells also grow more slowly and are more expensive than bacterial and yeast cells.

Mammalian cells, although costly, have recently become one of the most popular and valuable expression systems. Mammalian cells, such as Chinese

■ ■ ■

**TABLE 1-2**  COMPARISON OF EXPRESSION SYSTEMS

| Expression System | Advantages | Disadvantages |
|---|---|---|
| Bacteria | Short generation times<br>Large quantities of product<br>Low cost | Lack of posttranslational modifications<br>Formation of inclusion bodies<br>Unsuitable for large or complex proteins |
| Yeast | Some eukaryotic posttranslational modifications<br>Moderately short generation times | Product quantity limited by protease degradation<br>Overglycosylation<br>Vector instability<br>Product entrapment in periplasmic space |
| Baculovirus | Large quantities of product<br>Some eukaryotic posttranslational modifications<br>Proper protein folding | Difficult to handle<br>More expensive than bacteria and yeast<br>Long generation times<br>Unsuitable for proteins with repetitive sequences |
| Mammalian cells | Eukaryotic posttranslational modifications | Long generation times<br>Difficult to scale up<br>High cost |
| Transgenic animals | Enormous quantities of product<br>Eukaryotic posttranslational modifications<br>Can be cost-effective | Time-consuming |

Hamster Ovary (CHO) cells, produce necessary posttranslational modifications and recognize the same synthesis and processing signals found in the original organism. The major disadvantages of the mammalian system are low expression levels, long generation times, and high costs. Mammalian cell transfections are also less efficient than in bacteria or yeast, which further promote lower overall expression levels in the mammalian system.

Alternatively, the production of recombinant proteins in transgenic animals can achieve cost-effectiveness while maintaining favorable properties of the mammalian cell expression system. For example, transgenic goats express 1 to 3 g/L of tissue plasminogen activator (t-PA) in milk.[5] A major drawback of the transgenic animal expression system is that it takes months and sometimes years to raise the sufficient number of transgenic animals from the founder to produce the amount of proteins adequate for commercialization.

## RECOMBINANT PROTEIN DRUGS

### Nonmonoclonal Antibody Drugs

Most recombinant protein drugs currently on the market are naturally occurring human proteins, including coagulation factors, growth hormone, erythropoietin, colony-stimulating factors, t-PA, and insulin.[6] Furthermore, clinically useful proteins have been engineered to improve the original function toward specific therapeutic endpoints, and these engineered proteins account for a small portion of the recombinant protein drugs on the market. The functional improvements are accomplished through deletion/substitution of functional domains, site-specific point mutations, alteration of glycosylation sites, and/or fusion with other functional proteins. In addition to the traditional recombinant DNA technology, the phage display technology has allowed determination of effective domain sequences that possess higher binding affinity than the native proteins while retaining their normal bio-

logic function and pharmacokinetics (see the section on fully human monoclonal antibodies). This group of engineered proteins includes hepatitis vaccines, interferon variants, t-PA variants, and fusion proteins.

### Insulin

Insulin is a classic example of a naturally occurring protein produced by recombinant technology. Human insulin was the first recombinant protein commercially produced for therapeutic use. Before the availability of recombinant insulin, diabetic patients relied on insulin purified from the pancreases of pigs and cows, which occasionally resulted in serious immune reactions. Recombinant human insulin has dramatically improved the therapy for diabetes. Human insulin is expressed as a precursor form, single-chain prepro-insulin, which contains extra amino acids that are subsequently cleaved by proteases during the normal processing of this protein hormone. The mature insulin molecule consists of two short polypeptide chains A and B that are linked by two disulfide bonds. Recombinant human insulin was originally produced as the form of proinsulin that subsequently underwent enzymatic cleavage to form the active insulin molecule, but currently it is produced by expressing A and B chains separately, then refolding them into a mature insulin molecule (Figure 1-1).

### Somatropin

Somatropin is the recombinant human growth hormone (rhGH), identical to the pituitary-derived human growth hormone with respect to amino acid sequence (191 amino acids, 22 kDa). Somatropin is synthesized in E. coli as a precursor consisting of the GH molecule conjugated with a secretion signal from an E. coli protein, which directs the precursor to the plasma membrane of E. coli. The signal sequence is then removed, and the GH protein is secreted into the periplasm so that the protein is folded appropriately as it is expressed. Somatropin is indicated for the treatment of growth failure resulting

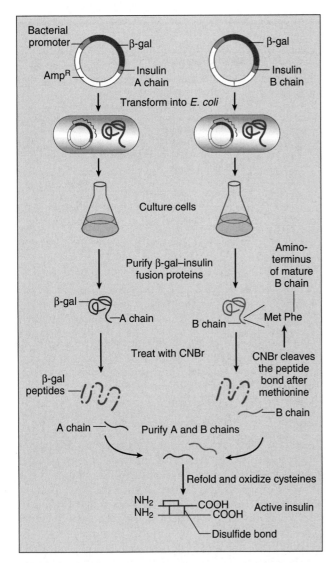

**FIGURE 1-1.** Expression of human insulin in *E. coli*. Recombinant insulin was first made by expressing the A and B chains separately, then refolding them into a mature insulin molecule. A DNA fragment encoding each insulin chain was made by annealing two complementary oligonucleotides that had been chemically synthesized. Each fragment was ligated into a bacterial expression vector so that, when translated, the insulin chain would be fused to the carboxy terminus of the enzyme β-galactosidase (β-gal). The expression vectors were transformed into *E. coli*, and the β-gal–insulin fusion proteins accumulated inside the bacterial cells. The cells were harvested, and each β-gal–insulin fusion protein was purified. The insulin-coding DNA was synthesized so that it started with a methionine codon. This setup provided a way to cleave off the β-gal part from the insulin polypeptide. Treatment of the fusion protein with the chemical cyanogen bromide (CNBr) resulted in cleavage of peptide bonds after all methionines. In this way, the natural insulin peptides were obtained. Because β-gal contains other methionine residues, CNBr treatment cleaved it into many small peptides. The insulin chains were not cleaved further because they did not contain internal methionines. The A and B chains were purified and then mixed together to form active recombinant insulin. *(From Recombinant DNA, by J.D. Watson, M. Gilman, J. Witkowski, M. Zoller ©1992, 1983 by J.D. Watson, M. Gilman, J. Witkowski, M. Zoller. Used with the permission of W.H. Freeman and Company, Cold Spring Harbor, NY.)*

from chronic renal insufficiency or endogenous growth hormone deficiency. Somatropin is also indicated for treatment of short stature associated with Turner's syndrome.

Recombinant human growth hormone has been investigated in clinical studies for patients with chronic heart failure. Serum levels of insulin-like growth factor (IGF)-I, reflecting endogenous GH secretion, are diminished in relation to the severity of heart failure in patients with dilated cardiomyopathy, and administration of rhGH increases the IGF-I levels, resulting in significant improvement of ejection fraction.[7] In patients with idiopathic dilated cardiomyopathy, rhGH increases myocardial mass and VO₂ max, while it reduces the left ventricular chamber size; myocardial sympathetic drive; serum levels of aldosterone; and proinflammatory cytokines including tumor necrosis factor (TNF)-α, its soluble receptors (sTNF-RI, sTNF-RII), interleukin-6 (IL-6), soluble IL-6 receptor (sIL-6R), and soluble Fas/FasL system. However, the results from randomized studies have been conflicting. In some studies, rhGH improved hemodynamics, myocardial energy metabolism, and clinical performance,[8-11] whereas other studies showed no benefits in improving clinical status, cardiac function, or neuroendocrine activation in patients with dilated cardiomyopathy, despite a significant increase in left ventricular mass.[12,13] These contradictory results may be the result of variable levels of IGF-I response to rhGH administration.[14]

### Recombinant Human Insulin-like Growth Factor-I

Recombinant human insulin-like growth factor (rhIGF)-I, which contains 70 amino acid residues (7.5 kDa), is produced in a variety of expression systems. Endogenous IGF-I may play a pivotal role in compensated heart failure, because the serum levels of IGF-I are elevated in mild to moderate heart failure (NYHA class I and II) but not in severe heart failure (NYHA class III and IV).[15] Although it has not been approved for clinical use, rhIGF-I has vasodilatory and positive inotropic effects and has been tested in human patients with heart failure. In healthy individuals, rhIGF-I significantly increases stroke volume, cardiac output, and ejection fraction without increasing heart rate at rest or during exercise.[16] In patients with chronic heart failure, rhIGF-I acutely increases stroke volume and cardiac index and decreases pulmonary artery wedge pressure and systemic vascular resistance.[17] A number of clinical studies of rhIGF-I and rhGH indicate significant potential of rhIGF-I as a drug to treat chronic heart failure. Further studies to establish long-term efficacy and safety of rhIGF-I are warranted.

### Nesiritide

Nesiritide is the recombinant human B-type natriuretic peptide (rhBNP) produced in *E. coli*. Nesiritide (32 amino acids, 3.5 kDa) is identical in amino acid sequence to the naturally occurring hBNP produced by ventricular cardiomyocytes. Not only does rhBNP have diuretic and natriuretic actions, but it also binds to the particulate guanylate cyclase receptors of vascular smooth muscle and endothelial cells, causing cyclic guanosine monophosphate (GMP)-mediated smooth muscle relaxation and vasodilation. Nesiritide is indicated for intravenous use in patients with acutely decompensated congestive heart failure with dyspnea at rest or minimal activity. In clinical trials, nesiritide reduced pulmonary capillary wedge pressure and improved dyspnea in this population.[18]

## Thrombolytic Agents

Thrombobolytic agents provide a classic example of the power of engineered recombinant proteins for human cardiovascular disease. Currently, there are three distinct generations of thrombolytic agents. The first-generation thrombolytics—streptokinase, anisteplase, and urokinase—are not fibrin-specific and activate plasminogen systemically, which may lead to a systemic lytic state. The second-generation thrombolytics include alteplase (rt-PA), saruplase (scu-PA), and duteplase; and the third-generation includes reteplase (r-PA), lanetoplase (n-PA), and tenecteplase (TNK-rt-PA). The second- and third-generation thrombolytics have also been designated as fibrinolytics, because they preferentially activate plasminogen at the fibrin clot, although systemic activation of plasminogen does occur with clinical doses.

### Alteplase (rt-PA)

Alteplase (rt-PA) is a recombinant protein of the naturally occuring t-PA. After human t-PA was cloned and expressed in *E. coli* and in mammalian cells,[19] it became the first commercially available recombinant protein drug that was entirely produced in mammalian cells (Figure 1-2). Since then, alteplase has been widely used as a fibrinolytic agent for patients with acute myocardial infarction.[20]

Human t-PA is a 527-amino-acid, single-chain serine protease (70 kDa) (Figure 1-3). It converts plasminogen into the active serine protease plasmin, which degrades fibrin meshwork in clots. By itself, t-PA is a weak enzyme, but fibrin remarkably enhances its enzymatic potency.[21] The t-PA molecule contains multiple distinct domains, and the functions of these domains have been identified by detailed structural-functional analysis with deletion mutagenesis.[22] The finger domain is the high-affinity binding site to fibrin, whereas the epidermal growth factor (EGF) and kringle 1 domains affect receptor binding in the liver and rapid serum clearance. The EGF domain interacts with calcium-dependent receptors on the liver parenchymal cells, and the kringle 1 domain contains the high mannose-type carbohydrate side-chain at Asn[117] that binds to mannose receptors on the liver endothelial cells. The glycosylation at Asn[117] is responsible for rapid clearance of t-PA by the liver. The kringle 2 domain binds to lysin and facilitates conversion of plasminogen to plasmin. The lysin-binding site of the kringle 2 domain, along with the finger domain, also mediates fibrin binding. The protease domain is a plasminogen-specific serine protease and contains the binding site for plasminogen activator inhibitor (PAI)-1.

As a therapeutic agent for acute myocardial infarction, t-PA has several unfavorable properties. Its short half-life (2 to 5 minutes) necessitates continuous intravenous infusion at relatively high doses for as long as 90 minutes, and its slow onset of action may allow for expansion of myocardial damage. The use of t-PA also requires adjunct heparin infusion to prevent reocclusion, which is caused by thrombin released during fibrinolysis. Moreover, its fib-

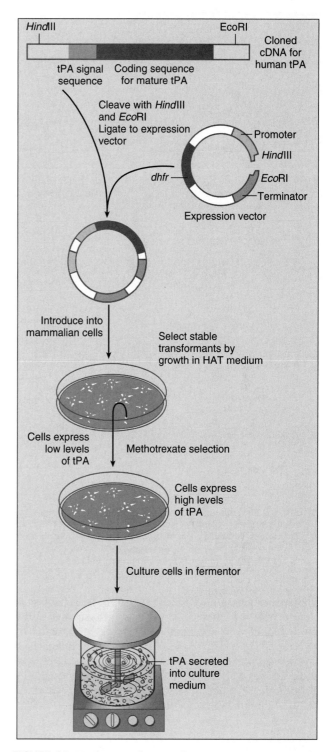

**FIGURE 1-2.** Production of tissue plasminogen activator (t-PA) by mammalian cell culture. The cloned cDNA for human t-PA is inserted into an expression vector that contains a promoter and terminator. The vector is transfected into a mammalian cell line (Chinese hamster ovary cells). The initial transformants secretes t-PA into the culture medium, but the level of expression is very low. Cell lines that express t-PA to high levels are obtained using methotrexate treatment, which selects for cells that have amplified the *dhfr* gene resident in the vector together with the linked t-PA expression cassette. High-expressing lines are grown in large fermentors and recombinant t-PA is purified from the culture medium. *(From Recombinant DNA by J.D. Watson, M. Gilman, J. Witkowski, M. Zoller ©1992, 1983 by J.D. Watson, M. Gilman, J. Witkowski, M. Zoller. Used with the permission of W.H. Freeman and Company, Cold Spring Harbor, NY.)*

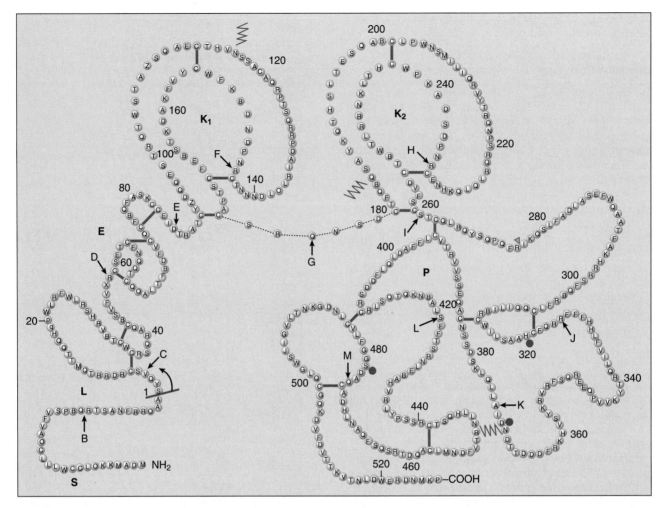

**FIGURE 1-3.** The amino acid sequence of tissue plasminogen activator showing domain organization and posttranslational modification. The letters in the circles represent the single-letter amino acid code. The intrachain and interchain disulphide bridges are indicated by bars. The zigzags denote positions of *N*-linked oligosaccharide. The open tailless arrow indicates the proteolytic cleavage site. The filled circles refer to the catalytic residues in the serine protease domain. The arrows B to M refer to the positions of intron-exon junctions determined from the gene structure. E, epidermal growth factor domain; F, fibronectin finger domain; $K_1$ and $K_2$, kringle structure; L, leader segment; P, serine proteinase domain; S, signal peptide. *(From Buckel P: Recombinant proteins for therapy. Trends Pharmacol Sci 1996;17:450.)*

rin-specificity is not clinically apparent. In a large-scale clinical trial, the rate of hemorrhagic stroke was significantly higher with accelerated t-PA versus streptokinase[23] (0.72% vs. 0.54%, P = 0.03). These shortcomings have prompted investigators to engineer the original t-PA molecule to create mutants with higher fibrin-specificity, more protease potency, slower clearance from the circulation, and more resistance to plasma inhibitors.

### Reteplase (r-PA)

Reteplase (r-PA, 39 kDa) is a single-chain nonglycosylated deletion mutant of human t-PA containing the kringle 2 and protease domains but lacking the kringle 1, finger, and EGF domains (Figure 1-4). Reteplase is designed to contain the minimum number of necessary functional domains and therefore has an improved solubility and is easily expressed in *E. coli.* Reteplase is isolated as inactive inclusion bodies from *E. coli,* converted into its active form by an *in vitro* folding process, and purified by chromatographic separation.

Compared with t-PA, reteplase has more fibrin-specificity, a longer half-life (14 to 18 minutes), enhan-

ced fibrinolytic potency, and a lower affinity for endothelial cells.[24-26] The low affinity for endothelial cells and monocytes is most likely because of the absence of the finger and EGF domains, which are apparently involved in the interaction with endothelial cell receptors.[27] Resistance to PAI-1 is not affected by these deletions. Development of anti-reteplase antibodies in patients treated with reteplace has not been reported.

In contrast to alteplace, reteplace is administered as a double-bolus injection at 30 minutes apart because its longer half-life. Each bolus is administered as an intravenous injection over 2 minutes. Based on a number of clinical trials, reteplace is considered therapeutically similar to alteplace, and the double-bolus administration is an advantage over alteplace.[28]

### Lanoteplase (n-PA)

Lanoteplase is a deletion mutant of t-PA that lacks the finger, EGF domains, and Asn[117] glycosylation. These modifications result in enhanced fibrin binding, more fibrinolytic potency, and a longer half-life[29] (23 minutes). Serum PAI activity is significantly lower with lanoteplase

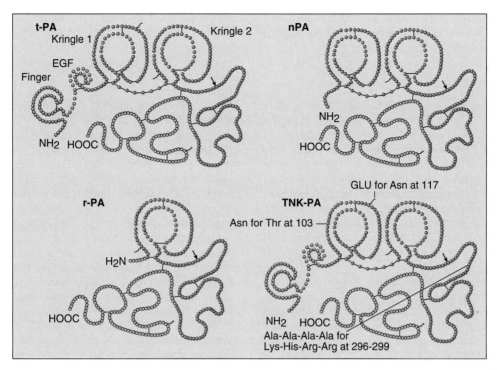

**FIGURE 1-4.** Molecular structures of tissue plasminogen activator (t-PA), reteplase (r-PA), lanetoplase (n-PA), and tenecteplase (TNK-rt-PA). *(From Topol EJ: Acute Coronary Syndrome. New York, Marcel Dekker, 1998, p. 169.)*

than t-PA (P < 0.01), which may contribute to its long half-life and potency.[30] Anti-lanoteplase antibodies have not been detected in various animal models. Despite its promising preliminary results, the development of lanoteplace was discontinued because of a higher incidence of intracranial hemorrhage than t-PA in a clinical trial[31] (1.12% vs. 0.64%, P = 0.004).

*Tenecteplase (TNK-rt-PA)*

Tenecteplase is a triple mutant of t-PA expressed in the CHO cells. The Asn[117] glycosylation site is deleted by substituting Asn[117] with Gln (N117Q), and another glycosylation site is created in the same domain by replacing Thr[103] with Asn (T103N). This change in the glycosylation locus significantly increases the fibrin binding and serum half-life[32] (10 to 24 minutes). In addition, the sequence Lys[296]-His[297]-Arg[298]-Arg[299] is replaced by four successive alanines, which increases resistance to PAI-1 and enhances fibrin specificity. This is accomplished through alanine-scanning mutagenesis, in which the amino acids located at randomly chosen points in the t-PA sequence are replaced with alanine with repeated analysis of the newly created mutant molecules.[33-35] Tenecteplase has more fibrinolytic potency than t-PA, and no immunogenic response has been reported.[36] These favorable properties give tenecteplace an advantage of a single bolus injection with the efficacy and safety comparable to that of accelerated t-PA.[32,37,38] A large-scale clinical trial has shown that for the tenecteplase and t-PA groups, the rates of 30-day mortality (6.18% vs. 6.15%), and intracranial hemorrhage (0.93% vs. 0.94%) were almost identical. The tenecteplase group had fewer noncerebral bleeding complications (26.43% vs. 28.95%,

P = 0.0003) and less frequent need for blood transfusion (4.25% vs. 5.49%, P = 0.0002) compared with the t-PA group.[39] The combination of tenecteplase plus enoxaparin or abciximab reduces the frequency of ischemic complications of acute myocardial infarction compared with that of tenecteplase plus unfractionated heparin.[40]

*Etanercept*

Etanercept is a dimeric fusion protein composed of the extracellular ligand-binding portion of the human TNF p75 receptor and the Fc portion of human IgG1. Each etanercept molecule (934 amino acids, 150 kDa) contains two TNF p75 receptors and one Fc portion. The Fc component of etanercept contains the hinge region, the $C_{H2}$ and $C_{H3}$ domains of $IgG_1$ (see the section on molecular structure of antibodies). Etanercept is produced in the CHO mammalian cell expression system.

Etanercept has been investigated for treatment of heart failure. The efficacy of etanercept to inhibit the negative inotropic effects of TNF-α shown in preclinical studies was confirmed in small, short-term clinical studies.[41-44] Based on these promising results, two large-scale randomized clinical trials, the RENAISSANCE trial in North America and the RECOVER trial in Europe and Australia, were initiated to evaluate the efficacy of etanercept in patients with moderate to severe heart failure. The primary end point of the RENAISSANCE and RECOVER was a clinical composite. The RENEWAL trial, which used the pooled data from the other two trials, evaluated the all-cause mortality and hospitalization for heart failure as the primary end point. These trials, however, were terminated prematurely because preliminary analysis of the data showed no benefit for etanercept on the clinical composite end point in RENAISSANCE and RECOVER and no benefit for all-cause mortality and heart failure hospitalization in RENEWAL.[45]

## Monoclonal Antibody Drugs

Since the 19th century, antibodies have been widely used for treatment and prophylaxis of disease in the form of animal-derived antisera. However, the efficacy of antiserum therapy was severely limited, because antiserum contains polyclonal antibodies, and only some of these antibodies bind to the target antigens. In addition, antiserum therapy was complicated by the symptoms of serum sickness, ranging from minor joint pain and fever to lethal anaphylactic shock. Serum sickness was caused by immune reactions against a number of animal-derived antibodies and nonantibody proteins present in the serum.

Over the last two decades, a series of technical breakthroughs have accelerated the evolution of antibody-based therapeutics. Recombinant DNA technology and hydridoma technology, both born in the mid-1970s, gave rise to antibody engineering, a highly specialized area of protein engineering devoted to the development of monoclonal antibodies (mAbs). Antibody engineering has resulted in the creation of fusion, chimeric, and humanized antibodies that are currently applied to the treatment of a wide spectrum of human diseases. Finally, phage display technology has replaced hybridoma technology, allowing construction of entirely human monoclonal antibodies with the desired antigenic specificity.

### Molecular Structure of Antibodies

Antibodies, also known as immunoglobulins (Igs), are large glycoprotein molecules produced by B lymphocytes. The most common human Ig, IgG, is shaped like the capital letter "Y" in which an antigen-binding site is at the end of the two arms, and an effector site is on the leg (Figure 1-5). The IgG is therefore bivalent. An IgG molecule consists of four protein chains, a pair of heavy chains and a pair of light chains, linked by disulfide bonds. Each chain consists of domains of approximately

110 amino acids in length; the light chain contains two domains, whereas the heavy chain has four. Antibodies can also be digested with proteases to release different fragments called Fv (variable fragment), Fab (antigen-binding fragment), and Fc (crystallization fragment). In addition, there are different isotypes of each chain: κ and λ in the light chain, and γ, α, δ, μ, and ε in the heavy chain. Depending on the isotype of the heavy chain, human Igs are divided into five different classes, $IgG_{1-4}$, $IgA_{1-2}$, IgD, IgM, and IgE. Each class of heavy chain can combine with either of the light chains. These different antibody classes are variations of IgG with a different number of chains or a different number of constant regions and sometimes with an additional J chain.

An antigen-binding site consists of the variable domains of both the light and heavy chains, created by somatic recombination and mutagenesis. The variable domains are highly diverse in amino acid sequence and thus confer specificity against a variety of antigenic epitopes. In contrast to the variable domains ($V_L$, $V_H$), the other domains contain a stable amino acid sequence, and are called constant domains ($C_L$, $C_{H1}$, $C_{H2}$, $C_{H3}$). Only a part of the amino acids in the variable region actually contacts the antigens, and these regions are called complementarity-determining regions (CDRs). The remaining components of the variable region serve as a scaffold to hold the CDRs in the right positions. There are three CDRs on the variable domain of each chain; therefore a total of six CDRs exist in an antigen-binding site ($CDR_{L1-3}$, $CDR_{H1-3}$). The length and composition of the amino acid sequence at the CDRs are hypervariable among different antibodies and are responsible for the specificity and affinity of the antibodies to their target antigens.

The effector functions are mediated by the constant (Fc) regions of the antibody. The Fc portion binds to the Fc receptors on the surface of the effector cells that induce antibody-dependent cellular cytotoxicity (ADCC). In addition, a different region of the Fc portion of the antibody molecule binds to C1q and initiates the classical complement pathway, which leads to complement-mediated cytolysis.

### Mouse Monoclonal Antibodies

The advent of the hybridoma technology (Figure 1-6) has revolutionized the scientific study of Igs, fostered their clinical application, and has set the ground for the development of antibody engineering.[46] The hybridoma technology has allowed large-scale production of mAbs that specifically bind to almost any target antigen of interest.

Although the hybridoma technology has provided mAbs that are currently playing a major role in biomedical research and clinical medicine, the application of hybridoma-derived mAbs for therapeutic use is limited by multiple difficulties. Because most hybridomas are of mouse origin, hybridoma-derived mAbs are not identical to human antibodies. When mouse mAbs are injected into humans, the patients develop anti-mouse mAb antibodies that accelerate their clearance. This human anti-mouse antibody (HAMA) response can occur within

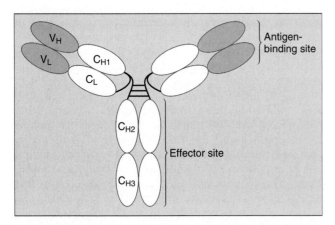

**FIGURE 1-5.** Structure of IgG. Gray ovals represent variable domains ($V_H$ and $V_L$), and white ovals represent constant domains ($C_L$, $C_{H1}$, $C_{H2}$, and $C_{H3}$).

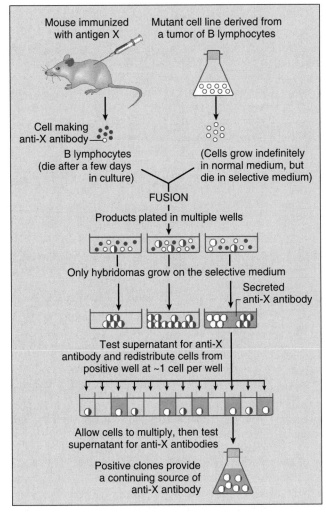

**FIGURE 1-6.** Hybridoma technology. A mouse is sensitized with an antigen of interest (antigen X). This stimulates the proliferation of B cells expressing antibodies against the antigen X. The spleen is removed, and the spleen cells, including B cells, are fused to myeloma cells to produce hybridomas by treatment with polyethylene glycol. This myeloma cell line does not produce antibodies of its own, and lacks hypoxanthine guanine phosphoribosyltransferase (HGPRT), thus it cannot synthesize purine nucleotides in the salvage pathway but only in the de novo pathway. The cells without HGPRT, therefore, will not survive in the presence of aminopterin, an inhibitor of *de novo* purine synthesis pathway. Aminopterin inhibits thymidine synthesis as well. Hybridomas are selected in the hypoxanthine, aminopterin, and thymidine (HAT) medium. A hybridoma consisting of a normal B cell and an HGPRT-deficient myeloma cell expresses HGPRT genes and, therefore, survives in the HAT medium, using hypoxanthine to produce purines. Unfused lymphocytes die in a few days in culture. Individual hybridomas are transferred to the wells of a microtiter dish and cultured for several days. Aliquots of the culture fluids are removed and tested for the presence of anti-X antibody using an enzyme-linked immunosorbent assay (ELISA) or radioimmunoassay (RIA). Cells that test positive are cultured for monoclonal antibody production. *(From Alberts B, Bray D, Lewis J, et al: Molecular Biology of the Cell, 4th ed. Reproduced by permission of Routledge, Inc., part of The Taylor & Francis Group.)*

a few weeks of the initiation of mAb treatment and precludes long-term therapy. The patients also form immune complexes that produce the symptoms of serum sickness. Furthermore, rodent antibodies are not as effective as human antibodies in recruiting effector functions of the immune system, because rodent Fc frag-

ments do not interact well with human Fc-dependent effector mechanisms.

### Muromonab-CD3

Muromonab-CD3 (OKT3) was the first therapeutic mAb in the history of medicine. Muromonab-CD3 is a mouse mAb against the CD3 molecules that form a portion of the human T cell antigen-receptor complex. Muromonab-CD3 binds to all mature T cells, functioning as an immunosuppressant. Although muromonab-CD3 is widely used in reversing rejection of transplanted organs, including heart, kidneys, and liver, the period of use is limited by the development of the HAMA response.

### Recombinant Antibody Fragments

Detailed sequence-structural analysis of antibody molecules has been made available through hybridoma and recombinant DNA technology, which has resulted in creation of antibody fragments of the smallest possible size that maintain the original antigen-binding capacity. Various recombinant antibody fragments with antigen-binding sites have been expressed in prokaryotes, including Fv, single-chain Fv (scFv), and Fab (Figure 1-7). The Fv module (25 kDa) is the smallest monovalent antigen-binding unit of an antibody and consists of $V_H$ and $V_L$ domains linked by disulfide bonds. The scFv module is an Fv module with an additional peptide that covalently links the $V_H$ and $V_L$ domains. The peptide linker is usually 15 to 20 amino acids long and is introduced at the cDNA level. These fragments are attached to a bacterial leader sequence that transports the protein to the periplasmic space, where the $V_H$ and $V_L$ domains fold into active protein with disulfide bond formation between the two domains.

Because of their small size (30 kDa), scFv fragments are easily expressed in bacterial cells and are subject to various engineering efforts using classic recombinant DNA techniques. Other fragments can be genetically combined with scFv fragments to produce *multivalent antibodies* (e.g., bivalent, trivalent, tetravalent antibodies) with increased affinity and tissue targeting or *multispecific antibodies* (e.g., bispecific, trispecific, tetraspecific antibodies) that recognize different antigens, thus allowing an antibody to bridge different antigens (see Figure 1-7). An example of a bispecific antibody is an anti-T cell receptor antibody fragment attached to a fragment with specificity for a viral, parasitic, or tumor antigen, which can bring the cytotoxic T cell directly to the antigens. Moreover, the antibody fragments can be fused genetically with toxins, enzymes, or cytokines to form *fusion antibodies* that may exhibit more potent effector functions than the Fc-dependent effector mechanisms, which are lacking in the small antibody fragments. Fusion antibodies that carry human TNF with specificity for colorectal carcinoma cell antigens are being developed.[47] Despite the potential significance of fusion antibodies for therapeutic use, the pharmacologic and pharmacokinetic properties of fusion antibodies *in vivo* are affected by various parameters and are often unpredictable. Another therapeutic application is the intracellular expression of antigen recognition

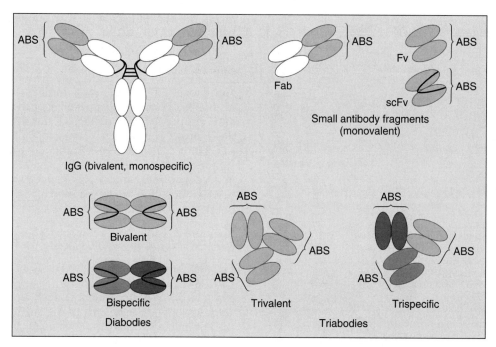

**FIGURE 1-7.** Recombinant antibody fragments. Intact IgG, monovalent antibody fragments (Fab, Fv, and scFv), diabodies (bivalent, bispecific), and triabodies (trivalent, trispecific) are shown. Gray ovals represent V-domains, whereas white ovals show C-domains. Black lines represent linkers. Different shading of the V-domains represents different target specificity at the antigen-binding sites (ABS).

domain of immunoglobulins to inhibit intracellular processes. The cDNA of these *intrabodies* are cloned into gene transfer vectors and are introduced in the target cells. The intrabodies can be directed to different intracellular compartments by adding various signal sequences and can be used to inhibit intracellular enzymes, transcription factors, and receptors.

### Chimeric Monoclonal Antibodies

To overcome the shortcomings of conventional mouse mAb therapy, hybrids of mouse and human antibodies have been produced *(chiemeric monoclonal antibodies)* (Figure 1-8). Chimeric mAbs are constructed by ligating the cDNA fragment that encodes the xenogenic (e.g., mouse) $V_L$ and $V_H$ domains to the fragment that encodes the Fc domain from a human antibody. In general, chimeric mAbs contain approximately 33% mouse protein and 67% human protein. Therefore, the final hybrid antibody products have the mouse variable regions that have the desired antigen specificity and the human constant regions that activate effector mechanisms. Construction of chimeric mAbs is relatively easy compared with constructing humanized mAbs. Chimeric mAbs exhibit reduced immunogenicity compared with mouse mAbs while retaining high binding affinity and specificity. However, some patients still experience variable degrees of human anti-chimeric antibody (HACA) immune response, which may reduce the efficacy of the mAb as a drug.

### Abciximab

Abciximab is the first human-murine chimeric mAb commercially produced for therapeutic use. Abciximab is the Fab fragment (48 kDa) of the mAbs that binds selectively to the glycoprotein (GP) IIb/IIIa receptors of human platelets. The GP IIb/IIIa ($\alpha_{IIb}\beta_3$) is a member of the integrin family of adhesion receptors and is the major platelet surface receptor involved in platelet aggregation. Abciximab inhibits platelet aggregation by preventing the binding of fibrinogen, von Willebrand factor, and other adhesive molecules to GPIIb/IIIa receptors on activated platelets. Abciximab also binds to the Mac-1 (CD11b/CD18) on leukocytes and the vitronectin ($\alpha_v\beta_3$) on platelets, vascular endothelial cells, and smooth muscle cells, although the relationship of binding characteristics to Mac-1 and vitronectin to clinical efficacy remains uncertain. Abciximab is devoid of the Fc fragment to decrease immunogenicity and, therefore, cannot activate effector mechanisms. Abciximab contains the murine $V_L$ and $V_H$ regions that confer antibody specificity, and the human $C_L$ and $C_{H1}$ regions derived from human IgG$_1$. Abciximab is produced by continuous perfusion in mammalian cell culture. The Fc fragment is cleaved with papain, and the Fab fragment is purified from the cell culture supernatant by column chromatography.

Abciximab is indicated as an adjunct to coronary angioplasty for the prevention of acute cardiac ischemic complications in patients at high risk for the sudden closure of the revascularized target vessel.

### Infliximab

Infliximab is a chimeric IgG$_1$ mAb with a molecular weight of 149 kDa. It is composed of human constant regions and murine variable regions that specifically bind to human TNF-α. Infliximab is produced by a recombinant cell line cultured by continuous perfusion and is purified by a series of steps that includes measures to inactivate and remove viruses.

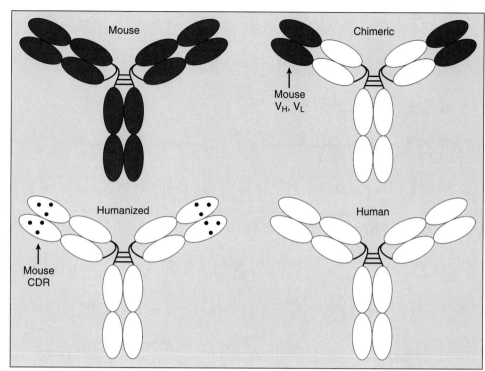

**FIGURE 1-8.** Engineered monoclonal antibodies. Mouse, chimeric, humanized, and human monoclonal antibodies. Black and white ovals represent the domains of mouse and human origin, respectively. In a chimeric monoclonal antibody, the variable domains ($V_H$ and $V_L$) derive from the mouse, and all the constant domains ($C_L$, $C_{H1}$, $C_{H2}$, and $C_{H3}$) derive from the human. In humanized antibody, only the complementarity-determining regions (CDRs) are of mouse origin.

The efficacy of infliximab was first tested in Crohn's disease. A randomized clinical study has shown that infliximab is effective in treatment of draining fistulas resulting from Crohn's disease.[48] Infliximab was also evaluated in active rheumatoid arthritis, and the combination of infliximab and methotrexate significantly and persistently reduced the signs and symptoms, improved the quality of life, and delayed the progression of joint damage compared with methotrexate therapy alone.[49] Infliximab was subsequently examined in a number of inflammatory diseases, including psoriatic arthritis, psoriasis, refractory sarcoidosis, ulcerative colitis, Sjögren's syndrome, and ankylosing spondylitis, and yielded favorable results. Nevertheless, results from clinical studies evaluating infliximab as a therapy for moderate to advanced heart failure have been disappointing. A randomized phase II clinical study (ATTACH trial) demonstrated a significant dose-related increase in death and heart failure hospitalizations with infliximab compared with a placebo.[45,50] The administration of infliximab is associated with serious infections, including bacterial pneumonia, sepsis, histoplasmosis, listeriosis, coccidiomycosis, pneumocystosis, and tuberculosis. In addition, treatment with infliximab can result in the formation of antibodies against infliximab. The development of anti-infliximab antibodies is associated with an increased risk of infusion reactions and a reduced duration of response to treatment. Concomitant immunosuppressive therapy may reduce the magnitude of the immunogenic response.[51]

## Humanized Monoclonal Antibodies

Humanized mAbs have been constructed to minimize the HAMA and HACA responses triggered with mouse and chimeric mAbs while maintaining high binding specificity to the desired antigen. In humanized mAbs, only the CDRs derive from mice or other xenogenic sources (5% to 10%), and the rest of the antibody domains (90% to 95%) are of human origin. Humanization requires grafting the CDR amino acid sequences from mouse mAbs into human antibodies using *in vitro* mutagenesis; therefore, humanized mAbs are also called CDR-grafted or reshaped mAbs. Although the recombinant DNA techniques to create humanized mAbs are relatively straightforward, mere grafting of the mouse CDRs into human antibodies does not always produce the antigen specificity and affinity of the original mouse mAb. The design of the engineered mAb has been found to be critical in reconstituting the properties of the original molecule. The designing process requires meticulous analysis of the sequence, structure, and glycosylations of the antigen-binding site of the original mouse mAb. An appropriate human framework that anchors mouse CDRs is selected out of numerous candidates, and the extent of mouse CDRs to be grafted into the human framework is determined following repeated construction and testing of different prototype antibodies. Therefore, the humanization process is technically challenging and often arduous and is still an area of active research efforts. To date, humanized mAbs were found to trigger minimal or no immune response in humans. However, all CDRs are unique and may contain components that are potentially antigenic regardless of production method. In fact, a small number of patients have developed human anti-human antibodies (HAHA) against a conformational antigenic determinant of the humanized monoclonal antibodies.

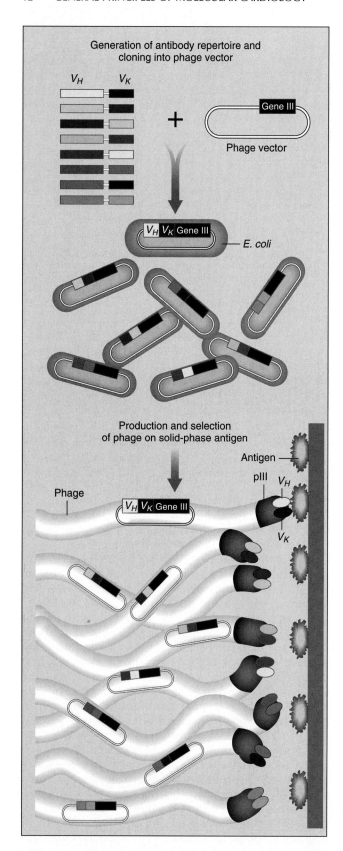

**FIGURE 1-9.** Phage display technology. In the top panel, a repertoire of single-chain Fv genes (*scFv*) is generated with a polymerase chain reaction. The repertoires are constructed either from $V_H$ and $V$ genes that have been rearranged *in vivo* or from *V* gene segments that are rearranged *in vitro* (not shown). The repertoire of *scFv* genes is cloned into a phage vector in a way that fuses the *scFv* gene to a gene (gene III) that encodes a protein (pIII) expressed on the phage surface. In the middle panel, the vector directs *E. coli* to produce phage antibodies, which have on their surface a functional scFv fused to pIII. Inside each phage antibody is the vector DNA containing the gene for the scFv. Phage antibodies binding a specific antigen can be separated from nonbinding phage antibodies by affinity chromatography on immobilized antigen *(bottom panel)*. A single round of selection increases the number of antigen-binding phage antibodies by a factor ranging from 20 to 1000, depending on the affinity of the antibody. Eluted phage antibodies are used to infect *E. coli*, which then produce more phage antibodies for the next round of selection. Repeated rounds of selection make it possible to isolate antigen-binding phage antibodies that were originally present at frequencies of less than 1 in a billion. *(From Marks C, Marks JD: Phage libraries: A new route to clinically useful antibodies. N Engl J Med 1996;335:730. Copyright © 1996 Massachusetts Medical Society. All rights Reserved.)*

## Daclizumab

Daclizumab is an immunosuppressive, humanized $IgG_1$ mAb (144 kDa) that binds specifically to the α subunit (p55α, CD25, or Tac subunit) of the human high-affinity IL-2 receptor that is expressed on the surface of activated lymphocytes. The human sequences derive from the constant regions of human $IgG_1$ and the variable regions of the Eu myeloma antibody. The murine sequences derive from the CDRs of a murine anti-Tac antibody. Daclizumab is currently indicated for prophylaxis of acute organ rejection in patients receiving renal transplants as part of an immunosuppressive regimen that includes cyclosporine and corticosteroids. In a randomized clinical trial, daclizumab significantly reduced the rate of biopsy-proven rejection in patients who received renal transplant compared with the placebo group[52] (28% vs. 47%, P = 0.001). Daclizumab was also evaluated in cardiac transplantation, and it significantly reduced the rate of acute rejection compared with a placebo[53] (18% vs. 63%, P = 0.04).

## Trastuzumab

Trastuzumab is a humanized mAb that selectively binds to the extracellular domain of the human epidermal growth factor receptor 2 protein, HER2 (ErbB2). The antibody is an $IgG_1$ that contains human framework regions with CDRs of a murine antibody that binds to HER2. Trastuzumab is produced by a CHO cell suspension culture in a nutrient medium. Trastuzumab is indicated for the treatment of HER2 overexpressing metastatic breast cancer, which composes 25% to 30% of breast cancers.

In patients with metastatic breast cancer, trastuzumab delayed the time to disease progression (median, 7.4 vs. 4.6 months, P < 0.001), increased the rate of objective response (50% vs. 32%, P < 0.001), prolonged the duration of response (median, 9.1 vs. 6.1 months, P < 0.001), decreased 1-year mortality (22% vs. 33%, P = 0.008), and improved survival (median survival, 25.1 vs. 20.3 months; P = 0.01). However, trastuzumab was complicated by a high rate of cardiac dysfunction (NYHA class III and IV). The incidence of cardiac dysfunction was 8% in patients treated with a conventional chemotherapy regimen including an anthracycline and increased to 27% in patients who received trastuzumab concurrently with the same regimen.[54] The cardiotoxicity of trastuzumab appears to be associated with the ErbB2/gp130-dependent cell-survival pathway.[55] Mice with a ventricular-restricted deletion of ErbB2 display no overt phenotype, but physiologic analysis has revealed the onset of dilated cardiomyopathy with chamber dilation, wall thinning, and decreased contractility. Moreover, cardiomyocytes isolated from these conditional mutants were more susceptible to anthracycline toxicity.[56]

## Fully Human Monoclonal Antibodies

Several technical advances have finally allowed construction of fully human mAbs. One of these technical breakthroughs is the phage display technology, which isolates fragments with desired specificity from the large and diverse libraries of small human mAb fragment genes *(Fab or scFv)*.[57] The human mAb fragment libraries can be produced from B lymphocytes in various organs of human donors either with *(immune library)* or without *(naive library)* prior immunization. Small antibody fragments against a wide variety of antigens have been isolated from naive libraries that possess high affinity comparable to those from immune libraries. Application of the phage display technology for human mAb selection is described in Figure 1-9. The affinity of a primary isolate can be further enhanced by mutagene-

sis, chain shuffling, or CDR walking, and repeated use of the phage display technology *(affinity maturation)*. The isolated fragment genes are then linked to the genes of the human constant region to create entirely human mAbs. Fully human mAbs can also be generated from transgenic mice carrying human immunoglobulin genes. These technical advances have almost obviated the classic hydridoma technology and the cumbersome humanization process in the production of therapeutic mAbs. Human mAbs are much less immunogenic than chimeric or humanized mAbs, reducing or even eliminating an immune response to these molecules during therapy. A number of fully human mAbs are undergoing preclinical and clinical trials, and the HAHA response has not been reported in humans. Because the technology is relatively new, there are no fully human mAb drugs available as yet for clinical use.

# FUTURE DIRECTIONS

As noted previously, recombinant protein and antibody therapy represent only a fraction of the current clinical applications of recombinant DNA technology. Although the list of sophisticated recombinant protein drugs will continue to expand, the biotechnology will become intertwined with novel cardiovascular devices that will deliver the protein of interest to an individual organ at a specific time in a variable dosing schedule. Tissue engineering, or cell-based therapy, is an advanced form of *ex vivo* gene therapy, and many successful studies have already been reported in various animal models. The engineering of genes, proteins, cells, and tissues represents different layers of biotechnology, which will evolve complementarily to foster a new era of molecular medicine.

## REFERENCES

1. Cohen SN, Chang AC, Boyer HW, et al: Construction of biologically functional bacterial plasmids in vitro. Proc Natl Acad Sci USA 1973;70:3240-3244.
2. Watson JD, Witkowski J, Gilman M, et al: Recombinant DNA, 2nd ed. New York, Scientific American Books, 1992.
3. Koths K: Recombinant proteins for medical use: The attractions and challenges. Curr Opin Biotechnol 1995;6:681-687.
4. Sambrook J, Russell DW: Molecular Cloning: A Laboratory Manual, 3rd ed. Cold Spring Harbor, NY, Cold Spring Harbor Laboratory Press, 2001.
5. Ebert KM, DiTullio P, Barry CA, et al: Induction of human tissue plasminogen activator in the mammary gland of transgenic goats. Biotechnology 1994;12:699-702.
6. Buckel P: Recombinant protein drugs. In Parnham MJ, Bruinvels J (eds): Milestones in Drug Therapy. Basel, Switzerland, Birkhauser Verlag, 2001.
7. Osterziel KJ, Ranke MB, Strohm O, et al: The somatotrophic system in patients with dilated cardiomyopathy: Relation of insulin-like growth factor-1 and its alterations during growth hormone therapy to cardiac function. Clin Endocrinol 2000;53:61-68.
8. Fazio S, Sabatini D, Capaldo B, et al: A preliminary study of growth hormone in the treatment of dilated cardiomyopathy. N Engl J Med 1996;334:809-814.
9. Capaldo B, Lembo G, Rendina V, et al: Sympathetic deactivation by growth hormone treatment in patients with dilated cardiomyopathy. Eur Heart J 1998;19:623-627.

10. Adamopoulos S, Parissis JT, Georgiadis M, et al: Growth hormone administration reduces circulating proinflammatory cytokines and soluble Fas/soluble Fas ligand system in patients with chronic heart failure secondary to idiopathic dilated cardiomyopathy. Am Heart J 2002;144:359-364.

11. Perrot A, Ranke MB, Dietz R, et al: Growth hormone treatment in dilated cardiomyopathy. J Card Surg 2001;16:127-131.

12. Osterziel KJ, Strohm O, Schuler J, et al: Randomised, double-blind, placebo-controlled trial of human recombinant growth hormone in patients with chronic heart failure due to dilated cardiomyopathy. Lancet 1998;351:1233-1237.

13. Isgaard J, Bergh CH, Caidahl K, et al: A placebo-controlled study of growth hormone in patients with congestive heart failure. Eur Heart J 1998;19:1704-1711.

14. Osterziel KJ, Blum WF, Strohm O, et al: The severity of chronic heart failure due to coronary artery disease predicts the endocrine effects of short-term growth hormone administration. J Clin Endocrinol Metab 2000;85:1533-1539.

15. Al-Obaidi MK, Hon JK, Stubbs PJ, et al: Plasma insulin-like growth factor-1 elevated in mild-to-moderate but not severe heart failure. Am Heart J 2001;142:E10.

16. Donath MY, Jenni R, Brunner HP, et al: Cardiovascular and metabolic effects of insulin-like growth factor I at rest and during exercise in humans. J Clin Endocrinol Metab 1996;81:4089-4094.

17. Donath MY, Sutsch G, Yan XW, et al: Acute cardiovascular effects of insulin-like growth factor I in patients with chronic heart failure. J Clin Endocrinol Metab 1998;83:3177-3183.

18. Colucci WS, Elkayam U, Horton DP, et al: Intravenous nesiritide, a natriuretic peptide, in the treatment of decompensated congestive heart failure. Nesiritide Study Group. N Engl J Med 2000;343: 246-253.

19. Pennica D, Holmes WE, Kohr WJ, et al: Cloning and expression of human tissue-type plasminogen activator cDNA in E. coli. Nature 1983;301:214-221.

20. Topol EJ, Morris DC, Smalling RW, et al: A multicenter, randomized, placebo-controlled trial of a new form of intravenous recombinant tissue-type plasminogen activator (activase) in acute myocardial infarction. J Am Coll Cardiol 1987;9:1205-1213.

21. Hoylaerts M, Rijken DC, Lijnen HR, et al: Kinetics of the activation of plasminogen by human tissue plasminogen activator: Role of fibrin. J Biol Chem 1982;257:2912-2919.

22. Brener SJ, Topol EJ: Third-generation thrombolytic agents for acute myocardial infarction. In Topol EJ (ed): Acute Coronary Syndromes. New York, Marcel Dekker, 1998, pp 167-192.

23. GUSTO I: An international randomized trial comparing four thrombolytic strategies for acute myocardial infarction. N Engl J Med 1993;329:673-682.

24. Martin U, von Mollendorff E, Akpan W, et al: Dose-ranging study of the novel recombinant plasminogen activator BM 06.022 in healthy volunteers. Clin Pharmacol Ther 1991;50:429-436.

25. Martin U, Sponer G, Strein K: Evaluation of thrombolytic and systemic effects of the novel recombinant plasminogen activator BM 06.022 compared with alteplase, anistreplase, streptokinase and urokinase in a canine model of coronary artery thrombosis. J Am Coll Cardiol 1992;19:433-440.

26. Hu CK, Kohnert U, Wilhelm O, et al: Tissue-type plasminogen activator domain-deletion mutant BM 06.022: Modular stability, inhibitor binding, and activation cleavage. Biochemistry 1994;33: 11760-11766.

27. Hajjar KA: The endothelial cell tissue plasminogen activator receptor: Specific interaction with plasminogen. J Biol Chem 1991;266:21962-21970.

28. Antman EM, Braunwald E: Acute myocardial infarction. In Braunwald E, Zipes DP, Libby P (eds): Heart Disease: A Textbook of Cardiovascular Medicine. Philadelphia, WB Saunders, 2001, pp 1114-1219.

29. Hansen L, Blue Y, Barone K, et al: Functional effects of asparagine-linked oligosaccharide on natural and variant human tissue-type plasminogen activator. J Biol Chem 1988;263:15713-15719.

30. Ogata N, Ogawa H, Ogata Y, et al: Comparison of thrombolytic therapies with mutant tPA (lanoteplase/SUN9216) and recombinant tPA (alteplase) for acute myocardial infarction. Jpn Circ J 1998;62:801-806.

31. Neuhaus KL: InTime-2 results. Presented at the Scientific Sessions of the American College of Cardiology, March 9, 1999, New Orleans.

32. Cannon CP, McCabe CH, Gibson CM, et al: TNK-tissue plasminogen activator in acute myocardial infarction. Results of the Thrombolysis in Myocardial Infarction (TIMI) 10A dose-ranging trial. Circulation 1997;95:351-356.

33. Paoni NF, Keyt BA, Refino CJ, et al: A slow clearing, fibrin-specific, PAI-1 resistant variant of t-PA (T103N, KHRR 296-299 AAAA). Thromb Haemost 1993;70:307-312.

34. Refino CJ, Paoni NF, Keyt BA, et al: A variant of t-PA (T103N, KHRR 296-299 AAAA) that, by bolus, has increased potency and decreased systemic activation of plasminogen. Thromb Haemost 1993;70:313-319.

35. Keyt BA, Paoni NF, Refino CJ, et al: A faster-acting and more potent form of tissue plasminogen activator. Proc Natl Acad Sci USA 1994;91:3670-3674.

36. Collen D, Stassen JM, Yasuda T, et al: Comparative thrombolytic properties of tissue-type plasminogen activator and of a plasminogen activator inhibitor-1-resistant glycosylation variant, in a combined arterial and venous thrombosis model in the dog. Thromb Haemost 1994;72:98-104.

37. Cannon CP, Gibson CM, McCabe CH, et al: TNK-tissue plasminogen activator compared with front-loaded alteplase in acute myocardial infarction: Results of the TIMI 10B trial. Thrombolysis in Myocardial Infarction (TIMI) 10B Investigators. Circulation 1998;98:2805-2814.

38. Van de Werf F, Cannon CP, Luyten A, et al: Safety assessment of single-bolus administration of TNK tissue-plasminogen activator in acute myocardial infarction: The ASSENT-1 trial. The ASSENT-1 Investigators. Am Heart J 1999;137:786-791.

39. ASSENT-2: Single-bolus tenecteplase compared with front-loaded alteplase in acute myocardial infarction: The ASSENT-2 double-blind randomised trial. Assessment of the Safety and Efficacy of a New Thrombolytic Investigators. Lancet 1999;354:716-722.

40. ASSENT-3: Efficacy and safety of tenecteplase in combination with enoxaparin, abciximab, or unfractionated heparin: The ASSENT-3 randomised trial in acute myocardial infarction. Lancet 2001;358:605-613.

41. Kapadia S, Torre-Amione G, Yokoyama T, et al: Soluble TNF binding proteins modulate the negative inotropic properties of TNF-alpha in vitro. Am J Physiol 1995;268:H517-H525.

42. Bozkurt B, Kribbs SB, Clubb FJ Jr, et al: Pathophysiologically relevant concentrations of tumor necrosis factor-alpha promote progressive left ventricular dysfunction and remodeling in rats. Circulation 1998;97:1382-1391.

43. Deswal A, Bozkurt B, Seta Y, et al: Safety and efficacy of a soluble P75 tumor necrosis factor receptor (Enbrel, etanercept) in patients with advanced heart failure. Circulation 1999;99:3224-3226.

44. Bozkurt B, Torre-Amione G, Warren MS, et al: Results of targeted anti-tumor necrosis factor therapy with etanercept (ENBREL) in patients with advanced heart failure. Circulation 2001;103: 1044-1047.

45. Mann DL: Inflammatory mediators and the failing heart: Past, present, and the foreseeable future. Circ Res 2002;91:988-998.

46. Kohler G, Milstein C: Continuous cultures of fused cells secreting antibody of predefined specificity. Nature 1975;256:495-497.

47. Xiang J, Moyana T, Qi Y: Genetic engineering of a recombinant fusion possessing anti-tumor F(ab')2 and tumor necrosis factor. J Biotechnol 1997;53:3-12.

48. Present DH, Rutgeerts P, Targan S, et al: Infliximab for the treatment of fistulas in patients with Crohn's disease. N Engl J Med 1999;340:1398-1405.

49. Lipsky PE, van der Heijde DM, St Clair EW, et al: Infliximab and methotrexate in the treatment of rheumatoid arthritis. Anti-Tumor Necrosis Factor Trial in Rheumatoid Arthritis with Concomitant Therapy Study Group. N Engl J Med 2000;343:1594-1602.

50. Anker SD, Coats AJ: How to RECOVER from RENAISSANCE? The significance of the results of RECOVER, RENAISSANCE, RENEWAL and ATTACH. Int J Cardiol 2002;86:123-130.

51. Baert F, Noman M, Vermeire S, et al: Influence of immunogenicity on the long-term efficacy of infliximab in Crohn's disease. N Engl J Med 2003;348:601-608.

52. Nashan B, Light S, Hardie IR, et al: Reduction of acute renal allograft rejection by daclizumab. Daclizumab Double Therapy Study Group. Transplantation 1999;67:110-115.

53. Beniaminovitz A, Itescu S, Lietz K, et al: Prevention of rejection in cardiac transplantation by blockade of the interleukin-2 receptor with a monoclonal antibody. N Engl J Med 2000;342:613-619.

54. Slamon DJ, Leyland-Jones B, Shak S, et al: Use of chemotherapy plus a monoclonal antibody against HER2 for metastatic breast cancer that overexpresses HER2. N Engl J Med 2001;344:783–792.
55. Chien KR: Stress pathways and heart failure. Cell 1999;98:555–558.
56. Crone SA, Zhao YY, Fan L, et al: ErbB2 is essential in the prevention of dilated cardiomyopathy. Nat Med 2002;8:459–465.
57. Marks C, Marks JD: Phage libraries: A new route to clinically useful antibodies. N Engl J Med 1996;335:730–733.

## EDITOR'S CHOICE

Ferrara N, Gerber HP, LeCouter J: The biology of VEGF and its receptors. Nat Med 2003;9:669–676.
*Overview of the key angiogenic growth factor (VEGF) that is a target for therapeutic coronary and peripheral angiogenesis and anti-angiogenesis in cancer.*
Heeschen C, Dimmeler S, Hamm CW, et al: Soluble CD40 ligand in acute coronary syndromes. N Engl J Med 2003;348:1104–1111.
*CD40 is a biomarker of acute coronary syndromes. Many new cytokines and receptors have been uncovered by the Genome Project, providing a basis for new biomarkers for many cardiovascular indications.*
Johansson SG, Haahtela T, O'Byrne PM: Omalizumab and the immune system: An overview of preclinical and clinical data. Ann Allergy Asthma Immunol 2002;89:132–138.
*Humanized antibodies to IgE represent a new therapeutic strategy for steroid-dependent asthma.*
Lebwohl M: Psoriasis. Lancet 2003;361:1197–1204.
*Humanized antibodies find wide applications in immune related disorders, including sporiasis.*

Leung DY, Sampson HA, Yunginger JW, et al: Effect of anti-IgE therapy in patients with peanut allergy. N Engl J Med 2003;348:986–993.
*Humanized IgE antibodies are effective in acute food allergies.*
Maisel AS, Krishnaswamy P, Nowak RM, et al: Rapid measurement of B-type natriuretic peptide in the emergency diagnosis of heart failure. N Engl J Med 2002;347:161–167.
*BNP is a sensitive biomarker for the diagnosis of acute decompensated heart failure.*
McCarthy M: Antiangiogenesis drug promising for metastatic colorectal cancer. Lancet 2003;361:1959.
*Humanized antibodies to VEGF (Avastin) represent a new anti-angiogenic therapy for colon cancer; could find wide usage as adjunctive therapy in other solid tumors.*
Waldmann TA, Levy R, Coller BS: Emerging therapies: Spectrum of applications of monoclonal antibody therapy. Hematology (Am Soc Hematol Educ Program) 2000;394–408.
*Three of the acknowledged leaders in immunotherapy via humanized antibodies summarize recent developments in the field.*
Wiseman GA, Gordon LI, Multani PS, et al: Ibritumomab tiuxetan radioimmunotherapy for patients with relapsed or refractory non-Hodgkin lymphoma and mild thrombocytopenia: A phase II multicenter trial. Blood 2002;99:4336–4342.
*A humanized antibody (Zevalin) can be engineered to deliver a radioactive payload to tumor cells; "armed" antibodies represent a new direction for immnotherapy.*
Wohrle J, Grebe OC, Nusser T, et al: Reduction of major adverse cardiac events with intracoronary compared with intravenous bolus application of abciximab in patients with acute myocardial infarction or unstable angina undergoing coronary angioplasty. Circulation 2003;107:1840–1843.
*Humanized antibodies directed against platelet receptors continue to show efficacy in a diverse group of coronary syndromes.*

# chapter 2

# Human Genome Project and Cardiovascular Disease Genes

*C.C. Liew*
*Victor J. Dzau*

## THE HUMAN GENOME PROJECT

With an allocated budget of more than $3 billion, the Human Genome Project (HGP) is the largest and most ambitious undertaking ever launched in the biomedical sciences. Now in its 12th year, the multidisciplinary, international HGP has linked thousands of researchers in fields such as medicine, biology, physics, chemistry, and computer science; the project has involved laboratories on every continent, including research centers in the United States, the United Kingdom, France, Germany, Canada, Japan, and China.

The formidable task of sequencing the 3 billion nucleotides of the human genome was first considered in the mid-1980s during meetings organized by the US Department of Energy (DoE) and the US National Institutes of Health (NIH). Completing the sequencing project and determining the location of the full complement of protein-encoding genes in the human genome was to lead to a new era in the biologic sciences. The leaders of the HGP hoped that the project would provide the tools for a better fundamental-level understanding of the approximately 4000 known human genetic diseases and provide new insights into complex polygenic diseases. At that time the ambitious proposal was highly controversial; it was viewed as impractical and even "quixotic."[1] The sequencing technology available at that time was relatively rudimentary, involving manual sequencing of only very short lengths of DNA—about 300 bases. Critics of the project argued that sequencing the entire genome would be a Herculean work and a "fishing expedition" of uncertain benefit. The huge predicted cost of the venture—$200 million a year for 15 years—led to worries that it would stifle other areas of scientific endeavor.[2]

Despite reservations, however, in 1990 DoE and NIH officially announced the beginning of the HGP. Initially led by James Watson, Nobel laureate and codiscoverer of the DNA double helix, the HGP was mandated to develop strategies for a sequencing operation to be completed by 2005, then considered a highly optimistic deadline.[3] The project was planned to develop in 5-year stages with clearly defined milestones to be achieved at each phase. The goals for the first 5 years included the development of a complete genetic map; a physical map with markers 100 kb apart; and the sequencing of the genomes of certain simple model organisms such as flies, worms, and yeast. In addition, a very important goal of the project was to develop novel technologies to drive future research.[4]

Scientific and technical success marked the first years of the HGP.[5] In 1990 Lipman and Myers published the sequence algorithm BLAST (Basic Local Alignment Search Tool)[6]; in 1991, Craig Venter, then with NIH, announced his strategy to obtain expressed sequence tags (EST) by partially sequencing randomly selected cDNA clones.[7] Between 1991 and 1993 the first physical chromosome maps (chromosome Y[8] and chromosome 21[9]) were completed, a genetic map of the mouse was completed,[10] and Cohen et al.[11] published a first-generation physical map of the human genome. By 1993, the project was considered so successful that NIH and DoE revised their plans, announcing as a second 5-year goal the sequencing of 80 Mb of DNA by 1998 and the completion of the entire human genome sequencing by 2005.[12]

The period from 1993 to 1998 was also a phase of rapid growth for HGP. In 1995 the first bacterial genome, the 1.8-Mb *Haemophilus influenzae,* was sequenced using the whole-genome shotgun approach, pioneered by Craig Venter and his scientific team.[13] Also in 1995, Hudson et al. published a physical map of the human genome with 15,000 markers.[14] By 1996, the sequencing of the 12 million base pairs of the yeast *Saccharomyces cerevisiae* was completed.[15] The first multicellular organism, the roundworm *Caenorhabditis elegans* (97 Mb), was sequenced by 1998.[16] In 1996, members of the Bermuda Second International Strategy Meeting on Human Genome Sequencing passed a resolution that all sequence data produced by the HGP should be in the public domain and freely accessible within 24 hours (GenBank: www.ncbi.nlm.nih.gov).[17]

At this time, there was a very low number of sequences available, and the story of the "race" between 1998 and 2000 to finish the HGP has been well documented.[18,19] In 1998 Celera, the Rockville, Maryland company founded by Venter, announced that it would finish the genome within 2 years (3 years in advance of the public genome project completion) and at a reduced cost. Venter's announcement galvanized the public consortium. In its new 5-year goals for 1998 to 2003, HGP increased funding and moved its own deadline up by 2 years, promising a blueprint by 2003.[20] The group renewed its commitment to technology development and added goals for studying human sequence variation (with a goal of mapping 100,000 single nucleotide polymorphisms [SNPs]) for completing the 180-Mb fruit fly genome, and for beginning the 3000-Mb mouse genome.[20] By 1999, 15% of the sequence was either wholly or partly completed, and NIH again advanced its completion date to 2000. In June 2000 both Celera and the international sequencing group announced the completion of an initial "draft" version of the human genome sequence.[18]

In February 2001, the two independent drafts of the genome, one produced by Venter's Celera group and the other by the International Human Genome Sequencing Consortium, were published simultaneously in the journals *Science*[21] and *Nature*.[22] The publication dates coincided with the anniversary of the birth of Charles Darwin.[23] The small number of genes estimated in the human genome, approximately 30,000 to 40,000, was far fewer than the original (and often quoted) 100,000 calculated by Walter Gilbert in the 1980s and came as a surprise to many.[24] Although incomplete, the drafts provide the first relatively accurate estimate of the total number of human genes in the genome. Data available as of May, 2003 suggests less than 30,000 genes, and gene prediction software estimates between 23,299 and 24,500.

In addition, our team was the first to describe the number of genes expressed in a single organ system. Using three independent approaches, we estimated the number of genes expressed in the cardiovascular system to range between 21,000 and 27,000.[26] This suggests that most genes in the human genome function in the normal maintenance and function of an organ regardless of its specific function, and only a small proportion are allocated to cell-specific functions. A brief chronology of events is presented in Table 2-1.

## Expressed Sequence Tags and the Human Genome Project

In the human context, a crucial first step, and a major challenge in the transition from structural to functional genomics, was the identification of the complete set of human genes, given that the large proportion of the genome (approximately 98%) does not code for any known functional gene product.

Perhaps the most promising approach to gene identification was the expressed sequence tag (EST) approach, proposed in 1991 by Dr. Mark Adams and Dr. J. Craig Venter and colleagues at NIH.[27] In this approach, as shown in Figure 2-1, individual clones are selected at random from cDNA libraries representing the genes expressed in a cell type, tissue, or organ of interest. Selected clones are amplified and sequenced in a single pass from one or both ends of the insert, yielding partial gene sequences known as ESTs. The EST sequences can then be compared against known gene sequences in existing nucleotide databases to determine whether they match to previously known genes or whether they represent uncharacterized genes. A similar approach had previously been taken by Putney et al.[28] several years earlier to identify 13 different muscle-specific proteins by sequencing 178 randomly selected cDNA clones from a rabbit muscle cDNA library. Venter and his colleagues took advantage of automated fluorescent DNA sequencing technology to dramatically increase the efficiency and scale of EST generation. In their pioneering paper, Venter's team described the rapid generation of ESTs representing more than 600 cDNA clones randomly selected from a human brain cDNA library[27] of which more than one half represented previously unknown human genes. Based on these findings, Venter argued that this strategy could, within a few years, lead to the identification and tagging of 80% to 90% of human genes, at a fraction of the cost of complete genome sequencing, a full decade before the proposed date of completion of the human genomic nucleotide sequence.[29] Similarly, the first human heart EST project was initiated in 1991 and began the monumental task of cataloguing the complete set of genes expressed in the cardiovascular system.[30-32]

Although initially met with significant skepticism[33,34] the EST approach ultimately gained widespread recognition

■ ■ ■

**TABLE 2-1** MAJOR TECHNOLOGIES AND ACHIEVEMENTS OF THE HUMAN GENOME PROJECT

| 1985 | Polymerase chain reaction (PCR) | K. Mullis, Cetus Corp. |
|---|---|---|
| 1987 | Yeast artificial chromosomes (YACs) | D. Burke, G. Carle, M. Olson |
| 1987 | First automated sequencer | Applied Biosystems |
| 1990 | Human Genome Project officially started | US Department of Energy and NIH |
| 1990 | BLAST published | D.J. Lipman and E.W. Myers |
| 1991 | Expressed sequence tags strategy | J. Craig Venter and M. Adams |
| 1992 | Institute for Genomic Research (TIGR) | J. Craig Venter |
| 1992 | Bacterial artificial chromosomes (BACs) | M. Simon, Cal. Tech. |
| 1995 | *Haemophilus influenza* genome | TIGR; H. Smith, Johns Hopkins |
| 1996 | Affymetrix DNA chips | Affymetrix |
| 1996 | *Saccharomyces cerevisiae* genome | International Consortium |
| 1998 | Celera founded | J. Craig Venter |
| 1998 | *Caenorhabditis elegans* genome | Sanger Center; Genome Sequencing Center |
| 1999 | Chromosome 22 sequenced | International Consortium |
| 2000 | *Drosophila melanogaster* genome | Celera; UC Berkeley |
| 2001 | Human Genome sequenced | Celera; NIH |
| 2001 | Cardiovascular genes estimated | A. Dempsey, C.C. Liew |

BLAST, Basic Local Alignment Search Tool; NIH, National Institutes of Health; TIGR, UC, University of California.

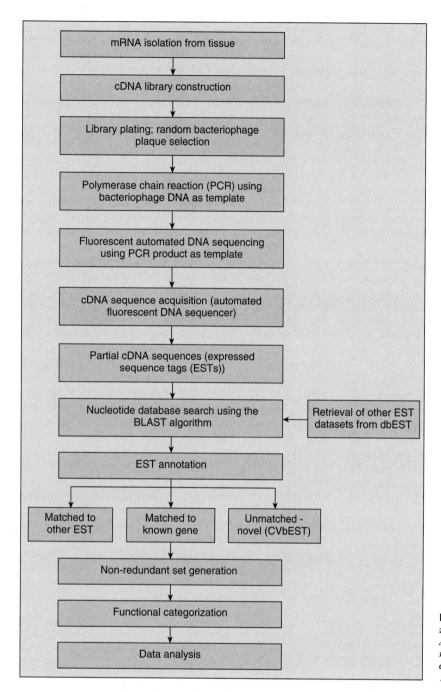

```
┌─────────────────────────────────────┐
│      mRNA isolation from tissue      │
└─────────────────────────────────────┘
                   │
                   ▼
┌─────────────────────────────────────┐
│      cDNA library construction       │
└─────────────────────────────────────┘
                   │
                   ▼
┌─────────────────────────────────────┐
│  Library plating; random bacteriophage │
│          plaque selection            │
└─────────────────────────────────────┘
                   │
                   ▼
┌─────────────────────────────────────┐
│ Polymerase chain reaction (PCR) using │
│     bacteriophage DNA as template    │
└─────────────────────────────────────┘
                   │
                   ▼
┌─────────────────────────────────────┐
│  Fluorescent automated DNA sequencing │
│      using PCR product as template   │
└─────────────────────────────────────┘
                   │
                   ▼
┌─────────────────────────────────────┐
│  cDNA sequence acquisition (automated │
│      fluorescent DNA sequencer)      │
└─────────────────────────────────────┘
                   │
                   ▼
┌─────────────────────────────────────┐
│  Partial cDNA sequences (expressed   │
│      sequence tags (ESTs))           │
└─────────────────────────────────────┘
                   │
                   ▼
┌─────────────────────────────────────┐     ┌──────────────────────┐
│  Nucleotide database search using the │◄────│ Retrieval of other EST │
│          BLAST algorithm             │     │  datasets from dbEST   │
└─────────────────────────────────────┘     └──────────────────────┘
                   │
                   ▼
┌─────────────────────────────────────┐
│            EST annotation            │
└─────────────────────────────────────┘
          │         │         │
          ▼         ▼         ▼
  ┌──────────┐ ┌──────────┐ ┌──────────┐
  │ Matched to│ │ Matched to│ │Unmatched -│
  │ other EST │ │known gene │ │novel (CVbEST)│
  └──────────┘ └──────────┘ └──────────┘
                   │
                   ▼
┌─────────────────────────────────────┐
│     Non-redundant set generation     │
└─────────────────────────────────────┘
                   │
                   ▼
┌─────────────────────────────────────┐
│      Functional categorization       │
└─────────────────────────────────────┘
                   │
                   ▼
┌─────────────────────────────────────┐
│            Data analysis             │
└─────────────────────────────────────┘
```

**FIGURE 2-1.** Flowchart of EST generation and analysis. *(Modified from Hwang DM, Dempsey AA, Wang RX, et al: A genome-based resource for molecular cardiovascular medicine: Toward a compendium of cardiovascular genes. Circulation 1997;96:4146–4203.)*

as an important and powerful strategy complementing complete genome sequencing for several reasons:

1. ESTs are an efficient vehicle for new gene discovery. Because each EST theoretically represents a single gene, generation of ESTs has proven to be a rapid and very efficient means to identify and isolate expressed genes from any tissue as well as to access large numbers of genes from virtually any organism (Table 2-2). Of the 609 cDNA clones first reported by Venter's group, 337 (or more than 50%) represented previously unknown human genes.[27] Subsequent publications reported similar or higher rates of novel gene discovery,[31,35-39] although this rate has diminished in recent years with increasing accumulation of EST data and the near completion of the human genome. Nevertheless, the impact made by ESTs on gene discovery is unquestionable. Only 7300 human DNA sequences, representing fewer than 3000 human genes, were known before 1991.[40] The generation of more than 3,700,000 human ESTs by various groups world-wide since 1991 has led to the identification of up to 30,000 to 40,000 additional human gene transcripts.[41] This explosion in sequence information necessitated the establishment of the database for expressed sequence tabs (dbEST), a division of GenBank devoted completely to EST data.[42] With the completion of the human genome sequence, the importance of ESTs in new gene discovery has diminished somewhat, although similar projects in other

## TABLE 2-2  SUMMARY OF HUMAN EST PROJECTS

| Tissue | | Tissue | | Tissue | |
|---|---|---|---|---|---|
| Multiple tissues | Adams et al., 1995<br>Camargo et al., 2001<br>Hillier et al., 1996<br>Kawamoto et al., 2000<br>Schaefer et al., 2001<br>Strausberg et al., 2000<br>Williamson, 1999 | Colon | Okubo et al., 1994<br>Frigerio et al., 1995 | Pancreas | Ferrer et al., 1997<br>Gress et al., 1996<br>Takeda et al., 1993 |
| | | Cornea | Nishida et al., 1996 | | |
| | | | | Prostate | Huang et al., 1999<br>Krizman et al., 1996<br>Liu AY et al., 2002<br>Nelson et al., 1998 |
| | | Embryo | Adjaye et al., 1997<br>Adjaye et al., 1998<br>Adjaye et al., 1999 | | |
| Adipose | Maeda et al., 1997 | Liver | Okubo et al., 1992<br>Choi et al., 1995<br>Kawamoto et al., 1996 | Retina | Agarwal et al., 1995<br>Gieser and Swaroop, 1992<br>Shimizu-Matsumoto et al., 1997 |
| Bone marrow | Jia et al., 2002 | | Jay et al., 1997<br>Morozov et al., 1998 | | |
| | | Eye trabecular network | Gonzalez et al., 2000 | | Xu et al., 2001<br>Yu et al., 2001 |
| Brain | Adams et al., 1991<br>Adams et al., 1992<br>Adams et al., 1993a<br>Adams et al., 1993b | | | | Sinha et al., 2000 |
| | | Hematopoietic cells | Claudio et al., 1998<br>Gubin et al., 1999<br>Mao et al., 1998 | | |
| | | | | Skeletal muscle | Houlgatte et al., 1995<br>Lanfranchi et al., 1996<br>Pallavicini et al., 1997 |
| | | Keratinocyte | Kita et al., 1996<br>Konishi et al., 1994 | | |
| | Hu et al., 2000 | Lung | Itoh et al., 1994<br>Schraml et al., 1994<br>Sudo et al., 1994 | | |
| | | | | Squamous cells | Leethanakul et al., 2000 |
| Granulocytoid cells | Itoh et al., 1998 | Mesangial cells | Murakawa et al., 1994<br>Okubo et al., 1995 | | |
| | | | | T-cell, CD34+ | Yang et al., 1996 |
| | Khan et al., 1992<br>Soares et al., 1994 | Multiple sclerosis brain lesions | Yasuda et al., 1998 | Testis | Affara et al., 1994<br>Pawlak et al., 1995<br>Sargent et al., 1993 |
| Breast | Dias Neto et al., 2000<br>Ji et al., 1997<br>Watson and Fleming, 1994 | Myoblasts | Becker et al., 1997<br>Genini et al., 1996 | | |
| Cartilage | Kumar et al., 2001 | Neuroblastoma | Yokoyama et al., 1996 | Thymus | Hwang MY et al., 1999<br>Lamerdin et al., 1995 |
| | Tanaka et al., 1996 | | Liew, 1993<br>Liew et al., 1994<br>Hwang et al., 1994<br>Hwang et al., 1995<br>Hwang et al., 1997 | | |
| Cochlea | Skvorak et al., 1999 | Osteoprogenitor cells | Candeliere et al., 1999 | | |

EST, expressed sequence tag.
Modified from Dempsey AA: Computational exploration of the human cardiovascular genome and its application to understanding human fetal heart development. PhD Thesis, University of Toronto. May, 2002.

organisms have now led to the deposition in dbEST of more than 8,600,000 ESTs (http://www. ncbi.nlm.nih.gov/dbEST/index.html), representing a resource of genetic information from nearly 350 different organisms (e.g., zebrafish; see reference 43) (Table 2-3).

2. ESTs provide information on gene expression levels in different cells/tissues. One of the early criticisms of the EST approach was that highly expressed genes would be encountered more often during random sequencing than low-expressed genes were and that this would markedly diminish the rate of new gene discovery. Although this was true, this redundancy nevertheless proved to have an important secondary benefit. Although disadvantageous to large-scale novel gene discovery, redundant sequencing of more highly expressed genes was found to be useful for characterizing patterns of gene transcription in different tissues. Because cDNA libraries are representative of the mRNA population used to construct the library, random sampling of a cDNA library by ESTs is a sampling of gene transcription in the tissue from which the library was constructed. EST data can, therefore, be used to generate detailed expression profiles, in which gene expression frequencies are estimated from relative numbers of ESTs corresponding to individual genes.[44] Such profiles are useful for genetic-level comparisons of different developmental or pathologic states of a tissue and for identifying genes that may be differentially expressed in such states. This strategy has been used to identify general differences in gene transcription between different tissues[31,32,36,37,45-47] and between different developmental and disease states.[32,46,48]

3. ESTs provide physical mapping and identification of disease genes. EST sequences can also be used to design PCR primers for physical mapping of a genome. To bypass problems of identifying intron and exon boundaries, only ESTs from three untranslated regions (3' UTR) that generally lack introns and are species specific are used.

ESTs are also becoming increasingly useful in the search for new genes involved in genetic disease. First, chromosomal localization of ESTs expedites the identification of novel disease genes, because ESTs within a region known to be associated with a certain disorder automatically become candidate genes for that disorder. The use of such "positional candidate" strategies has identified a novel candidate for a familial Alzheimer's disease gene.[49] Alternative strategies for disease gene identification have relied on computational methods to find potential disease-related genes in EST databases by homology to genes related to known phenotypes in other organisms.[50-52] Examples of successful uses of such computational strategies include the identification of genes causing hereditary colon cancer[53] and X-linked glycerol kinase deficiency[54] through sequence similarity of ESTs to bacterial sequences of known function and the identification of candidate genes for human retinopathies from ESTs exhibiting sequence similarity to genes responsible for retinal degeneration in *Drosophila*.[55,56]

The increasing availability of genomic sequence coupled with functional analysis from a number of organisms will continue to facilitate such cross-referencing between mutant genes in model organisms and their human homologues.[57]

Although ESTs have been useful for monitoring gene expression in different tissues or cells, now their primary use is to provide materials for other powerful methods emerging from the HGP for large-scale gene expression analysis such as cDNA microarrays.[58] By tagging and identifying thousands of genes, EST repositories presently serve as the primary source of cDNA clones for these microarrays. EST sequences have also historically been useful for identifying full-length transcripts generated by other large-scale expression analyses such as differential display and serial analysis of gene expression (SAGE),[59,60] although these techniques are now being largely superseded by microarray technology.

## The Human Genome Project and Microarray Technology

EST-based strategies for studying gene expression were initially both cost- and labor-intensive, requiring generation of large numbers of ESTs. ESTs have now become a necessary resource for microarrays. Microarrays allow for similar data to be produced simultaneously for thousands of genes in a single hybridization experiment. Two types of microarray systems are widely used. One involves the photolithographic synthesis of oligodeoxynucleotides directly onto silicon chips; the other uses an X-Y-Z robotic system to spot DNA directly onto coated standard glass microscope slides or nylon membranes.[58,61-63] To carry out transcript profiling using oligonucleotide arrays, biotin-labeled cDNA is generated from two mRNA pools of interest and hybridized independently to a single chip (i.e., two chips are used—one serving as a test and one as a reference). A streptavidin-erythromycin conjugate is hybridized to the biotin-labeled probe bound to the corresponding oligonucleotide on the chip. (Each gene is represented by approximately 20 unique oligonucleotide pairs.) The cDNA microarray system differs slightly. In this system, fluorescent tags, for example, Cy3 or Cy5, are incorporated directly into the cDNA probes and hybridized simultaneously to a single cDNA array. In both microarray systems the resulting fluorescent signal is read by a laser-mediated fluorescence scanner and a visual image is generated representing the signals obtained from the two fluorescent tags. After normalization of the two fluorescent signals and elimination of "uninformative spots" the ratio between the two signals for each "spot" is calculated. The differences in signal intensity are representative of differences in gene expression between the two transcript populations for each gene.

### Applications of DNA Microarrays

The advantage of DNA microarray technology lies in its capability to profile and compare thousands of genes simultaneously between mRNA populations (see Table 2-4). However, the DNA microarray is not only a novel

## TABLE 2-3 SUMMARY OF EST PROJECTS IN OTHER ORGANISMS

| Organism | Reference | Organism | Reference |
|---|---|---|---|
| *Acanthamoeba healyi* | Kong et al., 2001 | *Brugia malayi* (parasitic nematode) | Blaxter et al., 1999 |
| *Aedes aegypti* (yellow fever mosquito) | Severson and Zhang, 1996 | *Caenorhabditis elegans* (nematode) | Williams and Johnston, 1999 |
| *Agaricus bisporus* | Ospina-Giraldo et al., 2000 | | McCombie et al., 1992 |
| | Sonnenberg et al., 1996 | | Reboul et al., 2001 |
| *Amblyomma americanum* | Hill and Gutierrez, 2000 | | Waterston and Sulston, 1995 |
| *Anopheles gambiae* (African malaria mosquito) | Dimopoulos et al., 2000 | *Canis familiaris* (dog) | Lin and Sargan, 2001 |
| *Arabidopsis thaliana* (thale cress) | Asamizu et al., 2000b | *Cavia porcellus* (domestic guinea pig) | Oshima et al., 2000 |
| | Delseny et al., 1997 | *Chlamydomonas reinhardtii* | Asamizu et al., 1999 |
| | Hofte et al., 1993 | | Asamizu et al., 2000a |
| | Newman et al., 1994 | | Kusakabe et al., 2002 |
| | Rounsley et al., 1996 | *Ciona intestinalis* | Nishikata et al., 2001 |
| | White et al., 2000 | | Satou et al., 2001 |
| *Aspergillus nidulans* | Lee et al., 1996 | *Cryptomeria japonica* (Japanese cedar) | Ujino-Ihara et al., 2000 |
| *Blumeria graminis* f. sp. *hordei* | Thomas et al., 2001 | *Cryptosporidium parvum* | Strong and Nelson, 2000 |
| *Bombyx mori* (domestic silkworm) | Okano et al., 2001 | *Cyprinus carpio* (common carp) | Savan and Sakai, 2002 |
| *Bos taurus* (cattle) | Dorroch et al., 2001 | *Danio rerio* (zebrafish) | Clark et al., 2001 |
| | Grosse et al., 2000 | | Gates et al., 1999 |
| | Ma et al., 1998 | | Ton et al., 2000 |
| | Rebeiz and Lewin, 2000 | *Dictyostelium discoideum* | Morio et al., 1998 |
| | Smith TP et al., 2001a | *Drosophila melanogaster* (fruit fly) | Posey et al., 2001 |
| | Takasuga et al., 2001 | | Rubin et al., 2000 |
| *Branchiostoma belcheri* | Taniguchi et al., 2001 | *Echinostoma paraensei* | Adema et al., 2000 |
| *Brassica campestris* (field mustard) | Suzuki and Satoh, 2000 | *Eimeria tenella* | Wan et al., 1999 |
| | Kwak et al., 1997 | *Entamoeba dispar* | Sharma et al., 1999 |
| | Lim et al., 1996 | *Entamoeba histolytica* | Tanaka et al., 1997 |
| *Brassica napus* (oilseed rape) | Park et al., 1993 | | Willhoeft et al., 1999 |
| *Brassica rapa* subsp. *pekinensis* (Chinese cabbage) | Lim et al., 2000 | *Mastigamoeba balamuthi* | Bapteste et al., 2002 |
| *Equus caballus* (horse) | Lieto and Cothran, 2001 | *Medicago truncatula* (barrel medic) | Bell et al., 2001 |
| *Gallus gallus* (chicken) | Abdrakhmanov et al., 2000 | | Covitz et al., 1998 |
| | Carre et al., 2001 | | Gyorgyey et al., 2000 |
| | Li et al., 1998 | *Meleagris gallopavo* (common turkey) | Smith E et al., 2000 |
| | Smith EJ et al., 2001a | *Mus musculus + domesticus* (mouse) | Bain et al., 2000 |
| | Smith EJ et al., 2001b | | Chambers and Abbott, 1996 |
| | Spike et al., 1996 | | Kim et al., 1999 |
| | Tirunagaru et al., 2000 | | Ko et al., 2000 |
| *Glomus intraradices* (mycorrhizal fungus) | Sawaki and Saito, 2001 | | Marra et al., 1999 |
| *Haemonchus contortus* | Hoekstra et al., 2000 | | Neophytou et al., 1996 |
| *Halocynthia roretzi* | Kawashima et al., 2000 | | Nishiguchi et al., 1994 |
| | Makabe et al., 2001 | | Nishiguchi et al., 1996 |
| *Hordeum vulgare* (barley) | Druka et al., 2002 | | Sasaki et al., 1998 |
| | Bettini et al., 1994 | | Stewart et al., 1997 |
| *Ictalurus punctatus* (channel catfish) | Cao et al., 2001 | *Mycosphaerella graminicola* | Keon et al., 2000 |
| | Karsi et al., 1998 | *Neurospora crassa* | Nelson et al., 1997 |
| *Laminaria digitata* | Crepineau et al., 2000 | *Onchocerca volvulus* | Lizotte-Waniewski et al., 2000 |
| *Leishmania infantum* | Wincker et al., 1996 | *Oncorhynchus mykiss* (rainbow trout) | Kono et al., 2000 |
| *Lycopersicon esculentum* (tomato) | Ganal et al., 1998 | *Oryctolagus cuniculus* (rabbit) | Fujimaki et al., 1999 |
| *Lotus japonicus* | Endo et al., 2000 | *Oryza sativa* (rice) | Liu et al., 1995 |
| | Szczyglowski et al., 1997 | | |

*(Continued)*

**TABLE 2-3    SUMMARY OF EST PROJECTS IN OTHER ORGANISMS—cont'd**

| Organism | Reference | Organism | Reference |
|---|---|---|---|
| *Macaca fascicularis* (cynomolgus monkeys) | Osada et al., 2001 | *Oryzias latipes* (Japanese medaka) | Sasaki et al., 1994 |
| *Macropus eugenii* (tammar wallaby) | Collet and Joseph, 1994 | | Umeda et al., 1994 |
| *Malus x domestica* (apple tree) | Sung et al., 1998 | *Paralichthys olivaceus* (Japanese flounder) | Hirona and Aoki, 1997 |
| *Manihot esculenta* (cassava) | Suarez et al., 2000 | | Aoki et al., 1999 |
| *Marchantia polymorpha* (liverwort) | Nagai et al., 1999 | | Inoue et al., 1997 |
| | Nishiyama et al., 2000 | | Nam et al., 2000 |
| *Penaeus monodon* (black tiger shrimp) | Lehnert et al., 1999 | *Solanum tuberosum* (potato) | Crookshanks et al., 2001 |
| *Physcomitrella patens* | Machuka et al., 1999 | *Strongylocentrotus purpuratus* (purple urchin) | Cameron et al., 2000 |
| *Phytophthora sojae* | Qutob et al., 2000 | | Lee et al., 1999 |
| *Pisolithus tinctorius* | Tagu and Martin, 1995 | | Smith et al., 1996 |
| *Plasmodium falciparum* (malaria parasite) | Chakrabarti et al., 1994 | | Zhu X et al., 2001 |
| *Plasmodium yoelii* | Kappe et al., 2001 | *Suaeda maritima* subsp. salsa | Zhang et al., 2001 |
| *Pleuronectes americanus* (winter flounder) | Douglas et al., 1999 | *Sus scrofa* (pig) | Davoli et al., 1999 |
| *Polyandrocarpa misakiensis* | Kawamura et al., 1998 | | Davoli et al., 2002 |
| *Populus balsamifera* subsp. *trichocarpa* | Sterky et al., 1998 | | Jorgensen et al., 1997 |
| *Porphyra yezoensis* | Lee et al., 2000 | | Ponsuksili et al., 2001 |
| | Nikaido et al., 2000 | | Tosser-Klopp et al., 1997 |
| *Raphanus sativus* (radish) | Moon et al., 1998 | | Wang C et al., 2001 |
| *Rattus* sp. (rat) | Gebelein et al., 1996 | *Tortula ruralis* | Wood et al., 1999 |
| | Guo et al., 1999 | *Toxocara canis* | Tetteh et al., 1999 |
| | Harter et al., 1999 | *Toxoplasma gondii* | Ajioka, 1998 |
| | MacDonald, 1996 | | Hehl et al., 1997 |
| | Petkov et al., 2000 | | Manger et al., 1998 |
| | Sleeman et al., 2000 | | Wan et al., 1996 |
| | Soto-Prior et al., 1997 | *Trypanosoma brucei rhodesiense* | Djikeng et al., 1998 |
| *Salmo salar* | Davey et al., 2001 | | el-Sayed et al., 1995 |
| *Scherffelia dubia* | Becker et al., 2001 | *Trypanosoma cruzi* | Brandao et al., 1998 |
| *Schistosoma japonicum* (blood fluke) | Fan et al., 1998 | | Porcel et al., 2000 |
| *Schistosoma mansoni* (blood fluke) | Franco et al., 1995a | | Verdun et al., 1998 |
| | Franco et al., 1995b | *Xenopus laevis* (African clawed frog) | Blackshear et al., 2001 |
| | Franco et al., 1997 | | Shibata et al., 2001 |
| | Santos et al., 1999 | *Zea mays* (maize) | Davis et al., 1999 |
| | Williams and Johnston, 1999 | | |

EST, expressed sequence tag.

■ ▦ ■

## TABLE 2-4  APPLICATIONS OF MICROARRAYS

Identify differentially expressed genes between mRNA populations
  from different pathophysiologic conditions
Define genes in functional context
Fingerprint population traits and risk factors (e.g., phenotype,
  etiology, age, sex, blood pressure)
Identify disease genes or common *cis*-elements such as transcriptional
  factor binding sites and promoter regions
Identify drug targets
Predict natural history of disease
• DNA polymorphisms for prediction of drug response and side
  effects
• Expression profiling for prediction of drug response (e.g., cancer
  chemotherapy; tissue analysis)

tool for transcript profiling and identifying differences in expression between single genes on a large scale. The wealth of data generated from a series of transcript-profiling experiments can also be analyzed to determine the level of "relatedness" between genes or samples in multiple dimensions. Using a set of expression fingerprints (or profiles), similarities and differences in gene expression are capitalized on to group or cluster different mRNA populations or genes into discrete related sets or bins. This is extremely powerful because the clusters of coregulated genes often belong to the same biologic pathway or even to the same protein complex, whereas the clusters of mRNA populations are defined by their "expression fingerprint" providing a means to define differences between samples (e.g., tumors) that would otherwise not be possible.

Schena et al. in 1995 first reported the use of the cDNA microarray for transcript profiling of the mustard weed, *Arabidopsis thaliana*. They constructed custom-made arrays (containing 45 *A. thaliana* cDNAs) to compare differential gene expression between the mRNA population of the root and leaf tissues. The first human cDNA arrays were constructed to profile the heat shock response to phorbol ester in Jurkat T-cells (1046 unique genes) and tumorigenic (UACC-903) and nontumorigenic (UACC-903 [+6]) cell lines (1161 unique genes).[58,64] Since then, cDNA microarray systems have been employed in a range of experiments designed to compare transcript profiles in various cells and tissues. Current arrays contain approximately 10,000 to 15,000 cDNA clones.

The molecular basis of cancer has also been a subject for cDNA microarray analysis and is currently one of the most widely profiled human diseases. For example, in an attempt to classify breast tumors, Perou et al.[65] compared the transcript profiles from cultured human mammary epithelial cells and primary breast tumors subjected to a variety of growth factors or cytokines. Interestingly, a correlation between two subsets of genes with similar expression patterns *in vitro* and in the primary tumors was found, suggesting that these genes could be used for tumor classification.

A very interesting set of studies provided a profile of the time response of cultured human fibroblasts to serum.[66,67] The investigators compared the changes in gene expression that occurred over the course of fibroblast proliferation at 12 time points. The changes were readily observable. They revealed several clusters of genes with similar patterns of expression over time, including the clustering of numerous genes of unknown function with those of known function, thereby placing them into a functional context. Gene clustering between mRNA populations can be viewed from two perspectives. First, genes clustering over a time course can identify genes of similar function, because the expression of functionally related genes tend to be regulated and thus expressed in a similar manner (e.g., genes involved in $G_1$ phase of the yeast mitotic cell cycle). This is an important concept, because genes with no known function can now be placed into a biologic pathway. Second, clustering genes between several mRNA populations at a single time can identify a vast number of associations between the expression of a cluster of genes and the biologic phenotype. Since then, genetic modifiers in complex cardiovascular diseases such as heart failure have been investigated.[68]

Heart failure is a complex syndrome with various causes including hypertension, ischemic and congenital heart disease, cardiomyopathy, and myocarditis[69] (Fig. 2-2). The complex causes and secondary adaptations contributing to heart failure makes study of the underlying cellular and molecular mechanisms a challenging process. Microarrays are increasingly used to investigate patterns of gene expression in heart failure, and a few cardiovascular-based microarray studies have been published. Friddle et al.[70] used microarray technology in a mouse model to identify gene expression patterns altered during induction and regression of cardiac hypertrophy induced by administration of angiotensin II and isoproterenol. A total of 55 genes were identified during induction or regression of cardiac hypertrophy. They confirmed 25 genes or pathways previously shown to be altered by hypertrophy and further identified a larger set of 30 genes whose expression had not previously been associated with cardiac hypertrophy or regression. Among the 55 genes, 32 genes were altered only during induction, and 8 were altered only during regression. This study, using a genome-wide approach, demonstrated that a set of known and novel genes was involved in cardiac remodeling during regression and that these genes were distinct from those expressed during induction of hypertrophy. In the first reported human microarray study in end-stage heart failure, Yang et al.[71] examined gene expression in two failing human hearts using oligo-based arrays. The investigators used high-density oligonucleotide arrays to investigate failing and nonfailing human hearts (end-stage ischemic and dilated cardiomyopathy [DCM]). Similar changes were identified in 12 genes in both types of heart failure, which the authors maintain indicated that these changes may be intrinsic to heart failure. They found altered expression in cytoskeletal and myofibrillar genes; genes involved in degradation and disassembly of myocardial proteins, metabolism, and protein synthesis; and genes encoding stress proteins. Although the "Affychip" in this study offers a carefully controlled systematic method of analysis, its current lack of user flexibility in its design gives tissue-specific arrays an advantage because of the availability of a more defined set of genes present in the tissues of interest.

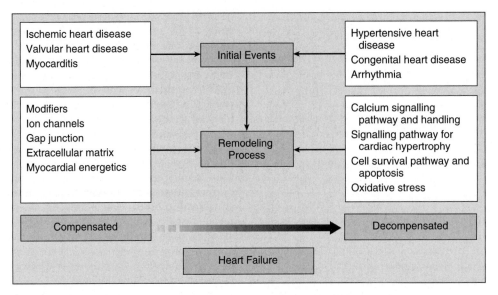

**FIGURE 2-2.** Molecular basis of heart failure. *(Modified from Hwang JJ, Dzau VJ, Liew CC: Genomics and the pathophysiology of heart failure. Curr Cardiol Rep 2001;3:198–207.)*

Most recently, the "CardioChip" microarray (Fig. 2-3) has proved to be a highly informative aid in elucidating some aspects of the complex of molecular and genetic events that lead to end-stage heart failure. Our group explored expression analysis in heart failure using the CardioChip, an in-house 10,848-element human cardiovascular-based EST glass slide cDNA microarray.[68,72] The group compared left ventricle heart transplant tissue and nonfailing heart controls. More than 100 transcripts proved to be consistently differentially expressed in DCM samples by more than one and a half times. Thus, through clustering the complete sets of gene expression data generated from heart failure samples, for example, several gene clusters can be identified and examined to determine the specific relationship with each particular mRNA population. Each unique heart failure phenotype profiled will have a specific gene expression fingerprint, based on the concept that the mRNA population defines the phenotype. However, these two perspectives are not necessarily mutually exclusive, and expression fingerprints can be identified for each time point over a time course and functional groups of genes defined for a single time point.

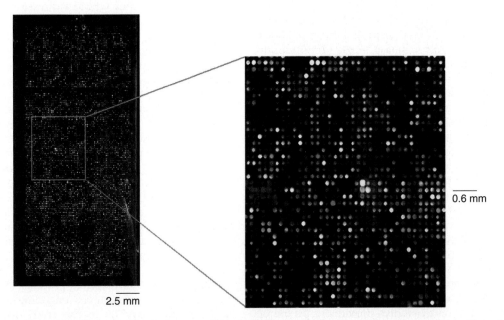

**FIGURE 2-3.** Representative full image and magnified section of the "CardioChip," a 10,368 element of cDNA microarray. Normal adult heart and normal fetal heart are each labeled with a differently colored fluorescent dye (typically green and red, respectively). Each dot in this image represents the superimposition of the two dyes for a specific gene; differential expression is measured by the intensity of one dye relative to the other (i.e., in a color image, each dot would have a color within the red-to-green spectrum). For example, a yellow dot would indicate that the gene in question is equally expressed in both types of tissue.

We observed a consistent upregulation of selected sarcomeric and extracellular matrix (ECM) proteins (e.g., β-myosin heavy chain, α-actinin, α-cardiac actin, troponin I, tropomyosin, collagen, etc.; see Figure 2-4). Evidence in knockout mice and human studies has offered insight into the putative role of these proteins in maintaining sarcomeric integrity.[73-79] Mutations of proteins associated with α-actinin, namely muscle lim protein (MLP), cardiac α-actin, desmin, and titin, have been shown to be present in certain forms of human DCM.[80-84] Ambiguities exist in the literature regarding the expression of collagen and other members of the ECM; nonetheless, regulation of the ECM is important in the formation of fibrosis and impaired contractile function.[85-87]

Calcium signaling has recently become an important area of interest in the investigation of heart failure.[88] A decrease in calcium-cycling genes has been shown to result in reduced contractility in mice whose β-adrenergic stimulation is blunted, leading to decreased phospholamban phosphorylation.[89] $Ca^{2+}$ATPase is key in regulating contractility, and its approximately twofold downregula-

tion in our DCM samples lends credence to its involvement. This is supported by a recent study in which the transfer of the $Ca^{2+}$ATPase gene into the rat myocardium prevents certain features of heart failure.[90] The presence of $Ca^{2+}$/calmodulin-dependent kinase in our analysis is particularly intriguing, because it is known to phosphorylate phospholamban.[91] In addition, inositol 1,4,5-triphosphate receptor (a member of the calcium channel family, which may be responsible for calcium release from intracellular stores)[92] was also significantly downregulated (1.86-fold). Inositol 1,4,5-triphosphate 3-kinase was recently cloned[93] and may be another key component in this regulation (with a 1.86-fold downregulation as well). Our findings suggest that the role of $Ca^{2+}$ signaling downregulation may be of crucial significance in the evolution of heart failure and warrants further investigation.

## HUMAN GENOME PROJECT AND CARDIOVASCULAR DISEASE GENES

The impact of the HGP and related ongoing HGP-related projects on the discovery of disease genes has been significant. Before the beginning of the HGP, disease genes were discovered by a laborious process, moving from identification of the relevant metabolic defect and distinguishing the protein involved, to gene cloning and mapping, and finally to searching for mutations in the sequence. This approach led to the discovery of genes for several diseases such as sickle cell anemia and Fabry's disease. However, this approach used tremendous amounts of time, labor, and effort to uncover genes. For example, almost a century of research was required to phenotype and then identify the gene involved in alkaptonuria, an inborn error of metabolism.[94] The ongoing development of technologies and techniques, and the research of the HGP provides the means to expedite the tedious process of gene finding.

### Mapping and Positional Cloning

From the outset, the HGP was devoted to constructing a research resource of genetic and physical maps of each chromosome. Mapping technologies developed include physical and transcriptional mapping, genomic cloning, and other mapping approaches.[95] Such maps are used for positional cloning gene discovery techniques.[96] This makes it possible to clone a disease gene by determining its position on the chromosomal map without knowing anything in advance about the putative function of the gene.[97] In 1990, at the beginning of the HGP, only about 10 disease genes had been identified. By 1999, more than 100 genes had been identified using positional cloning strategies.[5] More importantly, at least 26 disease genes were cloned as a direct result of the generation and public availability of the draft sequence of the human genome.[22]

As the project has progressed genome maps have become increasingly more detailed and enriched, providing tools for positional candidate cloning techniques[98] and, when combined with EST data, simplifying the search for genes.

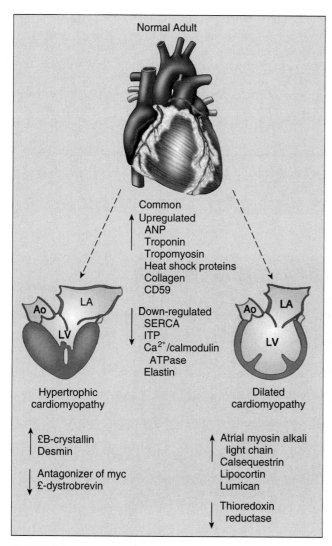

Normal Adult

Common
↑ Upregulated
ANP
Troponin
Tropomyosin
Heat shock proteins
Collagen
CD59

↓ Down-regulated
SERCA
ITP
$Ca^{2+}$/calmodulin
ATPase
Elastin

Ao LA
LV

Hypertrophic cardiomyopathy

↑ £B-crystallin
Desmin

↓ Antagonizer of myc
£-dystrobrevin

Ao LA
LV

Dilated cardiomyopathy

↑ Atrial myosin alkali light chain
Calsequestrin
Lipocortin
Lumican

↓ Thioredoxin reductase

**FIGURE 2-4.** Differentially expressed genes in heart failure—lessons from cDNA microarray analysis.

## Monogenic Cardiovascular Disease Genes

The technologies of the HGP have allowed researchers to explore the pathophysiology of several human diseases at the gene level. To date, the genes identified have been mainly genes in single-gene disorders, such as cystic fibrosis, polycystic kidney syndrome, familial hypertrophic cardiomyopathy (FHC), DCM, long QT syndrome, Marfan's syndrome, Becker's muscular dystrophy, and other relatively rare diseases. Such monogenic diseases (i.e., caused by single-gene mutations that affect the phenotype) have proved most amenable to the candidate gene approach and positional cloning techniques of gene discovery. Progress has been rapid and in some cases has had important prognostic and diagnostic implications. Despite new and exciting information, even monogenic disorders can be complex in their genetic heterogeneity. In the following section we very briefly discuss FHC, DCM, and long QT syndrome as examples of three monogenic cardiac diseases whose definition has been speeded up by technologies developed through the HGP.

### Familial Hypertrophic Cardiomyopathy

FHC, an inherited disorder of the myocardium affecting about 1 person in 500, was first described clinically in the 1950s.[99] Linkage analysis studies of a large kindred in 1989 localized the gene responsible to chromosome 14q2.[100] Further studies demonstrated links to other chromosomes and determined that the disease was related to mutations in genes encoding for sarcomeric proteins.[101,102] Studies have identified disease-causing gene mutations in a number of different sarcomeric proteins, and the disease has been defined as a sarcomyopathy (Table 2-5).[103,104]

FHC is a highly heterogenous disease. Its clinical manifestations range from few symptoms and normal life expectancy to severe symptoms and sudden death. Of prognostic interest, mutations in genes associated with FHC can potentially predict the clinical course of disease. For example, the Arg403-Gln mutation at position 403 of the β myosin heavy chain gene is associated with 40% risk of death by the age of 40. By contrast other mutations do not carry such a poor prognosis; the Val606-Met mutation is benign and associated with a normal life expectancy.[104,105] Thus, in the space of a very few years FHC evolved from a recognized hereditary disease of no phenotypically comprehensible etiology to a disorder localized to a specific protein, whose genes carry information with important diagnostic and prognostic implications.[106] Genetic testing for FHC is carried out only in specialized research centers; however, future genetic screening remains a possibility.

### Dilated Cardiomyopathy

DCM appears somewhat more heterogeneous than FHC, involving mutations in sarcomeric genes, such as α cardiac actin,[83] β-myosin heavy chain,[107] and cardiac troponin T,[107] in other nonsarcomeric structural genes such as desmin,[108] dystrophin,[109,110] and lamin A/C (a nuclear matrix protein[111,112]); and in genes encoding proteins

■ ■ ■

**TABLE 2-5   GENES INVOLVED IN HYPERTROPHIC CARDIOMYOPATHY, DILATED CARDIOMYOPATHY, AND LONG QT SYNDROME**

| Gene | Associated Protein | Protein Type | Chromosome |
|---|---|---|---|
| *Hypertrophic cardiomyopathy* | | | |
| MYH7 | β-myosin heavy chain | Sarcomeric protein | 14q11.2-q12 |
| MYL3 | Myosin ventricular light chain | Sarcomeric protein | 3p21.2-3p21.3 |
| MYL2 | Myosin ventricular regulatory light chain | Sarcomeric protein | 12q23-q24.3 |
| TNNT2 | Tropomyosin binding protein | Sarcomeric protein | 1q3 |
| TNN13 | Troponin inhibitory protein | Sarcomeric protein | 19p13.2-q13.2 |
| TPM1 | α-tropomyosin | Sarcomeric protein | 15q22 |
| MYBPC3 | Myosin binding protein | Sarcomeric protein | 11p11.2 |
| Unknown | Unknown | Unknown | 7q3 |
| ACTC | Actin | Cytoskeletal protein | 15q14 |
| *Dilated cardiomyopathy* | | | |
| DMD | Dystrophin | Cytoskeletal protein | Xp.21.2 |
| G4.5 | Tafazzin | Cytoskeletal protein | Xq28 |
| ACTC | Actin | Cytoskeletal protein | 15q14 |
| Unknown | Unknown | Unknown | 1q32 |
| Unknown | Unknown | Unknown | 2p31 |
| Unknown | Unknown | Unknown | 9q13-q21 |
| Unknown | Unknown | Unknown | 10q21-q23 |
| Unknown | Unknown | Unknown | 322-p25 |
| *Long QT syndrome* | | | |
| SCN5A | Cardiac sodium channel | Ion transporter | 3p21-24 |
| HERG | Potassium channel | Ion transporter | 7q35-q36 |
| KVLQT1 | α-subunit potassium channel | Ion transporter | 11p15.5 |
| MinK | Subunit potassium channel | Ion transporter | 21q22.1-p22 |
| Unknown | Unknown | Unknown | 4q25-q27 |

Modified from Ferrari P, Bianchi G: Genomics of cardiovascular disorders. Drugs 2000;59:1025–1042.

involved in metabolism (very long-chain acyl-CoA dehydrogenase).[113] Mutations of myosin binding protein C in mice[114] and various sarcoglycans, components of the dystrophin complex, in hamsters[115,116] have also been associated with DCM and hypertrophic cardiomyopathy (HCM). In addition to these mutations, however, overexpression or underexpression of a broad range of genes with a variety of functions in transgenic models recently have also been found to result in DCM. These include a number of genes involved in signaling pathways (G-α-q,[117] CREB* transcription factor,[118] tumor necrosis factor-α,[119] retinoic acid receptor-α,[120] bradykinin B2 receptor[121]), several structural genes (desmin,[122] tropomodulin,[84] muscle-specific LIM protein [MLP][123]), and various genes involved in metabolic processes (manganese superoxide dismutase,[124] mitochondrial-encoded genes [Table 2-5]).[125] In brief, DCM remains a syndrome of cardiomyopathy, and further exploration is required to define the cause of these disorders.

### Long QT Syndrome

Similar rapid progress has been made in elucidating the genes underlying long QT syndrome. This is a rare hereditary arrhythmic disorder, first described in the 1950s, that causes seizures, loss of consciousness, and death from repolarization-related ventricular tachyarrhythmias. One form is also characterized by congenital deafness. Long QT typically affects preadolescents and adolescents at a rate of about 1 in 10,000 to 15,000. Symptomatic untreated individuals have a 10-year mortality rate of about 50%. The candidate gene approach and positional cloning techniques have identified five genes that are associated with long QT syndrome: SCN5A on chromosome 3p21-24, HERG on chromosome 7q35-36, KVLQT1 on chromosome 11p15.5, KCNE1 (minK) on chromosome 21q22.1-q22.2, and KCNE2 on chromosome 21q22.1 (Table 2-5).

As a result of these studies, long QT syndrome is recognized as a cardiac ion channel disorder affecting either sodium channels or potassium channels. Furthermore, long QT shows differing responses to therapy depending on genotypic differences. For example, mexiletine, a sodium channel blocker, has been shown to be of benefit to those with sodium channel gene defects but not to those with potassium channel gene defects.[125] The long QT syndrome can now be predicted by genotype analysis.[126]

## Complex Diseases

Although much progress has been made in the characterization of monogenic disorders, the most common causes of cardiovascular (and total) morbidity and mortality today are not the relatively rare, single-gene diseases but rather the complex, polygenic, multifactorial disorders such as atherosclerosis, hypertension, and heart failure. Polygenic disorders can be defined as

diseases that involve two or more genes that interact with environmental influences or stochastic factors to cause phenotypic effects. Such diseases involve extremely complex interaction between conserved genetic elements and environmental factors, signaling factors and adaptive mechanisms, promotion, and inhibition. The molecular and genetic mechanisms of such diseases are far more difficult to discover than are the single-gene disorders. There may be 32,000 to 38,000 genes in the human genome, and any combination of these may contribute to phenotype in complex diseases. The complexity of common cardiovascular disorders can be illustrated by decompensation leading to heart failure as shown in Figure 2-2. For example, altered workload tends to increase efficiency or force of contraction and subsequently induce compensatory changes and alterations in gene expression at the molecular level. Heart failure is characterized by a series of cellular remodeling steps such as hypertrophic growth, modification of sarcomeres, ECM components exhibited by gene activation, and suppression as shown in Figure 2-4.

Linkage and association studies using candidate genes have contributed to the understanding of more complex diseases such as hypertension. However, early optimism among geneticists has been tempered because the techniques that were so remarkably successful in single-gene disorders have proved to be less useful in discovering the genetics of more complex polygenic diseases.[127] For the most part, the genes that contribute to more complex polygenic condition remain to be identified.[128]

Before polygenic diseases can be understood, new technologies and new strategies must be developed for interpreting and manipulating the data of the HGP. The output of data from the HGP has been enormous, and the rate of data accumulation has increased rapidly. In May 1999 about 700 million bases of the human genome were publicly available to researchers; by May 2000 there were 3 billion and by August 2000 the number increased to 4 billion.[129] Biology has been described as going from a "data-poor" science to a "data-rich" science.[130] Now that whole-genome information is available, the challenge is to understand the data in a functional context. Expression profiling has proven to be a successful means to discover candidate genes and pathways in various regulatory systems.

The first such gene expression profile of the cardiovascular system was generated from 3874 ESTs from an adult cardiac cDNA library.[31] The profile correlated well to expected patterns, based on known histologic characteristics and physiologic functions of the heart. For example, the high abundance of ESTs representing contractile proteins in the heart almost certainly relates to its contractile function, whereas the relatively abundant cytoskeletal elements and ECM proteins presumably compose the fibrous skeleton of the heart, which functions to transduce force generated by contractile components to produce useful mechanical work. This work places significant metabolic demands on the heart; thus, a significant proportion of transcripts encoding genes related to metabolic processes is required. Somewhat more surprising was the observation that transcripts encoding proteins involved in transcription

---

*cAMP (cyclic adenosine monophosphate) responsive element binding protein

and translation also constituted a large segment of gene expression. Although this could reflect the constant turnover of the large bulk of contractile proteins, it may also reflect basal activity associated with upkeep and maintenance of general cellular function.

This adult cardiac gene expression profile differed in several respects from one generated from fetal cardiac ESTs.[38,131] Most striking was the abundance of transcripts representing transcriptional and translational (TC/TL) apparatus and transcripts representing signal transduction or cell regulatory proteins in the fetal heart, compared with the relative lack of such proteins in the adult heart. In contrast, the fetal heart appeared to express lower levels of transcripts representing contractile elements than the adult heart.

Taken together, these findings appear to reflect on the overall physiologic status of the fetal heart. Rapid hyperplastic and hypertrophic growth of the heart under the influence of myriad different signals would demand not only increased protein synthesis, as evidenced by increases in TC/TL machinery, but also increased monitoring, regulation, and integration of growth signals, to allow for normal development and differentiation (hence, the increased expression of proteins responsible for signal transduction and cell regulation). Moreover, assuming that contractile proteins are markers of differentiation, expression of contractile proteins might be expected to be diminished when hyperplasia of myocytes occurs, as in the fetal heart. Thus, the differences in EST profiles of the fetal and adult hearts suggest a rapidly growing, relatively less differentiated state in the fetal heart, compared with a more stable, quiescent state in the adult.

Comparison of the cardiac profile to those of other tissues showed further correlation between the structure and function of tissues and the expected patterns of gene expression[131] (Table 2-6). Although the heart exhibited an abundance of ESTs representing contractile proteins, the brain, liver, and pancreatic islet did not. Furthermore, although the relative abundance of ECM proteins observed in the cardiac profile presumably compose the fibrous skeleton of the heart, much of the structural support in the brain appears to be derived not from ECM components but from intracellular structural proteins (26.3% of known transcripts) such as actin, tubulin, and glial fibrillary acidic protein, as evidenced by the numerous ESTs from the human brain representing such transcripts.[36] Also in agreement with predicted function, the pancreatic islet exhibited large proportions of ESTs representing both hormones and other secreted proteins, whereas almost one third of known hepatocyte transcripts also represented secreted proteins such as albumin. Interestingly, despite this high secretory activity, the pancreas appeared to express a similar proportion of ESTs for TC/TL proteins (approximately 19%) as the adult heart and brain do (organs not known for their protein synthetic or secretory capacity). In contrast, the rapidly growing fetal heart and hepatocyte cell line exhibited high levels of expression of TC/TL proteins. Another report also demonstrated very high levels of TC/TL protein expression in the fetal lung.[39] These data seem to indicate that genes related to TC/TL occupy a basal fraction of known cellular transcripts regardless of tissue and that this fraction is increased in relation to rapid growth, although not necessarily to specialization of function for protein synthesis and secretion. Similarly, genes related to metabolic processes occupied similar proportions of transcripts in the brain, pancreas, and adult heart (approximately 18%) but were slightly elevated in the fetal heart and hepatocyte, suggesting that rapid growth places higher metabolic demands on cells and tissues than normal function does. Taken together, these data support the notion that different cell types, regardless of their specific function, need to sustain certain basal activities associated with upkeep and maintenance of general cellular function, although these activities may be altered in response to special needs such as those imposed by rapid growth.

Although such analyses yielded some general insights into gene expression on a global level, more detailed *in silico* analyses of EST frequencies of individual genes have also suggested ubiquitous and tissue-restricted expression of specific genes in different tissues of the human body[45,132] and of the cardiovascular system.[32] Extension of this approach also identified a number of genes that were putatively overexpressed in heart fail-

■ ▦ ■

## TABLE 2-6   HUMAN HEART, BRAIN, HEPATOCYTE, AND PANCREATIC ISLET EST DISTRIBUTION DATABASE MATCHES BY FUNCTIONAL CATEGORIES*

| Category | Fetal Heart | Adult Heart | Brain | Hepatocyte | Islet |
|---|---|---|---|---|---|
| Contractile | 6.5 (50) | 21.0 (109) | 0.0 (0) | 0.0 (0) | 0.0 (0) |
| Cytoskeletal/structural | 8.1 (62) | 10.6 (55) | 26.3 (227) | 3.1(6) | 7.5 (27) |
| Extracellular matrix | 4.6 (35) | 8.1 (42) | 0.0 (0) | 0.0 (0) | 1.1 (4) |
| Energy metabolism | 11.9 (91) | 13.5 (70) | 6.1 (53) | 9.2 (18) | 2.8 (10) |
| Hormones/regulation | 4.3 (33) | 4.2 (22) | 0.7 (6) | 1.0 (2) | 7.7 (28) |
| Signal transduction/cell regulation | 16.6 (127) | 7.9 (41) | 19.9 (172) | 8.2 (16) | 11.0 (40) |
| Transcription/translation | 29.2 (223) | 18.7 (97) | 18.8 (162) | 31.8 (62) | 19.1 (69) |
| Membrane associated | 6.4 (49) | 8.8 (46) | 15.3 (132) | 2.1 (4) | 12.4 (45) |
| Metabolism | 11.0 (84) | 6.2 (32) | 11.7 (101) | 14.4 (28) | 14.9 (54) |
| Secreted protein | 1.3 (10) | 1.2 (6) | 1.3 (11) | 30.3 (59) | 23.5 (85) |
| Total | 100 (764) | 100 (520) | 100(864) | 100 (195) | 100 (362) |

*EST percentages per category (actual numbers of ESTs).
EST, expressed sequence tag.
Data from references 31, 37, 133, and 188.

ure, approximately one third of which had previously been implicated in processes leading to heart failure and the rest of which were not previously known to be involved (Table 2-7).[32,133] Together with the cDNA microarray, these two analyses of candidate genes related to complex diseases can be identified on the chromosomal loci. The validation of differential expression was also confirmed *in vitro* for a number of these genes by reverse-transcriptase polymerase chain reaction (RT-PCR) (Fig. 2-5), confirming the validity and potential power of such EST-based and microarray approaches to identifying genes potentially involved in developmental and disease processes.

Because of the new data available from the HGP, it has been necessary to develop new technology to understand the data.[130] Technologic achievements of the HGP include the development of automated sequencing instrumentation, high-throughput sequencing instruments for large-scale sequencing and robotics, and the development of EST strategies. These include improved vector systems for cloning large DNA fragments and assembling these clones into large overlapping sets that compose physical maps.

The advances made by the HGP so far have been significant. However, the completion of sequencing the human genome is only the beginning. Now research must focus on functional genomics. Researchers are optimistic that the availability of the complete human genome and new HGP-related technologies, such as computational microarray and other functional genomics technologies, will significantly accelerate the rate of gene discovery and the functional characterization of genes and gene complexes involved in more complex disorders. The field of pharmacogenomics should also benefit from the ideas, tools, and strategies of the HGP.

## PHARMACOGENOMICS AND THE HUMAN GENOME PROJECT

### Background

The term *pharmacogenetics* was coined by Friedrich Vogel in 1959 to describe a field that had been developing over the previous decade.[134] Researchers in the 1950s recognized and studied interesting hereditary individual variations in drug responses and traced the metabolic and genetic underpinnings of such interindividual variability. For example, respiratory paralysis, observed in some patients who were administered succinylcholine, a muscle relaxant used in electroshock therapy and surgery, was traced to an inherited cholinesterase deficiency.[135] Reporting a similar phenomenon, Hughes and coworkers in Cincinnati in 1954 noticed that approximately one third of patients exposed to the antituberculosis agent isoniazid developed painful neuropathies of the extremities, a reaction resulting from inherited deficiencies in isoniazid acetylation.[136,137] Complementary research reported inherited variability in responses to numerous other agents. For example, in a family study Mahgoub et al.[138] reported polymorphic hydroxylation of the hypertensive debrisoquine causing

variability in blood pressure response to this agent, and Eichelbaum et al.[139] found variability of response to the antiarrhythmia agent sparteine, suggesting phenotypic subtypes. Ideas stimulated by these and related studies formed the basis of present pharmacogenetics studies devoted to identifying important and clinically relevant polymorphisms and other sources of genetic variability in drug response.[140]

The next few years will likely lead to major developments in drug research and prescribing practice in cardiovascular medicine as the field known as pharmacogenomics begins to capitalize on the data and the technology of the HGP. It is thought that within 10 to 15 years, general physicians will have the capability to screen patients for drug interactive polymorphisms of clinical relevance. We conclude this chapter with a discussion of the present research in cardiovascular pharmacogenetics and pharmacogenomics and a look toward the future.

## Pharmacogenetics and Pharmacogenomics

Pharmacogenetics is the study of genetically based variations and how they relate to drug response. Although the terms are often used interchangeably, pharmacogenetics, strictly speaking, has to do with identification of single-gene variants, whereas pharmacogenomics is more holistically involved with large sets of genes and gene pathways that may contribute to drug effects.[141] Pharmacogenomics research is being driven by advances in high-throughput sequencing technology that enables rapid and efficient screening for large numbers of genetic variations and in expression profiling and bioinformatics, enabling the discovery of pathways and novel drug targets. Progress has been encouraging in pharmacogenetics studies in a number of medical specialties, and researchers are optimistic that clinically important developments will be obtained within 10 to 15 years. In this section we briefly outline the pharmacogenetics and pharmacogenomics field using examples relevant to cardiovascular medicine.

### Aims of Pharmacogenomics and Pharmacogenetics

It has long been apparent that many drugs, although effective in some patients, are ineffective, intolerable, and sometimes fatal in others. Despite best efforts in drug trial design and testing, adverse drug reactions remain a significant problem. A recent meta-analysis listed adverse drug reactions in hospitalized patients as between the fourth and sixth leading cause of death in the United States and a more common cause of death than diabetes and pneumonia.[142] The study underscores the fact that adverse reactions to drugs are a nontrivial and underappreciated source of morbidity and mortality. Multiple factors are involved in such adverse drug events, including environmental causes and individual patient features such as age and weight. Genetic variability is also well known as a major source of phenotypic idiosyncrasy. Variations at the level of the gene can have profound effects on drug pharmacokinetics (i.e., drug absorption, metabolism, distribution, and excretion) and

## TABLE 2-7 IDENTIFICATION OF GENES POTENTIALLY OVEREXPRESSED IN CARDIAC HYPERTROPHY

| Gene | Accession | Function | Fetal | Adult | Dis | p |
|---|---|---|---|---|---|---|
| Mitochondrial genome (consensus sequence) | X62996 | M | 7.85% | 8.13% | 22.99% | >1.0E-30 |
| Myoglobin | X00373 | C/OD | 0.02% | 0.01% | 0.82% | 6.6E-25 |
| Brain natriuretic peptide precursor | M25296 | CS/C | 0.01% | 0.00% | 0.67% | 4.3E-21 |
| Actin, α-skeletal | J00068 | CS/M | 0.00% | 0.03% | 0.53% | 8.1E-16 |
| Troponin I, cardiac | M64247 | CS/M | 0.01% | 0.04% | 0.40% | 8.6E-13 |
| Crystallin, α-B | S45630 | CS/M | 0.05% | 0.04% | 0.53% | 8.7E-12 |
| Myosin regulatory light chain | X54304 | CS/M | 0.05% | 0.03% | 0.33% | 4.0E-09 |
| Skeletal muscle LIM-protein SLIM1 | U60115 | U | 0.00% | 0.00% | 0.20% | 1.6E-08 |
| Tropomyosin, α skeletal muscle | M19715 | CS/M | 0.32% | 0.27% | 0.80% | 7.9E-08 |
| Atrial natriuretic factor* | M30262 | CS/C | 0.50% | 0.27% | 0.78% | 1.3E-07 |
| Myosin light chain-2* | S69022 | CS/M | 0.08% | 0.19% | 0.98% | 3.8E-07 |
| CD59 antigen | M34671 | U | 0.00% | 0.00% | 0.18% | 9.8E-07 |
| Lipoprotein lipase | M15856 | M | 0.00% | 0.01% | 0.18% | 2.2E-06 |
| Heat shock protein 70 (hsp70 protein 1) | M59830 | C/OD | 0.01% | 0.04% | 0.16% | 1.1E-05 |
| Plasminogen activator inhibitor-1 | X04429 | G/PE | 0.00% | 0.00% | 0.11% | 1.2E-05 |
| Creatine kinase (MtCK), sarcomeric mitochondrial | J05401 | C/OD | 0.01% | 0.03% | 0.18% | 1.4E-05 |
| Desmin* | U59167 | CS/M | 0.02% | 0.09% | 0.60% | 1.8E-05 |
| Ferritin L chain | M11147 | C/OD | 0.04% | 0.00% | 0.20% | 4.3E-05 |
| ATP/ADP translocator, heart/skeletal muscle (ANT1) | J04982 | M | 0.03% | 0.00% | 0.16% | 9.1E-05 |
| Troponin T, cardiac isoform | L40162 | CS/M | 0.25% | 0.23% | 0.55% | 9.5E-05 |
| Ubiquitin | M26880 | G/PE | 0.04% | 0.04% | 0.20% | 0.00011 |
| Troponin C, slow-twitch skeletal muscle* | X07897 | CS/M | 0.21% | 0.03% | 0.29% | 0.00015 |
| Metallothionein-II | V00594 | C/OD | 0.00% | 0.00% | 0.16% | 1.25E-07 |
| Decorin | L01131 | CS/M | 0.05% | 0.00% | 0.27% | 5.78E-07 |
| Ribosomal protein S11* | X06617 | G/PE | 0.14% | 0.00% | 0.22% | 2.14E-06 |
| HHCPA78, brain-expressed homologue | S73591 | U | 0.01% | 0.01% | 0.16% | 2.77E-05 |
| Heat shock protein 70B | X51758 | C/OD | 0.00% | 0.00% | 0.09% | 3.07E-05 |
| Calcyclin | J02763 | CS/C | 0.00% | 0.00% | 0.09% | 0.00010 |
| Glutathione peroxidase, plasma | X58295 | C/OD | 0.00% | 0.01% | 0.11% | 0.00016 |
| Metallothionein-Ie | M10942 | C/OD | 0.00% | 0.00% | 0.07% | 0.00025 |
| Myosin light chain 1, ventricular | X07373 | CS/M | 0.17% | 0.12% | 0.40% | 0.00026 |
| Prostaglandin D synthase | M61900 | M | 0.00% | 0.00% | 0.09% | 0.00028 |
| Ribosomal protein L39 | D79205 | G/PE | 0.00% | 0.00% | 0.09% | 0.00028 |
| Superoxide dismutase (SOD-2) (manganese) | X65965 | C/OD | 0.01% | 0.01% | 0.11% | 0.00030 |
| Enoyl-CoA hydratase-like protein, peroxisomal (HPXEL) | U16660 | M | 0.00% | 0.01% | 0.09% | 0.00030 |
| Gelsolin, plasma | X04412 | CS/C | 0.00% | 0.00% | 0.09% | 0.00030 |
| ATPase, calcium (HK2) | M23115 | M | 0.04% | 0.05% | 0.13% | 0.00031 |
| Ferritin heavy chain* | M97164 | C/OD | 0.09% | 0.01% | 0.18% | 0.00033 |
| P21 mouse homologue* | X64899 | CD | 0.19% | 0.06% | 0.33% | 0.00040 |
| Cytochrome c oxidase subunit VIIc* | X16560 | M | 0.10% | 0.00% | 0.13% | 0.00061 |
| CLP (LIM domain protein)* | U20324 | G/PE | 0.14% | 0.03% | 0.18% | 0.00061 |
| Ribosomal protein S8* | X67247 | G/PE | 0.13% | 0.03% | 0.16% | 0.00066 |
| Cell surface protein TAPA-1, 26 kDa | M33680 | U | 0.01% | 0.01% | 0.11% | 0.00069 |
| Ribosomal RNA, 28S | M11167 | G/PE | 0.19% | 0.30% | 0.42% | 0.00071 |
| Ribosomal protein S18* | X69150 | G/PE | 0.15% | 0.01% | 0.22% | 0.00092 |
| Cytochrome c, somatic | M22877 | M | 0.03% | 0.01% | 0.13% | 0.00095 |
| Prothymosin alpha | M14483 | CD | 0.05% | 0.03% | 0.13% | 0.00098 |
| Ribosomal protein S12 | X53505 | G/PE | 0.05% | 0.01% | 0.16% | 0.00099 |
| 26S proteasome subunit p31 | D38047 | G/PE | 0.00% | 0.00% | 0.07% | 0.0010 |
| Matrix Gla protein | X53331 | CS/M | 0.02% | 0.01% | 0.11% | 0.0012 |
| Ribosomal protein L9* | U09953 | G/PE | 0.17% | 0.00% | 0.16% | 0.0012 |
| Pyruvate dehydrogenase alpha subunit | M24848 | M | 0.02% | 0.01% | 0.09% | 0.0014 |
| Microglobulin, β-2* | M17987 | C/OD | 0.06% | 0.00% | 0.16% | 0.0017 |
| Prostaglandin D2 synthase | M98537 | M | 0.00% | 0.01% | 0.09% | 0.0023 |
| Ribosomal protein L26* | X69392 | G/PE | 0.15% | 0.00% | 0.09% | 0.0024 |
| Ribosomal protein L21* | U14967 | G/PE | 0.12% | 0.00% | 0.13% | 0.0026 |
| DS-1 | X81788 | U | 0.00% | 0.00% | 0.04% | 0.0028 |
| Long-chain acyl-CoA synthetase | D10040 | M | 0.00% | 0.00% | 0.04% | 0.0028 |
| Heterogeneous nuclear ribonucleoprotein E1 | X78137 | G/PE | 0.01% | 0.00% | 0.09% | 0.0032 |
| Glycogenin | U31525 | M | 0.02% | 0.01% | 0.09% | 0.0033 |
| RanBP2 (Ran-binding protein 2) | D42063 | CS/C | 0.01% | 0.00% | 0.07% | 0.0037 |
| Ribosomal protein L41* | S64030 | G/PE | 0.05% | 0.00% | 0.13% | 0.0044 |
| Ribosomal protein L27a* | U14968 | G/PE | 0.12% | 0.00% | 0.13% | 0.0044 |
| Phospholamban* | M63603 | CS/C | 0.13% | 0.01% | 0.11% | 0.0047 |

Genes represented by ESTs in at least two of three hypertrophic heart cDNA libraries were identified. Poisson probabilities were calculated as described in the text. Percentages indicate relative expression frequency of genes in pooled libraries. Asterisks (*) denote genes for which adult heart gene frequencies differed significantly from fetal heart frequencies, and for which p-values were determined using adult heart EST data alone as the reference value. Gene denotes the gene name; Accession denotes the Genbank accession number for each gene; Function denotes the functional category for each gene; Fetal denotes the expression frequency for the human fetal heart; Adult denotes the expression frequency for the human adult heart; Dis denotes the expression frequency for the human hypertrophic heart; p denotes the probability for differential expression in the hypertrophic against the normal heart. Functional categories are defined as follows: Cell Division (CD), Cell/Organism Defence (C/OD), Cell Signalling/Communication (CS/C), Cell Structure/Motility (CS/M), Gene/Protein Expression (G/PE), Metabolism (M), Unclassified (U).
Shading intensities, from darkest to lightest, reflect gene frequency and are defined as follows: >2.5%, 0.5–2.49%, 0.2–0.49%, 0.05–0.19%, <0.05%, and 0%, respectively. Modified from Hwang DM, Dempsey AA, Lee CY, et al: Identification of differentially expressed genes in cardiac hypertrophy by analysis of expressed sequence tags. Genomics 2000;66:1–14.

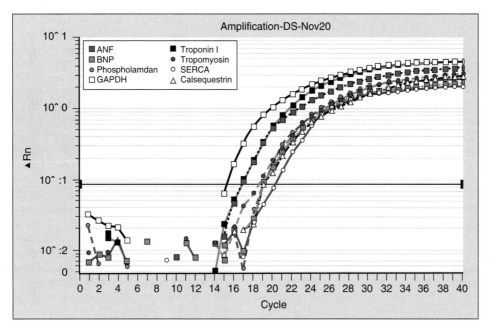

**FIGURE 2-5.** Validation of microarray expression profiles using real-time RT-PCR.

on drug pharmacodynamics (affecting drug activity and efficacy at the receptor level).

Pharmacogenetics and pharmacogenomics research aims to identify such drug-related genetic variations for clinically meaningful applications. For example, pharmacogenetics and pharmacogenomics information regarding whether a patient with a particular genetic profile will likely respond well to a given therapy or whether a drug is better avoided by the patient because of potential toxicity or side effects will enable physicians to tailor therapy. Pharmacogenomically based genome screening, DNA screening, or genetic signature technology is predicted to reach clinical relevance in cardiology and other medical disciplines within the next decade.

## Polymorphisms of Cardiovascular Relevance

Enzymes involved in drug metabolism have been the most extensively studied to date. Molecular and genomics studies beginning in the 1980s have identified polymorphisms in more than 20 human drug-metabolizing enzymes,[143] prominently the cytochrome P450 (CYP450) group of proteins, N-acetyltransferase, uridine diphosphate (UDP) glucuronosyl transferases, and the methyl transferases. Such gene polymorphisms have relevance in a range of pharmaceuticals used in various medical specialties; drugs in psychiatry and neurology are substrates of CYP2D6 (e.g., antidepressants, caffeine, and antipsychotics).[144] It is theorized that many polymorphisms that are involved in drug metabolism may have arisen during the course of evolution as defenses against various environmental chemicals and toxins to which organisms are exposed.[144]

### Cytochrome P450 Enzymes

Of particular relevance to cardiologists are polymorphisms in genes encoding for CYP450 enzymes. These enzymes are found mainly (although not exclusively) in the liver and have an important role in oxidative drug metabolism. Some 50 CYP450 proteins have been identified, many of which are involved in metabolism of a very wide range of drugs.[144] Cardiovascular drug metabolism has been shown to be crucially affected by polymorphisms in at least four CYP450 enzymes: CYP1A2, CYP2C9, CYP2D6, and CYP3A5.[145]

The most thoroughly researched of these enzymes is CYP2D6, also called debrisoquine hydroxylase, which carries about 70 alleles.[146] Large numbers of cardiovascular drugs use this enzyme for elimination, mainly by oxidative metabolism. CYP2D6 substrates include several β blockers, such as metoprolol, propanolol, bufuralol, and timolol; various antiarrhythmics, including flecainide and propafenone; and antihypertensives, including debriquosine and sparteine (now withdrawn).

Some CYP2D6 polymorphisms seem to impair or inactivate enzyme activity, leading to excessive plasma drug levels. The first report of a genetic polymorphism in the CYP enzymes was the study of Mahgoub et al.[138] London family study of debriquosine, which suggested that defective hydroxylation of this agent was inherited. "Poor metabolizers," that is, carriers who inadequately metabolize CYP2D6-selective drugs, may be subject to side effects, toxicity, and overdose. For example, the antihypertensive sparteine, a substrate of CYP2D6, causes diplopia, blurred vision, dizziness, and headaches in nonmetabolizers. This agent was also under investigation as an oxytocic during the 1950s, when it was withdrawn from the market because it was found to result in fetal death in 2% to 3% of cases. It has been suggested that fetal deaths may have occurred more commonly in sparteine nonmetabolizers.[139] Approximately 5% to 10% of whites and 1% to 2% of Asians carry polymorphisms that inactivate or inhibit CYP2D6. These represent substantial populations at increased risk of potentially dangerous and even fatal adverse drug reactions when prescribed any of the 40 or so known CYP2D6-substrate medications.[144]

Another subset of patients inherit an "amplification" polymorphism, which results in excessive metabolism of CYP2D6 substrate medications. For these patients, the "ultra-rapid metabolizers," very large doses of a drug are necessary before therapeutic efficacy can be reached.[143] Roden[141] speculates that because many β blockers are substrates of CYP2D6, the possibility exists that ultra-rapid metabolizers may be less cardioprotected by β blockers and thus more subject to sudden death. Ultrarapid metabolizers are found in 20% of Ethiopian populations, 7% of Spanish populations, and 1.5% of Scandinavian populations studied.[147]

Another interesting enzyme inactivating allele of cardiovascular relevance is the P450 gene, coding for CYP2C9. CYP2C9 is involved in warfarin metabolism, and it has long been known that patient variability of response to warfarin makes optimal dosage difficult to predict. Aithal et al.[148] found a strong association between patient sensitivity to this agent and a specific polymorphism in CYP2C9 (variant alleles CYP2C9 *2 and *3) Patients carrying this variant had low warfarin dose requirements and suffered more bleeding complications, including life-threatening bleeds. The complexities of warfarin pharmacogenetics have been recently reviewed.[149]

The potential clinical importance of preventing potential adverse reactions by identifying individuals with genetic variations affecting CYP450 enzyme substrate medications is clear. A simple, single DNA-based test to identify rapid or slow metabolizers that could be used to preventing drug overdose and minimize side effects or to guide drug dosage prescribing would be extremely useful. Practical pharmacogenomics-based applications for pharmacogenetic findings are beginning to be developed. A PCR-based method for genotyping poor metabolizers of debrisoquine has been developed.[150] Affymetrix (Santa Clara, California) has marketed a CYP2D6/ CYP2C19 GeneChip for potentially identifying poor drug metabolizers.[151] CYP2D6 genotype testing is offered in research centers in the Scandinavian countries where it is mainly offered to psychiatric patients who often suffer from debilitating drug-induced side effects.[151] Some researchers believe that research is adequate to support CYP2D6 polymorphism population-based pharmacogenetic testing,[151] and recently Kircheiner et al.[152] published the first CYP2D6 and CYP2C19 genotype-based average dose recommendations for 14 antidepressant medications.

## Other Cardiovascular Polymorphisms

Polymorphisms of cardiovascular interest also occur in N-acetyltransferase enzymes and may affect response to cardiovascular drugs including amrinone,[153] hydralazine,[154] and procainamide.[155] Rapid acetylators of these drugs may show a lack of response to drug doses that are effective in the majority of the population. By contrast slow acetylators may experience a range of side effects and toxicities. For example, long-term procainamide has been reported to trigger an autoimmune-like state and lupus-like syndrome in approximately one fifth of patients treated over the long term, with slow acetylators developing the disorder more rapidly than other patients.[156] Similarly, slow acetylators who have received hydralazine have been observed to develop a rheumatoid arthritis–like reaction and lupus.[157] In populations studied, up to 90% of North Africans and less than 10% of Orientals are slow acetylators.[145]

Several polymorphisms reportedly influence patients' response to anticholesteremic pravastatin therapy.[157] Kuivenhoven et al.[158] studied the Taq 1B polymorphism of the gene for cholesterol ester transferase protein (CETP). This is an enzyme that is involved in metabolizing high-density lipoprotein, which in turn is inversely and protectively linked to risk of coronary heart disease. The group found an association between a CETP gene variant (B1B1) and more rapidly progressing coronary atherosclerosis. Of potential therapeutic interest, pravastatin was observed to slow the atherosclerosis progression in B1B1 carriers. The genotype is also associated with better lipid profile response to diet therapy in patients with diabetes.[159]

In a recent study of patients with heart failure, McNamara et al.[160] reported that the D allele of the angiotensin-converting enzyme (ACE) gene was associated with increased risk for death or heart transplantation; in addition they reported that the allele was associated with improved response to β blocker therapy in ACE inhibitor treated patients with congestive heart failure.

## Polymorphisms in Hypertension

Hypertension is a complex multifactorial polygenic disease in which both genetic and environmental factors interact. Essential hypertension affects about 20% of the Western adult population, and genetically determined responses to hypertensive medications are attracting a great deal of pharmacogenomics research interest. About four different classes of antihypertensive medications are commonly used: diuretics, calcium antagonists, β blockers, and ACE inhibitors. However, many patients suffer considerable distress from side effects, antihypertensive medication often requires revision and adjustment, and poor patient compliance is an ongoing concern. In some studies it has been found that only 5% to 27% of hypertensives have their blood pressure adequately controlled by treatment,[161] making pharmacogenomic approaches to more rational therapy particularly desirable.[162]

Patients might be identified as better responders or warned if they are at higher risk of adverse reactions; this may help define and tailor the prescribing of antihypertensive medications.[161] Other important and potentially achievable pharmacogenomic goals are genotypically identifying subsets of stroke or myocardial infarction prone patients for more aggressive intervention or tailoring drug therapy to the patient's risk of end-organ failure.[163] The heterogeneity of essential hypertension, a complex multifactorial disease involving complex feedback mechanisms, makes study difficult. Drug responses to hypertensive medications are likely to be similarly polygenic, involving networks and clusters of interacting genes and gene pathways, and pharmacogenomic progress has been disappointingly slow.[164]

An important target for drug therapy in hypertension is the renin angiotensin system (RAS). This system controls systemic and renal blood pressure and sodium balance. A focus on genetic variants influencing RAS has a logical appeal for identifying gene-drug interaction responses. Plasma angiotensinogen concentrations and elevated blood pressure has been associated with the T235 allele of the angiotensinogen (AGT) gene.[165,166] Drugs targeted to this subset might be a productive aim in hypertension therapy. RAS, however, is a complex system, and evidence is inconclusive that an angiotensinogen genotype influences blood pressure response to RAS drugs. For example, in a 1995 treatment study by Hingorani et al.,[167] this polymorphism was associated with variations in response to ACE inhibition, with the best response associated with T235. Other studies have not, however, consistently shown decreases in blood pressure and association with ACE/angiotensin genetic variants. Dudley et al.[168] found that AGT or ACE polymorphisms failed to predict a consistent response to β blockers, ACE inhibitors, or calcium channel blockers. O'Toole et al.[169] studied ACE polymorphism in response to ACE therapy in patients with congestive heart failure in a double-blind crossover study of captopril and lisinopril. A significant relationship was discovered between ACE genotype and blood pressure with captopril but not with lisinopril. In another study, the 235T allele of the AGT gene was associated with greater blood pressure decrease after sodium restriction than was the 235M allele, an intriguing finding that leads to the possibility that such patients may benefit from sodium restriction.[170]

More consistent results have been obtained in studies of *ADD1* that encodes for adducin, a cytoskeletal protein possibly affecting regulation of ion transportation across the cell membrane.[171] In rats, α-adducin gene point mutations are linked to hypertension and kidney dysfunction in sodium transport.[172] In humans, variants of the *ADD1* gene associated with hypertension are found in some ethnic groups. A link between an α-adducin polymorphism (G460T) and essential hypertension was shown via salt sensitivity in whites,[173] but the polymorphism was not found to be a major genetic risk factor in Japanese.[174] *ADD1* variants have also been linked to response to diuretic therapy. A Trp460 variant in the adducin gene was studied in an Italian population Carriers of this variant showed a 70% to 100% fall in blood pressure in response to thiazide diuretics.[175] The Trp460 variant is not uncommon. Approximately 20% of European whites are carriers of this allele, and these findings could have considerable clinical significance in the treatment of hypertension if borne out in future studies.[176]

Also of interest in hypertension pharmacogenetics is a mutation in the β subunit of epithelial sodium channels, T594M. This polymorphism is known to be carried by blacks, and it is thought that the mutation may act on sodium channels in renal tubules to reduce sodium excretion, causing sodium retention and hypertension.

A case-control study carried out in London, England, found this T594M variant to be four times more common in black patients with hypertension than in black normotensives. In addition, subjects carrying this allele show evidence of sodium retention.[177] Because amiloride is a drug that acts as a sodium channel blocker, it is suggested that patients with this allele (e.g., 8% of black hypertensives in London according to Baker's study) may show good response to this drug in future studies.[176]

To date, pharmacogenetics studies in hypertension have led to intriguing possibilities for future studies but not yet to clear clinical implications. It is likely that HGP data and automated high-throughput technology coupled with bioinformatics strategies will lead to advances in therapeutic strategies for this complex polygenic disease.[178,179]

### Single-Nucleotide Polymorphisms

Cardiovascular and other pharmacogenomic studies of the future are likely to capitalize on newly available SNP maps now rapidly being developed and becoming publicly available through the HGP and the SNP consortium. Such a map will provide an important research resource by which drug responsive or nonresponsive phenotypes can be mapped by linkage disequilibrium.

SNP is the simplest form of DNA polymorphism, occurring when a single nucleotide is altered in the genome sequence. The approximately 1.5 to 3 million SNPs in the human genome are scattered 1 every 1000 to 2000 base pairs.[180] SNPs are evolutionarily stable in populations; are common, occurring at a rate of about 1% or more; and can differentiate individuals within that population. (By contrast gene mutations are rare differences occurring in much less than 1% of the population.[181]) Most SNPs occur in noncoding or "junk" areas of the genome; it is the biologically functioning coding SNPs that result in alterations of protein structure or expression and thus in disease or drug response and that are of greater interest in pharmacogenomics studies. There are currently 1.5 million human SNPs deposited in the dbSNP database (http//www.ncbi.nlm.nih.gov/SNP).

SNPs might be pharmacogenomically useful for identifying persons who may have potentially hazardous or beneficial genetic peculiarities in their responses to pharmaceuticals. The ultimate goal for laboratories and pharmaceutical companies is a simple, cheap, reliable DNA microarray chip or SNP profile that can be used to identify individual drug sensitivity or potential drug efficacy using a finger-prick blood test. Such a chip would provide a rapid screen of individual genetic variants providing physicians with clinically valuable information about patients' potential to react to specific drugs.[182] Drug prescribing at present is mostly empirical, with patients submitting to various—sometimes unpleasant—regimens before an appropriate and effective medication can be found. Abbreviated SNP profiles available on the DNA chip would reduce the time and difficulty involved and rationalize this process.[183]

Researchers are optimistic that clinically relevant SNP-based pharmacogenomics applications will begin to emerge at least within the next few decades. It has been estimated that the market for such applications may reach $800 million by 2005.[19] The rapidly developing technology and data accumulation of HGP are driving this optimism. High-throughput screening methods and databases will provide invaluable tools for future identification of drug idiosyncratic individuals. Some pharmaceutical companies reportedly now collect patient DNA samples during ongoing drug trials to conduct future pharmacogenomics investigations.[184]

A detailed and dense SNP map will greatly facilitate developments in pharmacogenomics. Most recently a group of pharmaceutical companies and academic centers, the SNP Consortium together with the International Human Genome Sequencing Consortium has published a publicly available comprehensive, high-density, genome-wide SNP map of 1.42 million SNPs with a density of one SNP every 1.9 kilobases.[180] The group estimates that it has identified 60,000 coding SNPs. Ten thousand of these have been validated by Orchid Biosciences Inc. (http://www.snp.cshl.org). The publication of these data is intended to make a valuable research tool publicly available. In addition, in the future, a detailed SNP map will likely serve as a standard for regulatory agencies such as the Food and Drug Administration (FDA).

Drug trial research is likely to undergo transformation as pharmacogenomics technologies come on line. Drugs take many years and millions of dollars before they can be marketed. Major and serious drug adverse effects may only be realized after the compound is in late-phase trials or even after marketing. Withdrawing or withholding such drugs represents not only a significant economic loss to the firms testing the compounds but also the loss of a valuable medication for many patients who would not be adversely affected. Pharmacogenomics studies may make it possible to streamline studies by stratifying more patients into potential responders (more appropriate for trials) and eliminating those who may do less well with certain medications. In addition, identifying patients potentially at risk of adverse events may make it possible to save products that would otherwise not be allowed on the market.[185] Some researchers consider it likely that detailed pharmacogenetic profiles of drugs will become a standard requirement for drug approval and regulation in future.[186]

Cardiovascular medicine and indeed all medicine is likely to undergo transformation in the future as pharmacogenomics technologies improve and the DNA signature chip becomes part of drug trials and prescribing. Pharmacogenomics of the future also will include the use of genotyping to understand the basis of disease to identify targets and also the use of expression profiling to identify pathways and novel drug targets. The overall benefits of this technology should be a reduction of patient morbidity and mortality from adverse drug events. Concerns have, however, been raised that it will be highly important to validate SNP profiles.[183] Genotype does not always cash out into clinically important phenotype, and false positives and false negatives could adversely affect patients. Rigorous research standards will be required to define phenotype.[185,186] In the future as in the past, good medicine will depend on assessing patients holistically, with regard not only to laboratory tests and DNA chips but also to the whole person.

## CONCLUSION

In this first decade of the 21st century, HGP and its associated technologies, discoveries, inventions, and methodologies is an ongoing project. Researchers must continue to refine the accuracy of the human sequences to discover individual characteristics in response to genetic disease, in particular, those related to complex diseases. The identification of SNPs in the coding sequences of each individual is crucial for developing a specialty in pharmacogenomics. In this chapter we have sketched the possibilities and potentials of the new genomic technologies for gene discovery and in pharmacogenomics. The search for genes is a voyage of discovery. It will be many years before the full implications of the HGP for cardiovascular medicine will result in improved diagnostic methods, prognostic methods (and perhaps prognosis), therapy, and treatments.

## Acknowledgments

Our special thanks to Isolde Prince for her assistance in thoroughly researching the literature to formulate this manuscript and to David Barrans, Adam Dempsey, and David Hwang for their critical evaluation and comments.

## REFERENCES

1. Lander E, Weinberg RA: Genomics: Journey to the center of biology. Science 2000;287:1777-1782.
2. Service RF: Big biology is bad biology. Science 2001;291:1182.
3. Collins FS, McKusik VA: Implications of the human genome project for medical science. JAMA 2001;285:540-544.
4. Department of Health and Human Services and Department of Energy: Understanding Our Genetic Inheritance. The US Human Genome Project: The First Five Years: 1991-1995. Washington DC, Government Printing Office (NIH publication #90-1590), 1990.
5. Collins FS: Medical and societal consequences of the human genome project. N Engl J Med 1999;341:28-37.
6. Altschul SF, Gish W, Miller W, et al: Basic local alignment search tool. J Mol Biol 1990;215:403-410.
7. Adams MD, Kelley JM, Gocayne JD, et al: Complementary DNA sequencing: Expressed sequence tags and the human genome project. Science 1991;252:1651-1656.
8. Vollrath D, Foote S, Hilton A, et al: The human Y chromosome: A 43-interval map based on naturally occurring deletions. Science 1992;258:52-59.
9. Chumakov I, Rigault P, Guillou S, et al: Continuum of overlapping clones spanning the entire human chromosome 21q. Nature 1992;359:380-387.
10. Dietrich W, Katz H, Lincoln SE, et al: A genetic map of the mouse suitable for typing intraspecific crosses. Genetics 1992;131:423-447.
11. Cohen D, Chumakov I, Weissenback J: A first generation physical map of the human genome. Nature 1993;366:698-701.
12. Collins F, Galas D: A new five-year plan for the U.S. Human Genome Project. Science 1993;262:43-46.
13. Fleischmann RD, Adams MD, White O, et al: Whole-genome random sequencing and assembly of Haemophilus influenzae. Science 1995;269:496-512.
14. Hudson T, Stein LD, Gerety SS, et al: An STS-based map of the human genome sequence. Science 1995;270:1945-1954.

15. Clayton RA, White O, Ketchum KA, et al: The first genome from the third domain of life. Nature 1997;387:459-462.

16. The C elegans Sequencing Consortium: Genome sequence of the nematode C. elegans: A platform for investigating biology. Science 1998;282:2012-2018.

17. Bentley DR: Genomic sequence information should be released immediately and freely in the public domain. Science 1996; 274:533-534.

18. Macilwain C: World leaders heap praise on human genome landmark. Nature 2000;405:983-984.

19. Brown K: The Human genome business today. Sci Am 2000; 283:50-55.

20. Collins FS, Patrinos A, Jordan E, et al: New goals for the US human genome project: 1998-2003. Science 1998;282:682-689.

21. Venter JC, Adams, MD, Myers EW: The sequence of the human genome. Science 2001;291:1304-1351.

22. Genome Sequencing Consortium: Initial sequencing and analysis of the human genome. Nature 2001;409:860-921.

23. Jasny B, Kennedy D: The human genome. Science 2001;291:1153.

24. Pennisi E: The human genome. Science 2001;291:1177-1180.

25. http://www.ornl.gov/TechResources/Human_Genome/faq/genenumber.html

26. Dempsey AA, Dzau VJ, Liew CC: Cardiovascular genomics: Estimating the total number of genes expressed in the human cardiovascular system. J Mol Cell Cardiol 2001;33:1879-1886.

27. Adams MD, Kelley JM, Gocayne JD, et al: Complementary DNA sequencing: Expressed sequence tags and human genome project. Science 1991;252:1651-1656.

28. Putney SD, Herlihy WC, Schimmel P: A new troponin T and cDNA clones for 13 different muscle proteins, found by shotgun sequencing. Nature 1983;302:718-721.

29. Roberts L: Gambling on a shortcut to genome sequencing. Science 1991;252:1618-1619.

30. Liew CC: A human heart cDNA library—the development of an efficient and simple method for automated DNA sequencing. J Mol Cell Cardiol 1993;25:891-894.

31. Liew CC, Hwang DM, Fung YW, et al: A catalogue of genes in the cardiovascular system as identified by expressed sequence tags (ESTs). Proc Natl Acad Sci USA 1994;91:10645-10649.

32. Hwang DM, Dempsey AA, Wang RX, et al: A genome-based resource for molecular cardiovascular medicine: Toward a compendium of cardiovascular genes. Circulation 1997;96:4146-4203.

33. Roberts L: Genome patent fight erupts. Science 1991;254:184-186.

34. Marshall E: The company that genome researchers love to hate. Science 1994;266:1800-1802.

35. Adams MD, Dubnick M, Kerlavage AR: Sequence identification of 2,375 human brain genes. Nature 1992:355:632-634.

36. Adams MD, Kerlavage AR, Fields C, Venter JC: 3,400 new expressed sequence tags identify a diversity of transcripts in human brain. Nat Genet 1993;4:256-267.

37. Adams MD, Soares MB, Kerlavage AR, et al: Rapid cDNA sequencing (expressed sequence tags) from a directionally cloned human infant brain cDNA library. Nat Genet 1993;4:373-380.

38. Hwang DM, Hwang WS, Liew CC: Single pass sequencing of a unidirectional human fetal heart cDNA library to discover novel genes of the cardiovascular system. J Mol Cell Cardiol 1994; 26:1329-1333.

39. Sudo K, Chinen K, Nakamura Y: 2058 Expressed sequence tags (ESTs) from a human fetal lung cDNA library. Genomics 1994;24:276-279.

40. Schmidtke J, Cooper DN: A comprehensive list of cloned human DNA sequences—1990 update. Nucleic Acids Res 1991;19(Suppl.): 2111-2126.

41. Miller G, Fuchs R, Lai E: IMAGE cDNA clones, UniGene clustering, and ACeDB: An integrated resource for expressed sequence information. Genome Res 1997;7:1027-1032.

42. Boguski MS, Lowe TM, Tolstoshev CM: dbEST: A database of expressed sequence tags. Nat Genet 1993;4:332-333.

43. Ton C, Hwang DM, Dempsey AA, et al: Identification, characterization and mapping of expressed sequence tags from an embryonic zebrafish heart cDNA library. Genome Res 2000;10:1915-1927.

44. Okubo K, Hori N, Matoba R, et al: Large scale cDNA sequencing for analysis of quantitative and qualitative aspects of gene expression. Nat Genet 1992;2:173-179.

45. Adams MD, Kerlavage AR, Fleischmann RD, et al: Initial assessment of human gene diversity and expression patterns based upon 83 million nucleotides of cDNA sequence. Nature 1995; 377(Suppl.):3-174.

46. Hwang DM, Fung YW, Wang RX, et al: Analysis of expressed sequence tags from a fetal human heart cDNA library. Genomics 1995;30:293-298.

47. Bortoluzzi S, d'Alessi F, Danieli GA: A novel resource for the study of genes expressed in the adult human retina. Invest Ophthalmol Vis Sci 2000;41:3305-3308.

48. Ji H, Liu YE, Jia T, et al: Identification of a breast cancer-specific gene, BCSG1, by direct differential cDNA sequencing. Cancer Res 1997;57:759-764.

49. Levy-Lahad E, Wasco W, Poorkaj P, et al: Candidate gene for the chromosome 1 familial Alzheimer's disease locus. Science 1995;269:973-977.

50. Banfi S, Borsani G, Rossi E, et al: Identification and mapping of human cDNAs homologous to Drosophila mutant genes through EST database searching. Nat Genet 1996;13:167-174.

51. Miklos GL, Rubin GM: The role of the genome project in determining gene function: Insights from model organisms. Cell 1996; 86:521-529.

52. Rawlings CJ, Searls DB: Computational gene discovery and human disease. Curr Opin Genet Dev 1997;7:416-423.

53. Papadopoulos N, Nicolaides NC, Wei YF, et al: Mutation of a *mutL* homolog in hereditary colon cancer. Science 1994;263:1625-1629.

54. Sargent CA, Affara NA, Bentley E, et al: Cloning of the X-linked glycerol kinase deficiency gene and its identification by sequence comparison to the Bacillus subtilis homologue. Hum Mol Genet 1993;2:97-106.

55. Banfi S, Borsani G, Rossi E, et al: Identification and mapping of human cDNAs homologous to Drosophila mutant genes through EST database searching. Nat Genet 1996;13:167-174.

56. Banfi S, Borsani G, Bulfone A, Ballabio A: Drosophila-related expressed sequences. Hum Mol Genet 1997;6:1745-1753.

57. Bassett DE Jr, Boguski MS, Spencer F, et al: Genome cross-referencing and XREFdb: Implications for the identification and analysis of genes mutated in human disease. Nat Genet 1997;15:339-344.

58. Schena M, Shalon D, Davis RW, et al: Quantitative monitoring of gene expression patterns with a complementary DNA microarray. Science 1995;270:467-470.

59. Velculescu VE, Zhang L, Vogelstein B, Kinzler KW: Serial analysis of gene expression. Science 1995;270:484-487.

60. de Waard V, van den Berg BM, Veken J, et al: Serial analysis of gene expression to assess the endothelial cell response to an atherogenic stimulus. Gene 1999;226:1-8.

61. Lockhart DJ, Dong H, Byrne MC, et al: Expression monitoring by hybridization to high-density oligonucleotide arrays. Nat Biotechnol 1996;14:1675-1680.

62. Bowtell DDL: Options available—from start to finish—for obtaining expression data by microarray. Nat Genet Suppl 1999;21:25-32.

63. Lipshutz RJ, Fodor SPA, Gingeras TR, et al: High density synthetic oligonucleotide arrays. Nat Genet Suppl 1999;21:20-24.

64. DeRisi J, Penland L, Brown PO, et al: Use of a cDNA microarray to analyse gene expression patterns in human cancer. Nat Genet 1996;14:457-460.

65. Perou CM, Jeffrey SS, vandeRinj M, et al: Distinctive gene expression patterns in human mammary epithelial cells and breast cancers. Proc Natl Acad Sci USA 1999;96:9212-9217.

66. Eisen MB, Spellman PT, Brown PO, Botstein D: Cluster analysis and display of genome-wide expression patterns. Proc Natl Acad Sci USA 1998;95:14863-14868.

67. Iyer VR, Eisen MB, Ross DT, et al: The transcriptional program in the response of human fibroblasts to serum. Science 1999;283:83-87.

68. Barrans JD, Stamatiou D, Liew CC: Construction of a human cardiovascular cDNA microarray: Portrait of a failing heart. Biochem Biophys Res Commun 2001;280:964-969.

69. Hwang JJ, Dzau VJ, Liew CC: Genomics and the pathophysiology of heart failure. Curr Cardiol Rep 2001;3:198-207.

70. Friddle CL, Koga T, Rubin EM, Bristo J: Expression profiling reveals distinct sets of genes altered during induction and regression of cardiac hypertrophy. PNAS 2000;97:6745-6750.

71. Yang J, Moravec CS, Sussman MA: Decreased SLIM1 expression and increased gelsolin expression in failing human hearts measured by high-density oligonucleotide arrays. Circulation 2000; 102:3046-3052.

72. Barrans JD, Sc MH, Allen PD, et al: Global gene expression profiling of end stage dilated cardiomyopathy using a human cardiovascular based cDNA microarray. Am J Pathol 2002;160:2035–2043.

73. Towbin JA, Bowles NE: Genetic abnormalities responsible for dilated cardiomyopathy. Curr Cardiol Rep 2000;2:475–480.

74. Towbin JA: The role of cytoskeletal proteins in cardiomyopathies. Curr Opin Cell Biol 1998;10:131–139.

75. Elliott K, Watkins H, Redwood CS: Altered regulatory properties of human cardiac troponin I mutants that cause hypertrophic cardiomyopathy. J Biol Chem 2000;275:22069–22074.

76. Kimura A, Harada H, Park JE, et al: Mutations in the cardiac troponin I gene associated with hypertrophic cardiomyopathy. Nat Genet 1997;16:379–82.

77. Redwood C, Lohmann K, Bing W, et al: Investigation of a truncated cardiac troponin T that causes familial hypertrophic cardiomyopathy: Ca(2+) regulatory properties of reconstituted thin filaments depend on the ratio of mutant to wild-type protein. Circ Res 2000;86:1146–1152.

78. Geisterfer-Lowrance AA, Kass S, Tanigawa G: A molecular basis for familial hypertrophic cardiomyopathy: A beta cardiac myosin heavy chain gene missense mutation. Cell 1990;62:999–1006.

79. Thierfelder L, Watkins H, MacRae C, et al: Alpha-tropomyosin and cardiac troponin T mutations cause familial hypertrophic cardiomyopathy: A disease of the sarcomere. Cell 1994;77:701–712.

80. Dalakas MC, Park KY, Semino-Mora C, et al: Desmin myopathy, a skeletal myopathy with cardiomyopathy caused by mutations in the desmin gene. N Engl J Med. 2000;342:770–780.

81. Satoh M, Takahashi M, Sakamoto T, et al: Structural analysis of the titin gene in hypertrophic cardiomyopathy: Identification of a novel disease gene. Biochem Biophys Res Commun 1999; 262:411–417.

82. Schonberger J, Seidman CE: Many roads lead to a broken heart: The genetics of dilated cardiomyopathy. Am J Hum Genet 2001;69:249–260.

83. Olson TM, Michels VV, Thibodeau SN, et al: Actin mutations in dilated cardiomyopathy, a heritable form of heart failure. Science 1998;280:750–752.

84. Arber S, Hunter JJ, Ross J Jr, et al: MLP-deficient mice exhibit a disruption of cardiac cytoarchitectural organization, dilated cardiomyopathy, and heart failure. Cell 1997;88:393–403.

85. Dempsey AA, Ton C, Liew CC: A cardiovascular EST repertoire: Progress and promise for understanding cardiovascular disease. Mol Med Today 2000;6:231–237.

86. Francis GS: Changing the remodeling process in heart failure: Basic mechanisms and laboratory results. Curr Opin Cardiol 1998;13:156–161.

87. Rao VU, Spinale FG: Controlling myocardial matrix remodeling: Implications for heart failure. Cardiol Rev 1999;7:136–143.

88. McKinsey TA, Olson EN: Cardiac hypertrophy: Sorting out the circuitry. Curr Opin Genet Dev 1999;9:267–274.

89. Chien KR: Genomic circuits and the integrative biology of cardiac diseases. Nature 2000;407:227–232.

90. Miyamoto MI, del Monte F, Schmidt U, et al: Adenoviral gene transfer of SERCA2a improves left ventricular function in aortic-banded rats in transition to heart failure. Proc Natl Acad Sci 2000;97;793–798.

91. Tada M, Yabuki M, Toyofuku T: Molecular regulation of phospholamban function and gene expression. Ann NY Acad Sci 1998;853:116–129.

92. Marks AR: Cardiac intracellular calcium release channels: Role in heart failure. Circ Res 2000;87:8–11.

93. Dewaste V, Pouillon V, Moreau C, et al: Cloning and expression of a cDNA encoding human inositol 1,4,5-trisphosphate 3-kinase C. Biochem J 2000;352:343–351.

94. Pyeritz RE: Genetic approaches to cardiovascular disease. In Chien K (ed): Molecular Basis of Cardiovascular Disease: A Companion to Braunwald's Heart Disease. Philadelphia, WB Saunders, 1999, pp 19–36.

95. Uddhav K, Ketan S: Advances in the human genome project. Mol Biol Rep 1998;25:27–43.

96. Collins FS: Positional cloning: Lets not call it reverse any more. Nat Genet 1992;1:3–6.

97. Royer-Pokora B, Kunkel LM, Monaco AP, et al: Cloning the gene for an inherited human disorder, chronic granulomatous disease, on the basis of its chromosomal location. Nature 1986;322:32–38.

98. Collins FS: Positional cloning moves from perdition to traditional. Nat Genet 1995;9:347–350.

99. Teare D: Asymmetrical hypertrophy of the heart in young patients. Br Heart J 1958;20:1–8.

100. Jarcho JA, McKenna W, Pare JA, et al: Mapping a gene for familial hypertrophic cardiomyopathy to chromosome 14Q2. N Engl J Med 1989;321:1372–1378.

101. Watkins H, MacRae C, Thierfelder L, et al: A disease locus for familial hypertrophic cardiomyopathy maps to chromosome 1q3. Nat Genet 1993;3:333–337.

102. Thierfelder L, MacRae C, Watkins H, et al: A familial hypertrophic cardiomyopathy locus maps to chromosome 15q2. Proc Natl Acad Sci USA 1993;90:6270–6274.

103. Ferrari P, Bianchi G: Genomics of cardiovascular disorders. Drugs 2000;59:1025–1042.

104. Bonne G, Carrier L, Richard P, et al: Familial hypertrophic cardiomyopathy from mutations to functional defects. Circ Res 1998;83:580–593.

105. Marian AJ, Roberts R: Molecular genetic basis of hypertrophic cardiomyopathy: Genetic markers for sudden cardiac death. J Cardiovasc Electrophysiol 1998;9:88–99.

106. Milewicz D, Seidman CE: Genetics of cardiovascular disease. Circulation 2000;102:103–111.

107. Kamisago M, Sharma SD, DePalma SR, et al: Mutations on sarcomere protein genes as a cause of dilated cardiomyopathy. N Engl J Med 2000;343:1688–1696.

108. Li D, Tapscott T, Gonzalez O, et al: Desmin mutation responsible for idiopathic dilated cardiomyopathy. Circulation 1999;100: 461–464.

109. Campbell KP: Three muscular dystrophies: Loss of cytoskeleton-extracellular matrix linkage. Cell 1995;80:675–679.

110. Muntoni F, Wilson L, Marrosu G, et al: A mutation in the dystrophin gene selectively affecting dystrophin expression in the heart. J Clin Invest 1995;96:693–699.

111. Brodsky GL, Muntoni F, Miocic S, et al: Lamin A/C gene mutation associated with dilated cardiomyopathy with variable skeletal muscle involvement. Circulation 2000;101:473–476.

112. Fatkin D, MacRae C, Sasaki T, et al: Missense mutations in the rod domain of the lamin A/C gene as causes of dilated cardiomyopathy and conduction-system disease. N Engl J Med 1999;341:1715–1724.

113. Mathur A, Sims HF, Gopalakrishnan D, et al: Molecular heterogeneity in very-long-chain acyl-CoA dehydrogenase deficiency causing pediatric cardiomyopathy and sudden death. Circulation 1999;99:1337–1343.

114. McConnell BK, Jones KA, Fatkin D, et al: Dilated cardiomyopathy in homozygous myosin-binding protein-C mutant mice. J Clin Invest 1999;104:1235–1244.

115. Sakamoto A, Ono K, Abe M, et al: Both hypertrophic and dilated cardiomyopathies are caused by mutation of the same gene, delta-sarcoglycan, in hamster: An animal model of disrupted dystrophin-associated glycoprotein complex. Proc Natl Acad Sci USA 1997;94:13873–13878.

116. Chien KR: Stress pathways and heart failure. Cell 1999; 98:555–558.

117. Mende U, Kagen A, Cohen A, et al: Transient cardiac expression of constitutively active Galphaq leads to hypertrophy and dilated cardiomyopathy by calcineurin-dependent and independent pathways. Proc Natl Acad Sci USA 1998;95:13893–13898.

118. Fentzke RC, Korcarz CE, Lang RM, et al: Dilated cardiomyopathy in transgenic mice expressing a dominant-negative CREB transcription factor in the heart. J Clin Invest 1998;101:2415–2426.

119. Kubota T, McTiernan CF, Frye CS, et al: Dilated cardiomyopathy in transgenic mice with cardiac-specific overexpression of tumor necrosis factor-alpha. Circ Res 1997;81:627–635.

120. Subbarayan V, Mark M, Messadeq N, et al: RXRalpha overexpression in cardiomyocytes causes dilated cardiomyopathy but fails to rescue myocardial hypoplasia in RXRalpha-null fetuses. J Clin Invest 2000;105:387–394.

121. Emanueli C, Maestri R, Corradi D, et al: Dilated and failing cardiomyopathy in bradykinin B(2) receptor knockout mice. Circulation 1999;100:2359–2365.

122. Sussman MA, Welch S, Cambon N, et al: Myofibril degeneration caused by tropomodulin overexpression leads to dilated cardiomyopathy in juvenile mice. J Clin Invest 1998;101:51–61.

123. Li Y, Huang TT, Carlson EJ, et al: Dilated cardiomyopathy and neonatal lethality in mutant mice lacking manganese superoxide dismutase. Nat Genet 1995;11:376-381.

124. Wang J, Wilhelmsson H, Graff C, et al: Dilated cardiomyopathy and atrioventricular conduction blocks induced by heart-specific inactivation of mitochondrial DNA gene expression. Nat Genet 1999;21:133-137.

125. Schwartz PJ, Priori, SG, Locali, EH, et al: Long QT syndrome patients with mutations of the SCN5A and HERG genes have differential responses to Na+ channel blockade and to increases in heart rate: Implications for gene-specific therapy. Circulation 1995;92:3381-3386.

126. Zareba W, Moss AJ, Schwartz PJ, et al: Influence of the genotype on the clinical course of the long QT syndrome. N Engl J Med 1998;339:960-965.

127. Risch NJ: Searching for genetic determinants in the new millennium. Nature 2000;405:847-856.

128. Rubin EM, Tall A: Perspectives for vascular genomics. Nature 2000;407:265-269.

129. Pennisi E: Genomics comes of age. Science 2000;290:2220-2221.

130. Vukmirovic OG, Tilghman SM: Exploring genome space. Nature 2000;405:820-822.

131. Hwang DM, Fung YW, Wang RX, et al: Analysis of expressed sequence tags from a fetal human heart cDNA library. Genomics 1995;30:293-298.

132. Matsubara K, Okubo K: cDNA analyses in the human genome project. Gene 1993;135:265-274.

133. Hwang DM, Dempsey AA, Lee CY, et al: Identification of differentially expressed genes in cardiac hypertrophy by analysis of expressed sequence tags. Genomics 2000;66:1-14.

134. Vogel F: Moderne Probleme der Humangenetik. Ergab inn Med Kinderheilkd 1959;12:52-125.

135. Kalow W: Familial incidence of low pseudocholinesterase level. Lancet 1956;2:576.

136. Hughes HB, Biehl J, Jones AP, et al: Metabolism of isoniazid in man as related to the occurrence of peripheral neuritis. Am Rev Tuberc 1954;70:266.

137. Evans DAP, Manley KA, McKusic VA: Genetic control of isoniazid in man. Br Med J 1960;2:485.

138. Mahgoub A, Idle JR, Dring LG, et al: Polymorphic hydroxylation of debrisoquine in man Lancet 1977;2:584-586.

139. Eichelbaum, M, Spannbrucker N, Steincke B, et al: Defective N-oxidation of sparteine in man: A new pharmacogenetic defect. Eur J Clin Pharm 1979;16:183-197.

140. Weber WW: Pharmacogenetics. New York, Oxford University Press, 1997.

141. Roden DM: Pharmacogenetics and drug-induced arrhythmias. Cardiovasc Res 2001;50:224-231.

142. Lazarou J, Pomeranz BH, Corey PN: Incidence of adverse drug reactions in hospitalized patients: A meta-analysis of prospective studies. JAMA 1998;279:1200-1205.

143. Kalow W: Pharmacogenetics in biological perspective. Pharmacol Rev 1997;49:369-379.

144. Nelson DR, Koymans L, Kamataki T, et al: P450 Superfamily: Update on new sequences gene mapping accession numbers and nomenclature. Pharmacogenetics 1996;6:1-42.

145. Nakagawa K, Ishizaki T: Therapeutic relevance of pharmacogenetic factors in cardiovascular medicine. Pharmacol Ther 2000;86:1-28.

146. Meyer UA: Pharmacogenetics and adverse drug reactions. Lancet 2000;356:1667-1671.

147. Wolf CR, Smith G: Pharmacogenetics. Br Med Bull 1999;55:367-384.

148. Aithal, GP, Day CP, Kesteven PJL, et al: Association of polymorphisms in the cytochrome P450 CYP 2C9 with warfarin dose requirement and the risk of bleeding complications. Lancet 1999;353:717-719.

149. Takashi H, Echizen H: Pharmacogenetics of warfarin elimination and its clinical implications. Clin Pharmacokinet 2001;40:587-603.

150. Heim M, Meyer UA: Genotyping of poor metabolisers of debrisoquine by allele-specific PCR amplification. Lancet 1990;336:529-532.

151. Wolf CR, Smith G, Smith RL: Science, medicine and the future: Pharmacogenetics. Br Med J 2000;320:987-990.

152. Kircheiner J, Brosen K, Dahl ML, et al: CYP2D6 and CYP2DC19 genotype-based dose recommendations for antidepressants: A first step towards subpopulation-specific dosages. Arch Psych Scand 2001;104:173-192.

153. Hamilton RA, Kowalsky SF, Wright EM: Effect of the acetylator phenotype on amrinone pharmacokinetics. Clin Pharmacol Ther 1986;40:615-619.

154. Perry HM, Tan EM, Carmody S, et al: Relationship of acetyl transferase activity to antinuclear antibodies and toxic symptoms in hypertensive patients treated with hydralazine. J Lab Clin Med 1970;76:114-125.

155. Drayer DE, Reidenberg MM: Clinical consequences of polymorphic acetylation of basic drugs. Clin Pharmacol Ther 1977;22:251-258.

156. Henningsen NC, Cederberg A, Hanson A, et al: Effects of long-term treatment with Procain Amide. Acta Med Scand 1975;198:475-482.

157. Jukema JW: Matching treatment to the genetic basis of lipid disorders in patients with coronary artery disease. Heart 1999;82:126-127.

158. Kuivenhoven JA, Jukema JW, Zwinderman AH, et al: The role of a common variant of the cholesteryl ester transfer protein gene in the progression of coronary atherosclerosis. N Engl J Med 1998;338:86-93.

159. Dullaart RP, Hoogenberg K, Riemens SC, et al: Cholesteryl ester transfer protein gene polymorphism is a determinant of HDL cholesterol and of the lipoprotein response to a lipid-lowering diet in type 1 diabetes. Diabetes 1997;46:2082-2087.

160. McNamara DM, Holubkov R, Janosko, K, et al: Pharmacogenic interactions between beta-blocker therapy and the angiotensin-converting enzyme deletion polymorphism in patients with congestive heart failure. Circulation 2001;103:1644-1648.

161. Ferrari P, Bianchi G: Genetic mapping and tailored antihypertensive therapy. Cardiovasc Drugs Ther 2000;14:387-395.

162. Dickerson JE, Hingorani AD, Ashby MJ, et al: Optimisation of antihypertensive treatment by crossover rotation of four major classes. Lancet 1999;353:2008-2013.

163. Pratt RE, Dzau VJ: Genomics and hypertension. Hypertension 1999;33:238-247.

164. Hamet P: Genes and hypertension: Where we are and where we should go. Clin Exp Hypertens 1999;21:947-960.

165. Jeunemaitre X, Soubrier F, Kotelevtsev, et al: Molecular basis of human hypertension. Cell 1992;71:169.

166. Schunkert H, Hense HW, Gimenez-Roqueplo AP, et al: The angiotensinogen T235 variant and the use of antihypertensive drugs in a population-based cohort. Hypertension 1997;29:628-633.

167. Hingorani AD, Jia H, Stevens PA, et al: Renin-angiotensin system gene polymorphisms influence blood pressure and the response to angiotensin converting enzyme inhibition. J Hypertens 1995;13:1602-1609.

168. Dudley C, Keavney B, Casadei B, et al: Prediction of patient responses to antihypertensive drugs using genetic polymorphisms: Investigation of renin-angiotensin system genes. J Hypertens 1996;14:259-262.

169. O'Toole L, Stewart M, Padfield P, et al: Effect of the insertion/deletion polymorphism of the angiotensin-converting enzyme gene on response to angiotensin-converting enzyme inhibitors in patients with heart failure. J Cardiovasc Pharmacol 1998;32:988-994.

170. Hunt SC, Geleijnse JM, Wu LL, et al: Enhanced blood pressure response to mild sodium reduction in subjects with the 235T variant of the angiotensinogen gene. Am J Hypertens 1999;12:460-466.

171. Ferrari P, Bianchi G: Genomics of cardiovascular disorders. Drugs 2000;59:1025-1042.

172. Bianchi G, Tripodi G, Casari G, et al: Two point mutations within the adducin genes are involved in blood pressure variation. Proc Natl Acad Sci USA 1994;91:3999-4003.

173. Cusi D, Barlassina C, Azzani T, et al: Polymorphisms of alpha-adducin and salt sensitivity in patients with essential hypertension. Lancet 1997;349:1353-1357.

174. Kato, N, Sugiyama, T, Nabika, T et al: Lack of association between the alpha-adducin locus and essential hypertension in the Japanese population. Hypertension 1998;31:730-733.

175. Glorioso N, Manunta P, Filigheddu F: The role of alpha-adducin polymorphism in blood pressure and sodium handling regulation may not be excluded by a negative association study. Hypertension 1999;34:649-654.

176. Samani NJ: Pharmacogenomics of hypertension: A realizable goal? Clin Sci 2000;99:231-232.

177. Baker EH, Dong YB, Sagnella, GA, et al: Association of hypertension with T594M mutation in beta subunit of epithelial sodium channels in black people resident in London. Lancet 1998;351:1388-1392.

178. Evans WE, Relling M: Pharmacogenomics: Translating functional genomics into rational therapeutics. Science 1999;286:487-491.

179. Turner ST, Schwartz GL, Chapman AB: Antihypertensive pharmacogenetics: Getting the right drug into the right patient. J Hypertens 2001;19:1-11.

180. The International SNP Map Working Group: A map of human genome sequence variation containing 1.42 million single nucleotide polymorphisms. Nature 2001;409:928-933.

181. Roses AD: Pharmacogenetics and the practice of medicine. Nature 2000;405:857-865.

182. Roses AD: Pharmacogenetics and future drug development and delivery. Lancet 2000;355:1358-1361.

183. Wilkins MR, Roses AD, Piers CC: Pharmacogenomics and the treatment of cardiovascular disease. Heart 2000;84:353-354.

184. Lindpaintner K: Genetics in drug discovery and development: Challenge and promise of individualizing treatment in common complex diseases. Br Med Bull 1999;55:471-491.

185. Ozdemir V, Shear NH, Kalow W: What will be the role of pharmacogenetics in evaluating drug safety and minimizing adverse effects? Drug Safety 2001;24:75-85.

186. Nebert DW: Pharmacogenetics and pharmacogenomics: Why is this relevant to the clinical geneticist? Clin Genet 1999; 56:247-258.

Brown PO, Botstein D: Exploring the new world of the genome with DNA microarrays. Nat Genet 1999;21:33-37.

Cheok MH, Yang W, Pui CH, et al: Treatment-specific changes in gene expression discriminate in vivo drug response in human leukemia cells. Nat Genet 2003;34:85-90.

Chi JT, Chang HY, Wang NN, et al: Genomewide view of gene silencing by small interfering RNAs. Proc Natl Acad Sci USA 2003; 100:6343-6346.

Collins FS, Green ED, Guttmacher AE, et al: A vision for the future of genomics research. Nature 2003;422:835-847.

Evans WE, McLeod HL: Pharmacogenomics: drug disposition, drug targets, and side effects. N Engl J Med 2003;348:538-549.

Gabriel SB, Schaffner SF, Nguyen H, et al: The structure of haplotype blocks in the human genome. Science 2002;296:2225-2229.

Gilman AG, Simon MI, Bourne HR, et al: Overview of the Alliance for Cellular Signaling. Nature 2002;420:703-706.

Hoffman SL, Subramanian GM, Collins FH, et al: Plasmodium, human and Anopheles genomics and malaria. Nature 2002;415:702-709.

Li J, Ning Y, Hedley W, et al: The molecule pages database. Nature 2002;420:716-717.

Mitsui K, Tokuzawa Y, Itoh H, et al: The homeoprotein Nanog is required for maintenance of pluripotency in mouse epiblast and ES cells. Cell 2003;113:631-642.

Roses AD: Genome-based pharmacogenetics and the pharmaceutical industry. Nat Rev Drug Discov 2002;1:541-549.

Sachidanandam R, Weissman D, Schmidt SC, et al: A map of human genome sequence variation containing 1.42 million single nucleotide polymorphisms. Nature 2001;409:928-933.

Waterston RH, Lander ES, Sulston JE: On the sequencing of the human genome. Proc Natl Acad Sci USA 2002;99:3712-3716.

## EDITOR'S CHOICE

Brenner S: Worms and science: An interview with Sydney Brenner, distinguished research professor at The Salk Institute, La Jolla, USA, and one of the winners of 2002 Nobel Prize for Physiology and Medicine. EMBO Rep 2003;4:224-226.

# Model Organisms for Cardiac Disease Gene Discovery

*Calum A. MacRae*
*Mark C. Fishman*

## GENETIC APPROACHES TO COMPLEX BIOLOGIC PROBLEMS

The attribution of gene function can be accomplished by two approaches: (1) through the definition of a heritable phenotype and subsequent identification of the gene or (2) by the targeted modification of specific genes, with characterization of the resultant phenotype in the model organism. The first approach requires no prior assumptions regarding mechanism and can be done on a large scale as part of a genetic screen (although the cloning of the causative gene may be laborious). The second approach is a potent experimental strategy but generally is limited to genes previously suspected to be involved in the process being studied.

We focus here on three genetic model organisms—the nematode *Caenorhabditis elegans,* the fruitfly *Drosophila melanogaster,* and the zebrafish *Danio rerio*—and their contributions to our understanding of cardiovascular development, biology, and disease. These three organisms are the first metazoans subjected to large-scale genetic screens, tractable to many types of genetic manipulation, each with a robust and growing genetic and genomic infrastructure. The adult nematode *C. elegans,* with only 1024 cells, is relevant to the human cardiovascular system through its spontaneously contractile pharyngeal tube, which expresses genes from families similar to those of mammalian cardiac muscle. *Drosophila* has a contractile heart tube and the molecular pathways leading to its generation have important parallels with those of mammals. Although they are of tremendous experimental utility, these invertebrates do not have a closed circulatory system, vascular endothelium, or a multichambered heart capable of generating high pressures. *D. rerio,* the zebrafish, provides these along with concomitant physiologic innovations, such as defined pacemaker sites and valves.

## Genetic Screens

Phenotype-initiated gene identification is the only feasible approach to genetic studies in humans. In this strategy, known as positional cloning (reviewed elsewhere in this volume), phenotypes of interest, which segregate within individual families as monogenic traits, are identified.[1,2] By mapping the chromosomal location of the mutated gene and refining the genetic interval, it is possible to define the minimal physical chromosomal segment that is sufficient to cause the phenotype. Ideally, this minimal interval contains only the disease gene. But in practice, the list of potential candidates is often only restricted, by physical location, to a manageable number, thus allowing identification of the disease-causing mutations. These techniques have been used to identify the gene defects responsible for several hundred spontaneously occurring human diseases (http://www3.ncbi. nlm.nih.gov/omim). The power of positional cloning was a major stimulus for the generation of genetic and genomic resources, both in humans (The Human Genome Project) and now in a host of model organisms (Table 3-1).

Although the positional cloning of human disease genes has been an incisive initial step in the study of many monogenic diseases, for most cardiovascular diseases with multifactorial causation and/or complex genetics the contributions of single genes are not identifiable by positional cloning.[3,4] Part of the logic for turning to model organisms for gene discovery is that even highly heritable illnesses in humans may be refractory to dissection using conventional genetic approaches. As putative human disease genes are identified in common cardiovascular disorders, it will be important to have experimental strategies for confirming or refuting the role of these genes and for exploring the interactions between multiple genes or between genes and the environment.[4,5] Another major contribution from genetic model organisms has been the provision of additional candidate genes.[6] Ever more important may be the model organism's ability to reveal molecular pathways of disease and, in time, molecular mechanism. Embryologic, physiologic, and genetic interactions all can thereafter be evaluated in model systems, ultimately with extrapolation back to humans.

Genetic screens are a means to scan the entire genome, defining the genes of interest by relying on phenotype and subsequently cloning these genes. The technique involves the random mutagenesis of gametes and screening subsequent offspring for particular phenotypes. Typically chemical mutagenesis is used. Once heritable phenotypes have been identified, it is possible to map and clone the responsible mutated genes. In principle, such genetic screens offer the potential to identify multiple components of the pathways that drive any phenotype. This was shown most elegantly in the

**TABLE 3-1    BASIC GENETIC AND GENOMIC RESOURCES BY SPECIES***

| Organism | SSR Genetic Map | SNP Project | RH Map | EST Project | Large Insert Libraries | Chr. No. (2n) | Genome Size (Mb) | Genome Sequencing Project | Transgenics | ES Cells Isolated | Homologous Recombination | Insertional Mutagenesis |
|---|---|---|---|---|---|---|---|---|---|---|---|---|
| Human | Yes | Yes | Yes | Yes | Yes | 46 | 3300 | Completed | No | Yes | No | No |
| Chimpanzee | No | No | No | No | No | 48 | 3600 | No | No | No | No | No |
| Baboon | No | No | No | No | No | 42 | 3600 | No | No | No | No | No |
| Pig | Yes | No | Yes | Yes | Yes | 38 | 3200 | Yes | No | No | No | No |
| Sheep | Yes | No | No | Yes | Yes | 54 | 3200 | No | Yes | No | No | No |
| Goat | No | No | No | No | No | 60 | 3200 | No | Yes | No | No | No |
| Dog | Yes | No | No | No | Yes | 78 | 3100 | Yes | No | No | No | No |
| Rabbit | No | No | No | No | No | 44 | 3500 | No | Yes | No | No | No |
| Rat | Yes | No | Yes | Yes | Yes | 42 | 3100 | Yes | Yes | Yes | No | No |
| Hamster | Yes | No | No | No | Yes | 22 | 3600 | No | No | No | No | No |
| Mouse | Yes | Yes | Yes | Yes | Yes | 40 | 3000 | Yes | Yes | Yes | Yes | Yes |
| Chicken | No | No | No | No | Yes | 78 | 1200 | Yes | No | No | No | No |
| *Xenopus* | No | Yes | No | Yes | Yes | 36 | 3100 | Yes | Yes | No | No | No |
| Zebrafish | Yes | Yes | Yes | Yes | Yes | 50 | 1700 | Yes | Yes | No | No | Yes |
| *Drosophila* | N/A | Yes | No | Yes | Yes | 8 | 136 | Completed | Yes | N/A | Yes | Yes |
| *Caenorhabditis elegans* | N/A | Yes | No | Yes | Yes | 12 | 97 | Completed | Yes | N/A | Yes | Yes |

The broad applicability of genetic techniques is illustrated by the proliferation of genome projects.
Chr. No., chromosome number (diploid); ES cells, embryonic stem cells; EST, expressed sequence tag; Mb, megabase; N/A, not applicable; RH, radiation hybrid; SNP, single nucleotide polymorphism; SSR, simple sequence repeat.

screens from *Drosophila* by Nuesslein-Volhard and Wieschaus, which revealed the molecular pathways regulating the assembly of body form. In much the same way, the pathways that drive the cell cycle were discovered in *Saccharomyces cerevisiae*, and the pathways of cell fate decisions, including programmed cell death, were discovered in *C. elegans*.[7] Once a pathway has been entered in this way, the causal interactions between genes can be defined by genetics or biochemistry.

Importantly, the pathways discovered in these genetic screens are conserved in higher organisms. Annotation of the human genome was in large part feasible by the conserved relationships between human and model organism genes.[8] Novel algorithms, comparing regulatory and intergenic sequences from multiple organisms, are being designed to expand this annotation beyond the limited scope of protein coding sequences.[9] Of course, despite similarities, each model organism species has evolved separately and gene function will be integrated in distinctive circuits, so extrapolations between species must be made cautiously. For example, *Drosophila* lacking *tinman* have no heart,[10] whereas mice homozygous for targeted mutations in the *tinman* homolog *nkx2.5* have a defective heart.[11,12] Unlike mice, humans who are haploinsufficient for *nkx2.5* have atrioseptal defects, conduction disturbances, and occasionally more complex congenital heart abnormalities.[13] These differences reflect in part the acquisition of additional homologs of *tinman* in the vertebrate.[14,15] Obviously the cardiovascular physiology and genetic makeup of the mouse is not identical to that of humans; thus, it should come as no surprise that changes in single genes play out very differently in each species.

## Caenorhabditis elegans

Sydney Brenner chose the nematode, *C. elegans*, as a genetic model organism in the early 1960s, seeking a multicellular organism sufficiently tractable to allow the study of complex behaviors.[16] *C. elegans* is transparent throughout its life cycle, so that each cell in the embryo can be traced to its final fate in the adult worm, and disruption of normal development can be observed using simple light microscopy. It is small and has a short (3-day) life cycle, which combined with self-fertilizing hermaphrodite forms facilitates genetics and large-scale screens. More recently other tools have been introduced for genetic studies of the nematode. For example, it is now possible to eliminate gene function using double-stranded RNA, or RNAi.[17] The phenomenon is dependent on a conserved processing pathway that results in the breakdown of the double-stranded RNA into 22 to 24 bp fragments; amplification of these fragments; and then, through interactions between these RNA fragments and the native mRNA, targeting for degradation of the transcripts containing the complementary sequences.[17,18] Simply feeding nematodes with bacteria expressing a particular double-stranded RNAi is sufficient to inactivate the cognate gene. Already, systematic inactivation of each of the genes on a single worm chromosome has been undertaken.[19]

## The Nematode Pharynx and Vertebrate Muscle Biology

Although the nematode has no heart or even a circulation *per se*, there is evidence that the pharynx of *C. elegans* shares many structural, molecular, and genetic parallels with the hearts of higher organisms (Figure 3-1). The pharynx, which is involved in nematode feeding behavior, spontaneously and continuously contracts[20] independent of any innervation.[21,22] Furthermore, the pharyngeal muscle, unlike the body wall muscles of the worm (but like vertebrate cardiac muscle), is not dependent on the MyoD family of muscle transcriptional regulators. The development of the nematode pharyngeal muscle requires a homeobox gene, *ceh-22*, which is homologous to the Drosophila *tinman* and vertebrate *nkx2.5* genes.[23] The gene *ceh-22* also is sufficient to activate pharyngeal muscle-specific transcription when expressed ectopically in the nematode body wall. The functional conservation is such that the zebrafish *nkx2.5* gene can rescue the *ceh-22* mutant phenotype when expressed in pharyngeal muscle.[24] This suggests that spontaneously contracting muscular organs, at least those recruited from anterior mesoderm, such as the

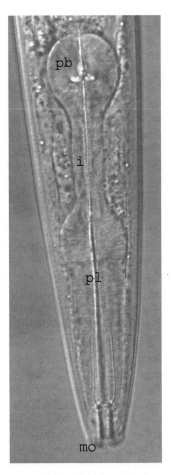

**FIGURE 3-1.** A Nomarski image of the adult *Caenorhabditis elegans* pharynx. This simple organ is composed of only 20 muscle cells, 20 neurons, 9 epidermal cells, and a few other glandular and structural cells. i, isthmus; mo, mouth opening; pb, posterior bulb; pl, pharyngeal lumen. *(Image courtesy Dr. William M. Winston, Department of Molecular and Cellular Biology, Harvard University, Cambridge, Massachusetts.)*

nematode pharynx, the *Drosophila* dorsal vessel, and the vertebrate heart, have a distinctive program of specification. It is not known whether this molecular similarity indicates true orthology between these structures, or rather convergent evolution. Also, it is clear from work in higher organisms that the NKX2 family serves several functions, only some of which overlap with *ceh-22* and *tinman*. It is of interest that recent work from mouse and chick suggests that the arterial pole of the heart forms from a subset of cells originating in pharyngeal mesoderm, anterior to the foregut.[25,26] These cells, within a secondary heart field, are distinguished by *fgf10* expression in the mouse, but, like primary myocardial cells, express *nkx2.5* and *gata4*.

### Body Wall Muscle

The tractability of the nematode also has been useful in the genetic dissection of sarcomere structure and function.[27,28] The basic components of the sarcomeres in the body wall muscle of *C. elegans* are very similar to those of skeletal and cardiac muscle in higher organisms. The uncoordinated movements and abnormal morphology of worms with mutations affecting their body wall muscles have led to the identification of many of the genes encoding these sarcomeric constituents. It has been possible, in this model, to dissect the roles of sarcomeric protein stoichiometry,[29] isoform splicing,[30] and extracellular matrix attachment[31] in the differentiation and maintenance of myocytes and to assess how these molecular changes impact the contractile function of the muscles.

## Drosophila

Since with the studies of T. H. Morgan in 1908, the fruitfly *D. melanogaster* has been used as a genetic model organism.[32,33] The chromosomal theory of inheritance and the physical mapping of genes both have their roots in early *Drosophila* work. The use of balancer chromosomes to suppress recombination and allow the maintenance of lethal mutations was also an innovation of fly geneticists. The cytogenetics of the large *Drosophila* chromosomes facilitated the first positional cloning of a gene.[34] The addition of insertional mutagenesis using transposable P-elements greatly increased the speed of mapping and cloning of the mutant genes, because it is only necessary to identify the sequences flanking the insertion.[35]

Many of these tools were combined in the first genome-wide mutational screen in a metazoan when Nusslein-Volhard and Wieschaus set out to identify all the genes involved in establishing the early embryonic body plan in *Drosophila*.[36] The success of this strategy defined not only the essential logical framework of development but also many of the critical signaling pathways required. It turns out, from subsequent work, that these pathways are conserved through evolution and are used in many different situations.[37,38] At a reductionist level the same pathways make fly wing and human bone. The single hedgehog gene of *Drosophila* may have duplicated to become three genes in vertebrates, but the key elements of molecular interactions using the *hedgehog* pathway are conserved.[39]

### Dorsal Vessel

A single vessel runs along the dorsal aspect of the *Drosophila* embryo throughout much of its length[40] (Figure 3-2). It pumps, by peristalsis, extracellular fluid (hemolymph) alternately backward and forward through the interstices of tissues rather than through an enclosed vascular tree. This is termed an "open" circulation. The dorsal vessel consists of groups of spontaneously contracting myocytes organized into a single tube. The dorsal vessel is known as the heart and is assembled from two groups of cells: muscular cells that pump hemolymph and cells that form openings called ostia through which hemolymph passively "leaks" into the organ. The anterior portion of the dorsal vessel has no openings and is referred to as the aorta. Also associated with the heart are alar muscle cells, which mechanically support the dorsal vessel, and pericardial cells that are believed to be stationary macrophages. There is also evidence of limited innervation of the dorsal vessel.[41]

This primitive structure undergoes substantial morphologic change during the transition from larval to adult form.[42] Evidence is accumulating that the adult organ is more complex than had previously been thought. Recent *in vitro* work has outlined a novel system of neuroamide and peptidergic regulation of *Drosophila* heart rate.[43,44] Exactly how these structures can be related, at a morphologic and molecular level, to the hearts of vertebrates is not known, but a remarkable conservation of some of the genetic programs involved in the process of cardial cell specification and dorsal vessel assembly is emerging.

### Cell Fate Specification

Mutations in the gene for the transcription factor *tinman* prevent formation of the dorsal vessel.[10] Before gastrulation, all cells of the presumptive mesoderm express *tinman,* but as the mesoderm spreads, expression becomes limited to the dorsal mesoderm. Dorsal vessel progenitors arise from a group of mesodermal cells defined by their persistent expression of *tinman*. The persistent expression of *tinman* in cardiomyocytes

DMef2

**FIGURE 3-2.** Immunohistochemical staining with anti-Dmef2 of a *Drosophila* embryo, demonstrating the cardiac and noncardiac muscle cells of the organism. The midline dorsal vessel is labeled (dv) and is known as the aorta anteriorly *(left)* and the heart posteriorly *(right)*. *(Image courtesy Dr Joseph Weiss, Oregon Health Sciences University, Portland.)*

reflects a subdivision of the mesoderm brought about in response to signals, some of which originate in another germ layer, the ectoderm. Maintenance of mesodermal *tinman* expression depends on expression of the BMP2/4-like gene *decapentaplegic (dpp)* in the adjacent ectoderm and on expression of the *dpp* receptor *thickvein* and the Smad4 homolog *medea* in the mesoderm.[45-47]

Although it is necessary, *tinman* alone is not sufficient to drive cardiogenesis.[48] One of the three known *Drosophila* GATA genes, *pannier,* also regulates heart formation. When either *tinman* or *pannier* is ectopically expressed in the mesoderm, each induces modest ectopic expression of downstream cardiac genes. However, when *tinman* and *pannier* are expressed together, the ectopic expression of cardiac genes is much stronger, and the expression domains extend to include the entire cephalic region and dorsal and ventral trunk mesoderm.[49] The *Drosophila* embryo externally appears as a series of simple highly similar repeated units. This periodic subdivision of the ectoderm is determined by segmentation genes, many of which, including *wingless* and *hedgehog,* are also involved in the subdivision of mesoderm. After gastrulation, *Drosophila* cardiac precursors form a series of sequentially repeated clusters of cells before coalescing to form the heart tube. These clusters are placed in the A parasegments of the trunk dorsal mesoderm, adjacent to the *wingless* expression domain in the ectoderm. Heart progenitors are missing in embryos mutant in *wingless* or in genes encoding components of the *wingless* signaling pathway (*dishevelled, zeste-white3, armadillo,* and *pangolin*).[50]

The clusters of six cardial cells that will generate the muscle of the heart form at the points of intersection of the *wingless* domain and the longitudinal *dpp* and *tinman* domains.[51] Combinatorial activation of downstream pathways subdivides the cells at the zones of intersection into small clusters of equivalent cells from which the individual progenitors arise.[52] It is these progenitor cells that then produce, through the asymmetric segregation of the product of the *numb* gene and the effects of identity genes such as *even skipped* and *ladybird,* the founder cells for dorsal muscle or cardiac lineages.

There are important parallels in cardiomyogenic cell fate regulation between *Drosophila* and vertebrates. Transcription factors of the *tinman* and *gata* families are essential for heart formation in the vertebrate, and they are regulated by similar mesodermal and ectodermal signals. However, unlike *tinman,* there is no single genetic defect that selectively and completely deletes the cardiomyogenic fate in vertebrates. This is probably a result of multiple redundancies in the vertebrate pathways generating heart cells. As noted earlier, not one but five *tinman* family genes (*Nkx2.3, Nkx2.5, Nkx2.6, Nkx2.7,* and *Nkx2.8*) are expressed in vertebrate cardiomyocyte precursors.[53] Thus, the fact that targeted mutation of *nkx2.5,* the *tinman* ortholog, perturbs only late heart maturation in vertebrates is predictable.[11] Further supporting a degree of redundancy, concomitant dominant inhibition of several members of this gene family prevents appearance of cardiomyogenic cells, at least in *Xenopus.*[54,55] Interestingly, heterozygous mutations in the human *Nkx2.5* gene appear to result in atrial septal defects and conduction system disease.[13] Similarly, only partly parallel GATA pathways exist in higher phyla, confirming that the extension of principles derived from one model system to others requires caution.

### Flight Muscle and Sarcomere Assembly

Although the range of functional muscle phenotypes in the nematode is somewhat restricted, in the fruitfly the demands of flight delineate a range of subtle phenotypic variants in various muscle groups. For obvious reasons flightless mutants were among the first to be identified and can readily be identified using a column "flight tester."[56] The cloning of several of these mutants has uncovered several remarkable features of myocyte biology. The critical role of component protein stoichiometry in the generation of the paracrystalline sarcomere proved amenable to dissection using a combination of recessive flightless mutants and compound heterozygotes.[57,58] Mutants with deficient myosin ATPase activity revealed the relationship between the function of the contractile apparatus and both sarcomere assembly and myocyte differentiation. New roles for the spatial organization of glycolytic enzymes within the sarcomere[59] and nonmuscle myosins in myogenesis have also been described.[60] Several myofilament proteins were first identified in the fruitfly, and insights gained from the specialized function of flight muscle sarcomeres have recently been incorporated into mouse models of cardiac function, shedding light on papillary muscle physiology and hypertrophic cardiomyopathy.[61]

### Disease Models and Drug Discovery

The generation of disease models in *Drosophila* has not yet been seen in cardiovascular biology, but the successful use of this tractable organism in the study of neurodegenerative diseases such as Parkinson's and Alzheimer's bodes well for the future.[62] It has proven possible to recapitulate the toxic effects of mutant alpha synuclein, first identified in monogenic variants of Parkinson's disease, in transgenic flies.[63] In these flies the mutant protein exhibits toxicity that is restricted to dopaminergic neurons, results in intranuclear filamentous inclusions containing the mutant protein (mimicking Lewy bodies), and produces locomotor dysfunction. This model is already being used, as are similar models of Alzheimer's disease, Huntington's chorea, and ataxia, to identify other genes in the disease pathway, including genes that ameliorate the phenotype.[64] Disease models in fruitflies are also being used to screen large chemical libraries for novel compounds that modify the phenotype, a direct form of drug discovery.

## Zebrafish

Many of the structures and physiologic functions disrupted in human disease are evolutionary innovations that first appear in the vertebrate. In the early 1980s,

Streisinger suggested that the zebrafish was a vertebrate potentially tractable to genetic screens, because the embryo is transparent, fertilization is external, offspring are numerous, and development is rapid.[65,66] The short generation time and relatively low maintenance and breeding costs of the zebrafish allow the generation of several thousand meioses, substantially increasing the resolution of genetic mapping. For genetic studies it is also important that the zebrafish is diploid (in contrast, e.g., *Xenopus* is tetraploid). By various manipulations, haploid or maternally homozygous diploid embryos can be generated, the former surviving only for brief periods, but their survival is sufficient to allow examination of very early developmental processes.

One of the most recent additions to the genetic armamentarium available for the zebrafish are morpholino antisense oligonucleotides.[67,68] These antisense oligonucleotides, using six-membered morpholine ring backbone moieties joined by nonionic linkages, afford substantially better antisense activity than do RNA, DNA, or their analogs, with five-membered ribose or deoxyribose backbone moieties joined by ionic linkages. These so-called morpholinos are highly stable and specific and can be delivered into cells in culture or injected into developing embryos such as those of zebrafish or xenopus. They may be targeted to the translational start site or to splice donor sites and, by disrupting translation or normal splicing, are capable of reproducibly knocking down in a specific manner the gene product for the first 36 to 72 hours of embryonic life.

Groups in Tubingen and Boston performed two large-scale screens for mutations affecting embryogenesis in the zebrafish.[69-71] One of the first discoveries from these screens was that the mutational approach is highly informative for organ development.[72,73] This came as a surprise to some, who had anticipated that late development would be intractable. The screens proved that single elements or functions of organs could be removed with relative specificity. These "modules," therefore, are tractable genetic units, just as segments in *Drosophila* are.[74] With regard to the cardiovascular system, mutations in individual genes selectively disrupt individual heart chambers, particular vessels, or specific functions such as pacemaking.[72,73]

### The Zebrafish Heart

The heart of the zebrafish at 24-hours postfertilization (hpf) is indistinguishable from that of the human embryo at 3 weeks' gestation.[75] It consists of a single atrium and single ventricle with an inner endocardial layer and outer myocardial layer. It is generated by fusion of bilateral primordia. By 24 hpf irregular peristaltic motions begin, flowing in a wave from the venous to arterial end and driving blood flow through the circulation. By 32 hpf contractions of the atrium are followed sequentially by the ventricle. The zebrafish can survive without a functioning heart, by diffusion from the water for several days. This fact combined with the informativeness of the mutations, the speed of cardiovascular development, and the ease of observation of heart or blood vessel structure and function have

made the fish particularly useful as a cardiovascular model system.

### Cell Fate Specification

In the zebrafish, as in other vertebrates, the heart field forms in the lateral mesoderm, from whence cells migrate medially to form a single heart tube.[76] Several mutations affect the heart field. Some might be predicted from signaling pathways known to be important in the generation of myocardial cells. Thus, *nkx 2.5, nkx 2.7, gata4,* and *fgf8* are all expressed in the region of the cardiac progenitors. Mutations in *bmp2 (swirl)* abolish both *nkx2.5* and *nkx2.7* expression.[77] Mutation of *fgf8 (acerebellar)* downregulates expression of both *nkx2.5* and *gata4.*[78]

Signals from the anterior end of the notochord appear to regulate the posterior border of the heart field. Hence notochord mutations, such as *no tail,* cause posterior expansion of *nkx2.5* expression.[79] Additional signals from the endoderm are essential for heart development. *Gata5, casanova,* and *one-eye-pinhead* (an epidermal growth factor [EGF] repeat containing protein that functions as a cofactor to *nodal*) are critical for normal endoderm development, and when mutated result in cardia bifida, with nonfused, beating, bilateral primordia.[77,80] Thus, both notochord and endoderm genes are among those essential for normal cardiac development.

### Modularity of Organogenesis-Form and Function

One of the most instructive results from the genetic screens performed in the zebrafish is the modular nature of organotypic components in vertebrates.[74] The heart of the fly is a relatively simple tube, whereas the vertebrate heart is a multichambered, physiologically complex organ. The structural innovations of the vertebrate heart serve to deliver blood through a specialized oxygenating interface (gills or lungs) and then to perfuse the tissues (at high pressure) through a distinctive vascular system. At least four elements are essential to ensure this unidirectional flow: the ventricle, a thick-walled high-pressure-generating chamber; valves, which prevent backflow of blood; endothelium, the single-cell lining of all vessels and of the heart; and a specialized conduction system, which coordinates the contraction of all the myocytes within each chamber. All have proved approachable in the genetic screens. When compared, similar modular units are evident in the mouse.

Embryos mutant in *dhand (hands off)* have cardiac precursors that express *nkx2.5,* but they fail to differentiate properly patterned myocardial tissue.[81] Indeed, ventricular tissue is nearly absent. Two other mutants, *pandora* and *lonely atrium,* display virtually complete, and selective removal of the ventricle.[72,73] In contrast, mutation in the *heart and soul (has)* gene (protein kinase C λ) affects the patterning of cardiac chambers but not the assumption of chamber-specific fates.[82,83] It is not known what controls the normal maturation pattern of ventricular wall growth, from growth along the longitudinal axis of the heart to concentric growth, with consequent wall thickening. Certainly, there are genes in noncardiac tissues that can change the orientation of cell division to accomplish similar purposes, such as *inscuteable* and *prospero* in the *Drosophila* sensory organ.[84,85] In zebrafish, mutations in three genes (*santa, valentine,* and *heart of glass*) prevent concentric thickening, such that the ventricle remains single layered.[73] Because there are normal numbers of cardiomyocytes, the ventricle becomes enormously dilated (Figure 3-3).

The contractile disturbances that result from mutations in the zebrafish resemble human diseases.[86] In fact, mutations in zebrafish may predict candidate genes for human disease. Mutation in the gene for titin causes a dilated cardiomyopathy both in zebrafish and in humans, although with differing inheritance patterns.[87,88] Zebrafish mutations are isolated as recessive, and the human disorder is dominant. The cloning of the many mutations affecting cardiac output likely will provide additional candidate genes for human diseases, both Mendelian and complex.

Valves form at the borders between the chambers of the heart, in a process dependent on site-specific interactions between endocardium and myocardium. From work in other systems, it is known that endocardial cells in both the atrioventricular canal and the outflow tract migrate away from the endocardial surface, forming mesenchymal components of the so-called cushions. This occurs, at least *in vitro,* under influence of signals from the myocardial layer, including transforming growth factor β1 (TGF-β1) and β3 (TGF-β3).[89] TGF-β1 and TGF-β2 both are expressed in the mouse heart, but only TGF-β2 null embryos have valvular and outflow tract defects.[90] Mice null for the *NF-ATc* gene have disrupted formation of aortic and pulmonic valves.[91,92] In the zebrafish, the *jekyll* mutation disturbs the formation of cardiac cushions and the initiation of atrioventricular

valve formation. The mutant gene is a uridine 5´-diphosphate-glucose dehydrogenase required for heparan sulfate, chondroitin sulfate, and hyaluronic acid production.[93] A particular population of endocardial cells located at the atrioventricular junction fails to differentiate in *jekyll* mutants, suggesting that the gene is required for a signaling event in this process.

Primitive hearts contract in a peristaltic fashion with oscillation in the origin of the primary pacemaker between ends of the heart. Clearly, more sophisticated controls are necessary for a system with a specialized vascular tree and a significant step-up in pressure across the heart. Components of such a system include a single atrial pacemaker site, a slowly conducting node at the atrioventricular junction that results in delayed onset of the ventricular beat, and a rapidly conducting system of specialized myocytes to guarantee organized synchronous contraction of the entire ventricle.[94] Primary disturbances of most aspects of normal rhythm and conduction have been described zebrafish cardiac conduction and rhythm.[72,73] Single-gene recessive mutations may result in isolated bradycardia *(slow mo),* exit block from the sinus venosus to the atrium *(reggae),* or atrioventricular block *(breakdance* and *hip hop)* or perturb intercellular conduction in different chambers *(island beat, polka,* and *tremblor). Slow mo* ablates the fast component of the hyperpolarization activated current Ih and provided the first *in vivo* proof that Ih actually regulates pacemaking.[95] The cloning of *slow mo* and the other mutations will help to identify the genes responsible for pacing and conduction and will provide candidate genes for human arrhythmias.

### Chemical Biology

The accessibility of the zebrafish embryo in its aqueous environment has already allowed scientists to explore the effects of libraries of small molecules on development.[96] Early insights have come from the discovery of phenocopies of genetic mutants.[82] These have allowed investigators to begin to access pathways from multiple points and at different times, enabling the temporal dissection of embryologic phenomena. The integration of large libraries of potential drugs or small molecules with a vertebrate that develops rapidly *in vitro* offers tremendous potential, particularly because it is adaptable to high-throughput screening. For example, in drug discovery, the zebrafish larvae have a full complement of functioning organs, enabling the net effects of multiple factors, such as drug absorption, metabolism, or excretion, to be addressed in the same assays used to detect the primary biologic effect.

## CONCLUSION

The model organisms described in this chapter offer the opportunity for phenotype-first, large-scale evaluation of the entire genome. Genetic screens reveal the logic of assembly. Each elemental unit is decipherable thereafter by cloning of the mutation. Once provided this entrance point, the remainder of the pathway is then accessible

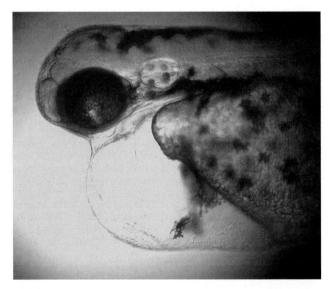

**FIGURE 3-3.** A *heart of glass* zebrafish larva, demonstrating the grossly dilated heart characteristic of this mutant. The heart is a single cell layer thick. Contractile function is significantly impaired. *(Image courtesy Dr John Mably, Cardiovascular Research Center, Massachusetts General Hospital, Boston.)*

by combinations of genetic and biochemical techniques. Conservation of genes, pathways, and modules through evolution means that extrapolation to human development and disease is quite direct.

## REFERENCES

1. Seidman JG, Seidman C: The genetic basis for cardiomyopathy: From mutation identification to mechanistic paradigms. Cell 2001;104:557-567.
2. Keating MT, Sanguinetti MC: Molecular and cellular mechanisms of cardiac arrhythmias. Cell 2001;104:569-580.
3. Risch NJ: Searching for genetic determinants in the new millennium. Nature 2000;405:847-856.
4. Risch N, Merikangas K: The future of genetic studies of complex human diseases. Science 1996;273:1516-1517.
5. Accili D, Kido Y, Nakae J, et al: Genetics of type 2 diabetes: Insight from targeted mouse mutants. Curr Mol Med 2001;1:9-23.
6. Bassett DE Jr, Boguski MS, Spencer F, et al: Genome cross-referencing and XREFdb: Implications for the identification and analysis of genes mutated in human disease. Nat Genet 1997;15:339-344.
7. Ledwich D, Wu YC, Driscoll M, et al: Analysis of programmed cell death in the nematode Caenorhabditis elegans. Methods Enzymol 2000;322:76-88.
8. Lander ES, Linton LM, Birren B, et al: Initial sequencing and analysis of the human genome. Nature 2001;409:860-921.
9. Mayor C, Brudno M, Schwartz JR, et al: VISTA: Visualizing global DNA sequence alignments of arbitrary length. Bioinformatics 2000;16:1046-1047.
10. Bodmer R: The gene tinman is required for specification of the heart and visceral muscles in Drosophila. Development 1993;118:719-729.
11. Lints TJ, Parsons LM, Hartley L, et al: Nkx-2.5: A novel murine homeobox gene expressed in early heart progenitor cells and their myogenic descendants. Development 1993;119:419-431.
12. Tanaka M, Chen Z, Bartunkova S, et al: The cardiac homeobox gene Csx/Nkx2.5 lies genetically upstream of multiple genes essential for heart development. Development 1999;126:1269-1280.
13. Schott JJ, Benson DW, Basson CT, et al: Congenital heart disease caused by mutations in the transcription factor NKX2-5. Science 1998;281:108-111.
14. Ranganayakulu G, Elliott DA, Harvey RP, et al: Divergent roles for NK-2 class homeobox genes in cardiogenesis in flies and mice. Development 1998;125:3037-3048.
15. Sparrow DB, Cai C, Kotecha S, et al: Regulation of the tinman homologues in Xenopus embryos. Dev Biol 2000;227:65-79.
16. Brenner S: The genetics of Caenorhabditis elegans. Genetics 1974;77:71-94.
17. Sharp PA: RNAi and double-strand RNA. Genes Dev 1999;13:139-141.
18. Maine EM: A conserved mechanism for post-transcriptional gene silencing? Genome Biol 2000;1(3):REVIEWS1018.
19. Barstead R: Genome-wide RNAi. Curr Opin Chem Biol 2001;5:63-66.
20. Raizen DM, Avery L: Electrical activity and behavior in the pharynx of Caenorhabditis elegans. Neuron 1994;12:483-495.
21. Albertson DG, Thomson JN: The pharynx of Caenorhabditis elegans. Philos Trans R Soc Lond B Biol Sci 1976;275:299-325.
22. Avery L, Horvitz HR. Pharyngeal pumping continues after laser killing of the pharyngeal nervous system of C. elegans. Neuron 1989;3:473-485.
23. Okkema PG, Fire A: The Caenorhabditis elegans NK-2 class homeoprotein CEH-22 is involved in combinatorial activation of gene expression in pharyngeal muscle. Development 1994;120:2175-2186.
24. Haun C, Alexander J, Stainier DY, et al: Rescue of Caenorhabditis elegans pharyngeal development by a vertebrate heart specification gene. Proc Natl Acad Sci USA 1998;95:5072-5075.
25. Waldo KL, Kumiski DL, Wallis KT, et al: Conotruncal myocardium arises from a secondary heart field. Development 2001;128:3179-3188.
26. Kelly RG, Brown NA, Buckingham ME: The arterial pole of the mouse heart forms from Fgf10-expressing cells in pharyngeal mesoderm. Dev Cell 2001;1:435-440.
27. Mackenzie JM Jr, Garcea RL, Zengel JM, et al. Muscle development in Caenorhabditis elegans: Mutants exhibiting retarded sarcomere construction. Cell 1978;15:751-762.
28. Francis GR, Waterston RH: Muscle organization in Caenorhabditis elegans: Localization of proteins implicated in thin filament attachment and I-band organization. J Cell Biol 1985;101:1532-1549.
29. Zengel JM, Epstein HF: Mutants altering coordinate synthesis of specific myosins during nematode muscle development. Proc Natl Acad Sci USA 1980;77:852-856.
30. Mullen GP, Rogalski TM, Bush JA, et al: Complex patterns of alternative splicing mediate the spatial and temporal distribution of perlecan/UNC-52 in Caenorhabditis elegans. Mol Biol Cell 1999;10:3205-3221.
31. Hammarlund M, Davis WS, Jorgensen EM: Mutations in beta-spectrin disrupt axon outgrowth and sarcomere structure. J Cell Biol 2000;149:931-942.
32. Sturtevant AH: Reminiscences of T. H. Morgan. Genetics 2001;159:1-5.
33. Rubin GM, Lewis EB: A brief history of Drosophila's contributions to genome research. Science 2000;287:2216-2218.
34. Sentry LW, Kaiser K: Progress in Drosophila genome manipulation. Transgenic Res 1995;4:155-162.
35. Cooley L, Berg C, Kelley R, et al: Identifying and cloning Drosophila genes by single P element insertional mutagenesis. Prog Nucleic Acid Res Mol Biol 1989;36:99-109.
36. Nusslein-Volhard C, Wieschaus E: Mutations affecting segment number and polarity in Drosophila. Nature 1980;287:795-801.
37. Leevers SJ: Growth control: Invertebrate insulin surprises! Curr Biol 2001;11:R209-212.
38. Scott M: Signalling and endocytosis: Wnt breaks down on back roads. Nat Cell Biol 2001;3:E185-186.
39. Ingham PW: Hedgehog signaling: A tale of two lipids. Science 2001;294:1879-1881.
40. Zaffran S, Astier M, Gratecos D, et al: Cellular interactions during heart morphogenesis in the Drosophila embryo. Biol Cell 1995;84:13-24.
41. Cantera R, Nassel DR: Segmental peptidergic innervation of abdominal targets in larval and adult dipteran insects revealed with an antiserum against leucokinin I. Cell Tissue Res 1992;269:459-471.
42. Curtis NJ, Ringo JM, Dowse HB: Morphology of the pupal heart, adult heart, and associated tissues in the fruit fly, Drosophila melanogaster. J Morphol 1999;240:225-235.
43. Johnson E, Ringo J, Dowse H: Modulation of Drosophila heartbeat by neurotransmitters. J Comp Physiol B 1997;167(2):89-97.
44. Johnson E, Sherry T, Ringo J, et al: Modulation of the cardiac pacemaker of Drosophila: Cellular mechanisms. J Comp Physiol B 2002;172(3):227-236.
45. Yin Z, Frasch M: Regulation and function of tinman during dorsal mesoderm induction and heart specification in Drosophila. Dev Genet 1998;22:187-200.
46. Riechmann V, Rehorn KP, Reuter R, et al: The genetic control of the distinction between fat body and gonadal mesoderm in Drosophila. Development 1998;125:713-723.
47. Xu X, Yin Z, Hudson JB, et al: Smad proteins act in combination with synergistic and antagonistic regulators to target Dpp responses to the Drosophila mesoderm. Genes Dev 1998;12:2354-2370.
48. Frasch M: Induction of visceral and cardiac mesoderm by ectodermal Dpp in the early Drosophila embryo. Nature 1995;374:464-467.
49. Gajewski K, Fossett N, Molkentin JD, et al: The zinc finger proteins Pannier and GATA4 function as cardiogenic factors in Drosophila. Development 1999;126:5679-5688.
50. Park M, Venkatesh TV, Bodmer R: Dual role for the zeste-white3/shaggy-encoded kinase in mesoderm and heart development of Drosophila. Dev Genet 1998;22:201-211.
51. Jagla T, Bidet Y, Da Ponte JP, et al: Cross-repressive interactions of identity genes are essential for proper specification of cardiac and muscular fates in Drosophila. Development 2002;129:1037-1047.
52. Carmena A, Gisselbrecht S, Harrison J, et al: Combinatorial signaling codes for the progressive determination of cell fates in

the Drosophila embryonic mesoderm. Genes Dev 1998;12: 3910-3922.

53. Tanaka M, Kasahara H, Bartunkova S, et al: Vertebrate homologs of tinman and bagpipe: Roles of the homeobox genes in cardiovascular development. Dev Genet 1998;22:239-249.

54. Fu Y, Yan W, Mohun TJ, et al: Vertebrate tinman homologues XNkx2-3 and XNkx2-5 are required for heart formation in a functionally redundant manner. Development 1998;125:4439-4449.

55. Grow MW, Krieg PA: Tinman function is essential for vertebrate heart development: Elimination of cardiac differentiation by dominant inhibitory mutants of the tinman-related genes, XNkx2-3 and XNkx2-5. Dev Biol 1998;204:187-196.

56. Koana T, Hotta Y: Isolation and characterization of flightless mutants in Drosophila melanogaster. J Embryol Exp Morphol 1978;45:123-143.

57. Beall CJ, Sepanski MA, Fyrberg EA: Genetic dissection of Drosophila myofibril formation: Effects of actin and myosin heavy chain null alleles. Genes Dev 1989;3:131-140.

58. Tansey T, Schultz JR, Miller RC, et al: Small differences in Drosophila tropomyosin expression have significant effects on muscle function. Mol Cell Biol 1991;11:6337-6342.

59. Wojtas K, Slepecky N, von Kalm L, et al: Flight muscle function in Drosophila requires colocalization of glycolytic enzymes. Mol Biol Cell 1997;8:1665-1675.

60. Bloor JW, Kiehart DP: Zipper nonmuscle myosin-II functions downstream of PS2 integrin in Drosophila myogenesis and is necessary for myofibril formation. Dev Biol 2001;239:215-228.

61. Davis JS, Hassanzadeh S, Winitsky S, et al: The overall pattern of cardiac contraction depends on a spatial gradient of myosin regulatory light chain phosphorylation. Cell 2001;107:631-641.

62. Link CD: Transgenic invertebrate models of age-associated neurodegenerative diseases. Mech Ageing Dev 2001;122:1639-1649.

63. Feany MB, Bender WW: A Drosophila model of Parkinson's disease. Nature 2000;404:394-398.

64. Auluck PK, Chan HY, Trojanowski JQ, et al: Chaperone suppression of alpha-synuclein toxicity in a Drosophila model for Parkinson's disease. Science 2002;295:865-868.

65. Streisinger G, Singer F, Walker C, et al: Segregation analyses and gene-centromere distances in zebrafish. Genetics 1986; 112:311-319.

66. Grunwald DJ, Streisinger G: Induction of recessive lethal and specific locus mutations in the zebrafish with ethyl nitrosourea. Genet Res 1992;59:103-116.

67. Ekker SC: Morphants: A new systematic vertebrate functional genomics approach. Yeast 2000;17:302-306.

68. Nasevicius A, Ekker SC: Effective targeted gene 'knockdown' in zebrafish. Nat Genet 2000;26:216-220.

69. Mullins MC, Hammerschmidt M, Haffter P, et al: Large-scale mutagenesis in the zebrafish: In search of genes controlling development in a vertebrate. Curr Biol 1994;4:189-202.

70. Solnica-Krezel L, Schier AF, Driever W: Efficient recovery of ENU-induced mutations from the zebrafish germline. Genetics 1994;136:1401-1420.

71. Haffter P, Granato M, Brand M, et al: The identification of genes with unique and essential functions in the development of the zebrafish, Danio rario. Development 1996;123:1-36.

72. Chen JN, Haffter P, Odenthal J, et al: Mutations affecting the cardiovascular system and other internal organs in zebrafish. Development 1996;123:293-302.

73. Stainier DY, Fouquet B, Chen JN, et al: Mutations affecting the formation and function of the cardiovascular system in the zebrafish embryo. Development 1996;123:285-292.

74. Fishman MC, Olson EN: Parsing the heart: Genetic modules for organ assembly. Cell 1997;91:153-156.

75. Hu N, Sedmera D, Yost HJ, et al: Structure and function of the developing zebrafish heart. Anat Rec 2000;260:148-157.

76. Serbedzija GN, Chen JN, Fishman MC: Regulation in the heart field of zebrafish. Development 1998;125:1095-1101.

77. Reiter JF, Verkade H, Stainier DY: Bmp2b and Oep promote early myocardial differentiation through their regulation of gata5. Dev Biol 2001;234:330-338.

78. Reifers F, Walsh EC, Leger S, et al: Induction and differentiation of the zebrafish heart requires fibroblast growth factor 8 (fgf8/acerebellar). Development 2000;127:225-235.

79. Goldstein AM, Fishman MC: Notochord regulates cardiac lineage in zebrafish embryos. Dev Biol 1998;201:247-252.

80. Reiter JF, Alexander J, Rodaway A, et al: Gata5 is required for the development of the heart and endoderm in zebrafish. Genes Dev 1999;13:2983-2995.

81. Yelon D, Ticho B, Halpern ME, et al: The bHLH transcription factor hand2 plays parallel roles in zebrafish heart and pectoral fin development. Development 2000;127:2573-2782.

82. Peterson RT, Mably JD, Chen JN, et al: Convergence of distinct pathways to heart patterning revealed by the small molecule concentramide and the mutation heart-and-soul. Curr Biol 2001; 11:1481-1491.

83. Horne-Badovinac S, Lin D, Waldron S, et al: Positional cloning of heart and soul reveals multiple roles for PKC lambda in zebrafish organogenesis. Curr Biol 2001;11:1492-1502.

84. Knoblich JA, Jan LY, Jan YN: Asymmetric segregation of Numb and Prospero during cell division. Nature 1995;377:624-627.

85. Kraut R, Chia W, Jan LY, et al: Role of inscuteable in orienting asymmetric cell divisions in Drosophila. Nature 1996;383:50-55.

86. Warren KS, Wu JC, Pinet F, et al: The genetic basis of cardiac function: Dissection by zebrafish (Danio rario) screens. Philos Trans R Soc Lond B Biol Sci 2000;355:939-944.

87. Xu X, Meiler SE, Zhong TP, et al: Cardiomyopathy in zebrafish due to mutation in an alternatively spliced exon of titin. Nat Genet 2002;30:205-209.

88. Gerull B, Gramlich M, Atherton J, et al: Mutations of TTN, encoding the giant muscle filament titin, cause familial dilated cardiomyopathy. Nat Genet 2002;30:201-204.

89. Potts JD, Dagle JM, Walder JA, et al: Epithelial-mesenchymal transformation of embryonic cardiac endothelial cells is inhibited by a modified antisense oligodeoxynucleotide to transforming growth factor beta 3. Proc Natl Acad Sci USA 1991;88:1516-1520.

90. Sanford LP, Ormsby I, Gittenberger-de Groot AC, et al: TGFbeta2 knockout mice have multiple developmental defects that are non-overlapping with other TGFbeta knockout phenotypes. Development 1997;124:2659-2670.

91. de la Pompa JL, Timmerman LA, Takimoto H, et al: Role of the NF-ATc transcription factor in morphogenesis of cardiac valves and septum. Nature 1998;392:182-186.

92. Ranger AM, Grusby MJ, Hodge MR, et al: The transcription factor NF-ATc is essential for cardiac valve formation. Nature 1998; 392:186-190.

93. Walsh EC, Stainier DY: UDP-glucose dehydrogenase required for cardiac valve formation in zebrafish. Science 2001;293:1670-1673.

94. Warren KS, Fishman MC: "Physiological genomics": Mutant screens in zebrafish. Am J Physiol 1998;275(1 Pt 2):H1-7.

95. Baker K, Warren KS, Yellen G, et al: Defective "pacemaker" current (Ih) in a zebrafish mutant with a slow heart rate. Proc Natl Acad Sci USA 1997;94:4554-4559.

96. Peterson RT, Link BA, Dowling JE, et al: Small molecule developmental screens reveal the logic and timing of vertebrate development. Proc Natl Acad Sci USA 2000;97:12965-12969.

## EDITOR'S CHOICE

Ashrafi K, Chang FY, Watts JL, et al: Genome-wide RNAi analysis of Caenorhabditis elegans fat regulatory genes. Nature 2003;421: 268-272.

*Documents the power of model organisms, in this case the worm, to rapidly dissect multiple control points in pathways for fat metabolism; this is one of the most powerful genetic systems to identify the function of genes.*

Bonini NM, Fortini ME: Human neurodegenerative disease modeling using Drosophila. Annu Rev Neurosci 2003; 26:627-656.

*Flies are used as a genetic system to study aging and human neurodegenerative diseases.*

Clark KA, McElhinny AS, Beckerle MC, et al: Striated muscle cytoarchitecture: An intricate web of form and function. Annu Rev Cell Dev Biol 2002;18:637-706.

*Studies in all creatures great and small support a critical role of the muscle cytoskeleton in general, and Z disc proteins in particular, in the maintenance of cardiac and skeletal muscle function.*

Hsu AL, Murphy CT, Kenyon C: Regulation of aging and age-related disease by DAF-16 and heat-shock factor. Science 2003;300:1142-1145.

*A recent chapter in a wonderful novel that chronicles the utility of worm genetics to study the biology of aging.*

MacRae CA, Fishman MC: Zebrafish: The complete cardiovascular compendium. Cold Spring Harb Symp Quant Biol 2002;67:301–307.

*A timely review by a pioneer in the development of the zebrafish as a system to find genes with physiological function; important implications for finding new genes and pathways for complex human biology and related diseases.*

Poss KD, Wilson LG, Keating MT: Heart regeneration in zebrafish. Science 2002;298:2188–2190.

*Cardiac regeneration occurs in fish, and studies like this form a basis to explore ways that it might in humans also.*

Uptain SM, Lindquist S: Prions as protein-based genetic elements. Annu Rev Microbiol 2002;56:703–741.

*Studies in yeast uncover the molecular mechanisms underlying prion diseases.*

Xu X, Meiler SE, Zhong TP, et al: Cardiomyopathy in zebrafish due to mutation in an alternatively spliced exon of titin. Nat Genet 2002;30:205–209.

*Studies in Zebrafish support a critical role of titin in cardiomyopathy; parallel studies in familial forms of human dilated cardiomyopathy document this to be the case.*

Zaffran S, Xu X, Lo PC, et al: Cardiogenesis in the Drosophila model: Control mechanisms during early induction and diversification of cardiac progenitors. Cold Spring Harb Symp Quant Biol 2002;67:1–12.

*Flies predict many of the key, early steps in heart mesoderm specification; these and related studies by Bodmer, Harvey, and Izumo document a critical early role of cardiac homeobox genes in the NKX2.5 gene family in cardiogenesis, and lead to identification of pathways for congenital heart disease.*

■ ■ ■ c h a p t e r **4**

# Generation and Cloning of Genetically Modified Animals

*Leon J. De Windt*
*Pieter A. Doevendans*
*Kenneth R. Chien*

## THE MOUSE AS THE PARADIGM OF MAMMALIAN GENETIC MODIFICATION

Currently, the mouse is the most important mammalian organism available for transgenic and gene targeting applications of integrative biology. Several considerations have led to the popularity of this particular model. The technology to manipulate the murine genome is well developed: mouse breeding time is rapid compared with breeding times of larger rodent or other mammalian species, the cost of maintenance and husbandry is relatively low, and the knowledge of mouse genetics has expanded enormously over the last decade. The mouse was selected as one of the model organisms for complete sequencing of its genome, an effort that has already led to practical and accessible databases (http://www.celera.com and http://www.ncbi.nlm.nih.gov). Although the mouse's small size often poses some challenges in designing instruments for physiologic measurements, these limitations have been largely overcome by ongoing global efforts to develop and optimize microsurgical techniques for this species and to miniaturize physiologic techniques.[1-3] These technical advances have significantly aided the acceptance and widespread use of mice for transgenic and gene-targeting experiments (Table 4-1).[4-18]

## Principles of Transgenesis

Transgenesis can be defined as the uncontrolled transfer of foreign DNA into the germline of an animal species. Transgenesis became possible only after significant advances were made in the understanding of developmental, reproductive, and molecular biologic principles of the mammalian genome. In addition, several techniques were developed simultaneously that played a fundamental role in the feasibility of introducing foreign DNA constructs into the murine genome. Methods were developed for handling fertilized mouse eggs at the one-cell stage, culturing mouse eggs to the blastocyst stage, and transferring eggs to the female reproductive system to ultimately obtain viable offspring.[19-23] In addition, rapid progress was made in recombinant DNA techniques, enabling molecular biologists to clone genes, create copy DNA constructs (accurate copies of DNA that encode a given protein), and transfer these DNA constructs into cultured eukaryotic cells via transfection approaches. These technologic advances led to the demonstration by Cappechi[24] that a cloned thymidine kinase (TK) cDNA construct could be injected directly into the nucleus of cultured cells by microinjection and achieve high transfection efficiency; most significantly, these cells contained TK activity.

Another revolutionary advance that significantly contributed to the advent of murine transgenesis was the demonstration that microinjected foreign DNA into germ cells resulted in the corresponding protein expression in the offspring somatic cell.[25] Brinster et al.[26] demonstrated that direct microinjection of β-globin mRNA into mouse oocytes and fertilized one-cell eggs resulted in translation of the corresponding gene product. It was not until 1974 that Jaenisch and Mintz[27] demonstrated that SV40 viral DNA microinjected into the murine blastocyst cavity resulted in identification of SV40 DNA in the genomic material of adult animals. In the early 1980s, several groups introduced DNA constructs into the male pronucleus of fertilized murine oocytes and observed stable integration of the constructs in the host chromosomal DNA, which was transferred to the offspring.[28-33] Although these initial reports clearly established the technical feasibility of all the critical steps involving murine transgenesis (stable integration, protein expression, stable germline transmission), the full significance of these findings was not fully appreciated until the report of Palmiter et al.[34] They were able to demonstrate that stable integration of the rat growth hormone (GH) gene into the murine genome produced dramatic increases in the size of GH transgenic mice, thereby demonstrating that the heterologous DNA construct transcribed, translated, and produced the expected physiologic response to the hormone in the whole animal. Since then transgenesis has become a cornerstone of modern integrative physiology. The number of reports involving genetically modified mice still increases exponentially, and transgenic approaches remain a significant proportion of these manipulative approaches in mice (Figs. 4-1 and 4-2).

In general, transgenic animals are used to address three fundamentally distinct topics: (1) to examine the physiologic consequence of a gain-of-function approach in which one overexpresses, or expresses ectopically, a protein to assess its physiologic and biologic function at

■ ■ ■

## TABLE 4-1   MINIATURIZED TECHNIQUES FOR MURINE PHENOTYPING

| Modality | Technique | Procedure | Advantages | Disadvantages | References |
|---|---|---|---|---|---|
| Noninvasive imaging | Echocardiography | 2D-guided echocardiography and Doppler | Rapid screening procedures, serial observations | Limited resolution | 4,5 |
| | Magnetic resonance imaging | Magnetic fields | High resolution, longitudinal examination vascular wall | Expensive | 6, 7 |
| | Fetal echocardiography | Ultrasound backscatter microscopy | High resolution | Specialized equipment, low frame rate | |
| | Magnetic resonance microscopy | High magnetic fields | Tomographic 3D imaging, high resolution | Motion artefacts | 8, 9 |
| | Real-time imaging | Annexin-V fluorescence | Noninvasive, high resolution | | 18 |
| Invasive imaging | Intravital microscopy | Microinjection of fluorescent probes in intraplacental circulation, high-speed video microscopy | Fetal heart imaging | Terminal experiment | 12 |
| | Contrast ventriculography | Densitometric method, digital data collection | Accurate assessment chamber volumes | X-ray based | 10 |
| *In situ* hemodynamics | Micromanometers | High fidelity | Pressure development during systole and diastole | Load-dependent | 10, 11, 13 |
| | Conductance catheter | High fidelity | Simultaneous pressure and volume assessments, load-independent | Volume calibration inaccurate | 17 |
| | Catheter-based telemetry | Chronic instrumentation | 24-hr blood pressure monitoring, conscious measurement | Low resolution | 11 |
| *Ex vivo* hemodynamics | Isolated, retrogradely perfused heart model (Langendorff) | Cannulation aorta excised heart, retrograde perfusion with oxygenated buffer | Load-independent, relative easy manipulation and setup | Terminal experiment, no accurate LV hemodynamics | 15, 16 |
| | Isolated, antegradely perfused heart model (working heart) | Cannulation LA and aorta, antegrade LV perfusion | Load-independent hemodynamics, LV volume calibration | Terminal experiment, highly specialized equipment | 15, 16 |

LA, left atrium; LV, left ventricle; 2D, two-dimensional; 3D, three-dimensional.

the cellular or subcellular, organ, or whole-animal level (this form of experimentation is the most common application of transgenesis); (2) to characterize the regulatory sequences in control of tissue-specificity of genes or gene families (in this approach, promoter constructs are placed upstream of reporter genes such as *β-galactosidase* or *luciferase* [Table 4-2] to trace the tissue distribution and extent of gene expression that correlates with that of the endogenous gene); or (3) to use transgene-induced insertions to identify new genetically important loci.[11,35-37]

## Consideration and Design of the Transgenic Construct

A key factor in the production of transgenic animals is the proper design of the transgenic construct, that is, the DNA sequence that contains the transgene of interest. Because of the widespread use and availability of plas-mids (bacterial, circular DNA that can be modified easily), most transgenic constructs are based on these self-replicating DNA molecules. In contrast to the high level of expression that can be obtained with cDNA constructs in transfection experiments of cultured cell systems, cDNA constructs with transgenes containing an open reading frame (ORF) larger than 2 kb tend to be expressed less efficiently when integrated into the murine genome, compared with genome sequence-based transgenic constructs.[38-40] This effect may be due to the presence of introns in the genomic sequence, which are absent in cDNA constructs. Introns have been shown to increase transcriptional efficiency, even when heterologous intron sequences are used.[41] Thus, a genomic sequence, or at least a so-called minigene, which consists of the ORF with several intron sequences, should be used. This approach proved to be superior when overexpressing the low-density lipoprotein (LDL) receptor gene in transgenic mice compared

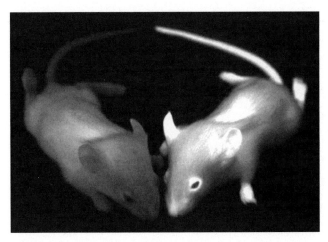

**FIGURE 4-1.** Green Fluorescent Protein (GFP) transgenic mice. GFP is responsible for the green bioluminescence of the jellyfish *Aequoria Victoria*. Transgenic mice were generated with an enhanced GFP cDNA under the control of a chicken beta-actin promoter and cytomegalovirus enhancer. All of the tissue from these eGFP transgenic mice, except for the hair and erythrocytes, were green under excitation light. The fluorescent nature of these cells from these eGFP transgenic mice would facilitate their use in many kinds of transplantation experiments. Also see the web site relating to these mice at http://kumikae01. gen-info.osaka-u.ac.jp/greenmouse.cfm. (See color plate.)

with an approach in which a pure cDNA LDL receptor is used for overexpression.[42]

## Large Transgenic Constructs: Yeast Artifical Chromosome, Bacterial Artificial Chromosome, or P1 Bacteriophage-Based Constructs

Conventionally, transgenic experiments were performed using DNA fragments up to 15 kb in length. However, this relatively small length may be suboptimal for many contemporary transgenesis experiments, because many mammalian genes span regions exceeding 40 kb. As a result, these fragments are inconvenient for cloning into conventional plasmids. To circumvent these problems, investigators are relying on Yeast Artificial Chromosome (YAC), Bacterial Artificial Chromosome (BAC), or P1 bacteriophage vectors to clone the relatively large genomic constructs. Schedl et al.[43] and Peterson et al.[44] were the first to report the generation of transgenic mice expressing tyrosinase and β-globin from 250- and 248-kb YACs, respectively. Similarly, an 80-kb P1 bacteriophage clone spanning the human apo-B lipoprotein gene was used to produce high levels of apo-B lipoprotein in transgenic mice.[45,46]

To generate transgenic mice with large fragments, one must avoid shearing DNA constructs during the purification process. Typically, the high molecular weight YAC DNA is removed from a pulsed-field agarose gel followed by digestion of agarose with agarase. Some investigators rely on the addition of spermidine, spermine, and 100 nM NaCl in all buffers, which force the DNA to aggregate, thereby reducing its vulnerability for shearing. Early studies demonstrated that the genomic DNA from

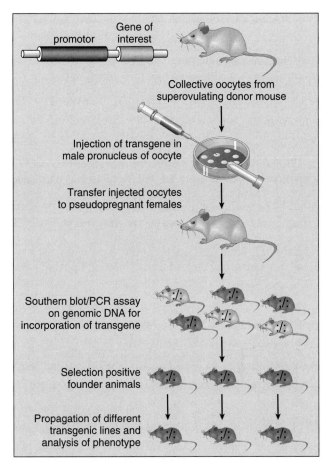

**FIGURE 4-2.** Overview of the generation of transgenic mice. The scheme is presented as a flow chart showing the animals and reagents required. First, a suitable transgenic DNA construct is generated using recombinant DNA procedures, consisting of a gene of interest placed downstream of a promoter sequence. Egg donor females are injected with gestyl and pregnyl, bred with males, and checked for copulatory plugs 24 hours later. Pregnant females are sacrificed and the fertilized eggs are collected (approximately 300) and microinjected with the transgenic vector suspension. Subsequently, the eggs are cultured to a two-cell stage and transferred to the oviduct of pseudopregnant recipient females and the eggs are brought to term. The pups are weaned on day 15, and a small piece of their tail or an ear punch is used for genotyping and identification of transgenic mice. Each of the transgenic animals (founders) are bred with nontransgenic animals to ensure transmittance of the transgene to the progeny and to establish an independent transgenic line.

■ ■ ■

## TABLE 4-2    REPORTER GENES AND METHODS OF DETECTION

| Reporter | Detection Methods |
| --- | --- |
| *LacZ* | 1, 2, 3, 5 |
| *Luciferase* | 1, 2, 5 |
| *CAT* | 1, 3, 5 |
| *GH* | 1, 2 |
| *GFP* | 1, 2, 4, 5 |

*CAT*, chloramphenicol transferase; *GFP*, green fluorescent protein; *GH*, growth hormone; *LacZ*, β-galactosidase; 1, *in situ* hybridization with nucleic acid probes; 2, immunocytochemistry; 3, *in situ* detection with histochemical strains; 4, *in situ* detection of fluorescence of the GFP; 5, measurements in cell lysates.

some transgenic animals generated with YACs carry fragmented rather than intact copies of the transgene.[44,47] Therefore, one must design strategies to assess the intactness of the constructs once they are integrated into the genome. One strategy is to find rare restriction endonucleases that cleave the microinjected DNA near its 5′ and 3′ ends and subsequently locate the inserted DNA in the genome of the animals via DNA blotting (Southern blot). Another strategy is to use PCR-based methods to scan the genomic DNA of transgenic animals for various regions of the inserted fragment, including the vector sequences at each end of the integrated segment. Unfortunately, PCR-based strategies cannot exclude the potential of two overlapping sheared fragments of DNA spanning the complete transgene, and, therefore, PCR methods should be used with caution.

Embryonic stem (ES) cell technology provides an alternative for constructing transgenic mice with large constructs. Cho et al. reported the generation of ES cell co-transfected with a YAC constructed and a neomycin resistance cassette. G418 resistant ES cell colonies that incorporated the YAC-based transgene were used to generate chimeric mice that transmitted the DNA to their progeny.[48] One advantage of ES cell technology is that the incorporation and intactness of the inserted DNA can be assessed before animals are generated and bred.

## Micromanipulation and Microinjection

Currently, all phases of the transgenic methodology are described in detail in laboratory handbooks. Therefore, this section is intended to provide a global overview of the methods required to generate transgenic mice.[49-51]

The first requirement is the availability of large numbers of high-quality eggs. The eggs are collected from females induced to superovulate by injections of gestyl and pregnyl hormone treatments and timed mating. One day after confirmation of the presence of copulatory plugs, the females are sacrificed and the eggs mechanically retrieved from the oviducts and enzymatically denuded from the associated cumulus cells.

Following egg collection, the single eggs are rotated on glass holding pipettes until the pronuclei are visible. Special glass micropipettes with long, tapered points are used for the injection of the solution containing the transgenic vector in a constant-flow mode. Normally, the total volume of the DNA solution used does not exceed a volume that expands the pronucleus by more than 50%, and the solution has a very low DNA concentration (2 to 5 ng/μL). Typically, several hundred eggs are injected simultaneously with one transgenic construct and the viability of the injected eggs exceeds 70% (Fig. 4-3).

After microinjection, the injected eggs (either at a single- or double-cell stage) are transferred immediately to the oviducts of pseudopregnant females, produced from matings with vasectomized males. The injected eggs are allowed to come to term in these foster mothers and, following weaning, the individual pups are tested for the integration of the injected DNA fragment, generally by obtaining genomic DNA from ear punches or tail clips. Typically three methods are used for the genotyping

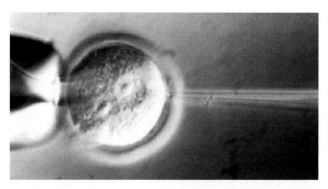

**FIGURE 4-3.** Microinjection of a fertilized mouse egg. The oocyte is held under suspension, free of underlying support, with a holding pipette, and the DNA suspension is injected into the male pronucleus with a microneedle. (See color plate.)

process: DNA dot blot analysis, Southern blot, or PCR-based technologies. The advantage of Southern blot is that this method provides information about the pattern of integration, the copy number, and the intactness of the DNA construct. DNA injected into rodent eggs is incorporated into the chromosomal genome in a random fashion and location, with occasional integration in Y or X chromosome. Often, multiple copies of the DNA constructs integrate into the same chromosomal location in a tandem head-to-tail array.

## Cardiac-Restricted Transgenesis

A major step forward in the transgenesis technology in recent years is the ongoing characterization of genomic sequences that control tissue-specific expression of genes.[52,53] For many genes, insight into the location of critical *cis*-acting regulatory sequences has been obtained by a combination of cell transfection and transgenic approaches. This approach for mapping regulatory sequences, which are critical for maintaining an expression pattern of reporter genes that resembles the endogenous gene, is elegantly illustrated by efforts to characterize the regulatory sequences for genes encoding ventricular regulatory myosin light chain-2 *(MLC-2v)*, fast skeletal myosin light chain-3f *(MLC-3f)*, and α- and β-myosin heavy chains *(αMyHC* and *βMyHC)*. Another reason that cardiac-selective promoters are identified is to achieve tissue-specificity (to prevent systemic expression of a transgene, which can seriously complicate the resultant phenotype). The development of promoters in which expression is largely restricted to the cardiac compartment has enhanced the utility of the transgenic approach for specifically remodeling cardiomyocyte physiology, without the confounding effects of other organ or muscle systems.[54]

The transgenic paradigm has been tested in detail using the characteristics of the cardiac *MLC-2* gene. *MLC-2* expression is developmentally and spatially controlled in the heart, and atrial- and ventricular-specific isoforms exist. Studies have further suggested a correlation between *MLC-2* isoform shifts and the development of dilated cardiomyopathy, hypertrophy, and altered myosin cycling kinetics in heart disease. Early studies have concentrated on the identification of the regulatory sequences and promoter region of the rat ventricular *MLC-2 (MLC-2v)* gene. The exon-intron structure is highly conserved between the ventricular and fast skeletal MLC isoform *(MLC-2f)* and among animal species. Nested 5′ deletions of the *MLC-2v* 5′-flanking region were fused to luciferase and tested for their ability to direct cardiac specific expression of the reporter gene in cultured cardiac myocytes and transgenic mice.[55-57] A small 250-bp region of the proximal *MLC-2* promoter region was sufficient to confer cardiac muscle-specific gene expression and characterize *cis*-regulatory sequences in detail (Fig. 4-4). Multiple regulatory sequences were identified in this small region, such as CarG- and E-box sites, MLE1, HF-1a/b and PRE B sites, which were demonstrated to coordinately control the expression of *MLC-2v*.[57] Finally, the truncated version of the MLC-2v promoter was used to express p21[ras] in a ventricular-specific manner and has generated a valuable model of cardiac hypertrophy and other transgenic mouse and rat models were generated using this promoter.[14]

Three cardiac MyHC isoforms exist; the relative amount depends on the species, developmental stage, hormonal status, and chamber. The isoforms termed $V_1$, $V_2$, and $V_3$ on the basis of their mobilities on polyacrylamide gels are the products of two genes α and β, with $V_1$ corresponding to an α,α dimer, $V_2$ to an α, β dimer, and $V_3$ to a β,β dimer. Interestingly, interspecies heart rate (speed of contraction) and ATPase activity of myosin correlate remarkably well. Compared with the α,α dimer, $V_2$, and $V_3$ show diminished ATPase activities.[58-61] The human ventricle, which is predominant $V_3$, has a resting heart rate of 60 to 80 beats per minute, whereas the murine adult heart, which contains only $V_1$, contracts at 500 to 550 beats per minute.

The ability of promoters (derived from the murine *α–MyHC* and *β-MYHC* genes) to drive transgene expression has been extensively characterized; initially these promoters were used to remodel the cardiac contractile apparatus.[62-65] Transgene expression closely mimics the expression of the endogenous gene product. For example, transgene expression derived from the *α-MyHC* promoter occurs in the primitive heart tube and in the developing atria throughout two thirds of gestation and is activated in the ventricular compartment just before birth (Fig. 4-4).[64]

One example of a transgenic contractile remodeling experiment concerned the replacement of the atrial with the ventricular isoform of *MLC-2* using the 5.5-kb fragment of the murine *α-MyHC* promoter to explore the functional consequence of *MLC-2a* replacement and atrial light chain functionality.[66-68] Although gene dosage effects were demonstrated to alter contractile protein levels with devastating effects on sarcomere structure and function in *Drosophila,* expression of the *MLC-2v* transgene had no effect on steady-state mRNA levels encoding related contractile proteins, including endogenous *MLC-2v* transcripts in the mouse. Although the

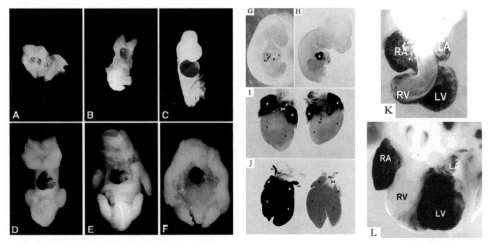

**FIGURE 4-4.** *(Left panel)* Whole mount staining of representative HF-1 LacZ transgenic embryos, using part of the MLC2v promoter driving LacZ expression. E 7-7.5. Late headfold stage/early foregut pocket; *A,* E 8-8.5; *B,* E 9-9.5; *C,* E 10-10.5; *D,* E 12-12.5; and *E,* E 14-14.5. In each case transgene expression was restricted to the heart with an anterior/posterior gradient similar to MLC2v (250 bp) LacZ transgenics. *(Middle panel)* Cardiac chamber-specific expression of an α-MyHC promoter-driven transgene. Whole-mount preparations of embryos *(G* and *H)* and postnatal hearts *(I* and *J)* are shown. *G,* Embryo at 9.5 days post coitum (dpc) shows *lacZ* expression in the primitive atrium (a) as it emerges from the sinus venosus (sv). *H,* By 10.5 dpc, *lacZ* staining is strong in the common atrium. *I,* Anterior *(left)* and posterior *(right)* views of the newborn animal's heart are shown. At birth, transgene expression is limited to the atria, the right superior vena cava (vc) as it enters the right atrium, and the pulmonary veins (out of the plane of focus). No expression is seen in the ventricles (v). *J,* Anterior view of *lacZ* expression in hearts from transgenic *(left)* and non-transgenic *(right)* littermates at 2 weeks of age. In the transgenic hearts, both atria and ventricles are intensely stained, as are the right and left superior vena cava and the pulmonary veins (not shown). ao, aorta; b, bulbus cordis; pa, pulmonary artery. *(Right panel)* Chamber specific nLacZ expression using the MLC3f transgene. Expression in E10.5 embryos *(K)* and in E14.5 embryos *(L),* showing confinement of expression to the right atrium and left ventricle. (See color plate.) *(Left panel modified from Ross et al. An HF-1a/HF-1b/MEF-2 combinatorial element confers cardiac ventricular specificity and establishes and anterior-posterior gradient of expression. Development 1996;122:1799-1809. Middle panel modified from Palermo, Gulick J, Colbert M, et al: Transgenic remodeling of the contractile apparatus in the mammalian heart. Circ Res 1996;78:504-509. Right panel modified from Franco et al: MLC3F transgene expression in iv mutant mice reveals the importance of left-right signaling pathways for the acquisition of left and right atrial but not ventricular compartment identity. Dev Dyn 2001;221:206-215).*

overall *MLC-2v* mRNA in the ventricle increased several fold, no commensurate increase in protein could be detected in either total protein or myofilament pool, indicating discordant messenger versus protein levels and suggesting that the protein synthesis or turnover rates of *MLC-2v* were altered to maintain the overall protein stoichiometry.[67] Complete replacement of the atrial *MLC-2* protein with the ventricular isoform was achieved in atria from transgenic mice. No overt pathology presented and ventricular function was not significantly affected; however, isoform function was demonstrated by examination of the contractile function of isolated transgenic atrial cardiomyocytes. In these cells the speed of shortening and relengthening at maximal $Ca^{2+}$ stimulation was increased, consistent with the higher contractile demands that are placed on the ventricle relative to the atrium.[67] Since the introduction of the *α-MyHC* promoter as a transgenic device, it has been used in numerous studies to drive (ectopic) expression of wild-type or mutated forms of ion channels, cytoplasmic signaling molecules, transcription factors, and mitochondrial components.[69]

Analysis of reporter gene expression in transgenic mice containing a nuclear-directed form of β-galactosidase *(nLacZ)* under transcriptional control of the *MLC-3f* promoter region confirmed strong *lacZ* expression in skeletal muscle and in cardiac muscle from E7.5.[70] Most strikingly, reporter gene in the myocardium was spatially restricted to the right atrial and left ventricular compartments (Fig. 4-4).[70] The heart is the first embryonic structure to display morphologic left-right asymmetry. Under normal conditions *(situs solitus)* the cardiac tube loops toward the right side of the developing embryo *(D-loop)*. Several genes are expressed asymmetrically in the lateral plate mesoderm before the looping event, suggesting that they are involved in embryonic left-right signaling. Abnormal specification of cardiac laterality has been associated with several human congenital cardiac malformations such as double outlet right ventricle, persistent truncus arteriosus, and atrial isomerism. The *MLC3f* transgenic reporter mice have been useful to perform fate-mapping experiments and to study the precise timing of the events that underlie specification of left and right atrial situs because they provided the first molecular markers that permit the examination of left and right identity during cardiogenesis.[71,72]

To date, numerous regulatory sequences have been identified and used to drive heterologous transgenes to specific target cell types and organs, allowing investigators to choose from a wide variety of promoter sequences to design their transgenic construct. Before proceeding with transgenic experimentation, one should analyze the specific characteristics of these available promoters and balance the disadvantages and advantages of a particular promoter. Internet-accessible databases are available to assist the investigator in these theoretical considerations (e.g., TBASE on http://tbase.jax.org./). In the cardiovascular field, a number of regulatory sequences have been successfully used to restrict expression of transgenes to cardiomyocytes, endothelial cells, and smooth muscle cells in the mouse (see Table 4-3).[14,64,65,70,73-82]

**TABLE 4-3    CARDIOVASCULAR TRANSGENIC PROMOTER CONSTRUCTS**

| Promoter | Tissue Distribution | Reference |
|---|---|---|
| Pax-3 | Neural crest | 73 |
| Wnt1 | Neural crest | 74 |
| α-Myosin heavy chain | Atrial and ventricular myocardium | 64, 65 |
| β-Myosin heavy chain | Embryonic atrial and ventricular myocardium | 75 |
| Myosin light chain 2v | Ventricular myocardium | 14 |
| Desmin | Heart, skeletal muscle | 76 |
| Myosin light chain 3f | Heart, skeletal muscle | 70 |
| Myosin light chain 1f | Skeletal muscle | 76 |
| Muscle creatine kinase | Skeletal muscle | 77 |
| MyoD | Skeletal muscle | 78 |
| SM22 | Smooth muscle | 79 |
| Tie-1 | Vascular endothelium | 82 |
| Tie-2 | Vascular endothelium | 81 |

## Consideration of Genetic Background for Transgenesis

Marked differences have been reported for physiologic parameters in various mouse strains, probably related to the genetic background. Few truly comparable studies are available because studies used mice of both sexes and various ages, and different anesthesia protocols have been applied. Furthermore, reports documenting improvements in the techniques to measure mouse cardiovascular physiology are reported on a regular basis. Despite these limitations, marked differences in values for electrocardiographic and hemodynamic function in wild-type mice with different genetic background have been reported.[83] The differences in ECG parameters are illustrative; the PR interval varies between 36 to 54 msec and the QT from 54 to 109 mseconds, constituting an almost 100% difference. If the expected phenotype involves QT prolongation the genetic background will determine the ease or difficulty in picking up changes in QT duration.

Similar variations have been reported for hemodynamic studies. It is, therefore, essential to perform control experiments with age- and gender-matched wild-type control animals. In addition, in the case of transgenic experiments several lines will have to be studied because of variation in the copy number of the transgene.[84] To reveal a phenotype it may be necessary to analyze the effect of the transgene in different mouse strains. Especially in transgenic experiments, the extent of expression is subject to the level of methylation and subsequent silencing of the construct introduced.[85] The genetic background is essential for the outcome of the transgenic experiment, and choosing the optimal strain helps to identify any phenotype, even after a challenge to the cardiovascular system (e.g., by transverse aortic banding) is introduced.

The differences observed after crossing a well-established mouse model to various strains can also be used to identify modifier genes that are either protective or detrimental for the phenotype studied. This approach has been successfully used in rats and mice for cardiovascular diseases such as hypertension, atherosclerosis, or dilated cardiomyopathy.[86]

Although mice and humans share many conserved genes that regulate several aspects of the cardiovascular system, the potential of interspecies differences is likely to become an increasingly important issue to define whether mice display fidelity to the clinical outcome. If interspecies differences are too large, the mouse may be "humanized" to display the response or phenotype of interest. Perhaps the most illustrative example consists of work from several laboratories that has led to engineering mouse models of atherosclerosis and lipoprotein metabolism. The wild-type mouse (with exception of the C57BL/6 inbred strain) is resistant to atherogenic diets and lacks several critical genes involved in lipoprotein metabolism. Nevertheless, several humanized mouse models have been generated that display critical analogies of human atherosclerosis, and, as a result, the mouse has become an important model system for increasing knowledge of human disease. In addition, by crossing C57BL/6j (atherosclerosis-resistant inbred strain) with C57BLKS/j mice (relatively vulnerable strain), changes in the susceptibility to atherosclerosis was demonstrated and a genetic region (quantitative trait locus) was identified on mouse chromosome 12 in an area that matches with human chromosome 2p24-25. By increasing the number of crossed animals the region can be more closely defined until the modifier gene has been pinpointed. Obviously, complete comparative maps between mouse, rat, and human are essential to fully use this form of genetic analysis.

This approach was followed to identify potential genetic modifier loci in mice with severe heart failure caused by cardiac-specific overexpression of the sarcoplasmatic reticulum $Ca^{2+}$-binding protein calsequestrin (CSQ).[87,88] CSQ transgenic mice recapitulate several phenotypic aspects of human dilated cardiomyopathy, including abnormal β-adrenergic responsiveness, cardiac enlargement, left ventricular dysfunction, and premature death. Similarly, the pathogenesis of human heart failure is complex, polygenetic, and multifactorial, with variable phenotypic penetrance in human subjects.[37,54,89] It was noted that the phenotypic outcome of the CSQ transgene was highly strain dependent, showing wide variation when crossed into different inbred mouse strains. To map modifier loci, parental CSQ transgenic mice in a dilute brown agouti (DBA) background were backcrossed for several generations with C57bl/6j and DBA wild-type mice. The progeny were phenotyped using variables such as echocardiographically determined function and survival, which showed remarkable deterioration in F1 DBA/B6 progeny compared with parental DBA mice. Thus far, two loci have been identified linked to survival (chromosome 2 and 3), and a separate locus on chromosome 3 was related to cardiac function, providing an excellent example of how variation in genetic background can be used to identify protective or disease-promoting genes.[86]

# Conditional Transgenesis: Tetracycline, Cre/loxP, and *lac* Operon

## Tetracycline-Inducible Systems

Transgenesis to achieve gain-of-function mutations in a systemic manner has yielded remarkable advances in understanding the roles of specific gene products in embryogenesis and later gene function. Nevertheless, inherent impediments include indirect systemic defects, which can complicate the elucidation of the role of genes in a specific pathophysiologic context. Aside from tissue-specific expression of transgenic gene products (see the section on micromanipulation and macromanipulation), a more refined strategy confers inducibility to the genetic alteration. One system that allows for inducible control of gene expression in transgenic mice is the tetracycline (*tet*) regulatory system developed by Bujard and colleagues.[90-92] The system consists of a transactivator that binds in a ligand-dependent manner to an engineered minimal promoter, thereby activating the transcription of a response gene. The transactivator (tTA) is a fusion protein composed of the bacterial tet-repressor and the transactivation domain of the viral VP16 protein. In the classical tet-system, the responder gene is expressed in the absence of the ligand and silenced on introduction of the ligand (e.g., tetracycline or doxycycline administered in the drinking water of the engineered mouse). In the reverse tet-system, a modified transactivator termed reverse tTA or rtTA is used that binds the promoter only in the presence of ligand. Therefore, the responder gene is normally silent but can be switched on by ligand administration (Fig. 4-5).[90-93]

Both tTA and rtTA-regulated binary systems have been shown to allow control over the expression of reporter genes in transgenic mice. Tissue-specificity can be obtained by placing the transactivator under the control of a suitable promoter, as shown by Kandel and coworkers. In their experiment, calmodulin-dependent protein kinase (*CamK*) II promoter drove expression of the tTA, and a dominant negative mutant of *CamKII* was used as the responder gene. In the absence of doxycycline, expression of the dominant mutant *CamKII* led to a loss of long-term potentiation and a deficit in spatial memory in the brain of mice, whereas doxycycline administration reversed both *CamKII* mutant expression and the phenotype.[94] In the heart, reporter gene expression has been demonstrated to be controllable by this system,[94,95] whereas tet-regulatory expression of a constitutively activated mutant of protein kinase Cβ was shown to signal either a severe dilated cardiomyopathy in young, postnatal mice or cardiac hypertrophy in the adult mouse heart.[96]

## Cre/loxP Mediated Conditional Overexpression System

Another strategy to achieve tissue-specific and conditional transgenesis exploits the Cre/loxP system derived from the bacteriophage P1. Cre recombinase is a 38-kDa P1 phage derived site-specific DNA recombinase, which specifically recognizes 34-bp nucleic acid sequences referred to as loxP (*locus* of *X*-ing over) sites. Because of

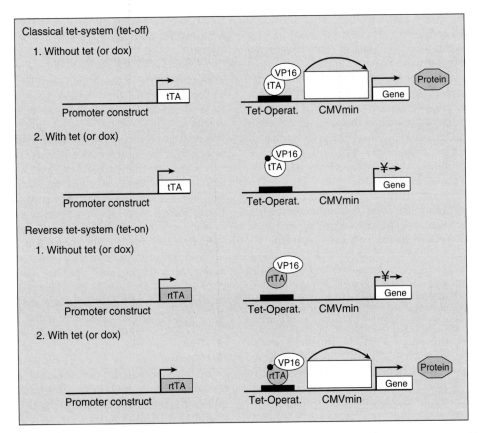

**FIGURE 4-5.** Schematic representation of the tetracycline-inducible system. *A,* The tetracycline system uses a tTA that is able to bind with high affinity and specificity to a minimal promoter containing multimerized *tet*-operators (*tetO* promoter), thereby activating gene expression. The tTA product itself consists of the *tet* repressor fused to the herpes simplex derived transcriptional activator domain VP16. In the classical system (also referred to as tet-off), in the presence of tetracycline or its derivative doxycycline the binding of tTA to *tet* operator sequences is blocked, preventing transcriptional activation of the gene of interest. *B,* In the alternative system, also referred to as the tet-on system, a mutated tTA transactivator protein is used (reverse tTA or rtTA). In the presence of tetracycline (or doxycycline) the rtTA transactivator binds to *tet* operator sequences, thereby inducing gene expression.

its ability to catalyze loxP-mediated recombination in the absence of cofactors or accessory proteins and optimal activity at 37˚C, the Cre/loxP system is well suited for genetic engineering in ES cells and mice (see also the section on conditional gene targeting).[97–99]

A loxP site consists of two 13-bp palindromic sequences flanking an 8-bp core sequence, which determines the orientation of the loxP site (Fig. 4-6). Cre-mediated recombination between two loxP sites results in the reciprocal exchange of DNA strands between these sites, such that when the two loxP sites are located in the same direction on a linear DNA molecule, Cre-mediated recombination results in the excision of the loxP-flanked DNA segment as a circular molecule leaving a single loxP site on each DNA product. When two loxP sites are orientated in opposite orientations, Cre mediates inversion of the loxP-flanked sequence.

Mating mice transgenic for a vector constructed such that a loxP flanked stuffer DNA sequence with its own poly A signal is placed immediately upstream of the actual transgene sequence, which renders the latter inactive; mice expressing Cre recombinase in a given tissue have Cre-mediated excision of the loxP sequences. Cre-mediated excision of such a stuffer sequence would result in the juxtaposition of the downstream intact cDNA sequence and the former promoter (Fig. 4-7).

Because the Cre/loxP system is entirely contingent on the exogenous recombinase, recombination can be regulated via timing and tissue specificity of Cre transgene expression.[100]

Recently, two independent research groups have demonstrated the possibility of achieving tissue-specificity and inducing Cre recombinase for the cardiac setting. Minamino et al.[101] placed a conditionally functional chimeric Cre recombinase, a fusion between Cre and the mutated ligand binding domain of the progesterone hormone receptor (CrePR1), under control of the murine *α-MyHC* promoter. After binding to the synthetic ligand RU486, these chimeric proteins become selective, allowing postmitotic recombination to occur in the adult heart because of the expression pattern of the *α-MyHC* promoter (tissue-specificity); this occurred only following administration of the synthetic hormone RU486 (inducibility).[101] In a similar manner, Sohal et al.[102] placed a Cre recombinase fusion with two mutated estrogen receptors (mER) at its N- and C-terminal ends (MerCreMer) under control of the murine *α-MyHC* promoter. Tamoxifen or RU486-regulated Cre recombination are temporaly feasible in the mouse heart by cross-breeding with ROSA-lacZ-flox-targeted mice (Fig. 4-8).[102] Both the CrePR1 and the MerCreMer transgenic mice will undoubtedly become valuable tools that permit tempo-

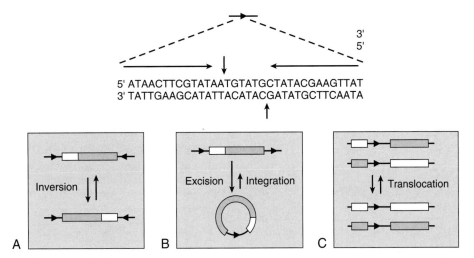

5' ATAACTTCGTATAATGTATGCTATACGAAGTTAT
3' TATTGAAGCATATTACATACGATATGCTTCAATA

**FIGURE 4-6.** The Cre/loxP system. Cre recombinase promotes site-specific recombination between two 34-bp loxP recognition sequences (indicated by the closed triangles). *A,* The loxP sequence itself consist of two 13 bp inverted repeats (horizontal arrows) flanking an 8 bp asymmetric core region that confers overall directionality. The two sites cleaved by Cre recombinase are indicated by vertical arrows. *B,* Recombination between two loxP sites inserted into the same DNA molecule (intramolecular recombination) in opposite direction leads to inversion of the intervening DNA segment. *C,* Whereas recombination between directly repeated loxP sites results in excision of the flanked region (circular product) leaving one loxP sequence behind. When the loxP sites are located on separate DNA molecules (intermolecular recombination), *(C)* DNA integration or *(D)* translocation can be achieved.

rally regulated activation or inactivation of a properly designed transgene or a loxP-targeted genetic locus exclusively within the heart, allowing dissection of putative disease-causing genes within the developing or adult heart.

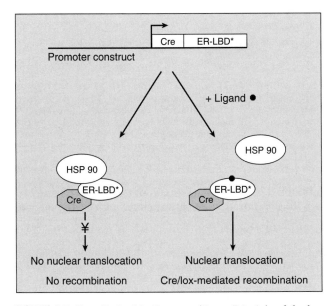

**FIGURE 4-7.** Ligand-inducible Cre recombinase. Principle of the hormone-regulated Cre-steroid receptor ligand binding domain (LBD) fusion protein. Cre is fused to a mutant LBD that is unresponsive to its natural ligand but can be activated by a synthetic ligand. The fusion protein is inactive and located cytoplasmically because it is bound by the ubiquitous heat shock protein 90 (HSP90) complex. On binding of the ligand (synthetic hormone) to the LBD, the fusion protein is released from the inactive state allowing nuclear translocation of Cre recombinase activity and subsequent recombination between two loxP sites.

### The lac Operator-Repressor Inducible System

A promising new system involves the functional transfer of the *lac* operator-repressor system (derived from *Escherichia coli*) into the murine genome. The bacterial *lac* operon consists of a set of genes coordinately regulated by the sugar lactose. The key regulatory components of this system are the *lac* repressor and the DNA-binding sequence (the *lac* operator). In the absence of lactose, the *lac* repressor occupies the *lac* operators and prevents transcription. Introduction of lactose induces a conformational change in the repressor, which vacates the operator sequences, and RNA polymerase accesses the promoter and can initiate transcription. Earlier attempts to introduce this system into the mammalian genome were hampered by heavy methylation and gene silencing. Cronin et al. were the first to report optimization of the codon usage of the *lacI* gene (designated *synlacI*), allowing efficient expression within the mammalian genome and further relieving a translation block by modifying the 3' region of the coding sequence. These efforts resulted in a correctly spliced and translated *synlacI* product in a series of transgenic mice *(LacI^R)* with a largely ubiquitous expression of the *lac* repressor, including the heart.[103]

The system was tested for its ability to reversibly induce expression of the tyrosinase gene. Tyrosinase is the protein encoded by the albino locus that catalyzes the first step in melanin biosynthesis. The target transgene consisted of the tyrosinase cDNA under control of the tyrosinase promoter, modified to contain several sets of the *lac* operator sequences *(Tyr^lacO)*. Mice containing only the modified tyrosinase transgene resembled pigmented animals. Cross breeding of *LacI^R* and *Tyr^lacO* transgenic mice resulted in binding of the *lac* operator sequences in the tyrosinase transgene and transcriptional repression of tyrosinase in *Tyr^lacO* transgenic mice,

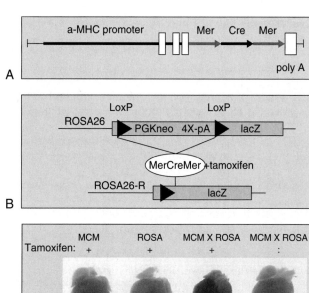

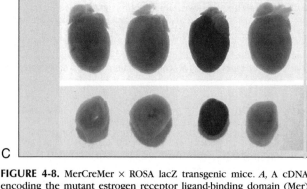

**FIGURE 4-8.** MerCreMer × ROSA lacZ transgenic mice. *A,* A cDNA encoding the mutant estrogen receptor ligand-binding domain (Mer) flanking the Cre recombinase was placed downstream of the 5.5 kb *α-MyHC* promoter to drive expression in the adult heart. *B,* Mice containing a single allele of the Cre recombinase-dependent lacZ gene knocked into the ROSA 26 locus were crossed with transgenic mice containing the MerCreMer transgene, permitting tamoxifen-inducible recombination within the heart. *C,* Assessment of tamoxifen-regulated Cre-mediated recombination in the heart of 6-week-old mice. Wholemount LacZ staining of the entire heart or a transverse section. The indicated experimental and control mice were treated with four injections of tamoxifen for 5 days or left untreated. (See color plate.) *(Modified from Sohal DS, Nghiem M, Crackower, et al: Temporally regulated and tissue-specific manipulations in the adult and embryonic heart using a tamoxifen-inducible Cre protein. Circ Res 2001;89:20–25.)*

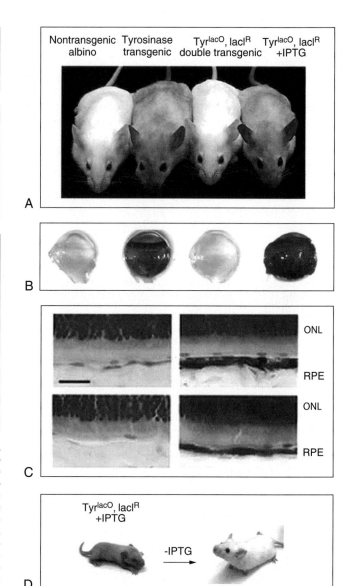

**FIGURE 4-9.** *Tyr^{lacO}-SynLacI^R* transgenic mouse. IPTG controls *LacI^R* repression of the *Tyr^{LacO}* target gene in the mouse. Mice *(A)*, dissected eyes *(B)*, and cross-sections through eyes *(C)*. Note the lack of pigmentation in the nontransgenic albino and the *Tyr^{LacO}, LacI^R* double transgenic mice, whereas the tyrosinase transgenic and the *Tyr^{LacO}, LacI^R* double transgenic mouse treated with IPTG are pigmented. ONL, outer nuclear layer; RPE, retinal pigment epithelium. *D,* Control of the *Tyr^{LacO}* target gene is reversible even after birth. Tyrosinase expression can be silenced after a period of derepression. Left and right panels show the same *Tyr^{LacO}, LacI^R* double transgenic animal, on the left as an infant (day 8) and on the right as an adult. IPTG was discontinued at day 9, causing reversion to an albino phenotype in the adult. If the animal was left treated with IPTG, a fully pigmented adult animal would have been generated. (See color plate.) *(Modified from Cronin CA, Gluba W, Scrable H, et al: The lac operator-repressor system is functional in the mouse. Genes Dev 2001;15:1506–1517.)*

which reverted single *Tyr^{lacO}* pigmented transgenic animals to albino. The absence of detectable leakiness of the system was demonstrated by adding 10 mM of the lactose analogue IPTG to the drinking water of *Tyr^{lacO}-LacI^R* double transgenic animals, resulting in pigmentation of the animals to a level comparable to single *Tyr^{lacO}* animals (Fig. 4-9).[103] The *lac* regulatory system also functioned during embryogenesis because IPTG is transplacentally functional. The pigmentation of the embryonic eye at E9.0 in single *Tyr^{lacO}* transgenic animals was prevented in *Tyr^{lacO}-LacI^R* double transgenic animals but presented again in double transgenic animals in which the mother was treated with IPTG (Fig. 4-9). Reversibility of the system was demonstrated by switching the tyrosinase transgene on after it had been switched off and vice versa, switching it off after it had been switched on (Fig. 4-9).

The conditional *lac* operator-repressor system has considerable advantages over alternative conditional sys-

tems such as the *tet* system or Cre-mediated excision. The *tet* system relies on viral promoter elements, which harbor the potential of erratic expression of downstream elements in the mammalian genome, whereas the VP16 activating domain has also been reported to be toxic to mammalian cells. Cre-mediated excision harbors the advantage of manipulation of endogenous genomic targets, but Cre-excision is a one-time, irreversible event. The *lac* system is fully reversible and may regulate expression of endogenous genes by introduction of *lac* operators in an endogenous promoter of target genes by homologous recombination. Thus, the *lac* system holds the future promise to create fully reversible mouse models of heart disease and to elucidate gene expression in their natural context.

## Limitations to the Transgenic Approach

Although transgenesis and the availability of well-characterized cardiac-specific promoters, particularly the *α-MyHC* promoter, has led to the generation of several informative transgenic mice, resulting in the identification of intrinsic cardiac myocyte pathways that regulate hypertrophy and contractility.

However, the potential for high level expression of transgene protein has cast some doubt about the theoretical validity of some transgenic studies, most specifically when it concerns cardiac hypertrophy studies. According to this view, the development of cardiac dysfunction and cardiomyopathy in some models could result from a more direct toxic effect of the transgenes expressed at unphysiologically high levels[104] and/or from (unwanted) toxic effects of the protein. One study reports that green fluorescent protein (GFP) overexpression can result in cardiomyopathy in a copy-number dependent manner, and this has raised considerable concern about the validity of this promoter for hypertrophy questions.[105] However, most transgenic mice with α-MyHC promoter driven reporter genes (chloramphenicol acyltransferase, β-galactosidase, luciferase)[65,106,107] have not displayed a discernible cardiac phenotype, whereas other transgenes with potentially deleterious effects on cellular homeostasis (such as Cre recombinase) were found to be identical to wild-type mice.[101,102] In fact, a subset of α-MyHC promoter-driven transgenes are potently antihypertrophic and resistant to cardiomyopathic stimuli, as would be expected from the nature of their transgenes.[108,109] As such, the cardiomyopathic GFP transgenic mouse most likely presents a strong case both for the suspicion that the GFP reporter is not as innocuous as previously expected and can negatively interfere with the normal relationship of cellular homeostasis and/or stoichiometric composition of the sarcomere.

In addition, the mosaic nature of transgene expression, line-to-line variations in the level of expression, effects of the genomic site of integration, and wide differences in the copy number of the transgene can make discrimination of primary versus secondary effects quite challenging. Finally, gain-of-function studies do not necessarily indicate an endogenous role for a given candidate gene in the naturally occurring biologic pathway, whereas the overexpression of dominant negatives are confounded by their nonspecific inhibitory effects. In short, transgenics have been valuable as a starting point for generating genetically modified mouse models of human disease, but the added value of gene ablation has become increasingly clear in identifying the role of endogenous genes in complex cardiac physiologic endpoints.

# GENE TARGETING: ES CELL MANIPULATION IN THE MOUSE

## Principles of Gene Targeting Approaches

The advent of gene targeting coincides with technologic advances in ES cell technology in the early 1980s. Gene targeting has been extensively used in the last decade as a tool to study gene function in the mouse as a mammalian model system. Initially, the technique referred only to the disruption of a target gene in the murine germline by insertional disruption of a target gene by a selectable marker, such as the neomycin gene. Many of these germline-mutated or "knock out" (KO) mice have provided valuable information on the biologic function of the studied gene. It has become possible to produce mice with designed genetic alterations ranging from simple gene disruptions and point mutations to large genomic deletions encompassing several centimorgans.[110-112] These diverse technologic potentials have since become an invaluable tool to dissect the function of individual components of complex biologic systems, namely to produce mouse models of human disease. The simplest model of gene targeting encompasses the genetic disruption of a single gene, which will be transferred into the germline. Because these animals can be bred to homozygosity to create a germline null allele, they represent an excellent model for inherited human disease. Somatic gene targeting leads to embryonic lethality or early postnatal mortality in about 30% of cases. Therefore, germline gene-targeted mice do not necessarily represent the best technical approach to study gene function, especially for those studies involving the pathology and physiology of the postnatal and adult animal (see the section on conditional gene targeting).[113]

Over time, the gene-targeting paradigm has evolved further to include more sophisticated technical procedures that allow the selective disruption of any given gene in a selectable and spatio-temporal fashion. Collectively, these relatively new techniques are referred to as conditional gene targeting (see the section on conditional gene targeting). Deletion of the gene of interest in conditional mutants involves the inactivation of the target gene by a expression of a site-specific DNA recombinase (Cre or FLP recombinase) in conjunction with the introduction of two recombinase-specific recognition sequences (loxP or FRT) into the noncoding regions adjacent to the coding exon(s) of the target gene. Practically, conditional mutagenesis involves the generation of two separate mouse strains: one mouse harboring a *loxP* or *FRT* flanked gene segment created by homologous recombination in cultured murine ES cells and a second strain expressing the DNA recombinase. The conditional mutant is generated by cross-breeding strategies between the two genetically modified strains such that inactivation of the target gene becomes either restricted to the organ of interest, restricted in temporal expression of the DNA recombinase, or both (see the section on conditional gene targeting).

## ES Cell Lines

Widely used ES cell lines are derived from pluripotent cells from the inner cell mass of preimplanted blastocysts, and these lines contribute to the generation of several somatic tissues after reintroduction into blastocysts after genetic manipulation. A crucial step for gene targeting experiments is to keep the (genetically manipulated) ES cells uncommitted and this depends on the culture conditions. Currently, this is achieved by culturing ES cells on feeder cells, which also serve as an extracellular matrix on which the ES cell adhere and/or the presence of leukemia inhibitory factor (LIF) in the culture medium[114-116] (Fig. 4-10).

One major issue that requires attention before designing a gene targeting experiment is making the decision on what genetic background the mutation is studied. The most available ES cell line has the Sv129 background, a mouse strain from which ES cells are relatively easily retrieved. In addition, coat color markers have usually been used for the detection of chimerism.[114] The host embryo has a different genotype for coat color than the genetically altered ES cells. If successful integration has been accomplished during the blastocyst injection, a certain level of chimerism can be easily detected in the pattern formation of the coat.[114] For example, when Sv129 ES cells (white coat color) are used for homologous recombination *in vitro* and injected into blastocysts derived from the inbred C57BL/6 mouse line (black coat color), successful transfer of genetic material from the ES will be reflected in the coat color of the offspring, which display bicolored chimerism (black derived from C57BL/6 wild-type blastocysts and agouti/white derived from the Sv129 ES cells) (Fig. 4-11).

Recently, efforts have been made to have ES cells available from a more wide variety of inbred mouse strains such as C57BL/6, Balb/c, and the hitherto nonpermissive CBA/Ca.[49] One advantage of the availability of more diverse cell lines is that after reimplantation of ES cells in blastocysts from the same background, the mutation can be immediately studied in a pure inbred mouse strain. This situation is opposed by the more common situation in which the mutation is initially available in a mixed Sv129 and C57BL/6 (or Sv129 and Balb/c) background. If cogenic ES cells are used, coat color identification for chimerism is no longer available in the resulting offspring.

## Vector Design for Germline Knockout Experiments

Generally the first step of gene targeting experimentation is to isolate genomic clones that encompass the gene of interest. Preferably, the targeting vector is constructed with isogenic DNA (i.e., genetic material that harbors the same genetic background as the ES cells that are to be manipulated) because this increases the frequency of homologous recombination process.[117] Targeting vectors can be classified as either replacement or insertional vectors (Fig. 4-12). A replacement vector is linearized in such a way that the vector sequences remain colinear with the target genomic sequences. Chromosomal sequences (e.g., a target exon) are replaced by vector sequences (typically a neomycin gene) by a double crossover event involving the homologous flanking regions. Most mouse null mutants have been generated with this type of vector. An insertion vector (Fig. 4-12) is linearized within the region of homology, and homologous recombination results in duplication of genomic sequences.[118,119]

Three factors determine the frequency of homologous recombination and the success rate of generating null mutants: First, during the design of the targeting vector the frequency of homologous recombination is critically dependent on the length of the homologous sequences. The length of total homology between the targeting

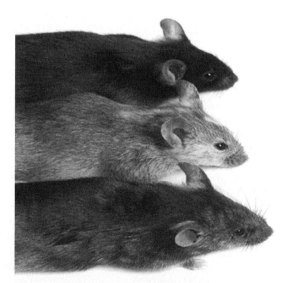

**FIGURE 4-11.** Chimeric mice. A chimeric mouse is created by mixing cells from a host embryo with ES cells and coat colors are used for the detection of chimerism. In this case, R1 ES cells were derived from 129/Sv-CP mice, which are agouti. The cells will give agouti coat color and dark eyes to the chimeras. When R1 cells are injected into C57BL/6 host blastocysts, the resulting chimera will be bicolored: black derived from the wild-type blastocyst and agouti derived from the R1 ES cells. In this picture, the top animal is not chimeric, the middle animal is 100% penetrant chimeric, and the bottom animal is partially chimeric. (See color plate.)

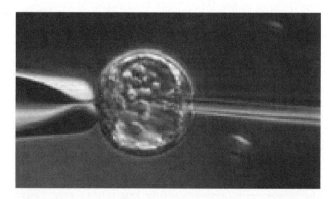

**FIGURE 4-10.** Microinjection of ES cells into the cavity of a mouse blastocyst. The blastocyst is held firmly with a holding pipette and the cavity of the blastocyst is punctured with a microneedle. In this photograph many ES cells have been deposited into the cavity and are resting on the inner cell mass of the blastocyst. (See color plate.)

vector and the genomic locus is typically at least 10 kb, with a minimal length for the short arm between 0.5 and 1 kb. Second, the exclusive use of isogenic DNA increases the frequency of homologous recombination. Third, absolute frequencies of homologous recombination seem to be locus dependent, probably because of differences in chromatin structure and accessibility for the enzymatic machinery involved.

The targeting vector carries several features, which allow for increased frequency of homologous recombination with the genomic sequences of interest (as opposed to chromosome insertion) and to select those ES cell populations with the mutated sequence. The most commonly used positive selection marker is a cassette carrying the neomycin resistance gene *(neo<sup>r</sup>)* under control of a viral promoter, which provides resistance against culture medium containing G418.[120] Alternatively, positive selection cassettes conferring resistance against the antibiotics hygromycin or puromycin have been reported.[121,122] Additional positive selection methods include the use of ES cells deficient for the hypoxanthine-phosphoribosyl-transferase *(HPRT)* gene.[123] As a result, the *HPRT* gene can be included in the targeting vector as an additional marker to screen transfectants in hypoxanthine aminopterin thymine (HAT)-medium.

An additional feature of many targeting vectors further enriches the process for clones that have undergone recombination as opposed to random chromosomal integration. This strategy, originally developed by Capecchi et al. is referred to as positive/negative selection and involves the addition of the *TK* gene from herpes simplex virus (HSV).[120] This gene is often inserted at the far end of the linearized targeting vector (Fig. 4-12). Because of this positioning of the negative marker, transfectants that have undergone true recombination with the chromosomal locus of interest have lost the *TK* gene, whereas cells that have the vector integrated randomly are vulnerable to elimination using toxins such as ganciclovir or 1-(2-deoxy-2-fluoro-β-D-arabino-furanosyl)-5-iodouracil (FIAU). These efforts for enrichments (*FIAU<sup>r</sup>/neo<sup>r</sup>* clones versus *neo<sup>r</sup>* clones) improve the efficiency of the system 3- to 10-fold.[120]

Finally, screening of correctly targeted clones is done by optimized Southern blot approaches and/or PCR strategies (Fig. 4-13). The latter strategy relies on one primer derived from the newly introduced selection cassette and the other primer hybridizing to genomic sequences outside the targeting constructs. To achieve this, the neo-flanking "short arm" is normally limited to 1 to 3 kb in length.[124]

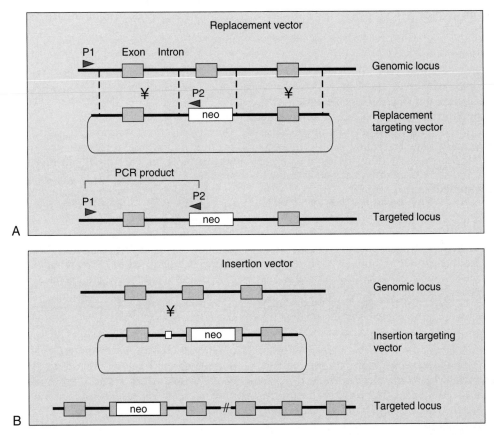

**FIGURE 4-12.** Replacement versus insertion targeting vectors. *A,* Sequence-replacement gene targeting vector for inactivating a gene of interest. Sequence replacement vectors are linearized outside the region of homology. A double crossover event involving the long and short arms of homology replaces the DNA sequences from the endogenous gene with those from the targeting vector. The *tk* gene is lost during this integration event and is degraded, allowing negative selection. Recombination of the indicated vector with the cognate gene would result in an allele lacking exon 2. *B,* Sequence-insertion gene targeting vector for inactivating a gene of interest. A sequence insertion vector is linearized before electroporation into ES cells and the site of linearization defines the site of integration into the genome. Insertion of the targeting vector into the cognate gene results in the duplication of exon 2 through 4 of the gene of interest, interfering with the transcription of the gene.

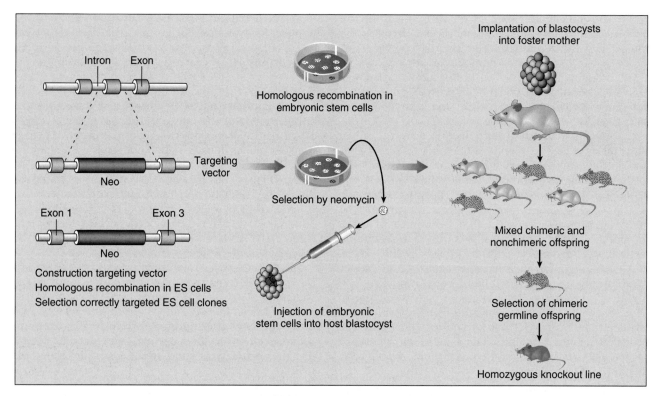

**FIGURE 4-13.** Overview gene targeting. Scheme for generating heterozygous and homozygous gene knockout mice by homologous recombination in mouse ES cells.

Although the generation of a simple somatic KO is often relatively straightforward (Fig. 4-13), several pitfalls in experimental design have only become apparent as the number of publications describing mouse mutants has increased. The following sections highlight some of these difficulties and shows how they may be avoided if the targeting vector is designed properly.

### Incomplete Knockouts

Following gene targeting the null mutant mouse should be checked for residual protein expressed from the targeted locus. Because in most cases large sections of coding sequences remain present in the genomic sequence with replacement or insertional vectors for the generation of null mutants, truncated or mutant forms of the protein may still be expressed. In many cases, the replacement sequence removes one or several internal exons, so that proteins truncated at the C-terminal part may still be formed, which may acquire new or even transdominant properties over other proteins. Examples of KO experiments in which residual protein expression resulting from exon skipping was observed include the DNA methyltransferase gene, the *CFTR* locus, the *L1* gene, and estrogen receptor alpha.[125,126] Although these studies were not intentionally designed this way, some of these mutants are allelic variants with interesting phenotypes of their own, showing partial rescue of a more severe null phenotype.

### Removal of Coding Regions or Regulatory Elements in Other Genes

One approach to circumvent residual protein expression or truncated protein formation may be to remove all coding exons. Significant pitfalls of this approach, however, are the possibilities to (1) create the unintended loss of, as yet, unidentified genes residing in introns or encoded by the opposite strand or (2) remove the regulatory elements governing expression of unrelated genes. The latter issue seems to be more relevant for clustered gene families, as was observed in the case of the myogenic regulatory factor 4 *(MRF4)* KOs, which were simultaneously carried out by independent groups. Three different alleles of similar design (deletions encompassing different parts of the *MRF4* genomic locus) resulted in phenotypes varying from complete viability to embryonic lethality. The differences in phenotype were subsequently demonstrated to be due to the deletion of positive regulatory elements that led to reduced expression of the neighboring *MRF5* gene. As such, the *MRF4* KO unexpectedly represented a functional *MRF4-/-/MRF5-/-* double KO.[127]

### Selection Cassette Interference

One concern associated with the design of replacement or insertional null targeting vectors is that transcription from strong promoters driving the selection marker may interfere with the expression of neighboring genes.

A series of experiments from Fiering et al.[128] confirmed this assumption: they targeted the 5'DNAse hypersensitive site 2 *(5'HS2)* of the locus control region (LCR) of the β-globin gene. A straightforward replacement technique to delete coding regions of the *5'HS2* gene by a PGK-neo cassette resulted in a considerable reduction of β-globin gene expression and homozygous mutant mice died *in utero* at the time point of fetal liver hematopoiesis. Removal of the selection marker by FLP-mediated site-specific recombination restored viability and globin expression was essentially normal, indicating a predominant phenotypic effect of the selection marker. Currently, it is generally accepted that (if possible) selection marker cassettes should be removed after homologous recombination.

## Introducing Subtle Mutations in the Murine Germline

Subtle mutations such as the insertion of stop codons or amino acid substitutions in the germline may be achieved by a number of strategies, which are outlined in Figure 4-14. The first approach is referred to as the "hit and run" technique (also called "in and out") during which a mutation is introduced in a two-step procedure.[129,130] The first step (the "hit" or "in") involves

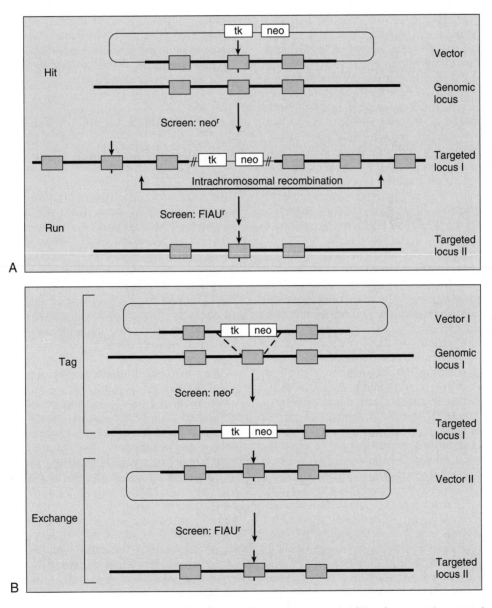

**FIGURE 4-14.** Targeting vectors for introducing a subtle mutation into the mouse genome. *A,* A hit and run targeting vector is a sequence insertion vector. The plasmid backbone contains both positive *(neo)* and negative *(tk)* selection markers. The segment of homology is modified, generally by site-directed mutagenesis, to contain a mutation of interest. In this example, a mutation is introduced in exon 2. In the "hit" step, the entire targeting vector is inserted into the genome at the site of interest. The ES cells are selected by the positive marker. In the "run" step, a correctly targeted ES cell clone is grown in the presence of FIAU, which selects for survival of clones that have undergone spontaneous intrachromosomal recombination, which results in the deletion of duplicated gene sequences, plasmid sequences, and the drug resistance markers. Depending on the precise site of the intrachromosomal recombination event, some ES cell clones retain the targeted point mutation and can be identified by further analyses. *B,* A highly similar, alternative approach to introduce subtle mutations in the mouse genome makes use of tag and exchange vectors.

homologous recombination using an insertional targeting vector designed so that recombination will lead to duplication of genomic sequences carrying the mutation and the concomitant integration of two selection markers (e.g., *neo* and *TK* as positive and negative markers, respectively). In the second step (the "run" or "out") selection against *TK* enriches for a rare intrachromosomal recombination event that excises the integrated vector sequences including the negative selection marker. Depending on the actual position of this crossover, the mutation introduced in the first step will remain incorporated in the genome, or the wild-type allele may be restored (Fig. 4-10).

The "tag and exchange" strategy involves two sequential recombination events using two separate targeting vectors (Fig. 4-14).[131] The first step involves the introduction of a positive and a negative selection marker, although only positive selection is applied in this stage. In the second round of gene targeting, a vector is used that carries a subtle mutation in the flanking region of homology, and negative selection is applied in this stage to enrich for clones that have undergone replacement of sequences introduced in the first round of recombination. The tag and exchange approach may save time if a series of subtle mutations within the same locus is envisioned. For example, Moore et al.[132] using the latter double-replacement strategy created a series of different mutants of the prion gene. Both strategies critically depend on the efficiency of negative selection for which either *TK* or *HPRT* (in *hprt*–ES cells) have been used as markers.

A modification of the tag and exchange protocol, termed "plug and socket," was developed to circumvent negative selection, which may be hampered by a background of clones that carry a nonfunctional negative marker gene without having undergone homologous recombination. In the plug and socket approach, the first step involves introduction of the *neo* gene together with a second positive but nonfunctional selection marker, such as a deletion mutant (Δ*hprt*) of the *hprt* gene. Via homologous recombination with the *HPRT* sequences, provided by the second targeting vector, functionality of the *HPRT* gene is restored allowing for positive selection in the second targeting step.[133] A disadvantage of this approach is that the *HPRT* selection cassette is cointroduced with the mutation.

Conventional gene targeting approaches have been especially valuable in identifying genes that are involved in critical aspects of embryogenesis, including *NKX 2.5*,[134] *GATA-4*,[135,136] *MEF-2*,[137] the *HAND* genes,[137-140] *RXRα*,[141] and several others.[142] Because the ablation occurs via a site-specific recombination event, issues of copy number, site of integration, and mosaicism are irrelevant. A subset of the most informative gene-targeted mouse models have been based on the KO of genes that are expressed in a cardiac muscle-restricted fashion, including mutations in cytoskeletal[143-145] and calcium-cycling genes.[146,147] However, gene targeting carries with it the risks of gene redundancy (particularly an issue for highly conserved transcription factors and signaling molecules that have several closely related family members that share overlapping expression patterns), inherent

costs of time and labor, and the difficulties of interpreting whether any adult phenotype that arises actually reflects an earlier developmental effect. Because many of the most intriguing candidate genes are widely expressed, it can also be unclear as to whether these genes are impacting cardiac physiology within cardiac myocytes or via secondary effects in neighboring cell types or integrative signals from other organ systems. Finally, and perhaps most important, early embryonic lethality in conventional gene-targeted animals can prevent an examination of the role of the gene of interest in the physiology of the postnatal heart.[113] These last two considerations formed the impetus for the development of new strategies to control the onset of the gene ablation in time and space (i.e., conditional gene targeting). Another advantage of conditional gene targeting is the availability of a more versatile strategy to introduce nonselectable mutations based on the Cre-loxP recombination system.[100] These and other considerations are outlined in the next section.

## CONDITIONAL GENE TARGETING

### Principle of Conditional Gene Targeting: The Cre/loxP Paradigm

Controllable chromosomal modification is a long-desired goal for DNA transfer systems. The low frequency of integration into active regions of chromosomes and the concomitant gene silencing that may occur are major problems with many gene expression paradigms. New techniques are now available that allow permanent modification of chromosomes at specific sites. The vast majority of these systems make use of site-specific recombinases, which catalyze the introduction or excision of DNA fragments. Currently, the crystal structure of four members of this family of enzymes (Cre, XerD, FLP, and HP1) illustrates their conservation in terms of three-dimensional structure and catalytic regions.[100]

Cre-mediated recombination between two loxP sites results in the reciprocal exchange of DNA strands between these sites, such that when the two loxP sites are located in the same direction on a linear DNA molecule, Cre-mediated recombination results in the excision of the loxP-flanked DNA segment as a circular molecule leaving a single loxP site on each DNA product. When two loxP sites are orientated in opposite orientations, Cre mediates inversion of the loxP flanked sequence. Cre contains amino acid sequences that direct its translocation into the eukaryotic nucleus, which is a requirement for genetic engineering in mammalian species, and addition of a nuclear localization signal did not increase its activity in mammalian cells. Only a few other recombinases besides Cre have been shown to exhibit activity in mammalian cells. Of these the yeast derived FLP recombinase is the best characterized example, and recognizes a short DNA target designated an FRT. FLP recombinase exhibits optimal activity at a temperature of 30°C (although mutational analysis of FLP has resulted in a mutant FLPe, which shows improved thermostability and activity at 37°C).[148] Accordingly, newer targeting vectors make use of dual site-specific recombination events to increase the efficiency of gene-targeting events in mice, involving an initial FLPe/FRT target-mediated early recombination event in ES cells and a later Cre-loxP mediated event in the gene-targeted mouse.[148,149]

Although recent reports have documented the successful use of the FLP/FRT system to create tissue-specific genomic deletions in mice and FLPe transgenic deleter mice have been reported,[149] most targeted gene modifications have made use of Cre deleter mice in conjunction with loxP carrying gene-targeted mice. In a landmark study by Gu et al.,[150] the Cre/loxP system was first used to knock out a gene in a tissue-specific manner. This specific characteristic of the Cre/loxP system to delete genes in a tissue-specific manner indicates the suitability of this system to study genes for which germline KO experiments have yielded an embryonic lethal phenotype. A general strategy for the Cre/loxP-mediated introduction of a nonselectable mutation is outlined in Figure 4-15. Using a replacement type of targeting vector, a positive selection marker followed by a negative selection marker is flanked by two loxP sites and the nonselectable mutation (e.g., a point mutation in an exon) is contained within one arm of the targeting vector. After homologous recombination and screening for the cotransfer of the mutation (e.g., by a newly introduced restriction site), Cre recombinase is introduced by transient transfection. ES cell clones that have excised the loxP-flanked markers can subsequently be enriched by negative selection (e.g., against *TK* or *HPRT*).

## Vector Design and Generation of loxP Flanked Alleles

The first requirement for Cre/loxP-base conditional mutants is the generation of an ES cell derived mouse strain that harbors a loxP-flanked DNA sequence in the gene of interest, typically a crucial exon for the protein product of that gene. Several strategies are in use to conditionally inactivate endogenous genes. One strategy employs Cre/loxP recombination for the conditional inactivation of the target gene and FLP/FRT recombination to remove the selection marker gene from the ES cell genome. Both recombinase-mediated steps can be performed in either ES cells by transient transfection with a recombinase expressing vector or more conveniently *in vivo* using Cre and FLP-deleter mouse strains.

The main objective in designing a conditional construct is that the expression of the target gene should not be disturbed by the loxP sites (as opposed to somatic gene targeting) but that it becomes inactivated (or otherwise modified) on Cre-mediated recombination *in vivo*. A conditional construct contains a positive selection marker (e.g., neomycin) flanked by two ~1- to 5-kb regions of homology to the target gene and optionally a *TK* negative selection marker. In contrast to conventional gene targeting, the positive/negative selection markers do not disrupt or displace one of the exons but are placed into an intron and flanked by two FRT sites next to a single loxP site. A second loxP site is placed into one of the homology arms such that both loxP sites are flanking one or more exons of the target gene (Fig. 4-15). Of course, careful sequencing of especially the exon homology sequences of the targeting construct should

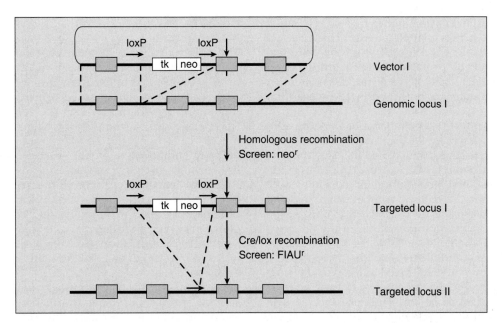

**FIGURE 4-15.** Cre/loxP mediated gene targeting. Tissue-specific gene inactivation is based on the excision of a loxP (triangle)-flanked exon in Cre-expressing cells. Cre-loxP strategy for tissue specific inactivation of a given gene in mice. A critical exon of the gene of interest is flanked by loxP sites by gene targeting in ES cells using a replacement vector. With the expression of Cre in the correctly targeted ES cells, the positive and negative selection markers are removed and a loxP flanked ("floxed") exon is obtained. From these floxed ES cells chimeric mice are generated. Crossing of these floxed mice with Cre deleter strains will result in deletion of the exon (and thereby disruption of gene function). Spatiotemporally controlled somatic mutagenesis is achieved by tissue-specific expression of a ligand-dependent Cre recombinase.

be performed to avoid the transfer of undesired mutations into the target gene. This double-loxP/double-FRT arrangement is introduced in ES cells through homologous recombination and transmitted though the germline of chimeric mice. On crossing with a FLP-deleter strain, the neomycin cassette is deleted during germline transmission resulting in a conditional, loxP flanked allele; crossing to a Cre deleter strain results in a conventional null allele.

Alternatively, both alleles can be obtained by transient transfection of the homologous recombined cells with a Cre or FLP expression vector, but later manipulation during tissue culture requires more effort and increases the chance that the targeted clones lose their germline potency.

One excellent cardiovascular example of the Cre/loxP system to avoid the issue of embryonic lethality involves the tissue-restricted deletion of the gp130 receptor.[151] Cytokines such as the individual members of the interleukin 6 (IL-6), LIF, ciliary neurotrophic factor (CNTF), or their downstream gp130-dependent signaling components play a critical signaling role in the regulation of mammalian physiology.[152,153] Germline KO mice with a complete deficiency in the cytokine signal transducer gp130 die prenatally because of defects in diverse embryonic compartments, making it hard to assess the role for gp130-mediated signaling in postnatal cardiac homeostasis. Hirota et al.[151] used the Cre/loxP strategy to achieve a ventricular chamber-restricted deletion of gp130 by creating gene-targeted mice harboring a loxP flanked gp130 locus (Fig. 4-16). In a separate study these authors created a line of mice that harbor the Cre coding sequence in the genomic locus of the myosin light chain 2v (MLC2v) gene by homologous recombination (MLC2v Cre knock in). Cross-breeding of the gp130 "floxed" allele mice with the MLC2v Cre knockin mice resulted in a unique line of mice, in which the expression of Cre is restricted to the ventricular cell lineage and leads to loss of gp130 from the cell membrane and a lack of responsiveness to gp130-related cytokine signaling. This allowed the assessment of gp130-mediated signaling in the postnatal myocardium (Fig. 4-16).

During the past few years, a number of Cre expressing mice have been described for the cardiovascular system. These mouse lines have been created by using different tissue-specific promoters that drive expression of the Cre recombinase; the possibilities for creating conditional mutant mice have now substantially expanded, depending on the spatial, developmental, and tissue-specific expression pattern characteristics of the promoter construct used (Table 4-4).[74,95,97,102,154-162] However, despite optimism about the Cre/loxP system, it is presently unclear whether floxed alleles can be completely deleted or whether incomplete KO will be more typical. In the example of the ventricular-specific deletion of the gp130 KO, near complete deletion of gp130 protein was observed yet this sufficed to detect the concomitant phenotype. However, incomplete Cre-mediated recombination might prove to be disappointing in cases in which minimal residual activity of the target gene may still interfere with the resulting phenotype.

Conditional mutants have been used to address various biologic questions that could not be resolved with germline mutants, often because a null allele results in an embryonic or neonatal lethal phenotype. If the main question to answer concerns the role of different cell types in a physiologic process, the use of noninducible, cell type-specific Cre strains is presently the most pragmatic choice because a collection of tissue-specific strains is already available (Table 4-4). A good example of this approach is the comparison of the cell type-specific inactivation of the insulin receptor in skeletal muscle, pancreas, and liver. Cell type specific gene targeting revealed a prime role for the liver and not the skeletal muscle in glucose homeostasis and insulin signaling in pancreatic insulin secretion. In the selection of a Cre transgenic strain for a particular experiment it is important to be aware of the developmental stage at which the chosen line starts to delete the target, because many promoter regions used to drive Cre recombinase expression are active before birth.

Inducible gene targeting may be especially of use to analyze gene function in the adult animals because it facilitates to perform gene inactivation studies in animals that have undergone normal embryonic development. Furthermore, it permits the investigation of the effect of gene inactivation after the onset of a chronic or acute disease. This aspect is of particular interest in the validation of genes for pharmaceutical drug development, because genes can be inactivated in the context of a fully developed disease. The use of inducible gene targeting in mouse models of human disease can provide an ideal surrogate for the treatment of patients with antagonistic drugs.

## PERSPECTIVE

The ability to modify the mouse genome by random integration of transgenes or at predetermined sites by homologous recombination in ES cells has greatly advanced the understanding of mammalian gene function in health and disease. The capacity to trigger site-specific gene recombination selectively in cardiac muscle cells using the Cre/loxP system, or in other defined components of the cardiovascular system, has obvious attractiveness as a means to circumvent irrelevant lethality resulting from extraneous organs. In addition, it allows one to preclude cardiovascular phenotypes that are merely the consequence of global or systemic defects and pinpoint intrinsic ("cell-autonomous") versus nonautonomous mechanisms for a given cell background in development or disease.[113]

Without doubt, the number of useful tissue-specific and/or inducible transgenic Cre mice will rapidly increase in the future. The Jackson Laboratory (http:// www.jax.org) and the European Mutant Mouse Archive (http://www.emma.rm.cnr.it) collect and distribute validated strains. A database for Cre-expressing lines is established (http://www.mshri.on.ca/nagy/cre.htm). Other site-specific recombinases, such as the yeast

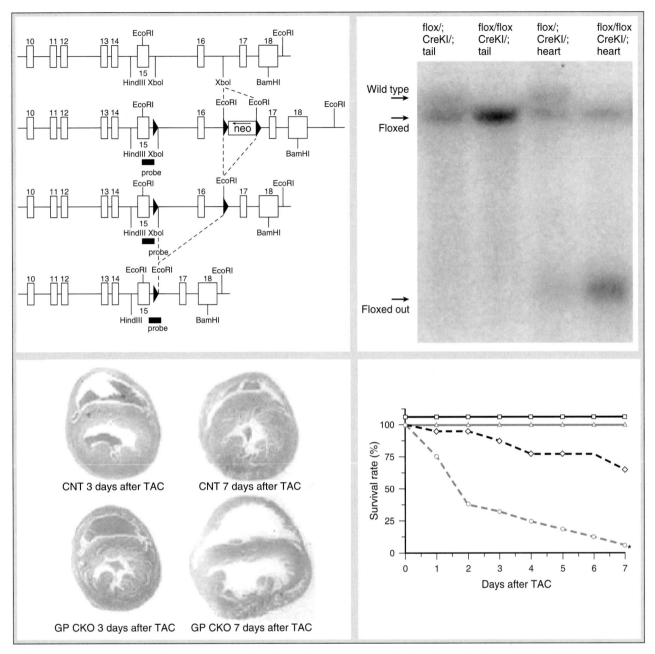

**FIGURE 4-16.** *MLC2v-Cre gp130lox.* Outline of the strategy to achieve ventricular chamber-restricted deletion of the *gp130* receptor gene. *A*, Schematic representation of exon structures in the part of the *gp130* gene encoding the transmembrane domain (exon 16). Targeting vector and mutant *gp130* gene are shown. The closed box (probe) corresponds to the sequence used for Southern hybridization in *(B)*. Exon numbers are indicated. *B*, Southern genotype analysis. The Southern blot, carrying adult mouse tail and ventricle DNA digested with EcoRI, hybridized with a probe that discriminates between the floxed, floxed out, and wild-type allele. The genotypes for the samples are *gp130flox/1, MLC2vCreKI/1,* tail (lane 1), *gp130flox/flox, MLC2vCreKI/1,* tail (lane 2), *gp130flox/1, MLC2vCreKI/1,* heart (lane 3), and *gp130flox/flox, MLC2vCreKI/1,* heart (lane 4). The position of the bands representing the *gp130 1* (wild-type), *gp130* flox (floxed allele), and *gp130* delta (floxed-out allele) alleles are shown. *C*, Phenotypic effects of biomechanical stress on gp130 conditional KO mice. Pathologic analysis of the *gp130* conditional KO hearts. Histologic sections of hearts from 3 days and 7 days after transmission attenuation correction (TAC) in concentrative nucleoside transporter (CNT) and glycoprotein (GP) conditional knockout (CKO) mice, demonstrating severe dilation of the left ventricular chamber following biomechanical stress. *D*, Survival analysis of *gp130* conditional KO mice after TAC. Each group started with 15 (CNT with TAC, diamonds), 21 (GP CKO with TAC, circles), 3 (CNT with sham-operation, squares), and 3 (GP CKO with sham-operation, triangles) mice. Differences in survival rates between the CNT and GP CKO groups after TAC were significant by Peto-Peto-Wilcoxon test (*, *p* < 0.001). *(Modified from Hirota H, Chen J, Betz UA, et al: Loss of a gp130 cardiac muscle cell survival pathway is a critical event in the onset of heart failure during biomechanical stress. Cell 1999;97:189–198.)*

FLP recombinase and the bacterial β-recombinase, are also active in mammalian cells and in mice. Mutated versions of FLP recombinase might have an efficiency comparable to Cre. Combined use of FLP and/or β-recombinase with Cre would theoretically permit highly flexible engineering strategies, allowing independently controlled genetic modifications. Future applications of genetic modification in mice may become limited merely by the scientist's imagination and by the capacity of animal facilities.

■ ■ ■

## TABLE 4-4   EXAMPLES OF (INDUCIBLE) CRE RECOMBINASE EXPRESSING MOUSE STRAINS

| System/Control Element | Site of Expression | References |
| --- | --- | --- |
| **Ubiquitous** | | |
| MX1 promoter | Ubiquitous, inducible | 97 |
| *Cre deleter strains* | | |
| LCK promoter | T cells | 155 |
| α-Crystallin promoter | Eye lens | |
| CD19 promoter | B cells | |
| CamKII promoter | Hippocampal neurons | 94, 95 |
| WAP promoter | Mammary gland | 156 |
| α-MyHC promoter | Cardiomyocytes | 157 |
| MLC-2v (knockin) | Ventricular myocytes | 158 |
| AP2 | Adipose tissue | 159 |
| *CreER (tamoxifen inducible)* | | |
| α-MyHC promoter | Cardiomyocytes | 102 |
| Wnt promoter | Embryonic neural tube | 74 |
| *CrePR (RU486 inducible)* | | |
| α-MyHC promoter | Cardiomyocytes | 101 |
| CamKII promoter | Brain | 161 |
| K14 promoter | Keratinocytes | 162 |

Ligand-activated recombination may also be useful to evaluate the real clinical potential of the disease pathways found in mouse models. The difficulty of germline gene manipulation in larger animals indicates the value of new investigative strategies that use peptide inhibitors, neutralizing antibodies, and somatic gene transfer with smart vectors that allow long-term gene expression. The many quantitatively different end points for complex *in vivo* cardiac phenotypes should drive us on to the next frontier that lies at the boundaries of genomic databases, physiology, and human disease. Given the difficulty of establishing cause-and-effect relationships between given complex genotypes and *in vivo* physiologic phenotypes in human populations, it is becoming increasingly likely that the molecular pathways will initially be identified in the mouse and subsequently corroborated in candidate gene studies in human populations.[113]

## REFERENCES

1. Chien KR: Genes and physiology: Molecular physiology in genetically engineered animals. J Clin Invest 1996;97:901–909.
2. Doevendans PA, Daemen MJ, de Muinck ED, Smits JF: Cardiovascular phenotyping in mice. Cardiovasc Res 1998;39:34–49.
3. James JF, Hewett TE, Robbins J: Cardiac physiology in transgenic mice. Circ Res 1998;82:407–415.
4. Tanaka N, Dalton N, Mao L, et al: Transthoracic echocardiography in models of cardiac disease in the mouse. Circulation 1996;94:1109–1117.
5. Gardin JM, Siri FM, Kitsis RN, et al: Echocardiographic assessment of left ventricular mass and systolic function in mice. Circ Res 1995;76:907–914.
6. Libby P: Lesion versus lumen. Nat Med 1995;1:17–18.
7. Lin MC, Rockman HA, Chien KR: Heart and lung disease in engineered mice. Nat Med 1995;1:749–1751.
8. Jacobs RE, Fraser SE: Magnetic resonance microscopy of embryonic cell lineages and movements. Science 1994;263:681–684.
9. Smith BR, Johnson GA, Groman EV, Linney E: Magnetic resonance microscopy of mouse embryos. Proc Natl Acad Sci USA 1994;91:3530–3533.
10. Rockman HA, Ono S, Ross RS, et al: Molecular and physiological alterations in murine ventricular dysfunction. Proc Natl Acad Sci USA 1994;91:2694–2698.
11. Chien KR: Molecular advances in cardiovascular biology. Science 1993;260:916–917.
12. Dyson E, Sucov HM, Kubalak SW, et al: Atrial-like phenotype is associated with embryonic ventricular failure in retinoid X receptor alpha -/- mice. Proc Natl Acad Sci USA 1995;92:7386–7390.
13. Milano CA, Allen LF, Rockman HA, et al: Enhanced myocardial function in transgenic mice overexpressing the beta 2-adrenergic receptor. Science 1994;264:582–586.
14. Hunter JJ, Tanaka N, Rockman HA, et al: Ventricular expression of a MLC-2v-ras fusion gene induces cardiac hypertrophy and selective diastolic dysfunction in transgenic mice. J Biol Chem 1995;270:23173–23178.
15. De Windt LJ, Willems J, Reneman RS, et al: An improved isolated, left ventricular ejecting, murine heart model: Functional and metabolic evaluation. Pflugers Arch 1999;437:182–190.
16. Grupp IL, Subramaniam A, Hewett TE, et al: Comparison of normal, hypodynamic, and hyperdynamic mouse hearts using isolated work-performing heart preparations. Am J Physiol 1993;265:H1401–1410.
17. Georgakopoulos D, Mitzner WA, Chen CH, et al: In vivo murine left ventricular pressure-volume relations by miniaturized conductance micromanometry. Am J Physiol 1998;274:H1416–1422.
18. Dumont EA, Reutelingsperger CP, Smits JF, et al: Real-time imaging of apoptotic cell-membrane changes at the single-cell level in the beating murine heart. Nat Med 2001;7:1352–1355.
19. Biggers JD, Whittingham DG, Donahue RP: The pattern of energy metabolism in the mouse oocyte and zygote. Proc Natl Acad Sci USA 1967;58:560–567.
20. Brinster RL: Lactate dehydrogenase activity in the preimplanted mouse embryo. Biochim Biophys Acta 1965;110:439–441.
21. Brinster RL: Cultivation of the mammalian embryo. In Rhothblat C (ed): Growth, Nutrition and Metabolism of Cells in Culture. New York, Academic Press, 1972, pp 251–286.
22. McLaren A: Studies on the transfer of fertilized mouse eggs to uterine foster-mothers. I. Factors affecting the implantation and survival of native and transferred eggs. J Exp Biol 1956;33:394–416.
23. McLaren A: Successful development and birth of mice cultivated in vitro as early embryos. Nature 1958;182:877–878.
24. Capecchi MR: High efficiency transformation by direct microinjection of DNA into cultured mammalian cells. Cell 1980;22:479–488.
25. Gurdon JB: The Croonian lecture, 1976: Egg cytoplasm and gene control in development. Proc R Soc Lond B Biol Sci 1977;198:211–247.
26. Brinster RL, Chen HY, Trumbauer ME, Avarbock MR: Translation of globin messenger RNA by the mouse ovum. Nature 1980;283:499–501.
27. Jaenisch R, Mintz B: Simian virus 40 DNA sequences in DNA of healthy adult mice derived from preimplantation blastocysts injected with viral DNA. Proc Natl Acad Sci USA 1974;71:1250–1254.
28. Gordon JW, Scangos GA, Plotkin DJ, et al: Genetic transformation of mouse embryos by microinjection of purified DNA. Proc Natl Acad Sci USA 1980;77:7380–7384.
29. Wagner EF, Stewart TA, Mintz B: The human beta-globin gene and a functional viral thymidine kinase gene in developing mice. Proc Natl Acad Sci USA 1981;78:5016–5020.
30. Wagner TE, Hoppe PC, Jollick JD, et al: Microinjection of a rabbit beta-globin gene into zygotes and its subsequent expression in adult mice and their offspring. Proc Natl Acad Sci USA 1981;78:6376–6380.
31. Costantini F, Lacy E: Introduction of a rabbit beta-globin gene into the mouse germ line. Nature 1981;294:92–94.
32. Brinster RL, Chen HY, Trumbauer M, et al: Somatic expression of herpes thymidine kinase in mice following injection of a fusion gene into eggs. Cell 1981;27:223–231.
33. Harbers K, Jahner D, Jaenisch R: Microinjection of cloned retroviral genomes into mouse zygotes: Integration and expression in the animal. Nature 1981;293:540–542.
34. Palmiter RD, Brinster RL, Hammer RE, et al: Dramatic growth of mice that develop from eggs microinjected with metallothionein-growth hormone fusion genes. Biotechnology 1992;24:429–433.

35. Palmiter RD, Brinster RL: Germ-line transformation of mice. Annu Rev Genet 1986;20:465-499.
36. Grosveld F, van Assendelft GB, Greaves DR, Kollias G: Position-independent, high-level expression of the human beta-globin gene in transgenic mice. Cell 1987;51:975-985.
37. Chien KR: Genomic circuits and the integrative biology of cardiac diseases. Nature 2000;407:227-232.
38. Yokode M, Hammer RE, Ishibashi S, et al: Diet-induced hypercholesterolemia in mice: Prevention by overexpression of LDL receptors. Science 1990;250:1273-1275.
39. Chiesa G, Hobbs HH, Koschinsky ML, et al: Reconstitution of lipoprotein(a) by infusion of human low density lipoprotein into transgenic mice expressing human apolipoprotein(a). J Biol Chem 1992;267:24369-24374.
40. Schaefer EM, Viard V, Morin J, et al: A new transgenic mouse model of chronic hyperglycemia. Diabetes 1994;43:143-153.
41. Brinster RL, Allen JM, Behringer RR, et al: Introns increase transcriptional efficiency in transgenic mice. Proc Natl Acad Sci USA 1988;85:836-840.
42. Hofmann SL, Russell DW, Brown MS, et al: Overexpression of low density lipoprotein (LDL) receptor eliminates LDL from plasma in transgenic mice. Science 1988;239:1277-1281.
43. Schedl A, Montoliu L, Kelsey G, Schutz G: A yeast artificial chromosome covering the tyrosinase gene confers copy number-dependent expression in transgenic mice. Nature 1993;362:258-261.
44. Peterson KR, Clegg CH, Huxley C, et al: Transgenic mice containing a 248-kilobase human beta locus yeast artificial chromosome display proper developmental control of human globin genes. Trans Assoc Am Physicians 1993;106:101-109.
45. McCormick SP, Linton MF, Young SG: Expression of P1 DNA in mammalian cells and transgenic mice. Genet Anal Tech Appl 1994;11:158-164.
46. Linton MF, Farese RV Jr, Chiesa G, et al: Transgenic mice expressing high plasma concentrations of human apolipoprotein B100 and lipoprotein(a). J Clin Invest 1993;92:3029-3037.
47. Frazer KA, Narla G, Zhang JL, et al: The apolipoprotein(a) gene is regulated by sex hormones and acute-phase inducers in YAC transgenic mice. Nat Genet 1995;9:424-431.
48. Choi TK, Hollenbach PW, Pearson BE, et al: Transgenic mice containing a human heavy chain immunoglobulin gene fragment cloned in a yeast artificial chromosome. Nat Genet 1993;4:117-123.
49. Hogan B, Beddington R, Constantini F, et al: Manipulating the mouse embryo: A laboratory manual. Plainview, NY, Cold Spring Harbor Laboratory Press, 1994.
50. Pinkert C: Transgenic Animal Technology. A Laboratory Handbook. San Diego, Academic Press, 1994.
51. Wassarman PM DM: Guide to Techniques in Mouse Development. San Diego, Academic Press, 1993.
52. Fuller SJ, Chien KR: Genetic engineering of cardiac muscle cells: In vitro and in vivo. Genet Eng 1994;16:17-31.
53. Hunter JJ, Zhu H, Lee KJ, et al: Targeting gene expression to specific cardiovascular cell types in transgenic mice. Hypertension 1993;22:608-617.
54. Chien KR, Shimizu M, Hoshijima M, et al: Toward molecular strategies for heart disease—past, present, future. Jpn Circ J 1997;61:91-118.
55. Navankasattusas S, Sawadogo M, van Bilsen M, et al: The basic helix-loop-helix protein upstream stimulating factor regulates the cardiac ventricular myosin light-chain 2 gene via independent cis regulatory elements. Mol Cell Biol 1994;14:7331-7339.
56. Shubeita HE, Martinson EA, Van Bilsen M, et al: Transcriptional activation of the cardiac myosin light chain 2 and atrial natriuretic factor genes by protein kinase C in neonatal rat ventricular myocytes. Proc Natl Acad Sci USA 1992;89:1305-1309.
57. Zhu H, Nguyen VT, Brown AB, et al: A novel, tissue-restricted zinc finger protein (HF-1b) binds to the cardiac regulatory element (HF-1b/MEF-2) in the rat myosin light-chain 2 gene. Mol Cell Biol 1993;13:4432-4444.
58. Ebrecht G, Rupp H, Jacob R: Alterations of mechanical parameters in chemically skinned preparations of rat myocardium as a function of isoenzyme pattern of myosin. Basic Res Cardiol 1982;77:220-234.
59. Jacob R, Kissling G, Ebrecht G, et al: Cardiac alterations at the myofibrillar level: Is a redistribution of the myosin isoenzyme pattern decisive for cardiac failure in haemodynamic overload? Eur Heart J 1984;5(Suppl. F):13-26.
60. Pagani ED, Julian FJ: Rabbit papillary muscle myosin isozymes and the velocity of muscle shortening. Circ Res 1984;54:586-594.
61. Schwartz K, Lecarpentier Y, Martin JL, et al: Myosin isoenzymic distribution correlates with speed of myocardial contraction. J Mol Cell Cardiol 1981;13:1071-1075.
62. Gulick J, Subramaniam A, Neumann J, Robbins J: Isolation and characterization of the mouse cardiac myosin heavy chain genes. J Biol Chem 1991;266:9180-9185.
63. Rindt H, Subramaniam A, Robbins J: An in vivo analysis of transcriptional elements in the mouse alpha- myosin heavy chain gene promoter. Transgenic Res 1995;4:397-405.
64. Subramaniam A, Jones WK, Gulick J, et al: Tissue-specific regulation of the alpha-myosin heavy chain gene promoter in transgenic mice. J Biol Chem 1991;266:24613-24620.
65. Subramaniam A, Gulick J, Neumann J, et al: Transgenic analysis of the thyroid-responsive elements in the alpha-cardiac myosin heavy chain gene promoter. J Biol Chem 1993;268:4331-4336.
66. Sanbe A, Gulick J, Hayes E, et al: Myosin light chain replacement in the heart. Am J Physiol Heart Circ Physiol 2000;279:H1355-1364.
67. Pawloski-Dahm CM, Song G, Kirkpatrick DL, et al: Effects of total replacement of atrial myosin light chain-2 with the ventricular isoform in atrial myocytes of transgenic mice. Circulation 1998;97:1508-13.
68. Palermo J, Gulick J, Colbert M, et al: Transgenic remodeling of the contractile apparatus in the mammalian heart. Circ Res 1996;78:504-509.
69. Robbins J, Palermo J, Rindt H: In vivo definition of a cardiac specific promoter and its potential utility in remodeling the heart. Ann NY Acad Sci 1995;752:492-505.
70. Kelly R, Alonso S, Tajbakhsh S, et al: Myosin light chain 3F regulatory sequences confer regionalized cardiac and skeletal muscle expression in transgenic mice. J Cell Biol 1995;129:383-396.
71. Kelly RG, Zammit PS, Mouly V, et al: Dynamic left/right regionalisation of endogenous myosin light chain 3F transcripts in the developing mouse heart. J Mol Cell Cardiol 1998;30:1067-81.
72. Franco D, Kelly R, Moorman AF, et al: MLC3F transgene expression in iv mutant mice reveals the importance of left-right signalling pathways for the acquisition of left and right atrial but not ventricular compartment identity. Dev Dyn 2001;221:206-215.
73. Chai Y, Jiang X, Ito Y, et al: Fate of the mammalian cranial neural crest during tooth and mandibular morphogenesis. Development 2000;127:1671-1679.
74. Li J, Liu KC, Jin F, et al: Transgenic rescue of congenital heart disease and spina bifida in Splotch mice. Development 1999;126:2495-2503.
75. Colbert MC, Hall DG, Kimball TR, et al: Cardiac compartment-specific overexpression of a modified retinoic acid receptor produces dilated cardiomyopathy and congestive heart failure in transgenic mice. J Clin Invest 1997;100:1958-1968.
76. Li Z, Marchand P, Humbert J, et al: Desmin sequence elements regulating skeletal muscle-specific expression in transgenic mice. Development 1993;117:947-959.
77. Donoghue MJ, Alvarez JD, Merlie JP, Sanes JR: Fiber type- and position-dependent expression of a myosin light chain- CAT transgene detected with a novel histochemical stain for CAT. J Cell Biol 1991;115:423-434.
78. Johnson JE, Wold BJ, Hauschka SD: Muscle creatine kinase sequence elements regulating skeletal and cardiac muscle expression in transgenic mice. Mol Cell Biol 1989;9:3393-3399.
79. Evans SM, Tai LJ, Tan VP, et al: Heterokaryons of cardiac myocytes and fibroblasts reveal the lack of dominance of the cardiac muscle phenotype. Mol Cell Biol 1994;14:4269-4279.
80. Kuhbandner S, Brummer S, Metzger D, et al: Temporally controlled somatic mutagenesis in smooth muscle. Genesis 2000;28:15-22.
81. Kisanuki YY, Hammer RE, Miyazaki J, et al: Tie2-Cre transgenic mice: A new model for endothelial cell-lineage analysis in vivo. Dev Biol 2001;230:230-242.
82. Gustafsson E, Brakebusch C, Hietanen K, Fassler R: Tie-1-directed expression of Cre recombinase in endothelial cells of embryoid bodies and transgenic mice. J Cell Sci 2001;114:671-676.

83. Blizard DA, Welty R: Cardiac activity in the mouse: Strain differences. J Comp Physiol Psychol 1971;77:337-344.

84. Bueno OF, De Windt LJ, Tymitz KM, et al: The MEK1-ERK1/2 signaling pathway promotes compensated cardiac hypertrophy in transgenic mice. Embo J 2000;19:6341-6350.

85. Garrick D, Fiering S, Martin DI, Whitelaw E: Repeat-induced gene silencing in mammals. Nat Genet 1998;18:56-59.

86. Suzuki M, Carlson KM, Marchuk DA, Rockman HA: Genetic modifier loci affecting survival and cardiac function in murine dilated cardiomyopathy. Circulation 2002;105:1824-1829.

87. Sato Y, Ferguson DG, Sako H, et al: Cardiac-specific overexpression of mouse cardiac calsequestrin is associated with depressed cardiovascular function and hypertrophy in transgenic mice. J Biol Chem 1998;273:28470-28477.

88. Loukianov E, Ji Y, Grupp IL, et al: Enhanced myocardial contractility and increased Ca2+ transport function in transgenic hearts expressing the fast-twitch skeletal muscle sarcoplasmic reticulum Ca2+-ATPase. Circ Res 1998;83:889-897.

89. Hunter JJ, Chien KR: Signaling pathways for cardiac hypertrophy and failure. N Engl J Med 1999;341:1276-1283.

90. Gossen M, Bonin AL, Freundlieb S, Bujard H: Inducible gene expression systems for higher eukaryotic cells. Curr Opin Biotechnol 1994;5:516-520.

91. Gossen M, Bonin AL, Bujard H: Control of gene activity in higher eukaryotic cells by prokaryotic regulatory elements. Trends Biochem Sci 1993;18:471-475.

92. Gossen M, Bujard H: Tight control of gene expression in mammalian cells by tetracycline- responsive promoters. Proc Natl Acad Sci USA 1992;89:5547-5551.

93. Valencik ML, McDonald JA: Codon optimization markedly improves doxycycline regulated gene expression in the mouse heart. Transgenic Res 2001;10:269-275.

94. Mansuy IM, Winder DG, Moallem TM, et al: Inducible and reversible gene expression with the rtTA system for the study of memory. Neuron 1998;21:257-265.

95. Tsien JZ, Chen DF, Gerber D, et al: Subregion- and cell type-restricted gene knockout in mouse brain. Cell 1996;87:1317-1326.

96. Bowman JC, Steinberg SF, Jiang T, et al: Expression of protein kinase C beta in the heart causes hypertrophy in adult mice and sudden death in neonates. J Clin Invest 1997;100:2189-2195.

97. Lakso M, Sauer B, Mosinger B Jr, et al: Targeted oncogene activation by site-specific recombination in transgenic mice. Proc Natl Acad Sci USA 1992;89:6232-6236.

98. Sauer B, Henderson N: Site-specific DNA recombination in mammalian cells by the Cre recombinase of bacteriophage P1. Proc Natl Acad Sci USA 1988;85:5166-5170.

99. Orban PC, Chui D, Marth JD: Tissue- and site-specific DNA recombination in transgenic mice. Proc Natl Acad Sci USA 1992; 89:6861-6865.

100. Metzger D, Feil R: Engineering the mouse genome by site-specific recombination. Curr Opin Biotechnol 1999;10:470-476.

101. Minamino T, Gaussin V, DeMayo FJ, Schneider MD: Inducible gene targeting in postnatal myocardium by cardiac-specific expression of a hormone-activated Cre fusion protein. Circ Res 2001;88:587-592.

102. Sohal DS, Nghiem M, Crackower MA, et al: Temporally regulated and tissue-specific gene manipulations in the adult and embryonic heart using a tamoxifen-inducible Cre protein. Circ Res 2001;89:20-25.

103. Cronin CA, Gluba W, Scrable H: The lac operator-repressor system is functional in the mouse. Genes Dev 2001;15:1506-1517.

104. Chien KR: Meeting Koch's postulates for calcium signaling in cardiac hypertrophy. J Clin Invest 2000;105:1339-1342.

105. Huang WY, Aramburu J, Douglas PS, Izumo S: Transgenic expression of green fluorescence protein can cause dilated cardiomyopathy. Nat Med 2000;6:482-483.

106. Knotts S, Rindt H, Robbins J: Position independent expression and developmental regulation is directed by the beta myosin heavy chain gene's 5' upstream region in transgenic mice. Nucleic Acids Res 1995;23:3301-3309.

107. Yu Z, Redfern CS, Fishman GI: Conditional transgene expression in the heart. Circ Res 1996;79:691-697.

108. De Windt LJ, Lim HW, Bueno OF, et al: Targeted inhibition of calcineurin attenuates cardiac hypertrophy in vivo. Proc Natl Acad Sci USA 2001;98:3322-3327.

109. Bueno OF, De Windt LJ, Lim HW, et al: The dual-specificity phosphatase MKP-1 limits the cardiac hypertrophic response in vitro and in vivo. Circ Res 2001;88:88-96.

110. Wurst W, Joyner AL: Production of targeted embryonic stem cell clones. In Joyner AL (ed): Gene Targeting: A Practical Approach. New York, Oxford University Press, 1993, pp 33-61.

111. Papaioannou V, Johnson R: Production of chimeras and genetically defined offspring from targeted ES cells. In Joyner AL (ed): Gene Targeting: A Practical Approach. New York, Oxford University Press, 1993, pp 107-146.

112. Hasty P, Bradley A: Gene targeting vectors for mammalian cells. In Joyner AL (ed): Gene Targeting. A Practical Approach. New York, Oxford University Press, 1993, 1-31.

113. Chien KR: To Cre or not to Cre: The next generation of mouse models of human cardiac diseases. Circ Res 2001;88:546-549.

114. McMahon AP, Bradley A: The Wnt-1 (int-1) proto-oncogene is required for development of a large region of the mouse brain. Cell 1990;62:1073-1085.

115. Smith AG, Heath JK, Donaldson DD, et al: Inhibition of pluripotential embryonic stem cell differentiation by purified polypeptides. Nature 1988;336:688-690.

116. Williams RL, Hilton DJ, Pease S, et al: Myeloid leukaemia inhibitory factor maintains the developmental potential of embryonic stem cells. Nature 1988;336:684-687.

117. te Riele H, Maandag ER, Berns A: Highly efficient gene targeting in embryonic stem cells through homologous recombination with isogenic DNA constructs. Proc Natl Acad Sci USA 1992;89:5128-532.

118. Thomas KR, Capecchi MR: Site-directed mutagenesis by gene - targeting in mouse embryo-derived stem cells. Cell 1987;51:503-512.

119. Hasty P, Rivera-Perez J, Bradley A: The length of homology required for gene targeting in embryonic stem cells. Mol Cell Biol 1991;11:5586-5591.

120. Mansour SL, Thomas KR, Capecchi MR: Disruption of the proto-oncogene int-2 in mouse embryo-derived stem cells: A general strategy for targeting mutations to non-selectable genes. Nature 1988;336:348-352.

121. Cruz A, Coburn CM, Beverley SM: Double targeted gene replacement for creating null mutants. Proc Natl Acad Sci USA 1991;88:7170-7174.

122. Taniguchi M, Sanbo M, Watanabe S, et al: Efficient production of Cre-mediated site-directed recombinants through the utilization of the puromycin resistance gene, pac: A transient gene integration marker for ES cells. Nucleic Acids Res 1998;26:679-680.

123. Thompson S, Clarke AR, Pow AM, et al: Germ line transmission and expression of a corrected HPRT gene produced by gene targeting in embryonic stem cells. Cell 1989;56:313-321.

124. Kim HS, Popovich BW, Shehee WR, et al: Problems encountered in detecting a targeted gene by the polymerase chain reaction. Gene 1991;103:227-233.

125. Moens CB, Auerbach AB, Conlon RA, et al: A targeted mutation reveals a role for N-myc in branching morphogenesis in the embryonic mouse lung. Genes Dev 1992;6:691-704.

126. Dorin JR, Dickinson P, Alton EW, et al: Cystic fibrosis in the mouse by targeted insertional mutagenesis. Nature 1992;359:211-215.

127. Olson EN, Arnold HH, Rigby PW, Wold BJ: Know your neighbors: Three phenotypes in null mutants of the myogenic bHLH gene MRF4. Cell 1996;85:1-4.

128. Fiering S, Kim CG, Epner EM, Groudine M: An "in-out" strategy using gene targeting and FLP recombinase for the functional dissection of complex DNA regulatory elements: Analysis of the beta-globin locus control region. Proc Natl Acad Sci USA 1993;90:8469-8473.

129. Hasty P, Ramirez-Solis R, Krumlauf R, Bradley A: Introduction of a subtle mutation into the Hox-2.6 locus in embryonic stem cells. Nature 1991;350:243-246.

130. Valancius V, Smithies O: Testing an "in-out" targeting procedure for making subtle genomic modifications in mouse embryonic stem cells. Mol Cell Biol 1991;11:1402-1408.

131. Askew GR, Doetschman T, Lingrel JB: Site-directed point mutations in embryonic stem cells: A gene-targeting tag-and-exchange strategy. Mol Cell Biol 1993;13:4115-4124.

132. Moore RC, Hope J, McBride PA, et al: Mice with gene targetted prion protein alterations show that Prnp, Sinc and Prni are congruent. Nat Genet 1998;18:118-125.

133. Lewis J, Yang B, Detloff P, Smithies O: Gene modification via "plug and socket" gene targeting. J Clin Invest 1996;97:3-5.

134. Lyons I, Parsons LM, Hartley L, et al: Myogenic and morphogenetic defects in the heart tubes of murine embryos lacking the homeo box gene Nkx2-5. Genes Dev 1995;9:1654-1666.

135. Molkentin JD, Lin Q, Duncan SA, Olson EN: Requirement of the transcription factor GATA4 for heart tube formation and ventral morphogenesis. Genes Dev 1997;11:1061-1072.

136. Kuo CT, Morrisey EE, Anandappa R, et al: GATA4 transcription factor is required for ventral morphogenesis and heart tube formation. Genes Dev 1997;11:1048-1060.

137. Lin Q, Schwarz J, Bucana C, Olson EN: Control of mouse cardiac morphogenesis and myogenesis by transcription factor MEF2C. Science 1997;276:1404-1407.

138. Firulli BA, Hadzic DB, McDaid JR, Firulli AB: The basic helix-loop-helix transcription factors dHAND and eHAND exhibit dimerization characteristics that suggest complex regulation of function. J Biol Chem 2000;275:33567-33573.

139. Riley P, Anson-Cartwright L, Cross JC: The Hand1 bHLH transcription factor is essential for placentation and cardiac morphogenesis. Nat Genet 1998;18:271-275.

140. Thomas T, Yamagishi H, Overbeek PA, et al: The bHLH factors, dHAND and eHAND, specify pulmonary and systemic cardiac ventricles independent of left-right sidedness. Dev Biol 1998; 196:228-236.

141. Sucov HM, Dyson E, Gumeringer CL, et al: RXR alpha mutant mice establish a genetic basis for vitamin A signaling in heart morphogenesis. Genes Dev 1994;8:1007-1018.

142. Srivastava D, Olson EN: A genetic blueprint for cardiac development. Nature 2000;407:221-226.

143. Arber S, Hunter JJ, Ross J Jr, et al: MLP-deficient mice exhibit a disruption of cardiac cytoarchitectural organization, dilated cardiomyopathy, and heart failure. Cell 1997;88:393-403.

144. Pashmforoush M, Pomies P, Peterson KL, et al: Adult mice deficient in actinin-associated LIM-domain protein reveal a developmental pathway for right ventricular cardiomyopathy. Nat Med 2001;7:591-597.

145. Coral-Vazquez R, Cohn RD, Moore SA, et al: Disruption of the sarcoglycan-sarcospan complex in vascular smooth muscle: A novel mechanism for cardiomyopathy and muscular dystrophy. Cell 1999;98:465-474.

146. Luo W, Grupp IL, Harrer J, et al: Targeted ablation of the phospholamban gene is associated with markedly enhanced myocardial contractility and loss of beta-agonist stimulation. Circ Res 1994; 75:401-409.

147. Minamisawa S, Hoshijima M, Chu G, et al: Chronic phospholamban-sarcoplasmic reticulum calcium ATPase interaction is the critical calcium cycling defect in dilated cardiomyopathy. Cell 1999;99:313-322.

148. Buchholz F, Angrand PO, Stewart AF: Improved properties of FLP recombinase evolved by cycling mutagenesis. Nat Biotechnol 1998;16:657-662.

149. Rodriguez CI, Buchholz F, Galloway J, et al: High-efficiency deleter mice show that FLPe is an alternative to Cre-loxP. Nat Genet 2000;25:139-140.

150. Gu H, Zou YR, Rajewsky K: Independent control of immunoglobulin switch recombination at individual switch regions evidenced through Cre-loxP-mediated gene targeting. Cell 1993; 73:1155-1164.

151. Hirota H, Chen J, Betz UA, et al: Loss of a gp130 cardiac muscle cell survival pathway is a critical event in the onset of heart failure during biomechanical stress. Cell 1999;97:189-198.

152. Wollert KC, Chien KR: Cardiotrophin-1 and the role of gp130-dependent signaling pathways in cardiac growth and development. J Mol Med 1997;75:492-501.

153. Pennica D, King KL, Shaw KJ, et al: Expression cloning of cardiotrophin 1, a cytokine that induces cardiac myocyte hypertrophy. Proc Natl Acad Sci U S A 1995;92:1142-1146.

154. Kuhn R, Schwenk F, Aguet M, Rajewsky K: Inducible gene targeting in mice. Science 1995;269:1427-1429.

155. Hennet T, Hagen FK, Tabak LA, Marth JD: T-cell-specific deletion of a polypeptide N-acetylgalactosaminyl-transferase gene by site-directed recombination. Proc Natl Acad Sci USA 1995;92: 12070-12074.

156. Wagner KU, Wall RJ, St. Onge L, et al: Cre-mediated gene deletion in the mammary gland. Nucleic Acids Res 1997;25:4323-4330.

157. Agah R, Frenkel PA, French BA, et al: Gene recombination in post-mitotic cells. Targeted expression of Cre recombinase provokes cardiac-restricted, site-specific rearrangement in adult ventricular muscle in vivo. J Clin Invest 1997;100:169-179.

158. Chen J, Kubalak SW, Chien KR: Ventricular muscle-restricted targeting of the RXRalpha gene reveals a non-cell-autonomous requirement in cardiac chamber morphogenesis. Development 1998;125:1943-1949.

159. Barlow C, Schroeder M, Lekstrom-Himes J, et al: Targeted expression of Cre recombinase to adipose tissue of transgenic mice directs adipose-specific excision of loxP-flanked gene segments. Nucleic Acids Res 1997;25:2543-2545.

160. Brocard J, Warot X, Wendling O, et al: Spatio-temporally controlled site-specific somatic mutagenesis in the mouse. Proc Natl Acad Sci USA 1997;94:14559-14563.

161. Kellendonk C, Tronche F, Casanova E, et al: Inducible site-specific recombination in the brain. J Mol Biol 1999;285:175-182.

162. Indra AK, Li M, Brocard J, et al: Targeted somatic mutagenesis in mouse epidermis. Horm Res 2000;54:296-300.

## EDITOR'S CHOICE

Crone SA, Zhao YY, Fan L, et al: ErbB2 is essential in the prevention of dilated cardiomyopathy. Nat Med 2002;8:459-465.
*Illustration of the power of tissue-specific mutations of genes to escape the embryonic lethality seen in complete, conventional knockout mice.*

Gitler AD, Zhu Y, Ismat FA, et al: Nf1 has an essential role in endothelial cells. Nat Genet 2003;33:75-79.
*A beautiful example of mapping the requirement of a single gene in a variety of different cell types in the developing heart using a fleet of Cre mice.*

King DP, Zhao Y, Sangoram AM, et al: Positional cloning of the mouse circadian clock gene. Cell 1997;89:641-53.
*Seminal paper that supports the feasibility of large scale ENU mutagenesis screens in mice to uncover unique genes for complex physiological phenotypes.*

Ruiz-Lozano P, Chien KR: Cre-constructing the heart. Nat Genet 2003;33:8-9.
*This review contains a list of Cre mouse lines for conditional mutagenesis in a wide variety of cardiovascular cell types.*

Smithies O: Forty years with homologous recombination. Nat Med 2001;7:1083-1086.
*Pioneer in the development of gene targeted mouse models summarizes work on mouse models of hypertension and the technology that allowed their development.*

Sohal DS, Nghiem M, Crackower MA, et al: Temporally regulated and tissue-specific gene manipulations in the adult and embryonic heart using a tamoxifen-inducible Cre protein. Circ Res 2001;89:20-25.
*An example of combining tissue-specific and temporal control of the onset of mutagenesis, increasingly critical in the study of cardiovascular physiological questions.*

# chapter 5

# Mouse Models of Human Cardiovascular Disease

*Geir Christensen*

*Ju Chen*

*John Ross Jr*

*Kenneth R. Chien*

Mouse models of cardiovascular disease have provided new and important insights into the pathobiology of human disease. The power of the mouse derives primarily from the ability to modify specific genes of interest. Novel strategies in mouse genetic engineering have allowed the development of mouse models with cell-specific gene modifications and mice designed to control the temporal onset of a given mutation using advanced techniques such as the Cre-loxP system (Chapter 4). The cardiovascular phenotype of these mouse models can be precisely assessed at the cellular and organ level using well-known and novel sophisticated methods *in vitro, ex vivo,* and *in vivo*.[1,2]

Over the last decade a large number of mouse models with phenotypes similar to human inherited or acquired cardiovascular disease have been developed. This chapter describes these mouse models and how they display similarity to human disease. It also indicates how mouse models have been used to increase the understanding of human disease, and in some cases how they have allowed examination of novel therapeutic approaches. The first section deals with congenital heart disease and a later section presents mouse models of human cardiomyopathy. These sections show the power of mouse models with regard to studies of inborn cardiovascular diseases. In addition, several sections of this chapter deal with acquired cardiovascular disease and illustrate how mouse models are being used to study common diseases such as atherosclerosis, myocardial ischemia, heart failure, and cardiac arrhythmias.

## MOUSE MODELS OF HUMAN HEART DISEASE

### Congenital Heart Disease

Congenital cardiovascular disease is defined as an abnormality in cardiocirculatory structure or function that is present at birth (Braunwald, Chapter 43). The complexity of the malformations has led to various types of classifications based on the anatomic malformations, hemodynamic alterations, or typical clinical features. Relatively little has been known regarding the cause of congenital heart diseases. Recently, it has been possible to study genes that regulate cardiogenesis. Mouse models have been particularly useful for examining genetic networks involved in the various stages of cardiac development,[3-7] and these models have increased the understanding of human congenital heart disease.

### *Hypoplasia of the Ventricular Wall*

In humans, hypoplasia of the right or left ventricle is a severe form of congenital heart disease. Familial occurrence is relatively frequent, and some of the syndromes have been linked to specific human mutations. Studies in genetically modified mice have revealed a genetic basis for development of the myocardial wall. Underdevelopment of the myocardial wall has been observed in genetically modified mice with mutations in genes encoding transcription factors, cytoskeletal components, receptors, cell adhesion molecules, and angiogenic factors (Table 5-1).

### *Transcription Factors*

In mice homozygous for a null mutation of *myocyte enhancer factor-2C (MEF2C)* a hypoplastic ventricular chamber was observed.[8] *MEF2C* is a member of the MEF2 family of transcription factors that bind a conserved A-T-rich sequence associated with most cardiac structural genes. In mutant embryos, the heart tube did not undergo rightward looping, and there was no morphologic evidence of the future right ventricle. A single hypoplastic ventricular chamber was fused directly to an enlarged atrial chamber. Studies indicate that *MEF2C* may co-operate with specific members of the basic helix-loop-helix transcription factors, such as *dHAND (deciduum, heart, autonomic nervous system, neural crest-derived)*. Mice homozygous for a null mutation in *dHAND*[9] exhibit a cardiac phenotype similar to the *MEF2C* mutant.

Mice with knockout of the *retinoic X receptor (RXR)α* gene displayed severe cardiac muscle defects.[10,11] Retinoid receptors are members of the steroid hormone receptor superfamily of ligand-dependent transcription factors. These receptors make up two subfamilies

■ ■ ■

**TABLE 5-1**   GENE MUTATIONS IN MICE WITH CONGENITAL HEART MALFORMATIONS

| Gene Mutated | Cardiovascular Manifestations | References |
|---|---|---|
| MEF2C | Hypoplastic ventricular chamber | 8 |
| RXRα | Thin myocardium, double-outlet right ventricle, persistent truncus arteriosus, VSD | 10–12 |
| N-myc | Thin myocardium | 15–18 |
| TEF-1 | Thin myocardium | 19 |
| NF1 | Thin myocardium, valvular defects, persistent truncus arteriosus, double-outlet right ventricle, VSD | 20, 21 |
| WF1 | Thin ventricular wall | 22 |
| Alp | Thinning of the right ventricle, right ventricular outflow tract dilation | 23 |
| Neuregulin/erbB2/erbB4 | Absent myocardial trabeculae | 24–26 |
| VCAM1 | Lack of epicardium, thin ventricular wall, VSD | 27, 28 |
| α4 integrin | Epicardial dissolution | 29 |
| VEGF | Thinning of the ventricular wall | 30 |
| Angiopoitin/TIE2 | Endocardial defects | 31, 32 |
| βARK1 | Thin myocardium | 398 |
| NF-ATc | Valve defects, VSD | 34 |
| Smad6 | Hyperplasia of cardiac valves | 35 |
| DiGeorge | Interrupted aortic arch, overriding aorta, pulmonary stenosis, VSD | 36 |
| ET/ECE/AT$_A$ | Interrupted aortic arch, double-outlet right ventricle, persistent truncus arteriosus, transposition of great arteries, VSD | 38–40 |
| NT3/trkC receptor | Aortic arch defects, persistent truncus arteriosus, valvular defects, pulmonary stenosis,  ASD, VSD, tetralogy of Fallot | 41, 42 |
| dHAND | Hypoplastic ventricular chamber, aortic arch defects, lethal at E 10.5 | 9 |
| box1.5 | Hypoplastic right ventricle, aortic and pulmonary valve defects, thin aorta | 43 |
| Sox4 | Common trunk, transposition of great arteries, valve defects, VSD | 44, 45 |
| rae28 | Pulmonary stenosis, aortic stenosis, tetralogy of Fallot, VSD | 46 |
| MFH-1 | Interruption of the aortic arch, VSD | 47 |
| neuropilin | Transposition of great vessels, persistent truncus arteriosus | 48 |
| Pax3 | Aortic arch defects, persistent truncus arteriosus, double-outlet right ventricle,  ASD | 49, 50 |
| Connexin43 | Pulmonary stenosis | 51 |
| NMHC-B | Myocardial hypertrophy, malposition of aorta, pulmonary stenosis,  ASD,  VSD | 52 |
| PBSF/SDF-1 | VSD | 55 |
| TGFβ-2 | Dual-outlet right ventricle, dual-inlet left ventricle, VSD | 56 |
| ActRIIB | Malposition of great arteries,  ASD,  VSD | 58 |
| NKX2.5 | ASD, lethal at E 9 | 62 |
| FOG-2 | Thin ventricular myocardium, coronary artery defects, tricuspid atresia | 59, 60 |

ASD, atrial septal defect; VSD, ventricular septal defect.

composed of three retinoic acid receptors (RARα, β, γ) and three RXRs (α, β, and γ). The mouse embryos lacking the *RXRα* gene died in midgestation from hypoplastic development of the myocardium of the ventricular chambers. Using microdissection and scanning electron microscopy, myocardial defects (in addition to a hypoplastic compact zone) were observed, such as ventricular septal defects, disorganized trabeculae, and dysplastic papillary muscles.[12] Also, atrioventricular (AV) cushion and conotruncal ridge defects with double-outlet right ventricle, aorticopulmonary window, and persistent truncus arteriosus were observed. Using video microscopy and *in vivo* microinjection of fluorescein-labeled albumin, depressed ventricular function was demonstrated.[13] The defects in the chamber morphogenesis did not appear to be cell autonomous for the cardiomyocyte lineage.[14]

Mice with null mutation in *N-myc,* a member of a family of nuclear proto-oncogenes, displayed poor development of the ventricular myocardium and the interventricular septum.[15-17] The mice died around E11, but a mouse model with two types of mutant alleles with 15% of normal levels of N-myc proteins lived longer and exhibited a deficient outer compact layer of the ventricular myocardium.[18] A mutation in *transcriptional*

*enhancer factor-1 (TEF-1)* has also been shown to affect normal myocardial development.[19] The homozygous embryos of this mouse model died between E11 and E12 and displayed an abnormal thinning of both the compact layer and the trabeculae of the ventricular wall leading to cardiac insufficiency. Mouse embryos homozygous for a mutation in the *neurofibromatosis (NF) type 1* gene died around E14 most likely because of cardiac failure.[20,21] This mouse model had a hypoplastic heart with disorganized muscle cells; septal defects, persistent truncus arteriosus, and valve abnormalities were also observed. A mutation in the *Wilms' tumor associated gene (WT-1)* resulted in epicardial dissolution and subsequent myocardial thinning.[22]

### Cytoskeletal Components

A phenotype similar to human right ventricular dysplasia was found in mice deficient in α-actinin-associated LIM-domain protein,[23] which is a member of the cytoskeletal LIM-domain protein superfamily. Analysis of mutant embryos revealed right ventricular dilation and right ventricular outflow-tract dilation with thinning of the right ventricular wall and septum (Figure 5-1). No evident defect was observed in the valves or aorta.

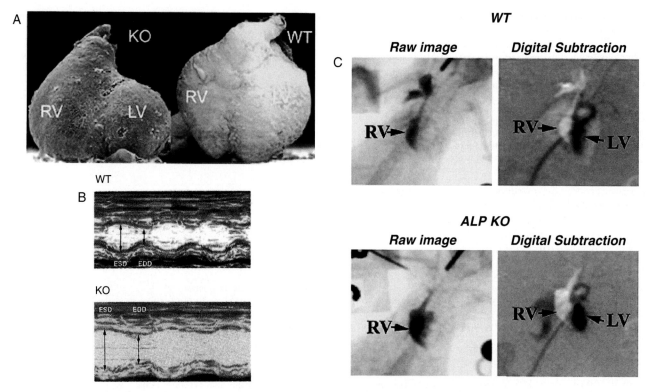

**FIGURE 5-1.** Mouse embryos deficient in α-actinin-associated LIM-domain protein show predominant right ventricular (RV) dilation similar to some forms of human right ventricular dysplasia. *A,* Scanning electron micrograph of knockout (KO) and wild-type (WT) hearts at embryonic day 12.5 showing marked RV and conotruncal dilation in the KO heart compared with the WT heart. *B,* Representative two-dimensional echocardiograms showing dilated cardiomyopathy in KO mice. Double arrowheads point to the end-diastolic (EDD) and the end-systolic (ESD) dimensions, respectively. *C,* Assessment of the *in vivo* RV chamber dilation in KO mice using digitized-subtraction microangiography. Raw images were obtained by injecting radiopaque dye into the superior vena cava. Following digitized subtraction, RV (light) and LV (dark) dimensions are contrasted. *(From Pashmforoush M, Pomies P, Peterson KL, et al: Adult mice deficient in actinin-associated LIM-domain protein reveal a developmental pathway for right ventricular cardiomyopathy. Nat Med 2001;7:591–597.)*

### Signaling Between Endocardium and Myocardium

Defects in the development of the ventricular trabeculae were observed in mice deficient in neuregulin[24] or its receptors, erbB2[25] and erbB4.[26] Neuregulin, which is expressed in the endocardium, induces growth and differentiation of epithelial, glial, and muscle cells in culture. It binds directly to erbB3 and erbB4 receptors, and receptor heterodimerization allows neuregulin-dependent activation of the erbB2 receptor. The mouse models with targeted mutation of *neuregulin,* *erbB2,* or *erbB4* genes die during embryogenesis most likely resulting from cardiac dysfunction. The mouse models indicate that signaling between endocardium and myocardium is important for growth of the ventricular wall.

### Cell Adhesion Molecules and Angiogenesis

In mice with mutations in genes encoding the vascular cell adhesion molecule-1[27,28] or a component of its receptor, α4 integrin,[29] a reduction in the thickness of the myocardium was observed. The mice often died around E12, and epicardial dissolution was a prominent defect.

Recently, thinned ventricular walls have been observed in a mouse model with cardiomyocyte-specific deletion of the gene encoding vascular endothelial growth factor A (VEGF-A).[30] The mice had dilated and hypovascular hearts with contractile dysfunction. This model of thin-walled ventricles and coronary hypovascularization did not show evidence of myocardial necrosis or replacement fibrosis. Other mouse models with disruption of angiogenic factors or their receptors also displayed cardiac defects. Embryos that lack angiopoietin-1[31] or the TIE2 receptor[32] have less complex ventricular endocardium and almost collapsed atrial endothelial lining. The mechanisms by which cell adhesion molecules and angiogenic factors affect ventricular wall development or their role in human syndromes of underdeveloped ventricles remain to be defined.

### Cardiac Valve Defects

In humans, a variety of congenital valvular lesions have been described (Braunwald, Chapter 43), but the cause of most of these is unknown. Children with trisomy 21 (Down's syndrome) have endocardial cushion defects and incomplete septation of the AV valves. Early in development, septation of the cardiac tube is achieved through regional swellings of extracellular matrix, often called cushions, that later develop into AV and ventriculoarterial valves. Genetically modified mouse models have revealed roles for some factors in this valvulogenesis.

Mice with a disruption in the *nuclear factor of activated T cells (NF-ATc)* gene fail to develop normal cardiac valves and die of circulatory failure.[33] NF-ATc is specifically expressed in the forming embryonic valves and belongs to a family of transcription factors that is controlled by the calcium-regulated phosphatase calcineurin. The mice displayed normal septation into right ventricular (pulmonary) and left ventricular (aortic) outflow tract, but both semilunar valves were underdeveloped. The tricuspid and mitral valves were also primitive and displayed no well-defined leaflets. A similar mouse model with targeted disruption of the *NF-ATc* gene was developed by another group of investigators.[34] Those mice displayed selective absence of the aortic and pulmonary valves. The tricuspid and mitral valve morphogenesis was normal.

Mice with mutations of the transcription factor *Smad6* display abnormally thickened and gelatinous valves,[35] similar to those observed in some human disorders. Smad proteins are intracellular mediators of signaling initiated by members of the transforming growth factor (TGF)-β superfamily.

## Defects in Cardiac Outflow Tract, Aortic Arch, and Pulmonary Artery

In humans, a large number of complex defects involving cardiac outflow tract, aortic arch, and the pulmonary artery have been described, based mainly on anatomic and physiologic features (Braunwald, Chapter 43). Although syndromes and familial cases with such malformations have been described, the pathogenesis of various malformations is unknown. Recently, mouse models (in conjunction with ongoing studies of chromosomal disorders and autosomal dominant syndromes with defects in the cardiac outflow tract, aortic arch, and the pulmonary artery) have provided new information. One example is a study of patients with DiGeorge's syndrome who have a heterozygous chromosome deletion within the band 22q11 and exhibit interrupted aortic arch, tetralogy of Fallot, and truncus arteriosus.

### DiGeorge's Syndrome

In the mouse, a region of chromosome 16 is highly similar in gene content and size to the deletion in humans with DiGeorge's syndrome. A mouse model was made carrying a deletion of most of that region using Cre-loxP chromosome engineering.[36] Heterozygous deletion of the region resulted in cardiovascular abnormalities of the same type as those associated with human DiGeorge's syndrome. When the mice were examined at 18.5 days post coitum it was found that 11 of the animals (26%) had cardiovascular abnormalities. Interrupted aortic

arch, infundibular pulmonary stenosis, aberrant origin of the right subclavian artery, overriding aorta, and ventricular septum defects were observed (Figure 5-2). Although tetralogy of Fallot, which is present in 17% of the 22q11 deleted human patients, was not observed, the structural components were present.

Mice lacking the *endothelin (ET)-1*,[37,38] *ET converting enzyme (ECE)-1*,[39] or *$ET_A$ receptor*[40] gene also displayed abnormalities associated with the 22q11 deletion in humans. In addition to morphologic abnormalities of the

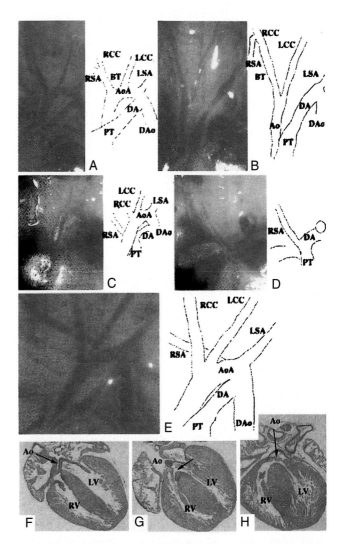

**FIGURE 5-2.** Examples of cardiovascular findings in embryos deficient for the DiGeorge's syndrome region (Df1/+). *A,* Normal anatomy in a wild-type embryo. *B,* Embryo with interrupted aortic arch type b, distal emergence of the right subclavian artery (RSA), and ventricular septal defect *(G, arrow)*. *C* and *D,* Embryo with aberrant origin of the RSA from the pulmonary trunk (aortic arch removed in *D*). *E,* Aberrant origin of the RSA from the descending aorta. *F,* Histologic section of heart from a wild-type 18.5 days post coitum embryo. *H,* Aberrant position of the emergence of the aorta from above the right and left ventricle (overriding aorta). Ao, aorta; AOA, aortic arch; BT, brachiocephalic trunk; DA, ductus arteriosus; DAo, descending aorta; LCC, left common carotid artery; LSA, left subclavian artery; PT, pulmonary trunk; RCC, right common carotid artery. *(From Lindsay EA, Botta A, Jurecic V, et al: Congenital heart disease in mice deficient for the DiGeorge syndrome region. Nature 1999;401:379-383.)*

pharyngeal arch–derived craniofacial tissues,[37] mice that lacked *ET-1* displayed interrupted aortic arch, aberrant right subclavian artery, and ventricular septal defect. Mice deficient for the *ET$_A$ receptor* also had severe craniofacial deformities and defects in the cardiovascular outflow tract, including interruption of the aorta, absent right subclavian artery, and right dorsal aorta with right-sided ductus arteriosus.[40] Ventricular septal defects with overriding aorta, double-outlet right ventricle, persistent truncus arteriosus, and transposition of the great arteries were also found. Mice with a null mutation in the *ECE-1*[39] exhibited craniofacial and cardiac malformations virtually identical to those observed in mice lacking *ET-1* and the *ET$_A$ receptor*. Altogether, these mouse models of congenital heart disease indicate that defects in the neural crest migration or differentiation underlie many of the cardiac outflow and aortic arch defects seen in human patients.

Homozygous *neurotrophin (NT)-3* null mutant mice displayed cardiovascular abnormalities including tetralogy of Fallot and septal defects.[41] NT-3 is one of five growth factors that has been shown to be involved in the regulation of neuronal survival and differentiation, and it effectively activates the trkC receptor tyrosine kinase. Histologic examination of *NT-3* null mice demonstrated defects associated with the aortic arch, ductus arteriosus, pulmonary artery, and valves. One mutant animal displayed all the defects associated with tetralogy of Fallot, including atrial septal defect, ventricular septal defect, pulmonary stenosis, and overriding aorta. In mice with a targeted mutation that disrupted the expression of all trkC receptor proteins,[42] the frequency, severity, and type of cardiovascular defects were similar to those described in the NT-3 deficient mice.

Other models with mutations that may affect the cardiac neural crest and vascular connections to the heart include mice with disruption in *dHAND*,[9] the homeobox gene *box1.5*,[43] the transcription factor *Sox4*,[44,45] the mouse homolog of *Drosophila polyhomeotic* gene called *rae28*,[46] winged helix transcription factor *mesenchyme fork head (MFH)-1*,[47] *NF-1*,[21] *neuropilin*,[48] *Pax 3*,[49,50] *RXRα*,[10-12] *connexin43*,[51] and *nonmuscle myosin heavy chain (NMHC)-B*.[52] The cardiovascular developmental defects in the outflow tract, aortic arch, and pulmonary artery in these mouse models are shown in Table 5-1.

## Ventricular Septal Defects

In humans, ventricular septal defects occur as isolated anomalies and in combination with other anomalies. Ventricular septal defects are characteristic of tetralogy of Fallot, double-outlet ventricle, and truncus arteriosus (Braunwald, Chapter 43) and may be seen as a result of malalignment during morphogenesis. Specific etiologic factors are mostly unknown, but heritable syndromes and particularly chromosomal abnormalities such as trisomy 21 (Down's syndrome) are associated with ventricular septal defects.

The mouse with trisomy 16 has been considered to be a genetic model for human trisomy 21, because

the murine chromosome 16 contains several genes whose homologs map to human chromosome 21. Hearts of these mice display deficient AV septation.[53] All hearts had ostium primum atrial septal defect and ventricular septal defect. Pulmonary stenosis and double-outlet ventricle is seen in trisomy 13, and discordant ventriculoarterial connections are observed in trisomy 14.[54]

Ventricular septal defects have also been described in mice with targeted disruption of single genes participating in various signaling pathways. Mice with targeted disruption of the gene encoding pre-B-cell growth-stimulating factor/stromal cell-derived factor (PBSF/SDF)-1, which is a member of the CXC group of chemokines,[55] died perinatally and had cardiac ventricular septal defect in addition to disturbances in B-cell lymphopoiesis. Large ventricular septal defects were found in mice lacking *TGFβ-2*.[56,57] These mice exhibited perinatal mortality and developmental defects commonly associated with disturbances in epithelial-mesenchymal interaction and in neural crest-derived components. The activins are also members of the TGF superfamily. Disruption of the *type IIB activin receptor (ActRIIB)* also resulted in cardiac defects with ventricular and atrial septal defects and malposition of the great arteries.[58]

Other mouse models with ventricular septal defect include the previously described mouse models with disruption of genes encoding RXRα,[12] VCAM-1,[28] NF-ATc,[33,34] friend of GATA (FOG)-2,[59,60] N-myc,[15,16] ET,[38] Sox4,[45,46] MFH1,[47] NT-3,[41] the trkC receptor,[42] and mouse models with disruption of the *NF1* gene.[20,21]

## Atrial Septal Defects

Atrial septal defects have typical anatomic locations and are classified as sinus venous defect, primum atrial defect, and secundum atrial defect. Each of these may result from disturbances in different parts of cardiac morphogenesis. Novel information regarding the cause of atrial septal defects has recently been obtained using human genetics and genetically modified mouse models. In families with atrial septal defects, point mutations in the gene encoding the homeobox transcription factor *NKX 2.5* were found.[61]

Mice with targeted disruption of *NKX2.5* displayed abnormal hearts at 8.5 days post coitum and died over the next 2 days, most likely from hemodynamic insufficiency.[62] A normal beating heart tube was formed, but the process of looping morphogenesis was not initiated. Looping is the start of a series of morphogenic events leading to chamber and valve formation. A cleft was observed between the atrial and ventricular chambers. Although the lethal defects observed in the NKX2.5-deficient mice are different from the human malformations caused by human NKX2.5 mutations, the mouse model indicates a role for a pathway involving NKX2.5 in atrial septation. Other mouse models with various types of atrial septal defects include *NT-3* null mutant mice[41] and mice with a disrupted expression of trkC receptor proteins.[42]

### Tricuspid Atresia

In humans, tricuspid atresia is characterized by absence of the tricuspid orifice, interatrial communication, hypoplasia of the right ventricle, and a large ventricular septal defect. Mice with disrupted *friend of gata (FOG)-2* gene displayed a cardiac phenotype similar to the human disease.[59] FOG-2 is cofactor for GATA transcription factors, which serve critical roles in development. *FOG-2* mutant mice demonstrated uniform and complete atresia of the tricuspid valve and a single, poorly formed common AV valve that connected both atria to the left ventricle. A large AV canal-type atrial septal defect, a large ventricular septal defect, and a hyperplastic pulmonic outflow tract were also observed. These mouse models suggest a genetic basis for human tricuspid atresia. In another study,[60] it was found that mice with disrupted *FOG-2* gene had absence of coronary vasculature and a thin ventricular myocardium in addition to a common AV canal and tetralogy of Fallot.

## Acute Myocardial Ischemia and Infarction

### Myocardial Ischemia

In humans, myocardial ischemia is usually a result of reduced coronary blood flow caused by atherosclerotic plaques and thrombi. Effects of reduced coronary blood flow have been assessed in humans and in various animal models (Braunwald, Chapter 34). However, important issues remain to be resolved. Among these issues are mechanisms involved in tissue injury during transient myocardial ischemia and reperfusion, the cardioprotective mechanisms involved in the phenomenon of ischemic preconditioning, and the molecular mechanisms of reversible contractile failure often termed *stunning*. Mouse models of myocardial ischemia allow detailed studies of these pathophysiologic processes or examination of new therapeutic strategies for myocardial protection.

### Ischemia and Reperfusion

Mouse models of short-term myocardial ischemia and reperfusion have been developed.[63,64] In the model developed by Michael et al.,[63] myocardial ischemia is induced in anesthetized and ventilated mice after opening the chest (Figure 5-3). Ligation of the left anterior descending branch of the left coronary artery is performed with a silk suture passed with a needle under the artery. A small piece of polyethylene tubing is placed on top of the vessel, and a knot is tied on top of the tubing to occlude the coronary artery. After occlusion for a prescribed period, cutting of the knot on top of the tubing with a surgical blade allows reperfusion of the formerly ischemic bed. Reperfusion can be determined by visual inspection, changes in ventricular function, and histopathologic characteristics. The area at risk and infarct size can be reliably assessed by Evans blue and triphenyltetrazolium chloride staining in combination with computerized planimetry.[63]

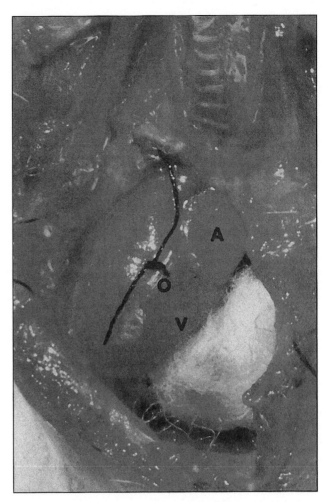

**FIGURE 5-3.** Mouse model of myocardial ischemia that allows reperfusion of the formerly occluded coronary bed. Photograph of open-chest mouse with occluder on left anterior descending coronary artery. A, left atrium; O, occluder V, free wall of left ventricle. *(From Michael LH, Entman ML, Hartley CJ, et al: Myocardial ischemia and reperfusion: A murine model. Am J Physiol 1995; 269: H2147-H2154.)*

The mouse model of transient ischemia has been used in combination with genetically modified mice to examine the impact of overexpression or absence of a gene product in progression of myocardial injury subsequent to myocardial ischemia and reperfusion. In one study,[65] a significant reduction in myocardial necrosis and infiltration of polymorphonuclear leukocyte infiltration was observed in CD18-deficient and intercellular adhesion molecule-1-deficient mice after short-term coronary ischemia and reperfusion. In other studies,[66,67] using similar experimental approaches, it was shown that mice with increased cardiac expression of heat shock proteins were protected against postischemic myocardial dysfunction. In one study,[66] regional myocardial function was assessed by an *in vivo* method for assessment of regional epicardial strain. Other studies have examined ischemia-reperfusion injury in endothelial nitric oxide (NO) deficient mice[68,69] or effects of hypercholesterolemia on ischemia-reperfusion injury in low-density lipoprotein receptor-deficient mice.[70]

*Ischemic preconditioning* is a powerful cardioprotective mechanism, and there is considerable interest in using this phenomenon to develop therapeutic strategies that can increase the tolerance of the human heart to ischemic injury. In mice, early- and late-phase ischemic preconditioning have been demonstrated using a balloon occluder[71] or a snare to occlude the coronary artery.[72] The mouse model of ischemic preconditioning has been used in conjunction with genetically engineered mice in which inducible NO synthase is selectively disrupted. One group[73] presented data suggesting that the late but not the early phase of ischemic preconditioning is mediated by inducible NO synthase. A transgenic mouse model with improved tolerance to ischemia-reperfusion similar to preconditioning has been developed by overexpression of cardiac A1 adenosine receptors.[74,75]

*Stunned myocardium* is a syndrome of reversible contractile failure associated with transient reduction in coronary flow. Myocardial stunning has been studied in the isolated mouse heart, and a technique has been developed to examine intracellular calcium dynamics in mouse hearts with reversible contractile failure.[76] Moreover, a transgenic mouse model has been developed that recapitulates the phenotype of stunned myocardium.[77] In that mouse model the major degradation product of troponin I ($TnI_{1-193}$) was expressed in the heart, because selective proteolysis of the thin filament protein troponin I has been correlated with stunned myocardium. The mice developed ventricular dilation, diminished contractility, and reduced myofilament calcium responsiveness, similar to what has been observed in stunned myocardium.

### Acute Myocardial Infarction

Although novel therapeutical strategies including thrombolytic agents and coronary angioplasty have led to a decline in myocardial infarction mortality, acute myocardial infarction is a fatal event in about one third of patients. During the initial phase after coronary occlusion, wall rupture and cardiac aneurysms may occur. Identification of pathways involved in repair of the infarcted region may allow specifically targeted therapy to reduce the complications.

Mouse models of coronary occlusion without reperfusion have been used to study the cardiac repair process after myocardial infarction. Most studies have used methods similar to that described by Michael et al.,[63] in which ligation of the coronary artery is performed with a silk suture passed with a needle under the artery and tied to occlude the coronary artery. Methods have been published for *in vivo* determination of risk area using myocardial contrast echocardiography[78] and for wall motion abnormalities using three-dimensional echocardiographic assessment.[79]

The cardiac repair process after myocardial infarction has been studied using genetically modified mice.[80-82] In one study,[80] a large collection of genetically modified mice were used. These mice had mutations in components of the plasminogen activator-metalloproteinase system, including tissue-type plasminogen activator, urokinase-type plasminogen activator, urokinase receptor, and the matrix metalloproteinases (MMPs) stromolysin-1 (MMP-3), gelatinase-B (MMP-9), and MMP-12. It was shown that within 4 days of infarct, 30% of wild-type mice died of cardiac rupture; a similar incidence occurred in mice lacking tissue-type plasminogen activator, urokinase-type plasminogen activator receptor, stromelysin, or MMP-12. The mice with disruption in either urokinase-type plasminogen activator or MMP-9 were protected against ventricular wall rupture. The urokinase-type plasminogen activator deficient mice had impaired scar formation and infarct revascularization. Administration of plasminogen activator inhibitor-1 or the matrix metalloproteinase-inhibitor-1 TIMP-1 completely protected wild-type mice against rupture but did not abort infarct healing. This study provides a clear rationale for further evaluation of MMPs as a therapeutical target to improve cardiac repair after myocardial infarction, and the experiments clearly demonstrate the power of genetically modified mouse models for identification of molecules involved in acquired forms of heart disease such as myocardial infarction.

Using the mouse model of acute myocardial infarction the role of tumor necrosis factor (TNF) was examined. A series of acute coronary occlusions were performed in mice lacking one or both TNF receptors.[83] Left ventricular infarct size was greater in the mice lacking TNF receptor type 1 and 2 than in wild-type mice, suggesting that TNF signaling gives rise to cytoprotective signals after acute ischemic injury.

## Myocardial Hypertrophy and Heart Failure

Myocardial hypertrophy is one of the principal mechanisms by which the heart compensates for increased load. In humans, increased cardiac load may be caused by congenital heart disease, valvular disease, myocardial infarction, or hypertension. Although initially compensatory, the process of myocardial hypertrophy often results in myocardial dysfunction and heart failure. Heart failure is a leading cause of mortality worldwide,[84] and the rates of morbidity and mortality are increasing. For development of new and more efficient therapeutic strategies, it is of great importance to identify the mechanisms involved in initiation and maintenance of myocardial growth and dysfunction.[85] To address these issues, mouse models have been developed that mimic various types of hypertrophy and heart failure found in humans. Surgical interventions to produce cardiac overload or myocardial infarction are particularly powerful when used in combination with genetically modified mice.

### Mechanical Overload Models of Myocardial Hypertrophy

Surgical interventions to produce mechanical overload models of myocardial hypertrophy include thoracic aortic banding,[86,87] pulmonary aortic banding,[88] arteriovenous fistula,[89] and induction of renal hypertension.[90]

## Left Ventricular Pressure Overload

To produce a model of left ventricular pressure overload in mice, the ascending aorta was constricted between the right innominate and left carotid arteries.[86,87] This model is characterized by a stable and reproducible hypertrophy 1 week after constriction of aorta. The severity of stenosis can be assessed by pressure measurements proximal and distal to the constriction site. An additional advantage with the site of constriction chosen in this model is that excessive overload is prevented because there is an outlet proximal to the constriction. The surgical procedure is performed on anesthetized and ventilated animals under a dissecting microscope.

The chest cavity is opened in the second intercostal space at the left sternal border, and aortic constriction is performed by tying a 7-0 nylon suture against a 27-gauge needle. This procedure produces a narrowing of the aortic diameter from 1.2 to 0.4 mm after removal of the needle. The method produced an acceptable constriction in about 70% of the mice operated on, and the perioperative mortality was about 15%. One week after aortic constriction a 41% increase in heart weight and an increase in the cross-sectional area of the cardiomyocytes were found.

This model of left ventricular pressure overload has been used in genetically modified mice to study pathways that mediate cardiac hypertrophy, and a few examples are presented. In one study,[91] the induction of mitogen-activated protein kinase activity was examined after aortic constriction in mice overexpressing a carboxyl-terminal peptide of $G\alpha_q$ that inhibits $G_q$-mediated signaling. In the transgenic mice with the $G_q$ inhibitor, the hypertrophic response was significantly attenuated. In another study,[92] it was shown that mice overexpressing $G\alpha_q$ responded to thoracic aortic banding with eccentric hypertrophy and ultimately heart failure. The model of left ventricular pressure overload has also been used in mice with mutations in receptors for either angiotensin II[93-95] or cytokines.[96] By using mice with ventricular restricted knockout of the gp130 cytokine receptor via Cre-LoxP-mediated recombination, the role for gp130-dependent pathways during pressure overload was examined.[96] The mutant mice have normal cardiac structure and function, but during aortic pressure overload the mice displayed dilated cardiomyopathy and massive induction of myocyte apoptosis; the control mice exhibited compensatory hypertrophy.

## Right Ventricular Pressure Overload

To produce a model of right ventricular pressure overload in mice, the pulmonary artery was constricted.[88] The animals were anesthetized and ventilated as described for aortic constriction. After opening the chest in the third intercostal space, a suture was tied around the pulmonary artery against a 25-gauge needle for a moderate degree of stenosis and against a 26-gauge needle for severe stenosis. Two weeks after pulmonary banding an increase in the weight of the right ventricle and myocyte cross-sectional area were found. To determine whether these animals develop right ventricular dysfunction, quantitative digital contrast microangiography was used for assessment of right ventricular function. Severe chronic pressure overload was shown to induce a reduction in ejection fraction and an increased end-diastolic volume, indicating right ventricular dysfunction. Thus, this mouse model mimics several features of right ventricular hypertrophy and failure similar to those found in human patients.

## Cardiac Volume Overload

A mouse model of cardiac volume overload has also been developed.[89] Overload was produced by creating an arteriovenous fistula between the infrarenal descending aorta and the inferior vena cava, as described for the rat.[97] In these mice, patent shunt flow was assessed by color flow mapping. When the heart was examined with echocardiography 1 week after surgery, findings consistent with an eccentric left ventricular hypertrophy were found. The thickness of the left posterior wall and the ventricular septum were mildly increased, and left end-diastolic diameter and left ventricular fractional shortening were elevated.

## Myocardial Hypertrophy and Heart Failure after Myocardial Infarction

Myocardial infarction induces changes in ventricular structure, shape, or size, a process usually termed ventricular remodeling. This process often leads to dilation of the left ventricular chamber and impaired systolic performance. The mouse model of myocardial infarction combined with genetically modified mouse strains should yield detailed insight into the pathogenesis of this common human disease.

The surgical procedure used in most studies to produce myocardial infarction is similar to that described in the section on myocardial ischemia.[63] In anesthetized animals a left thoracotomy is performed and either the main left coronary artery or the left anterior descending coronary artery is ligated. Ligation of the coronary artery usually results in an anteroapical infarction of the left ventricular wall (Figure 5-4). A model of coronary constriction in mice has also been described.[98] The surgical intervention used in that model provoked an average reduction in luminal diameter of 50%. Impaired pump function and eccentric hypertrophy was found after 7 days.

The structural and functional changes following myocardial infarction in the mouse model have been characterized.[99-101] Infarct size is usually about 40% of the left ventricular circumference. When examined 6 weeks after induction of infarction, an increase in left ventricular and lung weight to body weight ratios were reported[99] indicating hypertrophy of the noninfarcted region of the left ventricle and congestive heart failure. Mice with myocardial infarction demonstrated lower systolic blood pressure, lower left ventricular peak positive and negative dP/dt, and increased left ventricular end-diastolic pressure. Echocardiographic assessment of left ventricular dimensions and function revealed an increase in left ventricular end-diastolic diameter and end-systolic diameter, respectively, with

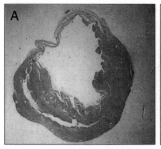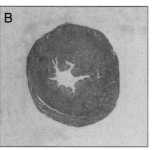

**FIGURE 5-4.** Mouse model of myocardial infarction and cardiac remodeling. Sections of hearts from mice obtained 7 days after ligation of the left anterior descending coronary artery *(A)* and sham-operated mice *(B)*. The myocardial infarction in the anterior-apical region is about 40% of the left ventricular circumference. Left ventricular chamber size is increased after myocardial infarction and hypertrophy of the noninfarcted region of the left ventricular myocardium has developed. *(Courtesy of PR Woldbaek, T Tønnessen, G Christensen, Institute for Experimental Medical Research, Ullevål University Hospital, Oslo, Norway.)*

decreased fractional shortening.[99,101] Functional consequences of left ventricular remodeling in the mouse after a myocardial infarction have been examined in the isovolumically contracting Langendorff preparation[102,103] up to 6 months after myocardial infarction. Myocardial infarction caused a rightward-shift of the diastolic pressure-volume relationship and reduced left ventricular contractile function, as evidenced by a decrease in developed pressure over a range of left ventricular volumes.

Studies have been performed using the mouse model of myocardial infarction to study the role of angiotensin II and the β-adrenergic system in the pathogenesis of ventricular remodeling and failure. In one study,[104] myocardial infarction was induced in angiotensin II type 1A receptor knockout mice and in wild-type mice. Four weeks after myocardial infarction, wild-type mice showed more marked remodeling than knockout mice, which indicates that angiotensin II type 1A signals play a role in the progression of left ventricular remodeling after myocardial infarction. In another study,[105] the effects of cardiac specific overexpression of β$_2$-adrenergic receptors on the development of heart failure were studied in wild-type and transgenic mice following myocardial infarction. β$_2$-Adrenergic receptor overexpression preserved left ventricular contractility following myocardial infarction without any adverse consequence.

### Genetically Modified Mouse Models of Myocardial Hypertrophy

#### Heptahelical Receptors and Angiotensin

Angiotensin II, α-adrenergic agonists, and endothelin bind to heptahelical receptors and are capable of inducing hypertrophic phenotypes in neonatal rat ventricular myocytes (Chapter 15). Transgenic mice were created that expressed high levels of a constitutively active mutant α$_{1B}$-adrenergic receptor.[106] These trans-

genic animals demonstrated a phenotype consistent with cardiac hypertrophy and had increased heart to body weight ratios and myocyte cross-sectional areas. In a later study,[107] it was shown that hearts from transgenic mice subjected to aortic constriction were larger than hearts from wild-type mice after 6 weeks. Assessment of lung weight and ventricular contractility implied decompensation and progression to heart failure, indicating a role for this receptor in transition from compensated hypertrophy to heart failure. Transgenic mice with overexpression of the rat angiotensinogen gene in the heart developed myocardial hypertrophy without signs of fibrosis independent of the presence of hypertension.[108] These mice demonstrated that local angiotensin II production may mediate a hypertrophic response *in vivo*.

#### Heterotrimeric Guanine Nucleotide-Binding Proteins

A hypertrophic phenotype similar to that observed during pressure overload was found in mice overexpressing the heterotrimeric guanine nucleotide-binding protein Gα$_q$.[109] The mice had increased heart weight, myocyte size, and apoptotic cell death.[110] Mice overexpressing Gα$_q$ also exhibited eccentric ventricular remodeling and left-ventricular contractile depression, indicating that this pathway is sufficient to cause progression to maladaptive cardiac hypertrophy. A mouse model was also developed with transient, modest cardiac expression of a hemagglutinin epitope-tagged, constitutively active mutant of the G$_q$ α subunit.[111] These mice developed hypertrophy and cardiac dilation that proceeded to death in heart failure. A role for G$_q$-mediated signaling during development of pressure overload hypertrophy was also shown using a mouse model with targeted expression of a carboxyl-terminal peptide of Gα$_q$.[112]

#### Low Molecular Weight GTPases

Mouse models with left ventricular hypertrophy have been created by overexpression of low molecular weight GTPases such as ras, RhoA, and rac1. Ras is activated by GDP-to-GTP exchange initiated by membrane bound receptors, which activate downstream signaling molecules such as raf-1 and all three mitogen activated protein kinase signaling branches (extracellular-signal-regulated kinases 1 and 2, cJun NH2-terminal kinases, and p38). The mice overexpressing the ras gene (targeted to the cardiac ventricular chambers)[113] displayed an increase in left ventricular mass and increased left ventricular thickness as determined by echocardiography.[114] A prolongation of cardiac relaxation and intraventricular pressure gradients were observed using a miniaturized catheter-micromanometer. Histologic examination revealed myofibrillar disarray in hearts from all ras mice. Other low molecular weight GTPases such as RhoA[115] and rac1[116] have been overexpressed in the mouse heart. Although mice with RhoA overexpression did not have ventricular hypertrophy, the animals that overexpressed the activated rac1 had cardiac hypertrophy and ventricular dilatation. No myofibril disarray was observed, and hypertrophic hearts were hypercontractile in working heart analysis.

## Protein Kinase C

Studies have indicated that some of the protein kinase C (PKC) isoforms are involved in hypertrophy signaling (Chapter 15). The PKC family consists of more than 10 isoenzymes encoded by different genes, and each of the isoforms exhibits distinct patterns of tissue-specific expression and agonist-mediated activation. The mouse model with overexpression of the PKCβ2 isoform in the heart had increased heart to body weight ratios, normal microscopic well-organized myocardial architecture without myofiber disarray, and diffuse myocyte hypertrophy with multifocal myocardial necrosis.[117] Echocardiographic assessments demonstrated thickening of the interventricular septal wall and the left ventricular posterior wall. Fractional shortening and left ventricular end-diastolic dimension were decreased, indicating impaired ventricular performance and reduced left ventricular chamber compliance. In a follow-up study,[118] it was demonstrated that the transgenic mice had decreased myofilament responsiveness to calcium. Using tetracycline-regulated expression of a mutationally activated PKCβ,[119] a mouse model was developed that displayed mild but progressive hypertrophy associated with impaired diastolic relaxation when the transgene was expressed in the adult mice. A mild concentric myocardial hypertrophy with normal left ventricular performance and no fibrosis was found in mice overexpressing the isoform PKCε.[120]

## Calcineurin

Profound cardiac hypertrophy that underwent transition to dilated heart failure within 2 months was observed in mice with overexpression of activated calcineurin in the heart.[121] The intracellular phosphatase calcineurin has been implicated as a regulator of the hypertrophic response in conjunction with the transcription factors NF-ATs.[122,123] When the constitutively active form of the calcineurin catalytic subunit was expressed in the heart, the heart to body weight ratio was two- to threefold greater than nontransgenic littermates. Histologic analysis showed concentric hypertrophy with a dramatic increase in cross-sectional areas of the ventricular walls and interventricular septum and extensive, primarily interstitial, deposits of collagen. The cardiomyocytes were disorganized and hypertrophic. Calcineurin dephosphorylates the transcription factor NF-AT3. Pathophysiologic changes similar to those found in human cardiac hypertrophy and failure were observed when constitutively active NF-AT3 was expressed in the mouse heart[121] (Figure 5-5). The mice displayed pronounced left and right ventricular concentric hypertrophy with extensive fibrosis, myofiber disarray, and cardiomyocyte enlargement. A parallel pathway operating through activation of the MEF 2 transcription factor also has been described, with overexpression in mice of Ca$^{2+}$/calmodulin-dependent protein kinase IV causing hypertrophy and dilated cardiomyopathy.[124]

## Gp130 Signaling

Transgenic mice with continuous activation of the gp130 signaling pathway exhibit cardiac hypertrophy. Gp130 is a transmembrane receptor that is activated by the ciliary neurotrophic factor/leukemia inhibitory factor/interleukin-6/cardiotrophin-1 family of cytokines. Downstream signaling molecules are members of a Janus kinase family of nonreceptor tyrosine kinases and a latent cytoplasmic transcription factor signal transducer and activator of transcription 3 (STAT3). To

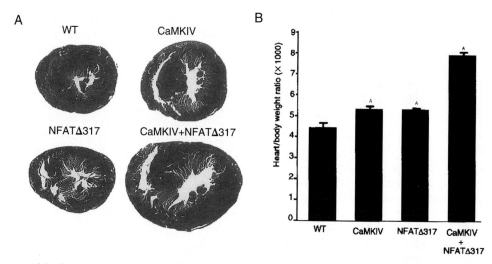

**FIGURE 5-5.** Mouse models of cardiac hypertrophy developed by overexpression of Ca$^{2+}$/calmodulin-dependent protein kinase IV (CaMKIV), overexpression of a constitutively activated form of the transcription factor NFAT3 (NFATΔ317), and intercross of the two lines of transgenic mice (CaMKIV+ NFATΔ317). *A,* Histologic sections obtained at 6 weeks of age and cut at the midsagittal level and parallel to the base. *B,* Heart weight to body weight ratio (× 1000) of wild-type (WT), CaMKIV, NFATΔ317, and CaMKIV+ NFATΔ317 at 6 to 8 weeks of age (*n* = 5 for each group). $^{A}p < 0.05$ versus WT animals. *(From Passier R, Zeng H, Frey N, et al: CaM kinase signaling induces cardiac hypertrophy and activates the MEF2 transcription factor in vivo. J Clin Invest 2000;105:1395–1406.)*

continuously activate the gp130 signaling pathway, transgenic mice that overexpressed both IL-6 and the IL-6 receptor were made.[125] These mice showed constitutive tyrosine phosphorylation of gp130 and STAT3 and exhibited a concentric hypertrophy, with an increase in left ventricular thickness and a reduction in the inner diameter of the left ventricle. An increase in cell volume was observed, but no evidence of disarray, ischemic necrosis, or fibrous scar formation was seen. In another study, STAT3 was overexpressed in the heart,[126] and the thickness of the left ventricle increased by about 20%. Cardiomyocyte width increased by about 30%, but no evidence of fibrosis or inflammation was found.

### Insulin-Like Growth Factor

Mice with activation of the insulin-like growth factor (IGF) signaling pathway by overexpressing human IGF-1B targeted to the cardiac ventricles with the α-myosin heavy chain (MHC) promoter were reported to have increased numbers of total myocytes without myocardial cell hypertrophy.[127] In another study,[128] IGF-1 was expressed in mice using a transgene containing α-skeletal actin promoter, human IGF-1 cDNA, and α-skeletal actin 3'UTR.[129] These mice exhibited increased cardiac mass early in life with an increase throughout life. Aortic-pulsed Doppler measurements showed an increase in peak aortic outflow velocity, a measure of systolic performance, at 10 weeks of age. However, by 52 weeks of age the peak aortic outflow was reduced. The hemodynamic measurements suggested that long-term effects of a loss of ventricular compliance were at least partially responsible for the changes in systolic performance. Histologic examination revealed myofiber hypertrophy, disarray, and increased fibrosis. Also, exogenous administration of recombinant human IGF-1 and recombinant human growth hormone produced cardiac hypertrophy in mice.[130]

### Transforming Growth Factor β-Activated Kinase

Transforming growth factor β-activated kinase (TAK1) has been considered to be a mediator of TGF signaling. A mouse model that expressed a constitutively active form of TAK1 in the myocardium exhibited myocyte hypertrophy, contractile dysfunction, interstitial fibrosis, apoptosis, and early lethality.[131]

## Cardiomyopathies

Cardiomyopathies are a group of diseases in which the dominant feature is involvement of the heart muscle (Braunwald, Chapter 48). Based on morphology and functional impairment three basic types of cardiomyopathies have been described: hypertrophic cardiomyopathy, dilated cardiomyopathy, and restrictive cardiomyopathy. Recently, progress has been made regarding the understanding of the molecular mechanisms involved in initiation and development of some types of cardiomyopathy. This progress has been possible because of insights from human genetics, molecular biology, and genetically modified animals. In particular,

involvement of components of the primary cardiac cytoarchitecture in the pathogenesis of cardiomyopathies has been recognized.[132-134]

### Hypertrophic Cardiomyopathy

Hypertrophic cardiomyopathy is characterized by inappropriate myocardial hypertrophy, often predominantly involving the interventricular septum (Chapter 16). Hemodynamically the disease is characterized by abnormal stiffness of the left ventricle with resultant impaired ventricular filling, which accounts for many of the symptoms associated with this disease. Systolic function is often normal or supranormal, but some patients with long-standing disease develop reduced contractile function and chamber dilation. Microscopic findings in these patients are usually strikingly abnormal, with myocyte hypertrophy and abnormalities of the cell-to-cell arrangements often termed *disarray*.

The discovery of a mutation in the *βMHC* gene that causes familial hypertrophic cardiomyopathy[135] provided the first evidence for a gene defect causing this disease. Since that initial discovery, mutations in genes coding for cardiac troponin T,[136] α tropomyosin,[137] myosin binding protein C,[138,139] cardiac actin,[140] troponin I,[141] essential and regulatory myosin light chains,[142] and titin[141] have been associated with hypertrophic cardiomyopathy. Mouse models with mutations in several of the genes coding for these proteins have been created.

### Myosin Heavy Chain

A mouse model was created using homologous recombination to introduce the Arg403-Gln mutation in the murine *αMHC* gene[143] (Figure 5-6). The murine α myosin isoform is highly homologous to the human β isoform and is the predominant myosin expressed in the adult ventricles of mice. Many features of the αMHC[403/+] mice resembled those found in human familial hypertrophic cardiomyopathy. Ventricular hypertrophy and atrial enlargement became evident by 15 weeks of age. Histologic examination revealed myocyte disarray, hypertrophy, and fibrosis that increased with age. The pathology was more pronounced in male mice. Hemodynamic studies also revealed that young mice lacking histopathologic features of hypertrophic cardiomyopathy had increased diastolic stiffness, delayed relaxation, and prolonged time to maximal filling,[144] indicating that diastolic dysfunction is a direct response to the sarcomere mutation. Hemodynamic measurements revealed that the kinetics of systole were accelerated. Single molecule mechanical assays performed on myocytes isolated from these mice demonstrated increases in actin-activated ATP hydrolysis and force generation.[145] Electrophysiologic examination revealed that these mice have prolonged repolarization, heterogeneous ventricular conduction properties, and inducible ventricular ectopy.[146] The variability of the cardiac phenotype in these mice indicates that modifying effects of background genes and environmental factors play important roles in hypertrophic cardiomyopathy.

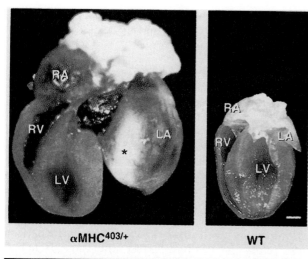

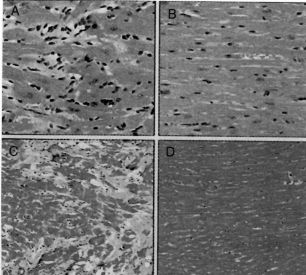

**FIGURE 5-6.** Hypertrophic cardiomyopathy in mice with Arg403-Gln mutation in the α-myosin heavy chain gene *(αMHC⁴⁰³/⁺)*. Upper panel shows hearts from exercised αMHC⁴⁰³/⁺ and wild-type (WT) mice. LA, left atrium; LV, left ventricle; RA, right atrium; RV, right ventricle. The sudden death αMHC⁴⁰³/⁺ mouse heart had fresh clot in all chambers and an organized thrombus (∗) in the markedly enlarged LA. Note the asymmetric hypertrophy of the LV. In the WT mouse normal cardiac anatomy was present after completing a 7-week swimming protocol. Scale bar, 1 mm. Lower panel shows myocyte hypertrophy and disarray in a 30-week-old male αMHC⁴⁰³/⁺ mouse *(A)* and normal histology in a heart from a WT mouse *(B)*. Progressive fibrosis, shown by collagen staining (light gray) of heart from a 30-week-old male αMHC⁴⁰³/⁺ mouse *(C)*, is absent in WT mice *(D)*. *(From Geisterfer-Lowrance AA, Christe M, Conner DA, et al: A mouse model of familial hypertrophic cardiomyopathy. Science 1996;272:731–734.)*

A transgenic mouse model of familial hypertrophic cardiomyopathy has been created by overexpressing rat αMHC cDNA containing the Arg403-Gln mutated residue and an additional deletion of amino acids 468 to 527 in the actin binding domain of the protein.[147] These mice recapitulated aspects of human disease, including foci of myocyte disarray, degenerating myofibrils, and fibrosis.[148] Transgenic mice overexpressing αMHC lacking the light-chain binding domain have

also been created.[149] These mice showed asymmetrically hypertrophied hearts with increased mass restricted to the anterior wall of the left ventricle. Histologic findings were similar to those observed in human disease.

### Myosin Binding Protein C

Several mutations in myosin binding protein C have been linked to familial hypertrophic cardiomyopathy. The function of this thick filament is not well understood, but it probably plays a role in thick filament assembly because it has both MHC- and titin-binding domains. Transgenic mice have been created that express a mutated protein mimicking a defined familial hypertrophic cardiomyopathy mutation in which both the myosin- and titin-binding sites were deleted.[150] Varying amounts of the mutant protein were incorporated. No effects on morbidity or mortality were observed, and no overt hypertrophy or dilation were detected. However, ultrastructural analysis showed a pattern of sarcomere disorganization. Kinetic studies on skinned fiber preparations showed increased calcium sensitivity and decreased maximum power output.

Using homologous recombination in embryonic stem cells, mice were created with replacement of MHC- and titin-binding domains of myosin binding protein C with novel amino acids.[151] Homozygous mice displayed histologic changes, left ventricular dilatation with impaired contractility, and diastolic dysfunction. The heterozygous mice demonstrated progressive left ventricular hypertrophy with increasing age but less severe than mice with *αMHC* gene mutations.[152]

### Myosin Light Chains

Mutations in the myosin light chains have been linked to familial hypertrophic cardiomyopathy. A Met49-Val mutation in the ventricular isoform of essential light chain 1 was associated with a hypertrophy that was largely restricted to the papillary muscle, resulting in midventricular obstruction.[142] Both the wild-type and the mutant genes were expressed in transgenic mice.[153] The mouse model expressing the mutant essential light chain 1 mimicked the human phenotype, demonstrating papillary muscle hypertrophy in aged adult animals.

### Troponin T

Several mutations in cardiac troponin T have been linked to familial hypertrophic cardiomyopathy. Patients with mutations in troponin T have less severe hypertrophy than patients with *MHC* mutations[136] but higher incidence of sudden death.[154] One transgenic mouse model[155] was made to mimic a human mutation that results in a protein that is missing 28 amino acids at the carboxyl terminus but has 7 amino acids that are not present in the normal peptide.[137] Mice that expressed the truncated troponin T at low levels (<5%) were viable and developed cardiomyopathy. The animals had smaller hearts, significant diastolic dysfunction, and milder systolic dysfunction as measured in the isolated work-performing heart model. Histologically the hearts from these animals demonstrated myocellular disarray.

A second human mutation was examined in transgenic mice that expressed troponin T with the missense mutation Arg92-Gln.[156] The expression level of the transgene proteins ranged from 1% to 10% of total cardiac troponin T. Echocardiography showed diastolic dysfunction but normal left ventricular dimensions and systolic function. Histologic examination revealed cardiac myocyte disarray and an increase in myocardial interstitial collagen content. The same mutant allele was examined by another group.[157] The transgenic mice expressed a higher level of total cardiac troponin T as missense allele. The animals had smaller left ventricles and significant fibrosis but no myocyte hypertrophy. Isolated working-heart preparations revealed hypercontractility and diastolic dysfunction.

## Tropomyosin

A mouse model was generated with cardiac expression of α-tropomyosin with a missense mutation associated with human familial hypertrophic cardiomyopathy.[158] These mice demonstrated myocyte disorganization and hypertrophy with impaired contractility and relaxation.

## Other Signaling Pathways

Although mutations in sarcomeric proteins initiate the development of familial hypertrophic cardiomyopathy, it is still not known how and why these mutations result in cardiac hypertrophy. As described earlier in this chapter several signaling pathways may be involved in hypertrophic cardiomyopathy, and genetically modified mice with alterations in these pathways display many of the phenotypic features of hypertrophic cardiomyopathy.

## Glucose Metabolism

Changes in glucose transport in the heart may contribute to myocardial dysfunction in diabetics. A mouse model was developed with cardiac-specific deletion of the GLUT4 glucose transporter using Cre-loxP-mediated recombination.[159] The mice developed modest cardiac hypertrophy with an increase in myocyte size and induction of atrial and brain natriuretic peptide gene expression in the ventricles. Cardiac dysfunction was not observed.

## Friedreich's Ataxia

Friedreich's ataxia is the most common autosomal recessive ataxia. The incidence of cardiac involvement exceeds 90%, and the most common echocardiographic finding is concentric hypertrophy. Through a conditional gene-targeting approach (Cre-loxP), neuron/cardiac frataxin deficient mice were developed.[160] These mice reproduced important features of human disease, including cardiac hypertrophy. The initial cardiac hypertrophy developed into a dilated hypertrophy, similar to what has been observed in humans.

## Dilated Cardiomyopathy

Dilated cardiomyopathy is characterized by ventricular dilation and impaired systolic function of one or both ventricles (Chapter 17). Although cardiac mass is often increased, ventricular wall hypertrophy is often mild. Histologic examination does usually not reveal substantial myocyte disarray, which is found in hypertrophic cardiomyopathy. However, myocyte hypertrophy, myocardial cell degeneration, and interstitial fibrosis are often observed. Dilated cardiomyopathy may be a result of a variety of cytotoxic, metabolic, immunologic, and infectious mechanisms. In about 25% of the patients with "idiopathic cardiomyopathy" the cause is hereditary.[161] Only a few gene mutations have been shown to be involved in causing human dilated cardiomyopathy, including *dystrophin* (associated with Duchenne's muscular dystrophy and X-linked muscular dystrophy),[162] *desmin, cardiac actin, δ-sarcoglycan,*[163] and *lamin A/C.* In addition, other loci for dilated cardiomyopathy genes have been identified by linkage analysis.

Although relatively few of the genes have been identified, recent molecular genetic studies have provided new insight into the pathogenesis of this disease,[132,133,164,165] linking mutations in the extrasarcomeric cytoskeleton to dilated cardiomyopathy. The extrasarcomeric cytoskeleton is composed of desmin- and lamin-containing filaments and subsarcolemmal proteins including dystrophin that provide a link between the sarcomere and the extracellular matrix. The sarcoglycan proteins are transmembrane proteins within the dystrophin-glycoprotein complex. A group of progressive skeletal muscle disorders is caused by mutations in the *dystrophin* or *δ-sarcoglycan* genes.[166] Mutations in dystrophin or its associated proteins can also cause familial forms of dilated cardiomyopathy. For example, patients with Duchenne's muscular dystrophy suffer a progressive muscle wasting of skeletal and cardiac muscle. The disease results from disruption of the gene that encodes dystrophin.

## Dystrophin

Humans with Duchenne's muscular dystrophy, which is caused by a mutation in the *dystrophin* gene, often die of heart failure resulting from dilated cardiomyopathy. However, mice lacking dystrophin have only mild skeletal muscle dystrophy, and they do not have any significant cardiomyopathy.[167] Mice lacking dystrophin and utrophin, which is a homolog of dystrophin, develop signs of cardiomyopathy in addition to skeletal muscle dystrophy. Utrophin may have substituted for dystrophin in mice lacking only dystrophin and hence prevented development of cardiomyopathy. In about half the hearts of older mice lacking dystrophin and utrophin, evidence of myocyte damage similar to that seen in patients with Duchenne's muscular dystrophy was observed.[167] In another mouse model, lacking dystrophin and the muscle-specific transcription factor

MyoD, a dilated cardiomyopathy was observed together with a severe skeletal myopathy.[168] Histologic analysis of sectioned hearts of affected animals revealed an apparent increase in ventricular diameter without a change in the thickness of the ventricular wall. Regions were found, especially in the left ventricle, in which individual cardiac myocytes were substantially enlarged. Because MyoD is not expressed in the heart, the myocardial changes may be secondary to other defects such as severe skeletal myopathy.

### Sarcoglycan

Mutations in sarcoglycan genes result in limb girdle muscular dystrophies, and these patients often have associated mild cardiomyopathy.[169] Moreover, a natural mutation of the δ-sarcoglycan gene in hamsters is associated with absence of this protein and other sarcoglycans and severe dilated cardiomyopathy.[165] Mice lacking γ-sarcoglycan[170] or δ-sarcoglycan[171] but not α-sarcoglycan have cardiomyopathy. In mice lacking γ-sarcoglycan, the right and left ventricular walls appeared thickened after 20 weeks, resulting in near obliterations of the ventricular cavities. The heart to body mass index was increased. Histology showed marked thickening of the ventricular walls, and fibrosis was observed. In another series of experiments, genetically engineered mouse models deficient for either α-sarcoglycan or δ-sarcoglycan were created.[171] Only mice lacking δ-sarcoglycan exhibited cardiomyopathy, but both types of mice developed skeletal muscle dystrophy. Myocardial tissue from mice lacking δ-sarcoglycan that were studied at 3 months revealed extensive alterations. Large and numerous foci of active cellular necrosis followed by fibrotic calcification and scarring were present. Ventricular excitation (QRS amplitude and duration) was markedly disturbed. Because lack of δ-sarcoglycan may lead to microvascular abnormalities, ischemia may be a participating factor.

### Muscle-Specific LIM Domain Protein

The muscle-specific LIM domain protein (MLP) knockout mouse[172] was one of the first genetically engineered mouse models of dilated cardiomyopathy. MLP is localized in the actin-based cytoskeleton in cardiac muscle cells. It is a conserved positive regulator of myogenic differentiation. Echocardiographic studies of MLP knockout mice demonstrated that the left ventricular chamber was enlarged, the walls were thinned, and left ventricular function was reduced. Although wall thinning was observed, the left ventricular weight to body weight ratio was increased indicating the presence of cardiac hypertrophy. Ultrastructural analysis revealed a dramatic disruption of cardiac myofibrillar organization. In addition to deficiency in the assembly of the myofibrillar apparatus, abnormal features included a pronounced increase in nonmyofibrillar space, ribosomes, sarcoplasmic reticulum, and extracellular space. The changes are qualitatively similar to alterations in ultrastructure described for the late phases of dilated cardiomyopathy in humans. The exact mechanism by which these mice develop dilated cardiomyopathy is not yet entirely clear, but the mice provide support for an intrinsic role of cardiomyocyte cytoskeletal proteins in dilated cardiomyopathy.

When MLP knockout mice were mated with phospholamban deficient mice, which have markedly enhanced myocardial contractility, the cardiac defects of the MLP knockout mice were rescued.[173] In that study, using recombinant adenoviruses and a protocol for in vivo murine cardiac gene transfer,[174] it was shown that myocytes that overexpress phospholamban with a point mutation that disrupted the inhibitory effect of phospholamban on sarcoplasmic reticulum $Ca^{2+}$ ATPase (SERCA2) displayed increased contractility. Also, transgenic overexpression of a peptide inhibitor of β-adrenergic receptor kinase (βARK1) was shown to prevent development of myocardial failure in MLP knockout mice.[175]

In a later study,[23] it was shown that adult mice deficient in actinin-associated LIM-domain protein displayed cardiomyopathy predominantly in the right ventricle, but a mild left ventricular cardiomyopathy was also observed. The actinin-associated LIM-domain protein is a member of the cytoskeletal LIM-domain protein superfamily. This mouse model mimics features found in human forms of right ventricular dysplasias.

### Desmin

Missense mutations in desmin have been associated with familial forms of dilated cardiomyopathy in humans.[176-178] Desmin is an intermediate filament protein that connects the sarcomere to the plasma membrane. A mouse model lacking desmin was developed before the previously mentioned observations were made.[179] The mice demonstrated a multisystem disorder involving cardiac, skeletal, and smooth muscle. Histologic and electron microscope analysis revealed severe disruption of muscle architecture, progressive degeneration, and necrosis of the myocardium accompanied by extensive calcification. Another mouse model with null mutation in the desmin gene[180,181] also developed cardiomyopathy. Transgenic mice overexpressing a seven amino acid deletion of desmin, a mutation linked to desmin-related cardiomyopathy, led to aberrant intrasarcoplasmic desmin aggregation, which is characteristic of human disease.[182] Also, a mutation (R120G) in αB-crystallin, a small heat shock protein, has been linked to desmin-related cardiomyopathy. Mice overexpressing mutant R120G-αB-crystallin displayed a phenotype with striking similarity to desminopathy in humans.

### Cardiac Actin

Although it has been suggested that mutations in the contractile apparatus primarily lead to hypertrophic cardiomyopathy, studies indicate that mutations in the force-generating intrasarcomeric cytoskeleton also may cause dilated cardiomyopathy. Mutations in the fixed end of the actin filament are associated with human hereditary dilated cardiomyopathy,[183] indicating that sarcomeric and cytoskeletal mutations can be responsible for this condition. α-Cardiac actin has been considered a component of the sarcomere, but it may also play a role in the intrasarcomeric cytoskeleton. Mice with disruption of the *cardiac α-actin* gene generally died within 2 weeks of birth.[184] Electron microscopic analysis showed a variable but extensive loss of thin filaments within the sarcomeres along with myofilament disarray.

### Lamin A/C

Mutations in the *lamin A/C* gene are responsible for Emery-Dreifuss muscular dystrophy, and recently mutations in the rod domain of the *lamin A/C* gene have been reported to cause dilated cardiomyopathy in humans.[185] Mice in which the *lamin A/C* gene was mutated developed to term with no overt abnormalities.[186] However, their postnatal growth was retarded and was characterized by muscular dystrophy. In the heart, the ventricular myocardium was severely compromised with nonuniform involvement of cardiomyocytes.

### Tropomodulin

Mice that overexpressed tropomodulin in the heart developed myofibril degeneration and dilated cardiomyopathy in juvenile animals.[187] Tropomodulin is a component of the thin filament complex in cardiac muscle, and the protein colocalizes where pointed ends of actin filaments are located. The mice showed cardiomyopathic changes between 2 and 4 weeks after birth. Contractile function was compromised severely as determined by echocardiographic analysis and in isolated Langendorff heart preparations. Histologic analysis showed widespread loss of myofibril organization.

### Other Pathways

In addition to mutations in the extrasarcomeric and intrasarcomeric cytoskeleton, several other pathways may potentially be involved in human dilated cardiomyopathy, including chemokines,[188] oncogenes,[189-192] mitochondrial function,[193] and transcription factors.[194-196]

### $G\alpha_q$ Signaling

Mice overexpressing the heterotrimeric guanine nucleotide-binding protein $G\alpha_q$ exhibited eccentric ventricular remodeling and left ventricular contractile depression,[109,110] indicating that this pathway can cause progression to dilated cardiomyopathy. After transverse aortic banding, the transgenic animals developed eccentric hypertrophy with progressively declining ventricular function, eventually resulting in functional decompensation and pulmonary edema.[92] Also, a mouse model with transient, modest cardiac expression of a hemagglutinin epitope-tagged, constitutively active mutant of the $G_q$ α subunit developed cardiac dilation that proceeded to death by heart failure.[111]

### $G_i$ Signaling

Using a tetracycline transactivator system and a modified $G_i$-coupled receptor,[197] it was demonstrated that increased $G_i$ signaling in mice can result in lethal heart failure.[198] In the heart, $G_i$-coupled receptors have been known to decrease intracellular cAMP levels, contractility, and heart rate. In adult mice, induced expression of the modified $G_i$-coupled receptor resulted in arrhythmias and a marked increase in mortality rate. Echocardiography after 8 weeks demonstrated increased left ventricular systolic chamber size and impaired left ventricular fractional shortening. No increase in heart weight was observed, but histology demonstrated patchy myocyte disarray and collagen deposition. This mouse model showed partial recovery of cardiac function after suppressing the expression of the modified $G_i$-coupled receptor.

### β-Adrenergic Signaling

During progression of heart failure, alterations take place in the β-adrenergic signaling system.[199] $\beta_1$-Adrenergic receptor density has been shown to be selectively reduced, and the remaining receptors appear desensitized.[200] Increased level of βARK1 represents a potential mechanism for β-adrenergic receptor desensitization. However, also other factors, such as increased levels of myocardial Gαi, are potential contributors to decreased β-adrenergic signaling in heart failure. Transgenic mice with overexpression of βARK1 demonstrated attenuation of isoproterenol stimulated contractility *in vivo,* dampening of myocardial adenylyl cyclase activity, and reduced functional coupling of β-adrenergic receptors.[201] These data support the concept that increased βARK1 may be a pathologic element in chronic heart failure. In the same study, a peptide inhibitor of βARK1 was expressed, and the mice exhibited enhanced contractility.

Several other genetically engineered mouse models of altered β-adrenergic signaling have been created, including models with overexpression of $\beta_1$-adrenergic receptor[202,203] and $\beta_2$-adrenergic receptor,[204] knockout of adrenergic receptors,[205] and overexpression of Gαs.[206] Mice with overexpression of $\beta_1$ receptor targeted to the ventricular myocardium had increased contractility at a young age but developed marked myocyte hypertrophy. This increase in myocyte area was followed by progressive heart failure with significant ventricular remodeling, including fibrosis.[203] Transgenic mice with overexpression of Gαs targeted to the myocardium[206,207] had augmented inotropic and chronotropic responses to sympathetic stimulation and develop myocardial damage characterized by cellular degeneration, necrosis, and replacement fibrosis; the remaining cells developed compensatory hypertrophy.

Mice with $\beta_2$ adrenergic receptor overexpression exhibited increased basal myocardial adenylyl cyclase activity, enhanced atrial contractility, and increased left ventricular function *in vivo*[204] but did not exhibit the deleterious effects on the heart seen with overexpression of $\beta_1$ receptor or Gαs. However, when transgenic mouse lines expressing various levels of $\beta_2$ adrenergic receptor were studied, the highest expressing line developed progressive fibrotic dilated cardiomyopathy.[208]

Because these studies demonstrated that it is possible to achieve enhanced contractility for a relatively long period without deleterious effects, they indicated that $\beta_2$ overexpression represents a therapeutic approach in heart failure. A transgenic mouse line over-expressing $\beta_2$-adrenergic receptors rescued the hypertrophy and basal ventricular function of the mouse model with $G\alpha_q$ overexpression.[209] However, over-expression of $\beta_2$-adrenergic receptor did not rescue the dilated cardiomyopathy and heart failure of the MLP knockout mouse.[175]

## Calcineurin

Progression to dilated cardiomyopathy within 2 months after birth was observed in transgenic mice over-expressing activated calcineurin in the heart.[121] The mice were also highly susceptible to sudden death. Pathophysiologic changes similar to those found in human cardiomyopathy were observed when constitutively active NF-AT3 was expressed in the heart.[121] Also, mice overexpressing $Ca^{2+}$/calmodulin-dependent protein kinase IV developed dilated cardiomyopathy.[124]

## Calcium Homeostasis

Heart failure has been associated with alterations in intracellular calcium homeostasis (Chapter 15). In particular, handling of calcium in the sarcoplasmic reticulum has been found to be depressed. Using homologous recombination the SERCA2 gene was eliminated, and heterozygous mutants expressed 65% of the protein level found in wild-type mice.[210] Homozygous SERCA2 null mutants were not observed. Mice with reduction in SERCA2 levels had decreased ventricular systolic pressure and lower absolute values of both positive and negative dP/dt than wild-type mice had. There was no evidence of cardiac hypertrophy in the heterozygous mutants.

Increasing the level of SERCA2 in the heart has been discussed as a therapeutic approach in heart failure, and hence transgenic mouse models with overexpression of SERCA2 have been created.[211-213] Increased levels of SERCA2 protein were associated with enhanced calcium pumping activity at the cellular level and accelerated rates of contraction and relaxation *in vivo*.

A mouse model with cardiac overexpression of phospholamban, which is the regulatory protein of SERCA2, exhibited decreased fractional shortening and mean velocity of circumferential fiber shortening.[214] At the cellular level, the amplitude of the calcium signal was decreased and the time for decay of the calcium signal was prolonged. No changes in heart weight or cardiomyocyte size were observed. Ablation of phospholamban has been proposed as a therapeutic strategy. Phospholamban-deficient mice exhibit no changes in gross cardiac morphology but have markedly enhanced myocardial contractility.[215]

Calsequestrin is a calcium binding protein in the sarcoplasmic reticulum[216] that is assumed to form a functional complex with junctin, triadin, and the ryanodine receptor.[217] Transgenic mouse models with overexpression of calsequestrin developed cardiac hypertrophy[218,219] with an increase in cardiomyocyte size. At the cellular level the frequency of spontaneous or calcium current triggered $Ca^{2+}$ sparks was reduced. Echocardiography demonstrated marked left ventricular hypertrophy and mild decrease in cardiac systolic function, which then rapidly deteriorated to left ventricular enlargement, severe cardiac dysfunction, and reduction in myocardial wall thickness.[220] Transgenic mice with overexpression of triadin 1 targeted to the heart exhibited cardiac hypertrophy and impaired relaxation.[221] The hypertrophy was relatively mild, as indicated by a moderate increase in heart weight, and the mice did not develop heart failure. FKBP-12 interacts with intracellular calcium release channels. Mutant mice deficient in FKBP-12 had severe dilated cardiomyopathy and ventricular septal defects.[222] A subgroup of these mice survived to weaning, and echocardiographic analysis of a 14-month-old mouse demonstrated a dilated left ventricular chamber. Finally, mice with overexpression of L-type calcium channels developed hypertrophy and severe cardiomyopathy.[223]

## Ischemic Cardiomyopathy

Impaired myocardial angiogenesis and ischemic cardiomyopathy were observed in mice lacking VEGF isoforms—$VEGF_{164}$ and $VEGF_{188}$.[224] VEGF is involved in embryonic and pathologic vascular development, and three isoforms are known: $VEGF_{120}$, $VEGF_{164}$, and $VEGF_{188}$. A mouse model was generated using the Cre-loxP technique, and the mice expressed only $VEGF_{120}$ isoform.[224] Depressed left ventricular contractility, enlarged systolic and diastolic dimensions, and impaired fractional shortening were found. Like patients with ischemic heart disease, the mice had prolonged QT interval, depression of the ST segment at rest, Pardee curve-like elevations of the ST segment during stress, and arrhythmias. Another mouse model of cardiac hypovascularity and contractile dysfunction was created by cardiac myocyte specific deletion of all VEGF isoforms using Cre-loxP technology.[30] This model demonstrated the role of myocyte-derived VEGF in cardiac morphogenesis. Examination of the mice revealed dilated thin-walled adult hearts but no evidence of cardiomyocyte necrosis or fibrosis. Function was assessed by echocardiography, MRI, and high-fidelity catheter-based hemodynamic evaluation, providing clear documentation of basal cardiac pump dysfunction and blunted response to $\beta$-adrenergic stimulation (Figure 5-7). It is possible that this model mimics aspects of "stunned" or "hibernating" human myocardium.

## Metabolic Cardiomyopathy

Mice have been developed that serve as a model for metabolic cardiomyopathy.[225] This mouse model was generated by cardiac overexpression of long-chain acyl CoA, which plays an important role in fatty acid transport across the plasma membrane. Lipid accumulation was observed in the heart, and the mice developed cardiac hypertrophy followed by development of left ventricular dysfunction and premature death.

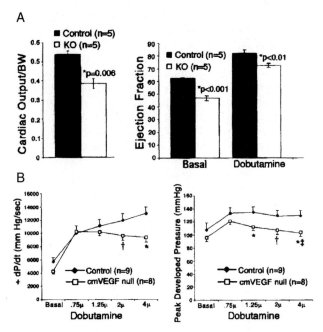

**FIGURE 5-7.** Cardiac function in a mouse model with reduced number of coronary microvessels and dilated thin-walled adult hearts resulting from cardiomyocyte-specific deletion of the vascular endothelial growth factor gene *(cmVEGF null)*. *A,* Magnetic resonance determination demonstrated reduced cardiac output per body weight (BW) *(left)* and reduced percent ejection fraction under basal conditions and with β-adrenergic stimulation (dobutamine) *(right)* in cmVEGF null (KO) compared with control hearts. *B,* Catheter-based hemodynamic assessments at baseline and with increasing doses of dobutamine. Rate of rise of left ventricular pressure during systole (+dP/dt in mm Hg/sec; $^*, p = 0.01$ and $\dagger, p = 0.09$) *(left)*. Peak developed left ventricular pressure in mm Hg ($^*, p < 0.05$; $\dagger, p = 0.07$; and $\ddagger, p < 0.001$ relative to peak pressure at 0.75-μg dobutamine dose) *(right)*. *(From Giordano FJ, Gerber HP, Williams SP, et al: A cardiac myocyte vascular endothelial growth factor paracrine pathway is required to maintain cardiac function. Proc Natl Acad Sci U S A 2001;98:5780-5785.)*

### Cell-Matrix Interaction

Mice that constitutively expressed the human collagenase MMP-1 in the heart reproduced changes observed in the progression of human heart failure.[226] MMPs are a family of proteolytic enzymes capable of degrading several extracellular matrix components. At 6 months of age, the mouse model with cardiac overexpression of MMP-1 demonstrated myocyte hypertrophy and an increase in collagen content resulting from increased transcription of type III collagen. At 12 months of age, loss of cardiac interstitial collagen and a marked deterioration of systolic and diastolic function were observed. Integrins are cell surface receptors that mediate cellular adhesion to the extracellular matrix. Mice with disruption of integrin function in the myocardium displayed perinatal lethality, fibrosis, and abnormal cardiac performance.[227]

### Tumor Necrosis Factor-α

Mice overexpressing TNF-α in the heart recapitulated the phenotype of congestive heart failure.[228,229] TNF-α is a proinflammatory cytokine with pleiotropic biologic effects. *In vivo,* ECG-gated MRI of symptomatic animals demonstrated severe impairment of cardiac function evi-

denced by biventricular dilation and depressed ejection fractions. Subgroups of transgenic animals died prematurely. Pathologic examination revealed myocyte apoptosis and myocarditis.

### Myocarditis

Myocarditis may lead to dilated cardiomyopathy by mechanisms that are currently not well known. Mouse models of viral myocarditis have been used for several years and are considered to be valid models for many aspects of the disease.[230] Encephalomyocarditis virus and coxsackievirus B are most often used. The virulence of murine infection is influenced by malnutrition, exercise, sex, age, and genetic background. Thus, depending on virus, mouse strain, and environmental factors, this mouse model may display ventricular dilation and congestive heart failure within a few days or may develop cardiac enlargement in the course of several months. Myocarditis and dilated cardiomyopathy can also be induced in susceptible mouse strains by immunization with purified cardiac myosin.[231] The mouse models of viral and autoimmune myocarditis have recently been used in combination with genetically modified mouse models to examine the pathogenesis of myocarditis and dilated cardiomyopathy.[232-234] Also, transgenic mice that express replication-restricted coxsackievirus genomes in the heart developed dilated cardiomyopathy.[235] This model indicates that persistent enteroviral nucleic acids, as has been observed in subgroups of patients with dilated cardiomyopathy, may play a pathogenetic role in this disease.

## Cardiac Arrhythmias

Cardiac arrhythmias are a leading cause of morbidity and mortality. The ability to predict, prevent, and treat individual cardiac arrhythmias has been limited, partly because of poor understanding of the molecular mechanisms involved. Several forms of cardiac arrhythmias are acquired, but inherited cardiac disorders with arrhythmias also occur.[236] Mouse models have been made to mimic these human mutations, allowing detailed assessment of physiology and testing of novel treatment strategies.

### Long QT Syndrome

Long QT syndrome is a group of disorders that is characterized by a prolonged QT interval on ECG. Clinically, it is associated with syncope and sudden death. Long QT syndromes can be inherited or acquired. Identification of specific genes encoding ion channels involved in inherited forms of long QT syndrome have provided insight into the molecular pathogenesis of cardiac arrhythmias (Chapter 19). The prolonged ventricular repolarization and dispersion of refractoriness in long QT syndrome is related to loss-of-function mutations in genes encoding subunits of voltage-gated potassium channels in the heart such as KvLQT, MinK, or HERG. Mutations in *SCN5A,* a gene encoding a subunit of sodium channels, have also been associated with long

QT syndrome. Mouse models mimicking several of these human forms of long QT syndrome have been made, and their cardiac electrophysiology has been studied using *in vivo* and *in vitro* electrophysiologic methods.[237]

### KVLQT1 (KCNQ1)

A mouse model of Jervell and Lange-Nielsen syndrome was created by targeted disruption of the *Kcnq1* gene.[238] Jervell and Lange-Nielsen syndrome is transmitted as a recessive trait and is associated with deafness in addition to prolonged QT interval. Mutations in *KVLQT1* (also called *KCNQ1*) or *minK* (also called *ISK*), which together form a K+ channel, can cause this disorder. The mice with targeted disruption of *Kcnq1* were deaf and had vestibular defects (Figure 5-8). ECG demonstrated abnormal T- and P-wave morphologies and prolongation of the QT and JT intervals when measured *in vivo* but not in isolated hearts. In another mouse model, a human cardiac isoform with a dominant negative effect on KvLQT1 channels was overexpressed in the heart.[239] These mice had a markedly prolonged QT interval associated with sinus node dysfunction. The prolonged QT interval correlated with prolonged action potential duration and with decreased K+ current density in patch-clamp experiments.

### ISK (minK)

Because Jervell and Lange-Nielsen syndrome also can result from mutations in the *ISK* (also called *minK*) gene, mice have been created with disruption of this gene.[240,241] Mice with disrupted ISK had bilateral deafness and inner ear defects strikingly similar to those observed in humans.[240] In a study by Drici et al.,[242] ECG recordings in these mice showed longer QT intervals at slow heart rates and shorter QT interval at fast heart rates. In another study,[241] in which the *minK* gene was replaced with *lacZ*, no QT prolongation was observed. The latter mouse model allowed assessment of the pattern of minK expression by staining for β-galactosidase.

### Kv1.1

Transgenic mice overexpressing the N-terminus and first transmembrane segment of the voltage-gated potassium channel Kv1.1 exhibited prolonged QT interval and ventricular tachycardia.[243] Cardiac myocytes from these mice have action potential prolongation caused by a significant reduction in the density of rapidly activating, slowly inactivating, 4-amino-pyridine sensitive outward K+ current. This mouse model of long QT syndrome is of particular interest because spontaneous ventricular arrhythmias have been observed.[244]

Prolonged QT interval has also been observed in mice with cardiac-specific expression of a mutant Kv2.1 subunit[245] or a mutant Kv4.2 subunit,[246] in mice lacking Kv1.4 and expressing a dominant negative Kv4 α subunit[247] and in mice overexpressing the human α3-isoform of the NaK-ATPase.[248] Also, mice lacking ankyrin(B), a

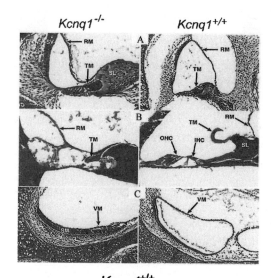

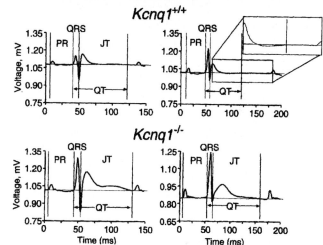

**FIGURE 5-8.** Mouse model of long QT syndrome (Jervell and Lange-Nielsen syndrome) developed by targeted disruption of the Kcnq1 gene (Kcnq1$^{-/-}$). Upper panel shows histology of inner ear structures of Kcnq1$^{-/-}$ and Kcnq1$^{+/+}$ mice. Note collapse of Reissner's membrane (RM) at postnatal day (P) 3 *(A)*, degeneration of inner (IHC) and outer hair cells (OHC) at P70 *(B)*, and collapse of the vesicular membrane (VM) at P0 *(C)*. TM, tectorial membrane. Lower panel shows representative surface ECG traces (lead II) recorded *in vivo* from two Kcnq1$^{+/+}$ mice *(upper two traces)* and two Kcnq1$^{-/-}$ mice *(lower two traces)*. The QT interval was measured from the beginning of the QRS complex to the end of the T-wave, where the end of the T-wave was defined as the point where the T-wave merges with the isoelectric line. To better illustrate how the end of the T-wave was measured, the indicated portion of the ECG trace *(upper right)* was magnified as shown *(inset)*. *(From Casimiro MC, Knollmann BC, Ebert SN, et al: Targeted disruption of the Kcnq1 gene produces a mouse model of Jervell and Lange-Nielsen Syndrome. Proc Natl Acad Sci U S A 2001;98:2526–2531.)*

cytoskeletal "adaptor" protein,[249] were found to have a prolonged QT interval.

### Arrhythmias in Familial Hypertrophic Cardiomyopathy

Typical features of familial hypertrophic cardiomyopathies have been described previously in this chapter. The patients are at risk for atrial and ventricular arrhythmias and sudden death. Unrecognized hypertrophic cardiomyopathy is considered to be the most common cause for sudden death in athletes.

Cardiac electrophysiology has been studied in mice with α-MHC Arg403-Gln missense mutation,[146,250,251] which results in histologic and hemodynamic abnormalities characteristic of familial hypertrophic cardiomyopathy.[143] Surface 12-lead ECG tracings from heterozygous male mice showed prolonged ventricular repolarization as measured by the JT and QT intervals.[146,250] Right axis deviation was seen in a subgroup of animals, which may be due to abnormal cardiac morphology or to left posterior hemiblock. The mice were also studied using a miniaturized *in vivo* epicardial electrophysiologic method allowing detailed analysis of cardiac conduction and electrophysiologic evaluation, including response to pacing and programmed stimulation.[252] Mice with α-myosin missense mutation demonstrated heterogenous ventricular conduction properties, prolonged sinus recovery time, and inducible ventricular ectopy.

### Arrhythmias in Myotonic Dystrophy

Myotonic dystrophy is the most common form of adult-onset muscular dystrophy, and patients with this disease develop AV conduction disturbances. The disorders of skeletal muscle and cardiac function occur as a consequence of a CTG repeat expansion located in the 3′ untranslated region of myotonic dystrophy protein kinase on human chromosome 19. A mouse model of this disease (lacking functional myotonic dystrophy protein kinase) developed late-onset skeletal myopathy.[253] Prolonged PR interval was observed on ECG in adult mice, indicating first-degree AV block.[254] Electrophysiologic assessment of the animals revealed conduction disturbances including second- and third-degree AV block. Thus, this mouse model of myotonic dystrophy is similar to the human phenotype, with age-related progression in AV conduction defects.

### Cardiac Conduction Defects and Ventricular Tachyarrhythmias

In humans, sudden cardiac death is often a result of cardiac conduction defects or ventricular tachyarrhythmias. Identification of molecular mechanisms involved in acquired forms of these disturbances and genes that contribute to arrhythmia susceptibility are essential for improved therapy and prevention in humans. Mouse models with phenotypes similar to conduction defects and arrhythmias found in humans are providing this insight.

### HF-1b Transcription Factor

Sudden cardiac death, severe defects in the conduction system, and spontaneous ventricular tachycardia were found in mice deficient in HF-1b.[255] HF-1b is a transcription factor preferentially expressed in the cardiac conduction system and ventricular myocytes in the heart. The mice deficient in HF-1b survive to term and have normal cardiac structure and function at birth. To examine the inducibility of life-threatening ventricular arrhythmias, an electrical stimulation protocol with a miniaturized ventricular electrode was designed.

Ventricular tachycardia was induced in all of the mutant mice, whereas none of the wild-type mice displayed ventricular tachycardia after a single extra stimulus. Continuous telemetric monitoring revealed sudden cardiac death resulting from conduction defects and ventricular arrhythmias. Single-cell electrophysiologic studies demonstrated prolonged action potential duration and greater transmural heterogeneity in myocytes from HF-1b mutant animals than from wild-type animals. A decrease and mislocalization of connexin40 and connexin43 gap junctional proteins were also observed. This mouse model of sudden cardiac death suggests a novel genetic pathway that implicates defects in the transition between ventricular and conduction system cell lineages.

### Connexin

Conduction slowing and sudden arrhythmic death were observed in mice with inactivation of connexin43.[256,257] Connexin43 is a major constituent of ventricular gap junctions, but connexin40 and connexin45 are also found in cardiac myocytes. In diseased myocardium, alterations in the gap junctional proteins have been observed,[258,259] and these changes may underlie arrhythmias associated with many forms of acquired heart disease.

Mice with targeted mutagenesis of connexin43 died at birth with cardiac malformations.[51] However, electrophysiologic studies have been performed in heterozygous connexin43 knockout mice. This mouse model has been found to have slower epicardial conduction; ECG showed prolongation of the QRS complex,[256] whereas atrial conduction was unaffected.[260] When acute ischemia was induced in isolated perfused hearts from this mouse model, the incidence, frequency, and duration of ventricular tachycardia were increased.[261] Some controversy exists, because another group[262] did not find any significant electrophysiologic differences when these heterozygous connexin43 knockout mice were compared with wild-type mice.

In a mouse model with cardiac-restricted inactivation of connexin43, sudden arrhythmic death and conduction slowing were observed.[257] To circumvent the lethal developmental phenotype, the Cre-loxP system was used to inactivate connexin43 expression only in the cardiomyocytes. The mice with cardiac-specific lack of connexin43 had normal heart morphology and contractile function. Nevertheless, by 2 months of age all of the 28 observed mice died of spontaneous ventricular arrhythmias. Optical mapping with a voltage-sensitive dye revealed markedly abnormal conduction parameters.

Connexin40 is expressed in atrial myocytes and in the His-Purkinje system in the mouse heart. Cardiac conduction anomalies characteristic of AV block and bundle branch block were observed in mice lacking connexin40.[263] These findings were supported by ECG findings in another study of connexin40-deficient mice demonstrating prolonged P-wave duration, PQ interval, and QRS duration.[264] In a subsequent study of these mice[265] sinoatrial, intra-atrial, and AV conduction disturbances were demonstrated. Moreover, it was shown that the connexin40-deficient mice had right bundle-branch block and impaired left bundle-branch conduction.[266]

### Mitochondrial Transcription Factor A

AV heart conduction block was observed in mice with mutation in the gene encoding mitochondrial transcription factor A (Tfam).[193] Using a loxP-flanked Tfam allele in combination with a Cre-recombinase transgene under control of the muscle creatine kinase promoter, Tfam was disrupted in heart and muscle. The mice also developed a mosaic cardiac-specific respiratory chain deficiency and dilated cardiomyopathy and died after 2 to 4 weeks. This mouse model reproduces the features of the dilated cardiomyopathy of Kearns-Sayre syndrome.

### $G_i$-Coupled Receptor

Conditional expression of a $G_i$-coupled receptor caused cardiomyopathy as described previously in this chapter.[197,198] These mice displayed ventricular conduction delay and a variety of arrhythmias.

### Angiotensin II Receptor

Mice with cardiac specific overexpression of the angiotensin II type 1 receptor displayed a lethal phenotype with heart block.[267] ECG revealed AV conduction block, as evidence by prolongation of the PR interval. Also, a widening of the QRS complex was observed, indicating a decrease in conduction velocity in these transgenic mice.

### Atrial Septal Defect

In humans, mutations in the cardiac transcription factor NKX2.5 is associated with atrial septal defects and cardiac conduction defects.[61] The mouse model with targeted disruption of NKX2.5 is lethal in embryos, whereas heterozygous mice survive. Electrophysiologic assessment of NKX2.5 haploinsufficient mice revealed atrial and ventricular arrhythmia vulnerability with programmed electrical stimulation.[237] Ventricular tachycardia was inducible in 6 of 10 heterozygous versus 0 of 9 wild-type mice.

### Atrial Fibrillation and Sinus Nodal Disturbances

Atrial fibrillation has been induced in the mouse.[268,269] Although it was possible to induce atrial fibrillation at basal conditions, the success rate was much higher after carbamyl choline injection. In addition, ventricular tissue from mice with an area as small as 100 mm² is capable of undergoing sustained reentrant activity and ventricular fibrillation.[270]

Sinoatrial node dysfunction was observed together with congenital deafness in mice lacking class D L-type $Ca^{2+}$ channels.[271] ECG and physical activity were simultaneously recorded by telemetry and showed that homozygotes had pronounced bradycardia and arrhythmia resulting from altered sinoatrial node pacemaker activity. Mice with cardiac-specific overexpression of

RhoA, a low molecular weight GTPase, displayed evidence of sinus and AV nodal dysfunction.[115] Ultimately, these mice developed lethal dilated cardiomyopathy associated with contractile failure.

## MOUSE MODELS OF HUMAN VASCULAR DISEASE

### Atherosclerosis

Atherosclerosis is a primary cause of morbidity and mortality. The atherosclerotic lesions develop from fatty streaks through several stages to become fibrous plaques (Braunwald, Chapter 30).[272] Although a number of environmental and genetic factors have been associated with atherogenesis, the specific role and relative importance of each of these factors must still be defined. The mouse models of atherosclerosis have provided an important *in vivo* system to study lesion pathogenesis and factors involved in development of atherosclerosis,[273-278] including dyslipidemias, diabetes, hypertension, and inflammation. Moreover, the development of well-characterized mouse models of atherosclerosis has provided opportunities to identify novel tools and targets for prevention and cure of cardiovascular disease.

#### Dyslipidemia

Wild-type mice are resistant to development of atherosclerosis, but studies starting in the late 1960s showed that susceptible strains develop atherosclerotic lesions when fed atherogenic diets.[279-282] When a series of inbred mouse strains were fed a high-fat, high-cholesterol, cholic acid containing diet,[281] the C57BL/6 strain developed foam cell lesions in the subendothelial space near the aortic valve leaflet. In subsequent studies this strain was used in attempts to identify genes responsible for increased susceptibility to atherosclerosis. However, the diet-induced mouse model of atherosclerosis has limitations. Although the mice were fed a diet containing about 10 times as much cholesterol as a Western diet, they had relatively small lesions that showed little evidence of progression to fibrous plaques, and lesion formation was limited to the aortic root in contrast to the lesions in humans.

Advanced atherosclerotic lesions were observed in genetically modified mouse models with targeted inactivation of apolipoprotein E (apoE)[283,284]; apoE acts as a ligand for receptor-mediated clearance of chylomicrons, very low density lipoproteins, and other lipoproteins. Consequently, apoE-deficient mice developed hypercholesterolemia that was primarily due to elevated levels of very low and intermediate density lipoproteins. Atherosclerotic lesions were observed after approximately 10 weeks and progressed over time from fatty streak to a complex lesion with a fibrous cap,[285,286] similar to the morphologic features of atherosclerosis in humans. Lesions were observed at sites typically affected in humans, such as the aortic root, lesser curvature of the thoracic aorta, and at branch points of several arteries.

When fed a high-fat Western-type diet the mice had marked hypercholesterolemia and accelerated development of atherosclerosis. Although the atherosclerosis resulted in extensive narrowing of the arterial lumen, lesions with thrombosis were not observed. In these mice, hypertension and endothelial dysfunction were observed, possibly resulting from atherosclerosis.[287] Heterozygous apoE-deficient mice developed fibrous lesions when fed a high-fat, high-cholesterol diet.[288,289]

The apoE-deficient mouse model has been used extensively to examine the influence of various environmental and genetic determinants on the development of atherosclerosis. Valuable information has been obtained by combining the apoE-deficient mouse model with mice engineered with modifications in other genes related to lipid metabolism (Chapter 21). Moreover, this mouse model has been used to study modifiers of atherosclerosis related to inflammation (Chapter 20), disturbances in glucose metabolism, hypertension, and coagulation.[275] Finally, the apoE-deficient mice have been used to test specific therapeutic approaches including viral transduction systems and known and novel pharmaceuticals.

Total absence of apoE is rare in humans. Type III hyperlipoproteinemia is more common; type III hyperlipoproteinemia is the presence of mutant forms of apoE that can lead to impaired clearance and accumulation of remnant lipoproteins. Transgenic mice overexpressing mutant forms of apoE (apoECys142 or apoE3-Leiden) had mild hyperlipidemia on a standard diet. However, when fed a high-cholesterol, high-fat diet these mouse models developed severe hypercholesterolemia and atherosclerotic lesions.[290-293]

Most humans with type III hyperlipoproteinemia are homozygous for the apoE2 isoform. Transgenic mouse models with overexpression of apoE2 have been generated[294,295] and have characteristics of the disease. More recently, mouse models have been generated in which the endogenous murine apoE was replaced with the human isoforms apoE2, apoE3, or apoE4.[296,297] Mice that expressed human apoE2 had virtually all characteristics of type III hyperlipoproteinemia and spontaneously developed atherosclerotic plaques. The mouse models expressing apoE3 or apoE4 recapitulated many of the phenotypic effects seen in humans with the same isoforms[297] and had less atherosclerosis than the apoE2-expressing mice.

LDL receptors play an important role in the regulation of plasma cholesterol by mediating cellular uptake of LDL and intermediate density lipoproteins. Defects in the human LDL receptor gene are known, and elevated plasma LDL cholesterol is a risk factor for atherosclerosis (Chapter 23). The mouse model lacking LDL receptor had twofold higher plasma cholesterol levels than wild-type mice, because of an increase in intermediate density lipoproteins and LDL.[298] Thus, this model has similarity to familial hypercholesterolemia. Moderate amounts of dietary cholesterol substantially increased the cholesterol content of intermediate density lipoproteins and LDL particles. Massive xanthomatosis and severe atherosclerotic lesions were observed in this mouse

model when fed high-cholesterol diets.[299] No such changes were seen in wild-type mice fed a high-fat diet or LDL receptor negative mice fed a normal diet. Since it was created in 1993 this mouse model[298] has been used in numerous studies examining environmental factors involved in atherogenesis, and it has been crossed with other genetically modified mice to examine the role of genetic modifiers of atherosclerosis.[275] Examples of mouse models with dyslipidemias that have been combined with LDL receptor deficient mice include mice with disruption of apoB mRNA editing catalytic polypeptide-1[300] and mice with transgene expression of apoCIII.[301] These mouse models developed severe atherosclerosis on a normal chow diet[300] or had increased susceptibility to atherosclerosis compared with the mouse model lacking only the LDL receptor.[301]

ApoB100 and apoB48 play important roles in lipoprotein metabolism, and high plasma levels of apoB100 are considered a risk factor for atherosclerosis in humans. Transgenic mice generated with a minigene expression vector had low expression of human apoB.[302] A mouse model with high levels of human apoB was developed using a P1 bacteriophage vector containing an insert with the entire human apoB gene.[303,304] The mice expressing the human apoB gene had mild hypercholesterolemia and no atherosclerosis when fed normal chow. On a high-fat diet, extensive atherosclerotic lesions were observed in the proximal aorta.[305] When mice expressing the human apoB gene were crossed with LDL-deficient mice, the mice had a lipoprotein profile similar to that observed in humans with familial hypercholesterolemia and exhibited severe atherosclerosis on a chow diet.[306]

Reduced levels of HDL cholesterol are associated with increased risk for atherosclerosis. A mouse model with transgenic expression of cholesteryl ester transfer protein resulted in lowering of HDL cholesterol and severe atherosclerosis.[307] Transgenic mice overexpressing apoAII (a structural protein of HDL) displayed increased atherosclerosis despite elevated HDL-cholesterol concentrations,[308] indicating a more complex relationship between HDL cholesterol and risk of atherosclerosis. In a subsequent study, it was suggested that overexpression of apoAII converts HDL to proinflammatory particles.[309]

Increased levels of lipoprotein(a) in humans have been associated with increased risk for atherosclerosis. Transgenic mice expressing human apolipoprotein(a) were more susceptible to lipid-staining lesions in the aorta when fed an atherogenic diet.[310] Transgenic mice fed normal chow or wild-type mice did not develop lipid-staining lesions in aorta.

### Other Risk Factors for Atherosclerosis

Diabetes mellitus and obesity are associated with increased risk for development of premature atherosclerosis. However, the specific pathogenetic mechanisms involved are not well understood. Mouse models with hyperglycemia,[311] hyperglycemia and hyperinsulinemia,[312] insulin resistance,[313,314] and obesity[315] have been developed, and novel mechanistic information regarding these risk factors is being gained by combining these models with mouse models of atherosclerosis, such as apoE or LDL receptor deficient mice.

A mouse model with hyperglycemia was established by treating the animals with multiple low-dose intraperitoneal injections of streptozotocin,[311] which is a toxin specific for insulin-producing cells. The mice had sustained hyperglycemia and a slight reduction in plasma insulin levels. When BALB/c streptozotocin-treated mice were fed an atherogenic diet they displayed an increase in atherosclerotic lesion area as compared with mice not treated with streptozotocin, supporting the concept that hyperglycemia contributes to increased risk of atherosclerosis. The streptozotocin model of hyperglycemia has been used in both apoE-deficient[316,317] (Figure 5-9) and LDL receptor deficient[318,319] mice. An increase in atherosclerotic lesions was observed in mice with combined hyperlipidemia and hyperglycemia compared with animals with only hyperlipidemia.[316,317,319]

Hypertension is assumed to be an independent risk factor for development of atherosclerosis. Mouse models with elevated blood pressure are described in the following section. Those mouse models alone or in combination with other mouse models are currently providing novel information regarding the role of hypertension in atherogenesis.[275]

Homocysteinemia is considered an independent risk factor for atherosclerosis, including coronary vascular disease, cerebrovascular disease, and peripheral vascular disease.[320] It has been suggested that endothelial injury is pathogenetically involved, but the mechanism by which homocysteine increases the predisposition for atherosclerosis is not well known. A mouse model with mild homocysteinemia resulting from heterozygous deficiency in the cystathionine β-synthase gene was developed.[321] This mouse model displayed endothelial

dysfunction in the absence of frank atherosclerotic lesions.[322] In another study,[323] it was shown that apoE-deficient mice with dietary induced hyperhomocysteinemia had increased atherosclerotic lesion area.

### Transplant-Associated Arteriosclerosis

Arteriosclerosis associated with transplantation limits the long-term survival of patients with organ transplantation. A mouse model of accelerated transplant arteriosclerosis was developed in which carotid arteries were transplanted between B.10A(2R) (H-2h2) donor mice and C57BL/6J (H-2b) recipients.[324] The carotid arteries from the donor mice were transplanted paratopically into the recipient in an end-to-side anastomosis. This model reproduced many features of human transplant arteriosclerosis and has subsequently been used in genetically modified mice.[325,326] In another model, a segment of donor thoracic aorta was used to replace a section of recipient abdominal aorta below the renal arteries.[327] Coronary artery disease in transplanted mouse hearts has been studied using models in which the hearts are transplanted heterotopically.[328,329]

## Vascular Injury and Thrombosis

### Vascular Injury

Percutaneous transluminal coronary angioplasty is often used for treatment of coronary atherosclerosis. The procedure causes injury of the arterial wall, and subsequent development of intimal hyperplasia and restenosis often occurs in these patients. To develop strategies for prevention and treatment of restenosis, better insight into the mechanisms causing intimal lesion growth is important. Mouse models have been developed in which vascular injury was induced by a flexible wire,[330] electric current,[331] photochemical induction of endothelial disruption,[332] desiccation and distension,[333] perivascular cuff,[334] and simple arterial ligature.[335] Several of these models have been used in conjunction with genetically modified mouse lines.

In the original model of mechanical injury,[330] a curved flexible wire was introduced into the common carotid artery, and under rotation the wire was passed along the vessel three times. Proliferation of smooth muscle cells in the media was maximal within 5 days after denudation. Subsequently, models were developed in which an angioplasty guidewire was introduced into the femoral arteries.[336,337] These models closely resembled balloon angioplasty, and rapid onset of medial cell apoptosis followed by reproducible neointimal hyperplasia was observed.

Vascular injury induced by perivascular delivery of electric current was shown to destroy all medial smooth muscle cells and denude the injured segment of intact endothelium.[331] Photochemical induction of endothelial disruption was achieved using green light and systemically administered rose bengal.[332] This model is suitable for studying smooth muscle replication and neointimal formation after endothelial injury. Endothelial denudation has also been achieved using a

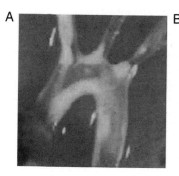 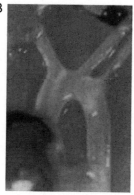

A          B

**FIGURE 5-9.** Model of accelerated and advanced atherosclerosis in diabetic mice deficient for apolipoprotein E. The mice were either made diabetic with streptozotocin *(A)* or treated with citrate buffer as control *(B).* After 6 weeks of diabetes or control treatment, the heart and aorta were dissected under microscopy and photographed. *(From Park L, Raman KG, Lee KJ, et al: Suppression of accelerated diabetic atherosclerosis by the soluble receptor for advanced glycation end-products. Nat Med 1998;4:1025-1031.)*

model of mechanical carotid artery dilation[333] based on a model previously described for the rat.[338] Mouse models with neointimal lesions in the presence of the endothelial lining have been developed by complete cessation of blood flow of the carotid artery[335] or placement of a perivascular cuff.[334]

### Thrombosis

Cardiovascular ischemic events, such as myocardial infarction and stroke, are often due to thrombotic occlusion of atherosclerotic arteries. In the mouse model of mechanical artery injury[330,339] mural thrombosis developed at the site of the endothelial lesion. The time course for the incidence of thrombosis in this model has been assessed, and the method has been used in genetically modified mice.[339] Also, perivascularly applied electric injury induces formation of a thrombus consisting mainly of platelets and fibrin.[331] A more controllable method for induction of arterial thrombosis in the mouse was established using topical application of a 1 × 2 mm strip of filter paper saturated with 10% ferric chloride solution.[340] The thrombus contained platelets, fibrin strands, and erythrocytes and was quantitated using computer-assisted planimetry. Other mouse models of arterial thrombosis includes transillumination of the carotid artery with green light after injection of rose bengal[341] and the use of laser.[342,343]

Mouse models of thromboembolism were established using injections of strong coagulation triggers such as thromboplastin, ADP, collagen, or thrombin alone or in combination with epinephrine.[344-347] In these models thromboembolic death was usually due to pulmonary clot formation. Mouse models of microvascular and venous thrombosis have also been developed.[274,348]

The number of mouse models with genetic modifications in the coagulation or fibrinolytic systems is increasing (Chapters 28/29), and several of these mouse lines display increased thrombogenicity. For example, a murine model of myocardial microvascular thrombosis was established by concomitant modifications of the tissue-type plasminogen activator and thrombomodulin, which resulted in myocardial necrosis and depressed cardiac function.[349]

## Mouse Models with Mutations in Elastic Fiber Proteins

### Marfan's Syndrome

Marfan's syndrome is an autosomal dominant disorder with manifestations that include aortic dilation, aortic dissection, dislocation of the ocular lens, and long bone overgrowth. The syndrome is caused by mutations in the gene that encodes fibrillin-1, a major constituent of the extracellular microfibrils. Mice homozygous for a targeted fibrillin-1 allele expressed very low levels of a centrally deleted monomer and died soon after birth with Marfan's syndrome-like vascular complications.[350] A mouse model homozygous for a hypomorphic allele expressed normal monomer at a level about 15% of normal.[351] The mice exhibited

overgrowth of bones and abnormalities in the vessel wall including elastic fiber calcification, excessive deposition of matrix elements, elastolysis, intimal hyperplasia, and aneurysmal dilatation. Concordant observations were made in elastic vessels from patients with Marfan's syndrome.[352]

### Supravalvular Aortic Stenosis

Supravalvular aortic stenosis is a congenital narrowing of the ascending aorta and is associated with hemizygosity of the elastin gene. Mice with disruption of the elastin gene were generated.[353] Homozygous mice developed a smaller and thicker aorta with narrowing of the arterial lumen and died postnatal day 4.5. Heterozygote mice had a 50% reduction in elastin mRNA and protein, and extensibility of aorta was reduced at pressures higher than 125 mm Hg.[354] An increase in the number of elastic lamellae and smooth muscle was observed in the arteries of these mice, similar to what was observed in the aortic wall of individuals with supravalvular aortic stenosis.[354]

## MOUSE MODELS OF HYPERTENSION

Hypertension is a principal risk factor for cardiovascular events. No specific cause is known for most hypertension, which is referred to as primary, in preference to essential, hypertension (Braunwald Ch. 28). There is substantial evidence for involvement of both environmental and genetic factors in the cause of hypertension. It has been proposed that most patients with primary hypertension have an unfortunate combination of several genetic variations (Chapter 31).[355] Genetically modified mice have provided the opportunity to test whether alterations in candidate genes cause elevated blood pressure *in vivo*.[356-359] In this section mouse models with mutations in genes associated with blood pressure regulation are presented. In addition to mice with gene disruption and transgenic overexpression, mouse models that have different number of copies of the candidate gene at its normal chromosomal location have been generated. Among secondary forms of hypertension, renovascular hypertension is the most common. Mouse models with surgically induced renovascular hypertension have been developed and will likely yield important information when used in combination with genetically modified mice.

## Renin Angiotensin System

The renin angiotensin system may be involved in the pathogenesis of human hypertension, and its role in blood pressure regulation has been examined in the mouse by overexpression or deletion of genes involved in the system. Angiotensinogen is secreted into the blood by the liver and is cleaved by renin to the inactive angiotensin I. Angiotensin II, which is produced by angiotensin-converting enzyme, induces vasoconstriction and synthesis of aldosterone.

Mice with one, two, three, or four functional copies of the angiotensinogen gene at its normal chromosomal location had increased blood pressure[360] (Figure 5-10). The mean arterial blood pressure in these mice increased linearly with about 8 mm Hg per gene copy. Plasma levels of angiotensinogen also increased with increasing gene copy number but not linearly. These mouse models of hypertension demonstrated a causal relationship between variations in the angiotensin genotype and blood pressure.

Transgenic mouse models with overexpression of both the human renin and the human angiotensinogen genes developed chronically increased blood pressure.[361,362] Transgenic mice with overexpression of either the human renin gene or the human angiotensinogen gene did not develop hypertension.[359] In the double transgenic mouse model, plasma angiotensin II was increased and renal lesions typical in hypertension were observed. Also, double transgenic mice with over-

expression of human renin systemically and human angiotensinogen intrarenally were chronically hypertensive, although the circulating levels of angiotensin II were normal.[363] A mouse model that may be useful for studies of pregnancy-associated hypertension has been developed using transgenic mice overexpressing human renin and angiotensinogen. After mating transgenic females expressing human angiotensinogen with transgenic males expressing the human renin gene, the pregnant females had transient increase in blood pressure during late pregnancy.[364]

Two classes of angiotensin II receptors have been identified, $AT_1$ and $AT_2$. These receptors have been modified in various mouse models. A mouse model with targeted disruption of the $AT_2$ receptor gene developed a significant increase in blood pressure.[365] Lack of hypertension reported by another group after disruption of the same gene[366] may be due to differences in genetic background.

## Natriuretic Peptide System

Atrial natriuretic peptide (ANP) is secreted from the atria. It affects blood pressure directly through its natriuretic and vasodilatory activities and indirectly by inhibiting the renin angiotensin system. Whether deficiencies in ANP activity play a role in hypertensive diseases is controversial. A mouse model with targeted homozygous disruption of the proANP gene had higher blood pressure than wild-type siblings.[367,368] Heterozygous animals developed hypertension when fed a high-salt diet, demonstrating that a genetically induced reduction in ANP production may cause salt-sensitive hypertension. Mice lacking the guanylate cyclase-A receptor (GC-A), which is thought to be the principal receptor for ANP, displayed chronic elevations of blood pressure.[369] Elevated blood pressure was not influenced by changes in salt intake, and thus this mouse model resembles human salt-insensitive forms of hypertension. In another study,[370] targeted disruption of the GC-A gene caused similar elevations in blood pressure but also marked cardiac hypertrophy with interstitial fibrosis and sudden death were observed. No reduction in cardiac performance was observed by echocardiography and left ventricular pressure measurements. A mouse model with only one copy of the GC-A gene had a blood pressure on average 9 mm Hg above normal.[371] In these mice, blood pressure was significantly higher when maintained on a high-salt rather than low-salt diet.

Brain natriuretic peptide (BNP) is produced by cardiomyocytes and has effects similar to ANP. Mice with targeted disruption of BNP did not develop hypertension on a standard or high-salt diet.[372] However, the hearts of these mice displayed multifocal fibrotic lesions similar to those observed in some models of cardiomyopathy, suggesting that BNP may act as an antifibrotic factor in cardiac remodeling.

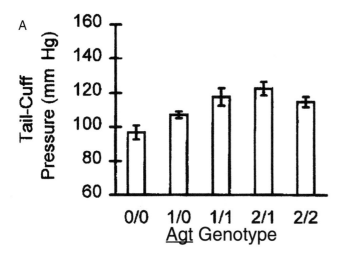

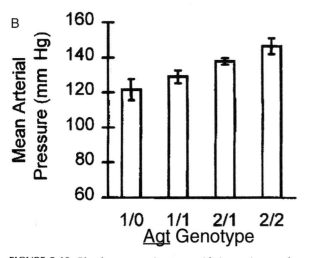

**FIGURE 5-10.** Blood pressures increase with increasing numbers of functional angiotensinogen (Agt) genes. *A,* Tail-cuff pressures of $F_2$ mice having zero (*n* = 3), one (*n* = 11), two (*n* = 10), three (*n* = 8), or four (*n* = 11) copies of the *Agt* gene. *B,* Mean arterial pressures of $F_2$ mice having one (*n* = 7), two (*n* = 9), three (*n* = 3), or four (*n* = 3) functional copies of the Agt gene. *(From Kim HS, Krege JH, Kluckman KD, et al: Genetic control of blood pressure and the angiotensinogen locus. Proc Natl Acad Sci U S A 1995;92:2735-2739.)*

## Endothelin-1

ET-1 has strong vasopressor properties. Surprisingly, heterozygous mice with disruption of ET-1 displayed an increase in blood pressure rather than a decrease.[37] These heterozygous mice had a mean arterial blood pressure of 116 mm Hg as compared with 105 mm Hg in wild-type mice. Homozygotes died soon after birth with craniofacial abnormalities. Elevated blood pressure was also observed in mice with disruption of the $ET_B$ receptor.[373]

## Nitric Oxide Synthase

NO is a potent vasodilator. It is produced in a variety of cell types by three NO synthase isoforms: endothelial NO synthase (eNOS), inducible NO synthase (iNOS), and neuronal NO synthase (nNOS). Elevated blood pressure of about 18 mm Hg was observed in mice lacking eNOS.[374,375] Endothelium-derived relaxing factor activity was absent in aortic rings from these eNOS mutant mice.[374] Homozygous mice were generally indistinguishable in appearance from wild-type mice, but a reduction in heart rate was observed. Despite hypertension and heart rate changes, normal cardiac histology and heart to body weight ratio were observed.[375] Plasma renin concentrations were increased in this mouse model of hypertension. Mice lacking iNOS or nNOS did not have significantly increased blood pressures.[376,377]

## Bradykinin

Bradykinin is a product of the action of kallikrein on kininogen, and it is able to induce vasodilation and natriuresis by releasing NO and prostaglandins. Most cardiovascular and renal actions are mediated by activation of the bradykinin $B_2$ receptors. A mouse model with targeted disruption of the gene encoding the $B_2$ bradykinin receptor has been generated.[378] Blood pressure was about 15 mm Hg higher in homozygous mice than in wild-type mice. Chronic salt loading increased the blood pressure by 34 mm Hg but was without effect on wild-type mice.[379] Clipping of the left renal artery[380] and administration of deoxycorticosterone[381] increased blood pressure more in this mouse model than in wild-type mice. After 360 days, myocardial hypertrophy, chamber dilation, and cardiac dysfunction were observed.[382] When these mice were examined by another group[383,384] significant increases in blood pressure were observed in homozygous mice only when they were fed a high-sodium diet.

## Prostaglandins

Prostaglandins are involved in several physiologic responses, including modulation of inflammation and regulation of vascular homeostasis. Prostaglandin $E_2$ mediates its effects through E-prostanoid (EP) receptors that have been divided into four pharmacologic classes: $Ep_1$ through $EP_4$. Mice with targeted disruption of the gene encoding the $EP_2$ receptor had slightly elevated baseline systolic blood pressure.[385] When fed a high-salt diet, these mice developed profound systolic hypertension. Baseline mean arterial blood pressures in mice with disruption of $EP_1$, $EP_3$, and $EP_4$ were not significantly different from wild-type mice.[386]

## Dopamine Receptors

Dopamine produced in the kidneys participates in regulation of sodium excretion. Activation of the $D_1$ receptor decreases renal sodium reabsorption and increases renin release and angiotensinogen gene expression. Thus, dysfunction in the dopaminergic system may be a genetic factor in hypertension. Mutant mice lacking functional $D_{1A}$ receptors were generated using homologous recombination.[387] The mice lacking both $D_{1A}$ alleles were growth retarded, but feeding with moistened food allowed growth to about 70% of wild-type mice. Both homozygous and heterozygous mice had increased blood pressures compared with wild-type mice.[388] The molecular mechanisms underlying hypertension in these mice remains to be fully defined. Disruption of the $D_3$ receptor also produced increased blood pressure.[389] The increased blood pressure in this model of hypertension was associated with increased renal renin activity.

## Sodium-Proton Exchanger

The $Na^+$-$H^+$ exchanger regulates intracellular pH and sodium reabsorption in renal tubules. Mice were generated overexpressing rabbit type 1 $Na^+$-$H^+$ exchanger under the control of human elongation factor 1 $\alpha$ promoter.[390] In these mice urinary excretion of water and sodium was significantly decreased, and systolic blood pressure was increased after salt loading. The blood pressure elevation may have been caused by impaired sodium excretion resulting from $Na^+$-$H^+$ overexpression in the renal tubules.

## Syndrome of Apparent Mineralocorticoid Excess

In humans, deficiency of 11$\beta$-hydroxysteroid dehydrogenase type 2 (11$\beta$-HSD2) causes the syndrome of apparent mineralocorticoid excess. The syndrome is associated with sodium retention, severe hypertension, and hypokalemia.[391] A mouse model of this disease with targeted disruption of the *11$\beta$-HSD2* gene has been generated.[392] The mice displayed many features of the human disease and had significantly elevated mean arterial blood pressure of 146 mm Hg compared with 121 mm Hg in wild-type mice. This model may allow more insight into other disorders such as Conn's and Liddle's syndromes and glucocorticoid-remediable hyperaldosteronism.

## Other Genetically Modified Mouse Models with High Blood Pressure

Increased blood pressure was observed in mice with deletion of the $\alpha$-calcitonin gene-related peptide.[393] Calcitonin gene-related peptide is a vasoactive neuropeptide that is found in the central and peripheral nervous system. This mouse model of hypertension indicates a role for calcitonin gene-related peptide in long-term regulation of resting blood pressure.

IGF-1 is a polypeptide that binds to the specific type I IGF-1 receptor present on many cell types. Vasoactive effects of IGF-1 suggested a role in blood pressure regulation. Mice deficient in IGF-1 were generated by site-specific insertion of a disrupted exon 3.[394] The mice had IGF-1 levels 30% of normal, sufficient for survival to adulthood. The severe IGF-1 deficiency resulted in elevated blood pressure and increased left ventricular contractility. This mouse model indicates that there is a role for IGF-1 in blood pressure regulation and that the components of this pathway are candidate genes for hypertension.

Elevated blood pressure has also been observed in mouse models lacking bombesin receptor subtype-3,[395] corticotropin-releasing hormone,[396] and adenosine $A_{2a}$ receptor.[397] In these mouse models the increases in blood pressures were observed in addition to relatively complex metabolic or neurologic dysfunctions.

## Surgically Induced Renovascular Hypertension

In humans, renovascular hypertension is the most common secondary form of hypertension. About two thirds of the cases are caused by atherosclerosis in the renal arteries, and about one third are caused by fibromuscular dysplasias (Braunwald, Chapter 28). Models of renovascular hypertension, known as two-kidney, one-clip and one-kidney, one-clip models, have been established in the mouse.[90] A mouse strain with a single renin gene was used. In anesthetized mice, the kidney was exposed and the renal artery of the left kidney individualized by blunt dissection. U-shaped stainless steel clips were used, and the appropriate size of the clip lumen was determined to be 0.12 mm. Right nephrectomy was performed without removal of the adrenal gland. Four weeks after clipping, two-kidney, one-clip hypertensive mice had a blood pressure approximately 20 mm Hg higher than sham-operated controls, and the increase was almost 35 mm Hg in the one-kidney, one-clip model. In the two-kidney, one-clip model, plasma renin levels were increased. These mouse models of renal hypertension developed cardiac hypertrophy, which was more pronounced in the one-kidney, one-clip model. Vascular hypertrophy was found in both models.

## REFERENCES

1. Hoit, Brian D, Richard A. Walsh: Cardiovascular Physiology in the Genetically Engineered Mouse. Boston, Massachusetts: Kluwer Academic Publishers, 1998.
2. Christensen G, Wang Y, Chien KR: Physiological assessment of complex cardiac phenotypes in genetically engineered mice. Am J Physiol 1997;272:H2513–H2524.
3. Srivastava D: Genetic assembly of the heart: Implications for congenital heart disease. Annu Rev Physiol 2001;63:451–469.
4. Srivastava D, Olson EN: A genetic blueprint for cardiac development. Nature 2000;407:221–226.
5. Chien KR: Genomic circuits and the integrative biology of cardiac diseases. Nature 2000;407:227–232.
6. Fishman MC, Chien KR: Fashioning the vertebrate heart: Earliest embryonic decisions. Development 1997;124:2099–2117.
7. Rossant J: Mouse mutants and cardiac development: New molecular insights into cardiogenesis. Circ Res 1996;78:349–353.
8. Lin Q, Schwarz J, Bucana C, Olson EN: Control of mouse cardiac morphogenesis and myogenesis by transcription factor MEF2C. Science 1997;276:1404–1407.
9. Srivastava D, Thomas T, Lin Q, et al: Regulation of cardiac mesodermal and neural crest development by the bHLH transcription factor, dHAND. Nat Genet 1997;16:154–160.
10. Sucov HM, Dyson E, Gumeringer CL, et al: RXR alpha mutant mice establish a genetic basis for vitamin A signaling in heart morphogenesis. Genes Dev 1994;8:1007–1018.
11. Kastner P, Grondona JM, Mark M, et al: Genetic analysis of RXR alpha developmental function: Convergence of RXR and RAR signaling pathways in heart and eye morphogenesis. Cell 1994;78:987–1003.
12. Gruber PJ, Kubalak SW, Pexieder T, et al: RXR alpha deficiency confers genetic susceptibility for aortic sac, conotruncal, atrioventricular cushion, and ventricular muscle defects in mice. J Clin Invest 1996;98:1332–1343.
13. Dyson E, Sucov HM, Kubalak SW, et al: Atrial-like phenotype is associated with embryonic ventricular failure in retinoid X receptor alpha –/–mice. Proc Natl Acad Sci USA 1995;92:7386–7390.
14. Chen J, Kubalak SW, Chien KR: Ventricular muscle-restricted targeting of the RXRalpha gene reveals a non-cell-autonomous requirement in cardiac chamber morphogenesis. Development 1998;125:1943–1949.
15. Charron J, Malynn BA, Fisher P, et al: Embryonic lethality in mice homozygous for a targeted disruption of the N-myc gene. Genes Dev 1992;6:2248–2257.
16. Stanton BR, Perkins AS, Tessarollo L, et al: Loss of N-myc function results in embryonic lethality and failure of the epithelial component of the embryo to develop. Genes Dev 1992;6:2235–2247.
17. Sawai S, Shimono A, Wakamatsu Y, et al: Defects of embryonic organogenesis resulting from targeted disruption of the N-myc gene in the mouse. Development 1993;117:1445–1455.
18. Moens CB, Stanton BR, Parada LF, Rossant J: Defects in heart and lung development in compound heterozygotes for two different targeted mutations at the N-myc locus. Development 1993;119:485–499.
19. Chen Z, Friedrich GA, Soriano P: Transcriptional enhancer factor 1 disruption by a retroviral gene trap leads to heart defects and embryonic lethality in mice. Genes Dev 1994;8:2293–2301.
20. Jacks T, Shih TS, Schmitt EM, et al: Tumour predisposition in mice heterozygous for a targeted mutation in Nf1. Nat Genet 1994;7:353–361.
21. Brannan CI, Perkins AS, Vogel KS, et al: Targeted disruption of the neurofibromatosis type-1 gene leads to developmental abnormalities in heart and various neural crest-derived tissues. Genes Dev 1994;8:1019–1029.
22. Kreidberg JA, Sariola H, Loring JM, et al: WT-1 is required for early kidney development. Cell 1993;74:679–691.
23. Pashmforoush M, Pomies P, Peterson KL, et al: Adult mice deficient in actinin-associated LIM-domain protein reveal a developmental pathway for right ventricular cardiomyopathy. Nat Med 2001;7:591–597.
24. Meyer D, Birchmeier C: Multiple essential functions of neuregulin in development. Nature 1995;378:386–390.
25. Lee KF, Simon H, Chen H, et al: Requirement for neuregulin receptor erbB2 in neural and cardiac development. Nature 1995;378:394–398.
26. Gassmann M, Casagranda F, Orioli D, et al: Aberrant neural and cardiac development in mice lacking the ErbB4 neuregulin receptor. Nature 1995;378:390–394.
27. Gurtner GC, Davis V, Li H, et al: Targeted disruption of the murine VCAM1 gene: Essential role of VCAM-1 in chorioallantoic fusion and placentation. Genes Dev 1995;9:1–14.
28. Kwee L, Baldwin HS, Shen HM, et al: Defective development of the embryonic and extraembryonic circulatory systems in vascular cell adhesion molecule (VCAM-1) deficient mice. Development 1995;121:489–503.
29. Yang JT, Rayburn H, Hynes RO: Cell adhesion events mediated by alpha 4 integrins are essential in placental and cardiac development. Development 1995;121:549–560.
30. Giordano FJ, Gerber HP, Williams SP, et al: A cardiac myocyte vascular endothelial growth factor paracrine pathway is required to maintain cardiac function. Proc Natl Acad Sci USA 2001;98:5780–5785.

31. Suri C, Jones PF, Patan S, et al: Requisite role of angiopoietin-1, a ligand for the TIE2 receptor, during embryonic angiogenesis. Cell 1996;87:1171–1180.

32. Sato TN, Tozawa Y, Deutsch U, et al: Distinct roles of the receptor tyrosine kinases Tie-1 and Tie-2 in blood vessel formation. Nature 1995;376:70–74.

33. de la Pompa JL, Timmerman LA, Takimoto H, et al: Role of the NF-ATc transcription factor in morphogenesis of cardiac valves and septum. Nature 1998;392:182–186.

34. Ranger AM, Grusby MJ, Hodge MR, et al: The transcription factor NF-ATc is essential for cardiac valve formation. Nature 1998;392:186–190.

35. Galvin KM, Donovan MJ, Lynch CA, et al: A role for smad6 in development and homeostasis of the cardiovascular system. Nat Genet 2000;24:171–174.

36. Lindsay EA, Botta A, Jurecic V, et al: Congenital heart disease in mice deficient for the DiGeorge syndrome region. Nature 1999; 401:379–383.

37. Kurihara Y, Kurihara H, Suzuki H, et al: Elevated blood pressure and craniofacial abnormalities in mice deficient in endothelin-1. Nature 1994;368:703–710.

38. Kurihara Y, Kurihara H, Oda H, et al: Aortic arch malformations and ventricular septal defect in mice deficient in endothelin-1. J Clin Invest 1995;96:293–300.

39. Yanagisawa H, Yanagisawa M, Kapur RP, et al: Dual genetic pathways of endothelin-mediated intercellular signaling revealed by targeted disruption of endothelin converting enzyme-1 gene. Development 1998;125:825–836.

40. Clouthier DE, Hosoda K, Richardson JA, et al: Cranial and cardiac neural crest defects in endothelin-A receptor-deficient mice. Development 1998;125:813–824.

41. Donovan MJ, Hahn R, Tessarollo L, Hempstead BL: Identification of an essential nonneuronal function of neurotrophin 3 in mammalian cardiac development. Nat Genet 1996;14:210–213.

42. Tessarollo L, Tsoulfas P, Donovan MJ, et al: Targeted deletion of all isoforms of the trkC gene suggests the use of alternate receptors by its ligand neurotrophin-3 in neuronal development and implicates trkC in normal cardiogenesis. Proc Natl Acad Sci USA 1997;94:14776–14781.

43. Chisaka O, Capecchi MR: Regionally restricted developmental defects resulting from targeted disruption of the mouse homeobox gene hox-1.5. Nature 1991;350:473–479.

44. Schilham MW, Oosterwegel MA, Moerer P, et al: Defects in cardiac outflow tract formation and pro-B-lymphocyte expansion in mice lacking Sox-4. Nature 1996;380:711–714.

45. Ya J, Schilham MW, de Boer PA, et al: Sox4-deficiency syndrome in mice is an animal model for common trunk. Circ Res 1998; 83:986–994.

46. Takihara Y, Tomotsune D, Shirai M, et al: Targeted disruption of the mouse homologue of the Drosophila polyhomeotic gene leads to altered anteroposterior patterning and neural crest defects. Development 1997;124:3673–3682.

47. Iida K, Koseki H, Kakinuma H, et al: Essential roles of the winged helix transcription factor MFH-1 in aortic arch patterning and skeletogenesis. Development 1997;124:4627–4638.

48. Kawasaki T, Kitsukawa T, Bekku Y, et al: A requirement for neuropilin-1 in embryonic vessel formation. Development 1999; 126:4895–4902.

49. Franz T: Persistent truncus arteriosus in the Splotch mutant mouse. Anat Embryol 1989;180:457–464.

50. Conway SJ, Henderson DJ, Copp AJ: Pax3 is required for cardiac neural crest migration in the mouse: Evidence from the splotch (Sp2H) mutant. Development 1997;124:505–514.

51. Reaume AG, de Sousa PA, Kulkarni S, et al: Cardiac malformation in neonatal mice lacking connexin43. Science 1995;267: 1831–1834.

52. Tullio AN, Accili D, Ferrans VJ, et al: Nonmuscle myosin II-B is required for normal development of the mouse heart. Proc Natl Acad Sci USA 1997;94:12407–12412.

53. Webb S, Brown NA, Anderson RH: Cardiac morphology at late fetal stages in the mouse with trisomy 16: Consequences for different formation of the atrioventricular junction when compared to humans with trisomy 21. Cardiovasc Res 1997;34:515–524.

54. Pexieder T, Miyabara S, Gropp A: Congenital heart disease in experimental (fetal) mouse trisomies: incidence. In Pexieder T (ed): Perspectives in Cardiovascular Research, vol. 5. New York, Raven Press, 1981:389–399.

55. Nagasawa T, Hirota S, Tachibana K, et al: Defects of B-cell lymphopoiesis and bone-marrow myelopoiesis in mice lacking the CXC chemokine PBSF/SDF-1. Nature 1996;382:635–638.

56. Sanford LP, Ormsby I, Gittenberger-de Groot AC, et al: TGFbeta2 knockout mice have multiple developmental defects that are non-overlapping with other TGFbeta knockout phenotypes. Development 1997;124:2659–2670.

57. Bartram U, Molin DG, Wisse LJ, et al: Double-outlet right ventricle and overriding tricuspid valve reflect disturbances of looping, myocardialization, endocardial cushion differentiation, and apoptosis in TGF-$\beta_2$-knockout mice. Circulation 2001;103: 2745–2752.

58. Oh SP, Li E: The signaling pathway mediated by the type IIB activin receptor controls axial patterning and lateral asymmetry in the mouse. Genes Dev 1997;11:1812–1826.

59. Svensson EC, Huggins GS, Lin H, et al: A syndrome of tricuspid atresia in mice with a targeted mutation of the gene encoding Fog-2. Nat Genet 2000;25:353–356.

60. Tevosian SG, Deconinck AE, Tanaka M, et al: FOG-2, a cofactor for GATA transcription factors, is essential for heart morphogenesis and development of coronary vessels from epicardium. Cell 2000; 101:729–739.

61. Schott JJ, Benson DW, Basson CT, et al: Congenital heart disease caused by mutations in the transcription factor NKX2-5. Science 1998;281:108–111.

62. Lyons I, Parsons LM, Hartley L, et al: Myogenic and morphogenetic defects in the heart tubes of murine embryos lacking the homeo box gene Nkx2-5. Genes Dev 1995;9:1654–1666.

63. Michael LH, Entman ML, Hartley CJ, et al: Myocardial ischemia and reperfusion: A murine model. Am J Physiol 1995;269: H2147–H2154.

64. Nossuli TO, Lakshminarayanan V, Baumgarten G, et al: A chronic mouse model of myocardial ischemia-reperfusion: Essential in cytokine studies. Am J Physiol Heart Circ Physiol 2000;278: H1049–H1055.

65. Palazzo AJ, Jones SP, Girod WG, et al: Myocardial ischemia-reperfusion injury in Cd18- and 1Cam-1 deficient mice. Am J Physiol 1998; 275:H2300–H2307.

66. Trost SU, Omens JH, Karlon WJ, et al: Protection against myocardial dysfunction after a brief ischemic period in transgenic mice expressing inducible heat shock protein 70. J Clin Invest 1998;101:855–862.

67. Hutter JJ, Mestril R, Tam EK, et al: Overexpression of heat shock protein 72 in transgenic mice decreases infarct size in vivo. Circulation 1996;94:1408–1411.

68. Yang XP, Liu YH, Shesely EG, et al: Endothelial nitric oxide gene knockout mice: Cardiac phenotypes and the effect of angiotensin-converting enzyme inhibitor on myocardial ischemia/reperfusion injury. Hypertension 1999;34:24–30.

69. Jones SP, Girod WG, Palazzo AJ, et al: Myocardial ischemia-reperfusion injury is exacerbated in absence of endothelial cell nitric oxide synthase. Am J Physiol 1999;276:H1567–H1573.

70. Girod WG, Jones SP, Sieber N, et al: Effects of hypercholesterolemia on myocardial ischemia-reperfusion injury in LDL receptor-deficient mice. Arterioscler Thromb Vasc Biol 1999;19: 2776–2781.

71. Guo Y, Wu WJ, Qiu Y, et al: Demonstration of an early and a late phase of ischemic preconditioning in mice. Am J Physiol 1998; 275:H1375–H1387.

72. Miller DL, Van Winkle DM: Ischemic preconditioning limits infarct size following regional ischemia-reperfusion in in situ mouse hearts. Cardiovasc Res 1999;42:680–684.

73. Guo Y, Jones WK, Xuan YT, et al: The late phase of ischemic preconditioning is abrogated by targeted disruption of the inducible NO synthase gene. Proc Natl Acad Sci USA 1999;96:11507–11512.

74. Matherne GP, Linden J, Byford AM, et al: Transgenic A1 adenosine receptor overexpression increases myocardial resistance to ischemia. Proc Natl Acad Sci USA 1997;94:6541–6546.

75. Morrison RR, Jones R, Byford AM, et al: Transgenic overexpression of cardiac A(1) adenosine receptors mimics ischemic preconditioning. Am J Physiol Heart Circ Physiol 2000;279:H1071–H1078.

76. Hampton TG, Amende I, Travers KE, Morgan JP: Intracellular calcium dynamics in mouse model of myocardial stunning. Am J Physiol 1998;274:H1821–H1827.

77. Murphy AM, Kogler H, Georgakopoulos D, et al: Transgenic mouse model of stunned myocardium. Science 2000;287:488–491.

78. Scherrer-Crosbie M, Steudel W, Ullrich R, et al: Echocardiographic determination of risk area size in a murine model of myocardial ischemia. Am J Physiol 1999;277:H986–H992.

79. Scherrer-Crosbie M, Steudel W, Hunziker PR, et al: Three-dimensional echocardiographic assessment of left ventricular wall motion abnormalities in mouse myocardial infarction. J Am Soc Echocardiogr 1999;12:834–840.

80. Heymans S, Luttun A, Nuyens D, et al: Inhibition of plasminogen activators or matrix metalloproteinases prevents cardiac rupture but impairs therapeutic angiogenesis and causes cardiac failure. Nat Med 1999;5:1135–1142.

81. Creemers E, Cleutjens J, Smits J, et al: Disruption of the plasminogen gene in mice abolishes wound healing after myocardial infarction. Am J Pathol 2000;156:1865–1873.

82. Ducharme A, Frantz S, Aikawa M, et al: Targeted deletion of matrix metalloproteinase-9 attenuates left ventricular enlargement and collagen accumulation after experimental myocardial infarction. J Clin Invest 2000;106:55–62.

83. Kurrelmeyer KM, Michael LH, Baumgarten G, et al: Endogenous tumor necrosis factor protects the adult cardiac myocyte against ischemic-induced apoptosis in a murine model of acute myocardial infarction. Proc Natl Acad Sci USA 2000;97:5456–5461.

84. Ho KK, Pinsky JL, Kannel WB, Levy D: The epidemiology of heart failure: The Framingham Study. J Am Coll Cardiol 1993;22(4 Suppl A):6A–13A.

85. Hunter JJ, Chien KR: Signaling pathways for cardiac hypertrophy and failure. N Engl J Med 1999;341:1276–1283.

86. Rockman HA, Ross RS, Harris AN, et al: Segregation of atrial-specific and inducible expression of an atrial natriuretic factor transgene in an in vivo murine model of cardiac hypertrophy. Proc Natl Acad Sci USA 1991;88:8277–8281.

87. Rockman HA, Knowlton J, Ross J Jr, Chien KR: In vivo murine cardiac hypertrophy: A novel model to identify genetic signaling mechanisms that activate an adaptive physiological response. Circulation 1993;87:VII 14–VII 21.

88. Rockman HA, Ono S, Ross RS, et al: Molecular and physiological alterations in murine ventricular dysfunction. Proc Natl Acad Sci USA 1994;91:2694–2698.

89. Tanaka N, Dalton N, Mao L, et al: Transthoracic echocardiography in models of cardiac disease in the mouse. Circulation 1996; 94:1109–1117.

90. Wiesel P, Mazzolai L, Nussberger J, Pedrazzini T: Two-kidney, one clip and one-kidney, one clip hypertension in mice. Hypertension 1997;29:1025–1030.

91. Esposito G, Prasad SV, Rapacciuolo A, et al: Cardiac overexpression of a G(q) inhibitor blocks induction of extracellular signal-regulated kinase and c-Jun NH(2)-terminal kinase activity in in vivo pressure overload. Circulation 2001;103:1453–1458.

92. Sakata Y, Hoit BD, Liggett SB, et al: Decompensation of pressure-overload hypertrophy in G alpha q-overexpressing mice. Circulation 1998;97:1488–1495.

93. Harada K, Komuro I, Zou Y, et al: Acute pressure overload could induce hypertrophic responses in the heart of angiotensin II type 1a knockout mice. Circ Res 1998;82:779–785.

94. Hamawaki M, Coffman TM, Lashus A, et al: Pressure-overload hypertrophy is unabated in mice devoid of AT1A receptors. Am J Physiol 1998;274:H868–H873.

95. Senbonmatsu T, Ichihara S, Price E Jr, et al: Evidence for angiotensin II type 2 receptor-mediated cardiac myocyte enlargement during in vivo pressure overload. J Clin Invest 2000; 106(3):R25–R29.

96. Hirota H, Chen J, Betz UA, et al: Loss of a gp130 cardiac muscle cell survival pathway is a critical event in the onset of heart failure during biomechanical stress. Cell 1999;97:189–198.

97. Lee S: Abdominal large vessel surgery. In Experimental Microsurgery. New York, Igaku Shoin, 1987: 105–127.

98. Li B, Li Q, Wang X, Jana KP, et al: Coronary constriction impairs cardiac function and induces myocardial damage and ventricular remodeling in mice. Am J Physiol 1997;273:H2508–H2519.

99. Patten RD, Aronovitz MJ, Deras-Mejia L, et al: Ventricular remodeling in a mouse model of myocardial infarction. Am J Physiol 1998;274:H1812–H1820.

100. Lutgens E, Daemen MJ, de Muinck ED, et al: Chronic myocardial infarction in the mouse: Cardiac structural and functional changes. Cardiovasc Res 1999;41:586–593.

101. Gao XM, Dart AM, Dewar E, et al: Serial echocardiographic assessment of left ventricular dimensions and function after myocardial infarction in mice. Cardiovasc Res 2000;45:330–338.

102. Eberli FR, Sam F, Ngoy S, et al: Left-ventricular structural and functional remodeling in the mouse after myocardial infarction: Assessment with the isovolumetrically-contracting Langendorff heart. J Mol Cell Cardiol 1998;30:1443–1447.

103. Sam F, Sawyer DB, Chang DL, et al: Progressive left ventricular remodeling and apoptosis late after myocardial infarction in mouse heart. Am J Physiol Heart Circ Physiol 2000;279: H422–H428.

104. Harada K, Sugaya T, Murakami K, et al: Angiotensin II type 1A receptor knockout mice display less left ventricular remodeling and improved survival after myocardial infarction. Circulation 1999;100:2093–2099.

105. Du XJ, Gao XM, Jennings GL, et al: Preserved ventricular contractility in infarcted mouse heart overexpressing beta(2)-adrenergic receptors. Am J Physiol Heart Circ Physiol 2000; 279:H2456–H2463.

106. Milano CA, Dolber PC, Rockman HA, et al: Myocardial expression of a constitutively active alpha 1B-adrenergic receptor in transgenic mice induces cardiac hypertrophy. Proc Natl Acad Sci USA 1994;91:10109–10113.

107. Wang BH, Du XJ, Autelitano DJ, et al: Adverse effects of constitutively active alpha(1B)-adrenergic receptors after pressure overload in mouse hearts. Am J Physiol Heart Circ Physiol 2000;279:H1079–H1086.

108. Mazzolai L, Nussberger J, Aubert JF, et al: Blood pressure-independent cardiac hypertrophy induced by locally activated renin-angiotensin system. Hypertension 1998;31:1324–1330.

109. D'Angelo DD, Sakata Y, Lorenz JN, et al: Transgenic Galphaq overexpression induces cardiac contractile failure in mice. Proc Natl Acad Sci USA 1997;94:8121–8126.

110. Adams JW, Sakata Y, Davis MG, et al: Enhanced Galphaq signaling: A common pathway mediates cardiac hypertrophy and apoptotic heart failure. Proc Natl Acad Sci USA 1998;95:10140–10145.

111. Mende U, Kagen A, Cohen A, et al: Transient cardiac expression of constitutively active Galphaq leads to hypertrophy and dilated cardiomyopathy by calcineurin-dependent and independent pathways. Proc Natl Acad Sci USA 1998;95:13893–13898.

112. Akhter SA, Luttrell LM, Rockman HA, et al: Targeting the receptor-Gq interface to inhibit in vivo pressure overload myocardial hypertrophy. Science 1998;280:574–577.

113. Hunter JJ, Tanaka N, Rockman HA, et al: Ventricular expression of a MLC-2v-ras fusion gene induces cardiac hypertrophy and selective diastolic dysfunction in transgenic mice. J Biol Chem 1995;270:23173–23178.

114. Gottshall KR, Hunter JJ, Tanaka N, et al: Ras-dependent pathways induce obstructive hypertrophy in echo-selected transgenic mice. Proc Natl Acad Sci USA 1997;94:4710–4715.

115. Sah VP, Minamisawa S, Tam SP, et al: Cardiac-specific overexpression of RhoA results in sinus and atrioventricular nodal dysfunction and contractile failure. J Clin Invest 1999;103: 1627–1634.

116. Sussman MA, Welch S, Walker A, et al: Altered focal adhesion regulation correlates with cardiomyopathy in mice expressing constitutively active rac1. J Clin Invest 2000;105:875–886.

117. Wakasaki H, Koya D, Schoen FJ, et al: Targeted overexpression of protein kinase C beta2 isoform in myocardium causes cardiomyopathy. Proc Natl Acad Sci USA 1997;94:9320–9325.

118. Takeishi Y, Chu G, Kirkpatrick DM, et al: In vivo phosphorylation of cardiac troponin I by protein kinase Cbeta2 decreases cardiomyocyte calcium responsiveness and contractility in transgenic mouse hearts. J Clin Invest 1998;102:72–78.

119. Bowman JC, Steinberg SF, Jiang T, et al: Expression of protein kinase C beta in the heart causes hypertrophy in adult mice and sudden death in neonates. J Clin Invest 1997;100:2189–2195.

120. Takeishi Y, Ping P, Bolli R, et al: Transgenic overexpression of constitutively active protein kinase C epsilon causes concentric cardiac hypertrophy. Circ Res 2000;86:1218–1223.

121. Molkentin JD, Lu JR, Antos CL, et al: A calcineurin-dependent transcriptional pathway for cardiac hypertrophy. Cell 1998;93: 215–228.

122. Molkentin JD: Calcineurin and beyond: Cardiac hypertrophic signaling. Circ Res 2000;87:731–738.

123. Molkentin J, Dorn IG: Cytoplasmic signaling pathways that regulate cardiac hypertrophy. Annu Rev Physiol 2001;63:391-426.

124. Passier R, Zeng H, Frey N, et al: CaM kinase signaling induces cardiac hypertrophy and activates the MEF2 transcription factor in vivo. J Clin Invest 2000;105:1395-1406.

125. Hirota H, Yoshida K, Kishimoto T, Taga T: Continuous activation of gp130, a signal-transducing receptor component for interleukin 6-related cytokines, causes myocardial hypertrophy in mice. Proc Natl Acad Sci USA 1995;92:4862-4866.

126. Kunisada K, Negoro S, Tone E, et al: Signal transducer and activator of transcription 3 in the heart transduces not only a hypertrophic signal but a protective signal against doxorubicin-induced cardiomyopathy. Proc Natl Acad Sci USA 2000;97:315-319.

127. Reiss K, Cheng W, Ferber A, et al: Overexpression of insulin-like growth factor-1 in the heart is coupled with myocyte proliferation in transgenic mice. Proc Natl Acad Sci USA 1996;93:8630-8635.

128. Delaughter MC, Taffet GE, Fiorotto ML, et al: Local insulin-like growth factor I expression induces physiologic, then pathologic, cardiac hypertrophy in transgenic mice. FASEB J 1999;13:1923-1929.

129. Coleman ME, DeMayo F, Yin KC, et al: Myogenic vector expression of insulin-like growth factor I stimulates muscle cell differentiation and myofiber hypertrophy in transgenic mice. J Biol Chem 1995;270:12109-12116.

130. Tanaka N, Ryoke T, Hongo M, et al: Effects of growth hormone and IGF-I on cardiac hypertrophy and gene expression in mice. Am J Physiol 1998;275:H393-H399.

131. Zhang D, Gaussin V, Taffet GE, et al: TAK1 is activated in the myocardium after pressure overload and is sufficient to provoke heart failure in transgenic mice. Nat Med 2000;6:556-563.

132. Seidman JG, Seidman C: The genetic basis for cardiomyopathy: From mutation identification to mechanistic paradigms. Cell 2001;104:557-567.

133. Chien KR: Stress pathways and heart failure. Cell 1999;98:555-558.

134. Robbins J: Remodeling the cardiac sarcomere using transgenesis. Annu Rev Physiol 2000;62:261-287.

135. Geisterfer-Lowrance AA, Kass S, Tanigawa G, et al: A molecular basis for familial hypertrophic cardiomyopathy: A beta cardiac myosin heavy chain gene missense mutation. Cell 1990;62:999-1006.

136. Watkins H, McKenna WJ, Thierfelder L, et al: Mutations in the genes for cardiac troponin T and alpha-tropomyosin in hypertrophic cardiomyopathy. N Engl J Med 1995;332:1058-1064.

137. Thierfelder L, Watkins H, MacRae C, et al: Alpha-tropomyosin and cardiac troponin T mutations cause familial hypertrophic cardiomyopathy: A disease of the sarcomere. Cell 1994;77:701-712.

138. Charron P, Dubourg O, Desnos M, et al: Clinical features and prognostic implications of familial hypertrophic cardiomyopathy related to the cardiac myosin-binding protein C gene. Circulation 1998;97:2230-2236.

139. Niimura H, Bachinski LL, Sangwatanaroj S, et al: Mutations in the gene for cardiac myosin-binding protein C and late-onset familial hypertrophic cardiomyopathy. N Engl J Med 1998;338:1248-1257.

140. Mogensen J, Klausen IC, Pedersen AK, et al: Alpha-cardiac actin is a novel disease gene in familial hypertrophic cardiomyopathy. J Clin Invest 1999;103(10):R39-R43.

141. Satoh M, Takahashi M, Sakamoto T, et al: Structural analysis of the titin gene in hypertrophic cardiomyopathy: Identification of a novel disease gene. Biochem Biophys Res Commun 1999;262:411-417.

142. Poetter K, Jiang H, Hassanzadeh S, et al: Mutations in either the essential or regulatory light chains of myosin are associated with a rare myopathy in human heart and skeletal muscle. Nat Genet 1996;13:63-69.

143. Geisterfer-Lowrance AA, Christe M, Conner DA, et al: A mouse model of familial hypertrophic cardiomyopathy. Science 1996;272:731-734.

144. Georgakopoulos D, Christe ME, Giewat M, et al: The pathogenesis of familial hypertrophic cardiomyopathy: Early and evolving effects from an alpha-cardiac myosin heavy chain missense mutation. Nat Med 1999;5:327-330.

145. Tyska MJ, Hayes E, Giewat M, et al: Single-molecule mechanics of R403Q cardiac myosin isolated from the mouse model of familial hypertrophic cardiomyopathy. Circ Res 2000;86:737-744.

146. Berul CI, Christe ME, Aronovitz MJ, et al: Electrophysiological abnormalities and arrhythmias in alpha MHC mutant familial hypertrophic cardiomyopathy mice. J Clin Invest 1997;99:570-576.

147. Vikstrom KL, Factor SM, Leinwand LA: A murine model for hypertrophic cardiomyopathy. Zeitschrift für Kardiologie 1995;84:49-54.

148. Vikstrom KL, Factor SM, Leinwand LA: Mice expressing mutant myosin heavy chains are a model for familial hypertrophic cardiomyopathy. Mol Med 1996;2:556-567.

149. Welikson RE, Buck SH, Patel JR, et al: Cardiac myosin heavy chains lacking the light chain binding domain cause hypertrophic cardiomyopathy in mice. Am J Physiol 1999;276:H2148-H2158.

150. Yang Q, Sanbe A, Osinska H, et al: A mouse model of myosin binding protein C human familial hypertrophic cardiomyopathy. J Clin Invest 1998;102:1292-1300.

151. McConnell BK, Jones KA, Fatkin D, et al: Dilated cardiomyopathy in homozygous myosin-binding protein-C mutant mice. J Clin Invest 1999;104:1235-1244.

152. McConnell BK, Fatkin D, Semsarian C, et al: Comparison of two murine models of familial hypertrophic cardiomyopathy. Circ Res 2001;88:383-389.

153. Vemuri R, Lankford EB, Poetter K, et al: The stretch-activation response may be critical to the proper functioning of the mammalian heart. Proc Natl Acad Sci USA 1999;96:1048-1053.

154. Moolman JC, Corfield VA, Posen B, et al: Sudden death due to troponin T mutations. J Am Coll Cardiol 1997;29:549-555.

155. Tardiff JC, Factor SM, Tompkins BD, et al: A truncated cardiac troponin T molecule in transgenic mice suggests multiple cellular mechanisms for familial hypertrophic cardiomyopathy. J Clin Invest 1998;101:2800-2811.

156. Oberst L, Zhao G, Park JT, et al: Dominant-negative effect of a mutant cardiac troponin T on cardiac structure and function in transgenic mice. J Clin Invest 1998;102:1498-1505.

157. Tardiff JC, Hewett TE, Palmer BM, et al: Cardiac troponin T mutations result in allele-specific phenotypes in a mouse model for hypertrophic cardiomyopathy. J Clin Invest 1999;104:469-481.

158. Muthuchamy M, Grupp IL, Grupp G, et al: Molecular and physiological effects of overexpressing striated muscle beta-tropomyosin in the adult murine heart. J Biol Chem 1995;270:30593-30603.

159. Abel ED, Kaulbach HC, Tian R, et al: Cardiac hypertrophy with preserved contractile function after selective deletion of GLUT4 from the heart. J Clin Invest 1999;104:1703-1714.

160. Puccio H, Simon D, Cossee M, et al: Mouse models for Friedreich ataxia exhibit cardiomyopathy, sensory nerve defect and Fe-S enzyme deficiency followed by intramitochondrial iron deposits. Nat Genet 2001;27:181-186.

161. McMinn TR Jr, Ross J Jr: Hereditary dilated cardiomyopathy. Clin Cardiol 1995;18:7-15.

162. Towbin JA, Hejtmancik JF, Brink P, et al: X-linked dilated cardiomyopathy: Molecular genetic evidence of linkage to the Duchenne muscular dystrophy (dystrophin) gene at the Xp21 locus. Circulation 1993;87:1854-1865.

163. Tsubata S, Bowles KR, Vatta M, et al: Mutations in the human delta-sarcoglycan gene in familial and sporadic dilated cardiomyopathy. J Clin Invest 2000;106:655-662.

164. Chen J, Chien KR: Complexity in simplicity: Monogenic disorders and complex cardiomyopathies. J Clin Invest 1999;103:1483-1485.

165. Ikeda Y, Ross J Jr: Models of dilated cardiomyopathy in the mouse and the hamster. Curr Opin Cardiol 2000;15:197-201.

166. Straub V, Campbell KP: Muscular dystrophies and the dystrophin-glycoprotein complex. Curr Opin Neurol 1997;10:168-175.

167. Grady RM, Teng H, Nichol MC, et al: Skeletal and cardiac myopathies in mice lacking utrophin and dystrophin: A model for Duchenne muscular dystrophy. Cell 1997;90:729-738.

168. Megeney LA, Kablar B, Perry RL, et al: Severe cardiomyopathy in mice lacking dystrophin and MyoD. Proc Natl Acad Sci USA 1999;96:220-225.

169. Melacini P, Fanin M, Duggan DJ, et al: Heart involvement in muscular dystrophies due to sarcoglycan gene mutations. Muscle Nerve 1999;22:473-479.

170. Hack AA, Ly CT, Jiang F, et al: Gamma-sarcoglycan deficiency leads to muscle membrane defects and apoptosis independent of dystrophin. J Biol Chem 1998;142:1279-1287.

171. Coral-Vazquez R, Cohn RD, Moore SA, et al: Disruption of the sarcoglycan-sarcospan complex in vascular smooth muscle: A novel mechanism for cardiomyopathy and muscular dystrophy. Cell 1999;98:465-474.

172. Arber S, Hunter JJ, Ross J Jr, et al: MLP-deficient mice exhibit a disruption of cardiac cytoarchitectural organization, dilated cardiomyopathy, and heart failure. Cell 1997;88:393-403.

173. Minamisawa S, Hoshijima M, Chu G, et al: Chronic phospholamban-sarcoplasmic reticulum calcium ATPase interaction is the critical calcium cycling defect in dilated cardiomyopathy. Cell 1999;99:313-322.

174. Christensen G, Minamisawa S, Gruber PJ, et al: High-efficiency, long-term cardiac expression of foreign genes in living mouse embryos and neonates. Circulation 2000;101:178-184.

175. Rockman HA, Chien KR, Choi DJ, et al: Expression of a beta-adrenergic receptor kinase 1 inhibitor prevents the development of myocardial failure in gene-targeted mice. Proc Natl Acad Sci USA 1998;95:7000-7005.

176. Goldfarb LG, Park KY, Cervenakova L, et al: Missense mutations in desmin associated with familial cardiac and skeletal myopathy. Nat Genet 1998;19:402-403.

177. Bonne G, Di Barletta MR, Varnous S, et al: Mutations in the gene encoding lamin A/C cause autosomal dominant Emery-Dreifuss muscular dystrophy. Nat Genet 1999;21:285-288.

178. Li D, Tapscoft T, Gonzalez O, et al: Desmin mutation responsible for idiopathic dilated cardiomyopathy. Circulation 1999;100: 461-464.

179. Milner DJ, Weitzer G, Tran D, et al: Disruption of muscle architecture and myocardial degeneration in mice lacking desmin. J Biol Chem 1996;134:1255-1270.

180. Thornell L, Carlsson L, Li Z, et al: Null mutation in the desmin gene gives rise to a cardiomyopathy. J Mol Cell Cardiol 1997; 29:2107-2124.

181. Li Z, Colucci-Guyon E, Pincon-Raymond M, et al: Cardiovascular lesions and skeletal myopathy in mice lacking desmin. Dev Biol 1996;175:362-366.

182. Wang X, Osinska H, Dorn GW, et al: Mouse model of desmin-related cardiomyopathy. Circulation 2001;103:2402-2407.

183. Olson TM, Michels VV, Thibodeau SN, et al: Actin mutations in dilated cardiomyopathy, a heritable form of heart failure. Science 1998;280:750-752.

184. Kumar A, Crawford K, Close L, et al: Rescue of cardiac alpha-actin-deficient mice by enteric smooth muscle gamma-actin. Proc Natl Acad Sci USA 1997;94:4406-4411.

185. Fatkin D, MacRae C, Sasaki T, et al: Missense mutations in the rod domain of the lamin A/C gene as causes of dilated cardiomyopathy and conduction-system disease. N Engl J Med 1999;341: 1715-1724.

186. Sullivan T, Escalante-Alcalde D, Bhatt H, et al: Loss of A-type lamin expression compromises nuclear envelope integrity leading to muscular dystrophy. J Cell Biol 1999;147:913-920.

187. Sussman MA, Welch S, Cambon N, et al: Myofibril degeneration caused by tropomodulin overexpression leads to dilated cardiomyopathy in juvenile mice. J Clin Invest 1998;101:51-61.

188. Kolattukudy PE, Quach T, Bergese S, et al: Myocarditis induced by targeted expression of the MCP-1 gene in murine cardiac muscle. Am J Pathol 1998;152:101-111.

189. Yee SP, Mock D, Maltby V, et al: Cardiac and neurological abnormalities in v-fps transgenic mice. Proc Natl Acad Sci USA 1989; 86:5873-5877.

190. Chow LH, Yee SP, Pawson T, McManus BM: Progressive cardiac fibrosis and myocyte injury in v-fps transgenic mice: A model for primary disorders of connective tissue in the heart? Lab Invest 1991;64:457-462.

191. Chalifour LE, Gomes ML, Wang NS, Mes-Masson AM: Polyomavirus large T-antigen expression in heart of transgenic mice causes cardiomyopathy. Oncogene 1990;5:1719-1726.

192. Huen DS, Fox A, Kumar P, Searle PF: Dilated heart failure in transgenic mice expressing the Epstein-Barr virus nuclear antigen-leader protein. J Gen Virol 1993;74:1381-1391.

193. Wang J, Wilhelmsson H, Graff C, et al: Dilated cardiomyopathy and atrioventricular conduction blocks induced by heart-specific inactivation of mitochondrial DNA gene expression. Nat Genet 1999;21:133-137.

194. Edwards JG, Lyons GE, Micales BK, et al: Cardiomyopathy in transgenic myf5 mice. Circ Res 1996;78:379-387.

195. Fentzke RC, Korcarz CE, Lang RM, et al: Dilated cardiomyopathy in transgenic mice expressing a dominant-negative CREB transcription factor in the heart. J Clin Invest 1998;101:2415-2426.

196. Colbert MC, Hall DG, Kimball TR, et al: Cardiac compartment-specific overexpression of a modified retinoic acid receptor produces dilated cardiomyopathy and congestive heart failure in transgenic mice. J Clin Invest 1997;100:1958-1968.

197. Redfern CH, Coward P, Degtyarev MY, et al: Conditional expression and signaling of a specifically designed Gi-coupled receptor in transgenic mice. Nat Biotechnol 1999;17:165-169.

198. Redfern CH, Degtyarev MY, Kwa AT, et al: Conditional expression of a Gi-coupled receptor causes ventricular conduction delay and a lethal cardiomyopathy. Proc Natl Acad Sci USA 2000;97: 4826-4831.

199. Koch WJ, Lefkowitz RJ, Rockman HA: Functional consequences of altering myocardial adrenergic receptor signaling. Annu Rev Physiol 2000;62:237-260.

200. Bristow MR, Ginsburg R, Minobe W, et al: Decreased catecholamine sensitivity and beta-adrenergic-receptor density in failing human hearts. N Engl J Med 1982;307:205-211.

201. Koch WJ, Rockman HA, Samama P, et al: Cardiac function in mice overexpressing the beta-adrenergic receptor kinase or a beta ARK inhibitor. Science 1995;268:1350-1353.

202. Bertin B, Mansier P, Makeh I, et al: Specific atrial overexpression of G protein coupled human beta 1 adrenoceptors in transgenic mice. Cardiovasc Res 1993;27:1606-1612.

203. Engelhardt S, Hein L, Wiesmann F, Lohse MJ: Progressive hypertrophy and heart failure in beta1-adrenergic receptor transgenic mice. Proc Natl Acad Sci USA 1999;96:7059-7064.

204. Milano CA, Allen LF, Rockman HA, et al: Enhanced myocardial function in transgenic mice overexpressing the beta 2-adrenergic receptor. Science 1994;264:582-586.

205. Rohrer DK: Physiological consequences of beta-adrenergic receptor disruption. J Mol Med 1998;76:764-772.

206. Iwase M, Bishop SP, Uechi M, et al: Adverse effects of chronic endogenous sympathetic drive induced by cardiac GS alpha overexpression. Circ Res 1996;78:517-524.

207. Iwase M, Uechi M, Vatner DE, et al: Cardiomyopathy induced by cardiac Gs alpha overexpression. Am J Physiol 1997;272: H585-H589.

208. Liggett SB, Tepe NM, Lorenz JN, et al: Early and delayed consequences of beta(2)-adrenergic receptor overexpression in mouse hearts: Critical role for expression level. Circulation 2000;101: 1707-1714.

209. Dorn GW, Tepe NM, Lorenz JN, et al: Low- and high-level transgenic expression of beta2-adrenergic receptors differentially affect cardiac hypertrophy and function in Galphaq-overexpressing mice. Proc Natl Acad Sci USA 1999;96:6400-6405.

210. Periasamy M, Reed TD, Liu LH, et al: Impaired cardiac performance in heterozygous mice with a null mutation in the sarco(endo)-plasmic reticulum Ca$^{2+}$-ATPase isoform 2 (SERCA2) gene. J Biol Chem 1999;274:2556-2562.

211. He H, Giordano FJ, Hilal-Dandan R, et al: Overexpression of the rat sarcoplasmic reticulum Ca$^{2+}$ ATPase gene in the heart of transgenic mice accelerates calcium transients and cardiac relaxation. J Clin Invest 1997;100:380-389.

212. Yao A, Su Z, Dillmann WH, Barry WH: Sarcoplasmic reticulum function in murine ventricular myocytes overexpressing SR CaATPase. J Mol Cell Cardiol 1998;30:2711-2718.

213. Baker DL, Hashimoto K, Grupp IL, et al: Targeted overexpression of the sarcoplasmic reticulum Ca$^{2+}$-ATPase increases cardiac contractility in transgenic mouse hearts. Circ Res 1998;83: 1205-1214.

214. Kadambi VJ, Ponniah S, Harrer JM, et al: Cardiac-specific overexpression of phospholamban alters calcium kinetics and resultant cardiomyocyte mechanics in transgenic mice. J Clin Invest 1996;97:533-539.

215. Luo W, Grupp IL, Harrer J, et al: Targeted ablation of the phospholamban gene is associated with markedly enhanced myocardial contractility and loss of beta-agonist stimulation. Circ Res 1994;75:401-409.

216. Mitchell RD, Simmerman HK, Jones LR: Ca$^{2+}$ binding effects on protein conformation and protein interactions of canine cardiac calsequestrin. J Biol Chem 1988;263:1376-1381.

217. Zhang L, Kelley J, Schmeisser G, et al: Complex formation between junctin, triadin, calsequestrin, and the ryanodine receptor: Proteins of the cardiac junctional sarcoplasmic reticulum membrane. J Biol Chem 1997;272:23389-23397.

218. Sato Y, Ferguson DG, Sako H, et al: Cardiac-specific overexpression of mouse cardiac calsequestrin is associated with depressed cardiovascular function and hypertrophy in transgenic mice. J Biol Chem 1998;273:28470-28477.

219. Jones LR, Suzuki YJ, Wang W, et al: Regulation of Ca$^{2+}$ signaling in transgenic mouse cardiac myocytes overexpressing calsequestrin. J Clin Invest 1998;101:1385-1393.

220. Cho MC, Rapacciuolo A, Koch WJ, et al: Defective beta-adrenergic receptor signaling precedes the development of dilated cardiomyopathy in transgenic mice with calsequestrin overexpression. J Biol Chem 1999;274:22251-22256.

221. Kirchhefer U, Neumann J, Baba HA, et al: Cardiac hypertrophy and impaired relaxation in transgenic mice overexpressing triadin 1. J Biol Chem 2001;276:4142-4149.

222. Shou W, Aghdasi B, Armstrong DL, et al: Cardiac defects and altered ryanodine receptor function in mice lacking FKBP12. Nature 1998;391:489-492.

223. Muth JN, Bodi I, Lewis W, et al: A Ca$^{2+}$-dependent transgenic model of cardiac hypertrophy: A role for protein kinase Calpha. Circulation 2001;103:140-147.

224. Carmeliet P, Ng YS, Nuyens D, et al: Impaired myocardial angiogenesis and ischemic cardiomyopathy in mice lacking the vascular endothelial growth factor isoforms VEGF164 and VEGF188. Nat Med 1999;5:495-502.

225. Chiu HC, Kovacs A, Ford DA, et al: A novel mouse model of lipotoxic cardiomyopathy. J Clin Invest 2001;107:813-822.

226. Kim HE, Dalal SS, Young E, et al: Disruption of the myocardial extracellular matrix leads to cardiac dysfunction. J Clin Invest 2000;106:857-866.

227. Keller RS, Shai SY, Babbitt CJ, et al: Disruption of integrin function in the murine myocardium leads to perinatal lethality, fibrosis, and abnormal cardiac performance. Am J Pathol 2001;158:1079-1090.

228. Bryant D, Becker L, Richardson J, et al: Cardiac failure in transgenic mice with myocardial expression of tumor necrosis factor-alpha. Circulation 1998;97:1375-1381.

229. Kubota T, McTiernan CF, Frye CS, et al: Dilated cardiomyopathy in transgenic mice with cardiac-specific overexpression of tumor necrosis factor-alpha. Circ Res 1997;81:627-635.

230. Kawai C: From myocarditis to cardiomyopathy: Mechanisms of inflammation and cell death: Learning from the past for the future. Circulation 1999;99:1091-1100.

231. Neu N, Rose NR, Beisel KW, et al: Cardiac myosin induces myocarditis in genetically predisposed mice. J Immunol 1987;139:3630-3636.

232. Knowlton KU, Badorff C: The immune system in viral myocarditis: Maintaining the balance. Circ Res 1999;85:559-561.

233. Bachmaier K, Neu N, Yeung RS, et al: Generation of humanized mice susceptible to peptide-induced inflammatory heart disease. Circulation 1999;99:1885-1891.

234. Wada H, Saito K, Kanda T, et al: Tumor necrosis factor-alpha (TNF-alpha) plays a protective role in acute viral myocarditis in mice: A study using mice lacking TNF-alpha. Circulation 2001;103:743-749.

235. Wessely R, Klingel K, Santana LF, et al: Transgenic expression of replication-restricted enteroviral genomes in heart muscle induces defective excitation-contraction coupling and dilated cardiomyopathy. J Clin Invest 1998;102:1444-1453.

236. Keating MT, Sanguinetti MC: Molecular and cellular mechanisms of cardiac arrhythmias. Cell 2001;104:569-580.

237. Gehrmann J, Berul CI: Cardiac electrophysiology in genetically engineered mice. J Cardiovasc Electrophysiol 2000;11:354-368.

238. Casimiro MC, Knollmann BC, Ebert SN, et al: Targeted disruption of the Kcnq1 gene produces a mouse model of Jervell and Lange-Nielsen syndrome. Proc Natl Acad Sci USA 2001;98:2526-2531.

239. Demolombe S, Lande G, Charpentier F, et al: Transgenic mice overexpressing human KvLQT1 dominant-negative isoform. I: Phenotypic characterisation. Cardiovasc Res 2001;50:314-327.

240. Vetter DE, Mann JR, Wangemann P, et al: Inner ear defects induced by null mutation of the isk gene. Neuron 1996;17:1251-1264.

241. Kupershmidt S, Yang T, Anderson ME, et al: Replacement by homologous recombination of the minK gene with lacZ reveals restriction of minK expression to the mouse cardiac conduction system. Circ Res 1999;84:146-152.

242. Drici MD, Arrighi I, Chouabe C, et al: Involvement of IsK-associated K$^{+}$ channel in heart rate control of repolarization in a murine engineered model of Jervell and Lange-Nielsen syndrome. Circ Res 1998;83:95-102.

243. London B, Jeron A, Zhou J, et al: Long QT and ventricular arrhythmias in transgenic mice expressing the N terminus and first transmembrane segment of a voltage-gated potassium channel. Proc Natl Acad Sci USA 1998;95:2926-2931.

244. Jeron A, Mitchell GF, Zhou J, et al: Inducible polymorphic ventricular tachyarrhythmias in a transgenic mouse model with a long Q-T phenotype. Am J Physiol Heart Circ Physiol 2000;278:H1891-H1898.

245. Xu H, Barry DM, Li H, et al: Attenuation of the slow component of delayed rectification, action potential prolongation, and triggered activity in mice expressing a dominant-negative Kv2 alpha subunit. Circ Res 1999;85:623-633.

246. Barry DM, Xu H, Schuessler RB, Nerbonne JM: Functional knockout of the transient outward current, long-QT syndrome, and cardiac remodeling in mice expressing a dominant-negative Kv4 alpha subunit. Circ Res 1998;83:560-567.

247. Guo W, Li H, London B, Nerbonne JM: Functional consequences of elimination of i(to,f) and i(to,s): Early afterdepolarizations, atrioventricular block, and ventricular arrhythmias in mice lacking Kv1.4 and expressing a dominant-negative Kv4 alpha subunit. Circ Res 2000;87:73-79.

248. O'Brien SE, Apkon M, Berul CI, et al: Phenotypical features of long Q-T syndrome in transgenic mice expressing human Na-K-ATPase alpha(3)-isoform in hearts. Am J Physiol Heart Circ Physiol 2000;279:H2133-H2142.

249. Chauhan VS, Tuvia S, Buhusi M, et al: Abnormal cardiac Na$^{+}$ channel properties and QT heart rate adaptation in neonatal ankyrin(B) knockout mice. Circ Res 2000;86:441-447.

250. Berul CI, Christe ME, Aronovitz MJ, et al: Familial hypertrophic cardiomyopathy mice display gender differences in electrophysiological abnormalities. J Interv Cardiol Electrophysiol 1998;2:7-14.

251. Bevilacqua LM, Maguire CT, Seidman JG, et al: QT dispersion in alpha-myosin heavy-chain familial hypertrophic cardiomyopathy mice. Pediatr Res 1999;45:643-647.

252. Berul CI, Aronovitz MJ, Wang PJ, Mendelsohn ME: In vivo cardiac electrophysiology studies in the mouse. Circulation 1996;94:2641-2648.

253. Reddy S, Smith DB, Rich MM, et al: Mice lacking the myotonic dystrophy protein kinase develop a late onset progressive myopathy. Nat Genet 1996;13:325-335.

254. Berul CI, Maguire CT, Aronovitz MJ, et al: DMPK dosage alterations result in atrioventricular conduction abnormalities in a mouse myotonic dystrophy model. J Clin Invest 1999;103(4):R1-R7.

255. Nguyen-Tran VT, Kubalak SW, Minamisawa S, et al: A novel genetic pathway for sudden cardiac death via defects in the transition between ventricular and conduction system cell lineages. Cell 2000;102:671-682.

256. Guerrero PA, Schuessler RB, Davis LM, et al: Slow ventricular conduction in mice heterozygous for a connexin43 null mutation. J Clin Invest 1997;99:1991-1998.

257. Gutstein DE, Morley GE, Tamaddon H, et al: Conduction slowing and sudden arrhythmic death in mice with cardiac-restricted inactivation of connexin43. Circ Res 2001;88:333-339.

258. Peters NS, Green CR, Poole-Wilson PA, Severs NJ: Reduced content of connexin43 gap junctions in ventricular myocardium from hypertrophied and ischemic human hearts. Circulation 1993;88:864-875.

259. Johannsson E, Lunde PK, Heddle C, et al: Upregulation of the cardiac monocarboxylate transporter MCT1 in a rat model of congestive heart failure. Circulation 2001;104:729-734.

260. Thomas SA, Schuessler RB, Berul CI, et al: Disparate effects of deficient expression of connexin43 on atrial and ventricular conduction: Evidence for chamber-specific molecular determinants of conduction. Circulation 1998;97:686-691.

261. Lerner DL, Yamada KA, Schuessler RB, Saffitz JE: Accelerated onset and increased incidence of ventricular arrhythmias induced by ischemia in Cx43-deficient mice. Circulation 2000;101:547-552.

262. Morley GE, Vaidya D, Samie FH, et al: Characterization of conduction in the ventricles of normal and heterozygous Cx43 knockout mice using optical mapping. J Cardiovasc Electrophysiol 1999; 10:1361-1375.

263. Simon AM, Goodenough DA, Paul DL: Mice lacking connexin40 have cardiac conduction abnormalities characteristic of atrioventricular block and bundle branch block. Curr Biol 1998;8: 295-298.

264. Kirchhoff S, Nelles E, Hagendorff A, et al: Reduced cardiac conduction velocity and predisposition to arrhythmias in connexin40-deficient mice. Curr Biol 1998;8:299-302.

265. Hagendorff A, Schumacher B, Kirchhoff S, et al: Conduction disturbances and increased atrial vulnerability in connexin 40-deficient mice analyzed by transesophageal stimulation. Circulation 1999;99:1508-1515.

266. van Rijen HV, van Veen TA, van Kempen MJ, et al: Impaired conduction in the bundle branches of mouse hearts lacking the gap junction protein connexin40. Circulation 2001;103:1591-1598.

267. Hein L, Stevens ME, Barsh GS, et al: Overexpression of angiotensin AT1 receptor transgene in the mouse myocardium produces a lethal phenotype associated with myocyte hyperplasia and heart block. Proc Natl Acad Sci USA 1997;94:6391-6396.

268. Zhao ZY, Guo YM: CaCl$_2$-Ach induced atrial fibrillation (flutter) in mice. Zhongguo Yao Li Xue Bao 1982;3(3):185-188.

269. Wakimoto H, Maguire CT, Kovoor P, et al: Induction of atrial tachycardia and fibrillation in the mouse heart. Cardiovasc Res 2001;50:463-473.

270. Vaidya D, Morley GE, Samie FH, Jalife J: Reentry and fibrillation in the mouse heart. A challenge to the critical mass hypothesis. Circ Res 1999;85:174-181.

271. Platzer J, Engel J, Schrott-Fischer A, et al: Congenital deafness and sinoatrial node dysfunction in mice lacking class D L-type Ca$^{2+}$ channels. Cell 2000;102:89-97.

272. Lusis AJ: Atherosclerosis. Nature 2000;407:233-241.

273. Breslow JL: Mouse models of atherosclerosis. Science 1996;272: 685-688.

274. Carmeliet P, Moons L, Collen D: Mouse models of angiogenesis, arterial stenosis, atherosclerosis and hemostasis. Cardiovasc Res 1998;39:8-33.

275. Knowles JW, Maeda N: Genetic modifiers of atherosclerosis in mice. Arterioscler Thromb Vasc Biol 2000;20:2336-2345.

276. Faraci FM, Sigmund CD: Vascular biology in genetically altered mice: Smaller vessels, bigger insight. Circ Res 1999;85:1214-1225.

277. Fazio S, Linton MF: Mouse models of hyperlipidemia and atherosclerosis. Front Biosci 2001;6:D515-D525.

278. Reardon CA, Getz GS: Mouse models of atherosclerosis. Curr Opin Lipidol 2001;12(2):167-173.

279. Vesselinovitch D, Wissler RW: Experimental production of atherosclerosis in mice. II. Effects of atherogenic and high-fat diets on vascular changes in chronically and acutely irradiated mice. J Atheroscler Res 1968;8:497-523.

280. Thompson JS: Atheromata in an inbred strain of mice. J Atheroscler Res 1969;10:113-122.

281. Paigen B, Morrow A, Brandon C, et al: Variation in susceptibility to atherosclerosis among inbred strains of mice. Atherosclerosis 1985;57:65-73.

282. Paigen B, Morrow A, Holmes PA, et al: Quantitative assessment of atherosclerotic lesions in mice. Atherosclerosis 1987;68:231-240.

283. Plump AS, Smith JD, Hayek T, et al: Severe hypercholesterolemia and atherosclerosis in apolipoprotein E-deficient mice created by homologous recombination in ES cells. Cell 1992;71:343-353.

284. Zhang SH, Reddick RL, Piedrahita JA, Maeda N: Spontaneous hypercholesterolemia and arterial lesions in mice lacking apolipoprotein E. Science 1992;258:468-471.

285. Reddick RL, Zhang SH, Maeda N: Atherosclerosis in mice lacking apo E. Evaluation of lesional development and progression. Arterioscler Thromb 1994;14:141-147.

286. Nakashima Y, Plump AS, Raines EW, et al: ApoE-deficient mice develop lesions of all phases of atherosclerosis throughout the arterial tree. Arterioscler Thromb 1994;14:133-140.

287. Yang R, Powell-Braxton L, Ogaoawara AK, et al: Hypertension and endothelial dysfunction in apolipoprotein E knockout mice. Arterioscler Thromb Vasc Biol 1999;19:2762-2768.

288. Zhang SH, Reddick RL, Burkey B, Maeda N: Diet-induced atherosclerosis in mice heterozygous and homozygous for apolipoprotein E gene disruption. J Clin Invest 1994;94:937-945.

289. van Ree JH, van den Broek WJ, Dahlmans VE, et al: Diet-induced hypercholesterolemia and atherosclerosis in heterozygous apolipoprotein E-deficient mice. Atherosclerosis 1994;111:25-37.

290. Fazio S, Sanan DA, Lee YL, et al: Susceptibility to diet-induced atherosclerosis in transgenic mice expressing a dysfunctional human apolipoprotein E(Arg 112,Cys142). Arterioscler Thromb 1994;14: 1873-1879.

291. Fazio S, Lee YL, Ji ZS, Rall SC Jr: Type III hyperlipoproteinemic phenotype in transgenic mice expressing dysfunctional apolipoprotein E. J Clin Invest 1993;92:1497-1503.

292. van Vlijmen BJ, van den Maagdenberg AM, Gijbels MJ, et al: Diet-induced hyperlipoproteinemia and atherosclerosis in apolipoprotein E3-Leiden transgenic mice. J Clin Invest 1994;93: 1403-1410.

293. van den Maagdenberg AM, Hofker MH, Krimpenfort PJ, et al: Transgenic mice carrying the apolipoprotein E3-Leiden gene exhibit hyperlipoproteinemia. J Biol Chem 1993;268:10540-10545.

294. van Vlijmen BJ, van Dijk KW, van't Hof HB, et al: In the absence of endogenous mouse apolipoprotein E, apolipoprotein E*2(Arg-158 -> Cys) transgenic mice develop more severe hyperlipoproteinemia than apolipoprotein E*3-Leiden transgenic mice. J Biol Chem 1996;271:30595-30602.

295. Huang Y, Schwendner SW, Rall SC Jr, Mahley RW: Hypolipidemic and hyperlipidemic phenotypes in transgenic mice expressing human apolipoprotein E2. J Biol Chem 1996;271:29146-29151.

296. Sullivan PM, Mezdour H, Quarfordt SH, Maeda N: Type III hyperlipoproteinemia and spontaneous atherosclerosis in mice resulting from gene replacement of mouse Apoe with human Apoe*2. J Clin Invest 1998;102:130-135.

297. Knouff C, Hinsdale ME, Mezdour H, et al: Apo E structure determines VLDL clearance and atherosclerosis risk in mice. J Clin Invest 1999;103:1579-1586.

298. Ishibashi S, Brown MS, Goldstein JL, et al: Hypercholesterolemia in low density lipoprotein receptor knockout mice and its reversal by adenovirus-mediated gene delivery. J Clin Invest 1993;92: 883-893.

299. Ishibashi S, Goldstein JL, Brown MS, Herz J, Burns DK: Massive xanthomatosis and atherosclerosis in cholesterol-fed low density lipoprotein receptor-negative mice. J Clin Invest 1994;93: 1885-1893.

300. Powell-Braxton L, Veniant M, Latvala RD, et al: A mouse model of human familial hypercholesterolemia: Markedly elevated low density lipoprotein cholesterol levels and severe atherosclerosis on a low-fat chow diet. Nat Med 1998;4:934-938.

301. Masucci-Magoulas L, Goldberg IJ, Bisgaier CL, et al: A mouse model with features of familial combined hyperlipidemia. Science 1997;275:391-394.

302. Chiesa G, Johnson DF, Yao Z, et al: Expression of human apolipoprotein B100 in transgenic mice: Editing of human apolipoprotein B100 mRNA. J Biol Chem 1993;268:23747-23750.

303. Linton MF, Farese RV Jr, Chiesa G, et al: Transgenic mice expressing high plasma concentrations of human apolipoprotein B100 and lipoprotein(a). J Clin Invest 1993;92:3029-3037.

304. Callow MJ, Stoltzfus LJ, Lawn RM, Rubin EM: Expression of human apolipoprotein B and assembly of lipoprotein(a) in transgenic mice. Proc Natl Acad Sci USA 1994;91:2130-2134.

305. Purcell-Huynh DA, Farese RV Jr, Johnson DF, et al: Transgenic mice expressing high levels of human apolipoprotein B develop severe atherosclerotic lesions in response to a high-fat diet. J Clin Invest 1995;95:2246-2257.

306. Sanan DA, Newland DL, Tao R, et al: Low density lipoprotein receptor-negative mice expressing human apolipoprotein B-100 develop complex atherosclerotic lesions on a chow diet: No accentuation by apolipoprotein(a). Proc Natl Acad Sci USA 1998;95:4544-4549.

307. Marotti KR, Castle CK, Boyle TP, et al: Severe atherosclerosis in transgenic mice expressing simian cholesteryl ester transfer protein. Nature 1993;364:73-75.

308. Warden CH, Hedrick CC, Qiao JH, et al: Atherosclerosis in transgenic mice overexpressing apolipoprotein A-II. Science 1993;261: 469-472.

309. Castellani LW, Navab M, Lenten BJ, et al: Overexpression of apolipoprotein AII in transgenic mice converts high density

lipoproteins to proinflammatory particles. J Clin Invest 1997;100:464-474.

310. Lawn RM, Wade DP, Hammer RE, et al: Atherogenesis in transgenic mice expressing human apolipoprotein(a). Nature 1992;360: 670-672.

311. Kunjathoor VV, Wilson DL, LeBoeuf RC: Increased atherosclerosis in streptozotocin-induced diabetic mice. J Clin Invest 1996;97: 1767-1773.

312. Stenbit AE, Tsao TS, Li J, et al: GLUT4 heterozygous knockout mice develop muscle insulin resistance and diabetes. Nat Med 1997;3:1096-1101.

313. Bruning JC, Winnay J, Bonner-Weir S, et al: Development of a novel polygenic model of NIDDM in mice heterozygous for IR and IRS-1 null alleles. Cell 1997;88:561-572.

314. Kido Y, Burks DJ, Withers D, et al: Tissue-specific insulin resistance in mice with mutations in the insulin receptor, IRS-1, and IRS-2. J Clin Invest 2000;105:199-205.

315. Robinson SW, Dinulescu DM, Cone RD: Genetic models of obesity and energy balance in the mouse. Annu Rev Genet 2000;34: 687-745.

316. Park L, Raman KG, Lee KJ, et al: Suppression of accelerated diabetic atherosclerosis by the soluble receptor for advanced glycation endproducts. Nat Med 1998;4:1025-1031.

317. Tse J, Martin-McNaulty B, Halks-Miller M, et al: Accelerated atherosclerosis and premature calcified cartilaginous metaplasia in the aorta of diabetic male Apo E knockout mice can be prevented by chronic treatment with 17 beta-estradiol. Atherosclerosis 1999; 144:303-313.

318. Reaven P, Merat S, Casanada F, et al: Effect of streptozotocin-induced hyperglycemia on lipid profiles, formation of advanced glycation endproducts in lesions, and extent of atherosclerosis in LDL receptor-deficient mice. Arterioscler Thromb Vasc Biol 1997;17:2250-2256.

319. Keren P, George J, Shaish A, et al: Effect of hyperglycemia and hyperlipidemia on atherosclerosis in LDL receptor-deficient mice: Establishment of a combined model and association with heat shock protein 65 immunity. Diabetes 2000;49:1064-1069.

320. Clarke R, Daly L, Robinson K, et al: Hyperhomocysteinemia: An independent risk factor for vascular disease. N Engl J Med 1991;324:1149-1155.

321. Watanabe M, Osada J, Aratani Y, et al: Mice deficient in cystathionine beta-synthase: Animal models for mild and severe homocyst(e)inemia. Proc Natl Acad Sci USA 1995;92:1585-1589.

322. Eberhardt RT, Forgione MA, Cap A, et al: Endothelial dysfunction in a murine model of mild hyperhomocyst(e)inemia. J Clin Invest 2000;106:483-491.

323. Hofmann MA, Lalla E, Lu Y, et al: Hyperhomocysteinemia enhances vascular inflammation and accelerates atherosclerosis in a murine model. J Clin Invest 2001;107:675-683.

324. Shi C, Russell ME, Bianchi C, et al: Murine model of accelerated transplant arteriosclerosis. Circ Res 1994;75:199-207.

325. Shi C, Lee WS, He Q, et al: Immunologic basis of transplant-associated arteriosclerosis. Proc Natl Acad Sci USA 1996;93: 4051-4056.

326. Shi C, Lee WS, Russell ME, Zhang D, et al: Hypercholesterolemia exacerbates transplant arteriosclerosis via increased neointimal smooth muscle cell accumulation: Studies in apolipoprotein E knockout mice. Circulation 1997;96:2722-2728.

327. Koulack J, McAlister VC, Giacomantonio CA, et al: Development of a mouse aortic transplant model of chronic rejection. Microsurgery 1995;16(2):110-113.

328. Russell PS, Chase CM, Winn HJ, Colvin RB: Coronary atherosclerosis in transplanted mouse hearts. I. Time course and immunogenetic and immunopathological considerations. Am J Pathol 1994;144:260-274.

329. Hirozane T, Matsumori A, Furukawa Y, Sasayama S: Experimental graft coronary artery disease in a murine heterotopic cardiac transplant model. Circulation 1995;91:386-392.

330. Lindner V, Fingerle J, Reidy MA: Mouse model of arterial injury. Circ Res 1993;73:792-796.

331. Carmeliet P, Moons L, Stassen JM, et al: Vascular wound healing and neointima formation induced by perivascular electric injury in mice. Am J Pathol 1997;150:761-776.

332. Kikuchi S, Umemura K, Kondo K, et al: Photochemically induced endothelial injury in the mouse as a screening model for inhibitors of vascular intimal thickening. Arterioscler Thromb Vasc Biol 1998;18:1069-1078.

333. Simon DI, Dhen Z, Seifert P, et al: Decreased neointimal formation in Mac-1(−/−) mice reveals a role for inflammation in vascular repair after angioplasty. J Clin Invest 2000;105:293-300.

334. Moroi M, Zhang L, Yasuda T, et al: Interaction of genetic deficiency of endothelial nitric oxide, gender, and pregnancy in vascular response to injury in mice. J Clin Invest 1998;101:1225-1232.

335. Kumar A, Lindner V: Remodeling with neointima formation in the mouse carotid artery after cessation of blood flow. Arterioscler Thromb Vasc Biol 1997;17:2238-2244.

336. Roque M, Fallon JT, Badimon JJ, et al: Mouse model of femoral artery denudation injury associated with the rapid accumulation of adhesion molecules on the luminal surface and recruitment of neutrophils. Arterioscler Thromb Vasc Biol 2000;20:335-342.

337. Sata M, Maejima Y, Adachi F, et al: A mouse model of vascular injury that induces rapid onset of medial cell apoptosis followed by reproducible neointimal hyperplasia. J Mol Cell Cardiol 2000;32:2097-2104.

338. Fishman JA, Ryan GB, Karnovsky MJ: Endothelial regeneration in the rat carotid artery and the significance of endothelial denudation in the pathogenesis of myointimal thickening. Lab Invest 1975;32:339-351.

339. Cheung WM, D'Andrea MR, Andrade-Gordon P, Damiano BP: Altered vascular injury responses in mice deficient in protease-activated receptor-1. Arterioscler Thromb Vasc Biol 1999;19: 3014-3024.

340. Farrehi PM, Ozaki CK, Carmeliet P, Fay WP: Regulation of arterial thrombolysis by plasminogen activator inhibitor-1 in mice. Circulation 1998;97:1002-1008.

341. Matsuno H, Kozawa O, Niwa M, et al: Differential role of components of the fibrinolytic system in the formation and removal of thrombus induced by endothelial injury. Thromb Haemost 1999;81:601-604.

342. Rosenblum WI, Nelson GH, Povlishock JT: Laser-induced endothelial damage inhibits endothelium-dependent relaxation in the cerebral microcirculation of the mouse. Circ Res 1987;60:169-176.

343. Rosen ED, Raymond S, Zollman A, et al: Laser-induced noninvasive vascular injury models in mice generate plat. Am J Pathol 2001; 158:1613-1622.

344. Kumada T, Dittman WA, Majerus PW: A role for thrombomodulin in the pathogenesis of thrombin-induced thromboembolism in mice. Blood 1988;71:728-733.

345. Broersma RJ, Kutcher LW, Heminger EF: The effect of thrombin inhibition in a rat arterial thrombosis model. Thromb Res 1991;64:405-412.

346. Roba J, Claeys M, Lambelin G: Antiplatelet and antithrombogenic effects of suloctidil. Eur J Pharmacol 1976;37:265-274.

347. DiMinno G, Silver MJ: Mouse antithrombotic assay: A simple method for the evaluation of antithrombotic agents in vivo: Potentiation of antithrombotic activity by ethyl alcohol. J Pharmacol Exp Ther 1983;225:57-60.

348. Dorffler-Melly J, Schwarte LA, Ince C, Levi M: Mouse models of focal arterial and venous thrombosis. Basic Res Cardiol 2000; 95:503-509.

349. Christie PD, Edelberg JM, Picard MH, et al: A murine model of myocardial microvascular thrombosis. J Clin Invest 1999;104: 533-539.

350. Pereira L, Andrikopoulos K, Tian J, et al: Targetting of the gene encoding fibrillin-1 recapitulates the vascular aspect of Marfan syndrome. Nat Genet 1997;17:218-222.

351. Pereira L, Lee SY, Gayraud B, et al: Pathogenetic sequence for aneurysm revealed in mice underexpressing fibrillin-1. Proc Natl Acad Sci USA 1999;96:3819-3823.

352. Bunton TE, Biery NJ, Myers L, et al: Phenotypic alteration of vascular smooth muscle cells precedes elastolysis in a mouse model of Marfan syndrome. Circ Res 2001;88:37-43.

353. Li DY, Brooke B, Davis EC, et al: Elastin is an essential determinant of arterial morphogenesis. Nature 1998;393:276-280.

354. Li DY, Faury G, Taylor DG, et al: Novel arterial pathology in mice and humans hemizygous for elastin. J Clin Invest 1998;102: 1783-1787.

355. Smithies O, Kim HS, Takahashi N, Edgell MH: Importance of quantitative genetic variations in the etiology of hypertension. Kidney Int 2000;58:2265-2280.

356. Takahashi N, Smithies O: Gene targeting approaches to analyzing hypertension. J Am Soc Nephrol 1999;10:1598-1605.

357. Garbers DL, Dubois SK: The molecular basis of hypertension. Annu Rev Biochem 1999;68:127-155.

358. Lifton RP, Gharavi AG, Geller DS: Molecular mechanisms of human hypertension. Cell 2001;104:545-556.

359. Cvetkovic B, Sigmund CD: Understanding hypertension through genetic manipulation in mice. Kidney Int 2000;57:863-874.

360. Kim HS, Krege JH, Kluckman KD, et al: Genetic control of blood pressure and the angiotensinogen locus. Proc Natl Acad Sci USA 1995;92:2735-2739.

361. Fukamizu A, Sugimura K, Takimoto E, et al: Chimeric renin-angiotensin system demonstrates sustained increase in blood pressure of transgenic mice carrying both human renin and human angiotensinogen genes. J Biol Chem 1993;268:11617-11621.

362. Merrill DC, Thompson MW, Carney CL, et al: Chronic hypertension and altered baroreflex responses in transgenic mice containing the human renin and human angiotensinogen genes. J Clin Invest 1996;97:1047-1055.

363. Davisson RL, Ding Y, Stec DE, et al: Novel mechanism of hypertension revealed by cell-specific targeting of human angiotensinogen in transgenic mice. Physiol Genomics 1999;1(1):3-9.

364. Takimoto E, Ishida J, Sugiyama F, et al: Hypertension induced in pregnant mice by placental renin and maternal angiotensinogen. Science 1996;274:995-998.

365. Ichiki T, Labosky PA, Shiota C, et al: Effects on blood pressure and exploratory behaviour of mice lacking angiotensin II type-2 receptor. Nature 1995;377:748-750.

366. Hein L, Barsh GS, Pratt RE, et al: Behavioural and cardiovascular effects of disrupting the angiotensin II type-2 receptor in mice. Nature 1995;377:744-747.

367. John SW, Krege JH, Oliver PM, et al: Genetic decreases in atrial natriuretic peptide and salt-sensitive hypertension. Science 1995;267:679-681.

368. Melo LG, Veress AT, Chong CK, et al: Salt-sensitive hypertension in ANP knockout mice: Potential role of abnormal plasma renin activity. Am J Physiol 1998;274:R255-R261.

369. Lopez MJ, Wong SK, Kishimoto I, et al: Salt-resistant hypertension in mice lacking the guanylyl cyclase-A receptor for atrial natriuretic peptide. Nature 1995;378:65-68.

370. Oliver PM, Fox JE, Kim R, et al: Hypertension, cardiac hypertrophy, and sudden death in mice lacking natriuretic peptide receptor A. Proc Natl Acad Sci USA 1997;94:14730-14735.

371. Oliver PM, John SW, Purdy KE, et al: Natriuretic peptide receptor 1 expression influences blood pressures of mice in a dose-dependent manner. Proc Natl Acad Sci USA 1998;95:2547-2551.

372. Tamura N, Ogawa Y, Chusho H, et al: Cardiac fibrosis in mice lacking brain natriuretic peptide. Proc Natl Acad Sci USA 2000;97:4239-4244.

373. Ohuchi T, Kuwaki T, Ling GY, et al: Elevation of blood pressure by genetic and pharmacological disruption of the ETB receptor in mice. Am J Physiol 1999;276:R1071-R1077.

374. Huang PL, Huang Z, Mashimo H, et al: Hypertension in mice lacking the gene for endothelial nitric oxide synthase. Nature 1995;377:239-242.

375. Shesely EG, Maeda N, Kim HS, et al: Elevated blood pressures in mice lacking endothelial nitric oxide synthase. Proc Natl Acad Sci USA 1996;93:13176-13181.

376. Laubach VE, Shesely EG, Smithies O, Sherman PA: Mice lacking inducible nitric oxide synthase are not resistant to lipopolysaccharide-induced death. Proc Natl Acad Sci USA 1995;92:10688-10692.

377. Huang PL, Dawson TM, Bredt DS, et al: Targeted disruption of the neuronal nitric oxide synthase gene. Cell 1993;75:1273-1286.

378. Borkowski JA, Ransom RW, Seabrook GR, et al: Targeted disruption of a B2 bradykinin receptor gene in mice eliminates bradykinin action in smooth muscle and neurons. J Biol Chem 1995;270:13706-13710.

379. Madeddu P, Varoni MV, Palomba D, et al: Cardiovascular phenotype of a mouse strain with disruption of bradykinin B2-receptor gene. Circulation 1997;96:3570-3578.

380. Madeddu P, Milia AF, Salis MB, et al: Renovascular hypertension in bradykinin B2-receptor knockout mice. Hypertension 1998;32:503-509.

381. Emanueli C, Fink E, Milia AF, et al: Enhanced blood pressure sensitivity to deoxycorticosterone in mice with disruption of bradykinin B2 receptor gene. Hypertension 1998;31:1278-1283.

382. Emanueli C, Maestri R, Corradi D, et al: Dilated and failing cardiomyopathy in bradykinin B(2) receptor knockout mice. Circulation 1999;100:2359-2365.

383. Alfie ME, Sigmon DH, Pomposiello SI, Carretero OA: Effect of high salt intake in mutant mice lacking bradykinin-B2 receptors. Hypertension 1997;29:483-487.

384. Alfie ME, Yang XP, Hess F, Carretero OA: Salt-sensitive hypertension in bradykinin B2 receptor knockout mice. Biochem Biophys Res Commun 1996;224:625-630.

385. Kennedy CR, Zhang Y, Brandon S, et al: Salt-sensitive hypertension and reduced fertility in mice lacking the prostaglandin EP2 receptor. Nat Med 1999;5:217-220.

386. Audoly LP, Tilley SL, Goulet J, et al: Identification of specific EP receptors responsible for the hemodynamic effects of PGE2. Am J Physiol 1999;277:H924-H930.

387. Drago J, Gerfen CR, Lachowicz JE, et al: Altered striatal function in a mutant mouse lacking D1A dopamine receptors. Proc Natl Acad Sci USA 1994;91:12564-12568.

388. Albrecht FE, Drago J, Felder RA, et al: Role of the D1A dopamine receptor in the pathogenesis of genetic hypertension. J Clin Invest 1996;97:2283-2288.

389. Asico LD, Ladines C, Fuchs S, et al: Disruption of the dopamine D3 receptor gene produces renin-dependent hypertension. J Clin Invest 1998;102:493-498.

390. Kuro-o M, Hanaoka K, Hiroi Y, et al: Salt-sensitive hypertension in transgenic mice overexpressing Na+-proton exchanger. Circ Res 1995;76:148-153.

391. Ulick S, Levine LS, Gunczler P, et al: A syndrome of apparent mineralocorticoid excess associated with defects in the peripheral metabolism of cortisol. J Clin Endocrinol Metab 1979;49:757-764.

392. Kotelevtsev Y, Brown RW, Fleming S, et al: Hypertension in mice lacking 11beta-hydroxysteroid dehydrogenase type 2. J Clin Invest 1999;103:683-689.

393. Gangula PR, Zhao H, Supowit SC, et al: Increased blood pressure in alpha-calcitonin gene-related peptide/calcitonin gene knockout mice. Hypertension 2000;35:470-475.

394. Lembo G, Rockman HA, Hunter JJ, et al: Elevated blood pressure and enhanced myocardial contractility in mice with severe IGF-1 deficiency. J Clin Invest 1996;98:2648-2655.

395. Ohki-Hamazaki H, Watase K, Yamamoto K, et al: Mice lacking bombesin receptor subtype-3 develop metabolic defects and obesity. Nature 1997;390:165-169.

396. Coste SC, Kesterson RA, Heldwein KA, et al: Abnormal adaptations to stress and impaired cardiovascular function in mice lacking corticotropin-releasing hormone receptor-2. Nat Genet 2000;24:403-409.

397. Ledent C, Vaugeois JM, Schiffmann SN, et al: Aggressiveness, hypoalgesia and high blood pressure in mice lacking the adenosine A2a receptor. Nature 1997;388:674-678.

398. Jaber M, Koch WJ, Rockman H, et al: Essential role of β-adrenergic receptor kinase 1 in cardiac development and function. Proc Natl Acad Sci USA 1996;93:12974-12979.

## EDITOR'S CHOICE

Bruneau BG., Nemer G, Schmitt JP, et al: A murine model of Holt-Oram syndrome defines roles of the T-box transcription factor Tbx5 in cardiogenesis and disease. Cell 2001;106: 709-721.

*Mouse model of human congenital heart disease uncovers pathway that leads to arrythmogenesis, MRI can be used to assess septal defects in living mouse embryos.*

Chutkow WA, Pu J, Wheeler MT, et al: Episodic coronary artery vasospasm and hypertension develop in the absence of Sur2 K(ATP) channels. J Clin Invest 2002;110:203-208.

*Prinzmetal's angina in a mouse model that is related to the loss of a single channel gene.*

Crackower MA, Oudit GY, Kozieradzki I, et al: Regulation of myocardial contractility and cell size by distinct PI3K-PTEN signaling pathways. Cell 2002;110:737-749.

*A new pathway for the control of cardiac contractility via PI-3 kinase, comprehensive characterization of the in vivo cardiac phenotype that sets a standard for the field.*

Hoshijima M, Pashmforoush M, Knoll R, and Chien KR: The MLP family of cytoskeletal Z disc proteins and dilated cardiomyopathy: a stress pathway model for heart failure progression. Cold Spring Harb Symp Quant Biol 2002;67:399-408.

*A review of the MLP mutant mouse story shows the utility of genetically engineered mouse models to not only elucidate disease pathways, but also to identify new human mutations and to validate new therapeutic targets for both genetic and acquired forms of cardiac disease.*

Knoll R, Hoshijima M, Hoffman HM, et al: The cardiac mechanical stretch sensor machinery involves a Z disc complex that is defective in a subset of human dilated cardiomyopathy. Cell 2002;111: 943-955.

*The MLP mutant mouse model identifies the first molecular glimpse of the cardiac muscle stretch sensor that triggers heart muscle growth in response to mechanical stress.*

Kuo HC, Cheng CF, Clark RB, et al: A defect in the Kv channel-interacting protein 2 (KChIP2) gene leads to a complete loss of I(to) and confers susceptibility to ventricular tachycardia. Cell 2001;107: 801-813.

*A mouse model that results in the complete loss of ITO current has marked susceptibility to polymorphic ventricular tachycardia that resembles Brugada syndrome; provides links with acquired forms of ventricular arrythmias.*

Lambrechts D, Storkebaum E, Morimoto M, et al: VEGF is a modifier of amyotrophic lateral sclerosis in mice and humans and protects motoneurons against ischemic death. Nat Genet 2003;34:383-394.

*Mouse model of a deficiency in a key angiogenic gene suggests unsuspected links to neurodegenerative diseases.*

Li S, Wang DZ, Wang Z, et al: The serum response factor coactivator myocardin is required for vascular smooth muscle development. Proc Natl Acad Sci USA 2003;100:9366-9370.

*Although initially thought to be linked to cardiogenesis, a muscle specific transcriptional co-factor is shown to be more critical for smooth muscle than cardiac muscle formation; highlights the importance of exploring functional roles of genes in vivo using mouse knockout model systems.*

Lindsay EA, Vitelli F, Su H, et al: Tbx1 haploinsufficiency in the DiGeorge syndrome region causes aortic arch defects in mice. Nature 2001;410:97-101.

*Landmark study that creates a deletion in the mouse genome that corresponds to the DiGeorge chromosome 22 microdeletion; leads to the ultimate identification of TBX 1 as the most critical gene that is deleted that is responsible for the cardiac defects.*

Rentschler S, Vaidya DM, Tamaddon H, et al: Visualization and functional characterization of the developing murine cardiac conduction system. Development 2001;128:1785-1792.

*First clear visualization and tracking of conduction system formation in the embryonic mammalian heart; uses a marker that is inserted into a gene locus that leads to specific expression in the conduction system myocytes in the embryonic heart.*

Wang YX, Lee CH, Tiep S, et al: Peroxisome-proliferator-activated receptor delta activates fat metabolism to prevent obesity. Cell 2003;113:159-170.

*Mouse knockout models uncover new functions for nuclear hormone receptors in metabolic diseases; similar strategies beginning to "de-orphanize" other members of this large superfamily.*

Zhang Y, Proenca R, Maffei M, et al: Positional cloning of the mouse obese gene and its human homologue. Nature 1994;372:425-432.

*A technical tour de force leads to the positional cloning of leptin in a naturally occurring mutant mouse model; has widespread implications for obesity pathways in mammalian systems and highlights the importance of neural circuits that control appetite.*

# Toward Stem Cell Therapy

*Pieter A. Doevendans*
*Kenneth R. Chien*
*Christine Mummery*

Mending a "broken" heart by introducing juvenile cells from embryos is a challenging idea. To many it may sound more like magic than medicine. The idea behind the use of stem cells for cardiac repair is simple. When cardiomyocyte loss is the major cause of cardiac remodeling and failure, then replacing cells is a potential solution. Unfortunately, however, the heart is a difficult organ to repair. It requires contractile units, and these units must be organized in such a way that they increase contractile force. Even more crucial is an improvement in the hemodynamic profile of the heart. This can only be achieved if the architectural blueprint of the heart is restored. Furthermore, adequate nourishment of new cells is required and this depends on adequate blood flow and tight regulation of the fiber-to-capillary ratio. After repairing the damaged heart, the arrhythmogenic substrate should also be reduced. However, implanting functional tissue fragments could either transiently or permanently provide a new substrate for slow conduction and, therefore, reentry tachycardias. Before stem cells can meet all of these criteria and can be safely implemented in cardiac repair, a considerable body of basic cell biologic research and tissue engineering will have to be carried out. Nevertheless, recognition of the potential applications of stem cells in cardiovascular research and therapy is one of the most exciting recent breakthroughs in cardiology and will certainly occupy a prominent position in the field in the decade ahead.

The existence of stem cells in humans was recognized many decades ago. The identification of stem cells in bone marrow formed the basis for developing radical treatments for hematologic disease by destruction of the diseased cells and their complete replacement by bone marrow from a matched donor. The potential use of undifferentiated stem cells from other adult tissues for tissue repair and as a source of differentiated myocytes is a more recent finding. Apart from providing a potential source of myocytes for myocardial tissue repair, it also appears that some stem cells can differentiate into vascular cells and support vasculogenesis and angiogenesis; thus, one and the same stem cell could give rise to new cardiomyocytes and vascular networks in the failing heart or after myocardial infarction. Although the most important developments in stem cell therapy are based on experimental work *in vitro* and in animal models, there is no fundamental reason to doubt that human applications are feasible. Early embryos are an obvious and proven source of stem cells with the capacity to form all somatic cell types, because (at least in mammals) a complete new individual develops from only a few rapidly proliferating virtually naïve cells present at the blastocyst stage of development. In addition, the stem cells that have been uncovered in a variety of adult tissues, such as the brain, have demonstrated an unexpected capacity of these tissues to repair and the capacity to transdifferentiate to cell types of other tissues. Exceptionally, the heart appears to contain no resident stem cell population and is, thus, unable to recruit such cells from within the heart for repair. Major challenges that must be met if other stem cell sources are to be used in this particular context include identification of the best stem cell source (adult vs. embryonic), tissue type, development of the optimal conditions for transplantation (surgical, intravenous local injection), integration with host tissue, and methods to ensure the long-term survival of the transplanted cells. Only then will therapy become available to the general cardiovascular patient.

## DEFINITION AND TERMINOLOGY IN STEM CELL BIOLOGY

A brief outline of early embryonic development in mammals, including humans, is useful for the purpose of defining the stem cell terminology used in this chapter. In the first week of development, the fertilized ovum (totipotent cell) cleaves and divides, until at about the 16- to 32-cell stage a blastocyst starts to form; a fluid-filled (blastocoelic) cavity can then be distinguished with an excentrically placed group of cells at one pole, known as the inner cell mass, that will later give rise to all somatic tissues of the fetus and the adult. The outer cells of the blastocyst, known as the trophoblast stem (TS) cells, give rise to extraembryonic tissues and membranes and are important for placenta formation (Fig. 6-1*A*). Embryonic stem (ES) cells are derived from the inner cell mass; because they are generally regarded as having lost the capacity to form trophectoderm and hence the extraembryonic tissues necessary to support mammalian development, they are not considered as equivalent to embryos despite their pluripotency. In the following days (in mice) or weeks (2 to 3 weeks in humans), three different germ layers, the endoderm, ectoderm, and, a little later, the mesoderm, form from the

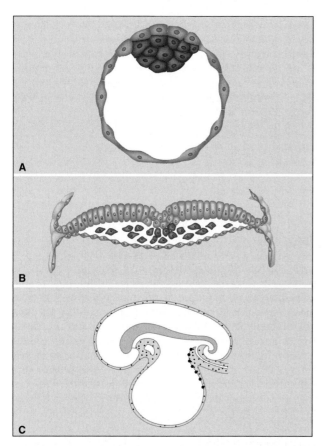

**FIGURE 6-1.** Development of the embryo. *A,* Blastocyst showing the inner cell mass at the top and the trophoblast of one cell layer. *B,* Formation of mesoderm. *C,* Migration of primordial germ cells *(black circles).*

inner cell mass (Fig. 6-1*B*). This requires implantation in the uterine wall to take place in an orderly fashion with correct axis formation. Around this time, the first primordial germ cells (PGCs) can be found in the dorsal part of the embryo; between weeks 3 to 6 these migrate through the mesentery of the hind gut to the gonads, where they give rise to the gametes (Fig. 6-1*C*). One key question is how is differentiation of cells from the different germ layers controlled; knowing the answer to this question in normal embryonic development could lead to the development of essential strategies that are needed to drive the differentiation of (embryonic) stem cells into the cell types required for transplantation. When cells have the potential to differentiate into more than one cell type within one germ layer they are called multipotent. For example, hematopoietic stem or precursor cells, which form all derivatives of the blood lineage, are considered multipotent.[1] At the other end of the spectrum are cells such as skeletal myoblasts. Myoblasts or satellite cells still have self-renewal potential but are very limited in their differentiation potential; they are nullipotent because they are destined to become only skeletal myocytes.[2] However, some apparently committed stem cells have been shown to be more plastic in their differentiation potential and develop into cells of unexpected lineages or even other germ layers (blood-to-bone, brain-to-blood). This process has been defined as transdifferentiation.

Because ES cells can give rise to all cell types and layers of embryonic tissue, including PGCs, they are considered pluripotent. This pluripotency has been clearly documented in mice in which microinjection of ES cells into the blastocyst (which can provide the trophoblast) results in a normal embryo with ES cell contributions to all tissues. For obvious reasons, this method of demonstrating pluripotency of ES cells in chimeric individuals is applicable in animals but not in humans. A human ES cell line must meet all of the following criteria: immortality, the expression of specific sets of marker genes, and the capacity to form derivatives of all three embryonic germ layers either in culture or in teratocarcinoma (a particular type of tumor that can develop from ES cells in immunodeficient mice). Teratocarcinomas, which can occur spontaneously in both mice and humans and became known to many through its most famous victim (Lance Armstrong, the cyclist), contain many tissue types, including hair, teeth, and nerve and a dividing stem cell population known as embryonal carcinoma (EC). Teratocarcinoma resembles a disorganized embryo; thus it is useful in testing for pluripotency. Other (adult) stem cells that fulfill (some of) these criteria include stromal cells from adult bone marrow and selected cells from liver, brain, and fat. These cells can also give rise to various cell types of different germ layers such as myocytes, bone, cartilage, tendon, adipose cells, and neurons.[3,4] Until recently adult stem cells were thought only to give rise to cell types associated with their tissue of origin but it has now been shown that most exhibit a more remarkable degree of plasticity. They are now regarded as multipotent although not pluripotent, because, for example, induction of their differentiation to pancreatic islet cells for the treatment of diabetes has remained elusive.

Although there are some similarities between embryonic and adult stem cells, there are also important differences. Adult stem cells, for example, particularly from humans, are very difficult to grow in culture. Furthermore, it is very difficult to distinguish them on the basis of specific markers from among hundreds, perhaps many thousands, of other cell types present, and their differentiated phenotype can be difficult to maintain long term. However, their potential to provide a perfect tissue match for a patient undergoing cell transplantation therapy certainly could make efforts to overcome these technical problems worthwhile. Ethics aside, it is not possible simply on scientific grounds to decide on the relative merits of embryonic versus adult stem cells for tissue transplantation. The research still has to be carried out, but the likely outcome is that, for some diseases, ES cells will represent the best cellular source for therapy; in other diseases, the best source will be stem cells from adult tissues.

The two most important characteristics of stem cells are their indefinite renewal potential and lack of differentiation. The self-renewal capacity refers to the ability of the cell to divide without changing its characteristics. Classically a stem cell undergoes asymmetric division, with one daughter cell identical to the mother and the other developing the differentiated phenotype of the lineage from which the stem cell derives. Exceptionally, ES cells divide into two identical daughters, either both resembling the mother or both resembling differentiated progeny. In addition, there should be no signs of ageing or senescence indicated by shortening of the telomeres (high telomerase activity). This criterion of immortality is certainly met by both mouse and human ES cells, as mentioned previously, but recent evidence is suggesting that adult stem cells may have telomerase activity and, therefore, exhibit some capacity for indefinite growth. Independent of telomerase activity, the growth capacity of stem cells in culture *(in vitro)* depends very much on the specific culture conditions. The cells have a continuous tendency to differentiate so that special culture conditions are required to maintain self-renewal and to prevent activation of a gene program for differentiation. Both mouse and human ES cells require maintenance with a so-called feeder layer of embryonic fibroblasts to maintain their undifferentiated state (Fig. 6-2). In mouse ES cells the feeder cell layer can be replaced by leukemia inhibitory factor (LIF). If ES cells are cultured in the presence of LIF, cells grow in colonies indefinitely, and, on removal of LIF, differentiation starts. In human ES cells, LIF is not effective in maintaining the undifferentiated state. Thus far, no pharmacologic or genetic procedures are known to either prevent or control human ES cell differentiation, although one report has described propagation of undifferentiated human ES (hES) cells using fibroblast-feeder conditioned medium on a specific extracellular matrix coated substrate.[4] Improving and defining culture conditions for undifferentiated hES cell is presently an area of active research. Until large numbers of undifferentiated cells can be generated rapidly and efficiently, transfer of cell therapies from small experimental animals to humans will be difficult. A similar argument is also pertinent for adult stem cells.

## EMBRYONAL CARCINOMA CELLS

Before ES cells became available from mice in 1981 and from humans in 1998, many studies on the control of early differentiation, including differentiation to cardiomyocytes, was carried out on teratocarcinoma (or EC) cells. These cells are the pluripotent stem cells of

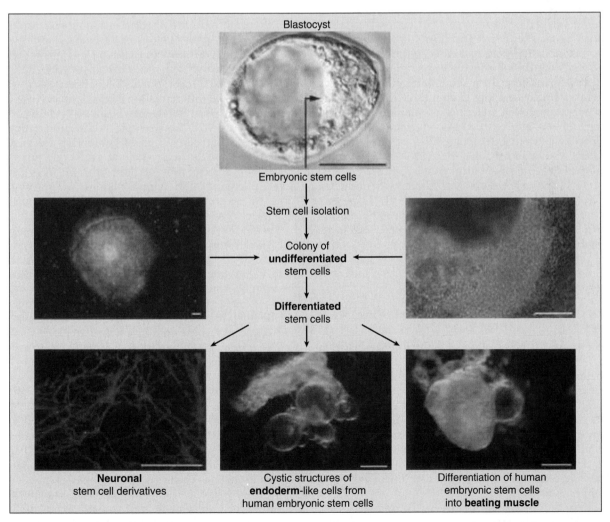

Blastocyst

Embryonic stem cells

Stem cell isolation

Colony of **undifferentiated** stem cells

**Differentiated** stem cells

**Neuronal** stem cell derivatives

Cystic structures of **endoderm**-like cells from human embryonic stem cells

Differentiation of human embryonic stem cells into **beating muscle**

**FIGURE 6-2.** Different stages of stem cell isolation and culture. Cells are isolated from the inner cell mass and cultured on feeder cells to maintain the undifferentiated phenotype. Different differentiation pathways can then be followed by the stem cells, resulting in cells with different morphologies and phenotypes representative of all three embryonic germ layers. (See color plate.)

teratocarcinomas, as described previously; the presence of this rapidly dividing cell population in the tumor is the reason for its malignancy. In teratocarcinomas, cells are found at various stages of maturation and the organization of an embryo is lacking, but extensive organization into more complex tissues is present. The malignancy of the tumor is determined by undifferentiated cells with maintained self-renewal potential. These are the EC cells.[5] When these cells are introduced into a mouse blastocyst, they become part of the inner cell mass and can contribute to the formation of all normal embryonic tissues except the germ line.[6] This research on EC cells and the growth factor or hormone-activated signal transduction pathways that control their differentiation in culture has provided an invaluable basis for developing stem cell therapies using ES cells in animal models. One of these cell lines, P19EC from a mouse teratocarcinoma, has a particular predisposition to differentiate to neuronal cell types and to cardiomyocytes. These EC cells grown as aggregates in suspension are called embryoid bodies (EBs).[7] Treatment of P19EC EBs with high doses of retinoic acid causes them to form visceral endoderm-like cells; at lower doses they form cells with neuronal characteristics (neurons, glial cells, astrocytes), and at very low doses they form cells of mesodermal origin including beating cardiomyocytes.[8,9] Cardiomyocyte differentiation can alternatively be induced by dimethylsulfoxide treatment. Retinoic acid-induced differentiation of P19EC cells to cardiomyocytes is accompanied by visceral endoderm-like cells in the culture. Reasoning that the heart normally develops from mesoderm adjacent to the visceral endoderm during normal development, in the Hubrecht laboratory a visceral endoderm-like cell line was cloned from differentiated P19 cultures (END2). Coculture studies showed that these END2 cells secreted a factor crucial for muscle formation in undifferentiated P19 cells.[10] The exact nature of this myocyte-inducing soluble factor is still unknown, although electrophysiologic studies and analysis of ion channel profiles indicate that the cardiomyocyte derived from P19EC cells has a fetal rather than adult phenotype.

# EMBRYONIC STEM CELLS

## Mouse

The first successful isolation of ES cells was made in mice.[11-13] This was a major breakthrough that formed the basis of functional genomics and gene targeting in the mouse over the last 20 years; however, the usefulness of these cells as a system to study early differentiation was largely underexploited. Exceptionally, a few research groups did characterize these cells in terms of their differentiation capacity in culture, using methods similar to those developed for EC cells.[14-20] EBs from mouse ES cells differentiate spontaneously to a variety of cell types in culture; this is most evident if they are replated and allowed to attach to a substrate. Cardiomyocytes, hematopoietic cells, and vascular networks of endothelial cells form particularly easily, and if retinoic acid is present, a spectrum of neuronal cell types will form, just

as in P19EC cells. The aggregates may form cystic bodies, in which the cyst mimics the proamniotic cavity of the egg cylinder stage embryo just after implantation; when cardiomyocytes develop they may start to beat in a regular fashion mimicking the fetal heartbeat. The EBs can be maintained floating in culture or as hanging drops on a culture dish.

From these artificial in vitro models of cardiogenesis we learned several important facts. There is a conserved temporal regulation of gene expression during development of the cardiogenic lineage whether this occurs in vivo or in vitro. New proteins and genes that have an important function in normal heart development in vivo were identified during these in vitro studies. An example is cardiotrophin, which is discussed in more detail later in the chapter.

Detailed immunocytologic analysis of isolated cardiomyocytes from the EBs showed a mixture of undifferentiated, atrial, and ventricular cardiomyocytes at the RNA and protein levels.[21] An important lesson from these studies was that cardiac genes are expressed early in development, preceding the expression of the dominant transcription factors for skeletal muscle development. By electrophysiologic analysis it was also possible to show the presence of cells with pacemaker current $(I_h)$.[22] Furthermore, the activation and modulation of various currents in the myocytes resembles in vivo fetal development, with respect to timing and current characteristics.[23,24] However, the cardiomyocytes that form retain fetal characteristics and do not mature to the adult phenotype. The differentiation of cardiomyocytes occurs independent of spontaneous beating. Even when the EBs do not reveal macroscopic contractions, they still show the same pattern of differentiation. Because the cell population is heterogenous, single-cell analysis is important; this can now be done at the RNA or protein level in combination with functional assays, which if done by electrophysiology are often by definition single-cell measurements[25] (Fig. 6-3).

The finding that ventricular differentiation occurred in the EB despite the lack of positional cues is important. Apparently cells can go through the genetic program of ventricular differentiation without the development of a heart tube and axis formation. Because differentiation was observed even in nonbeating EBs there seems to be no definite requirement for electrical stimulation. The implication of these findings was that ES cell systems could potentially be used as a source of ventricular cardiomyocytes.[26] Because cardiomyocytes were documented to be the first cells in the muscle lineage, ES-derived muscle cells could be harvested and used for transplantation experiments in rodents.

During studies with mouse EBs, a secreted factor inducing hypertrophy was identified and designated cardiotrophin 1.[27] Cardiotrophin is a cytokine that belongs to the interleukin-6 family and interacts through the gp130 signaling pathway. The protein is involved in hypertrophy and cell survival. The importance of this pathway for development and in pathologic conditions was further demonstrated through gene targeting experiments.[28,29] Mutant mice with ventricular-specific inducible cardiotrophin deficiency have normal cardiac

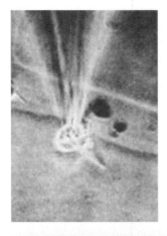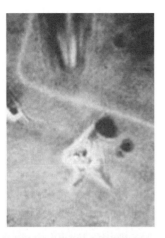

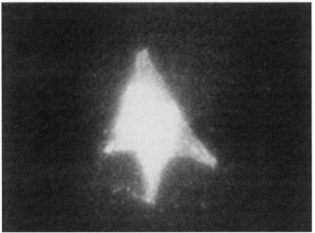

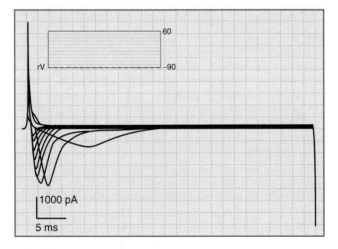

FIGURE 6-3. Single-cell analysis of mouse stem cell–derived cardiomyocyte. Cell was stained with the atrial myosin light chain 2 antibody. The sarcomeric structure is condensed possible through the preceding patch clamp procedure. The lower panel shows a family of current tracings induced by depolarizing pulses recording $I_{Na}$. *(From Doevendans PA, Kubalak SW, An RH, et al: Differentiation of cardiomyocytes in floating embryoid bodies is comparable to fetal cardiomyocytes. J Mol Cell Cardiol 2000;32:839–851. With permission.)*

structure and function, but, during aortic pressure overload, they display rapid onset of dilated cardiomyopathy and massive induction of myocyte apoptosis compared with wild-type mice, which exhibit compensatory hypertrophy.

Although there may be no difference in the ability of stem cell lines to contribute cells in a chimeric embryo, experiments in mice showed that not all stem cell lines have the same differentiation potential or capacity *in vitro*. For instance, the D3 ES cell line is particularly efficient in its differentiation to cardiomyocytes,[30,31] whereas E14 ES cells form endothelial cells that will undergo extensive vasculogenesis in culture so that complex blood-filled vascular networks appear on the surface of EBs.[32] The E14 cells form cardiomyocytes relatively inefficiently. For other cell types other lines are preferred and it is not unlikely that, when extensive comparisons are available with human ES cells (see later), significant differences will be observed in their differentiation capacity *in vitro* and even *in vivo*. Nevertheless, from a variety of mouse ES cell lines, it is possible to induce differentiation, select out the required subpopulation of differentiated cells, and transplant these either to normal rodents or disease models in rodents. Examples include rats with spinal cord lesions that have been able to move after transfer of mouse EBs to the lesion site, diabetic mice that have received ES-derived pancreatic islet cells and can produce insulin in response to glucose elevation, and ES-derived neurons that have been shown to survive and produce dopamine in a mouse model of Parkinson's disease.[33-35] Long-term survival of ES-derived cardiomyocytes in a mouse model of myocardial infarction has not been possible. This is an area actively being researched.

## Human

Successful isolation of human ES cells was, in part, made possible by technologic improvements. Supernumerary human embryos remaining after *in vitro* fertilization can now be stored in liquid nitrogen for future use. Immunosurgery from mouse embryology was adapted to remove the trophoblast without damaging the inner cell mass; thus, it became possible to harvest and culture first primate then human ES cell lines.[36] In these latter experiments, antibodies against BeWo cells, a human choriocarcinoma cell line, were allowed to bind to the TS of human blastocysts grown from embryos frozen and thawed at the eight-cell stage. Complement was then added, which lyses the antibody-labeled TS cells.[37] The isolated inner cell mass cells were then grown on irradiated mouse embryonic fibroblasts in a relatively standard culture medium. In these initial experiments it was impossible to replate a single-cell suspension or individual cells (clonal growth). The best results were obtained by passing clumps of cells (50 to 100).[38,39] Recent developments showed that it is possible to circumvent the fibroblast feeder cells for some hES cell lines that used feeder-conditioned medium as described earlier; under these conditions, clonal growth is also achievable, which will be essential if genetic manipulation and selection of stable transfected cells is to become possible. After several passages under feeder-free conditions the cells maintain their growth potential, telomerase activity, normal karyotype, and pluripotency, as evidenced by their ability to form teratomas containing multiple cell types in immunodeficient mice.[40] Currently most of the published work has been on cell lines from a group of researchers in Wisconsin (lines designated H1, H7, H9, H13, and H14 and subclones of H9, H9.1, and 9.2) and another from a group active in Singapore, Australia, Israel, and the Netherlands (lines designated hES 1 to 6). However, a total of 64 lines have been registered as verified by National Institutes of Health (NIH) and are eligible for NIH funding. Development of many of the cell lines has been funded by biotechnology companies so that they are not freely available without a signed material transfer agreement, which varies in the degree of restriction imposed but generally covers commercial exploitation of hES-derived products and patents.

As predicted by the mouse studies, there are some differences in the behavior of the different stem cell lines. For instance spontaneous EB formation and contractions were observed in H9.1 cell lines but never in the uncloned hES cells. From H9.1 EBs, cardiomyocytes were isolated and immunostained. Contracting cells were shown to be positive for α myosin heavy chain, α actinin, desmin, cardiac troponin I, and atrial natriuretic factor.[41] Interestingly, in undifferentiated H9.1 stem cell, subclone activity of the atrial myosin light chain 2 was reported, suggesting some kind of selection of a potential cardiac lineage. Both action potentials and calcium transients supported the phenotypic appearance of cardiomyocytes.

Molecular pathways that lead to specification and terminal differentiation of cardiomyocytes from embryonic mesoderm during development are not entirely clear, but data largely derived from different species have suggested that signals emanating from endoderm in the early embryo may be involved in both processes. Tissue recombination experiments have shown that, for example, in the chick, the primitive hypoblast (endoderm) induces cardiogenesis in the posterior epiblast (ectoderm), whereas in *Xenopus,* endoderm and Spemann organizer synergistically induce cardiogenesis in embryonic mesoderm undergoing erythropoiesis.[42,27] In addition, the zebrafish mutant *casanova*, which lacks endoderm, also exhibits severe heart anomalies. When undifferentiated P19 EC cells are plated onto a confluent monolayer of the visceral-endoderm such as END-2 cells, they aggregate spontaneously and within a week differentiate to cultures containing areas of beating muscle at high frequency.[10] Differentiation to beating muscle was observed also when aggregates of P19 EC cells were grown in conditioned medium from END-2 cells. Comparable effects were demonstrated by coculturing END-2 and hES cells including the appearance of beating muscle.[38,43] By contrast, in a pluripotent hEC cell line GCT27X, aggregation took place in the coculture, but no evidence of beating muscle was found.[44] Characterization of the hES-derived cardiomyocytes formed following END-2 coculture characterization have recently been reported (http://www.translational-med.nl/moleculaire-cardio.nl).[45]

During the first week of coculture of hES and END-2 cells, small aggregates of cells gradually spread and differentiated into cells with mixed morphology. By the second week, these swelled to fluid-filled cysts. Between the cysts, distinct patches of cells that began to beat became evident a few days later. Between 12 and 21 days, more of these beating patches appeared. Overall, 15% to 20% of the wells contained one or more areas of beating muscle. Beating rate was approximately 60 beats per minute and was highly temperature sensitive, compared with mouse ES-derived cardiomyocytes. These cells stained positively with α-actinin, confirming their muscle phenotype. In contrast to mES and P19EC-derived cardiomyocytes, however, the sarcomeric banding patterns were poorly defined. It may be assumed that hES culture conditions are not optimal for cardiomyocytes so that the hES-derived cardiomyocytes exhibit an incomplete sarcomere assembly. It will be essential to optimize these conditions to obtain fully functional cardiomyocytes from stem cells in culture. Despite the absence of a perfect sarcomeric structure, hES-derived cardiomyocytes continue to beat rhythmically over several weeks and action potentials can be recorded by current clamp electrophysiology (Fig. 6-4). However, carrying out electrophysiology in this manner, that is, in aggregates rather than single cells, yields action potentials that are the accumulated effects of groups of cells. They are, therefore, difficult to interpret and to attribute to either ventricular, atrial, or pacemaker cells.[43]

## TROPHOBLAST STEM CELLS

To form an embryo, inner cell mass and TS interactions are crucial. Although the potential of ES cells is impressive and covers endoderm, ectoderm, and mesoderm lineages, mouse ES cells are unable to form TS cells, which are required for the extraembryonic tissues like placenta (Fig. 6-5). Undifferentiated stem cells derived from the TS can give rise to all cell types that are important for placenta formation.[46] Fibroblast growth factor (FGF)-4 plays an important role in TS formation. One of the genes linked to the undifferentiated phenotype of ES is the transcription factor Oct 4. In the absence of Oct 4 no inner cell mass can develop. If expression of Oct 4 is downregulated in cultured mouse ES cells, giant cells are found reminiscent of TS. By contrast, upregulation of Oct 4 appears to favor visceral endoderm differentiation.[47,48] Thus, by modifying gene expression in ES cells, TS formation is apparently induced. Currently no dominant transcription factors for TS formation have been described. Although various genes have been described that are expressed specifically in the developing TS, they are not mandatory for trophectoderm formation. Thus far, it has not been possible to force TS cells into the ES cell lineage. Most of these experiments have been performed in mice. On differentiation of human ES cells some cells express human chorionic gonadotrophin, indicating a spontaneous formation of TS-like cells.[46,49] There is no evidence in mice that recombination of ES cells with TS cells reconstitutes an embryo.

## PRIMORDIAL GERM CELLS

The PGCs are among the most fascinating cells in an embryo. These cells form the gametes and, thus, deter-

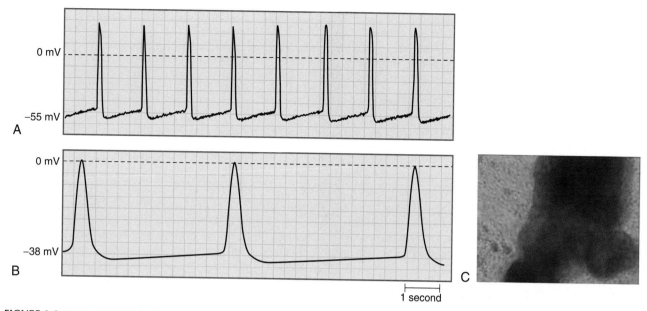

**FIGURE 6-4.** Electrophysiologic characteristics of cardiomyocytes from stem cells. Repetitive action potentials recorded from spontaneously beating areas. *A,* In mouse P19 EC cell-derived cardiomyocytes. *B,* In an aggregate of human embryonic stem–derived cardiomyocytes. *C,* Phase contrast image of the beating area in the hES culture from which the recording showed in *B* was derived. (Note the height of the protruding structure where the beating region is located, 20× objective). *(From Mummery C, Ward D, van den Brink CE, et al: Towards human embryonic stem cell derived cardiomyocytes. In Doevendans PA, Kaab S (eds): Cardiovascular Genomics: New Pathophysiological Concepts. Dordrecht, Kluwer, 2002.)*

mine the genetic information for the next generation. An unresolved issue is how PGCs migrate from the site where they originate in the dorsal part of the embryo via the mesentery of the hindgut to the gonads (Fig. 6-1*C*). Furthermore, these are the only cells expressing Oct 4

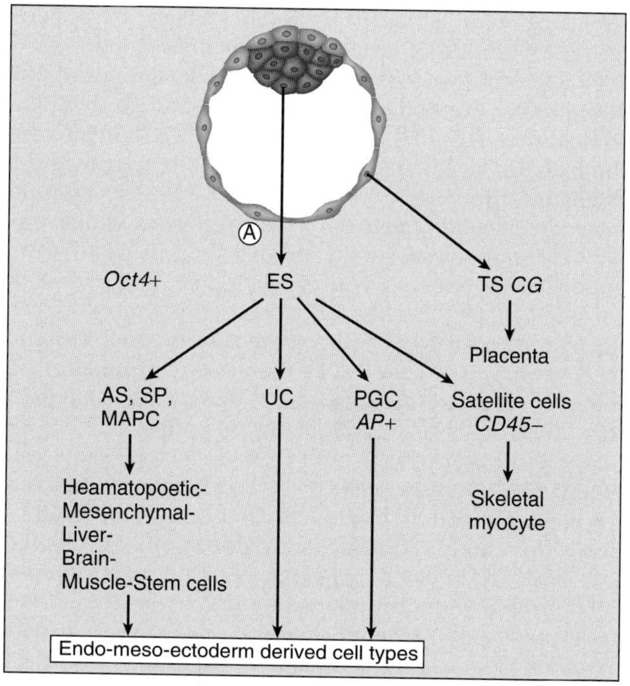

**FIGURE 6-5.** Simplified scheme of stem cell source and documented differentiation potential *in vitro* and *in vivo*. AS, adult stem cells; CG, chorion gonadotrophin; ES, embryonic stem cells; MAPC, multipotent adult progenitor cells; PGC, primordial germ cells; SP, side population; TS, trophoblast stem cells; UC, umbilical cord;.

after gastrulation, indicative of pluripotency as outlined previously.

These features suggested that it might be possible to obtain PGCs from developing embryos at postimplantation stages and grow cells from them in culture comparable to ES cells. Under normal developmental conditions PGCs will not contribute to somatic cell lineages. However, it turned out that on isolation of these cells from the embryo and growth under specific culture conditions, these cells will proliferate as pluripotent stem cells resembling ES cells; they have been termed embryonic germ (EG) cells. EG cells can differentiate (just as ES cells can) *in vitro* into somatic cells and *in vivo* in chimeric mice to somatic and germ cells. Recently it has also been possible to establish similar pluripotent EG cell lines in humans. The PGCs were isolated from gonadal ridges and mesenteries 5 to 9 weeks postfertilization. The PGCs were cultured on mouse fibroblast feeder layers in the presence of human recombinant LIF and bFGF. Over a period of 7 to 21 days, the PGCs gave rise to large multicellular colonies resembling those of mouse EG cells. Throughout the culture period most cells within the colonies continued to be alkaline phosphatase positive and tested positive against a panel of four immunologic markers (SSEA-1, SSEA-4, TRA-1-60, and TRA-1-81) (Table 6-1) that were used to characterize hES in previous studies.[50] The positive staining shown in the human PGCs (hPGCs) and human EG (hEG) cells for SSEA-1 has not been found in hES. These cells form EBs *in vitro,* and cells from all three germ layers were shown to be present, including endothelium and myocytes. They have also been cloned. However, these results have thus far only been reported by one group and not independently verified. Nevertheless, they may represent another source of stem cells, but because they

■ ■ ■

**TABLE 6-1**

| Cell type | Gene expression | Species | Ref |
|---|---|---|---|
| SP | Lin−, CD34−, SCA+, CD45+ | M,H | (70) |
| EPC | CD34+ | M,H | (56) |
| PGC | SSEA-1, SSEA-4, TRA-1−60, TRA-1−81, alkaline phosphatase, Oct4 | M,H | (50, 125) |
| EC | SSEA3, SSEA4, TRA-1-60, TRA-1-81 | | (36) |
| ES | Oct4, SSEA1, CD34 | M,H | (4;50) |
| TS | Chorionic gonadotrophin | M,H | (36) |
| Skeletal myoblast | SCA1+, CD45− | M,H | (82) |
| HSC | c-kit+, MDR1+, SCA1+ | H | (74) |

M, Mouse; H, human

are obtained from aborted fetuses the EG cells raise a different set of ethical, legal, and social questions.

## UMBILICAL CORD BLOOD DERIVED STEM CELLS

Another interesting option to obtain stem cells is to isolate cells from umbilical vessel blood taken shortly after birth. The blood can be obtained without invasive procedures, and stem cells can be enriched by centrifugation methods or selected on the basis of cell surface markers and stored for years in liquid nitrogen.[28,51] After cryopreservation, these stem cells have been demonstrated to maintain their proliferation and differentiation potential *in vivo*. Thus far, most studies have focused on their potential application as an alternative for bone marrow transplants to treat hematologic disease. In several clinical studies of acute leukemia the use of umbilical cord derived stem cells of nonrelated individuals was tested and proven to be successful.[52,53] The potential of umbilical cord derived stem cells to replace bone marrow seems favorable when compared with hematopoietic stem cells (HSCs) derived from adult tissues. *In vitro* HSCs from the umbilical cord have a higher turnover rate, form more colonies, and have a greater telomere length.[54,55] With respect to the cardiovascular system, the recognition of endothelial progenitor cells (EPCs) is a fascinating development.[56] HSCs and EPCs have a common ancestor—the hemangioblast. Many interesting features of EPCs have been described. In culture these cells can make capillary-like structures and express the endothelial nitric oxide synthase (eNOS) gene and produce NO in response to VEGF stimulation, all characteristics of functional endothelial cells.[57,58] *In vivo* human umbilical cord derived EPCs have also been shown to be functional and to contribute to postnatal vasculogenesis in immunodeficient animals. For these experiments CD34-positive cells were isolated, cultured, and injected into an experimentally induced ischemic hindlimb in rat. The fluorescently labeled EPCs were integrated into the vascular network and improved blood flow in the affected limb.[59] Thus far, the development of cardiomyocytes or other lineages from umbilical cord stem cells has not been reported. However, the ease with which stem cells can be harvested directly after birth has raised interest worldwide in storing these cells on a commercial basis, in anticipation

of possible developments in the future when not only hematologic diseases but also other diseases may be treatable with these cells. However, experimental evidence is still required. Whether research will lead to broader applications of these stem cells is unknown.[60]

## STEM CELLS FROM ADULT TISSUES

### Bone Marrow Stromal Cells

Stem cells exist not only in embryonic tissue and cord blood but also in many adult tissues that can undergo renewal or repair (Fig. 6-5). Of all adult tissues, these cells are most prominent in the stroma of bone marrow, where cells giving rise to HSCs and EPCs can be found. In addition, stromal cells have been found in bone marrow that have the characteristics of multipotent or even pluripotent stem cells, with the apparent ability to give rise to a wide range of cell types. They have been termed multipotent adult precursor cells (MAPCs).[61,62] Very few of these cells can be retrieved from peripheral blood under physiologic conditions. Although there are some differences in the behavior of MAPCs derived from the marrow versus peripheral blood, both appear to differentiate extensively.[63] For adult stem cells derived from mice spectacular results have been reported, which suggest extreme plasticity. In stromal cells isolated from bone marrow treated with 5′azacitidine, acetylation of DNA and subsequently gene expression is altered. Thus, Fukuda et al., for example, were able to establish cell lines with a high rate of cardiomyocyte formation on repeated 5′azacitidine treatment. Fukada et al. suggested that these cells are cardiomyocyte precursor cells or possibly cardiomyoblasts and have designated them cardiomyogenic (CMG) cells.[3,64] CMG cells start expressing β-adrenergic and muscarinic receptors on differentiation.[64] In addition, these cells can be stably transfected and have been used in transplantation experiments. CMG cells expressing green fluorescent protein (GFP) driven by a CMV promoter were shown to survive, couple with neighboring cells, and contract for more than 3 weeks postinjection.[65,66] Injection of fetal and neonatal cardiomyocytes in cryoinjured murine hearts showed similar results, including the expression of cadherin and connexin43. Despite these promising results, cell growth was uncontrollable, and also long-term cell survival *in vivo* has not been achieved.[67] Currently, no human CMG-like cells have been identified. However, both in mouse and man the multipotent CD45+ glycophorin A+ cells from bone marrow (MAPCs) have been kept in culture for many passages, without changes in karyotype or loss of their high telomerase activity.[61,62] Most importantly despite tedious culture demands, once established they will differentiate to somatic cells of most lineages in culture including cardiomyocytes. MAPCs represent one of the several potential sources of tissue-matched donor cells for patients. Definitive proof of their value, however, will require transplant experiments.

Among the other stem cell and precursor populations in adult bone marrow is one that is lin−, cKit+; several transplantation experiments with these cells have been reported in rodents. Using a model of mouse myocardial infarction, for example, the selected stromal stem cells (lin−, cKit+) from adult mouse bone marrow were injected into the border zone after myocardial infarction. The injected cells contributed to the regeneration of myocardial tissue including cardiomyocytes, fibroblasts, and endothelial cells. The histologic evidence of myocardial regeneration was further supported by increased survival of the mice and recovery of cardiac function.[68] However, relatively short-term survival data were reported and cell numbers for successful autologous transplantation were limited. The numbers of stem cells in peripheral blood can be increased by cytokine stimulation of the animal or patient. The response to cytokine treatment in potential human bone marrow donors can be such that sufficient cells become available from peripheral blood to make transplantation feasible. A similar noninvasive approach was followed in mice after myocardial infarction was treated with stem cell factor and granulocyte colony stimulating factor.[69] Again, a marked improvement histologically and functionally was documented, which was combined with enhanced survival of the mice.

Another approach to obtain stem cells from bone marrow was discovered by Goodell and coworkers. The selection depends solely on dual-wavelength flow cyto-metric analysis of bone marrow cells stained with the fluorescent DNA-binding dye Hoechst 33342. This method, which appears to rely on the differential ability of stem cells to efflux the Hoechst dye, defines an extremely small and homogeneous population of cells (termed side population [SP] cells, based on their position in the spectrum; Figure 6-6). This method has been used to produce transplantable cells in mice, apes, and man.[70,71] SP cells have been shown to contribute to regeneration of ischemic myocardial tissue in mice by differentiating into endothelial cells and cardiomyocytes.[72] The relevance of these findings was substantiated by a recent study in human transplanted hearts in which the presence of recipient-derived cardiomyocytes and vascular cells was demonstrated in the atrium and ventricle. Up to 10% of the cells in the donor heart were from the recipient, with higher levels in the atria compared with the ventricles. The primitive cells identified expressed c-kit, MDR-1, and SCA-1, and a subpopulation also was positive for cardiomyocyte proteins.[73] The cells presumably derived from the bone marrow/peripheral blood of the donor of the heart.[74] The signals involved in stem cell differentiation are unclear. Indeed, it has been questioned whether the expression tissue markers by a transplanted stem cell actually represents transdifferentiation or dedifferentiation or is based on a rare fusion event between the stem cells and adjacent somatic cells. This phenomenon of cell fusion has recently been described in culture between mES cells and bone marrow or neural cells.[75,76] Fusion results in tetraploid hybrid cells with the hybrid cells expressing somatic cell markers.

## Mesenchymal Cells

The connective and supporting tissues of the body develop from mesoderm. Mesodermal cells form a loose cellular network known as mesenchyme between the epithelial organs. Within connective tissue the relatively undifferentiated mesenchymal cells differentiate into fibroblasts, cartilage, and a number of other specialized cell types. These mesenchymal stem cells are also present in the liver and brain in mice and even in lipoaspirates from human fat. Like their counterparts in bone marrow, these lipoaspirate-derived cells have been shown to be multipotential and to differentiate into a skeletal muscle lineage (MyoD and myosin heavy chain expression) within 6 weeks.[77]

From human liver biopsies CD34-positive cells that differentiated into cellular blood components (±2%) were isolated.[78] Pluripotent cells derived from rat liver were also shown to differentiate into cardiomyocytes following injection into healthy tissue. The genetically marked transplanted cells were detected by X-gal staining, and their origin was confirmed by Y chromosome detection in female hearts. Furthermore, the cardiomyocyte phenotype was confirmed by immunohistochemistry and ultrastructural analysis.

In specific regions of the brain of adult mice, including the hippocampus and the olfactory region, cells have also been recovered from adult mice that appear to be pluripotent.[79-81] Earlier studies had revealed the self-

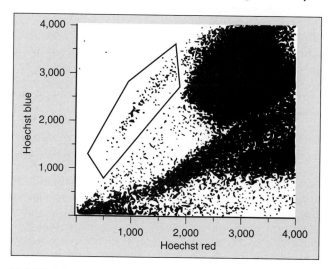

**FIGURE 6-6.** SP of bone marrow cells. Cells were stained with Hoechst 33342. The cells indicated in the upper left field are the multipotent cells from adult bone marrow.

renewal and migratory potential of ependymal cells. Following injury, ependymal cells start to divide and migrate to the site of injury, where they differentiate into astrocytes.[33] Together, these studies support the notion that throughout the adult body there are pools of stem cells with limited damage repair potential that may have the capacity (under nonhomeostatic conditions) to transdifferentiate to cell types not characteristic of their tissue of origin. Whether this leads to fully functional cells in a new tissue or is simply adaptation of the phenotype to the local environment is at present unclear.

## Skeletal Muscle

The potential of skeletal muscle to repair damage has been recognized for many years. Skeletal muscle contains satellite cells (or myoblasts), a unique population of cells that have self-renewal potential and are destined to replace injured myofibers. Thus far, there is little evidence that these cells can switch to an alternative cell type or transdifferentiate into another lineage. Satellite cells and SP (HSC-like stem) cells have been isolated from skeletal muscle and compared. They are clearly different with respect to gene expression and differentiation potential. The satellite cells express SCA-1 but not CD45, whereas the SP cells express both.[82] Furthermore, the SP/HSC-like stem cells appear to be pluripotent in contrast to the satellite cells.[83] Only under specific culture conditions or after treatment with specific growth factors, bone morphogenetics proteins (BMPs), have satellite cells been shown to exhibit some degree of multipotency. Satellite cells have, however, been used for transplantation experiments in rabbits, large animals, and even in patients in phase I clinical trials. For this purpose, they are first harvested from muscle biopsies, cultured, expanded *in vitro*, and injected into myocardial scar tissue.[2,84,85] Histologically this results in isolated islands of skeletal muscle, phenotypically resembling skeletal myocytes.[86] Injection of these myoblasts did prove beneficial for systolic and diastolic cardiac function, but, surprisingly, injection of cultured fibroblasts with a nonmyoblastic phenotype also improved diastolic function. Experiments in rats showed that the baseline function of the heart and the number of cells injected are related to the level of recovery.[87] However, overinterpretation of data showing apparent functional recovery must be avoided; the duration of the recovery is the crucial determinant of success rather than the immediate degree of recovery.

## Endothelium and Angiogenesis

A seminal paper on the feasibility of stem cells to form capillaries *in vitro* was published by J. Isner's group in 1997.[56] In this study, human cells were selected for CD34 expression and designated as EPCs or angioblasts based on tube formation in culture conditions. Furthermore, the homing and integration of EPCs in areas of angiogenesis in response to injury was shown in animal models. Moreover, improvement of vascularization, reduction of infarct size, and preserved cardiac function was shown in rats injected with cultured EPCs, compared with animals injected with culture medium.[88] Similar findings were reported in an ischemic pig model. Here, nonselected labeled bone marrow was injected and compared with the effects of endothelial cell injections. In this study the safety and efficacy of bone marrow injection to promote angiogenesis was demonstrated.[89]

Recently, the idea emerged that during treatment with HMG-CoA reductase enzyme inhibitors (statins), initiated to lower cholesterol levels, EPCs could play a role in functional recovery of the endothelium. Mononuclear cells (MNCs) derived from peripheral blood in healthy volunteers were shown to differentiate into EPCs on statin treatment.[90] Another important observation is the activation and mobilization of EPCs in gene therapy of patients treated with VEGF. VEGF has many functions important for endothelial growth and function, such as the induction of NO release.[58] Previously, VEGF was considered to induce angiogenesis based on endothelial cell division, but it can apparently also stimulate EPC formation and migration to the site of angiogenesis.[91] In patients suffering from a myocardial infarction a peak in VEGF was detected 7 days after the insult, which correlated with an increase in EPCs (MNCcd34+) in peripheral blood. In addition, these cells from myocardial infarction patients revealed a marked increase in the potential for cell cluster formation in culture.[92]

## GROWTH FACTORS AND STEM CELL DIFFERENTIATION

Production and selection of a transplantable cell is the prerequisite for implementation of stem cell therapies for cardiomyopathies. At present we do not know at which stage in the differentiation pathway, from inner cell mass, to epiblast to nascent then precardiac mesoderm and finally to a terminally differentiated cardiomyocyte, that a cell will be most suitable for (surgical) transfer to a damaged heart. Clearly, transfer of an undifferentiated cell would represent the highest (but still undetermined) risk of teratocarcinoma or teratoma development. At the other extreme, a terminally differentiated cell with the properties of a mature, adult cardiomyocyte would probably have the least chance of surviving transfer to the ischemic areas of an infarcted heart and establishing functional connections with surrounding viable cells of the host tissue. The ideal cell for transplantation would probably be intermediate between these extremes, with the capacity to develop de novo gap junctions with host cells, a (limited) capacity to divide and increase in cell number in the host, and preferably with some resistance to ischemia, to avoid extensive apoptosis presently observed during cell transfer. Mouse ES cells can be induced to differentiate to many different cell types by growth as EBs, and there is evidence that a variety of growth factors and growth conditions can promote toward cardiomyocytes[43,45,93-97] with a fetal phenotype. Maturation to an adult phenotype with appropriate morphology and ion channel expression does not appear to occur *in vitro.*[98-100] Whether the phenotype of cardiomyocytes formed by hES is fetal or adult is unknown, largely because of the lack of data on primary human cardiomyocytes for reference.[41,45] In the first differentiation step of mES to epiblast-like cells, medium conditioned by HepG2 liver cells appears to secrete factor(s) that induce expression of *fgf 5* and repress Rex-1 (markers of epiblast and stem cells, respectively)[101,102] and *oct-4* (a transcription factor expressed in all stem cells) remains constant. Evidence from mES cells and studies of heart development in zebrafish and *Xenopus* suggest a complex interplay between wnt signaling via the frizzled/α-catenin/GSK3 pathway and BMPs via their receptors, and downstream Smads 1, 5, and 8 may be involved in the subsequent steps toward cardiomyocyte formation (Fig. 6-7). Johansson and Wiles,[103] for example, showed that in chemically defined medium, mES cells showed little of their normal tendency to form mesoderm in EBs. However, when BMP4 or activin were also present at low concentration, mesoderm markers were upregulated and areas of beating muscle developed.[103] At high concentrations, this effect was repressed. In serum-containing medium, cardiomyocyte differentiation appeared to be promoted at higher concentrations,[104] although this has also been reported to promote chondrocyte differentiation.[97] In avian embryos, FGF-4 and BMP signaling have been shown to be required for full cardiac differentiation of non-precardiac mesoderm, but the dose regimen (first short FGF exposure followed by long BMP exposure) appeared to determine the efficiency with which this process occurred. Thus, the dose of each factor was critical; high BMP doses typically result in a noncardiac phenotype.[105] BMP and FGF, respectively, induce expression of chick Nkx2.5[106,107] and serum response factor,[108-110] heterodimers of which strongly promote cardiac gene expression.[111] It was shown that both FGF and BMP were necessary in addition to serum response factor and Nkx2.5 in chick non-precardiac mesoderm. Both factors are present in the early chick and mouse embryo at the right time and place for such interaction to be conceivable. The evidence suggests that FGF may be acting as a survival factor, and BMP is cardiac specification.

Another growth factor required for cardiogenesis is cripto. This factor has an epidermal growth factor domain and, based on the expression pattern, is related to mesoderm formation.[112] Functional studies revealed that the gene was crucial for the development of beating muscle in EBs.[113]

Establishing the exact sequence of developmental signals induced by growth factor ligands that lead to cardiomyocyte differentiation is essential for increasing the efficiency of differentiation to fetal cardiomyocytes. We have much to learn from developmental studies in a variety of vertebrate species.

## TRANSCRIPTION FACTORS AND CARDIOMYOCYTE FORMATION

Whether dominant transcription factors (that can change precursor, fibroblast, or stem cells into cardiomyocytes in a manner analogous to the skeletal myogenic factors) are important in the heart is unknown.[114,115] An intense search for the cardiomyocyte "master gene" revealed that many factors are involved in cardiogenesis; *dHAND* and *eHAND,* for example, were candidates because they belong to the same family of genes as *MyoD* (helix-loop-helix genes), the master gene for the skeletal muscle lineage.[116,117] However, although several genes are essential for early cardiogenesis and others are required for septation (*TBX5, NKX2.5*), valve formation (*NFATc, Smad6, TGF-β*), and atrial versus ventricular differentiation *(Irx4),*[118-120] there are no genes that drive all susceptible cells to adopt a cardiac phenotype (for review see references 121 and 122). This is one of the most important pitfalls for large-scale differentiation of pluripotent cells to the cardiogenic lineage. There appears to be a panel of transcription factors that determine the ultimate phenotype, although there are certainly newly identified genes with a powerful effect on cardiac gene expression, such as *myocardin* (cofactor to serum response factor) and *midori,* a gene that promotes cardiomyocyte differentiation in EC cells (P19EC subclone 6).[123,124] The fact that pluripotent cells go through the various differentiation steps provides a model to uncover key alterations in gene expression and activation. This is one of the most challenging fields in stem cell research today. The most important limitation in these studies is the definition and recognition of an intermediate phenotype like a cardioblast or cardiomyocyte precursor cell. To define the phenotype of these cells, EC cells such as P19 and mouse EBs are still extremely valuable tools. It seems likely that the phenotype will have to be defined on proteins expressed on the cell surface (http://www.nih.gov/news/stemcell/scireport.htm/appendixE) or by promoter activation of reporter or selection genes. Unfortunately, we are far

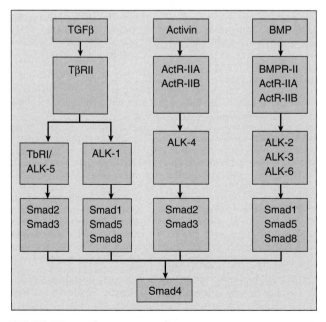

**FIGURE 6-7.** TGF-β signaling. TGFβ family members signal through a distinct set of type I and type II receptors resulting in the phosphorylation of specific Smad molecules.

from resolving the puzzle of transcriptional regulation going from stem cell to cardioblast.

## PERSPECTIVE

There is a good reason for the current excitement surrounding the discovery of pluripotency in stem cells, irrespective of their source. Although the future applications and options for cell-based transplant therapy are promising, it is essential to move ahead carefully without overinterpretation of results and unjustified extrapolation of data from rodents to humans. In the long term this could bring stem cell research into discredit if patients' hopes remain unfulfilled. The signals controlling stem cell activation, migration, and differentiation are just beginning to be discovered. Whether cells should be expanded and modified to differentiate terminally *ex vivo* or introduced in a relatively primitive state into the damaged tissue remains to be established. The ability to integrate into and cooperate with the host tissue under relatively oxygen-poor conditions are likely to determine the success of cardiomyocyte transplantation. Scientific breakthroughs are most likely to come from expression profiling during cardiogenesis and angiogenesis that will provide the genome-wide basis for understanding genetic control of differentiation. Robust research efforts will be required to apply these new options in the clinic. It is in the interest of scientists, industry, and, most of all, patients to develop therapeutic potential in the years to come.

## GLOSSARY (For an extensive glossary see http://www.nih.gov/news/stemcell/scireport.htm /appendixF)

**Embryoid body:** Aggregate of ES cells grown in suspension
**Embryonal carcinoma cells:** The stem cell of teratomas
**Embryonic stem cells:** Pluripotent cell derived from the inner cell mass of a blastocyst-stage embryo
**Transdifferentiation:** Differentiation from one somatic cell type to the other
**Multipotent:** Cells that can give rise to more than one cell type, but associated with one germ layer
**Nullipotent:** Giving rise to one cell type only
**Pluripotent:** Cells that can differentiate into all somatic cells and germ cells of the adult organism
**Totipotent:** Cells that can differentiate into all cell types including inner cell mass, trophoblast, and their derivatives

## REFERENCES

1. McCulloch EA, Till JE, Siminovitch L: The role of independent and dependent stem cells in the control of hemopoietic and immunologic responses. Wistar Inst Symp Monogr 1965;4: 61-68.
2. Taylor DA, Atkins BZ, Hungspreugs P, et al: Regenerating functional myocardium: Improved performance after skeletal myoblast transplantation. Nat Med 1998;4:929-933.
3. Makino S, Fukuda K, Miyoshi S, et al: Cardiomyocytes can be generated from marrow stromal cells in vitro. J Clin Invest 1999;103:697-705.
4. Pera MF: Human pluripotent stem cells: A progress report. Curr Opin Genet Dev 2001;11:595-599.
5. Stevens LC, Hummel KP: A description of spontaneous congenital testicular teratomas in strain 129 mice. J Natl Cancer Inst 1957;18:179.
6. Papaioannou VE: Experimental chimaeras and the study of differentiation. Prog Clin Biol Res 1981;45:77-91.
7. Rudnicki MA, McBurney MW: In Robertson E (ed): Embryonic Stem Cells. Oxford, IRL Press, 1986.
8. Jones-Villeneuve EM, McBurney MW, Rogers KA, Kalnins VI: Retinoic acid induces embryonal carcinoma cells to differentiate into neurons and glial cells. J Cell Biol 1982;94:253-262.
9. Mummery CL, Weima SM: Growth factors and receptors during differentiation: A comparison of human and murine embryonal carcinoma cell lines. Recent Results Cancer Res 1991;123:165-182.
10. Mummery CL, Van Achterberg TA, Eijnden-van Raaij AJ, et al: Visceral-endoderm-like cell lines induce differentiation of murine P19 embryonal carcinoma cells. Differentiation 1991; 46:51-60.
11. Evans MJ, Kaufman MH: Establishment in culture of pluripotential cells from mouse embryos. Nature 1981;292:154-156.
12. Martin GR: Isolation of a pluripotent cell line from early mouse embryos cultured in medium conditioned by teratocarcinoma stem cells. Proc Natl Acad Sci U S A 1981;78:7634-7638.
13. Martin GR: Teratocarcinomas and mammalian embryogenesis. Science 1980;209:768-776.
14. Keller GM: In vitro differentiation of embryonic stem cells. Curr Opin Cell Biol 1995;7:862-869.
15. Wiles MV: Embryonic stem cell differentiation in vitro. Methods Enzymol 1993;225:900-918.
16. Wiles MV, Keller G: Multiple hematopoietic lineages develop from embryonic stem (ES) cells in culture. Development 1991;111:259-267.
17. Hescheler J, Meyer R, Plant S, et al: Morphological, biochemical, and electrophysiological characterization of a clonal cell (H9c2) line from rat heart. Circ Res 1991;69:1476-1486.
18. Hescheler J, Fleischmann BK, Lentini S, et al: Embryonic stem cells: A model to study structural and functional properties in cardiomyogenesis. Cardiovasc Res 1997;36:149-162.
19. Smith AG: Mouse embryo stem cells: Their identification, propagation and manipulation. Semin Cell Biol 1992;3:385-399.
20. Heath JK, Smith AG: Regulatory factors of embryonic stem cells. J Cell Sci Suppl 1988;10:257-266.
21. Miller Hance WC, LaCorbiere M, Fuller SJ, et al: In vitro chamber specification during embryonic stem cell cardiogenesis: Expression of the ventricular myosin light chain-2 gene is independent of heart tube formation. J Biol Chem 1993; 268:25244-25252.
22. Maltsev VA, Wobus AM, Rohwedel J, et al: Cardiomyocytes differentiated in vitro from embryonic stem cells developmentally express cardiac-specific genes and ionic currents. Circ Res 1994;75:233-244.
23. An RH, Davies MP, Doevendans PA, et al: Developmental changes in beta-adrenergic modulation of L-type Ca2+ channels in embryonic mouse heart. Circ Res 1996;78:371-378.
24. Davies MP, An RH, Doevendans P, et al: Developmental changes in ionic channel activity in the embryonic murine heart. Circ Res 1996;78:15-25.
25. Doevendans PA, Kubalak SW, An RH, et al: Differentiation of cardiomyocytes in floating embryoid bodies is comparable to fetal cardiomyocytes. J Mol Cell Cardiol 2000;32:839-851.
26. Klug MG, Soonpaa MH, Koh GY, Field LJ: Genetically selected cardiomyocytes from differentiating embryonic stem cells form stable intracardiac grafts. J Clin Invest 1996;98:216-224.
27. Yatskievych TA, Ladd AN, Antin PB: Induction of cardiac myogenesis in avian pregastrula epiblast: The role of the hypoblast and activin. Development 1997;124:2561-2570.
28. Pafumi C, Zizza G, Pernicone G, et al: Two enrichment methods to obtain CD34+ stem cells from umbilical cord blood. Bratisl Lek Listy 2001;102:183-186.

29. Wollert KC, Chien KR: Cardiotrophin-1 and the role of gp130-dependent signaling pathways in cardiac growth and development. J Mol Med 1997;75:492-501.

30. Doetschman TC, Eistetter H, Katz M, et al: The in vitro development of blastocyst-derived embryonic stem cell lines: Formation of visceral yolk sac, blood islands and myocardium. J Embryol Exp Morphol 1985;87:27-45.

31. Hescheler J, Fleischmann BK, Lentini S, et al: Embryonic stem cells: A model to study structural and functional properties in cardiomyogenesis. Cardiovasc Res 1997;36:149-162.

32. Goumans MJ, Zwijsen A, van Rooijen MA, et al: Transforming growth factor-beta signalling in extraembryonic mesoderm is required for yolk sac vasculogenesis in mice. Development 1999;126:3473-3483.

33. Johansson CB, Momma S, Clarke DL, et al: Identification of a neural stem cell in the adult mammalian central nervous system. Cell 1999;96:25-34.

34. McDonald JW, Liu XZ, Qu Y, et al: Transplanted embryonic stem cells survive, differentiate and promote recovery in injured rat spinal cord. Nat Med 1999;5:1410-1412.

35. Park KI, Liu S, Flax JD, et al: Transplantation of neural progenitor and stem cells: Developmental insights may suggest new therapies for spinal cord and other CNS dysfunction. J Neurotrauma 1999;16:675-687.

36. Thomson JA, Kalishman J, Golos TG, et al: Isolation of a primate embryonic stem cell line. Proc Natl Acad Sci U S A 1995;92:7844-7848.

37. Kojima K, Kanzaki H, Iwai M, et al: Expression of leukaemia inhibitory factor (LIF) receptor in human placenta: A possible role for LIF in the growth and differentiation of trophoblasts. Hum Reprod 1995;10:1907-1911.

38. Reubinoff BE, Pera MF, Fong CY, et al: Embryonic stem cell lines from human blastocysts: Somatic differentiation in vitro. Nat Biotechnol 2000;18:399-404.

39. Thomson JA, Itskovitz-Eldor J, Shapiro SS, et al: Embryonic stem cell lines derived from human blastocysts. Science 1998;282:1145-1147.

40. Amit M, Carpenter MK, Inokuma MS, et al: Clonally derived human embryonic stem cell lines maintain pluripotency and proliferative potential for prolonged periods of culture. Dev Biol 2000;227:271-278.

41. Kehat I, Kenyagin-Karsenti D, Snir M, et al: Human embryonic stem cells can differentiate into myocytes with structural and functional properties of cardiomyocytes. J Clin Invest 2001;108:407-414.

42. Nascone N, Mercola M: An inductive role for the endoderm in Xenopus cardiogenesis. Development 1995;121:515-523.

43. Mummery C, Ward D, van den Brink CE, et al: Towards human embryonic stem cell derived cardiomyocytes. In Doevendans PA, Kaab S (eds): Cardiovascular Genomics: New Pathophysiological Concepts. Dordrecht, Kluwer, 2002.

44. Pera MF, Cooper S, Mills J, Parrington JM: Isolation and characterization of a multipotent clone of human embryonal carcinoma cells. Differentiation 1989;42:10-23.

45. Mummery C, Ward-van Oostwaard D, van den Brink CE, et al: Cardiomyocyte differentiation of mouse and human embryonic stem cells. J Anat 2002;200:233-242.

46. Rossant J: Stem cells from the mammalian blastocyst. Stem Cells 2001;19:477-482.

47. Nichols J, Zevnik B, Anastassiadis K, et al: Formation of pluripotent stem cells in the mammalian embryo depends on the POU transcription factor Oct4. Cell 1998;95:379-391.

48. Pesce M, Scholer HR: Oct-4: Gatekeeper in the beginnings of mammalian development. Stem Cells 2001;19:271-278.

49. Odorico JS, Kaufman DS, Thomson JA: Multilineage differentiation from human embryonic stem cell lines. Stem Cells 2001;19:193-204.

50. Shamblott MJ, Axelman J, Wang S, et al: Derivation of pluripotent stem cells from cultured human primordial germ cells. Proc Natl Acad Sci U S A 1998;95:13726-13731.

51. Wang SY, Hsu ML, Huang MZ, et al: The activity in ex vivo expansion of cord blood myeloid progenitor cells before and after cryopreservation. Acta Haematol 2001;105:38-44.

52. Rocha V, Cornish J, Sievers EL, et al: Comparison of outcomes of unrelated bone marrow and umbilical cord blood transplants in children with acute leukemia. Blood 2001;97:2962-2971.

53. Laughlin MJ, Barker J, Bambach B, et al: Hematopoietic engraftment and survival in adult recipients of umbilical-cord blood from unrelated donors. N Engl J Med 2001;344:1815-1822.

54. Vaziri H, Dragowska W, Allsopp RC, et al: Evidence for a mitotic clock in human hematopoietic stem cells: Loss of telomeric DNA with age. Proc Natl Acad Sci U S A 1994;91:9857-9860.

55. Mayani H, Lansdorp PM: Thy-1 expression is linked to functional properties of primitive hematopoietic progenitor cells from human umbilical cord blood. Blood 1994;83:2410-2417.

56. Asahara T, Murohara T, Sullivan A, et al: Isolation of putative progenitor endothelial cells for angiogenesis. Science 1997;275:964-967.

57. Murohara T, Horowitz JR, Silver M, et al: Vascular endothelial growth factor/vascular permeability factor enhances vascular permeability via nitric oxide and prostacyclin. Circulation 1998;97:99-107.

58. van der Zee R, Murohara T, Luo Z, et al: Vascular endothelial growth factor/vascular permeability factor augments nitric oxide release from quiescent rabbit and human vascular endothelium. Circulation 1997;95:1030-1037.

59. Murohara T, Ikeda H, Duan J, et al: Transplanted cord blood-derived endothelial precursor cells augment postnatal neovascularization. J Clin Invest 2000;105:1527-1536.

60. Ballen K, Broxmeyer HE, McCullough J, et al: Current status of cord blood banking and transplantation in the United States and Europe. Biol Blood Marrow Transplant 2002;7:635-645.

61. Reyes M, Verfaillie CM: Characterization of multipotent adult progenitor cells, a subpopulation of mesenchymal stem cells. Ann N Y Acad Sci 2001;938:231-233.

62. Reyes M, Lund T, Lenvik T, et al: Purification and ex vivo expansion of postnatal human marrow mesodermal progenitor cells. Blood 2001;98:2615-2625.

63. Verfaillie CM, Almeida-Porada G, Wissink S, Zanjani ED: Kinetics of engraftment of CD34(−) and CD34(+) cells from mobilized blood differs from that of CD34(−) and CD34(+) cells from bone marrow. Exp Hematol 2000;28:1071-1079.

64. Hakuno D, Fukuda K, Makino S, et al: Bone marrow-derived regenerated cardiomyocytes (CMG Cells) express functional adrenergic and muscarinic receptors. Circulation 2002;105:380-386.

65. Fukuda K: Development of regenerative cardiomyocytes from mesenchymal stem cells for cardiovascular tissue engineering. Artif Organs 2001;25:187-193.

66. Doevendans PA, Becker DA, An R, Kass RS: The utility of fluorescent in vivo reporter genes in molecular cardiology. Biochem Biophys Res Comm 1996;222:352-358.

67. Reinecke H, Zhang M, Bartosek T, Murry CE: Survival, integration, and differentiation of cardiomyocyte grafts: A study in normal and injured rat hearts. Circulation 1999;100:193-202.

68. Orlic D, Kajstura J, Chimenti S, et al: Bone marrow cells regenerate infarcted myocardium. Nature 2001;410:701-705.

69. Orlic D, Kajstura J, Chimenti S, et al: Mobilized bone marrow cells repair the infarcted heart, improving function and survival. Proc Natl Acad Sci U S A 2001;98:10344-10349.

70. Goodell MA, Rosenzweig M, Kim H, et al: Dye efflux studies suggest that hematopoietic stem cells expressing low or undetectable levels of CD34 antigen exist in multiple species. Nat Med 1997;3:1337-1345.

71. Goodell MA: Introduction: Focus on hematology. CD34(+) or CD34(−): Does it really matter? Blood 1999;94:2545-2547.

72. Goodell MA, Jackson KA, Majka SM, et al: Stem cell plasticity in muscle and bone marrow. Ann N Y Acad Sci 2001;938:208-218.

73. Anversa P, Nadal-Ginard B: Myocyte renewal and ventricular remodelling. Nature 2002;415:240-243.

74. Quaini F, Urbanek K, Beltrami AP, et al: Chimerism of the transplanted heart. N Engl J Med 2002;346:5-15.

75. Terada N, Hamazaki T, Oka M, et al: Bone marrow cells adopt the phenotype of other cells by spontaneous cell fusion. Nature 2002;416:759-763.

76. Ying Q, Nichols J, Evans EP, Smith A: Changing potency by spontaneous fusion. Nature 2002;416:545-548.

77. Mizuno H, Zuk PA, Zhu M, et al: Myogenic differentiation by human processed lipoaspirate cells. Plast Reconstr Surg 2002; 109:199-209.

78. Crosbie OM, Reynolds M, McEntee G, et al: In vitro evidence for the presence of hematopoietic stem cells in the adult human liver. Hepatology 1999;29:1193-1198.

79. Uchida N, Buck DW, He D, et al: Direct isolation of human central nervous system stem cells. Proc Natl Acad Sci U S A 2000; 97:14720-14725.

80. Clarke D, Frisen J: Differentiation potential of adult stem cells. Curr Opin Genet Dev 2001;11:575-580.

81. Clarke DL, Johansson CB, Wilbertz J, et al: Generalized potential of adult neural stem cells. Science 2000;288:1660-1663.

82. McKinney-Freeman SL, Jackson KA, Camargo FD, et al: Muscle-derived hematopoietic stem cells are hematopoietic in origin. Proc Natl Acad Sci USA 2002;99:1341-1346.

83. Seale P, Asakura A, Rudnicki MA: The potential of muscle stem cells. Dev Cell 2001;1:333-342.

84. Menasche P, Hagege A, Scorsin M, et al: [Autologous skeletal myoblast transplantation for cardiac insufficiency: First clinical case]. Arch Mal Coeur Vaiss 2001;94:180-182.

85. Menasche P, Hagege AA, Scorsin M, et al: Myoblast transplantation for heart failure. Lancet 2001;357:279-280.

86. Atkins BZ, Lewis CW, Kraus WE, et al: Intracardiac transplantation of skeletal myoblasts yields two populations of striated cells in situ. Ann Thorac Surg 1999;67:124-129.

87. Pouzet B, Vilquin JT, Hagege AA, et al: Factors affecting functional outcome after autologous skeletal myoblast transplantation. Ann Thorac Surg 2001;71:844-850.

88. Kawamoto A, Gwon HC, Iwaguro H, et al: Therapeutic potential of ex vivo expanded endothelial progenitor cells for myocardial ischemia. Circulation 2001;103:634-637.

89. Kamihata H, Matsubara H, Nishiue T, et al: Implantation of bone marrow mononuclear cells into ischemic myocardium enhances collateral perfusion and regional function via side supply of angioblasts, angiogenic ligands, and cytokines. Circulation 2001;104:1046-1052.

90. Dimmeler S, Aicher A, Vasa M, et al: HMG-CoA reductase inhibitors (statins) increase endothelial progenitor cells via the PI 3-kinase/Akt pathway. J Clin Invest 2001;108:391-397.

91. Kalka C, Tehrani H, Laudenberg B, et al: VEGF gene transfer mobilizes endothelial progenitor cells in patients with inoperable coronary disease. Ann Thorac Surg 2000;70:829-834.

92. Shintani S, Murohara T, Ikeda H, et al: Mobilization of endothelial progenitor cells in patients with acute myocardial infarction. Circulation 2001;103:2776-2779.

93. Slager HG, Freund E, Buiting AM, et al: Secretion of transforming growth factor-beta isoforms by embryonic stem cells: Isoform and latency are dependent on direction of differentiation. J Cell Physiol 1993;156:247-256.

94. Kramer R, Bucay N, Kane DJ, et al: Neuregulins with an Ig-like domain are essential for mouse myocardial and neuronal development. Proc Natl Acad Sci USA 1996;93:4833-4838.

95. Guan K, Chang H, Rolletschek A, Wobus AM: Embryonic stem cell-derived neurogenesis: Retinoic acid induction and lineage selection of neuronal cells. Cell Tissue Res 2001;305:171-176.

96. Prelle K, Wobus AM, Krebs O, et al: Overexpression of insulin-like growth factor-II in mouse embryonic stem cells promotes myogenic differentiation. Biochem Biophys Res Commun 2000;277:631-638.

97. Kramer J, Hegert C, Guan K, et al: Embryonic stem cell-derived chondrogenic differentiation in vitro: Activation by BMP-2 and BMP-4. Mech Dev 2000;92:193-205.

98. Maltsev VA, Rohwedel J, Hescheler J, Wobus AM: Embryonic stem cells differentiate in vitro into cardiomyocytes representing sinus nodal, atrial and ventricular cell types. Mech Dev 1993;44:41-50.

99. van der Heyden MA, Veltmaat JM, Hendriks JA, et al: Dynamic connexin43 expression and gap junctional communication during endoderm differentiation of F9 embryonal carcinoma cells. Eur J Cell Biol 2000;79:272-282.

100. van der Heyden MA, Rook MB, Hermans MM, et al: Identification of connexin43 as a functional target for Wnt signalling. J Cell Sci 1998;111:1741-1749.

101. Lake J, Rathjen J, Remiszewski J, Rathjen PD: Reversible programming of pluripotent cell differentiation. J Cell Sci 2000;113:555-566.

102. Rathjen J, Lake JA, Bettess MD, et al: Formation of a primitive ectoderm like cell population, EPL cells, from ES cells in response to biologically derived factors. J Cell Sci 1999;112:601-612.

103. Johansson BM, Wiles MV: Evidence for involvement of activin A and bone morphogenetic protein 4 in mammalian mesoderm and hematopoietic development. Mol Cell Biol 1995;15:141-151.

104. Doevendans PA, Mummery C: Pluripotent stem cells: Biology and applications. Neth Heart J 2001;9:103-107.

105. Barron M, Gao M, Lough J: Requirement for BMP and FGF signaling during cardiogenic induction in non-precardiac mesoderm is specific, transient, and cooperative. Dev Dyn 2000;218: 383-393.

106. Frasch M: Induction of visceral and cardiac mesoderm by ectodermal Dpp in the early Drosophila embryo. Nature 1995; 374:464-467.

107. Schultheiss TM, Burch JB, Lassar AB: A role for bone morphogenetic proteins in the induction of cardiac myogenesis. Genes Dev 1997;11:451-462.

108. Schneider MD, McLellan WR, Black FM, Parker TG: Growth factors, growth factor response elements, and the cardiac phenotype. Basic Res Cardiol 1992;87(Suppl 2):33-48.

109. Moss JB, McQuinn TC, Schwartz RJ: The avian cardiac alpha-actin promoter is regulated through a pair of complex elements composed of E boxes and serum response elements that bind both positive- and negative-acting factors. J Biol Chem 1994; 269:12731-12740.

110. Parker TG, Chow KL, Schwartz RJ, Schneider MD: Positive and negative control of the skeletal alpha-actin promoter in cardiac muscle: A proximal serum response element is sufficient for induction by basic fibroblast growth factor (FGF) but not for inhibition by acidic FGF. J Biol Chem 1992;267:3343-3350.

111. Chen CY, Schwartz RJ: Recruitment of the tinman homolog Nkx-2.5 by serum response factor activates cardiac alpha-actin gene transcription. Mol Cell Biol 1996;16:6372-6384.

112. Dono R, Scalera L, Pacifico F, et al: The murine cripto gene: Expression during mesoderm induction and early heart morphogenesis. Development 1993;118:1157-1168.

113. Xu C, Liguori G, Adamson ED, Persico MG: Specific arrest of cardiogenesis in cultured embryonic stem cells lacking Cripto-1. Dev Biol 1998;196:237-247.

114. Weintraub H, Tapscott SJ, Davis RL, et al: Activation of muscle-specific genes in pigment, nerve, fat, liver, and fibroblast cell lines by forced expression of MyoD. Proc Natl Acad Sci USA 1989;86:5434-5438.

115. Sumariwalla VM, Klein WH: Similar myogenic functions for myogenin and MRF4 but not MyoD in differentiated murine embryonic stem cells. Genesis 2001;30:239-249.

116. Srivastava D, Thomas T, Lin Q, et al: Regulation of cardiac mesodermal and neural crest development by the bHLH transcription factor, dHAND. Nat Genet 1997;16:154-160.

117. Srivastava D, Cserjesi P, Olson EN: A subclass of bHLH proteins required for cardiac morphogenesis. Science 1995;270: 1995-1999.

118. Bao ZZ, Bruneau BG, Seidman JG, et al: Regulation of chamber-specific gene expression in the developing heart by Irx4. Science 1999;283:1161-1164.

119. Ranger AM, Grusby MJ, Hodge MR, et al: The transcription factor NF-ATc is essential for cardiac valve formation. Nature 1998;392:186-190.

120. Schott JJ, Benson DW, Basson CT, et al: Congenital heart disease caused by mutations in the transcription factor NKX2-5. Science 1998;281:108-111.

121. Doevendans PA, van Bilsen M: Transcription factors and the cardiac gene programme. Int J Biochem Cell Biol 1996;28:387-403.

122. Srivastava D, Olson EN: A genetic blueprint for cardiac development. Nature 2000;407:221-226.
123. Wang D, Chang PS, Wang Z, et al: Activation of cardiac gene expression by myocardin, a transcriptional cofactor for serum response factor. Cell 2001;105:851-862.
124. Hosoda T, Monzen K, Hiroi Y, et al: A novel myocyte-specific gene Midori promotes the differentiation of P19CL6 cells into cardiomyocytes. J Biol Chem 2001;276:35978-35989.

## EDITOR'S CHOICE

Alonso L, Fuchs: E Stem cells in the skin: Waste not, Want not. Genes Dev 2003;17:1189-1200.

*Growing role for Wnt signaling in the boilogy of stem cells of diverse origins. Skin stem cells serve a paradigm for the renewal and recruitment of tissue specific progenitors.*

Anderson DJ, Gage FH, Weissman IL: Can stem cells cross lineage boundaries? Nat Med 2001;7:393-395.

*Pivotal discussion of the difficulties in unequivocally establishing whether stem cells in vivo can transdifferentiate into other cell types that originally lie outside of their normal programmed lineages; establishes rigorous criteria, many of which have yet to be fully met with regard to the vast and growing literature on the in vivo injection of cardiovascular stem cells.*

Brivanlou AH, Gage FH, Jaenisch R, et al: Stem cells. Setting standards for human embryonic stem cells. Science 2003;300:913-916.

*Human ES cells are political and ethical hot potato, but hold great long-term potential for understanding human biology and disease, although stem cell therapy appears to be a very long-term prospect*

Cavaleri F, Scholer HR: Nanog: A new recruit to the embryonic stem cell orchestra. Cell 2003;113:551-552.

Chambers I, Colby D, Robertson M, et al: Functional expression cloning of Nanog, a pluripotency-sustaining factor in embryonic stem cells. Cell 2003;113:643-655.

*Beautiful story of the discovery of a factor that is critical for allowing embryonic stem cells to maintain their pluripotency during self renewal; critical question for both stem cells and progenitor cells, the latter usually having more limited renewal capability.*

Dowell JD, Rubart M, Pasumarthi KB, et al: Myocyte and myogenic stem cell transplantation in the heart. Cardiovasc Res 2003;58:336-350.

*Critical, thoughtful, and comprehensive review from one of the thought leaders in the in vivo grafting of cardiac myocytes into the in vivo heart; not as easy as it seems, given difficulties of electrical coupling, long-term stability, and ability to procure and deliver a sufficient number of cells to the intact heart to exert a global therapeutic effect.*

Hochedlinger K, Jaenisch R: Nuclear transplantation, embryonic stem cells, and the potential for cell therapy. N Engl J Med 2003;349:275-286.

*A leader in embryonic stem cell biology describes a vision for correcting genetic defects via nuclear transplantation in embryonic stem cells, based on breakthrough studies in the mouse.*

Hubner K, Fuhrmann G, Christenson LK, et al: Derivation of oocytes from mouse embryonic stem cells. Science 2003; 300:1251-1256.

*Creating germ line cells (oocytes) from embryonic stem cells; technology moving ahead rapidly, implications for fertility disorders.*

Kim J, Lo L, Dormand E, Anderson DJ: SOX10 maintains multipotency and inhibits neuronal differentiation of neural crest stem cells. Neuron 2003;38:17-31.

*This study and others by this lab establish neural crest stem cells as a paradigm for understanding the principles and pathways that guide stem cell renewal and differentiation.*

Kumano K, Chiba S, Kunisato A, et al: Notch1 but not Notch2 is essential for generating hematopoietic stem cells from endothelial cells. Immunity 2003;18:699-711.

*Notch signaling appears critical for hematopoietic stem cell renewal.*

Leobon B, Garcin I, Menasche P, et al: Myoblasts transplanted into rat infarcted myocardium are functionally isolated from their host. Proc Natl Acad Sci USA 2003; 100:7808-7811.

*Myoblasts have difficulty in electrical coupling with neighboring cardiac muscle cells during in vivo injection studies; may be important limitation for myoblast therapy for heart failure.*

Menasche P: Skeletal muscle satellite cell transplantation. Cardiovasc Res 2003;58:351-357.

*Pioneer of myoblast therapy for heart failure provides intellectually stimulating and rigorous description of the past, present, and future challenges and opportunities for this therapeutic approach.*

Mitsui K, Tokuzawa Y, Itoh H, et al: The homeoprotein Nanog is required for maintenance of pluripotency in mouse epiblast and ES cells. Cell 2003;113:631-642.

*Companioin paper to Chambers et al (see above) from independent Japanese group that identifies crucial gene to maintain "stem-cell like" nature of ES cells.*

Murry CE, Whitney ML, Laflamme MA, et al: Cellular therapies for myocardial infarct repair. Cold Spring Harb Symp Quant Biol 2002;67:519-526.

*Open discussion of the perils of interpreting and designing studies of bone marrow stem cell implantation and its efficacy in heart failure.*

Olson EN, Schneider MD: Sizing up the heart: Development redux in disease. Genes Dev. in press

*Comprehensive review from leaders in the field of cardiac myocyte biology on the growth, death hypertrophy, and renewal of heart muscle cells; comprehensive review of the literature.*

Park IK, Qian D, Kiel M, et al: Bmi-1 is required for maintenance of adult self-renewing haematopoietic stem cells. Nature 2003;423:302-305.

*Recent uncovering of new pathways for hematopoietic stem cell renewal.*

Passier R, Mummery C: Origin and use of embryonic and adult stem cells in differentiation and tissue repair. Cardiovasc Res 2003;58:324-335.

*Nice Review of potential and problems of human ES cells for tissue repair by experienced scientists in the field.*

Perin EC, Dohmann HF, Borojevic R, et al: Transendocardial, autologous bone marrow cell transplantation for severe, chronic ischemic heart failure. Circulation 2003;107:2294-2302.

*Describes a Brazilian based study of the in vivo injection of autologous bone marrow cells into the myocardium of patients with severe heart failure following myocardial infarction, a daring clinical approach, but caution is warranted before concluding that this represents a viable therapeutic path.*

Polesskaya A, Seale P, Rudnicki MA: Wnt signaling induces the myogenic specification of resident CD45+ adult stem cells during muscle regeneration. Cell 2003;113:841-852.

*Beautiful work on the mechanisms that restore and maintain the number of satellite cells (myoblasts) during muscle regeneration.*

Poss KD, Wilson LG, Keating MT: Heart regeneration in zebrafish. Science 2002;298:2188-2190.

*Model organisms can be used to study heart regeneration.*

Reya T, Duncan AW, Ailles L, et al: A role for Wnt signalling in self-renewal of haematopoietic stem cells. Nature 2003;423:409-414.

*More evidence of the crucial role of Wnt signaling in stem cell renewal.*

Rosenthal N: Prometheus's vulture and the stem-cell promise. N Engl J Med 2003;349:267-274.

*Engaging review of a timely topic.*

Sampaolesi M, Torrente Y, Innocenzi A, et al: Cell therapy of alpha-sarcoglycan null dystrophic mice through intra-arterial delivery of mesoangioblasts. Science 2003; 301:487-492.

*Arterial delivery of muscle stem cells; homing of cells may be a new approach to gain tissue specificity of delivery.*

Song H, Stevens CF, Gage FH: Astroglia induce neurogenesis from adult neural stem cells. Nature 2002;417:39-44.

*Glial cells trigger neurogenesis, raise question of the potential parallel role of endogenous cardiac mesenchymal cells in the heart.*

Tanaka EM: Regeneration: if they can do it, why can't we? Cell 2003;113:559–562.

*Intriguing review of differences between lower organisms and mammals with regard to tissue regeneration.*

Willert K, Brown JD, Danenberg E, et al: Wnt proteins are lipid-modified and can act as stem cell growth factors. Nature 2003;423:448–452.

*Wnts are triggers for stem cell growth.*

Wurmser AE, Gage FH: Stem cells: Cell fusion causes confusion. Nature 2002;416:485–487.

*Growing body of work documents that many of the previously described transdifferentiation events following in vivo injections of stem cells is due to fusion with host cells; makes clear argument for direct assessment of fusion events with genetically based tools.*

# chapter 7

# Cardiovascular Signaling Pathways

*Susan F. Steinberg*
*Michael Karin*
*Joan Heller Brown*

The goal of this chapter is to provide a working vocabulary for understanding the major signal transduction pathways implicated in cardiovascular control. We have chosen to reference not only reviews but also primary literature that establishes the principles of involvement of these mediators in cellular response of cardiomyocytes and in physiologic responses of the heart and vasculature. Although the referencing is extensive, it is not inclusive, and we apologize for any major oversights.

The chapter is organized from outside in: first, the relevant cell surface receptors and their ligands (e.g., adrenergic receptors, TNFα receptors) are discussed; then, their interacting partners (e.g., G-proteins) and the downstream effectors (e.g., phospholipase C [PLC], PI3 kinase) responsible for generation of second messengers that regulate protein kinases (e.g., protein kinase C, IKK kinase) are presented. Figures have been included to illustrate the pathways discussed. These are simplified to represent the generic features of the pathway, leaving aside the multitude of cell-specific variations and interactions with other pathways.

The scope of topics included here is very broad. For that reason the details of signaling beyond protein kinase activation are not covered. Much of this information is, however, provided in other chapters in this book. Clearly one of the most critical effects of protein kinase activation is on transcription factors and expression of particular genes; transcriptional control mechanisms in regulation of hypertrophy are detailed in Chapter 10. The role of protein kinases in phosphorylating $Ca^{2+}$ regulatory proteins and controlling $Ca^{2+}$ handling and contractile function is also critical to physiologic regulation of ventricular function and heart failure; these issues are covered in Chapter 15. Finally, pathways for apoptosis and cell survival are targets for regulation by the kinase pathways described in this chapter; these responses, central to ischemic damage and heart failure, are considered in Chapter 15.

## RECEPTORS

### β-Adrenergic Receptors

β-Adrenergic receptors (β-ARs) are seven transmembrane spanning domain (TMD) G-protein coupled receptor (GPCR) prototypes with widespread expression and cardiovascular functions. Under normal physiologic conditions, cardiac contractility (rate, amplitude, and kinetics of force generation and relaxation) is regulated by the predominant cardiomyocyte $\beta_1$-AR subtype, whereas the vasodilatory $\beta_2$-AR contributes to blood pressure control. However, direct cardiac actions of cardiomyocyte $\beta_2$- and $\beta_3$-ARs also have been identified more recently. On balance, the pathways activated by $\beta_2$-ARs provide inotropic support and promote cardiomyocyte survival during ischemic stresses. $\beta_3$-ARs, which have prominent noncardiac actions in adipose tissue and the gastrointestinal tract, are present in human cardiomyocytes where, in contrast to $\beta_1$- and $\beta_2$-ARs, they are relatively refractory to agonist-induced desensitization and *depress* contractile function via a pathway that involves a PTX-sensitive G-protein and the activation of nitric oxide synthase.[1,2] $\beta_2$- and $\beta_3$-receptors are viewed as ancillary catecholamine-activated mechanisms that assume increased functional importance in heart failure, in which $\beta_1$-receptors are downregulated.

$\beta_2$-ARs (the first GPCRs to be cloned) have been used as a model to explore the structural basis of ligand-dependent GPCR activation. The prevailing model depicts a network of intramolecular interactions that align the receptor's TMDs, forming a pocket or receptacle for ligand (extracellular and intracellular loops are not required for ligand binding to β-ARs). The β-AR agonist-binding site is buried within the membrane structure; contact points for the *meta-* and *para-*hydroxyl groups of the catecholamine ring are on serine residues (Ser204 and Ser207) in the fifth TMD, whereas the cationic amino group (at the other end of classical catecholamine agonists such as norepinephrine [NE] or epinephrine) electrostatically interacts with the carboxylate side chain of Asp-113 in the third TMD.[3] The intracellular loops of the β-AR (and in particular, juxtamembrane regions of the third intracellular loop and C-tail) form a binding surface for G-proteins. However, recent studies have identified additional structural features that regulate β-AR trafficking. An interaction between a proline-rich region in the third cytoplasmic loop, the $\beta_1$-AR, and endophilins controls receptor internalization.[4] Interactions between the C-terminal PDZ domain-interacting motif and the $Na^+/H^+$ exchanger regulatory factor (NHERF, an inhibitor of $Na^+/H^+$ exchanger type 3) regulates recycling of internalized $\beta_2$-ARs.[5] A similar interaction between a C-terminal PDZ-domain interacting motif and PSD-95 or membrane-associated guanylate kinase inverted-2 (MAGI-2) exerts reciprocal control on the internalization of $\beta_1$-AR.[5,6]

Adrenergic receptors exist in equilibrium between at least two structurally and functionally distinct states: an inactive conformation (generally designated R) and an active conformation capable of activating G-proteins (designated R*). Studies in transgenic mice that overexpress $\beta$-ARs in the heart have identified spontaneous transition of $\beta$-ARs from R to R*, even in the absence of activating ligand[7]; the equilibrium between R and R* sets the basal level of receptor activation. Agonists are compounds that promote the formation of R*, whereas inverse agonists are compounds that prevent the spontaneous transition to R*. This property is distinct from classical antagonists, which bind receptors with high affinity and simply prevent further agonist binding and receptor activation.

$\beta_1$-AR stimulation leads to the activation of the stimulatory G-protein ($G_s$), activation of adenylyl cyclase (AC), accumulation of cAMP, stimulation of protein kinase A (PKA), and phosphorylation of key target proteins (including L-type calcium channels, phospholamban [PLB], ryanodine receptors, and troponin I) (Fig. 7-1). Although $\beta_2$-ARs also couple to the $G_s$-AC pathway, their acute effects on cardiomyocyte contraction and long-term effects on cardiac muscle cell biology are quite distinct from those identified for $\beta_1$-ARs. The most dramatic evidence for distinct $\beta_1$- and $\beta_2$-AR actions comes from studies of transgenic mice, in which cardiac $\beta_2$-AR overexpression at relatively high levels (50- to 200-fold higher than total $\beta$-ARs in nontransgenic mice) leads to enhanced contractile function without deleterious effects, unless $\beta_2$-AR overexpression is maintained at very high levels or for protracted intervals.[8] In contrast, even low levels (5- to 15-fold) of transgenic $\beta_1$-AR overexpression lead to an aggressive cardiomyopathy that is not tolerated.[9,10]

$\beta_1$-AR actions are largely confined to signals emanating from $G_s$ proteins.[11] In contrast, $\beta_2$-ARs heterologously expressed in undifferentiated cell lines couple to several G-proteins ($G_s$, $G_i$, $G_{12}$) and effectors (AC, ERK, PI3-K, p38-MAPK).[11] There is growing evidence that $\beta_2$-AR activation of growth regulatory pathways such as the ERK cascade can be highly contextual (likely reflecting differences in the endogenous signaling machinery in different cell types). In some cells, $\beta_2$-AR activation of ERK is via a mechanism that involves the sequential coupling of the $\beta_2$-AR to Gs followed by $G_i$. According to this scenario, $\beta_2$-AR activation of the cAMP/PKA pathway leads to PKA-dependent phosphorylation of the $\beta_2$-AR, which shifts its coupling preference from Gs to $G_i$; $G_i$ is a major source of $\beta\gamma$ dimers and can activate the ERK cascade via Src and Ras proteins.[12–14] However, $\beta_2$-AR activation of ERK can result from other mechanisms, including epidermal growth factor receptor (EGFR) transactivation or from the recruitment of $\beta$-arrestin, which serves as a scaffold to bind Src and other proteins.[15]

$\beta_1$-ARs activate the $G_s$/cAMP pathway and increase the amplitude and relaxation kinetics of the twitch (i.e., induce positive inotropic and lusitropic responses) in cardiomyocytes (Fig. 7-1). $\beta_2$-ARs also provide important catecholamine-dependent inotropic support, particularly in the neonatal and failing adult heart.

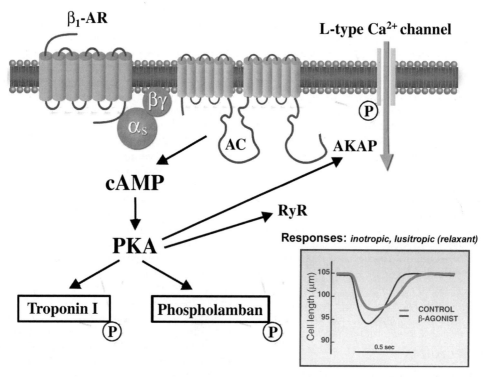

**FIGURE 7-1.** $\beta$-Adrenergic receptor signaling pathway. Catecholamines stimulate coupling of the $\beta_1$AR to $G_s$, increasing cAMP formation. Activated PKA phosphorylates substrates in the sarcomere, SR, and plasma membrane (organized through scaffolding proteins called AKAPs) lead to increased contractile function.

However, $\beta_2$-ARs act via distinct signaling mechanisms in various cardiac preparations. In neonatal rat cardiomyocytes, $\beta_2$-ARs promote cAMP accumulation and exert positive inotropic and lusitropic responses; these responses are not influenced by PTX-sensitive G-proteins.[16] The limited available studies on human tissues (largely from failing ventricles or normal atrium) identify a similar cAMP-dependent (PTX-insensitive) pathway for $\beta_2$-ARs in human cardiomyocytes.[17-19] There is general consensus that $\beta_2$-AR agonists also increase the amplitude of the twitch in adult rat cardiomyocytes and that this occurs without any associated acceleration in the kinetics of relaxation.[20-23] Some authors report no detectable $\beta_2$-AR-dependent rise in intracellular cAMP levels in adult cardiomyocytes; this cannot be attributed to a $\beta_2$-AR-$G_i$ protein linkage (offsetting the effects of the stimulatory $G_s$ pathway), because $\beta_2$-ARs do not elevate cAMP levels in cells pretreated with PTX.[16] Although a functionally important increase in cAMP that is localized to the sarcolemma has not been excluded, an effect of $\beta_2$-ARs to promote intracellular alkalinization (which enhances myofibrillar calcium sensitivity) has been identified as a cAMP-independent pathway for $\beta_2$-AR-dependent inotropic support.[24]

Other investigators espouse a model that considers cAMP an obligate downstream effector for all $\beta$-AR responses (both $\beta_1$- and $\beta_2$-ARs) in all cardiomyocyte preparations including adult rat cardiomyocytes.[25] According to this model, the cAMP signal emanating from $\beta_1$-ARs is broadcast throughout the cell, whereas a localized cAMP signal emanating from $\beta_2$-ARs is confined to effectors at the sarcolemma as a result of simultaneous $\beta_2$-AR activation of Gs and an opposing PTX-sensitive G-protein that stimulates an intracellular phosphatase and thereby counteracts the stimulatory effects of PKA at intracellular substrates such as PLB.[25] The precise mechanisms that distinguish the signaling phenotypes of cardiomyocyte $\beta_1$- and $\beta_2$-ARs remains an active area of investigation, with recent interest in roles for lipid rafts or caveolae (as sites that compartmentalize $\beta_2$-ARs and cardiac AC isoforms[26-28]) and phosphoinositide 3-kinase-$\gamma$, which regulates signaling by $\beta_2$-ARs, but not $\beta_1$-ARs.[29]

Scattered reports over the past decade have variably described effects of $\beta$-ARs to induce features of the hypertrophic growth program or to promote cardiomyocyte apoptosis.[30-33] Attempts to discriminate the independent actions of $\beta_1$- and $\beta_2$-ARs are recent. There is evidence that $\beta_1$-ARs induce hypertrophy in cultured neonatal rat cardiomyocytes and apoptosis (but not hypertrophy) in cardiomyocytes cultured from adult rat ventricles.[32,34,35] In contrast, $\beta_2$-ARs generally protect cardiomyocytes from apoptosis induced by a variety of stresses.[34,36,37] Differences in growth regulation by $\beta_1$-(proapoptotic) and $\beta_2$-ARs (antiapoptotic) are predicted to be the consequence of differences in $\beta$-AR subtype signaling to cAMP and other effector pathways that regulate cardiomyocyte growth and survival including p38-MAPK, phosphoinositide 3'-kinase (PI3-K)/AKT, calcineurin, Src, and Rac.[31,38-40]

Polymorphisms in the genes encoding human $\beta_1$- and $\beta_2$-ARs have been identified as disease modifiers. A poly-morphism of the $\beta_1$-AR gene results in either a glycine or an arginine at amino acid position 389 within the $G_s$-coupling domain; the $\beta_1$Arg389 receptor couples to AC better that the $\beta_1$Gly389 receptor in recombinant cell-based assays. Recent studies indicate that the $\beta_1$Arg389 receptor acts synergistically with a hypofunctional polymorphic $\alpha_{2C}$-adrenergic receptor ($\alpha_{2C}$Del322-325) to increase the risk of heart failure in black populations.[41] Polymorphisms of the $\beta_2$-AR also appear to influence cardiac function. The most common $\beta_2$-AR polymorphisms involve a Arg→Gly substitution at position 16 and a Gln→Glu substitution at position 27 of the extracellular N-terminus.[42] Although both of these polymorphic variants of the $\beta_2$-AR activate AC similar to wild-type, their trafficking and downregulation phenotypes are quite distinct. The Arg16→Gly $\beta_2$-AR undergoes enhanced agonist-promoted downregulation and is associated with severe or nocturnal asthma.[43,44] In contrast, the Gln27→Glu $\beta_2$-AR displays attenuated downregulation during long-term agonist exposure; the Gln27 allele is associated with hyperresponsive lower airways in asthmatic patients.[45] A much less prevalent polymorphism (heterozygous frequency ~5%) involves an isoleucine for threonine substitution at position 164 in the fourth transmembrane spanning domain; the Thr164→Ile polymorphism displays reduced high-affinity ligand binding and impaired coupling to the Gs/AC pathway. Individuals with heart failure harboring the hypofunctioning Ile-164 $\beta_2$-AR polymorphism are reported to have poorer survival.[46]

## $\alpha$–Adrenergic Receptors

Like the $\beta$-adrenergic receptors described previously, the seven transmembrane spanning $\alpha$-adrenergic receptors ($\alpha$-ARs) GPCRs are part of the superfamily of receptors that mediate cellular responses to the endogenous catecholamines (NE and epinephrine). The concept of distinct family members of adrenergic receptors was initially proposed by Ahlquist in 1948.[47] The heterogeneity among these receptors was recognized long before the subtypes were isolated by cloning. Initially they were divided into the so-called stimulatory $\alpha$-adrenergic receptor and inhibitory $\beta$-adrenergic receptors based on potency differences seen with sympathomimetic amines.[47] It was not until 1974 that $\alpha$-adrenergic receptors were further subdivided into $\alpha$ ($\alpha_1$-AR) and $\alpha_2$ ($\alpha_2$-AR).[48] The existence of these receptor subtypes was postulated based on anatomic criteria; $\alpha_1$-AR was suggested to represent the postsynaptic form of the receptor, and $\alpha_2$-AR was considered to represent presynaptic form of the receptor.[49] Although the $\alpha_1$-ARs continues to be considered largely as a postsynaptic receptor, the $\alpha_2$-ARs are located both presynaptically and postsynaptically. The $\alpha_2$-AR, when located presynaptically, inhibits the release of NE. The functional relevance of this response may be most evident when sympathetic drive is elevated. For example, these receptors appear to play a more important role in enhancing catecholamine release in patients with congestive heart failure than in those with normal LV function.[50] Heart failure patients with dysfunctional $\alpha_2$-AR have a worse clinical status, and $\alpha_2$-AR knockout mice show reduced survival following banding.[51] There is also evidence for $\alpha$-AR mediated inhibition of acetylcholine release.[52] In contrast, $\alpha_1$-AR mediated cellular responses are primarily effected at the end organ and include stimulation of VSMC contraction, cardiac contractility, and hypertrophic cardiomyocyte growth. The postsynaptic $\alpha_2$-ARs generally show a tissue distribution like that of the $\alpha_1$-AR but elicit a response opposite to that of the $\alpha_1$-AR (depending on the tissue). These responses are discussed in more detail following.

Both the $\alpha_1$-AR and $\alpha_2$-AR receptor families have now been further subdivided. The subdivision was predicable based on observed differences in the rank order of potency of antagonist affinity among tissues and the heterogeneity (i.e., high- and low-affinity states) in radioligand binding. The cloning and expression of these AR subtypes in the late 1980s and early 1990s confirmed the existence of what are now three distinct $\alpha_1$-AR (A/C, B, and D) and three distinct $\alpha_2$-AR (A, B, and C) AR. A putative $\alpha_{2D}$-AR was ultimately recognized to be a species variation (ortholog) of the $\alpha_{2A}$.[53] The terminology now used for the $\alpha_2$-AR, ($\alpha_{2A}$ and $\alpha_{2B}$, $\alpha_{2C}$) is logical and not contentious. In contrast the terminology used for the $\alpha_1$-AR subtypes requires some explanation. The gene that was cloned and initially named $\alpha_{1C}$ was subsequently determined to represent the previously characterized $\alpha_{1A}$ receptor subtype and its nomenclature was adjusted accordingly (some still use the term $\alpha_{1A/C}$ to refer to this subtype). In addition, the receptor initially assumed to be the $\alpha_{1A}$ when initially cloned is now recognized as the $\alpha_{1D}$. The tissue distribution of the $\alpha$-receptors subtypes reveals extensive species variation.[54] Because of the lack of sufficiently selective ligands and antibodies to discriminate among the subtypes, studies can suggest a predominate subtype in the control of a particular function but cannot rule out contributions from the other subtypes.

The mRNA for all three $\alpha_1$-AR subtypes is present in cardiomyocytes from the adult rat heart. There is some question, however, regarding whether $\alpha_{1D}$ is expressed as a functional protein. This is supported by recent studies from the $\alpha_{1D}$-AR knockout in which the $\alpha_1$-AR density was unchanged in the mouse heart,[55] suggesting, at best, that the $\alpha_{1D}$-AR is a very minor component of the heart $\alpha_1$-AR pool. However, these studies are also difficult to perform, because the density of $\alpha_1$-ARs in the mouse heart is in the 30 to 50 fentomolar range. In regard to cardiac parameters, the $\alpha_{1D}$-AR knockout displayed no changes in either heart rate or cardiac function as assessed by echocardiography. In the human heart it appears that the $\alpha_{1A}$ subtype predominates, whereas in the rat heart the predominant subtype is $\alpha_{1B}$. The subtypes may also be differentially localized at the cell surface versus in intracellular compartments, as observed in both stably transfected fibroblasts and cultured VSMCs (see reference 56 for review). For example, although $\alpha_{1B}$ was expressed predominantly on the cell surface the $\alpha_{1D}$ receptor was found to be highly localized in intracellular compartments. This may reflect internalization of the $\alpha_{1D}$-receptor subtype. The high degree of internalization may reflect a compensatory mechanism because this receptor shows a high degree of constitutive activity.[56] The localization may also explain why this subtype appears to couple poorly to the expected signaling cascades.[57]

The $\alpha_2$-AR couple predominantly to the $G_i$ protein and hence to inhibition of adenylate cyclase. In contrast the predominant coupling of the $\alpha_1$-AR is through $G_q$ and activation of PLC (Fig. 7-2). Subsequent hydrolysis of $PIP_2$ generates $InsP_3$, which mobilizes intracellular $Ca^{2+}$ and increases diacylglycerol, thus activating protein kinase C. There is also evidence that the $\alpha_1$-AR can activate voltage-sensitive calcium channels[56] and signal through PTX-sensitive G-proteins ($G_i$ and $G_o$). Activation of $Ca^{2+}$ dependent kinases and protein kinase C (PKC) serves to further transduce signals from these receptors to cellular responses. In cells other than cardiomyocytes, $InsP_3$-induced $Ca^{2+}$ mobilization is clearly evident and provides a pathway for activation of kinase cascades (e.g., CaMK, PKC, MLCK) that underlie increases in contraction and secretion. VSMCs are richly endowed with $\alpha_1$-AR of all three subtypes.[58] Although the extent to which each subtype mediates vascular contractility in humans is not known, pharmacologic studies in rats and data available from transgenic and knockout mice suggest differences in the roles of the $\alpha_1$ A/C, B, and D receptors in vascular control. Most clearly, the $\alpha_{1B}$ receptor does not appear to play a role in controlling contraction of blood vessels because deletion of the receptor does not alter the resting mean arterial pressure or significantly diminish adrenergic agonist induced contractility.[59] Consistent with these findings, overexpression of the $\alpha_{1B}$ receptor in transgenic mice did not elevate blood pressure, and analysis of individual superior mesenteric arteries in both the overexpressed and knockout models revealed no change in their contractile properties.[60] On the other hand, studies in mice in which the $\alpha_{1A/C}$ or the $\alpha_{1D}$-receptor is deleted demonstrate decreases in both resting blood pressure and in the pressor response to $\alpha$ agonists.[55,61]

The role of the $\alpha_1$-AR in regulating calcium levels and contractile function in the heart is far less prominent than that in blood vessels. Clearly it is the $\alpha$-AR not the $\alpha_1$-AR that provide the major driving force for the increase in intracellular calcium in response to sympathetic activation. Although $InsP_3$ receptors are present in cardiomyocytes, a major role for $InsP_3$ in $Ca^{2+}$ release in the myocardium is controversial. In some species and cardiac cell types, $\alpha_1$-AR stimulation causes well documented albeit subtle changes in calcium transients preparations.[62-64] These are thought to contribute to the inotropic response to $\alpha$-AR stimulation, a response observed in numerous species including the human ventricle.[65] Additional mechanisms also contribute to the $\alpha_1$-AR enhancement of cardiac contractility; a change in myofilament calcium sensitivity is the most evident mechanism. This has been postulated to result from cellular alkalization mediated by the $Na^+/H^+$ exchanger and/or from phosphorylation of myofilament proteins.[66,67] The phenomenon of calcium sensitization is well described in smooth muscle, and a series of recent studies have demonstrated that this occurs in vascular

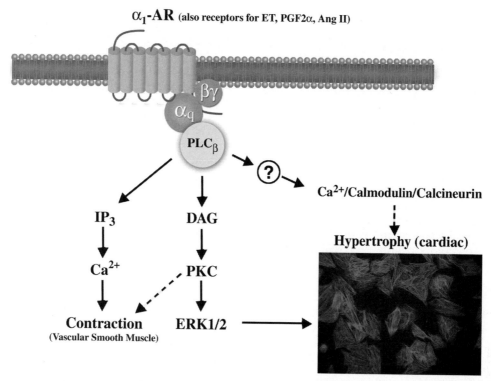

**FIGURE 7-2.** $\alpha_1$-Adrenergic receptor signaling pathway. Agonist-stimulated coupling of the $\alpha_1$ AR to Gq activates PLC. The formation of the second messengers IP$_3$ and DAG regulate intracellular Ca$^{2+}$ and PKC, which modulate contraction of smooth muscle. ERK activation contributes to cardiac hypertrophy in response to Gq-coupled agonists; calcium-activated enzymes may also mediate effects of these receptors on cardiac hypertrophy.

smooth muscle through the small G-protein (smg) Rho and changes in myosin phosphorylation effected by Rho kinase (discussed later). Interestingly, recent reports suggest that Rho and Rho kinase also mediate increases in $\alpha_1$-AR mediated myofilament Ca sensitivity observed in failing hearts.[68] In the mouse, in contrast to rat myocardium, the response to $\alpha_1$-AR stimulation is a negative inotropic affect, associated with decreased Ca$^{2+}$ transients.[69]

Studies carried out in the early 1980s by Simpson and coworkers demonstrated that NE effects changes in hypertrophic growth of neonatal rat cardiac myocytes. Initially changes in cell volume and protein content were described, and it was demonstrated that this occurred through an $\alpha_1$-AR[70] (Fig. 7-2). Subsequently adrenergic stimulation was shown to induce the expression of various immediate early genes (cfos, cmyc, egr1)[71] and to increase the expression of embryonic genes or isoforms (e.g., ANF, β-myosin heavy chain, skeletal α-actin).[72] Stimulation of the $\alpha_1$-AR activates PLC in rat cardiomyocytes,[73-75] and this occurs through the PTX-insensitive G-protein G$_q$. A variety of other GPCRs that regulate PLC also induce the aforementioned hypertrophic response in neonatal rat cardiomyocytes. PKC and MAP kinases are among the downstream kinases that are activated by α-AR agonists and implicated as mediators of hypertrophic growth.[76,77] The specific $\alpha_1$-AR subtype suggested to mediate phenylephrine-induced hypertrophy in isolated cardiomyocytes is the $\alpha_{1A/C}$ receptor,[75] although studies using constitutively activated α receptors implicate $\alpha_{1A}$ and $\alpha_{1B}$.[78] Surprisingly, overexpression of the $\alpha_{1A}$-AR in

transgenic mice does not induce hypertrophy as assessed by echocardiographic, histologic, or morphologic criteria or by changes in gene expression. Interestingly, contractility is markedly enhanced in these mice.[79] In earlier seminal studies the Lefkowitz group had demonstrated that the $\alpha_{1B}$ receptor, expressed in transgenic mice under the control of the same promoter (α-MHC), led to development of many of the expected hypertrophic changes.[80] Notably however, these studies were carried out using a constitutively active form of the receptor, and subsequent work from this laboratory using the wild-type receptor indicated no hypertrophy.[81] This is consistent with more recent work in which wild-type and activated forms of the receptor were expressed at relatively low levels, using an isogenic promoter (i.e., the mouse $\alpha_{1B}$ gene promoter). In these studies, prominent hypotension (resulting from central autonomic failure) was observed, and there were modest increases in heart to body weight ratio without molecular changes indicative of hypertrophic growth.[60] In $\alpha_{1B}$-receptor knockout mice, the pressor response to catecholamines was lost, but there was no loss of the hypertrophic response to banding.[82] Most recently, double-knockout mice lacking $\alpha_{1A/C}$ and $\alpha_{1B}$-AR were generated.[83] Decreased developmental hypertrophy and exercise tolerance were evident, but only in males, and banding-induced hypertrophy did not appear to be diminished. In light of these data and the complexities of comparing species, *in vitro* studies, transgenic models, and different sexes, it remains difficult to reach a final consensus regarding the α-AR subtype that mediates hypertrophy.

## Muscarinic Receptors

Acetylcholine, the neurotransmitter of the parasympathetic nervous system, effects cellular responses (mAChR) in glands, smooth muscle, and cardiac muscle cells via activation of muscarinic cholinergic receptors. In contrast with the nicotinic cholinergic receptors, which are ligand-gated ion channels that mediate skeletal muscle and ganglionic depolarization, the mAChR are G-protein coupled. These seven transmembrane spanning receptors couple to G-proteins of the $G_i$ and $G_q$ families to inhibit adenylate cyclase and activate PLC, respectively (Fig. 7-3). The receptors were cloned in the late 1980s, and five distinct gene products were identified.[84] These receptors are designated as the $M_1$, $M_2$, $M_3$, $M_4$, and $M_5$ receptors. The $M_5$ receptor is largely confined to the central nervous system and is the least studied. The $M_1$ and $M_3$ receptors couple preferentially to the activation of $G_{q/11}$ proteins, leading to PTX-insensitive PLC activation. The $M_2$ and $M_4$ receptors couple primarily to the PTX-sensitive $G_i$ or $G_o$ proteins and via this route inhibit adenylate cyclase and regulate ion channels. Studies using mutagenesis and generation of chimeric receptors led to the identification of specific regions in the third intracellular loop (and regions in the second loop) that showed high homology between the $G_q$ coupled $M_1$ and $M_3$ receptors and between the $G_i$ coupled $M_2$ and $M_4$ receptors but not across the groups.[85-87] The determinants of selectivity in coupling to effectors responsible for downstream responses have been unusually well defined for the mAChR family.

Stimulation of mAChR exerts prominent stimulatory effects on glandular secretion and leads to contraction of muscles of the eye, urinary bladder, and gastrointestinal tract (Fig. 7-3). These responses are primarily mediated by $M_1$ and $M_3$ receptors, which couple to $G\alpha q$ to directly activate PLC and consequently increase intracellular $Ca^{2+}$ and activate PKC. Stimulation of mACh on blood vessels causes vessel relaxation rather than contraction resulting from indirect mAChR-mediated release of EDRF/NO from endothelial cells.[88] If endothelial cells are absent, ACh can induce vasoconstriction through direct activation of $M_3$ or $M_1$ receptors located on vascular smooth muscle cells.[89] Peripheral vascular resistance is not under muscarinic cholinergic control, however, because the vasculature is not innervated by the parasympathetic nervous system.

The major mAChR subtype in the heart is the $M_2$ mAChR.[50] Activation of cardiac mACR inhibits adenylate cyclase[90-93] and can thereby antagonize stimulatory effects of β-adrenergic receptor activation mediated through cAMP formation. In isolated ventricular myocytes one can observe $M_2$ mAChR mediated inhibition of isoproterenol-stimulated calcium currents and contractility; these effects are mediated via $G_o$ and or $G_i$ protein subunits.[94-96] The ventricular myocardium receives little parasympathetic innervation, however; thus contractile function *in vivo* is markedly stimulated via βAR and cyclic AMP but minimally affected via cholinergic stimulation.[50]

The mAChR regulation of cardiac function is most evident in nodal and conducting tissue. Vagal tone domi-

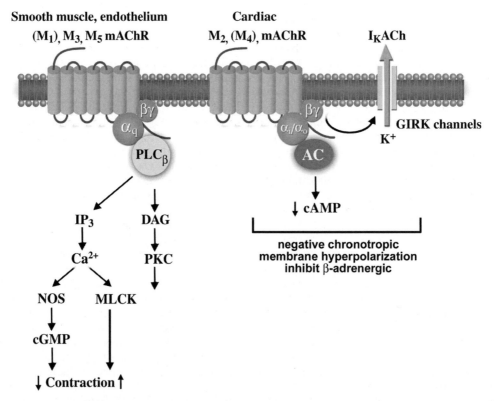

**FIGURE 7-3.** Muscarinic receptor signaling pathway. Receptors of the $M_1$, $M_3$, and $M_5$ subtypes couple to Gq and PLC activation and regulate contraction as detailed in the legend to Figure 7-2. The predominant cardiac mAChR, the $M_2$ and $M_4$ isoforms, couple to $G_i$ to inhibit cAMP formation and to $G_o$ to regulate $K^+$ channels, altering cardiac function.

nates in the control of resting heart rate by stimulating muscarinic receptors in the SA node. Conduction of impulses through the AV node is also inhibited, with excessive cholinergic stimulation leading to AV block. One of the most thoroughly studied molecular effects of cardiac mAChR stimulation is regulation of inward-rectifying $K^+$ channels, also referred to as GIRK channels, in atrial and pacemaker cells. Regulation of this channel is also mediated via the $M_2$ muscarinic receptor and its coupling to PTX-sensitive G-proteins, either $G_i$ or $G_o$. Considerable controversy arose over the issue of whether the $K^+$ channel regulation occurred through effects of the $\alpha$ or of the $\beta\gamma$ subunits derived from these proteins.[97,98] It appears that the consensus has favored the latter, in particular now that myriad other effectors of $\beta\gamma$ signaling have been described. Activation of $K^+_{ACh}$ channels hyperpolarizes cells and retards cellular excitability, contributing to the negative chronotropic response to vagal stimulation and to changes in action potential conduction that contribute to arrhythmias. In human atria, $M_2$ muscarinic receptors regulate ACh release from parasympathetic nerves and this may be altered under pathophysiologic conditions.[99] Changes in mAChR function are also observed in patients with Chagas' disease, in which autoantibodies are formed that interact with an extracellular loop of the $M_2$ mAChR.[100]

In neonatal rat ventricular myocytes the endogenous mAChR is only weakly coupled to phosphoinositide hydrolysis, relative to $\alpha$-adrenergic, endothelin (ET), or other $G_q$-coupled receptors.[101,102] Although MAP kinase is activated through the $M_2$ mAChR[101,103] there is no activation of the hypertrophic gene program.[102,103] This is consistent with the central role for $G_q$-coupled rather than $G_i$-coupled receptors in initiating hypertrophic responses.[104,105] Notably following heterologous expression of the $G_q$-coupled $M_1$ mAChR, or of chimeric mAChRs that couple to $G_q$, cardiomyocytes develop hypertrophic responsiveness to cholinergic receptor agonists.[102]

In isolated cardiomyocytes some unanticipated effects of mAChR stimulation have been observed. For example, mAChR stimulation increases phosphoinositide hydrolysis in murine atria and in chick and rat cardiomyocytes via a PTX-insensitive pathway.[106-110] These findings are at odds with the notion that only $M_2$ receptors, which couple to $G_{i/o}$, are present in the heart. Positive inotropic effects of mAChR stimulation via $G_{i/o}$ independent pathways are also observed (albeit at agonist concentrations above those causing negative inotropy), and this has been suggested to result from increased intracellular sodium.[111-113] The presence of $M_1$ mAChR in the heart also has been suggested as the basis for these responses.[50,110,114]

All five of the mAChR genes have been deleted, and the knockout mice extensively examined. Loss of the $M_1$ mAChR resulted in altered sympathetic ganglionic transmission and CNS susceptibility to seizures, but no cardiovascular changes were evident, in keeping with the absence of this receptor subtype in the heart.[115,116] $M_2$ receptor knockout mice exhibited a host of peripheral and centrally mediated effects; most strikingly, isolated atria from wild-type mice showed marked bradycardia in

response to the stable ACh analog carbachol, and this response was lost in the $M_2$ knockout mice.[117,118] As described previously, the $M_3$ receptor is necessary for salivary secretion, pupil constriction, and bladder contraction, all responses that are no longer observed in the $M_3$ mAChR knockout.[119] Studies with $M_4$ mAChR knockout mice suggest that this receptor has more limited functions than the homologous $M_2$ receptor,[118,120] although this may be different in the rat.[120] An interesting central cardiovascular effect of the $M_5$ receptor is suggested by studies on $M_5$ mAChR knockout mice in which cholinergic dilation of cerebral but not peripheral blood vessels was compromised.[121]

## Endothelin Receptors

ET, originally isolated as a factor derived from vascular endothelial cells, acts as a potent vasoconstrictor. The gene sequence for this contracting factor was identified in 1987, and the factor was named endothelin.[122] ET-1 is a 21 amino acid peptide and is the predominant form of ET in the vasculature. It is structurally related to the snake venom sarafotoxins, which have actions in common with ET-1.[123] ET-2 and ET-3 are 21 amino acid peptide products of separate genes that differ from ET-1 by three and six amino acids, respectively. ET-1 is formed through the actions of endothelin converting enzyme (ECE) on its substrate the 39 amino acid big ET. ECE-1 is a member of the metalloprotease family and is found in a variety of cells, where it catalyzes the formation of ET-1 at the cell surface and intracellularly. In contrast, the related ECE-2 seems only to form ET-1 within the cell.[124] ECE-1 and ECE-2 are the major enzymes responsible for ET formation, but other mechanisms must exist because considerable amounts of ET-1 are present in ECE-1 and ECE-2 knockout mice.[125]

The primary site of ET synthesis is the endothelial cell.[122] A variety of other cell types including vascular smooth muscle and cardiomyocytes also synthesize ET-1.[124,126] The availability of ET-1 is controlled primarily through changes in mRNA expression, specifically that of the precursor 203 amino acid prepro-endothelin. Interestingly, a recent study suggests that ET-1 synthesis in endothelial cells is suppressed by small amounts of red wine extract.[127] This gene is transcriptionally regulated by a number of factors integrally involved in cardiac physiology and pathology. These include interleukins, TNF, angiotensin II (AngII), and thrombin. Increases or decrease in ET-1 mRNA are also observed in response to stretch, hypoxia, and nitric oxide. Vascular remodeling after injury is also regulated via this receptor.[128] The circulating levels of ET-1 and big ET are extremely low but are increased in pathologic conditions such as heart failure.[129-131] Enzymatic mechanisms for ET-1 degradation contribute to its clearance, as does binding to the one subtype of the ET receptor (the $ET_B$ receptor) discussed later.

The effects of ET are mediated through activation of seven transmembrane spanning receptors. Two receptor subtypes, $ET_A$ and $ET_B$, show about 50% homology at the amino acid level; $ET_A$ has high (subnanomolar) affinity for ET1 and ET2 but far lower affinity for ET3.

The $ET_B$ receptor has similar high affinities for all three ET forms, consistent with its suggested function in ET clearance. The $ET_A$ receptor is present on VSMCs. This is the receptor that is largely responsible for ET-1 induced vasoconstriction. There are also $ET_B$ receptors on some vascular smooth muscle, but the predominant vascular location of the $ET_B$ receptor is on endothelial cells where they mediate vasodilation through formation of mediators such as nitric oxide. Vascular remodeling after injury is also regulated via this receptor.[128] Infused ET has clearly observable and pronounced effects on blood pressure. On the other hand the question of whether $ET_A$ antagonists lower resting blood pressure is more controversial, as might be expected based on the low level of circulating ET-1.[124] There is nonetheless considerable support for a physiologic role for ET-1 in vascular regulation because resting blood pressure is significantly lower in mice in which the ET-1 gene is deleted.[131] In addition, a role for ET-1 in pathologic control of the vasculature (i.e., in hypertension) is suggested by animal studies, although it is unproved in humans.[124,131]

The $ET_A$ receptor is also present as the predominant receptor subtype in atrial and ventricular myocytes.[131,132] Both positive inotropic and chronotropic effects of ET-1 can be demonstrated.[133-137] The mechanism for the positive inotropic response is not clear because intracellular $Ca^{2+}$ is not significantly elevated by ET-1 and $ET_A$ receptor activation in cardiomyocytes. However, as suggested for the $\alpha_1$-AR, activation of the $Na^+/H^+$ exchanger and alkalinization in response to ET-1 may lead to altered myofibrillar $Ca^{2+}$ sensitivity.[138] Activation of PLC also appears to be important for $ET_A$ receptor regulated inotropy.[139] ET is a key candidate for a neurohumoral factor involved in the development of cardiac hypertrophy.[140,141] In the isolated neonatal rat ventricular myocyte model, ET is highly effective at inducing hypertrophic responses. In particular increases in MAP kinase activation, protein synthesis, ANF gene expression, myofibrillar organization, and cell size have been demonstrated.[140,142-145] In addition, many of the kinase pathways mediating hypertrophic responses including PKC and the MAP kinases, discussed later in this chapter, are activated in response to ET-1.[143,145-147] Cardiac fibroblasts and endothelial cells also express $ET_A$ receptors that may regulate changes in the extracellular matrix, suggesting involvement in remodeling. ET receptor antagonists are effective in animal models of heart failure and are considered to have promise as a therapeutic modality for human disease. Currently, there are few classes of agents with proven efficacy in heart failure.[131,137,141,148]

## Lysophospholipid (LPA and S-1P) or Edg Receptors

One of the newest additions to the family of G-protein coupled receptors, the Edg receptors are now acknowledged to be the long-sought cell surface receptors for the bioactive lipids lysophosphatidic acid (LPA) and sphingosine-1-phosphate (S-1P, also known as S-1P). The first of the receptors for LPA, *edg2*, was cloned from mice and was characterized in Chun's laboratory in 1996.[149] The human *edg2* receptor gene was subsequently isolated.[150] The Edg2 receptor is now referred to as $LPA_1$. The *edg1* gene product was subsequently demonstrated to be a lysophospholipid receptor activated not by LPA but by S-1P and this receptor is referred to as $S-1P_1$.[151,152] Additional members have been added to both of the lysophospholipid receptor families, and currently there are three LPA receptors (edg 2, 4, and 7) and five S-1P receptors (edg 1, 3, 5, 6, and 8). The approved nomenclature for these receptors is $LPA_{1,2,3}$ and $S-1P_{1-5}$.[153] A significant amount of information has accrued in the last 5 years concerning these receptors and their signaling pathways, and there are several excellent reviews on this topic[154-159] including several related to cardiovascular systems.[160-163]

The ligands for the LP receptors are the bioactive lipids LPA and S-1P. Both S-1P and LPA are present at high concentrations in blood and are the principle growth factors in unconditioned serum.[154,159,164,165] LPA can be formed from phosphatidic acid (PA) the product of phospholipase D mediated phospholipid breakdown. Ceramide and sphingosine, which serve as precursors for S-1P, are products of sphingomyelin hydrolysis by the enzyme sphingomyelinase. Both of these mediators are thought to work within the cell, and in particular ceramide has been considered to mediate apoptotic cell death in cardiomyocytes and other cells,[166,167] whereas S-1P can suppress ceramide-induced apoptosis.[168] Sphingosine kinase, which is rate limiting in catalyzing formation of S-1P from sphingosine, is activated by $Ca^{2+}$ and GPCR stimulation, creating a potential feedforward loop in which S-1P concentrations can rise.[169-171] TNF$\alpha$ can regulate sphingomyelinase activity and production of sphingosine and ceramide.[172-174] Recent evidence suggests that sphingosine kinase not only is active in the intracellular compartment but also is exported from cells.[175] Thus, S-1P may be formed outside the cell and contribute (along with S-1P released from mast cells, monocytes, and platelets) to S-1P receptor activation. The contribution of intracellular S-1P versus released S-1P and receptor activation remains uncertain.[159] In the heart, sphingosine appears to be released from cardiomyocytes during hypoxia and converted to S-1P by platelets or other blood components.[174]

The LPA and S-1P receptors couple to virtually all of the well-described G-protein effector systems. Thus, activation of $G_q$ and PLC, of $G_{12/13}$ and Rho-dependent cytoskeletal responses and of $G_i$ and cyclase inhibition, MAP kinase cascades, and ion channel regulation have all been described.[157,159,176,177] Selectivity in receptor subtype coupling to particular G-proteins has been suggested based on heterologous expression.[178,179] Such selectivity is better demonstrated from experiments examining G-protein activation[180,181] and in experiments using knockout cells.[177,182,183] For example, using murine embryonic fibroblasts (MEFs) from the $S-1P_3$ (EDG3) knockout mouse, it was demonstrated that PLC activation ($G_q$ signaling) was markedly impaired, whereas cyclase inhibition ($G_i$ signaling) and Rho activation ($G_{12/13}$) were intact.[182] In $S-1P_{2/3}$ double knockouts, Rho activation was lost.[183] These data are consistent with the notion that $S-1P_1$ couples to $G_i$, $S-1P_2$ that couples primarily to $G_{12/13}$ and Rho, and S-1P$_3$ couples to $G_q$ and PLC.

The lysophospholipid receptors are remarkable in their robust coupling to the actin cytoskeleton, mediated at least in part through activation of $G_{12/13}$ and Rho signaling pathways.[184-193] In zebrafish, migration of heart precursors to the midline is mediated through S-IP and an S-IP receptor.[194] Endothelial cell migration is stimulated via S-1P receptor activation, suggesting a role of S-1P in angiogenesis and chemotaxis.[160,195-197] LPA also stimulates chemotaxis.[196] The S-1P$_1$ receptor knockout is embryonic lethal, a phenotype that appears to result from lack of proper vascular maturation.[161,185] Recent studies have implicated the S-1P$_1$ receptor in cell motility induced by PDGF, suggesting that tyrosine kinase activation contributes to the effects of the S-1P receptor on activation of Rac and subsequent changes in cell motility.[197] In other studies, phosphorylation of the S-1P receptor by AKT has been implicated in activation of Rac and downstream effects on chemotaxis.[198]

The LPA$_1$ gene is highly expressed in the mouse heart,[158] human atrial cardiomyocytes,[199] and rat cardiomyocytes. In contrast, there are only low levels of the LPA$_3$ receptor transcript in the mouse heart[158] or neonatal rat ventricular myocytes (NRVMs). The LPA$_2$ receptor appears to be absent from the mouse heart by Northern analysis[158] but not by RT-PCR (Means and Brown, unpublished observation), although this may depend on culture conditions[200]). Regarding the S-1P receptors, the S-1P$_1$, S-1P$_2$, and S-1P$_3$ are consistently seen in mouse, cat, and human hearts and in isolated rat atrial and ventricular myocytes.[164,182,199-202] Thus, it is clear that this receptor family must play an important and conserved role in cardiovascular control.

There is a multitude of documented actions of both LPA and S-1P on cardiac function. LPA activates MAP kinase, PI-3 kinase, and p70 S6 kinase in neonatal rat cardiomyocytes[203] and increases protein synthesis and SRE-luciferase gene expression in these cells.[200] S-1P causes bradycardia when injected into rats[204] and activates an inwardly rectifying $K^+$ channel in rabbit SA nodal cells[205] and in guinea pig, mouse, and human atrial myocytes.[199,206,207] S-1P also decreases excitability by reducing $I_{Na}$ in rat ventricular cells[208] and dysregulates calcium cycling in NRVMs.[201] Both LPA and S-1P have been shown to induce hypertrophy,[202,209] although these response are not particularly robust in comparison to those of the well-described $G_q$-coupled receptor agonists such as phenylephrine, ET, and PGF$_{2\alpha}$. The possibility that the effects of S-1P is protective (i.e., that it promotes cardiomyocyte survival) is more intriguing, and recently S-1P was shown to inhibit apoptosis induced by hypoxia in NRVMs.[210] A role for activation of these receptors under physiologic or pathologic conditions is suggested by the myriad sources of S-1P. S-1P and related compounds are components of serum,[164] platelets are sources of S-1P that accumulate in areas of infarcts, sphingomyelinase is activated by cytokines such as TNFα[173] and during hypoxia-reoxygenation of cardiomyocytes,[211] and sphingosine is released from ischemic cardiomyocytes.[174]

## Angiotensin Receptors

AngII is a biologically active octapeptide that transduces its actions through AngII receptors (AT). AngII is formed from its precursor, angiotensinogen, by the actions of renin and ACE, which leaves two amino acids. Recently ACE2, another carboxypeptidase that may antagonize ACE activity has been described and disrupted.[212] AngII acts in both an endocrine fashion, as a systemic or circulating hormone, and an autocrine or paracrine fashion. In addition to the well-known circulating renin angiotensin system (RAS), tissues including the vasculature and heart are capable of generating AngII, which acts on local receptors to mediate cellular responses.[213,214] In the cardiovascular system, the involvement of AngII in the control of vascular tone and blood pressure is indisputable. In the heart, AngII effects on fibroblasts clearly contribute to fibrosis.[215] The role of AngII and its receptors in the development of cardiac hypertrophy is more controversial. In the context of heart failure, ACE inhibitors and AT$_1$ receptor blockers are effective therapies.

There are two types of angiotensin receptors—AT$_1$ and AT$_2$. The AT$_1$ receptor was isolated by molecular cloning in 1991[216] and is a seven transmembrane spanning receptor belonging to the family of G-protein coupled receptors. The AT$_1$ receptor is highly expressed in the adrenal, vasculature, kidney, and heart. In rodents, there are two receptor subtypes termed AT$_{1A}$ and AT$_{1B}$ in the AT$_1$ family. These are products of separate genes, but they are highly homologous. The AT$_{1A}$ receptor is the major subtype in the cardiovascular system,[217] and in humans there appears to be only one AT$_1$ receptor.[218] Nonetheless, to analyze the function of the AT$_1$ receptor in transgenic and knockout mice it has been necessary to delete (or express) both AT$_{1A}$ and AT$_{1B}$ receptors. These studies, which are described in the following, have suggested functional differences in these subtypes. The AT$_2$ receptor shows only 34% homology to the AT$_1$ receptor. It is expressed at lower levels in adult tissue than in fetal tissue, and its expression appears to be regulated in pathologic conditions such as heart failure, vascular injury, and myocardial infarction.[219-221] A role of the AT$_2$ receptor in fetal development has been suggested; however, development is not abnormal in the AT$_2$ receptor knockout mice.[222-224]

Signaling pathways used by the AT$_1$ receptor are those associated with receptor coupling to $G_q$- and $G_i$-coupled receptors. AngII, acting through AT$_1$ receptors, stimulates phosphatidylinositol hydrolysis and PKC activation in guinea pig hearts and rat ventricular myocytes[225-227] and in vascular smooth muscle.[228] AngII is released during stretch and is a key mediator of the effects of stretch on cardiomyocyte hypertrophy.[226,229] In addition to the activation of PLC, AngII effects on cardiomyocytes include activation of tyrosine kinases, MAP kinases, and p90S6 kinase[230] and activation of Jak/Stat pathways.[231] Cross talk between AT$_1$ receptors and tyrosine kinase growth factor receptors (e.g., PDGF, EGF receptors) has been widely demonstrated, and transactivation of these receptors is considered to play a key role in mediating AngII signaling.[232] The signaling properties of the AT$_2$ receptor appear, in general, to be opposite those of the AT$_1$ receptor. Thus, there is evidence for activation of specific phosphatases (MKP-1, SHP-1, PP2A) that would diminish signaling through MAP kinase, tyrosine kinase, and serine threonine kinase cascades.[219,220,233-235]

Knockout and transgenic strategies have been extensively applied to study AT receptor function. These studies are discussed in detail in the review by Brede and Hein.[217] As expected, based on the profound pressor response to AngII and localization of the AT$_{1A}$ receptor in vascular smooth muscle, mice in which the AT$_{1A}$ receptor gene is disrupted have decreased resting blood pressure, and pressor responses to infused AngII are attenuated.[236,237] These findings indicate that the AT$_{1B}$ receptor does not play a redundant role in mediating AngII vasoconstriction. Indeed, the AT$_{1B}$ knockout mouse has normal blood pressure, and the pressor response to AngII is not lost.[238] However, in the double knockout, basal and AngII pressor response were more fully diminished.[217,239,240]

The ability of these animals to respond to pressure overload hypertrophy has also been examined. Earlier studies using mouse models of pressure overload hypertrophy had demonstrated that the AT$_1$ receptor antagonist losartan attenuated the increases in heart to body weight and ANF gene expression seen in this model.[241] However, in mice devoid of AT$_{1A}$ receptors, hypertrophy was still induced by pressure overload.[242-244] In addition, cardiomyocytes isolated from AT$_{1A}$ knockout mice developed hypertrophy in response to stretch, despite elimination of the AT$_{1A}$ receptor; involvement of a tyrosine kinase pathway was suggested.[245] Transgenic mice overexpressing AT$_1$ receptors show hypertrophy, although there is a range of observed phenotypes depending perhaps on which species of receptor is expressed.[217] Thus, although transgenic overexpression of the AT$_1$ receptor may induce cardiac hypertrophy *in vivo*,[246] as can adenoviral overexpression of the receptor in isolated cardiomyocytes,[247] studies from the knockout mice imply that this receptor does not mediate physiologic hypertrophy.

AT$_2$ receptor knockout mice develop normally, as mentioned previously, and only subtle phenotypic changes are observed under basal conditions. There is either no change or an increase in arterial blood pressure.[222-224] Interventions reveal more remarkable alterations in function. These include enhanced vasoconstrictor response to AngII and other agonists, exaggerated VSMC growth, and enhanced neointimal formation following balloon injury.[222-224,248,249] These are consistent with removal of growth inhibitory pathways. Inhibitory effects of AT$_2$ receptor on cardiac growth have also been suggested; for example, blockade of AT$_2$ receptors amplifies the LV growth response to AngII.[250]

On the other hand, there is a body of evidence implicating the AT$_2$ receptor in growth promoting pathways, albeit through as yet unclear mechanisms.[219] A growth stimulatory role of the AT$_2$ receptor may be indicated by the effects of AT$_2$ receptor knockout on cardiac hypertrophy. In the basal state these mice showed

reduced LV wall thickness. Most importantly, after 10 weeks of aortic banding, the mice show practically no hypertrophy relative to wild-type mice.[251] Failure to hypertrophy was also observed following chronic AngII infusion.[252] Thus, it is possible that upregulation of AT$_2$ receptors occurs in and contributes to the development of pressure overload hypertrophy. Of note, many of the well-known markers of ventricular hypertrophy including β-MHC and ANF were increased in the knockout and wild-type mice.[251] The distinguishing feature differentiating wild-type from knockout mice was the ability to activate p70$^{s6k}$, which plays a pivotal role in controlling protein synthesis and may be a critical mediator of AngII/AT$_2$ receptor effects on hypertrophy.

## Protease-Activated Receptors

Protease-activated receptors (PARs) are specialized ubiquitously expressed peptide GPCRs that carry a tethered ligand.[253] PAR-1, the prototype for this receptor family, is activated on cleavage of its extracellular N-terminus by thrombin to expose a new N-terminal sequence (SFLLRN, human; SFFLRN, rodent) that binds intramolecularly to the body of the cleaved receptor.[253] PAR-1 also is activated (independent of proteolysis) by synthetic peptides corresponding to the N-terminal tethered peptide ligand exposed by thrombin's actions.

PARs display certain unique features as a result of their distinctive proteolytic cleavage mechanism. First, a proteolytically activated PAR in theory would be able to signal indefinitely because the ligand is physically attached and cannot diffuse away. Platelets are not likely to require mechanisms for PAR desensitization and resensitization because once they are incorporated into a clot, they are not reused. However, "single-use" PARs present a problem in signal regulation for other cell types. Here, signal termination for PAR-1 is accomplished through rapid phosphorylation-dependent uncoupling from G-proteins, internalization, and targeting to lysosomes for degradation (rather than recycling to the surface like other GPCRs). In endothelial cells and fibroblasts, resensitization results from the rapid delivery of intracellularly stored intact receptor to the cell surface; in megakaryoblastic erythroleukemia cells that lack intracellular stores of PAR-1, resensitization requires new receptor synthesis and is much slower. The second unique feature of PARs relates to their susceptibility to activation by any serine protease capable of cleaving the N-terminus at the site that exposes the tethered ligand sequence (i.e., selectivity is influenced by the nature of the enzymes released in the cell's microenvironment). Cleavage of PARs at proximal sites that amputate the tethered ligand sequence also render them unresponsive to subsequent activation by thrombin. Cathepsin G, which is released by activated neutrophils during vascular injury and inflammation, generates such a cleavage product of PAR-1 and inhibits the biologic actions of thrombin in cells that express PAR-1. The pathophysiologic importance of this alternate mechanism to downregulate PAR signaling has not been fully explored.

PAR-1 expression is widespread; PAR-1 couples to several heterotrimeric G-proteins ($G_q$, $G_i$, $G_{12}$) and a host of cellular responses that influence cell shape, growth, and differentiation. The potential cardiovascular actions of PAR-1 are profound, because thrombin is one of the most potent stimuli for platelet activation and PAR-1 exerts a range of actions in the vasculature and heart. Thrombin-dependent activation of PAR-1 has been implicated in changes in endothelial cell shape that lead to increased monolayer permeability and edema; the regulation of blood vessel diameter through endothelial-dependent vasodilation (or in denuded vessels, smooth muscle cell contraction); and mitogenesis in endothelial cells, smooth muscle cells, and fibroblasts (i.e., vascular remodeling at sites of injury). Proliferative responses to PAR-1, including responses in cardiac fibroblasts, require tyrosine kinase activity; this reflects a pathway involving EGF receptor transactivation, which links PAR-1 to the activation of kinases (ERK, p38-MAPK, and AKT) implicated in mitogenesis.[254] In cardiomyocytes, PAR-1 influences the rate and rhythm of contraction and activates a hypertrophic growth program that induces fetal gene expression and alters cardiomyocyte morphology.[255-258] Of note, recent studies indicate that PAR-1 induces cell elongation (with less of an increase in cell width), which is reminiscent of the changes identified in volume-overload hypertrophy. This is quite distinct from $\alpha_1$-AR activation by NE, which leads to a uniform increase in cell dimensions that is more typical of the morphologic phenotype observed in the setting of pressure-overload hypertrophy. Activation of PAR-1 on the surface of cardiomyocytes and cardiac fibroblasts is predicted to be pertinent at sites of cardiac injury (hemorrhagic infarction in which cardiomyocytes would come into direct contact with bloodborne coagulation factors) and/or inflammation (myocarditis, the border zone of a myocardial infarction). Finally, PAR-1 has been implicated in critical function during development because PAR-1 null mice display high partial lethality at E9 to 10 (a period of fetal development that is characterized by widespread expression of PAR-1 mRNA and is critical for cardiovascular development). Although PAR-1 null mice that survive to birth display no obvious phenotype as adults under normal conditions, a phenotype becomes manifest during pathologic injury of the kidney or vessels.[259-261]

Since the initial cloning of PAR-1, three additional structurally homologous PARs have been identified. PAR-2 is expressed by many cell types (including cardiomyocytes and endothelial cells) and is the only known PAR not activated by thrombin. PAR-2 is activated by trypsin, mast cell tryptase, coagulation factors VIIa and Xa, or by short synthetic peptides corresponding to the newly exposed N-terminus after receptor cleavage (SLIGVK, human; SLIGRL, mouse[262,263]). PAR-2 cleavage by trypsin is believed to be important in the gastrointestinal tract and in airway epithelium; PAR-2 is a potent inhibitor of bronchoconstriction, a property that could be exploited for the therapy of asthma and bronchitis.[264-266] Mast cell tryptase may be the pathophysiologically important activator of PAR-2 in the vasculature,

where PAR-2 induces endothelium-dependent relaxation of arterial rings and endothelial cell mitogenesis.[267-269] PAR-2 activation by tryptase also may be pertinent in cardiomyocytes, where mast cell infiltration can be identified between muscle fibers in normal ventricles and in increased density in idiopathic and dilated cardiomyopathies.[267,270] Because cytokines induce PAR-2 mRNA expression in endothelium and in coronary vessels, PAR-2 also may play a role in inflammation.[271,272] PAR-2 mimics the effect of PAR-1 to induce cardiomyocyte hypertrophy and also may contribute to cardiac remodeling.[273]

PAR-3 and PAR-4 are thrombin receptors whose function has been studied almost exclusively in the context of platelet aggregation; PAR antagonists potentially offer a strategy to interfere with thrombin's actions in platelets, without increasing bleeding diathesis by inhibiting fibrin formation. PAR-4 is activated by thrombin or a synthetic peptide that mimics its tethered ligand (GYPGKF). In human platelets, PAR-1 and PAR-4 account for most (if not all) of thrombin's actions. PAR-1 induces rapid and robust platelet responses; PAR-1 contains a hirudin-like domain adjacent to the thrombin cleavage site, binds thrombin with high affinity, and mediates platelet activation at low thrombin concentrations. PAR-4 is not necessary for platelet activation when PAR-1 is intact. However, PAR-4 can substitute for PAR-1 when its function is impaired, although PAR-4 lacks the thrombin-binding hirudin-like domain and is activated only at high concentrations of thrombin. Recent studies identify differences in the tempo and nature of PAR-1 versus PAR-4 responses, suggesting that PAR-4 and PAR-1 are not entirely redundant or that PAR-4 might mediate responses to proteases other than thrombin.[274] In fact, recent studies show that the effect of thrombin to Src in cardiomyocytes (including in cardiomyocytes cultured from PAR-1 null mice) is via PAR-4 and not PAR-1.[275] Finally, PAR-3 acts in a manner that is distinct from other PAR family members. PAR-3 does not confer responsiveness to thrombin when heterologously expressed alone; when coexpressed with PAR-4, the extracellular N-terminal thrombin-binding domain of PAR-3 acts as a cofactor that enables PAR-4 to respond to low concentrations of thrombin.

## Receptor Tyrosine Kinases

Receptor tyrosine kinases (RTKs) constitute a multi-member family of growth factor receptors that display distinctive structural organization and functional features. RTKs are polypeptides that transverse the membrane once. The extracellular ligand-binding domains contain highly conserved structural motifs, such as immunoglobulin (Ig)-like domains, cysteine-rich regions, and fibronectin repeats; these motifs confer specific high-affinity ligand binding. Because many growth factors are bivalent molecules, binding promotes the formation of receptor dimers. The insulin receptor, which exists as a receptor dimer in the absence of ligand, is the sole variation on this model. The transmembrane domain of RTKs is primarily $\alpha$-helical in structure. Its primary role is to anchor the receptor in the correct orientation within the membrane, but mutations in the transmembrane domains of two RTKs produce receptors that constitutively dimerize in the absence of ligand. This suggests RTK transmembrane domains can also function to stabilize the dimeric conformation of the receptor.

RTKs contain a highly conserved intracellular kinase domain. Activation and dimerization places two RTK molecules in close proximity to each other; activation is the result of autophosphorylation of tyrosine residues in trans. Autophosphorylation potentiates the intrinsic tyrosine kinase activity of the receptor and creates docking sites for signaling molecules that contain Src homology 2 (SH2) or phosphotyrosine-binding (PTB) domains (motifs that interact with phosphotyrosines). SH2 domains are highly conserved ~100 residue motifs that bind phosphotyrosyl targets and display essentially no binding affinity for the nonphosphorylated sequence. SH2 domain-containing proteins include molecules with intrinsic catalytic activity (PLC-$\gamma$, Src, Ras-GAP, etc.) and molecules devoid of known catalytic activity that function as adapters to bring other modular signaling proteins into the macromolecular receptor complex (Grb2, the p85 regulatory subunit of PI3-kinase). PTB domains represent an alternative phosphotyrosyl recognition motif found in Shc and certain other signaling proteins. Recent studies indicate that in addition to transducing signals from their individual ligands, RTKs also are phosphorylated in response to activation of certain GPCRs and in the context of stimulation by certain cytokines, cell adhesion, and cellular stresses. Hence, RTKs function in many cells as a central relay station to integrate signals from environmental physiologic and pathologic inputs to growth regulatory networks including the Ras/MAPK cascade, PLC$\gamma$, and the PI3-kinase/AKT pathway.

Many RTKs have been implicated in inherited and acquired human disease syndromes.[276] The EGF (or ErbB) subfamily of RTKs has been the focus of particular research interest because of their contribution to the development and progression of many human cancers and their importance in normal cardiac development. The ErbB family consists of four receptor subtypes: EGFR (also termed ErbB1 or HER1), ErbB2 (HER2; c-neu), ErbB3, and ErbB4. ErbB1, ErbB3, and ErbB4 are activated by a family of epidermal growth factor-related growth factors. Epidermal growth factor, transforming growth factor-$\alpha$ (TGF-$\alpha$), and heparin-binding-EGF-like growth factor (HB-EGF) are ligands that directly activate ErbB1. Glial growth factor (GGF), heregulin, and neuregulins are ligands that directly bind and activate ErbB3 and/or ErbB4 (and activate ErbB2 only indirectly, through actions at ErbB2-containing receptor heterodimers). ErbB2 is an orphan receptor; no ligand has been identified. High levels of ErbB2 expression support ligand-independent homodimerization, presumably as a result of spontaneous dimer formation. ErbB2 also is the preferred heterodimerization partner for other ErbB family members. Heterodimerization with ErbB2 leads to a high affinity for ligand and deceleration in the rate of ligand dissociation. The resultant prolongation in the kinetics of signaling enhances the transforming potential of the ErbB2-containg heterodimer. Heterodimerization

also provides a mechanism for signal specificity and diversity, because the combinatorial interactions produce receptors with signaling properties that are unique and not simply the sum of the signaling properties of the individual dimerization partners. Finally, heterodimerization is particularly critical for activation of ErbB3, which lacks intrinsic kinase activity and only signals when complexed with another family member. Current literature suggests that a heterodimer comprised of ligandless-ErbB2 and kinase-defective-ErbB3 is the most potent ErbB signaling complex.

ErbB receptors are critical for normal cell differentiation during fetal development; null mutations of any of the four ErbB family member results in an embryonic lethal phenotype. Of note, disruption of the genes encoding ErbB2, Erb4, or their ligand neuregulin results in fetal demise at day 10 to 11, with almost identical defects in the heart and brain. Loss of neuregulin in the endocardium or ErbB2/ErbB4 in the myocardium results in defective cardiomyocyte differentiation and poor ventricular wall trabeculation. Although the precise mechanisms for the ErbB receptor-dependent cardiac actions remain largely unknown, recent studies identify an effect of endocardial-derived neuregulin to induce embryonic cardiomyocyte differentiation into cells of the conduction system.[277] In vitro studies also identify an effect of neuregulin-ErbB to activate MAPK and p70[S6K], suppress apoptosis, and promote myocyte proliferation and survival.[278,279]

ErbB overexpression, or activating mutants of ErbB receptors, have been implicated in neoplastic transformation and tumors in animal models. The oncogenes v-erbB and c-neu are constitutive mutants of ErbB1 and ErbB2, respectively. ErbB signaling is increased in certain human tumors because of amplification of the gene. Overexpression of ErbB2 is particularly common in breast and ovarian cancer, where it correlates with poor prognosis and has come to be identified as a promising target for cancer therapy. Trastuzumab (Herceptin), a specific monoclonal antibody against the extracellular domain of ErbB2, has been developed as a ErbB2 inhibitor. Trastuzumab has been approved by the FDA for the treatment of metastatic breast cancer on the basis of clinical trials demonstrating that it improves the chemotherapeutic response rate and the median duration of responses when used in combination with other chemotherapeutic agents. However, reports that 28% of women receiving trastuzumab in combination with an anthracycline develop heart failure, with 19% developing class III to IV symptoms (class III to IV symptoms develop in only 3% of patients treated with doxorubicin alone), have raised serious concerns that trastuzumab may inhibit important cardiac functions mediated by ErbB2 and that the risk-to-benefit ratio of this drug deserves further analysis.[280]

## TNF and Toll-Like Receptors

Two important families of cell surface receptors that are crucial for the activation of cellular and organismic responses to infection and tissue injury are the TNF receptor (TNFR) family and the Toll-like receptor (TLR) family. Members of both families can play critical roles in the pathogeneses of cardiovascular diseases including chronic heart failure, myocardial infarction, ischemia-reperfusion injury, myocarditis, and atherosclerosis.[281-287] TNFα signaling pathways and their role in cardiac physiology and pathology have recently been extensively reviewed.[288-291] TNFα signaling pathways involved in both hypertrophy and apoptosis in isolated cardiomyocytes have also been delineated.[292]

The TNFR family derives its name from TNF, the founding member of a family of cytokines that are produced by many different cell types in response to inflammation, infection, tissue injury, and other forms of stress.[293] In addition to TNF, this family includes cytokines such as lymphotoxin (LT) α and β, Fas-ligand (FasL), CD40-ligand (CD40L), receptor activator of NF-κB (RANK)-ligand (RANKL), TNF-related apoptosis-inducing ligand (TRAIL), and many others.[294] Unlike other cytokines and growth factors, members of the TNF family function as trimers binding to trimeric receptors.[294,295] TNF family members exhibit 25% to 30% sequence similarity, mostly in residues responsible for trimerization and formation of disulfide bridges.[295] The external surfaces of the trimers, which mediate receptor selectivity, are more divergent. TNF can elicit an unusually wide spectrum of biologic responses including inflammation, fever, lymphocyte and leukocyte migration, acute phase response, cell proliferation, differentiation, and death.[293] Through its potent proinflammatory effects, TNFα has been suggested to play a critical role in the cause of chronic heart failure.[281,296] However, targeted approaches to neutralize TNFα have often worsened heart failure, and several lines of evidence suggest that TNFα signaling might serve a beneficial homeostatic role.[289,297]

By comparison, other TNFα family members have more limited functions. For instance, TRAIL and FasL induce apoptosis and no inflammation.[298] Activation of only a subset of the biochemical responses elicited by TNFα may explain the more restricted biologic responses elicited by other members of the TNF family. Instead of discussing the signaling mechanisms used by each family member, we focus on the type 1 TNFR (TNFR1) because it is the most diverse in its biochemical and biologic activities. Like all its relatives, TNFR1 is a type 1 transmembrane protein whose extracellular domain (ECD) contains several (three for TNFR1) cysteine-rich domains (CRD), which are 40 amino acid pseudorepeats responsible for ligand binding (mostly CRD2 and CRD3).[294,295] Soluble forms of the ECD and anti-TNFα antibodies exhibit potent anti-inflammatory effects and have been evaluated for the treatment of chronic heart failure.[281,283] The binding of a trimeric ligand stabilizes the TNFR1 trimer and allows the formation of 3:3 complexes between the intracellular domain (IRD) of the receptor and various signaling molecules.[299] The IRD of TNFR1 contains a death domain (DD), which is a 60 amino acid protein sequence motif that forms a globular α helix bundle used for interaction with other DD-containing proteins.[298] Instead of a DD, which is also present in Fas and several other death receptors (DR 3 to 6), the IRD of TNFR2 and other family members contain a TNF (tumor necrosis factor) receptor-associated factor (TRAF) binding motif, used for direct interactions with members of the TRAF family of signaling molecules.[299]

The DD of TNFR1 mediates recruitment of TNFR1-associated DD protein (TRADD), which serves as a platform that recruits at least three more signaling proteins: receptor-interacting protein 1 (RIP1), Fas-associated DD protein (FADD), and TNFR-associated factor 2 (TRAF2)[299-304] (Fig. 7-4). RIP1 and FADD are both DD proteins, but other than that they share no structural or functional similarities. FADD was originally identified as a DD protein that is directly recruited by the IRD of the liganded (trimerized) form of Fas to mediate the activation of caspases through its death effector domain (DED).[302] The DED of FADD interacts with the prodomains of caspase 8 or 10 and elicits their activation through an induced proximity mechanism that is highly dependent on receptor oligomerization.[298] The activation of caspases 8 and 10 results in activation of "executor" caspases, such as caspase 3, leading to the cleavage of many cellular proteins followed by apoptotic cell death.[298]

RIP1 is a protein kinase, which is essential for TNFα-mediated NF-κB activation, but it has no role in MAPK activation.[305] Although RIP1 kinase activity is not essential for NF-κB activation, it is possible that the catalytically inactive mutant of RIP1 used to reconstitute signaling in *rip1*[−/−] cells may interact with and thereby activate other RIP-like kinases—RIP2 and RIP3.[299] Both RIP2 and RIP3 can activate NF-κB on overexpression,[306] but their exact functions in TNF signaling remain to be defined. TRAF2 is a member of the TRAF family, which is characterized by the presence of a highly conserved C-terminal TRAF domain and a more variable N-terminal TRAF domain that contains a RING finger and several Zn fingers.[307] Although the recruitment of TRAF2 to TNFR1 is dependent on TRADD, it can be recruited directly to TNFR2 because of the presence of a TRAF binding motif in the latter.[308] TRAF2, however, has higher affinity to TRADD than to either TNFR1 or TNFR2,[309] which may explain why TNFα is a more potent activator of TRAF2. Overexpression of TRAF2 or oligomerization of its N-terminal domain are sufficient for activation of the IKK to NF-κB and MAPK to AP-1 signaling pathways.[299] Although the knockout of TRAF2 abolishes TNFα-induced JNK activation, it only results in a partial loss of IKK or NF-κB activation.[310] The residual response is due to TRAF5, which can be recruited to TNFR1 in the absence of TRAF2 and thereby allows weak activation of NF-κB.[310] As discussed later, TRAF2 recruits IKK to TNFR1, and RIP1 is responsible for IKK activation.[311] The mechanism by which TRAF2 oligomerization results in activation of MAPK cascades is not very clear. Although several MAP3Ks were proposed to be involved in TNFα-induced MAPK activation, none of them was found to be essential in knockout experiments.[299]

A second family of cell surface receptors that mediate responses to infection and tissue injury is the TLR family.[312] The founding member of the family is the IL-IR receptor (IL-1R), but the family actually derives its name from the *Drosophila* Toll protein, which was first identified as necessary for establishment of dorso-ventral

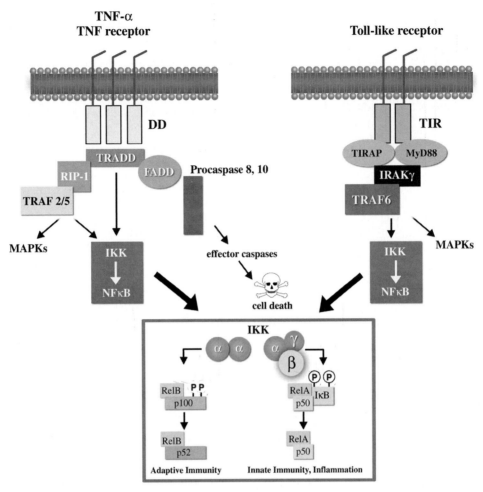

**FIGURE 7-4.** TNF-α and Toll-like receptor signaling pathway. TNF-α and Toll-like receptors, when engaged by ligand, nucleate multiprotein complexes that result in activation of caspases, MAP kinases, and IKK. Activation of NFκB proceeds through IKK-mediated phosphorylation, which releases inhibition and leads to NFκB-mediated responses.

polarity in the *Drosophila* embryo.[313] Toll achieves its developmental function through activation of one of the *Drosophila* NF-κB proteins—Dorsal.[314] In addition, Toll is required for the activation of innate immunity in response to fungal infections, which depends on synthesis of NF-κB-dependent antifungal peptides.[315] With the exception of IL-1R and IL-18R, which are activated by cytokines, the TLRs are activated by a diverse collection of pathogen-associated molecular patterns (PAMPs), which are molecules such as lipopolysaccharides (LPSs), lipoteichoic acids (LTAs), or nonmethylated CpG-containing DNA that are relatively unique to microbes or viruses.[312] In addition, there are indications that some TLRs may be activated by normal cytoplasmic or nuclear proteins that are released to the extracellular milieu following cell and tissue injury.[316,317]

Members of the TLR family are type 1 transmembrane proteins characterized by an extracellular leucine-rich repeat (LRR) and an intracellular Toll/IL-1R (TIR) domain[318] (Fig. 7-4). TLRs 2, 4, and 6 have been detected in the heart, although their function is not known with certainty. Instead of an LRR, the IL-1R and IL-18R have three Ig-like domains that are directly involved in ligand binding.[312] Interestingly, many if not most members of

this family are either unable to bind ligands with high affinity on their own or cannot transduce an effective signal and require interactions with a variety of accessory proteins. For instance, IL-IR heterodimerizes with IL-1RAcP to form a competent signal transducing complex.[319] IL-1RAcP, however, is not required for ligand binding. By contrast, CD14 is a high-affinity receptor for LPS that together with MD-2 facilitates the recognition and activation of TLR4 by LPS.[320] The activation of TLR4 signaling by LPS eventually lends to production of TNFα or other inflammatory mediators. Recently Toll-like receptor 4 has been shown to be necessary for the development of LPS-induced LV dysfunction in a sepsis model.[321]

Following ligand binding, the TIR domains interact with the adaptor protein MyD88, which contains an N-terminal DD and a C-terminal TIR domain.[319,322] MyD88 recruitment is absolutely essential for signaling by IL-1R, TLR2, and TLR9.[323,324] MyD88, however, is required only for some of TLR3- and TLR4-mediated responses,[312] suggesting the existence of an MyD88-independent pathway. Indeed a second adapter protein called TIRAP or MAL (MyD88 adaptor-like) was recently identified that interacts with the TIR domain of TLR4 and mediates

MyD88 independent signaling.[325,326] TIRAP also contains a TIR domain but lacks a DD and instead has a serine- and proline-rich domain at its N-terminus. Once MyD88 is recruited to the receptor, it mediates the recruitment of additional signaling proteins: a protein kinase called IRAK (IL-1R associated kinase) and TRAF6.[319,322,327,328] Like RIP, IRAK contains a DD in addition to its protein kinase domain, which interacts with the DD of MyD88.[328] Although IRAK is autophosphorylated following IL-1R occupancy, its kinase activity is not required for activation of effector pathways.[329] IRAK may simply provide for more efficient recruitment of TRAF6, or alternatively its kinase activity may be redundant with that of other IRAK-like proteins.[330] Like TRAF2/5 in the case of TNFα signaling, TRAF6 is an essential intermediate in IL-1 and LPS signaling, required for activation of the IKK-NF-κB pathway and the different MAPK cascades.[331] TRAF6 has also been suggested to be activated in response to ligation of the leukocyte integrin Mac-1, a molecule that plays an important role in blood vessel inflammation.[285]

# G-PROTEINS

## G-Proteins and Their βγ Subunits

G-proteins have evolved as a family of signaling intermediates that are strategically located to regulate GPCR activation of effectors. Heterotrimeric G-proteins are composed of an α subunit that is loosely bound to a tightly associated dimer of β and γ subunits. GPCR activation catalyzes the exchange of GDP for GTP on the α subunit, which results in the dissociation of GTP-liganded α from βγ dimers. Effectors are regulated by the actions of both the freed α subunit and βγ dimers. The signal is terminated by the hydrolysis of GTP to GDP, because the GDP-liganded α subunit is unable to activate effectors and inactivates the βγ dimer by binding to it. Because Gα subunits are relatively inefficient GTPases, an additional family of proteins termed regulators of G-protein signaling (RGS) proteins play a key role to accelerate the hydrolysis of GTP by the Gα subunit and thereby hasten the termination of Gα subunit activation.[332]

G-protein α and γ subunits undergo covalent lipid modifications that are critical for proper plasma membrane targeting and are required for efficient signaling by GPCRs. All α subunits are reversibly, post-translationally palmitoylated at their N-termini, PTX-sensitive α subunits are myristoylated at their N-termini, and γ subunits are isoprenylated at their C-termini.[333] The α subunit anchoring to the plasma membrane also requires stable binding to βγ dimers. The identity of the G-protein heterotrimer is defined by the α subunit. However, recent studies indicate that the βγ dimer also contributes to the specificity of heterotrimeric G-protein interactions with GPCRs and effectors. Molecular cloning studies identify 5 β subunits and more than 12 γ subunits. The β subunits are structurally characterized as WD40 repeat motif proteins. The β1 to β4 subunits share more than 80% identity with

one another in their primary amino acid sequence; although originally believed to be functionally interchangeable (based largely on in vitro reconstitution studies), recent studies of G-protein function in intact cell preparations suggest that β subunits may contribute to signaling specificity.[334] This may be pertinent because a polymorphism of the $\beta_3$ subunit gene (the GNB3 825T allele) encodes an alternatively spliced (41 amino acid shorter) variant of the $\beta_3$ subunit that lacks one WD repeat domain and is associated with essential hypertension.[335] Although the precise signaling function of this $\beta_3$ subunit variant has not been identified, it has been associated with enhanced signaling via PTX-sensitive G-proteins, enhanced coronary vascular reactivity, and increased neutrophil chemotactic responses.[336,337] The most recently identified family member $\beta_5$ is expressed largely in brain and is an outlier by structural and functional criteria. The γ subunits display considerable structural divergence and have been divided into three classes largely based on their amino acid structures and post-translational modifications (the identity of the isoprenoid lipid added to an invariant cysteine residue in a CAAX motif four residues from the C-terminus). Subclass I includes $\gamma_1$, $\gamma_{11}$, and $\gamma_{14}$ and is modified by a 15-carbon farnesyl group. Subclass II includes $\gamma_2$, $\gamma_3$, $\gamma_4$, $\gamma_7$, and $\gamma_{12}$ and is modified by a 20-carbon geranylgeranyl group. Subclass III includes $\gamma_5$ and $\gamma_{10}$. These also are geranylgeranylated, but $\gamma_5$ (which associates with βγ at the membrane and also is found in focal adhesions) displays distinct C-terminal processing.[338] Studies to date suggest that βγ dimer composition in heart involves $\beta_1$, $\beta_2$, $\gamma_5$, $\gamma_7$, $\gamma_{11}$, and $\gamma_{14}$ (each γ subunit class is represented) and that βγ dimer expression changes during cardiac development.[339-341]

## Gα$_s$

Gα$_s$ proteins are stimulatory regulators of AC, linking β-AR stimulation to the accumulation of the second messenger cAMP. A disease-associated abnormality of Gα$_s$ underlies the watery diarrhea induced by the exotoxin of Vibrio cholerae (or the toxin produced by pathogenic strains of Escherichia coli that cause travelers' diarrhea); this toxin attaches an ADP-ribose moiety from intracellular NAD to the side chain of a key arginine residue in Gα$_s$. ADP-ribosylation of Gα$_s$ markedly slows GTP hydrolysis, locking Gα$_s$ in an active GTP-bound form that persistently stimulates AC; the elevated intracellular cAMP levels induce profuse watery diarrhea.

Although GPCR-dependent activation of AC requires intact Gα$_s$ function, recent studies identified an additional effect of βγ dimers to direct the fidelity and specificity of this pathway. Depletion of $\gamma_7$ using a ribozyme approach results in the selective loss of $\beta_1$ subunits and not other β subunits and a defect in AC activation by $\beta_2$-AR but not PGE$_1$[342,343]; these studies implicate $\beta_1\gamma_7$ dimers in AC activation by $\beta_2$-ARs. $\beta_1\gamma_7$ dimers also selectively support Kir 3.2 activation by $\beta_2$-ARs (and not $\beta_1$-ARs, when these components are coexpressed in Xenopus oocytes[344]) providing further evidence that βγ dimers cooperate with α subunits to contribute to G-protein specificity.

Genetic gain- or loss-of-function mutations of $G\alpha_s$ have been implicated in the rare endocrine disorders of McCune-Albright syndrome and pseudohypoparathyroidism, respectively. The consequences of chronic $\alpha$s activation (resulting from catecholamine stimulation of $\beta$-ARs, typical of heart failure) has been examined using murine models of cardiac-specific $G\alpha_s$ overexpression.[345] These studies show that enhanced $G\alpha_s$ expression leads to increased $\beta$-AR responsiveness with normal cardiac architecture in young adult animals. However, as the animals age, they develop a cardiomyopathy characterized by chamber dilation, reduced ejection fraction, interstitial fibrosis, cellular hypertrophy and apoptosis, ventricular arrhythmias, and sudden death. Importantly, administration of $\beta$-AR blocker therapy (from 9 to 10 months when the cardiomyopathy first becomes manifest to 15 to 17 months when the cardiomyopathy is fully expressed) completely prevents the development of contractile dysfunction and arrests the progression of ventricular fibrosis and cardiomyocyte apoptosis. These results provide strong evidence that chronically enhanced $\beta$-AR signaling mediates the cardiomyopathic phenotype in $G\alpha_s$ mice and that chronic catecholamine stimulation of $\beta$-AR is deleterious. The assumption is that pathologic changes in this model can be attributed to $\alpha$s activation of AC and enhanced formation of cAMP and activation of PKA. However, cAMP-independent targets of $G\alpha_s$ (including Src family tyrosine kinases, recently identified as potential alternate direct—cAMP-independent—effectors of the $\beta$-AR-$G\alpha_s$ pathway[346,347]) also may contribute to the cardiomyopathic phenotype.

## $G\alpha_{i/o}$

The $G\alpha_{i/o}$ protein family consists of structurally related proteins first identified as inhibitors of $\beta$-AR-activated AC. Three forms of $G\alpha_i$ ($G\alpha_{i1}$, $G\alpha_{i2}$, and $G\alpha_{i3}$) and two forms of $G\alpha_o$ have been identified; all of these proteins are targets for ADP-ribosylation by the bacterial PTX. ADP-ribosylation prevents $G\alpha_{i/o}$ subunit interactions with their cognate receptors (i.e., inhibits signaling via $G\alpha_{i/o}$-mediated pathway).

In the heart, the major substrates for PTX-catalyzed ADP-ribosylation include $G\alpha_{i2}$, $G\alpha_{i3}$, and $G\alpha_o$; however, $G\alpha_o$ is largely confined to atrial tissue. PTX treatment inhibits the $G\alpha_i$-dependent anti-$\beta$-AR actions of mAChRs in cardiomyocytes. The genes encoding individual PTX-sensitive $G\alpha$ subunits have been disrupted in ES cells and in mice as a strategy to distinguish the individual roles of $\alpha_{i2}$, $\alpha_{i3}$, and $\alpha_o$ in mAChR signaling. The $\alpha_{i2}$, $\alpha_{i3}$, and $\alpha_o$ null mice are viable, and ventricular myocytes from these animals display normal baseline contractility and isoproterenol-dependent (largely $\beta_1$-AR-dependent) stimulation of L-type calcium current and contractility.[95,94,348] In keeping with the observation that $G\alpha_o$ makes up 0.2% to 0.5% of brain particulate protein and 10% of the growth cone membrane, mice lacking $G\alpha_o$ suffer tremors and occasional seizures, although surprisingly the nervous system is grossly intact. $G\alpha_o$ null mice have a defect in mAChR regulation of L-type calcium channels in cardiomyocytes but not in

mAChR regulation of atrial K+ channels in cardiomyocytes. The L-type calcium channel responds normally to isoproterenol, but there is no inhibition by mAChRs; mAChR-dependent inhibitory modulation of AC also is intact, indicating that $G\alpha_o$-dependent inhibition of calcium channels is not via changes in cAMP.[94,349] Targeted ablation of $G\alpha_{i2}$ has been shown to blunt mAChR-dependent inhibition of $\beta$-AR-dependent activation of AC in heart homogenates, mAChR-dependent inhibition of $\beta$-AR stimulation of contractility and calcium currents in ventricular myocytes, and mAChR activation of $I_K+_{Ach}$ in ES cells.[95,96,350,351] Targeted ablation of $G\alpha_{i3}$ also disrupts mAChR-dependent activation of $I_K+_{Ach}$ in ES cells, but mAChR inhibition of $\beta$-AR-dependent stimulation of contractility and calcium currents is preserved in ventricular myocytes.[95] The negative chronotropic response to carbachol, which is mediated by $I_f$ (a channel thought to be regulated by $G\alpha_o$ and not $G\alpha_i$), is preserved in $G\alpha_{i2}$ and $G\alpha_{i3}$ null mice.[351,352]

Recent studies in model systems suggest that aberrant $G_i$ signaling contributes to the cause of idiopathic dilated cardiomyocytes (IDCM) in humans. Patients with IDCM display activating autoantibodies to $G_i$-linked mAChRs and increase $G\alpha_i$ mRNA, protein, and function.[353] To determine whether increased $G\alpha_i$ signaling represents a mechanism that contributes to the cause of IDCM rather than a compensatory response to the hyperadrenergic state of heart failure, the Conklin laboratory generated mice that express a modified human $G_i$-linked $\kappa$-opioid receptor that is activated solely by a synthetic ligand (RASLL, opioid 1). Prolonged high levels of RASLL expression causes hyperactive $G_i$ signaling and a lethal dilated cardiomyopathy with wide QRS complex arrhythmias and abnormalities in systolic function.[354] Although $G_i$ signals inhibit AC in this model, the role of AC versus other effectors (ion channels, kinase cascades) in the development of ventricular remodeling and dilatation has not been addressed.

## $G\alpha_q$

The $G\alpha_q$ subunit is a member of a class of G-proteins, which also includes $G\alpha_{11}$, $G\alpha_{14}$, and $G\alpha_{15/16}$. The $G\alpha_q$ and $G\alpha_{11}$ subunits were first cloned in 1990[355] and shown to be highly homologous (88%). $G\alpha_q$ and $G\alpha_{11}$ are ubiquitously expressed, whereas expression of the other family members $G\alpha_{14}$ and particularly $G\alpha_{15}$ is more limited to hematopoietic cell lineages.[356] All members of this family lack sites for ADP-ribosylation, distinguishing them from members of the $G\alpha i$ family and rendering $G\alpha_{q/11}$-mediated responses PTX insensitive. Expression of $G\alpha_q$ and $G\alpha_{11}$ in the atria and ventricle of both the adult and neonatal rat heart has also been examined by Western blotting.[339] Interestingly, $G\alpha_q$ appears to be downregulated in adult ventricle.

The $G\alpha_q$ protein isolated from brain has been reconstituted with purified PLC $\beta$. Addition of the G-protein stimulates PLC enzymatic activity in a GTP-dependent manner.[357,358] This observation demonstrates that PLC is a direct effector of $G\alpha_q$ much as adenylate cyclase is an effector of $G\alpha_s$. Other members of the $G\alpha_q$ family share the ability to activate PLC that, as discussed later, is responsible for the generation of inositol tris phosphate and diacylglycerol. Mutations in particular regions of $G\alpha_q$ have been determined to prevent coupling to PLC.[359] There is an interesting reciprocal relationship between PLC and $G\alpha_q$ in that the enzyme also serves as a GTPase activator (GAP) that "turns off" activated $G\alpha_q$ by enhancing GTP hydrolysis.[360]

Many of the receptors discussed previously including the $\alpha_1$-adrenergic, $M_1$ and $M_3$ muscarinic, ET S-1P, and AT1 have been shown to regulate PLC in a PTX-insensitive manner. This is generally taken as evidence for the receptor coupling to $G\alpha_q$. What would constitute more direct evidence for coupling of a receptor to $G\alpha_q$ would be the ability of the receptor agonist to increase GTP/GDP exchange and thereby increase the GTP loading or labeling of $G\alpha_q$. In limited cases this type of direct experiment has been done, confirming, for example, that the $S1P_2$ and $S1P_3$ receptors causes activation of $G\alpha_q$.[180] The function subserved by an activated $G\alpha_q$-coupled GPCR (i.e., increasing the fraction of $G\alpha_q$ in the GTP-liganded state) can be mimicked by mutations in $G\alpha_q$ that render them resistant to GTP hydrolysis. Two such mutants have been widely studied—an R183C substitution in the murine cDNA[361] and Q209L.[362] These constitutively active mutants activate PLC continuously and cause exaggerated cellular responses. A toxin from *Pasteurella* can also stimulate $G\alpha_q$ activity,[363] although its effects are not confined to activation of this pathway.[364]

Stimulation of receptors that couple to $G\alpha_q$ and its downstream targets leads to secretion from glands and contraction of smooth muscle throughout the body. These responses are initiated in large part through increases in intracellular calcium, initiated by its release from the $InsP_3$-sensitive endoplasmic reticular stores in these tissues. In contrast, in the heart, changes in contractile function and $Ca^{2+}$ release from the sarcoplasmic reticulum (SR) are not primarily controlled by $G\alpha_q$ but rather by $G\alpha_s$ activation with antagonism through the $G\alpha_i$ system. Heart rate and pacemaker activity are likewise regulated through $G\alpha_s$ and $G\alpha_i$ pathways. In contrast to the acute responses, however, $G\alpha_q$-mediated signaling events are critical to the development of cardiomyocyte hypertrophy and appear to contribute to the development of apoptosis and heart failure as well, as detailed later.[104,365]

A number of different lines of evidence implicate activation of $G\alpha_q$ and/or its counterpart $G\alpha_{11}$ in hypertrophic growth. This topic is discussed in detail in several reviews.[104,365] Briefly, in the neonatal rat cardiomyocyte used as a model for hypertrophic growth, a number of receptors that act through $G\alpha_q$ induce features of hypertrophy, whereas those that couple to $G\alpha_i$ do so poorly if it all. Antibodies directed against the C-terminal region of $G\alpha_q$ (the region that couples to the receptor) block PLC activation and, when microinjected into myocytes, prevent phenylephrine-mediated hypertrophy.[366] Studies with transgenic mice extend these conclusions to the *in vivo* setting and to pressure-overload induced hypertrophy. Thus, expression of wild-type $G\alpha_q$ in the heart leads to ventricular hypertrophy and the accompanying changes in gene expression and function.[367] Expression of a constitutively active form of $G\alpha_q$

also induces hypertrophy and ultimately death from heart failure.[368] Complementing the observation that $G\alpha_q$ expression leads to hypertrophy, the ability of aortic constriction to induce hypertrophy is attenuated by expression of a peptide derived from the C-terminal of $G\alpha_q$.[369] Similarly, expression of a regulator of G-protein signaling (RGS) with specificity for $G\alpha_q$ (RGS4) blocked pressure overload hypertrophy.[370] Mice in which $G\alpha_q$ is deleted show ataxia[371] and defective platelets aggregation,[372] but most physiologic functions are normal presumably because they can be subserved by $G\alpha_{11}$ or other $G\alpha_q$ family members of $G\alpha_q$. Knockout of $G\alpha_q$ and $G\alpha_{11}$ is embryonic lethal; those with one intact allele show cardiac malformation and die shortly after birth.[373] Therefore, knockout mice in which both $G\alpha_q$ and $G\alpha_{11}$ were conditionally deleted using a tissue-specific (CRE-lox) strategy have been generated. In mice lacking both $G\alpha q$ and $G\alpha_{11}$ in heart, pressure overload induced by aortic constriction is unable to increase heart to body weight or activate the expected compliment of genes normally upregulated as part of the hypertrophic gene program.[374]

A striking observation made in studies with the $G\alpha q$ expressing transgenic mice was the development of a dilated cardiomyopathy and a high level of mortality in the peripartum period. Approximately 70% of the female mice died in the days following delivery of their first or second litter, and a high degree of apoptosis was evident based on TUNEL staining and DNA laddering. Expression of a constitutively activated form of $G\alpha_q$ (Q209L) in cardiomyocytes similarly induced initial hypertrophy, which was rapidly followed by apoptosis.[105] The underlying mechanism leading to apoptosis is mitochondrial dysfunction with loss of mitochondrial membrane potential and cytochrome C release.[375] Membrane phosphoinositide and AKT activation are also compromised.[376] Caspase inhibition decreases both the amount of apoptotic cell death and the severity of peripartum failure (Hayakawa et al, Circulation, In press, 2003). The data support the hypothesis that prolonged or sustained stimulation of $G\alpha_q$-signaling pathways may contribute to the decompensation that leads hypertrophy to heart failure.

## Small G-Proteins

The low molecular weight G-proteins, or smgs, are 20-to 25-kd proteins that are activated by binding GTP. Although there are regions of considerable homology between these proteins and the $\alpha$ subunit of the heterotrimeric G-proteins, the smgs are far smaller than their 38- to 41-kd relatives. In addition Ras and Rho family smgs do not associate with $\beta\gamma$ subunits, which serve to anchor the heterotrimeric G-proteins to the membrane. Rather the smgs are membrane targeted by isoprenylation, either farnestylation (for Ras) or geranylgeranylation (for Rho). Farnestylation inhibitors have been exploited to prevent membrane targeting and, thus, activation of Ras, a smg found in its activated form in a wide range of tumor cells. Inhibition of prenylation is also one of the significant non–cholesterol-lowering effects of the statins (lovastatin and simvastatin).

The mechanisms of activation for Ras and Rho proteins are similar and quite distinct from those used by the heterotrimeric G-proteins. Whereas ligand binding to a GPCR is the signal that induces GDP-release from (and GTP binding to) the α subunit of the heterotrimeric G-protein, Ras and Rho do not associate with agonist-occupied GPCRs. Instead the release of GDP from Ras and Rho is effected through activation of guanine nucleotide exchange factors (GEFs). The molecular interactions involved in Ras activation by tyrosine kinase growth factors was unraveled and eloquently described by a series of studies carried out in the early 1990s. A sequence of protein-to-protein interactions is instigated by binding of PH domains to tyrosine phosphorylated growth factor receptors or adaptor proteins. Among these proteins is the Ras exchange factor, son of sevenless (SOS). Activated Ras in turn binds Raf, leading to initiation of the mitogen activated kinase cascade discussed later. It is now clear that GPCRs and tyrosine kinase growth factors can activate Ras and downstream MAP kinase cascades. $G_i$-coupled receptors activate Ras through effects of released βγ subunits, which lead to formation of scaffolds containing tyrosine kinases (e.g., src) and tyrosine phosphorylated proteins (e.g., shc).[377] $G_q$-coupled receptors probably activate MAP kinases through effects on PKC and perhaps on PYK2 or other tyrosine kinases.[377,378]

There are several members of the Ras family including Ha-Ras, $K_1$-Ras, and N-Ras. The first evidence that Ras was involved in cardiac signaling pathways relevant to hypertrophy came from studies demonstrating that a mutant Ras protein, which functions as a dominant negative inhibitor by virtue of its ability to bind Ras exchangers, blocked the hypertrophic effects of $α_1$-AdrR stimulation in neonatal rat ventricular myocytes.[366,379] Ras is activated by hypertrophic agonists in this model system,[380-382] and MAP kinase (ERK) activation is inhibited by dnRas expression or antibodies.[380,383] One of the first cardiac specific transgenic mouse lines generated was one in which the expression of Ras in ventricle was driven by the MLC2-V promoter.[384] The development of hypertrophy provided evidence that Ras is not only critical for but sufficient to induce cardiac growth. The extent of hypertrophy in this model is relatively mild, but echo-selected lines show many features of human hypertrophic cardiomyopathy.[385] A unique feature of this model for cardiac hypertrophy is that hypertrophy does not progress to failure.

The Rho family proteins are divided into subfamilies Rho, Rac, Rnd, and Cdc42. Within each of these there are further subtypes. The Rnd proteins lack GTPase activity. Little is known about the function of Cdc42 in the cardiovascular system. Cdc42 like the other Rho family proteins plays a prominent role in regulation of the actin cytoskeleton in particular control of filopodia formation.[386,387] Members of the Rho subfamily include RhoA, RhoB, RhoC, RhoD, and others. Virtually all of the experimental work that has been done examining Rho activation and involvement in the cardiac and vascular system has focused on RhoA or has not distinguished among the various Rho members. Rho is a target for ribosylation by the C3 exoenzyme from *Clostridium botulinum* and other bacterial toxins.[388] The C3 exoenzyme has been used, either through extracellular application or cellular expression, to inhibit Rho functions. Studies using C3 toxin and those using dominant negative inhibitors of Rho demonstrate a requirement for Rho in agonist- and stretch-induced hypertrophic growth and gene expression in neonatal rat ventricular myocytes.[389-392] In addition, expression of activated Rho in neonatal cardiomyocytes causes cell enlargement, myofilament organization, and increased ANF and MLC-2 expression.[390] Rho function can also be inhibited by treatment with statins to prevent its geranylation. Recent studies indicate that this intervention, which also targets Ras, leads to loss of agonist induced hypertrophy responses *in vitro* and *in vivo*.[393-395]

A variety of potential Rho effectors have been identified based on their ability to bind activated Rho. Several well-characterized enzymes that are modulated by Rho, including phospholipase D and PI 4,5 kinase.[396-400] Other enzymes that are downstream targets of Rho are Rho kinase (ROCK), rhotekin, and protein kinase N (PKN). Rho kinase is the best studied of these.[401] An important substrate for Rho kinase is the myosin binding subunit of the phosphatase that regulates myosin light chain kinase. Accordingly, Rho activation enhances myosin light chain phosphorylation, and this mechanisms underlies the G-protein dependent $Ca^{2+}$ sensitization of smooth muscle.[402,403] Thus, activation of Rho facilitates contraction in the absence of $Ca^{2+}$ mobilization. Rho kinase inhibitors such as Y-27632 have been demonstrated to lower blood pressure in several models of hypertension,[404] implicating hyperactivity of the Rho pathway in the dysregulation of vascular tone. Myofibrillar $Ca^{2+}$ sensitivity is also increased by phenylephrine in cardiomyocytes from failing hearts, a response sensitive to inhibition by Y-27632.[68] Inhibition of Rho kinase (by expression of dn ROK) also attenuates agonist-induced hypertrophic cardiomyocyte growth.[390,405]

Rho is activated by exchange of GDP for GTP, catalyzed by a Rho GEF. A number of exchange factors with specificity for Rho have been identified. Several of these (e.g., lbc, LARG) were initially identified as genes responsible for cell transformation. A molecular mechanism for Rho activation by GPCR agonists was recently described based on the finding that p115, a Rho GEF, interacts with the α subunit for the G-proteins $G_{12}$ and $G_{13}$. The p115 RhoGEF serves as a regulator of G-protein signaling (RG5) for $Gα_{12/13}$ by increasing their GTPase activity. Independent of its RGS activity, p115 RhoGEF stimulates Rho GTP exchange and this function is apparently increased by its interaction with activated $Gα_{12}$. A number of GPCR ligands cause Rho activation, in particular those that appear to act through receptors that activate $Gα_{12}$ and $Gα_{13}$ (reviewed in references 406 and 407). Thrombin, thromboxane $A_2$, LPA, and S-1P are the best studied. In neonatal cardiomyocytes, Rho is activated by some of these same ligands. The hypertrophic agonists, ET, phenylephrine, and angiotensin are effective in this regard.[382,408] Interestingly, overexpression of wild-type RhoA in myocardium induced hypertrophy that rapidly progressed to heart failure and was associated with pronounced bradycardia.[409] In vascular smooth muscle, thrombin is a highly efficacious Rho activator that also stimulates VSMC proliferation and migration.[410] In several models of hypertension, VSMC Rho expression and its activation are increased, providing a potential mechanism for enhanced cell proliferation and migration.[411]

Rac was initially described as an activator of NADPH, which generated superoxide in phagocytic cells. A protein kinase called PAK is the most clearly identified target for activated Rac and mediates the effects of chemoattractants on neutrophils.[412,413] Rac also regulates MAP kinase cascades, in particular activation of JNK,[414-416] at least in part via PAK. This may underlie the involvement of Rac, like Rho, in Ras-mediated cell transformation.[417-419] In addition, Rac, like cdc42 and Rho, has a prominent effect on the actin cytoskeleton, inducing membrane ruffing in fibroblasts[420] and lamellipodia formation in neuroblastoma cells.[421] Rac activation increases focal contacts associated with cell adhesion and attachment.[387] The coordinated regulation of cell adhesion and spreading at the leading edge of cells is associated with activation of Rac, whereas Rho-driven contractility at the back of the cell helps to propel the cell forward.[422] In the neonatal rat cardiomyocyte, expression of an activated Rac leads to sarcomere organization and to increases in ANF secretion and protein synthesis. Conversely, N17 Rac attenuates the effects of phenylephine.[423] ET and phenylephrine cause activation of Rac in neonatal rat cardiomyocytes.[382] A transgenic mouse line in which Rac is overexpressed in myocardium was generated and demonstrated a dilated cardiomyopathy associated with altered focal adhesions.[424] The roles of Rho and Rac in cardiac hypertrophy are considered in a recent review.[425]

# EFFECTORS

## Adenylyl Cyclase

The synthesis of cAMP from ATP is catalyzed by a family of structurally related AC enzymes. Although each of the nine ~120-kDa AC isoforms (AC1 to AC9) that have been cloned from mammalian cells displays unique patterns of cofactor regulation, they share a common general topology; a highly variable cytosolic N-terminus is followed by a hydrophobic domain (with six membrane-spanning helices, designated M1) and a large (~40 kDa) cytoplasmic domain (C1). This motif is repeated (with a second set of six membrane-spanning helices [M2] and a second cytoplasmic domain [C2]) to form a pseudosymmetric integral membrane protein. C1 and C2 domains are subdivided into C1a/C1b and C2a/C2b; because C2b is vanishingly short in some isoforms (and has as yet no known function), C2a and C2 are used synonymously. C1a and C2a sequences are highly homologous to each other and are highly conserved across AC family members; similar domains are found in membrane-bound and soluble guanylyl cyclases. C1a and C2a, from the same or different isoforms, heterodimerize with each other in solution and form $G\alpha_s$-activated soluble enzymes.

Mutagenesis studies and the solution of the crystal structure of C1a/C2 complexed with $G\alpha s$ and forskolin, a diterpene activator of AC, have yielded a detailed structural map of the C1a/C2 catalytic core. As anticipated from their high degree of sequence homology, C1a and C2a have almost identical tertiary structures. These structures are precisely aligned in a head-to-tail fashion such that residues from C1a and C2a that are critical for ATP binding and catalysis are juxtaposed.

There is still relatively little information on the structural or function features of AC transmembrane domains. The marked sequence diversity of M1 and M2, which are not sufficiently conserved to be aligned, either suggests a lack of evolutionary pressure to maintain a specific structural and functional motif or (the diametrically opposite conclusion) that the 12 transmembrane domains (rather than one or two) subserve isoform-specific functions beyond their role as simple membrane anchors. Fluorescence resonance energy transfer (FRET) and co-immunoprecipitation techniques have been used to demonstrate that the two transmembrane clusters of AC8 form a tight complex, which is essential for proper plasma membrane targeting and alignment of the cytosolic catalytic domains of the enzyme. A common feature of AC isoforms is a consensus N-glycosylation site in extracellular loop 5 (and/or loop 6) of M2. Splice variants of AC8, including one that lacks the N-glycosylated loop 5, have been identified.[426] An M2 construct based on the structure of this naturally occurring AC8 splice variant displays only a weak interaction with M1 and is retained in the ER.[427] The observation that a chimeric construct with M1 from AC5 and M2 from AC7 or vice versa drives expression of a membrane-bound catalytically inactive enzyme has been taken as evidence that isoform-delimited pair-like interactions between M1 and M2 domains may be required for precise alignment of the catalytic core.[428] Other studies identify homomeric interactions for the M2 transmembrane cluster; this raises the intriguing notion that M2 directs the formation of higher ordered multimeric structures; this is consistent with early target size analysis suggesting that AC is part of a higher order complex and the more recent evidence that recombinant WT and mutant AC1 co-immunoprecipitate.

Sequence analysis and functional studies suggest certain AC subgroupings (AC1; AC3; AC8—AC2, AC4, and AC7; AC5; and AC6). Most cells coexpress multiple AC isoforms with distinct regulatory features; cAMP responses reflect signal integration by the endogenous repertoire of AC isoforms and will vary with cell type. Studies of AC isoforms expression and subcellular localization have been limited by the lack of highly selective antibodies that discriminate individual isoforms. Based on mRNA studies, some isoforms are considered ubiquitous (AC2, AC4, and AC6), whereas others appear to be expressed in a highly localized fashion (AC1 and AC5 are detected largely in brain or heart, respectively). The calcium/calmodulin-sensitive brain AC1 has been disrupted in mice. AC1 null mice manifest no gross anatomic defects but display abnormalities in certain forms of synaptic plasticity and memory. An analogous phenotype is detected in the spontaneous loss-of-function mutation in the AC1 gene in "barrelless" mice.[429,430]

The major mechanism for AC activation is via Gαs proteins. Current structural models place Gαs binding at a cleft in the C2a domain of the catalytic core. Only certain AC isoforms (AC1, AC5, and AC6) are inhibited by Gαi. There is evidence that Gαi interacts with a site on C1a that is homologous to the Gαs site on C2a (i.e., that the duplicated pseudosymmetrical structure of the catalytic core provides for bidirectional regulation of AC by Gα subunits). βγ dimers inhibit AC1; alone, βγ has little effect on other isoforms. However, βγ dimers conditionally activate AC2 and AC4 in the context of stimulation by Gαs. Stimulatory concentrations of Gαs and βγ dimers are vastly different. Gαs stimulates AC at picomolar concentrations; coliberated βγ dimers would not influence AC, because βγ stimulation of AC requires nanomolar concentrations. Hence, AC2 and AC4 are considered coincidence detectors for $G_s$ and $G_{i/o}$ pathways (particularly in brain, where $G_o$ proteins are abundant sources of βγ dimers).

AC1 to AC8 are activated by the diterpene forskolin, which binds to a highly conserved hydrophobic pocket at the C1a/C2a interface, which stabilizes the C1a/C2a interaction. The only known forskolin-insensitive isoform is AC9; it is rendered forskolin-sensitive by a single tyr→leu substitution in the forskolin-binding hydrophobic pocket. Surprisingly, overexpression of AC9 in chick cardiomyocytes leads to a marked increase in forskolin-dependent cAMP accumulation.[431] This has been construed as evidence that AC9 dimerizes (or oligomerizes) with a forskolin-sensitive AC isoform in cardiomyocytes.

Changes in intracellular calcium have profound effects on cAMP accumulation that depend on the AC isoform composition of the cell. In cells that express AC1 or AC8, agonists that elevate intracellular calcium markedly increase cAMP accumulation through the stimulatory actions of calcium/calmodulin; calmodulin binding to AC1 has been mapped to a helical region of C1b. Although all AC isoforms are inhibited by high, nonphysiologic submillimolar concentrations of calcium (likely as a result of competition with the magnesium required for catalysis), AC5 and AC6 are inhibited by low micromolar calcium. This calcium must come from capacitive calcium entry channels; calcium release from intracellular stores or nonspecific ionophore-mediated calcium entry through the plasma membrane does not inhibit AC5 and AC6. Recent studies indicate that tonic AC6 inhibition results from its close spatial proximity with capacitive calcium entry channels in functional subdomains of the plasma membrane (caveolae). Several other AC isoforms have been localized to lipid rafts (AC3, AC4, and AC5), including in cell types that lack caveolin expression.[432] This argues that AC isoforms target to lipid rafts via a mechanism that does not require a AC-caveolin interaction. Nevertheless, there is evidence that AC-caveolin interactions in caveolae serve to inhibit enzyme activity.

AC isoforms are desensitized by PKA. PKA phosphorylates a functionally relevant site in the C1b domain of AC6; the molecular basis for PKA regulation of other AC isoforms has not been examined. Some AC isoforms also are regulated by PKC. PKCα and PKCζ phosphorylate and markedly activate AC5 in vitro, although the in vivo relevance of this process has not been explored in any detail; PKC also phosphorylates AC6 (at Ser10 in its large cytosolic N-terminal domain) leading to diminished catalytic activity.[433] Of note, AC6 cDNA clones that lack Ser10 have been isolated in some studies, suggesting that alternative splicing of the AC6 gene might generate forms of AC6 that are not regulated by PKC.[434]

Most studies have focused on AC5 and AC6 as the predominant isoforms in cardiomyocytes. These isoforms are termed the cardiac subclass, based on their structural homology and similar pattern of regulation by cofactors (stimulation by Gαs and forskolin, inhibition by Gαi and calcium, insensitivity to βγ subunits). However, it is worth noting that AC5 and AC6 mRNAs also are detected in other tissues and the heart expresses mRNAs encoding other AC isoforms with distinct regulatory properties. Expression of AC4 and presumably AC7 provide for conditional stimulation by βγ dimers.

Studies in cardiomyocytes lend support to the concept that certain GPCRs selectively target to the activation of specific AC isoforms. Purinergic receptor stimulation with ATP leads to an increase in cAMP that is additive with the response to isoproterenol (combined $β_1$-AR/$β_2$-AR agonist) in neonatal rat cardiomyocytes. The response to isoproterenol is inhibited by mAChR signaling through $G_i$, whereas cAMP accumulation in response to ATP (or the selective $β_2$-AR agonist zinterol) is not.[435-437] The distinct patterns of cAMP regulation by different Gs-coupled GPCRs could be due to specificity in GPCR coupling to individual AC isoforms or GPCR localization to distinct domains of the plasma membrane. Studies in HEK293 cells show that AC5 is stimulated by both ATP and isoproterenol, whereas AC4 and AC6 are stimulated only by isoproterenol not ATP; this suggests that purinergic receptors preferentially link to AC5 (rather than AC4 and AC6). Other studies indicate that $β_2$-ARs colocalize in caveolae with cardiac AC isoforms (AC5 and/or AC6, because these are not distinguished by available antibodies). In contrast, the bulk of the $β_1$-AR and mAChRs reside in noncaveolae membranes. Hence, spatial constraints would restrict $G_i$-coupled mAChR interactions with $β_2$-ARs and facilitate mAChR interactions with $β_1$-ARs.

One of the best described examples of an ontogenic change in AC expression is in cardiomyocytes, where steady state levels of mRNAs encoding AC5 increases with age, whereas the abundance of transcripts for AC6 decreases during the normal development of the heart.[438] The physiologic implications of this reciprocal developmental change in cardiac AC isoforms expression remain uncertain. Cardiac-specific AC5 or AC6 overexpression in transgenenic mice results in different cardiac phenotypes. Overexpression of AC5, the predominant isoform in adult hearts, increases basal AC and KA activity and enhances baseline heart rate and fractional shortening but has no effect on signaling by β-ARs as assessed using a range of biochemical and functional endpoints.[439] Although cardiac AC5 and AC6 isoforms display very similar regulatory properties *in vitro*, AC6 overexpression in the heart results in a completely different phenotype. AC6 overexpression (~20-fold over endogenous levels) has no effect on baseline cAMP levels, intrinsic heart rate, or contractile function but markedly increases β-AR responsiveness; a similar biochemical phenotype is observed in neonatal cardiomyocyte cultures. These results have been interpreted as evidence that AC6 sets the limit on transmembrane β-AR signaling, whereas AC5 does not. However, arguments regarding stoichiometry traditionally have not taken into account domain-specific differences in the relative densities of β-AR subtypes, G-protein subunits, and potentially distinct AC isoforms that likely also set the efficiency and specificity of signal transduction. Because AC6 appears to increase recruitable adrenergic responsiveness without inducing a deleterious phenotype (in contrast to β-AR or Gαs overexpression, in which the sustained elevations in cAMP levels lead to cardiac fibrosis and dilated cardiomyopathy as the animals age), it has been viewed as a therapeutic target to improve LV contractile function in heart failure.

Reasoning that cardiac AC5 and AC6 isoforms are inhibited by calcium and, therefore, prone to negative feedback by elevations in calcium during catecholamine stimulation and/or heart failure, other investigators have targeted the calcium/calmodulin-activatable AC8 to the hearts of transgenic mice.[440] The studies suggest that the overexpressed AC8 isoform senses elevated calcium, but it is not responsive to β-AR activation. AC8 overexpression does not induce any changes in cardiac morphology (up to 2 months of age). Other features of this model include normal heart and contractility in the context of an intact autonomic nervous system; however, elevated cardiac function, which is unresponsive to further β-AR stimulation, is seen after bilateral vagotomy. Studies to determine the relative merit of this novel approach with calcium-sensing AC isoforms as a mechanism to deliver inotropic support to the failing heart are ongoing.[441]

## Phospholipase C

More than 50 years ago, Hokin and Hokin[442] observed that the incorporation of labeled phosphate into inositol-containing phospholipids was stimulated by hormones such as acetylcholine. The primary hormonally regulated step was determined several decades later to be the breakdown rather than the synthesis of the inositol phospholipids. More specifically, phosphatidylinositol 4,5-bisphosphate ($PI(4,5)P_2$), a highly phosphorylated but relatively minor component of the total membrane inositol phospholipids was shown to decrease rapidly and transiently in membranes from cells treated with appropriate agonists.[443] Phosphoinositide-specific PLC is the enzyme that catalyzes the removal of the polar inositol phosphate ring from the phospholipid backbone. The eukaryotic enzymes all show a preference for $PI(4,5)P_2$ over PI4P or PI as substrate. The products generated by this hydrolysis are the second messengers inositol trisphosphate ($InsP_3$) and diacylglycerol (DAG).[444,445] The latter is a key activator of all except the atypical isoforms of PKC (see the section on PKC). In landmark studies carried out 20 years ago, inositol trisphosphate was demonstrated to release calcium from intracellular stores,[446] a finding that linked the calcium-mobilizing effects of hormones to their ability to activate PLC.[444,445]

Three isoforms of PLC were cloned and sequenced in the 1980s and 1990s and a fourth was discovered in the last year. The beta, gamma, and delta isoforms have been extensively studied and reviewed.[447-451] The most recently isolated PLC, the epsilon isoform, has only recently come under scrutiny.[452-456] All of the PLCs are products of a single gene, but each has a myriad of potential regulatory domains that differ among the isoforms. The smallest of the enzymes is PLC δ; the mammalian enzyme is a protein of approximately 85 kd. In contrast, the epsilon isoform has an estimated mass of 255 kd. Two regions termed the X and Y domains are common to all of the isoforms and are believed to form the catalytic domain, based on the crystallographic structure obtained with PLC δ.[457] Calcium binds to this region and regulates catalytic activity of PLC δ, with a $K_{act}$ for calcium in the micromolar range. In the case of the beta and gamma isoforms of PLC, the $K_{act}$ values for calcium are lower, suggesting that these isoforms would be active at the resting level of cytoplasmic calcium rather than regulated by increases in cell calcium as may occur for PLC δ.[450] In addition to the X and Y domains, all of the isoforms have PH domains that bind the headgroup of polyphosphoinositides ($PIP_2$ and $PIP_3$) and bind WD40 proteins. Furthermore, all contain C2 domains that appear to act in concert with other regions to bind key regulators.

The primary feature that distinguishes PLC β from the other isoforms is the relatively long extension of the carboxyl terminal following the C2 domain. PLC γ is distinguished by a large region between the X and Y domains that contains SH2 and $SH_3$ domains. The newly discovered epsilon isoform contains a unique Ras-guanine nucleotide exchange factor domain and Ras binding domains. These domains can be related to the specific mechanisms by which each isoform is regulated. Thus, only PLC β is regulated by binding of G-protein α or βγ subunits, whereas PLC γ regulation results from binding of the enzyme to tyrosine phosphorylated receptors or adaptors. The regulation of PLC δ has not been well elucidated, but clearly calcium plays a role in its regulation and Ras or other small GTPases appear to participate in the control of PLC ε. The regulation and physiologic functions of these isoforms are described in more detail later.

The ability of agonists to stimulate phosphoinositide hydrolysis in isolated atria, ventricles, and cardiomyocytes was first described in studies from our laboratory and those of others in the mid-1980s, as summarized in several reviews and papers.[107,458-461] The question of whether and when $InsP_3$ is formed and whether it plays a role in agonist-mediated calcium responses in the heart has been extensively reviewed.[460-462] It is now clear that there are specific receptors for $InsP_3$ in the myocardium.[463-465] Recent studies suggest that InsP$_3$ formation may occur under conditions in which calcium is elevated and that InsP$_3$ generation may relate to the development of arrhymias.[466-468] Roles for InsP$_3$ in causing spontaneous calcium release[469] and in regulating calcium flow between the SR and mitochondria[470] are also consistent with a physiologic or pathologic role for InsP$_3$ in the control of cardiac automaticity.

The involvement of a G-protein in agonist-mediated PLC activation in the heart was suggested by early studies examining phosphoinositide hydrolysis.[107,113,458,459,471] In subsequent studies the G-protein mediating this response to α-adrenergic agonists was shown to be G$_q$.[366] PLC β isoforms that are regulated by G-proteins are clearly present in the heart. Studies using immunoblot analysis to examine PLC isoforms in the adult and neonatal rat heart and cardiac myocytes identified PLC β$_3$ as the predominant beta isoform, and failed to detect PLC β$_1$.[339] In contrast, studies using RT-PCR to analyze PLC β isoforms in human myocardium pointed to the predominance of the PLC β$_1$ isoform, although these authors also failed to detect PLC β$_1$ when immunochemical techniques were applied.[472] In more recent studies, both PLC β$_1$ and β$_3$ were shown to be expressed under basal conditions in neonatal rat cardiomyoctyes.[473] Interestingly when overexpressed through infection with adenovirus, PLC β$_1$ enhanced the α-AdR mediated inositol phosphate response to NE, whereas PLC β$_3$ expression enhanced the purinergic receptor mediated response to ATP.[473]

The PLC β$_1$ and β$_3$ isoforms are regulated by the α subunit of G-protein subunits from the G$_q$ family, as elegantly demonstrated in reconstitution experiments using purified G-protein subunits and phospholipases.[357,358,451] An interesting feature of PLC β is that it shows a reciprocal relationship with its activator Gα$_q$. This G-protein has a slow rate of GTP hydrolysis, which is stimulated by its interaction with PLC β.[360] In contrast to Gαq, the α subunits of G$_i$, G$_o$, and other G-proteins fail to regulate PLC. In addition PLC β$_2$, which is largely confined to hematopoietic cells, is relatively insensitive to regulation by the α subunit of G$_q$ family proteins. For PLC β$_2$ the primary mechanism of regulation is via G-protein βγ subunits. The βγ subunits are highly effective activators of PLC β$_2$, but PLC β$_3$ can also be activated by βγ subunits at least *in vitro*.[450] The ability of βγ subunits to stimulate PLC explains the observation that regulation of inositol phosphate formation can occur in a PTX-sensitive manner and in response to GPCRs that couple to G$_i$ rather than to G$_q$. PLC β$_2$ or β$_3$ activation in these cases would arise from the release of βγ subunits from the relatively abundant G$_i$ proteins.

All of the PLC β isoforms have been disrupted by gene targeting, and very different phenotypes are observed. In one report, PLC β$_3$ appeared to be essential for life, with embryonic lethality developing in homozygous knockout animals between embryonic days 2 and 3.[474] However, studies from another laboratory using a different targeting vector, resulted in the generation of viable homozygous PLC β$_3$ knockout mice. These workers were then able to test the involvement of this isoform in PLC activation and calcium mobilization in aortic smooth muscle cells.[475,476] As predicted based on the regulatory pathways described previously, PLC activation by G$_i$-coupled receptors was abolished, consistent with the role of PLC β$_3$ in mediating responses to βγ subunits. In contrast, responses to G$_q$-coupled receptors, which could regulate PLC β$_1$, were unaffected.[476] PLC β$_2$ knockout mice show no obvious phenotypic difference from wild-type animals, but isolated neutrophils showed altered superoxide production and chemotaxis in response to chemokines.[477,478] Mice lacking PLC β$_1$ show seizure disorders,[479] whereas those lacking PLC β$_4$ show motor coordination defects[479] and defects in visual responses.[480]

PLC γ is regulated in an entirely different manner than PLC β. This isoform is not directly regulated by GPCRs but rather by RTKs. Recruitment of PLC γ, by binding of its SH2 domains to tyrosine phosphorylated sites on the RTK, leads to phosphorylation of PLC γ. This is a necessary but not sufficient step for PLC γ activation. It now appears that the activation of PI3-kinase, which is also be regulated through RTK binding, generates PIP3 that in turn contributes to the control of PLC γ activity.[481] PLC is highly expressed in rat cardiomyoctyes in the heart.[339,473,482] A specific role for PLC γ in cardiac puringergic signaling was suggested by the observation that this PLC isoform was translocated and tyrosine phosphorylated in response to ATP.[482] Further studies demonstrated that Src family kinases and PI3-kinase were activated and that these kinases mediated the translocation and activation of PLC γ by ATP. PLC activation in turn contributed to InsP$_3$ generation and spontaneous spiking induced by ATP in cardiac cells.[483] These observations are surprising because the effects of ATP on phospholipase activity were assumed to be mediated through its interaction with one of the purinergic GPCRs, not with an RTK. However, there is also considerable evidence that another GPCR that, for AngII, stimulates PLC gamma in a tyrosine kinase dependent manner in vascular smooth muscle.[484,485] Activation of PLC γ by GPCRs may complement the more rapid, calcium-mobilizing responses mediated through activation of PLC β and contribute to more sustained calcium or PKC signaling. It is also of interest, albeit not unexpected, that agonists such as FGF or IGF1, which are known to act at RTKs, lead to PLC γ translocation or activation in the heart or in cardiac-derived cells.[486,487] It is likely that one of the most important role of PLC γ is in development, as gleaned from studies with PLC γ knockout mice.[450,488] In this context growth factors such as those cited previously and PDGF, NGF, EGF, and others may depend on PLC γ signaling to activate signaling cascades necessary for appropriate gene expression and cell division.

PLC δ is widely expressed, and at least four isoforms (δ$_1$ to δ$_4$) and several splice variants exist in mammals. Despite a great deal of investigation and elucidation of the enzymes crystal structure,[457,489] the biologic mechanisms regulating this enzyme are poorly understood. Most evidence points to a role of calcium, because PLC δ activity can be increased by elevating intracellular calcium in permeabilized cells or by addition of thapsigargin or hormones such as thrombin and bradykinin.[490-492]

A Rho GAP has also been found to associate with and activate PLC δ, but the significance of this interaction is unclear.[493] Neither α nor βγ subunits of the heterotrimeric G-protein subunits function as regulators of PLC. However, Gh, an atypical G-protein that also functions as a transglutaminase, was demonstrated to associate with PLC δ and regulate its activity.[494,495] The importance of this association in coupling receptors to PLC is questionable because the extent of adrenergic receptor coupling to PLC δ via Gh is poor relative to its coupling to PLC β via $G\alpha_q$.[496,497] As an additional test of the hypothesized role of Gh in regulating PLC activity, the Gh protein was expressed *in vivo* in the mouse heart under control of the αMHC promoter. In contrast to the observations made with Gαq, mice expressing Gh did not show biochemical evidence of PLC activation nor did they demonstrate cardiac hypertrophy, as observed with Gαq expression.[498]

PLC ε was recently identified as a fourth class of PLC enzymes following cloning of rat and human genes.[453,454,499,500] As the largest form of PLC, the enzyme also contains multiple putative regulatory sites. The physiologic significance of the various control mechanisms described to date remains to be determined, because all have been examined in heterologous expression or *in vitro* assays. Notably and relevant to GPCR regulation, the α subunits of $G_{12}$ and $G_{13}$ (currently known largely for coupling to Rho activation) have been shown to regulate PLC ε.[454,452] Regulation by βγ subunits is also marked.[452] Also unexpected are the regulation of the enzyme by binding to Ras[453,499] and its regulation by Rap, another smg whose activation is modulated via cAMP.[455,456,500] The ultimate resolution of the regulatory pathways and functional significance of PLC ε will be necessary to determine whether this enzyme expressed in the heart[453,454] subserves any specific function.

## KINASES AND PHOSPHATASES

### PI3 Kinase and Akt

Phosphoinositide 3 kinases (PI3-Ks) catalyze the phosphorylation of the 3′ position on the inositol ring of various phosphoinositides. The PI3-K family is divided into classes based on substrate specificity. Class I PI3-Ks predominantly phosphorylate $PI(4,5)P_2$ in cells to form $PI(3,4,5)P_3$. Class II PI3-Ks phosphorylate PI and $PI(4)P$ *in vitro*, but their function in cells is still largely undetermined. Class III PI3-Ks phosphorylate PI to form $PI(3)P$, which is thought to play an important role in membrane trafficking. Only the class I PI3-Ks are thought to be involved in the receptor-mediated increase of $PIP_3$, either through tyrosine kinase receptors or G-protein coupled receptors (Fig. 7-5). Class I PI3-Ks are further subdivided into A and B classes. Class IA PI3-Ks are composed of a p110α, β, or δ catalytic subunit, in association with a p85 regulatory protein. The p110α and β subunits are present in the heart.[483] Activation occurs by direct interaction of the regulatory p85 subunit with phosphotyrosyl residues on tyrosine phosphorylated growth factor receptors and adaptor proteins with YXXM motifs or by Ras activation. Class IB PI3-K contain a p110γ catalytic subunit in association with a p101 adaptor molecule. PI3-K-γ has also been reported to be abundant in the heart.[501] Activation of this PI3-K has been shown to occur through interaction with G-protein βγ subunits released by GPCR stimulation.[501,502]

*In vivo*, βγ subunits derived from the heterotrimeric G-protein $G_q$ are responsible for the specific activation of PI3-K-γ in response to pressure overload-induced hypertrophy.[503] The majority of the PI3-K knockout animals exhibit defects in the hematopoietic system.[504] However, the p110γ-deficient mice exhibit enhanced cardiac contractility, without any changes in heart or cell size.[29] This is in stark contrast with mice overexpressing constitutively active p110α in a heart-specific manner, which exhibit cardiac enlargement without altering hemodynamic parameters.[505] Accordingly, the dominant negative p110α transgenic mouse exhibits reduced myocyte cell size and heart size, altered function, or basal levels of cardiomyocyte apoptosis.[505]

$PIP_3$, the product of PI3-K, makes up only a very small proportion of the total cellular phospholipid, but as a signaling lipid it is involved in varied cellular processes from development to cell adhesion to apoptosis.[506] Not surprisingly, the synthesis of $PIP_3$ is tightly regulated by the activity of PI3-kinases, and, on its production, $PIP_3$ is rapidly dephosphorylated by lipid

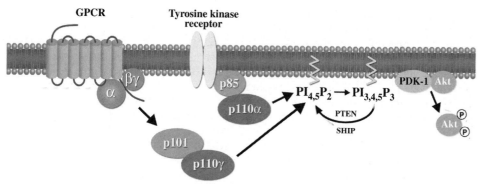

**FIGURE 7-5.** PI-3 kinase signaling pathway. PI-3 kinases catalyze formation of $PIP_3$. Distinct isoforms of $PIP_3$ kinase are activated by GPCRs and RTKs. $PIP_3$ regulates PDK1 and Akt activation. Lipid phosphatases (PTEN, SHIP) reverse the pathway.

phosphatases. PTEN, one of the $PIP_3$-phosphatases, hydrolyses the 3-position to form $PI(4,5)P_2$.[507] SHIP-1 and SHIP-2 are 5-phosphatases that cleave $PIP_3$ to form $PI(3,4)P_2$ but also hydrolyze $PI(4,5)P_2$ to $PI(4)P$.[508,509] SHIP-1 expression is restricted primarily to hematopoietic cells, whereas SHIP-2 is more ubiquitously expressed.[510] The lipid phosphatases are a growing family, with regulatory mechanisms and specificities that have yet to be elucidated. PTEN overexpression by adenoviral expression has been reported to induce apoptosis in neonatal rat cardiomyocytes.[511] Conversely, expressing a dominant negative PTEN was found to induce hypertrophy in these cells.[511] *In vivo*, muscle-specific ablation of PTEN resulted in increased myocyte size and diminished contractility of the heart, which did not decompensate to failure or exhibit signs of apoptosis.[29] Crossing the PTEN deficient mice with $p110\alpha$ transgenic mice resulted in normal cell size without affecting the contractile parameters, whereas the $p110\gamma$ knockout was able to rescue the contractile dysfunction without affecting cell size.[29] This finding reinforces the idea that different PI3-K isoforms may have different cellular functions through $PIP_3$ generation, but more experiments are needed to fully understand the mechanisms involved.

As a signaling phospholipid, $PIP_3$ initiates the activation of numerous downstream pathways. Generation of $PIP_3$ at the plasma membrane can recruit many PH-domain containing proteins to the membrane. $PIP_3$ targets the phosphoinositide dependent kinase-1 (PDK-1) to the membrane and is required for phosphorylation of some PDK-1 substrates (Fig. 7-5). Although the mechanisms of PDK-1 activation are still under investigation, it appears that generation of $PIP_3$ causes the translocation of PDK-1 to the membrane, where it is presumably colocalized with substrates such as Akt[512] or $PKC\delta$.[513] PDK-1 has a number of other substrates, including some PKC family members, PAK, $p70^{S6K}$, RSK, and PRK, which do not appear to exhibit $PIP_3$-dependent phosphorylation. Clearly, PDK-1 can affect multiple pathways and cellular responses.

The PDK-1 substrate Akt, also known as PKB, has been extensively examined and used as an indicator of PI3-K activation. Members of this family of serine and threonine kinases (Akt 1, 2, and 3) are phosphorylated by PDK-1 at Thr308; Akt subsequently autophosphorylates at Ser473 for complete activation.[514] On activation, Akt can phosphorylate a number of targets in different cell types, including transcription factors, mitochondrial proteins involved in apoptosis, enzymes utilized in glucose metabolism, and regulators of protein synthesis.[515,516]

Several stimuli lead to activation of Akt in cardiomyocytes. These include ligands for RTKs (e.g., insulin and IGF-1),[517,518] cytokines (e.g., cardiotrophin-1 and LIF[519-521]), estrogen,[522] and oxidative stress.[517] In cultured cardiomyocytes, Akt overexpression blocked the apoptosis caused by hypoxia[523] and serum deprivation.[518] Intracoronary injection of adenovirus expressing a membrane-targeted, activated form of Akt was shown to protect against the cell death, wall thickening, and development of cardiomyopathy caused by ischemia-

reperfusion.[518,524,525] *In vivo* gene transfer of membrane-targeted Akt also blocked the development of heart failure caused by doxorubicin, an antineoplastic agent that is known to cause cardiomyopathies in rats and humans.[526]

The role of Akt *in vivo* has also been addressed by several studies using transgenic mice. Three different activated forms of Akt have been overexpressed in a cardiac-restricted manner, all resulting in increased heart size because of enlargement of individual cardiomyocytes. The T308D/S473D Akt mice were examined for changes in signaling pathways to determine which of the many putative Akt substrates were modulated in the heart. This study revealed that $p70^{S6K}$ phosphorylation was increased, whereas $GSK-3\beta$ phosphorylation was unchanged. However, these mice also showed signs of heart failure and died prematurely.[527] Overexpression of the membrane targeted Akt (myr-Akt) resulted in increased $p70^{S6K}$ phosphorylation, without any changes in ERK, JNK, p38, or $GSK-3\beta$ activation. This chronic Akt activation was still able to protect against the damage caused by ischemia-reperfusion.[528] Microarray analysis was also performed using ventricular tissue from these mice and demonstrated changes at the transcriptional level in about 40 genes.[529] Unlike the other transgenic Akt mice, overexpression of the E40K mutant Akt caused an increase in $GSK-3\beta$ phosphorylation. These mice were extensively examined for hemodynamic parameters and were found to exhibit enhanced contractility, suggesting that Akt can affect calcium handling in the cardiomyocyte.[530] Despite all these detailed studies, it is still not clear which Akt substrates mediate the protective effect of Akt in cardiomyocytes.

## G-Protein Regulated Kinases and β-Arrestins

Desensitization is the process whereby GPCR signaling is attenuated during prolonged agonist exposure. An important initial event in this process is phosphorylation of the receptor by two families of kinases. Second messenger activated kinases (PKA and PKC) phosphorylate receptors in the absence or presence of agonist (heterologous desensitization). In contrast, GPCR kinases (GRKs, GRK1-7) specifically bind and phosphorylate the agonist-occupied conformation of GPCRs—a process termed homologous desensitization. GRKs display an overall topology that is characterized by a highly conserved central catalytic domain flanked by a 183 to 188 amino acid N-terminal domain and a C-terminal regulatory domain that is both variable in length and structural architecture. The mechanism whereby GRKs localize or translocate to the plasma membrane is largely encoded by features in the C-terminus. For some GRKs (notably ones not detected in appreciable amounts in cardiomyocytes), membrane anchoring or lateral mobility in membranes results from C-terminal post-translational lipid modifications; GRK1 (rhodopsin kinase) is farnesylated, GRK4 and GRK6 are palmitoylated, and GRK7 is geranylgeranylated. In contrast, GRK2 (βARK1) and its structural homologue GRK3 (βARK2) are expressed by cardiomyocytes and are primarily cytosolic in resting cells;

GRK2 and GRK3 are recruited to the membrane as a result of interactions between their C-terminal pleckstrin-homology domains and membrane PIP$_2$ and membrane-anchored G-protein βγ dimers. The requirement for freed G-protein βγ dimers ensures GRK activation only during active GPCR signaling (i.e., properly timed GPCR phosphorylation by GRKs). The βγ dimer-dependence also in theory can provide a mechanism for the observed *in vivo* specificity of GRKs, because GRK2 desensitizes β-ARs and AngII type 1A receptors (but not α$_{1B}$-ARs and protease-activated receptor-1), whereas the structurally homologous GRK3 desensitizes α$_{1B}$-ARs and protease-activated receptor-1 (but not β-ARs.[531-533] Because GRK2 and GRK3 are most divergent in their Gβγ-binding domains, some have speculated that specificity in GPCR-GRK interactions is dictated by the structurally distinguishable Gβγ dimers released on GPCR activation that recruit different GRK isoforms to the plasma membrane.[534] Cardiomyocytes also express the structurally distinct GRK5 enzyme that phosphorylates agonist-occupied GPCRs, but does not require membrane translocation for activation; it is constitutively membrane anchored through a highly basic region in the C-terminus that binds phospholipids. GRK5 desensitizes cardiomyocyte β$_1$-ARs, PAR-1, and to a lesser extent α$_{1B}$-ARs but not AngII receptors.[535,536]

The N-termini of all GRKs contain a ~120-residue region that displays substantial homology to the regulatory domain of regulators of G-protein signaling (RGS) family proteins, proteins that serve as GTPase-activating proteins (GAP) by binding to the transition state of Gα subunits and limit their half-lives of activation by accelerating intrinsic rates of GTP hydrolysis. There is evidence that GRK2 and GRK3 can bind and sequester Gα$_{q/11}$ but not Gα$_i$, Gα$_{12/13}$, or Gα$_s$; the ability of GRK2 and GRK3 to act as a GAP appears to be more dubious.[537,538] Nevertheless, these studies suggest that GRK2 and GRK3 exert multidomain regulation of GPCR signaling, through the phosphorylation of agonist-occupied GPCRs (via the catalytic domain) and phosphorylation-independent binding interactions that could sequester Gαq subunits (via the C-terminus) and Gβγ dimers (via the N-terminus). Consensus RGS domain can be identified throughout the GRK family, but the effects of other GRKs to bind and modulate Gα subunits have not been explored.

GRK-dependent phosphorylation of the agonist-occupied GPCRs facilitates β-arrestin binding, which serves as a molecular switch. β-Arrestin sterically hinders interactions between agonist-occupied GPCRs and their cognate G-proteins, thereby initiating agonist-induced receptor desensitization and internalization. This process terminates GPCR signaling via the classical G-protein-dependent pathways. However, β-arrestins function as adapter proteins to promote the stable association of other molecules with GPCRs. β-Arrestin docks Src tyrosine kinases, thereby conferring tyrosine kinase activity on the GPCR.[539] β-Arrestin acts as a scaffold for elements in the ERK and JNK cascades and binds components of the endocytic machinery (AP-2, clathrin). Collectively, these functions of β-arrestin are critical for GPCR trafficking, desensitization and resensi-

tization, and the initiation and regulation of a "second-wave" of effector responses through the ERK and JNK cascades that are independent of G-proteins. Tethering signaling components, which display little substrate specificity when analyzed *in vitro*, into discrete β-arrestin-scaffolded GPCR-controlled signaling complexes provides a mechanism to regulate the outcome of signaling. For example, β-arrestins form complexes with internalized PAR2, Raf-1, and ERK1/2.[540] The PAR-2-β-arrestin-scaffolded ERK complex is sequestered in the cytoplasm where it promotes the nonproliferative effects of PAR2 agonists; cytosolic retention prevents nuclear accumulation of active ERK, which is required for gene induction and proliferative signaling. Recent studies identify the AngII 1A receptor-β-arrestin2 complex as a scaffold for the assembly of a signaling module containing JNK3 and ASK1 (MAPKKK[541]). There is increasing evidence that MAPK modules engaged by GPCR-β-arrestin complexes influence the balance of proliferative versus apoptotic signaling.

GRK2 is elevated in conditions associated with elevated circulating catecholamines, including a wide range of human and animal models of cardiac dysfunction, where it acts to diminish β-AR responses, including the activation of AC and the modulation of contractile function.[542] There is substantial evidence that catecholamines regulate GRK2 activity and expression. β-ARs activation results in increased GRK2 mRNA, protein, and activity[543]; α$_1$-AR activation results in GRK2 activation, by recruiting it to the plasma membrane.[544] This effect may largely be mediated by PKC, which phosphorylates GRK2 and enhances its activity and membrane association.[545] The role of GRK2 in the pathogenesis of heart failure has been the focus of recent investigation. Citing clinical trails demonstrating that long-term β-AR blockade reduces the combined risk of morbidity and mortality in heart failure, some investigators have viewed depressed β-AR signaling as cardioprotective in heart failure.[546] According to this formulation, β-AR activation contributes to the progression of heart failure; pharmacologic strategies to intervene at the level of β-AR signaling provide clinical benefit. However, there is evidence that strategies that increase β$_2$-AR activity or reverse β-AR desensitization by reducing GRK levels improve myocardial performance and prolong survival in experimental models of heart failure. βARKct (a peptide that contains the Gβγ binding domain and competes with endogenous GRK for binding and Gβγ-mediated translocation to the membrane) has been used to prevent the development of heart failure in the genetic murine dilated cardiomyopathy caused by ablation of the muscle LIM protein or rescue mice from heart failure resulting from cardiac overexpression of the SR calcium-binding protein calsequestrin.[547,548] Adenoviral delivery of βARKct into the left circumflex marginal artery via a percutaneous catheter 3 weeks after myocardial infarction has been reported to reverse the abnormalities in β-AR signaling and LV systolic function.[549] However, in some models of heart failure, GRK2 inhibition with βARKct restores β-AR responsiveness and inotropic reserve but does not prevent the development of hypertrophy.[550,551] Hence, the relative importance of GRK2 as a mediator of hypertrophy and/or a modulator of contraction remains the focus of continued study.

## Protein Kinase A

PKA holoenzyme is a heterotetramer composed of two regulatory (R) subunits that maintain two catalytic (C) subunits in a dormant state; cAMP binding to two tandem sites on each R subunit results in C subunit dissociation. The freed C subunit phosphorylates serine or threonine residues on target proteins in the nucleus and cytoplasm leading to changes in cell metabolism, ion channel function, synaptic transmission, gene expression, growth, and differentiation. Although cAMP is generated in response to many different hormones and neurotransmitters, cells have a mechanism to discriminate the cAMP signals that emanate from different external stimuli. For example, $PGE_2$ and isoproterenol elevate cAMP to similar levels in cardiomyocytes, but only isoproterenol activates glycolytic enzymes and enhances contractility.[552] One way to ensure proper localization and timing of the cAMP signal is to produce gradients of cAMP through the cell via opposing actions of AC and phosphodiesterases. Alternatively, specificity for PKA signaling can arise as a result of differences in the composition of the PKA holoenzyme. The C subunit exists as three gene products ($\alpha$, $\beta$, and $\gamma$) in mammalian cells with virtually indistinguishable biochemical properties, but PKA holoenzymes are classified as type I or type II according to their distinct R subunits, which exist as RI and RII (each with two distinct gene products termed $\alpha$ and $\beta$). RI and RII subunits differ in their tissue distribution, subcellular localization, and affinity for cAMP. RI subunits reside primarily in the cytoplasm, whereas a substantial component of RII associates with particulate structures as a result of interactions with specific anchoring proteins; cAMP binds to RI with higher affinity than to RII. Accordingly, holoenzymes containing RI or RII subunits decode cAMP signals that differ in duration and intensity. RI-containing holoenzymes are activated transiently by weak cAMP signals, whereas RII-containing holoenzymes (primarily expressed in neurons and endocrine cells) respond to persistently high concentrations of cAMP. These biochemical differences explain at least in part the observation that certain hormone receptors preferentially activate either type I or type II PKA holoenzymes and that PKAI and PKAII holoenzymes play distinct roles in mediating cAMP-dependent regulation of gene transcription.[553-555]

PKA isoform-specific function has most recently been investigated in gene knockout models in mice. Targeted disruption of the RII$\alpha$ gene yields viable mice with no detectable physiologic abnormality. In contrast, RI$\beta$ or C$\beta$1 subunit ablation results in similar defects in hippocampal function and memory consolidation, and RII$\beta$ null mice have defects in neuronal learning, behavior, and metabolism. Although compensatory changes in regulatory proteins and functional redundancy make it difficult to decipher the precise molecular basis for each phenotype, these models validate the notion that structural heterogeneity of the PKA holoenzymes encodes specificity in the cAMP pathway.

Recent studies indicate that specificity in cyclic AMP signaling also can be orchestrated by PKA interactions with AKAPs, which provide a mechanism to direct PKA to discrete subcellular sites to ensure rapid enzyme activation and selective substrate phosphorylation. AKAPs comprise a large family of more than 50 structurally distinct proteins that have been named according to their apparent molecular weights on SDS-PAGE. AKAPs typically have two structural domains; a conserved amphipathic helix acts as a R subunit binding motif and separate targeting motifs that direct the PKA holoenzyme-AKAP complex to discrete subcellular locations (structural proteins, membranes, or cellular organelles[556]). Peptides mimicking the AKAP amphipathic helix (Ht31) bind RII with nanomolar affinity. When introduced into cells, these peptides act as competitive antagonists, disrupt RII-AKAP interactions, and provide a useful strategy to elucidate the functional consequences of PKA-AKAP anchoring in cells. Some AKAPs (such as AKAP79, the first AKAP to be cloned) act as multivalent scaffolds. The interaction of AKAP79 with a range of kinases (including PKA, PKC, PP2B, and GRK2) represents a mechanism to assemble and tether enzyme complexes at the plasma membrane. Early studies demonstrated that this tethering is critical for the coordinate regulation of the phosphorylation state and hence the activity of AMPA/kainate type glutamate receptors in hippocampal neurons.[556,557] Recent studies also place $\beta_2$-ARs in this multiprotein complex and implicate AKAP79 as a targeting mechanism that promotes agonist-dependent phosphorylation of $\beta_2$-ARs by both PKA and GRK2.[557] Although $\beta_2$-AR-AKAP79 interactions are constitutive, $\beta_2$-ARs also are reported to interact with another AKAP protein AKAP250, or gravin, in an agonist-regulated manner. $\beta_2$-AR association with gravin coordinates interactions with PKA, PKC, and PP2B that regulate agonist-induced $\beta_2$-AR desensitization, resensitization, and internalization.[558,559] It has been speculated that certain GPCRs may interact with more than one AKAP (each with its distinct but overlapping set of signaling partners) as a mechanism to physically separate modules that fulfill distinct functions in signaling pathways. For example, a recent study demonstrated that the $\beta_2$-AR C-terminal tail specifically associates with a multiprotein signaling complex containing G$\alpha$ and G$\beta$ subunits, AC, PKA, PP2A, and the pore forming $\alpha_{1c}$ subunit of the L-type calcium channel and that assembly of this multiprotein complex at postsynaptic membranes of excitatory neurons critically ensures specific local signal propagation.[560] AKAP79, which resides in these membranes and can bind each element in this signaling cascade, would be an obvious candidate regulatory element in this pathway but was not examined in this study. AKAP79 is reported to nucleate the pathway for $\beta_2$-AR activation of the ERK cascade.[557] Finally, other AKAPs have been identified as nucleation centers for other combinations of kinases (PKA, Rho-dependent kinase, PKN) and phosphatases (PP1, PP2A) at various intracellular sites (centrosomes, Golgi).[556-559]

AKAPs are not merely passive carriers of kinases and phosphatases. Rather, binding to AKAPs leads to functionally important changes in enzyme activity. The catalytic subunits of PKA and PKC are inactive when bound to AKAPs. In contrast, PP1 binds to yotiao, an adapter protein that complexes PKA and PP1 with NMDA receptors in its active state and functionally limits NMDA ion channel activity under resting conditions state when cAMP levels are low.

AKAP expression and regulation of cAMP/PKA signaling in muscle cells including cardiomyocytes has been the focus of studies in several laboratories. Gao et al.[561] first demonstrated that a peptide corresponding to the AKAP RII binding motif can inhibit PKA-dependent regulation of L-type calcium channel activity during β-AR stimulation in dissociated adult ventricular cardiomyocytes. AKAP79 or AKAP15/18 is required for PKA regulation of calcium channels activity in heterologous expression systems[561]; AKAP15/18 (not AKAP79) is expressed by cardiomyocytes and would be the more physiologic regulator. Another AKAP detected in cardiomyocytes is mAKAP (formerly called AKAP100[562]); mAKAP is unusual in that it targets RII to multiple intracellular compartments (nucleus, intercalated discs, and T-tubule/junctional SR), whereas other AKAPs typically target RII to a single class of intracellular membrane. This is speculated to reflect the actions of auxiliary proteins that might provide additional targeting information or other factors and requires further study.[562] The mAKAP targeting of PKA to the SR has been implicated in PKA regulation of ryanodine receptors.

## Protein Kinase C

The PKC family of serine and threonine kinases transduce signals that arise as a result of receptor activated phospholipid hydrolysis.[563] The prototypical activation pathway involves PLC-dependent hydrolysis of inositol phospholipids to generate inositol trisphosphate, which mobilizes intracellular calcium, and diacylglycerol. Diacylglycerol also can be generated from phosphatidylcholine via the sequential actions of phospholipase D and phosphatidic acid phosphohydrolase. The basic primary structure of all PKC isozymes consists of a single polypeptide chain with amino-terminal regulatory and carboxyl-terminal catalytic domains (Fig. 7-6). Based on structural homology and sensitivity to activators, PKC isozymes are grouped into three general classes. Classical or calcium-sensitive cPKC isoforms—α, βI, βII, and γ—contain four conserved domains (C1 to C4) interspaced with variable domains that are unique to each isoform. The regulatory N-terminal half of cPKCs contains two functional modules; a C1 domain consists of tandem cysteine-rich Zn-binding domains that represent the site of diacylglycerol-binding or tumor-promoting phorbol ester-binding and a C2-domain that binds calcium. The C1-domain is preceded by a short basic sequence that surrounds an alanine residue termed the autoinhibitory pseudosubstrate domain; peptides based on this sequence, but with a serine for alanine substitution, are good PKC substrates. The catalytic C-terminal half of cPKC contains the C3/C4 sites for ATP and substrate binding. Novel PKC isoforms (nPKC: δ, ε, η, and θ) are structurally homologous to cPKC isoforms but lack the calcium-sensitive C2 domain; as a result, nPKC isoforms are maximally activated by diacylglycerol/phorbol ester, in the absence of calcium. Members of the atypical PKC (aPKC; ς, λ/ι) subfamily lack both the C2-domain and one cysteine-rich Zn-binding motif in the C1-domain and are not activated by calcium, diacylglycerol, or phorbol

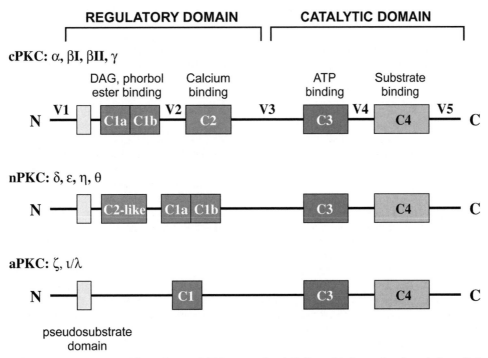

**FIGURE 7-6.** PKC isoform domain structure. Three classes of PKC, conventional (Ca²⁺ sensitive), novel, and atypical are distinguished largely by membrane-targeting modules in their regulatory domains.

esters; the distinct mode of aPKC regulation has been the focus of numerous recent studies.

Mechanisms for PKC isoform activation and regulation were first elucidated for the cPKC isoforms. Inactive cPKC isoforms partition to the soluble fraction of the cell. The cPKC activation is via the combined actions of calcium (which increases the affinity of the enzyme for lipids) and DAG (which anchors the enzyme in its stable conformation to membrane structures, where it gains access to substrate). Individual PKC isoforms display only limited substrate specificity *in vitro* but subserve distinct roles *in vivo* as a result of isoform-selective interactions with membrane-associated anchoring proteins termed *receptors for activated C-Kinase* (RACKs); RACKs act as targeting signals by binding specifically and saturably to only activated conformations of PKC isoforms. To date, two RACKs have been cloned and characterized; both display the seven repeat WD40 motifs first identified in G-protein β subunits. RACK1 is a PKCβII-selective RACK; its binding site on PKCβII maps at least in part to a portion of the C2 domain (a common sequence in cPKC isoforms) and a region in the V5 domain that is distinct in PKCβI and PKCβII. RACK1 colocalizes with PKCβII to the perinuclear areas of neonatal rat cardiomyocytes.[564] β'-COP, a coatomer COPI protein necessary for Golgi budding and trafficking of vesicles, has been characterized as a PKCε-selective RACK; β'-COP specifically interacts with a unique sequence (amino acids 14 to 21) within the V1 region of PKC and colocalizes with PKCε to the Golgi complex.[565] Current models hold that PKC activation leads to a conformational change that exposes the RACK binding domain to direct membrane targeting and removes the pseudosubstrate domain from the catalytic core. Recent studies also identify a series of "priming" phosphorylations, which are completed during the synthesis of the enzyme, in the catalytic domain (one in the activation loop and two in the C-terminal V-5 domain). These phosphorylations maintain the enzyme in a closed, stabilized, protease-resistant conformation and contribute to catalytic activity; this constitutes a separate mechanism to regulate the activity and subcellular localization of PKC isoforms.[441] Although these phosphorylations are "priming" events for cPKC isoforms, activation loop and hydrophobic motifs phosphorylations are highly regulated events that control nPKC isoform catalytic activity and the kinetics of nPKC downregulation in cardiomyocytes.[566]

PKC isoforms activate a spectrum of adaptive and maladaptive responses in the heart, including cardiac hypertrophy and failure and cardioprotection. Cardiomyocytes coexpress multiple PKC isoforms, including member of the cPKC, nPKC, and aPKC categories, with many displaying developmental downregulation. There is general consensus that cPKCs are the most abundant isoforms; some estimates place PKCα expression at ~75% of total PKC protein. There is controversy regarding whether cardiomyocytes express PKCβ; this deserves resolution because a specific PKCβ inhibitor (LY333531) has been developed to ameliorate the vascular complications of diabetes, in which PKCβ expression and activity is reported to be elevated and could exert direct cardiac actions.[567] The presence of multiple PKC isoforms in cardiomyocytes, as in most cells, has fueled speculation that individual PKC isoforms mediate unique functions in the heart. Most of the evidence for PKC isoform-specific function has come from overexpression studies, first in cultured cardiomyocytes and more recently in transgenic mice. The initial studies focused on PKCβ, which transcriptionally activates the fetal gene program in cardiac cultures.[568] Cardiac overexpression of wild-type PKCβ *in vivo* (at levels 10- to 20-fold higher than the endogenous proteins, driven by the α-MHC promoter) induces concentric pathologic hypertrophy, fetal gene expression, and contractile dysfunction.[569,570] Conditional overexpression of low levels of constitutively active PKCβ in the adult heart results in a mild progressive hypertrophic phenotype with contractile dysfunction but little fibrosis or fetal gene induction; this model displays cardioprotection during ischemia. However, the conditional PKCβ overexpression model has emphasized the contextual nature of signaling by even a single PKC isoforms, because cardiac overexpression of the constitutively active PKCβ transgene from birth leads to abnormalities in the regulation of intracellular calcium and sudden death in neonates.[571] Other studies have focused on PKCε, which has been implicated as an upstream regulator of calcium and the Ras/Raf-ERK cascade.[147,572] Overexpression of constitutively active PKCε in cardiac cultures leads to cellular remodeling (elongation), without a significant increase in overall surface area or total protein accumulation[573]; transgenic cardiac overexpression of constitutively active PKCε leads to mild concentric cardiac remodeling with partial recapitulation of the fetal gene program, but no evidence of fibrosis, and normal *in vivo* contractile performance.[574] Although these studies have been taken as evidence that PKCs (which are typically upregulated or activated during hypertrophy and ischemia) contribute to the induction of the hypertrophic phenotype, recent studies reveal that targeted disruption of PKCβ or PKCε in mice does not interfere with normal neonatal cardiac development and growth[575,576]; a null mutation of PKCβ does not block the development of pathologic hypertrophy in adult mice.[577] These results argue that PKCβ or PKCε are not required for cardiac growth or that there is redundancy in these signaling pathways.

Although targeted overexpression of individual PKC isoforms has been the major strategy used to unravel PKC isoform-specific function in the heart, transgenesis alters the natural stoichiometry between PKC isoforms and its upstream activators and downstream substrate effectors; PKC overexpression at levels that are not likely to be encountered even in human disease can lead to nonphysiologic phenotypes. In keeping with the notion that PKC signaling requires proper anchoring to RACKs, peptides corresponding to the RACK binding site on PKC isozymes (or PKC binding site on RACKs) have been used as translocation inhibitors. Similarly, peptides that displace intramolecular RACK-binding site interactions (pseudo-RACKs) have been used as PKC agonists to stabilize the open conformation, expose the catalytic site, and promote PKC anchoring to RACKs.

Translocation inhibitor peptides corresponding to the C2 domain of cPKC (the contact points for cPKC interaction with RACK1) are reported to block PMA-dependent regulation of L-type calcium channel activity in cardiomyocytes. Although this initially was interpreted as evidence that a cPKC isoforms (possibly PKCβII) regulates L-type calcium channel function in cardiomyocytes, subsequent studies with peptides that modulate PKCε translocation also suggest a role for PKCε. This paradigm also was used recent to implicate PKCε in ethanol-dependent cardioprotection.[578,579] Translocation modulator peptides have been used *in vivo*. Cardiac-specific transgenic expression of the PKCε peptide translocation inhibitor induces a lethal dilated cardiomyopathy; it converts the nonfailing hypertrophy phenotype of Gαq mice to a lethal dilated cardiomyopathy. Transgenic overexpression of the PKCε peptide translocation activator produces concentric ventricular remodeling with decreased cardiomyocyte size and normal contractile function; it provides protection against ischemic injury.[580] When coexpressed with Gαq, it improves cardiac contractile function. These studies have fueled speculation that PKCε induces an adaptive physiologic cardiomyocyte growth pattern, which differs from the pathologic maladaptive hypertrophy induced by other growth stimuli. However, other recent studies indicate that a nPKC isoform (PKCδ or PKCε) represses AKT phosphorylation, prevents its activation by EGF receptors, and enhances susceptibility to apoptosis.[581] This identifies a continuum of PKC-dependent responses that span compensated hypertrophy to decompensated heart failure. Hence, PKC isoforms hold enormous promise as therapeutic targets for the therapy of heart failure and ischemia.

## Ca²⁺/Calmodulin-Dependent Protein Kinase

The Ca$^{2+}$/calmodulin-dependent protein kinases (CaM kinases or CaMKs) are critical transducers of Ca$^{2+}$ signals.[582] These multifunctional serine and threonine kinases have been shown to phosphorylate a large number of substrates *in vitro* and *in situ*, and, therefore, have the potential to affect a diverse array of cellular functions. The CaM kinase family consists of CaM kinases I, II, and IV. An enzyme originally termed CaMKIII is now known to be a kinase dedicated to the phosphorylation of just one substrate eEF2, and, therefore, called eEF2 kinase.[583] Both CaMKI and CaMKIV are monomeric enzymes and are activated by CaM kinase kinase[584,585]; both are expressed at very low levels in the heart.[586,587] In contrast, CaMKII is a multimer of 6 to 12 subunits consisting of α, β, γ, or δ subunits, each encoded by a separate gene.[582,588] Expression of α and β subunits is mainly restricted to neuronal tissues, whereas there is a broad spectrum of tissue expression for γ and δ subunits.[589] Several laboratories have identified the δ subunit of CaM kinase II as the predominant isoform in the heart.[586,587,590-592] Furthermore, the heart contains several distinct splice variants of the δ subunit ($\delta_B$, $\delta_C$, etc.), characterized by the presence of a second variable domain.[586,592] The $\delta_B$ subunit contains an 11 amino acid nuclear localization signal (NLS) that is absent from $\delta_C$.

Thus, CaMKII, comprised predominantly of $\delta_B$ subunits, localizes to the nucleus, and CaMKII, comprised of $\delta_C$ subunits, localizes to the cytoplasm.[586,593,594] Binding of Ca$^{2+}$/CaM to CaMKII leads to its autophosphorylation,[582] which produces a state of CaMKII that retains enzymatic activity even in the absence of Ca$^{2+}$/CaM, a form of activity known as Ca$^{2+}$/CaM-independent activity (autonomous activity).

CaMKII has been implicated in the modulation of several key aspects of acute cellular Ca$^{2+}$ regulation related to cardiac excitation-contraction (E-C) coupling in ventricular myocytes. CaM kinase has the potential to regulate cardiac function through phosphorylation of SR proteins including ryanodine receptors (RyR) and PLB[595-599] (Fig. 7-7). Phosphorylation of RyR has been suggested to alter the channel open probability,[599,600] and phosphorylation of PLB has been suggested to regulate SR Ca$^{2+}$ uptake.[599] It is also likely that CaMKII phosphorylates the L-type Ca$^{2+}$ channel complex or an associated regulatory protein and, thus, mediates Ca$^{2+}$ current ($I_{Ca}$) facilitation[601-604] and the development of early afterdepolarizations (EADs) and arrhythmias.[605-608] Thus, CaMKII has significant acute effects on E-C coupling and cellular Ca$^{2+}$ regulation.

The role of CaMKII in Ca$^{2+}$ signal transduction and regulation of cardiac function appears to be determined by its subcellular localization. Transient expression of $\delta_B$ isoform of CaMKII in neonatal rat ventricular myocytes induces ANF gene expression and results in an enhanced response to phenylephrine as assessed by transcriptional activation of an ANF-luciferase reporter gene.[594] The nuclear localization signal of CaMKII$\delta_B$ was shown to be required for this response because transfection of CaMKII$\delta_C$ did not result in enhanced ANF expression.[594] Several transgenic mouse models subsequently confirmed a role for CaMKII in the development of hypertrophy. Transgenic mice overexpressing calmodulin develop severe cardiac hypertrophy,[609] which is associated with an increase in the autonomous activity of CaMKII *in vivo*.[610] Like CaMKII$\delta_B$, CaMKI and CaMKIV induce a hypertrophic response in cardiomyocytes *in vitro*.[611] Pronounced hypertrophy develops in transgenic mice that overexpress CaMKIV,[611] and this is associated with specific changes in gene expression. However, CaMKIV knockout mice are still able to develop hypertrophy after transverse aortic constriction (TAC).[612] Although CaMKI and CaMKIV are not present at significant levels in the heart,[586,587] they have, in common with the cardiac CaMKII$\delta_B$ (but not the $\delta_C$ isoform), the ability to enter the nucleus. Not surprisingly, transgenic mice that overexpress the $\delta_B$ isoform of CaMKII in the heart were shown to develop hypertrophy.[613] In these mice, the CaMKII$\delta_B$ transgene was present and highly concentrated in the cardiomyocyte nucleus. In light of the different subcellular localization of CaMKII$\delta_B$ and $\delta_C$ isoform, CaMKII $\delta_C$ was predicted to have specificity for phosphorylating cytoplasmic substrates. Most recently, transgenic mice that expressed the cytoplasmic $\delta_C$ isoform of CaMKII have been generated.[614] It has been demonstrated that CaMKII$\delta_C$ can phosphorylate RyR2 and PLB and induce dilated cardiomyopathy and heart failure when expressed *in vivo*,[614]

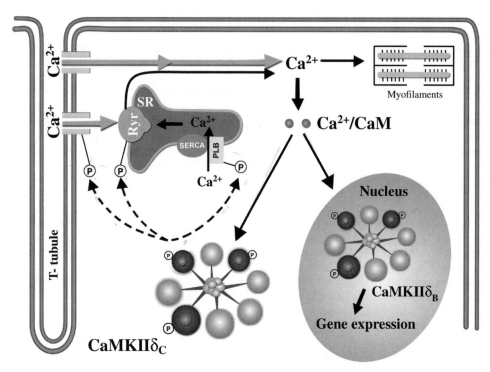

**FIGURE 7-7.** $Ca^{2+}$/CaM kinase signaling pathway. The predominant cardiac CaMKII isoform CaMKII$\delta$ has nuclear ($\delta_B$) and cytoplasmic ($\delta_C$) splice variants. $Ca^{2+}$ binding to CaM activates CaMKII, which is then activated by autophosphorylation. Cardiac CaMKII substrates include PLB, the RyR, and the L-type $Ca^{2+}$ channel.

associated with $Ca^{2+}$ handling defects evident in cardiomyocytes isolated from these mice.[615] This suggests that CaMKII$\delta_C$ plays an important role in the pathogenesis of dilated cardiomyopathy and heart failure and that this occurs at least in part via alterations in $Ca^{2+}$ handling proteins.

The contractile dysfunction that develops with hypertrophy and characterizes heart failure is associated with changes in the ability of cardiomyocytes to properly regulate $Ca^{2+}$ homeostasis.[616] It has been reported that cardiac CaMKII expression and activity are altered in animal models of cardiac hypertrophy[614,617-619] and of heart failure[620,621] and in cardiac tissue from patients with dilated cardiomyopathy.[622,623] Studies in hypertrophied myocardium from a variety of animal models including hypertensive rat hearts, coronary artery ligated rabbit hearts, and transverse aortic constrictive mouse hearts all showed increased CaMKII expression and activity.[614,617-619] Studies of human failing hearts secondary to dilated cardiomyopathy[622,623] showed increased CaMKII activity and protein expression. In contrast, in failure induced by myocardial infarction[620] and in a canine model of heart failure produced by intracoronary microembolizations[621] there is reduced CaMKII activity and expression. The possibility that different isoforms of CaMKII$\delta$ are differentially regulated and play distinct roles in cardiac pathophysiology is intriguing. Two reports examined changes in CaMKII$\delta$ expression and showed that in a spontaneously hypertensive rat (SHR) model of cardiac hypertrophy the transcript levels of $\delta_B$ and $\delta_C$ were unchanged, whereas the embry-

onic $\delta_4$ and the minor $\delta_9$ variants were upregulated.[617,624] On the other hand, the expression of the $\delta_B$ isoform appeared to be increased at both the transcript and protein levels in failing human myocardium.[623] In pressure-overload induced hypertrophy, the expression of CaMKII$\delta_C$ isoform is selectively increased in adult mouse hearts as early as 1 day after TAC.[614] In addition, the activation of CaMKII$\delta_B$ and of CaMKII$\delta_C$, as indexed by autophosphorylation, increases as early as 2 days after TAC.[614] The increase in CaMKII$\delta_B$ activation is consistent with previous work indicating its role in hypertrophy.[586,611] The observation that both the expression and activation of CaMKII$\delta_C$ increase several days before the development of cardiac hypertrophy suggested that the increased expression and activation of this CaMKII$\delta_C$ isoform could play a critical role in the response to pressure overload.

Apoptosis is now considered to be a hallmark and likely causal mechanism for development of heart failure. Some evidence suggests that CaMKII mediates signal transduction in apoptosis. Selective inhibitors of CaMKII have been reported to significantly inhibit apoptotic effects induced by TNF$\alpha$, UV-irradiation, and the natural toxin microcystin in noncardiac cells.[625,626] Most recently, $\beta_1$ adrenergic stimulation was found to induce apoptosis in adult cardiomyocyte, and this response was demonstrated to occur through CaMKII rather than PKA.[627] However, all of these studies were carried out using CaMKII inhibitors; thus, it is still not clear whether activation or overexpression of CaMKII can directly induce cardiomyocyte apoptosis.

## Calcineurin

Calcineurin (calcium/calmodulin-dependent protein phosphatase 2B, or PP2B) is a serine- and threonine-specific phosphatase that has been studied intensively in T cells, where it dephosphorylates nuclear factor of activated T cells (NFAT) proteins that then translocate to the nucleus and activate immune response genes. The active calcineurin holoenzyme consists of the calcineurin A catalytic subunit, the calcium binding protein calcineurin B, and calmodulin. Of the three mammalian calcineurin A genes cloned ($\alpha$, $\beta$, and $\gamma$), only the ubiquitously expressed calcineurin A$\alpha$ and A$\beta$ gene products are detected in cardiomyocytes. Structurally, calcineurin A proteins contain a catalytic domain, calcineurin B and calmodulin-binding domains, and a C-terminal autoinhibitory domain. Calmodulin binding displaces the adjacent autoinhibitory domain from the catalytic region and results in activation.

A role for calcineurin in cardiomyocyte hypertrophy was first identified on the basis of evidence that cardiac-specific overexpression of an activated calcineurin mutant leads to hypertrophy that transitions to dilated failure by 2 to 3 months of age.[628] Adenoviral-mediated calcineurin expression is also sufficient to induce hypertrophy *in vitro* in neonatal cardiomyocyte cultures. The original studies focused on NFAT3 dephosphorylation, nuclear translocation, and interaction with the cardiac-restricted zinc finger transcription factor GATA4 as the mechanism whereby calcineurin induces cardiomyocyte hypertrophy. Although mRNAs for all five NFAT genes have been detected in the heart, nuclear translocation of NFAT protein has never been identified. This could be attributed to technical factors, such as the lack of antibodies capable of detecting the low levels of NFAT expression. Alternatively, calcineurin is a physiologically relevant phosphatase for Elk-1,[629] NF-$\kappa$B, and myocyte enhancer factor-2 (MEF2) and may induce hypertrophy independent of NFAT. Finally, calcineurin dephosphorylation of BCL2 antagonist of cell death (BAD) has been implicated in calcium-induced apoptosis in neurons.[630] However, there is evidence that calcineurin's contribution to the decision to commit to apoptosis may depend on cell context (i.e., the contribution of other costimulated pathways). In cardiomyocytes, where calcineurin is upstream of an array of signals (JNK, ERK, and PKC isoforms), calcineurin generally is reported to be cytoprotective.[631]

The cellular actions of calcineurin typically have been identified with cyclosporin A or FK506, which inhibit calcineurin catalytic activity by complexing with cyclophilins and FKBP12, respectively. Given their widespread use as immunosuppressives in humans, many studies attempted to use these drugs to evaluate the role of calcineurin in cardiac hypertrophy with contradictory results (in some cases, even ostensibly the same model). This has been attributed to a variety of factors, ranging from differences in the nature of the hypertrophy model studied; drug regimen (effectiveness of calcineurin inhibition vs. toxicity of cyclosporin A when administered at high doses for prolonged intervals), age, sex, and strain of the animals; or effects of cyclosporin A to inhibit other enzymes (JNK, p38-MAPK).[632] These drugs may be particularly ill-suited to define the role of calcineurin in hypertrophic signaling pathways, given the high calcineurin levels in cardiomyocytes (relative to lymphocytes) and the difficulty in attaining inhibitory concentrations of systemically delivered cyclosporin A. Accordingly, recent studies have circumvented this concern by examining the effects of cellular proteins that bind calcineurin and inhibit its ability to dephosphorylate substrates. Five classes of calcineurin inhibitors have been identified.[633] Myocyte-enriched calcineurin-interacting protein (MCIP1) was first annotated as DSCR1, based on its location within the Down's syndrome critical region of human chromosome 21. Cardiac-specific overexpression of MCIP1 at levels that inhibit calcineurin signaling produces a minimal reduction in cardiac mass but no obvious deleterious effects on the unstressed normal heart.[634] However, MCIP1 prevents the hypertrophic response to calcineurin overexpression, isoproterenol infusion, and exercise. Because MCIP1 expression is abundant in myocardium and is upregulated by calcineurin activity, it represents a negative feedback mechanism to limit calcineurin activity and holds promise as a clinical target. Hypertrophic responses also have been blocked by other classes of calcineurin inhibitors, including Cain/Cabin (a noncompetitive inhibitor with a submicromolar $K_i$) and AKAP79. These results argue for the functional importance of calcineurin in hypertrophic signaling pathways.

## The IKK-NF-$\kappa$B Pathway

An important target for TNFR and TLR signaling is the NF-$\kappa$B transcription factor. In mammals there are five NF-$\kappa$B proteins: RelA (p65), RelB, c-Rel, NF-$\kappa$B1/p50, and NF-$\kappa$B21/p52 that can associate to form a variety of homodimers and heterodimers that recognize a common DNA sequence—the $\kappa$B site.[635] There is evidence that NF-$\kappa$B dimers are activated in heart failure,[636] and blocking the binding of NF-$\kappa$B proteins to their natural binding sites through the use of $\kappa$B site decoy oligonucleotides can reduce the severity of myocarditis,[282] myocardial infarction,[637] and ischemia-reperfusion injury.[638] On the other hand, NF-$\kappa$B has been shown to be required for cardiac hypertrophy,[639,640] and the question of whether it is friend or foe in ischemia-reperfusion has been raised.[641]

The NF-$\kappa$B proteins contain a common domain—the Rel homology domain (RHD), which is responsible for their dimerization and binding to DNA.[635,642,643] Although RelA, RelB, and c-Rel do not require any processing, NF-$\kappa$B1/p50 and NF-$\kappa$B2/p52 are synthesized as larger precursors—p105 and p100, respectively—whose C terminal domains must be removed to produce the mature proteins that are capable of DNA binding.[644] The most common form of NF-$\kappa$B is the p50:RelA heterodimer, but p50:c-Rel and p52:RelB heterodimers and p50:p50 and RelA:RelA homodimers are also present. The p50-containing heterodimers are present in the cytoplasm of nonstimulated cells because they are complexed with specific inhibitors—the IκBs, which contain six ankyrin repeats that bind to the RHD and mask the nuclear translocation sequence (NLS) present within it[635] (Fig. 7-4). The C-terminal domains of NF-κB1/pl05 and NF-κB2/p100 also contain a series of ankyrin repeats very similar to those present in IκBs and can, therefore, function as IκB-like proteins that are excluded from the nucleus.[645] Interestingly, the p52:RelB dimer does not bind regular IκB proteins, and p100 binds specifically to RelB but not to RelA or c-Rel.[646] Thus, p100:RelB heterodimer present in the cytoplasm gives rise after proteolytic processing that removes the inhibitory C-terminal domain of p100[647] to p52:RelB heterodimers that translocate to the nucleus.[646]

In a similar manner, the IκBs need to be removed from standard NF-κB dimers (e.g., p50:RelA) before the latter can enter the nucleus. The removal of IκBs is the essence of NF-κB signaling. This process occurs in several steps. First, the IκBs are phosphorylated at two serine residues (S32 and S36 in IκBα) that are located in their N-terminal regulatory domain, which is not involved in NF-κB binding.[644] This phosphorylation, which is stimulus-dependent, is carried out by the IκB kinase (IKK) complex.[648,649] Next, the phosphorylated IκBs, still attached to NF-κB dimers, are recognized by an E3 ubiquitin ligase of the SCF (Skip-Cullin-F box) type that uses an F box protein called βTrCP or E3R^IκB as a recognition subunit that specifically interacts with the two phosphorylated serines at the N-terminal regulatory domain of IκB.[644,650] This results in recruitment of a specific E2 ubiquitin conjugating enzyme that transfers activated ubiquitin chains from E1-ubiquitin to lysine residues located in the N-terminus of IκB. The polyubiquitinated IκB is recognized and rapidly degraded by the 26S proteasome; the liberated NF-κB dimers translocate to the nucleus, bind to target gene promoters, and stimulate their transcription.[644]

Of the many proteins involved in the process, the key regulatory role lies on the shoulders of IKK (Fig. 7-4), because it is the only enzymatic activity in this pathway whose activity is stimulus dependent, and once the IκBs are N-terminally phosphorylated, the rest of the events spontaneously follow. IKK is a complex composed of three subunits: IKKα (IKK1), IKKβ (IKK2), and IKKγ (NEMO, IKKAP-1). IKKα and IKKβ are the catalytic subunits of the complex, sharing 52% overall sequence identity, whereas IKKγ is the regulatory subunit.[648] In vitro, IKKα and IKKβ exhibit similar substrate specificity, targeting the two serines in the N-terminal regulatory domain of IκB proteins.[651] However, IKKβ is a more potent IκB kinase than IKKα. Like NF-κB, IKK activity is responsive to proinflammatory stimuli and various byproducts of microbial and fungal infections. As discussed later, IKK activity is essential for NF-κB activation during inflammatory and immune responses.

Gene-targeting experiments have shown that IKKβ and IKKγ are required for proper NF-κB activation by all known proinflammatory stimuli, including LPS, negative-strand RNA viruses, dsRNA, ISS-DNA, TNFα, IL-1, and antigens.[652-659] All of these stimuli lead to IKK activation, whose kinetics and magnitude are directly related to those of NF-κB activation. How do all of these diverse stimuli converge to activate a single signaling enzyme? Although the mechanistic details regarding IKK activation are still being unraveled, most of the currently available results, those that have been verified genetically, point to one general mechanism based on IKK phosphorylation.

Both IKKα and IKKβ can be produced as active recombinant proteins using baculovirus or yeast expression systems.[651,660] However, in mammalian cells their activation depends on association with the IKKγ regulatory subunit.[648,655,661] The activity of IKKα and IKKβ also depends on their ability to form either homodimers or heterodimers through their leucine zipper motifs.[662-664] Once IKKα and IKKβ dimerize they can associate with IKKγ through a short interaction motif located at the very C-terminus of either catalytic subunit.[665,666] Short peptide mimics of this interaction motif can be used to disrupt the IKK complex and prevent its activation.[666] Interestingly, these peptides show anti-inflammatory activity in vivo and should, therefore, be examined for their effectiveness in models of cardiovascular inflammation. The association of IKKα and IKKβ dimers (usually IKKα:IKKβ heterodimers) with IKKγ results in formation of a large complex, composed of IKKα:IKKβ heterodimers held together via dimeric interactions between two IKKγ molecules.[660,667] Assembly of this complex is essential for stimulus-dependent IKK activation.[648] In addition to its assembly function, IKKγ serves an important regulatory function by connecting the IKK complex to upstream activators through its C terminus, which contains a Zn finger motif. Truncation of the IKKγ C terminus does not affect assembly of the large IKK holoenzyme but compromises its activation.[667] Mutations affecting the C terminus of IKKγ have been linked to two inherited disorders associated with either inflammation or immunodeficiency.

Apart from assembly of this large IKK holocomplex, activation of IKK by all proinflammatory and innate immune stimuli depends on phosphorylation of either the IKKβ or IKKα catalytic subunits at two conserved serines located within their activation loops.[663,668,669] Regulation of protein kinase activity through phosphorylation of specific sites within the activation loop is one of the most common mechanisms of protein kinase regulation.[670] Such phosphorylation can be achieved either through the action of an upstream kinase or through trans-autophosphorylation brought about by induced proximity between two catalytic subunits within the same complex.

Cell stimulation with either TNFα or IL-1 results in a rapid increase in IKKα and IKKβ phosphorylation.[668] In the case of IKKβ, the first sites to be phosphorylated are the activation loop serines, whose replacement with alanines generates a mutant form of IKKβ that, when incorporated into IKK holocomplexes, prevents activation by TNFα, IL-1, or LPS.[668] Curiously, the substitution of the same two serines in the IKKα activation loop, whose sequence is almost identical to that of IKKβ, does not interfere with activation of the IKK holocomplex assembled around the mutant IKKα^AA form.[668,671] Similar results were obtained using catalytically inactive (i.e., defective in ATP binding) mutants of IKKα and IKKβ.

These findings provided the first indication that despite their structural similarity, IKKα and IKKβ may not be functionally equivalent. Thanks to gene-targeting experiments,[652,653,672] it is now well-established that IKKβ and not IKKα is the subunit required for IKK and NF-κB activation by proinflammatory stimuli. These findings raised the question of whether IKKα is completely dispensable for IKK and NF-κB activation or whether it mediates a response to a different set of agonists. Recent results strongly argue that, although IKKα is dispensable for the response to proinflammatory stimuli, it is essential for IKK activation by a set of signals that do not affect the IKKβ subunit.[671] Mammary epithelial cells and B lymphocytes that express the IKKα[AA] form instead of the wt protein exhibit defective IKK and NF-κB activation in response to two members of the TNF cytokine family: RANKL and B lymphocyte stimulator (Blys/BAFF), respectively.[671] Because of the presence of a wt IKKβ subunit, IKK complexes that contain the IKKα[AA] subunit display normal responses to TNFα, IL-1, and LPS. Thus, certain signals activate IKK via IKKα, whereas most proinflammatory stimuli target IKK through the IKKβ subunit.

Exactly how any given signaling pathway targets the IKK complex is still a matter of debate. It was suggested that cell stimulation with TNFα results in recruitment of IKK complexes to the TNFR1 signaling complex.[311,673] Although the amount of recruited IKK is relatively small, it may be sufficient to activate the remainder of the IKK pool via IKK-mediated *trans*-autophosphorylation. Both IKKα and IKKβ are efficiently autophosphorylated within the activation loop when overexpressed, and this autophosphorylation is required for their activation.[651,660] As mentioned previously, gene-targeting experiments have established the involvement of the protein kinase RIP1 and the two interchangeable TRAF proteins TRAF2 and TRAF5[305,311,674] in IKK activation. It was proposed that TRAF2 and presumably TRAF5 recruit the IKK complex to the receptor, whereas RIP1 is responsible for IKK activation.[311] Curiously, however, the kinase activity of RIP1 is dispensable, suggesting that RIP1 most likely acts through protein-protein interactions either with IKK or a yet-to-be identified IKK-kinase. A similar signaling mechanism may be used by IL-1 and certain forms of LPS (from *Leptospira interrogans* and *Porphyromonas gingivalis*), whose receptors recruit the adaptor molecule MyD88, the protein kinase IRAK1, and the TRAF protein TRAF6.[675] Gene-targeting experiments have shown that all three of these proteins are involved in IKK and NF-κB activation. Like RIP1, the kinase activity of IRAK1 is not required for IKK activation.[329] Another protein kinase involved in IKK activation whose protein kinase is not required for the activation function is PKR, which is activated by dsRNA and mediates the response to viral infection.[657] It is possible that PKR, IRAK1, and RIP1 activate IKK directly via an induced proximity mechanism. In this case no IKK kinase is involved.

Regardless of the mechanisms involved in its activation, it is clear that the IKK complex plays a central role in regulation of NF-κB activity. Therefore, IKK activation is essential for the successful mounting of innate immune responses, but its overactivation can result in chronic or acute inflammation. A major challenge for future research entails the identification of all the different situations in which deregulation IKK activation is a key contributor to pathogenesis; then safe IKK inhibitors can be developed to ameliorate these conditions.

## Non-Receptor Tyrosine Kinases

Src-family non-RTKs are a family of related enzymes that participate in growth factor signaling and share a highly conserved domain architecture and mode of regulation. C-Src, Fyn, and Yes are the three most widely expressed Src family members. Structurally, from their N-terminus, these proteins contain a short N-terminal region with one or two acylation sites (required for membrane attachment and targeting to detergent-resistant liquid-ordered microdomains such as caveolae), a unique domain that defines each family member, a SH3 domain, a SH2 domain, the catalytic domain, and a C-terminal regulatory sequence. Tyrosine phosphorylation of Src mediates both positive and negative regulation of enzyme activity. Src phosphorylation at a tyrosine residue in the C-tail regulatory sequence (present in c-Src but not in oncogenic v-Src) by C-Src kinase (Csk) maintains the enzyme inactive in the basal state as a result of an intramolecular interaction between the C-terminal catalytic domain and cognate SH2 and SH3 domains. Autophosphorylation of a tyrosine residue in the catalytic domain increases the activity of the enzyme.

Src family kinases are activated in many cell types, including cardiomyocytes, in response to a variety of physiologic and pathologic stimuli. Most studies have focused on their role in mitogenic signaling by growth factors; Src kinases bind to receptors that are themselves tyrosine kinases and also physically associate with and confer tyrosine kinase activity on receptors that lack intrinsic kinase activity (i.e., GPCRs). Src kinases also are activated during cell adhesion and in response to certain cellular stresses.

Another major class of non-RTKs is the structurally related FAK family members (FAK and PYK2). These proteins have unique N-termini, centrally located catalytic domains that resemble known protein tyrosine kinases, and two proline-rich regions in their C-termini. Although FAK and PYK2 lack modular SH2 and SH3 domains, the proline-rich motifs in their C-termini bind SH3-domain containing proteins. FAK is recruited to focal adhesion contacts during integrin-engagement and cell attachment, and it becomes autophosphorylated at Tyr397 in the N-terminal domain. This creates a docking site for the SH2 domain of Src and the formation of a bipartite FAK/Src complex that propagates signals through further Src-dependent phosphorylation of FAK at Tyr576/577 in the kinase domain activation loop (which increases the intrinsic tyrosine kinase activity of FAK) and at Tyr925 in the C-terminus. The activated noncatalytic C-terminus of FAK contains docking sites for SH2- and SH3-containing proteins (Grb2, p130[Cas], paxillin, the p85 regulatory subunit of PI3-kinase) and plays a critical role in the assembly of the multimeric signal transduction complex leading to cellular activation. In some cells, the C-terminal domain of FAK is expressed as a separate protein termed FAK-related non-kinase (FRNK), which acts as a biologic inhibitor of FAK signaling. Heterologous expression of FRNK or FAK gene knockout results in profound abnormalities in cell migration.

There is recent evidence that FAK and the related PYK2 are rapidly phosphorylated in response to activation of certain GPCRs and play a broad role in cell signaling. PYK2 was originally identified in cells of neural origin, but recent reports indicate that it also is expressed by VSMCs and cardiomyocytes. PYK2 is reported to display a generalized distribution throughout the cytoplasm and/or in the perinuclear region, where it is postulated to link calcium/PKC signaling (downstream from GPCRs) to protein tyrosine kinase pathways. Like FAK, PYK2 phosphorylation leads to complex formation with other SH2-containing signaling molecules (Src, Shc, and Grb2), which stimulates signaling via MAPK cascades (ERK, p38-MAPK, JNK).

Non-RTKs have been implicated in hypertrophic signaling pathways in cardiomyocytes. Several Src family kinase members (Src, Fyn, Yes) are activated during hypertrophic signaling by AngII, ET, or ATP; each of these proteins transcriptionally activates ANF, although individual family members display differences in their activity.[676-678] ET and phenylephrine also increase the tyrosine phosphorylation of FAK, PYK2, and paxillin; tyrosine phosphorylation of focal adhesion proteins is particularly prominent in cardiomyocytes grown on extracellular matrix proteins such as fibronectin.[679,680]

Pharmacologic studies suggest a role for tyrosine kinases in the regulation of ion channel function, but direct tyrosine phosphorylation of channel proteins generally has not been demonstrated. In rat cardiomyocytes, ATP strongly activates Src/Fyn and induces the tyrosine phosphorylation of FAK; Fyn and FAK association with the anion $Cl^-/HCO_3^-$ exchanger; AE1 leads to intracellular acidification. Studies with pharmacologic inhibitors suggests that tyrosine kinases regulate L-type calcium channels and the $I_f$ pacemaker channel in cardiomyocytes.[681] Other studies demonstrate that PYK2 phosphorylation plays a role in the inhibition of delayed rectifier $K^+$ channels by mAChR agonists.[682] This mecha-

nism could be pertinent to the modulation of vascular tone, in which AngII-dependent activation of PYK2 also leads to the inhibition of $K^+$ currents and VSMC membrane depolarization.[683]

## MAP Kinases

The family of serine threonine kinases referred to collectively as the MAP kinases subserves a myriad of function in control of gene transcription, cell proliferation, and cell survival. The common feature of these enzymes is that they are activated by concomitant tyrosine and threonine phosphorylation within a conserved Thr-x-Tyr motif located in the activation loop of all of the family members. Numerous excellent reviews detail the development and current state of understanding of these key signaling cascades.[684-687] Perhaps the greatest difficulty for those not thoroughly versed in this field is to sort out the terminology used to refer to these enzymes and their upstream activators. Not only are there a large number of distinct players that make up the various MAP kinase signaling modules but also historical precedent has led to the unfortunate continued use of multiple names for the same kinases. Therefore, a catalog of these names and some historical perspective is required, and some of the most common nomenclature is indicated in Table 7-1.

The first member of the MAP kinase family was identified as mitogen activated protein kinase and hence given the acronym of MAP kinase. Another group working on the same enzyme considered it to be an extracellular signal regulated kinase (ERK). In light of the fact that the notation *MAP kinases* is now used to refer to any of a family of enzymes, the term ERK is most useful for distinguishing this first family member. The second MAP kinase family member was identified as the kinase responsible for phosphorylation of the transcription factor cJun, hence the term cJun N-terminal kinases (Jun kinases), from which the acronym JNK derives. Another group identified these same enzymes as being activated by stress, hence stress activated protein kinases (SAP kinase) are synonymous with the JNK family. Because it appears that the third family, the p38 MAP kinases, are largely activated by stress and have also been referred to as SAP kinases by some, the use of JNK (rather than SAP

■ ■ ■

**TABLE 7-1**    SOME TERMINOLOGY USED FOR MITOGEN ACTIVATED PROTEIN (MAP) KINASES AND THEIR UPSTREAM ACTIVATORS

| MAP 3K (MKKK) | | MAP kinase kinase (MKK) | | MAP kinase |
|---|---|---|---|---|
| **Raf** | ⇒ | **MKK1 (MEK1)** | ⇒ | **ERK1 (p44 MAPK)** |
| | | MKK2 (MEK2) | | ERK2 (p42 MAPK) |
| | | MKK4 (MEK4) | ⇒ | JNK1 (SAPKα or 1c) |
| MEKK1 | | MKK 7 (MEK7) | | JNK2 (SAPKα or 1a) |
| MLK 2,3 | ⇒ | | | JNK3 (SAPKβ or 1b) |
| MEKK4 | | | | |
| ASK1 | | MKK3 (MEK3) | ⇒ | p38α (SAPK2a) |
| | | MKK6 (MEK6) | | p38α (SAPK 2b) |
| | | | | p38δ (SAPK 3) |
| | | | | P38δ (SAPK 4) |

kinase) is the least confusing and most generally applied way of referring to this second family. The third MAP kinase family, the p38 kinases, were first described as 38-kD proteins that were tyrosine phosphorylated in response to osmotic shock. Although sometimes referred to as SAP kinases, as noted previously, the current literature is now largely in agreement on the use of the p38 terminology.

There are 2 isoforms of ERK, 15 isoforms of JNK, and 4 isoforms of p38.[685] There is some evidence for differential cellular effects of the isoforms on cellular function, but clearly there is also redundancy as indicated by studies in which the individual gene products are deleted by gene targeting. The enzymes responsible for phosphorylating the tyrosine and threonine and activating the MAP kinases are termed MAP kinases (or ERK) kinases, hence MKKs or MEKs. Activation of the ERK signaling pathway by tyrosine kinase growth factors defined the paradigm that applies to all of the MAP kinases. In the case of the ERK family, extracellular stimuli such as tyrosine kinase growth factors lead to the activation of the smg Ras, which initiates the activation a MAP kinase kinase kinase, which then activates a MAP kinase kinase, which then activates the MAP kinase ERK. Table 7-1 lists the terminology commonly used for the kinases in this cascade. The upstream kinases activating p38 and JNK are also listed in Table 7-1. The most diverse group of enzymes in these cascades are the MKKKs or more simply the MAP3Ks. The knowledge of the role the various kinase cascades in the cardiac system is extensive but incomplete. Most of what has been done has focused on delineating the stimuli leading to activation of the ERK, JNK, or p38 cascades and the role of these kinases in ventricular hypertrophy and cardiomyocyte responses to stress. The details on differential effects of the various MAP kinase isoforms and the delineation of the particular MKKs and MKKKS involved in these responses has barely been explored and is an area ripe for investigation by the intrepid.

There is now abundant evidence that various members of the MAP kinase family are activated and participate in the development of cardiac hypertrophy.[687] Sugden and Bogyovitch were the pioneers in this field, demonstrating that the p44 and p46 ERKs were activated in neonatal rat ventricular myocytes and perfused hearts by GPCR agonists known to induce hypertrophic growth.[101,145,146] Interestingly, ERK is activated not only by the $G_q$-coupled agonists that stimulate hypertrophy but also by agonists for GPCRs linked to $G_i$, such as carbachol and bradykinin. The observation that these agonists cause ERK activation but do not induce hypertrophy[103] indicates that ERK activation is not a sufficient stimulus to signal hypertrophic growth of cardiomyocytes. Studies using inhibitors of ERK activation, specifically PD 098059 or U0126, to inhibit MEK (the MKK upstream of ERK) reach disparate conclusions, suggesting that some but not all hypertrophic effects of some but not all agonists require ERK activation.[103,383,679]

On the other hand, other observations provide strong evidence that activation of ERK is required to induce hypertrophy. Studies using ERK antisense to downregulate ERK1 and ERK2 demonstrate inhibition of

PE-induced sarcomere assembly and attenuation of the increases in ANF mRNA.[688] Expression of MKP-1, which dephosphorylates ERK, blocks both *in vivo* and *in vitro* hypertrophy, although the mechanistic basis for this may be complicated because the other MAP kinases are also substrates for this phosphatase.[689] Some of the upstream activators of ERK, notably Ras, Raf, and MEK1, have been tested for their ability to induce hypertrophy both in cardiomyocytes and in transgenic animals (see references 690 and 691). Hunter and Chien used cardiac specific expression of Ras in one of the earliest demonstrations that hypertrophy could be induced by cardiac specific transgenic overexpression of signaling molecules.[384,385] More recently Molkentin's group used MEK expression in transgenic animals to demonstrate that hypertrophy could be induced through activation of the MEK1/ERK signaling pathway.[692] Notably in both the Ras and MEK models, compensated hypertrophy developed that did not lead to decompensation and failure over time.

Regulation of the stress-activated kinases p38 and JNK in the heart is discussed in several comprehensive reviews.[691,693-695] These kinases are also activated by hypertrophic agonists, stretch, and pressure overload.[76,696-698] However, these MAP kinases are far more effectively activated by osmotic stress, $H_2O_2$, or hypoxia and reoxygenation interventions that mimic ischemia or ischemia-reperfusion.[699-704] Several investigators have demonstrated that p38 is activated in ischemia and that this state remains activated or increases further with reperfusion.[702,705] JNK activation is more confined to the reperfusion period.[702,703]

Although less widely accepted than the role of ERK, there is also evidence for a role of JNK in hypertrophy. In the isolated cardiomyocyte model, JNK was selectively activated (vs. other MAP kinases) and hypertrophic responses were induced by expression of MEKK1[381] and by MKK7,[706] which stimulated both ANF expression and myofilament organization. In addition, Choukroun et al.[144] showed that dn MKK4 (SEK1) blocked ET-1 induced hypertrophy in myocytes and subsequently reported inhibition of pressure-overload hypertrophy (as indicated by echocardiography and ANF expression) by *in vivo* gene transfer of the KR mutant of MKK4.[707] MEKK1 is a highly selective upstream activator of JNKs. An MEKK1 knockout mouse generated in Gary Johnson's laboratory has been used by two groups to assess the requirement for JNK activation in the development of hypertrophy. In one study the MEKK1 knockout mice were crossed with mice that developed hypertrophy because of G$\alpha$q overexpression; deletion of the JNK pathway was shown to abrogate G$\alpha_q$-induced myocyte and cardiac enlargement and ANF expression, concomitant with loss of agonist and G$\alpha_q$-mediated MEKK and JNK activation in mice and isolated ES cells. These findings are consistent with earlier evidence that dnMEKK or JIP-1 (an inhibitor of JNK) prevents hypertrophy in response to G$\alpha_q$-coupled receptor agonists *in vitro*.[381,708] In striking contrast to these findings, work from Sadoshima and Vatner, using the same knockout animals (also generated by G. Johnson) that were subjected to transverse aortic banding, demonstrated no significant attenuation of the banding-induced increase in LV weight, ANF expression, or myocyte cell size.[709] Thus, it appears that the $G\alpha_q$-signaling pathway leading to hypertrophy is more highly dependent on JNK activation than are the pathways elicited by TAC.

Several laboratories have also suggested that p38 activation may be involved in hypertrophy *in vitro*.[696-698] Much of this data derives from the ability of MKK6, a specific activator of p38, to increase ANF, BNP, and αSk actin expression and sarcomere organization *in vitro*. These responses are also sensitive to the p38 inhibitor SB 203580.[696,697] Interestingly, effects of the p38 isoforms may differ because p38β appears to be involved in hypertrophy, whereas the α isoform mediates apoptosis.[698] TAK, an upstream activator of p38 is prominently activated by pressure overload and can induce hypertrophy decompensating to failure when expressed in its activated form in transgenic mice.[710] This response appears to involve p38 and additional mediators altered by TAK activation. On the other hand, some groups report limited effects of p38 inhibitors on agonist-induced hypertrophy.[711]

ERK has been shown to have protective effects on cardiomyocyte survival,[692,712,713] and this may contribute to the ability of the Ras/ERK pathway to stimulate hypertrophic growth without transition to failure. Much more emphasis has been focused on the role of JNK and p38 in cardiomyocyte survival and apoptosis. One of the first studies relevant to cardiomyocyte function demonstrated that the absence of MEKK1 (in myocytes derived from MEKK1 null ES cells) increases $H_2O_2$-induced apoptosis.[714] Because JNK is no longer activated by $H_2O_2$ in the MEKK null mice (although p38 is activated) these findings suggest that JNK is normally protective. However, the basis for the protection is complex, because it appears to result at least in part from enhanced TNFα production (p38 upregulates and JNK normally suppresses TNFα expression). Another publication consistent with this report demonstrated that pressure overload induces apoptosis (increases TUNEL positive cells) at 7 days in the MEKK1 knockout but not control mice. There is also higher mortality, enhanced ventricular dilation, and decreased ventricular function as assessed by echocardiographic analysis in the MEKK1-/-mice 2 weeks after banding. Thus, these findings support a protective role for JNK activation. Although the protective effect of JNK in both of the previous studies was related to TNF α expression, others have demonstrated cardioprotection in isolated myocytes independent of cytokine release.[715,716] There are a number of sites at which JNK could affect apoptosis, including effects on mitochondrial regulatory proteins. In fact there is evidence that JNK is proapototic rather than protective, at least in adult rat myocytes.[704]

The proapoptotic versus antiapoptotic effects of p38 are complicated by the existence of different p38 isoforms, by the involvement of mitochondrial versus other apoptotic pathways, and in particular by the release of cytokines. Wang et al.[698] showed that in isolated myocytes MKK3/6 induces apoptosis via p38 alpha, whereas p38 beta has opposing effects, enhancing hypertrophy and promoting cell survival. Studies examining apoptosis in neonatal rat cardiomyocytes presented evidence that p38 activation was protective, and the mechanism was found to involve changes in release of IL-6, a protective cytokine.[717] On the other hand, studies in a rabbit ischemia-reperfusion model indicate that p38 appears to contribute to apoptosis because blocking p38 blunts apoptosis, decreases creatine kinase loss, and decreases infarct size.[705] Daunomycin-induced apoptosis was likewise improved by p38 inhibition with SB203580.[713] These data suggest that p38 activation is maladaptive rather than protective.

## FUTURE DIRECTIONS

As is evident from the details provided in this chapter, the pathways by which cells transduce signals from extracellular mediators to effect changes in cell function are extraordinarily complex. Not only are there molecular complexes between interacting signaling proteins but also, for each of the receptors, G-proteins, effectors, and kinases considered in this chapter, multiple subtypes and isoforms are present. This complexity and apparent redundancy must serve a biologic function, however, and although it interferes with full elucidation of mechanisms, it provides great opportunity. Thus, if one considers that the rationale for understanding these signaling pathways is to ultimately identify potential sites of therapeutic intervention, then the richness of targets and the possibility that they might be selectively inhibited or activated is indeed useful. The pathways described in this chapter evolved to serve physiologic roles in maintaining tissue homeostasis. There can be little doubt, however, that alterations in the molecular players occur at the level of gene polymorphisms, altered gene expression, or post-translational modification and that these contribute to pathophysiologic changes in cell and organ function that underlie cardiovascular disease. Research into signal transduction pathways continues at a rapid pace, and more complexities and players are certain to emerge, particularly as information from the human genome and microarray studies is incorporated into the knowledge base. For those interested in consolidating and validating information concerning signal transduction, the Alliance for Cell Signaling generates molecule pages and pathways, which will serve as rich and timely sources for extending the information contained in this chapter. These pages and pathways are in the public domain and can be found at www.afes.org.

## REFERENCES

1. Gauthier C, Tavernier G, Charpentier F, et al: Functional β3-adrenoceptor in human heart. J Clin Invest 1996;98:556–562.
2. Gauthier C, Leblais V, Kobzik L, et al: The negative inotropic effect of β3-adrenoceptor stimulation is mediated by activation of a nitric oxide synthase pathway in human ventricle. J Clin Invest 1998;102:1377–1384.
3. Strader CD, Fong TM, Tota MR, et al: Structure and function of G protein-coupled receptors. Ann Rev Biochem 1994;63:101–132.

4. Tang Y, Hu LA, Miller WE, et al: Identification of the endophilins (SH3p4/p8/p13) as novel binding partners for the β$_1$-adrenergic receptor. Proc Natl Acad Sci U S A 1999;96:12559-12564.

5. Hall RA, Premont RT, Chow CW, et al: The β$_2$-adrenergic receptor interacts with the Na$^+$/H$^+$-exchanger regulatory factor to control Na$^+$/H$^+$ exchange. Nature 1998;392:626-630.

6. Xu J, Paquet M, Lau AG, et al: β$_1$-adrenergic receptor association with the synaptic scaffolding protein membrane-associated guanylate kinase inverted-2 (MAGI-2): Differential regulation of receptor internalization by MAGI-2 and PSD-95. J Biol Chem 2001;276:41310-41317.

7. Milano CA, Allen LF, Rockman HA, et al: Enhanced myocardial function in transgenic mice overexpressing the β$_2$-adrenergic receptor. Science 1994;264:582-586.

8. Liggett SB, Tepe NM, Lorenz JN, et al: Early and delayed consequences of β$_2$-adrenergic receptor overexpression in mouse hearts: Critical role for expression level. Circulation 2000; 101:1707-1714.

9. Bisognano JD, Weinberger HD, Bohlmeyer TJ, et al: Myocardial-directed overexpression of the human β$_1$-adrenergic receptor in transgenic mice. J Mol Cell Cardiol 2000;32:817-830.

10. Engelhardt S, Hein L, Wiesmann F, et al: Progressive hypertrophy and heart failure in β$_1$-adrenergic receptor transgenic mice. Proc Natl Acad Sci U S A 1999;96:7059-7064.

11. Barr AJ, Brass LF, Manning DR: Reconstitution of receptors and GTP-binding regulatory proteins (G proteins) in Sf9 cells: A direct evaluation of selectivity in receptor-G protein coupling. J Biol Chem 1997;272:2223-2229.

12. Okamoto T, Murayama Y, Hayashi Y, et al: Identification of a G$_s$ activator region of the β$_2$-adrenergic receptor that is autoregulated via protein kinase A-dependent phosphorylation. Cell 1991;67:723-730.

13. Daaka Y, Luttrell LM, Lefkowitz RJ: Switching of the coupling of the β$_2$-adrenergic receptor to different G proteins by protein kinase A. Nature 1997;390:88-91.

14. Zamah AM, Delahunty M, Luttrell LM, et al: Protein kinase A-mediated phosphorylation of the β$_2$-adrenergic receptor regulates its coupling to G$_s$ and G$_i$: Demonstration in a reconstituted system. J Biol Chem 2002;277:31249-31256.

15. Maudsley S, Pierce KL, Zamah AM, et al: The β$_2$-adrenergic receptor mediates extracellular signal-regulated kinase activation via assembly of a multi-receptor complex with the epidermal growth factor receptor. J Biol Chem 2000;275:9572-9580.

16. Rybin VO, Pak E, Alcott S, et al: Developmental changes in β$_2$-Adrenergic receptor signaling in ventricular myocytes: The role of Gi proteins and caveolae microdomains. Mol Pharmacol 2003;63:1338-1348.

17. Kaumann AJ, Sanders L, Lynham J, et al: β$_2$-adrenoceptor activation by zinterol causes protein phosphorylation, contractile effects and relaxant effects through a cAMP pathway in human atrium. Mol Cell Biochem 1996;163/164:113-123.

18. Kaumann A, Bartel S, Molenaar P, et al: Activation of β$_2$-adrenergic receptors hastens relaxation and mediates phosphorylation of phospholamban, troponin I and C-protein in ventricular myocardium from patients with terminal heart failure. Circulation 1999;99:65-72.

19. Stamatelopoulou SI, Mittmann C, Eschenhagen T: β-Adrenergic stimulation of azidoanilido [$^{32}$P]-GTP binding to Gs and Gi/Go proteins in human myocardial membranes. Circulation 1999;100: I-487.

20. Kuznetsov V, Pak E, Robinson RB, et al: β$_2$-Adrenergic receptor actions in neonatal and adult rat ventricular myocytes. Circ Res 1995;76:40-52.

21. Steinberg SF: The molecular basis for distinct β-adrenergic receptor subtype actions in cardiomyocytes. Circ Res 1999;85: 1101-1111.

22. Steinberg SF: The cellular actions of β-adrenergic receptor agonists: Looking beyond cAMP. Circ Res 2000;87:1079-1082.

23. Laflamme MA, Becker PL: Do β$_2$-adrenergic receptors modulate Ca$^{2+}$ in adult rat ventricular myocytes? Am J Physiol 1998;274: H1308-H1314.

24. Jiang T, Steinberg SF: β$_2$-adrenergic receptors enhance contractility by stimulating HCO$_3$-dependent intracellular alkalinization. Am J Physiol 1997;273:H1044-H1047.

25. Xiao RP, Cheng H, Zhou YY, et al: Recent advances in cardiac β$_2$-adrenergic signal transduction. Circ Res 1999;85:1092-1100.

26. Rybin VO, Xu X, Lisanti MP, et al: Differential targeting of beta-adrenergic receptor subtypes and adenylyl cyclase to cardiomyocyte caveolae: A mechanism to functionally regulate the cAMP signaling pathway. J Biol Chem 2000;275: 41447-41457.

27. Ostrom RS, Gregorian C, Drenan RM, et al: Receptor number and caveolar co-localization determine receptor coupling efficiency to adenylyl cyclase. J Biol Chem 2001;276:42063-42069.

28. Xiang Y, Rybin VO, Steinberg SF, et al: Caveolar localization dictates physiologic signaling of beta 2-adrenoceptors in neonatal cardiac myocytes. J Biol Chem 2002;277:34280-34286.

29. Crackower MA, Oudit GY, Kozieradzki I, et al: Regulation of myocardial contractility and cell size by distinct PI3K-PTEN signaling pathways. Cell 2002;110:737-739.

30. Iwaki K, Sukhatme VP, Shubeita HE, et al: α- and β-adrenergic stimulation induces distinct patterns of immediate early gene expression in neonatal rat myocardial cells. J Biol Chem 1990;265: 13809-13817.

31. Morisco C, Zebrowski D, Condorelli G, et al: The Akt-glycogen synthase kinase 3 β pathway regulates transcription of atrial natriuretic factor induced by β-adrenergic receptor stimulation in cardiac myocytes. J Biol Chem 2000;275:14466-14475.

32. Morisco C, Zebrowski DC, Vatner DE, et al: β-Adrenergic cardiac hypertrophy is mediated primarily by the β$_1$-subtype in the rat heart. J Mol Cell Cardiol 2001;33:561-573.

33. Shizukuda Y, Buttrick PM, Geenen DL, et al: Beta-adrenergic stimulation causes cardiocyte apoptosis: Influence of tachycardia and hypertrophy. Am J Physiol 1998;275:H961-968.

34. Communal C, Singh K, Sawyer DB, et al: Opposing effects of β$_1$- and β$_2$-adrenergic receptors on cardiac myocyte apoptosis: Role of a pertussis toxin-sensitive G protein. Circulation 1999; 100:2210-2212.

35. Zaugg M, Xu W, Lucchinetti E, et al: β-adrenergic receptor subtypes differentially affect apoptosis in adult rat ventricular myocytes. Circulation 2000;102:344-350.

36. Communal C, Colucci WS, Singh K: p38 Mitogen activated protein kinase pathway protects adult rat ventricular myocytes against β-adrenergic receptor stimulated apoptosis: Evidence for Gi dependent activation. J Biol Chem 2000;275:19395-19400.

37. Chesley A, Lundberg MS, Asai T, et al: The β$_2$-adrenergic receptor delivers an anti-apoptotic signal to cardiac myocyte through G$_i$-dependent coupling to phosphatidylinositol 3′-kinase. Circ Res 2000;87:1172-1179.

38. Sabri A, Pak E, Alcott SA, et al: Coupling function of endogenous α$_1$- and β-adrenergic receptors in mouse cardiomyocytes. Circ Res 2000;86:1047-1053.

39. Zheng M, Zhang SJ, Zhu WZ, et al: β$_2$-adrenergic receptor-induced p38 MAPK activation is mediated by protein kinase A rather than by G$_i$ or Gβγ in adult mouse cardiomyocytes. J Biol Chem 2000; 275:40635-40640.

40. Sadoshima J, Zebrowski DC: Stimulation of the β-adrenergic receptor activates transcription of ANF through Ca$^{2+}$-dependent mechanisms. Circulation 1998;98:I-624.

41. Small KM, Wagoner LE, Levin AM, et al: Synergistic polymorphisms of β$_1$- and α$_{2C}$-adrenergic receptors and the risk of congestive heart failure. N Engl J Med 2002;347:1135-1142.

42. Liggett SB: Polymorphisms of the β$_2$-adrenergic receptor and asthma. Am J Respir Crit Care Med 1997;156:S156-S162.

43. Reihsaus E, Innis M, MacIntyre N, et al: Mutations in the gene encoding for the β$_2$-adrenergic receptor in normal and asthmatic subjects. Am J Respir Cell Mol Biol 1993;8:334-339.

44. Turki J, Pak J, Green SA, et al: Genetic polymorphisms of the β$_2$-adrenergic receptor and nocturnal asthma. J Clin Invest 2002; 95:1635-1641.

45. Hall IP, Wheatly A, Wilding P, et al: Association of Glu 27 b2-adrenoceptor polymorphism with lower airway reactivity in asthmatic subjects. Lancet 1995;345:1213-1214.

46. Liggett SB, Wagoner LE, Creaft LL, et al: The Ile 164 β$_2$-adrenergic receptor polymorphism adversely affects the outcome of congestive heart failure. J Clin Invest 1998;102:1532-1539.

47. Ahlquist RP: A study of adrenoceptors. Am J Physiol 1948;153: 586-600.

48. Langer SZ: Presynaptic regulation of catecholamine release. Biochem Pharmacol 1974;23:1788–1800.

49. Starke K: Alpha-adrenoceptor subclassification. Rev Physiol Biochem Pharmacol 1981;88:199–236.

50. Brodde O-E, Michel MC: Adrenergic and muscarinic receptors in the human heart. Pharmacol Rev 1999;51:651–689.

51. Brede M, Wiesmann F, Jahns R, et al: Feedback inhibition of catecholamine release by two different alpha2-adrenoceptor subtypes prevents progression of heart failure. Circulation 2002;106:2491–2496.

52. Wetzel GT, Brown JH: Presynaptic modulation of acetylcholine release from cardiac parasympathetic neurons. Am J Physiol 1985; 248:H33–H39.

53. O'Rourke MF, Iversen LJ, Lomasney JW, et al: Species orthologs of the alpha-2A adrenergic receptor: The pharmacological properties of the bovine and rat receptors differ from the human and porcine receptors. J Pharmacol Exp Ther 1994;271: 735–740.

54. Sun LS, Huber F, Robinson RB, et al: Muscarinic receptor heterogeneity in neonatal rat ventricular myocytes in culture. J Cardiovasc Pharmacol 1996;27:455–461.

55. Tanoue A, Nasa Y, Koshimizu T, et al: The alpha(1D)-adrenergic receptor directly regulates arterial blood pressure via vasoconstriction. J Clin Invest 2002;109:765–775.

56. Piascik MT, Perez DM: Alpha1-adrenergic receptors: New insights and directions. J Pharmacol Exp Ther 2001;298:403–410.

57. Theroux TL, Esbenshade TA, Peavy RD, et al: Coupling efficiencies of human $\alpha_1$-adrenergic receptor subtypes: Titration of receptor density and responsiveness with inducible and repressible expression vectors. Mol Pharmacol 1996;50:1376–1387.

58. Guimaraes S, Moura D: Vascular adrenoceptors: An update. Pharmacol Rev 2001;53:319–356.

59. Cavalli A, Lattion A-L, Hummler E, et al: Decreased blood pressure response in mice deficient of the $\alpha_{1b}$-adrenergic receptor. Proc Natl Acad Sci U S A 1997;94:11589–11594.

60. Zuscik MJ, Chalothorn D, Hellard D, et al: Hypotension, autonomic failure, and cardiac hypertrophy in transgenic mice overexpressing the alpha 1B-adrenergic receptor. J Biol Chem 2001;276: 13738–13743.

61. Rokosh DG, Simpson PC: Knockout of the alpha 1A/C-adrenergic receptor subtype: The alpha 1A/C is expressed in resistance arteries and is required to maintain arterial blood pressure. Proc Natl Acad Sci U S A 2002;99:9474–9479.

62. Endoh M: Regulation of myocardial contractility via adrenoceptors: differential mechanisms of alpha- and beta-adrenoceptors-mediated actions. In Grobecker H, Philippu A, Starke K (eds): New Aspects of the Role of Adrenoceptors in the Cardiovascular System. Heidelberg, Springer-Verlag Berlin, 1986, pp 78–104.

63. Bayer K-U, Koninck PD, Leonard AS, et al: Interaction with the NMDA receptor locks CaMKII in an active conformation. Nature 2001;411:801–805.

64. O'Rourke B, Reibel DK, Thomas AP: Alpha-adrenergic modification of the $Ca^{2+}$ transient and contraction in single rat cardiomyocytes. J Mol Cell Cardiol 1992;24:809–820.

65. Bruckner R, Meyer W, Mugge A, et al: Alpha-adrenoceptor-mediated positive inotropic effect of phenylephrine in isolated human ventricular myocardium. Eur J Pharmacol 1984;99:345–347.

66. Terzic A, Puceat M, Clement O, et al: $\alpha$1-Adrenergic effects on intracellular pH and calcium and on myofilaments in single rat cardiac cells. J Physiol (Lond) 1992;447:275–292.

67. Fedida D: Modulation of cardiac contractility by alpha 1 adrenoceptors. Cardiovasc Res 1993;27:1735–1742.

68. Suematsu N, Satoh S, Kinugawa S, et al: Alpha1-adrenoceptor-Gq-RhoA signaling is upregulated to increase myofibrillar $Ca^{2+}$ sensitivity in failing hearts. Am J Physiol Heart Circ Physiol 2001; 281:H637–H646.

69. McCloskey DT, Rokosh DG, O'Connell TD, et al: Alpha(1)-adrenoceptor subtypes mediate negative inotropy in myocardium from alpha(1A/C)-knockout and wild type mice. J Mol Cell Cardiol 2002;34:1007–1017.

70. Simpson P: Norepinephrine-stimulated hypertrophy of cultured rat myocardial cells is an $\alpha_1$-adrenergic response. J Clin Invest 1983;72:732–738.

71. Simpson PC: Proto-oncogenes and cardiac hypertrophy. Annu Rev Physiol 1988;51:189–202.

72. Chien KR, Zhu H, Knowlton KU, et al: Transcriptional regulation during cardiac growth and development. Annu Rev Physiol 1993;55:77–95.

73. Clerk A, Sugden PH: Regulation of phospholipases C and D in rat ventricular myocytes: Stimulation by endothelin-1, bradykinin and phenylephrine. J Mol Cell Cardiol 1997;29:1593–1604.

74. McDonough PM, Brown JH, Glembotski CC Phenylephrine and endothelin differentially stimulate cardiac PI hydrolysis and ANF expression. Am J Physiol 1993;264:H625–H630.

75. Knowlton KU, Michel MC, Itani M, et al: The $\alpha$1a-adrenergic receptor subtype mediates biochemical, molecular, and morphologic features of cultured myocardial cell hypertrophy. J Biol Chem 1993;268:15374–15380.

76. Lazou A, Sugden PH, Clerk A: Activation of mitogen-activated protein kinases (p38-MAPKs, SAPKs/JNKs and ERKs) by the G-protein-coupled receptor agonist phenylephrine in the perfused rat heart. Biochem J 1998;332:459–465.

77. Bogoyevitch MA, Andersson MB, Gillespie-Brown J, et al: Adrenergic receptor stimulation of the mitogen-activated protein kinase cascade and cardiac hypertrophy. Biochem J 1996;314:115–121.

78. McWhinney C, Wenham D, Kanwal S, et al: Constitutively active mutants of the alpha1a-and the alpha1b-adrenergic receptor subtypes reveal coupling to different signaling pathways and physiological responses in rat cardiac myocytes. J Biol Chem 1999;275:2087–2097.

79. Lin F, Owens WA, Chen S, et al: Targeted alpha(1A)-adrenergic receptor overexpression induces enhanced cardiac contractility but not hypertrophy. Circ Res 2001;89:343–350.

80. Milano CA, Dolber PC, Rockman HA, et al: Myocardial expression of a constitutively active $\alpha_{1B}$-adrenergic receptor in transgenic mice induces cardiac hypertrophy. Proc Natl Acad Sci U S A 1994; 91:10109–10113.

81. Akhter SA, Milano CA, Shotwell KF, et al: Transgenic mice with cardiac overexpression of $\alpha_{1B}$-adrenergic receptors. In vivo $\alpha_1$-adrenergic receptor-mediated regulation of $\beta$-adrenergic signaling. J Biol Chem 1997;272:21253–21259.

82. Vecchione C, Fratta L, Rizzoni D, et al: Cardiovascular influences of alpha1b-adrenergic receptor defect in mice. Circulation 2002;105:1700–1707.

83. O'Connell TD, Ishizaka S, Nakamura A, et al: The $\alpha_{1A/C}$-and $\alpha_{1B}$-adrenergic receptors are required for physiological cardiac hypertrophy in the double-knockout mouse. J Clin Invest 2003;111: 1783–1791.

84. Bonner TI, Buckley NJ, Young AC, et al: Identification of a family of muscarinic acetylcholine receptor genes. Science 1987; 237:527–532.

85. Wess J, Bonner TI, Dorje F, et al: Delineation of muscarinic receptor domains conferring selectivity of coupling to guanine nucleotide-binding proteins and second messengers. Mol Pharmacol 1990;38:517–523.

86. Wess J: Molecular biology of muscarinic acetylcholine receptors. Crit Rev Neurobiol 1996;10:69–99.

87. Caulfield MP, Birdsall NJ: International Union of Pharmacology. XVII. Classification of muscarinic acetylcholine receptors. Pharmacol Rev 1998;50:279–290.

88. Furchgott RF: Endothelium-derived relaxing factor: Discovery, early studies, and identification as nitric oxide. Biosci Rep 1999; 19:235–251.

89. Eglen RM, Hegde SS, Watson N: Muscarinic receptor subtypes and smooth muscle function. Pharmacol Rev 1996;48:531–565.

90. Fleming JW, Watanabe AM: Muscarinic cholinergic-receptor stimulation of specific GTP hydrolysis related to adenylate cyclase activity in canine cardiac sarcolemma. Circ Res 1988;64:340–350.

91. Brown JH: Depolarization-induced inhibition of cyclic AMP accumulation: Cholinergic-adrenergic antagonism in murine atria. Mol Pharmacol 1979;16:841–850.

92. Hilal-Dandan R, Kanter JR, Brunton LL: Characterization of G-protein signaling in ventricular myocytes from the adult mouse heart: Differences from the rat. J Mol Cell Cardiol 2000; 32:1211–1221.

93. Brown JH: Cholinergic inhibition of catecholamine-stimulable cyclic AMP accumulation in murine atria. J Cyclic Nucleotide Res 1979;5:423–433.

94. Valenzuela D, Han X, Mende U, et al: $G\alpha_o$ is necessary for muscarinic regulation of $Ca^{2+}$ channels in mouse heart. Proc Natl Acad Sci U S A 1997;94:1727–1732.

95. Nagata K, Ye C, Jain M, et al: $G\alpha_{12}$ but not $G\alpha_{13}$ is required for muscarinic inhibition of contractility and calcium currents in adult cardiomyocytes. Circ Res 2000;87:903-909.

96. Chen F, Spicher K, Jiang M, et al: Lack of muscarinic regulation of $Ca^{2+}$ channels in $G_{i2}\alpha$ gene knockout mouse hearts. Am J Physiol Heart Circ Physiol 2001;280:H1989-H1995.

97. Wickman K, Clapham DE: Ion channel regulation by G proteins. Physiol Rev 1995;75:865-885.

98. Yamada M, Inanobe A, Kurachi Y: G protein regulation of potassium ion channels. Pharmacol Rev 1998;50:723-760.

99. Oberhauser V, Schwertfeger E, Rutz T, et al: Acetylcholine release in human heart atrium: Influence of muscarinic autoreceptors, diabetes, and age. Circulation 2001;103:1638-1643.

100. Sterin-Borda L, Joensen L, Bayo-Hanza C, et al: Therapeutic use of muscarinic acetylcholine receptor peptide to prevent mice chagasic cardiac dysfunction. J Mol Cell Cardiol 2002;34:1645-1654.

101. Bogoyevitch MA, Clerk A, Sugden PH: Activation of the mitogen-activated protein kinase cascade by pertussis toxin-sensitive and -insensitive pathways in cultured ventricular cardiomyocytes. Biochem J 1995;309:437-443.

102. Ramirez MT, Post GR, Sulakhe PV, et al: $M_1$ muscarinic receptors heterologously expressed in cardiac myocytes mediate Ras-dependent changes in gene expression. J Biol Chem 1995;270:8446-8451.

103. Post GR, Goldstein D, Thuerauf D, et al: Dissociation of p44 and p42 mitogen-activated protein kinase activation from receptor-induced hypertrophy in neonatal rat ventricular myocytes. J Biol Chem 1996;271:8452-8457.

104. Dorn GW, Brown JH: Gq signaling in cardiac adaptation and maladaptation. Trends Cardiovasc Med 1999;9:26-34.

105. Adams JW, Sakata Y, Davis MG, et al: Enhanced $G\alpha_q$ signaling: A common pathway mediates cardiac hypertrophy and apoptotic heart failure. Proc Natl Acad Sci USA 1998;95:10140-10145.

106. Jackowski S, Rettenmier CW, Sherr CJ, et al: A guanine nucleotide-dependent phosphatidylinositol 4,5-bisphosphate phospholipase C in cells transformed by the v-fms and v-fes oncogenes. J Biol Chem 1986;261:4978-4985.

107. Brown JH, Buxton IL, Brunton LL: $\alpha$1-Adrenergic and muscarinic cholinergic stimulation of phosphoinositide hydrolysis in adult rat cardiomyocytes. Circ Res 1985;57:532-537.

108. Masters SB, Martin MW, Harden TK, et al: Pertussis toxin does not inhibit muscarinic-receptor-mediated phosphoinositide hydrolysis or calcium mobilization. Biochem J 1985;227:933-937.

109. Yang CM, Chen F-F, Sung T-C, et al: Pharmacological characterization of muscarinic receptors in neonatal rat cardiomyocytes. Am J Physiol 1993;265:C666-C673.

110. Colecraft HM, Egamino JP, Sharma VK, et al: Signaling mechanisms underlying muscarinic receptor-mediated increase in contraction rate in cultured heart cells. J Biol Chem 1998;273:32158-32166.

111. Kohl C, Schmitz W, Scholz H: Positive inotropic effect of carbachol and inositol phosphate levels in mammalian atria after pretreatment with pertussis toxin. J Pharmacol Exp Ther 1990;254:894-899.

112. Korth M, Kuhlkamp V: Muscarinic receptor-mediated increase of intracellular $Na^+$-ion activity and force of contraction. Pflugers Arch 1985;403:266-272.

113. Tajima T, Tsuji Y, Brown JH, et al: Pertussis-toxin insensitive phosphoinositide hydrolysis, membrane depolarization, and positive inotropic effect of carbachol in chick atria. Circ Res 1987;61:436-445.

114. Sharma VK, Colecraft HM, Wang DX, et al: Molecular and functional identification of $m_1$ muscarinic acetylcholine receptors in rat ventricular myocytes. Circ Res 1996;79:86-93.

115. Hamilton SE, Loose MD, Qi M, et al: Disruption of the m1 receptor gene ablates muscarinic receptor-dependent M current regulation and seizure activity in mice. Proc Natl Acad Sci USA 1997;94:13311-13316.

116. Hardouin SN, Richmond KN, Zimmerman A, et al: Altered cardiovascular responses in mice lacking the M(1) muscarinic acetylcholine receptor. J Pharmacol Exp Ther 2002;301:129-137.

117. Gomeza J, Shannon H, Kostenis E, et al: Pronounced pharmacologic deficits in M2 muscarinic acetylcholine receptor knockout mice. Proc Natl Acad Sci U S A 1999;96:1692.-1697

118. Stengel PW, Gomeza J, Wess J, et al: M(2) and M(4) receptor knockout mice: Muscarinic receptor function in cardiac and smooth muscle in vitro. J Pharmacol Exp Ther 2000;292:877-885.

119. Matsui M, Motomura D, Karasawa H, et al: Multiple functional defects in peripheral autonomic organs in mice lacking muscarinic acetylcholine receptor gene for the M3 subtype. Proc Natl Acad Sci U S A 2000;97:9579-9584.

120. Shapiro MS, Loose MD, Hamilton SE, et al: Assignment of muscarinic receptor subtypes mediating G-protein modulation of Ca(2+) channels by using knockout mice. Proc Natl Acad Sci USA 1999;96:10899-10904.

121. Yamada M, Lamping KG, Duttaroy A, et al: Cholinergic dilation of cerebral blood vessels is abolished in M(5) muscarinic acetylcholine receptor knockout mice. Proc Natl Acad Sci USA 2001;98:14096-14101.

122. Yanagisawa M, Kurihara H, Kimura S, et al: A novel potent vasoconstrictor peptide produced by vascular endothelial cells. Nature 1988;332:411-415.

123. Kloog Y, Ambar I, Sokolovsky M, et al: Sarafotoxin, a novel vasoconstrictor peptide: phosphoinositide hydrolysis in rat heart and brain. Science 1988;242:268-270.

124. Kedzierski RM, Yanagisawa M: Endothelin system: The double-edged sword in health and disease. Annu Rev Pharmacol Toxicol 2001;41:851-876.

125. Yanagisawa H, Hammer RE, Richardson JA, et al: Disruption of ECE-1 and ECE-2 reveals a role for endothelin-converting enzyme-2 in murine cardiac development. J Clin Invest 2000; 105:1373-1382.

126. Iijima Y, Laser M, Shiraishi H, et al: c-Raf/MEK/ERK pathway controls protein kinase C-mediated p70S6K activation in adult cardiac muscle cells. J Biol Chem 2002;277:23065-23075.

127. Corder R, Douthwaite JA, Lees DM, et al: Endothelin-1 synthesis reduced by red wine. Nature 2001;414:863-864.

128. Murakoshi N, Miyauchi T, Kakinuma Y, et al: Vascular endothelin-B receptor system in vivo plays a favorable inhibitory role in vascular remodeling after injury revealed by endothelin-B receptor-knockout mice. Circulation 2002;106:1991-1998.

129. Stewart DJ, Kubac G, Costello KB, et al: Increased plasma endothelin-1 in the early hours of acute myocardial infarction. J Am Coll Cardiol 1991;18:38-43.

130. Zolk O, Quattek J, Sitzler G, et al: Expression of endothelin-1, endothelin-converting enzyme, and endothelin receptors in chronic heart failure. Circulation 1999;99:2118-2123.

131. Giannessi D, Del Ry S, Vitale RL: The role of endothelins and their receptors in heart failure. Pharmacol Res 2001;43:111-126.

132. Woodcock EA, Land SL, Andrews RK, et al: A low-affinity, low-molecular-mass endothelin-A receptor in neonatal rat heart. Biochem J 1994;304(Pt 1):113-119.

133. Ishikawa T, Yanagisawa M, Kimura S, et al: Positive inotropic action of novel vasoconstrictor peptide endothelin on guinea pig atria. Am J Physiol 1988;255:H970-H973.

134. MacCarthy PA, Grocott-Mason R, Prendergast BD, et al: Contrasting inotropic effects of endogenous endothelin in the normal and failing human heart: Studies with an intracoronary ET(A) receptor antagonist. Circulation 2000;101:142-147.

135. Ishikawa T, Yanagisawa M, Kimura S, et al: Positive chronotropic effects of endothelin, a novel endothelium-derived vasoconstrictor peptide. Pflugers Arch 1988;413:108-110.

136. Kelly RA, Eid H, Krämer BK, et al: Endothelin enhances the contractile responsiveness of adult rat ventricular myocytes to calcium by a pertussis toxin-sensitive pathway. J Clin Invest 1990;86:1164-1171.

137. Sakai S, Miyauchi T, Kobayashi M, et al: Inhibition of myocardial endothelin pathway improves long-term survival in heart failure. Nature 1996;384:353-355.

138. Krämer BK, Smith TW, Kelly RA: Endothelin and increase contractility in adult rat ventricular myocytes. Role of intracellular alkalosis induced by activation of the protein kinase C-dependent $Na^+$-$H^+$ exchanger. Circ Res 1991;68:269-279.

139. Kelso EJ, McDermott BJ, Silke B, et al: Endothelin(A) receptor subtype mediates endothelin-induced contractility in left ventricular cardiomyocytes isolated from rabbit myocardium. J Pharmacol Exp Ther 2000;294:1047-1052.

140. Yamazaki T, Komuro I, Kudoh S, et al: Endothelin-1 is involved in mechanical stress-induced cardiomyocyte hypertrophy. J Biol Chem 1996;271:3221-3228.

141. Luscher TF, Barton M: Endothelins and endothelin receptor antagonists: Therapeutic considerations for a novel class of cardiovascular drugs. Circulation 2000;102:2434-2440.

142. Shubeita HE, McDonough PM, Harris AN, et al: Endothelin induction of inositol phospholipid hydrolysis, sarcomere assembly, and cardiac gene expression in ventricular myocytes: A paracrine mechanism for myocardial cell hypertrophy. J Biol Chem 1990;265:20555–20562.

143. Hilal-Dandan R, Ramirez MT, Villegas S, et al: Endothelin ETA receptor regulates signaling and ANF gene expression via multiple G protein-linked pathways. Am J Physiol 1997;272:H130–H137.

144. Choukroun G, Hajjar R, Kyriakis JM, et al: Role of the stress-activated protein kinases in endothelin-induced cardiomyocyte hypertrophy. J Clin Invest 1998;102:1311–1320.

145. Bogoyevitch MA, Glennon PE, Andersson MB, et al: Endothelin-1 and fibroblast growth factors stimulate the mitogen-activated protein kinase signaling cascade in cardiac myocytes. J Biol Chem 1994;269:1110–1119.

146. Bogoyevitch MA, Glennon PE, Sugden PH: Endothelin-1, phorbol esters and phenylephrine stimulate MAP kinase activates in ventricular cardiomyocytes. FEBS Lett 1993;317:271–275.

147. Clerk A, Bogoyevitch MA, Andersson MB, et al: Differential activation of protein kinase C isoforms by endothelin-1 and phenylephrine and subsequent stimulation of p42 and p44 mitogen-activated protein kinases in ventricular myocytes cultured from neonatal rat hearts. J Biol Chem 1994;269:32848–32857.

148. Remuzzi G, Perico N, Benigni A: New therapeutics that antagonize endothelin: Promises and frustrations. Nat Rev Drug Discov 2002;1:986–1001.

149. Hecht JH, Weiner JA, Post SR, et al: *Ventricular Zone Gene-1* (*vzg-1*) encodes a lysophosphatidic acid receptor expressed in neurogenic regions of the developing cerebral cortex. J Cell Biol 1996;135:1071–1083.

150. An S, Bleu T, Huang W, et al: Identification of cDNAs encoding two G protein-coupled receptors for lysosphingolipids. FEBS Lett 1997;417:279–282.

151. Zondag GC, Postma FR, Etten IV, et al: Sphingosine 1-phosphate signalling through the G-protein-coupled receptor Edg-1. Biochem J 1998;330(Pt 2):605–609.

152. Lee MJ, Van Brocklyn JR, Thangada S, et al: Sphingosine-1-phosphate as a ligand for the G protein-coupled receptor EDG-1. Science 1998;279:1552–1555.

153. Chun J, Goetzl EJ, Hla T, et al: International Union of Pharmacology. XXXIV. Lysophospholipid receptor nomenclature. Pharmacol Rev 2002;54:265–269.

154. Goetzl EJ, An S: Diversity of cellular receptors and functions for the lysophospholipid growth factors lysophosphatidic acid and sphingosine 1-phosphate. FASEB J 1998;12:1589–1598.

155. Fukushima N, Ishii I, Contos JJ, et al: Lysophospholipid receptors. Annu Rev Pharmacol Toxicol 2001;41:507–534.

156. Goetzl EJ: Pleiotypic mechanisms of cellular responses to biologically active lysophospholipids. Prostaglandins 2001;64:11–20.

157. Pyne S, Pyne N: Sphingosine 1-phosphate signalling via the endothelial differentiation gene family of G-protein-coupled receptors. Pharmacol Ther 2000;88:115–131.

158. Contos JJ, Ishii I, Chun J: Lysophosphatidic acid receptors. Mol Pharmacol 2000;58:1188–1196.

159. Hla T, Lee MJ, Ancellin N, et al: Lysophospholipids–receptor revelations. Science 2001;294:1875–1878.

160. Levade T, Auge N, Veldman RJ, et al: Sphingolipid mediators in cardiovascular cell biology and pathology. Circ Res 2001;89:957–968.

161. Allende ML, Proia RL: Sphingosine-1-phosphate receptors and the development of the vascular system. Biochim Biophys Acta 2002;1582:222–227.

162. Karliner JS: Lysophospholipids and the cardiovascular system. Biochim Biophys Acta 2002;1582:216–221.

163. Kluk MJ, Hla T: Signaling of sphingosine-1-phosphate via the S1P/EDG-family of G-protein-coupled receptors. Biochim Biophys Acta 2002;1582:72–80.

164. Liliom K, Sun G, Bunemann M, et al: Sphingosylphosphocholine is a naturally occurring lipid mediator in blood plasma: A possible role in regulating cardiac function via sphingolipid receptors. Biochem J 2001;355:189–197.

165. Yatomi Y, Igarashi Y, Yang L, et al: Sphingosine 1-phosphate, a bioactive sphingolipid abundantly stored in platelets, is a normal constituent of human plasma and serum. J Biochem (Tokyo) 1997;121:969–973.

166. Cuvillier O, Pirianov G, Kleuser B, et al: Suppression of ceramide-mediated programmed cell death by sphingosine-1-phosphate. Nature 1996;381:800–803.

167. Bielawska AE, Shapiro JP, Jiang L, et al: Ceramide is involved in triggering of cardiomyocyte apoptosis induced by ischemia and reperfusion. Am J Pathol 1997;151:1257–1263.

168. Cuvillier O, Pirianov G, Kleuser B, et al: Suppression of ceramide-mediated programmed cell death by sphingosine-1-phosphate. Nature 1996;381:800–803.

169. Meyer zu HD, Lass H, Kuchar I, et al: Stimulation of intracellular sphingosine-1-phosphate production by G-protein-coupled sphingosine-1-phosphate receptors. Eur J Pharmacol 2001;414:145–154.

170. Young KW, Bootman MD, Channing DR, et al: Lysophosphatidic acid-induced Ca²⁺ mobilization requires intracellular sphingosine 1-phosphate production: Potential involvement of endogenous EDG-4 receptors. J Biol Chem 2000;275:38532–38539.

171. Young KW, Challiss RA, Nahorski SR, et al: Lysophosphatidic acid-mediated Ca²⁺ mobilization in human SH-SY5Y neuroblastoma cells is independent of phosphoinositide signalling, but dependent on sphingosine kinase activation. Biochem J 1999;343(Pt 1):45–52.

172. Schutze S, Potthoff K, Machleidt T, et al: TNF activates NF-kappaB by phosphatidylcholine-specific phospholipase C-induced "acidic" sphingomyelin breakdown. Cell 1992;71:765–776.

173. Oral H, Dorn GW, Mann DL: Sphingosine mediates the immediate negative inotropic effects of tumor necrosis factor-alpha in the adult mammalian cardiac myocyte. J Biol Chem 1997;272:4836–4842.

174. Cavalli AL, Ligutti JA, Gellings NM, et al: The Role of TNFα and sphingolipid signaling in cardiac hypoxia: evidence the cardiomyocytes release TNFα and sphingosine. Basic Appl Myol 2002;12:167–175.

175. Ancellin N, Colmont C, Su J, et al: Extracellular export of sphingosine kinase-1 enzyme: Sphingosine 1-phosphate generation and the induction of angiogenic vascular maturation. J Biol Chem 2002;277:6667–6675.

176. Kranenburg O, Moolenaar WH: Ras-MAP kinase signaling by lysophosphatidic acid and other G protein-coupled receptor agonists. Oncogene 2001;20:1540–1546.

177. Contos JJ, Ishii I, Fukushima N, et al: Characterization of lpa(2) (Edg4) and lpa(2) (Edg2/Edg4) lysophosphatidic acid receptor knockout mice: signaling deficits without obvious phenotypic abnormality attributable to lpa(2). Mol Cell Biol 2002;22:6921–6929.

178. Ancellin N, Hla T: Differential pharmacological properties and signal transduction of the sphingosine 1-phosphate receptors EDG-1, EDG-3, and EDG-5. J Biol Chem 1999;274:18997–19002.

179. Takuwa Y, Okamoto H, Takuwa N, et al: Subtype-specific, differential activities of the EDG family receptors for sphingosine-1-phosphate, a novel lysophospholipid mediator. Mol Cell Endocrinol 2001;177:3–11.

180. Windh RT, Lee M-J, Hla T, et al: Differential coupling of the sphingosine 1-phosphate receptors Edg-1, Edg-3, and h218/Edg-5 to the $G_i$, $G_q$, and $G_{12}$ families of heterotrimeric G proteins. J Biol Chem 1999;274:27351–27358.

181. Siehler S, Manning DR: Pathways of transduction engaged by sphingosine 1-phosphate through G protein-coupled receptors. Biochim Biophys Acta 2002;1582:94–99.

182. Ishii I, Friedman B, Ye X, et al: Selective loss of sphingosine 1-phosphate signaling with no obvious phenotypic abnormality in mice lacking its g protein-coupled receptor, lpb3/edg-3. J Biol Chem 2001;276:33697–33704.

183. Ishii I, Ye X, Fredman B, et al: Marked perinatal lethality and cellular signaling deficits in mice null for the two sphingosine 1-phosphate receptors, S1P₂/LP_{B2}/EDG-5 and S1P₃/LP_{B3}/EDG-3. J Biol Chem 2002;277:25152–25159.

184. Garcia JG, Liu F, Verin AD, et al: Sphingosine 1-phophate promotes endothelial cell barrier integrity by Edg-dependent cytoskeletal rearrangement. J Clin Invest 2001;108:689–701.

185. Liu Y, Wada R, Yamashita T, et al: Edg-1, the G protein-coupled receptor for sphingosine-1-phosphate, is essential for vascular maturation. J Clin Invest 2000;106:951–961.

186. Fukushima N, Kimura Y, Chun J: A single receptor encoded by *vzg-1/lp_{A}/edg-2* couples to G proteins and mediates multiple cellular responses to lysophosphatidic acid. Proc Natl Acad Sci U S A 1998;95:6151–6156.

187. Lee MJ, Thangada S, Claffey KP, et al: Vascular endothelial cell adherens junction assembly and morphogenesis induced by sphingosine-1-phosphate. Cell 1999;99:301–312.

188. Postma FR, Jalink K, Hengeveld T, et al: Sphingosine-1-phosphate rapidly induces Rho-dependent neurite retraction: Action through a specific cell surface receptor. EMBO J 1996;15:2388-2395.

189. Tigyi G, Fischer DJ, Sebok A, et al: Lysophosphatidic acid-induced neurite retraction in PC12 cells: Control by phosphoinositide-$Ca^{2+}$ signaling and Rho. J Neurochem 1996;66:537-548.

190. Gohla A, Harhammer R, Schultz G: The G-protein $G_{13}$ but not $G_{12}$ mediates signaling from lysophosphatidic acid receptor via epidermal growth factor receptor to Rho. J Biol Chem 1998; 273:4653-4659.

191. Gohla A, Offermanns S, Wilkie TM, et al: Differential involvement of $G_{\alpha12}$ and $G_{\alpha13}$ in receptor-mediated stress fiber formation. J Biol Chem 1999;274:17901-17907.

192. Kranenburg O, Poland M, van Horck FPG, et al: Activation of RhoA by lysophosphatidic acid and $G\alpha_{12/13}$ subunits in neuronal cells: Induction of neurite retraction. Mol Biol Cell 1999;10:1851-1857.

193. Takuwa Y: Subtype-specific differential regulation of Rho family G proteins and cell migration by the Edg family sphingosine-1-phosphate receptors. Biochim Biophys Acta 2002;1582:112-120.

194. Kupperman E, An S, Osborne N, et al: A sphingosine-1-phosphate receptor regulates cell migration during vertebrate heart development. Nature 2000;406:192-195.

195. Morales-Ruiz M, Lee MJ, Zollner S, et al: Sphingosine 1-phosphate activates Akt, nitric oxide production, and chemotaxis through a Gi protein/phosphoinositide 3-kinase pathway in endothelial cells. J Biol Chem 2001;276:19672-19677.

196. Panetti TS, Nowlen J, Mosher DF: Sphingosine-1-phosphate and lysophosphatidic acid stimulate endothelial cell migration. Arterioscler Thromb Vasc Biol 2000;20:1013-1019.

197. Hobson JP, Rosenfeldt HM, Barak LS, et al: Role of the sphingosine-1-phosphate receptor EDG-1 in PDGF-induced cell motility. Science 2001;91:1800-1803.

198. Lee MJ, Thangada S, Paik JH, et al: Akt-mediated phosphorylation of the G protein-coupled receptor EDG-1 is required for endothelial cell chemotaxis. Mol Cell 2001;8:693-704.

199. Himmel HM, Meyer zu HD, Graf E, et al: Evidence for Edg-3 receptor-mediated activation of I(K.ACh) by sphingosine-1-phosphate in human atrial cardiomyocytes. Mol Pharmacol 2000; 58:449-454.

200. Goetzl EJ, Lee H, Azuma T, et al: Gelsolin binding and cellular presentation of lysophosphatidic acid. J Biol Chem 2000;275:14573-14578.

201. Nakajima N, Cavalli AL, Biral D, et al: Expression and characterization of Edg-1 receptors in rat cardiomyocytes: Calcium deregulation in response to sphingosine 1-phosphate. Eur J Biochem 2000;267:5679-5686.

202. Robert P, Tsui P, Laville MP, et al: Edg1 receptor stimulation leads to cardiac hypertrophy in rat neonatal myocytes. J Mol Cell Cardiol 2001;33:1589-1606.

203. Xu YJ, Ouk KS, Liao DF, et al: Stimulation of 90- and 70-kDa ribosomal protein S6 kinases by arginine vasopressin and lysophosphatidic acid in rat cardiomyocytes. Biochem Pharmacol 2000; 59:1163-1171.

204. Sugiyama A, Aye NN, Yatomi Y, et al: Effects of sphingosine 1-phosphate, a naturally occurring biologically active lysophospholipid, on the rat cardiovascular system. Jpn J Pharmacol 2000;82:338-342.

205. Gohla A, Schultz G, Offermanns S: Role for $G_{12}/G_{13}$ in agonist-induced vascular smooth muscle cell contraction. Circ Res 2000; 87:221-227.

206. van Koppen C, Meyer zu HM, Laser KT, et al: Activation of a high affinity Gi protein-coupled plasma membrane receptor by sphingosine-1-phosphate. J Biol Chem 1996;271:2082-2087.

207. Bunemann M, Brandts B, zu Heringdorf DM, et al: Activation of muscarinic $K^+$ current in guinea-pig atrial myocytes by sphingosine-1-phosphate. J Physiol 1995;489(Pt 3):701-777.

208. MacDonell KL, Severson DL, Giles WR: Depression of excitability by sphingosine 1-phosphate in rat ventricular myocytes. Am J Physiol 1998;275:H2291-H2299.

209. Sekiguchi K, Yokoyama T, Kurabayashi M, et al: Sphingosylphosphorylcholine induces a hypertrophic growth response through the mitogen-activated protein kinase signaling cascade in rat neonatal myocytes. Circ Res 1999;85:1000-1008.

210. Karliner JS, Honbo N, Summers K, et al: The lysophospholipids sphingosine-1-phosphate and lysophosphatidic acid enhance survival during hypoxia in neonatal rat cardiac myocytes. J Mol Cell Cardiol 2001;33:1713-1717.

211. Hernandez OM, Discher DJ, Bishopric NH, et al: Rapid activation of neutral sphingomyelinase by hypoxia-reoxygenation of cardiac myocytes. Circ Res 2000;86:198-204.

212. Crackower MA, Sarao R, Oudit GY, et al: Angiotensin-converting enzyme 2 is an essential regulator of heart function. Nature 2002; 417:822-828.

213. Dinh DT, Frauman AG, Johnston CI, et al: Angiotensin receptors: Distribution, signalling and function. Clin Sci (Lond) 2001; 100:481-492.

214. Unger T: The role of the renin-angiotensin system in the development of cardiovascular disease. Am J Cardiol 2002;89:3A-9A.

215. Schnee JM, Hsueh WA: Angiotensin II, adhesion, and cardiac fibrosis. Cardiovasc Res 2000;46:264-268.

216. Sasaki K, Yamano Y, Bardhan S, et al: Cloning and expression of a complementary DNA encoding a bovine adrenal angiotensin II type-1 receptor. Nature 1991;351:230-233.

217. Brede M, Hein L: Transgenic mouse models of angiotensin receptor subtype function in the cardiovascular system. Regul Pept 2001;96:125-132.

218. Yoshida H, Kakuchi J, Guo DF, et al: Analysis of the evolution of angiotensin II type 1 receptor gene in mammals (mouse, rat, bovine and human). Biochem Biophys Res Commun 1992; 186:1042-1049.

219. Inagami T, Senbonmatsu T: Dual effects of angiotensin II type 2 receptor on cardiovascular hypertrophy. Trends Cardiovasc Med 2001;11:324-328.

220. Stoll M, Unger T: Angiotensin and its AT2 receptor: New insights into an old system. Regul Pept 2001;99:175-182.

221. Matsubara H: Pathophysiological role of angiotensin II type 2 receptor in cardiovascular and renal diseases. Circ Res 1998;83:1182-1191.

222. Ichiki T, Labosky PA, Shiota C, et al: Effects on blood pressure and exploratory behaviour of mice lacking angiotensin II type-2 receptor. Nature 1995;377:748-750.

223. Hein L, Barsh GS, Pratt RE, et al: Behavioural and cardiovascular effects of disrupting the angiotensin II type-2 receptor in mice. Nature 1995;377:744-747.

224. Brede M, Hadamek K, Meinel L, et al: Vascular hypertrophy and increased P70S6 kinase in mice lacking the angiotensin II AT(2) receptor. Circulation 2001;104:2602-2607.

225. Baker KM, Singer HA: Identification and characterization of guinea pig angiotensin II ventricular and atrial receptors: coupling to inositol phosphate production. Circ Res 1988;62: 896-904.

226. Paul K, Ball NA, Dorn GW, et al: Left ventricular stretch stimulates angiotensin II-mediated phosphatidylinositol hydrolysis and protein kinase C ε isoform translocation in adult guinea pig hearts. Circ Res 1997;81:643-650.

227. Lokuta AJ, Cooper C, Gaa ST, et al: Angiotensin II stimulates the release of phospholipid-derived second messengers through multiple receptor subtypes in heart cells. J Biol Chem 1994; 269:4832-4838.

228. Ushio-Fukai M, Griendling KK, Akers M, et al: Temporal dispersion of activation of phospholipase C-beta1 and -gamma isoforms by angiotensin II in vascular smooth muscle cells. Role of alphaq/11, alpha12, and beta gamma G protein subunits. J Biol Chem 1998;273:19772-19777.

229. Sadoshima J-I, Xu Y, Slayter HS, et al: Autocrine release of angiotensin II mediates stretch-induced hypertrophy of cardiac myocytes in vitro. Cell 1993;75:977-984.

230. Sadoshima J, Qiu Z, Morgan JP, et al: Angiotensin II and other hypertrophic stimuli mediated by G protein-coupled receptors activate tyrosine kinase, MAP kinase and 90-kD S6 kinase in cardiac myocytes: The critical role of $Ca^{2+}$-dependent signaling. Circ Res 1995;76:1-15.

231. McWhinney CD, Hunt RA, Conrad KM, et al: The type I angiotensin II receptor couples to Stat1 and Stat3 activation through Jak2 kinase in neonatal rat cardiac myocytes. J Mol Cell Cardiol 1997;29:2513-2524.

232. Saito Y, Berk BC: Transactivation: A novel signaling pathway from angiotensin II to tyrosine kinase receptors. J Mol Cell Cardiol 2001;33:3-7.

233. Fischer TA, Singh K, O'Hara DS, et al: Role of AT1 and AT2 receptors in regulation of MAPKs and MKP-1 by ANG II in adult myocytes. Am J Physiol 1998;275:H906-H916.

234. Bedecs K, Elbaz N, Sutren M, et al: Angiotensin II type 2 receptors mediate inhibition of mitogen-activated protein kinase cascade and functional activation of SHP-1 tyrosine phosphatase. Biochem J 1997;325(Pt 2):449-454.

235. Huang XC, Richards EM, Sumners C: Mitogen-activated protein kinases in rat brain neuronal cultures are activated by angiotensin II type 1 receptors and inhibited by angiotensin II type 2 receptors. J Biol Chem 1996;271:15635-15641.

236. Ito M, Oliverio MI, Mannon PJ, et al: Regulation of blood pressure by the type 1A angiotensin II receptor gene. Proc Natl Acad Sci USA 1995;92:3521-3525.

237. Sugaya T, Nishimatsu S, Tanimoto K, et al: Angiotensin II type 1a receptor-deficient mice with hypotension and hyperreninemia. J Biol Chem 1995;270:18719-18722.

238. Chen X, Li W, Yoshida H, et al: Targeting deletion of angiotensin type 1B receptor gene in the mouse. Am J Physiol 1997;272:F299-F304.

239. Oliverio MI, Kim HS, Ito M, et al: Reduced growth, abnormal kidney structure, and type 2 (AT2) angiotensin receptor-mediated blood pressure regulation in mice lacking both AT1A and AT1B receptors for angiotensin II. Proc Natl Acad Sci USA 1998; 95:15496-15501.

240. Tsuchida S, Matsusaka T, Chen X, et al: Murine double nullizygotes of the angiotensin type 1A and 1B receptor genes duplicate severe abnormal phenotypes of angiotensinogen nullizygotes. J Clin Invest 1998;101:755-760.

241. Rockman HA, Wachhorst SP, Mao L, et al: ANG II receptor blockade prevents ventricular hypertrophy and ANF gene expression with pressure overload in mice. Am J Physiol 1994;266:H2468-H2475.

242. Harada K, Komuro I, Shiojima I, et al: Pressure overload induces cardiac hypertrophy in angiotensin II type 1A receptor knockout mice. Circulation 1998;97:1952-1959.

243. Harada K, Komuro I, Zou Y, et al: Acute pressure overload could induce hypertrophic responses in the heart of angiotensin II type 1a knockout mice. Circ Res 1998;82:779-785.

244. Hamawaki M, Coffman TM, Lashus A, et al: Pressure-overload hypertrophy is unabated in mice devoid of AT1A receptors. Am J Physiol 1998;274:H868-H873.

245. Kudoh S, Komuro I, Hiro Y, et al: Mechanical stress induces hypertrophic responses in cardiac myocytes of angiotensin II type 1a knockout mice. J Biol Chem 1998;273:24037-24043.

246. Paradis P, Dali-Youcel N, Paradis FW, et al: Overexpression of angiotensin II type I receptor in cardiomyocytes induces cardiac hypertrophy and remodeling. Proc Natl Acad Sci USA 2000;97:931-936.

247. Thomas WG, Brandenburger Y, Autelitano DJ, et al: Adenoviral-directed expression of the type 1A angiotensin receptor promotes cardiomyocyte hypertrophy via transactivation of the epidermal growth factor receptor. Circ Res 2002;90:135-142.

248. Akishita M, Ito M, Lehtonen JY, et al: Expression of the AT2 receptor developmentally programs extracellular signal-regulated kinase activity and influences fetal vascular growth. J Clin Invest 1999;103:63-71.

249. Akishita M, Horiuchi M, Yamada H, et al: Inflammation influences vascular remodeling through AT2 receptor expression and signaling. Physiol Genomics 2000;2:13-20.

250. Bartunek J, Weinberg EO, Tajima M, et al: Angiotensin II type 2 receptor blockade amplifies the early signals of cardiac growth response to angiotensin II in hypertrophied hearts. Circulation 1999;99:22-25.

251. Senbonmatsu T, Ichihara S, Price E, et al: Evidence for angiotensin II type 2 receptor-mediated cardiac myocyte enlargement during in vivo pressure overload. J Clin Invest 2000;106:R25-R29.

252. Ichihara S, Senbonmatsu T, Price E Jr, et al: Angiotensin II type 2 receptor is essential for left ventricular hypertrophy and cardiac fibrosis in chronic angiotensin II-induced hypertension. Circulation 2001;104:346-351.

253. Coughlin SR: How the protease thrombin talks to cells. Proc Natl Acad Sci U S A 1999;96:11023-11027.

254. Sabri A, Short J, Guo J, et al: Protease-activated receptor-1-mediated DNA synthesis in cardiac fibroblast is via epidermal growth factor receptor transactivation: distinct PAR-1 signaling pathways in cardiac fibroblasts and cardiomyocytes. Circ Res 2002;91:532-539.

255. Steinberg SF, Robinson RB, Lieberman HB, et al: Thrombin modulates phosphoinositide metabolism, cytosolic calcium, and impulse initiation in the heart. Circ Res 1991;68:1216-1229.

256. Jiang T, Kuznetsov V, Pak E, et al: Thrombin receptor actions in neonatal rat ventricular myocytes. Circ Res 1996;78:553-563.

257. Glembotski CC, Irons CE, Krown KA, et al: Myocardial α-thrombin receptor activation induces hypertrophy and increases atrial natriuretic factor gene expression. J Biol Chem 1993;268:20646-20652.

258. Yasutake M, Haworth RS, King A, et al: Thrombin activates the sarcolemmal Na$^+$-H$^+$ exchanger: Evidence for a receptor-mediated mechanism involving protein kinase C. Circ Res 1996;79:705-715.

259. Connolly AJ, Ishihara H, Kahn ML, et al: Role of the thrombin receptor in development and evidence for a second receptor. Nature 1996;381:516-519.

260. Darrow AL, Fung-Leung WP, Ye RD, et al: Biological consequences of thrombin receptor deficiency in mice. Thrombosis Haemostasis 1996;76:860-866.

261. Cheung WM, D'Andrea MR, Andrade-Gordon P, et al: Altered vascular injury responses in mice deficient in protease-activated receptor-1. Arterioscler Thromb Vasc Biol 1999;19:3014-3024.

262. Molino M, Barnathan ES, Numerof R, et al: Interactions of mast cell tryptase with thrombin receptors and PAR-2. J Biol Chem 1997;272:4043-4049.

263. Dery O, Corvera CU, Steinhoff M, et al: Proteinase-activated receptors: Novel mechanisms of signaling by serine proteases. Am J Physiol 1998;274:C1429-C1452.

264. Kong W, McConalogue K, Khitin LM, et al: Luminal trypsin may regulate enterocytes through proteinase-activated receptor 2. Proc Natl Acad Sci USA 1997;94:8884-8889.

265. Corvera CU, Dery O, McConalogue K, et al: Mast cell tryptase regulates rat colonic myocytes through proteinase-activated receptor 2. J Clin Invest 1997;100:1383-1393.

266. Cocks TM, Fong B, Chow JM, et al: A protective role for protease-activated receptors in the airways. Nature 1999;398:156-160.

267. Konanen PT, Kaartinen M, Paavonen T: Infiltrates of activated mast cells at the site of coronary atheromatous erosion or rupture in myocardial infarction. Circulation 1995;92:1084-1088.

268. Mirza H, Yatsula V, Bahou WF: The proteinase activated receptor-2 (PAR-2) mediates mitogenic responses in human vascular endothelial cells: Molecular characterization and evidence for functional coupling to the thrombin receptor. J Clin Invest 1996; 97:1705-1714.

269. Hwa JJ, Ghibaudi L, Williams P, et al: Evidence for the presence of a proteinase-activated receptor distinct from the thrombin receptor in vascular endothelial cells. Circ Res 1996;78:581-588.

270. Patella V, Marino I, Arbustini E, et al: Stem cell factor in mast cells and increased mast cell density in idiopathic and ischemic cardiomyopathy. Circulation 1998;97:971-978.

271. Nystedt S, Ramakrishnan V, Sundelin J: The proteinase-activated receptor 2 is induced by inflammatory mediators in human endothelial cells. Comparison with the thrombin receptor. J Biol Chem 1996;271:14910-14915.

272. Hamilton JR, Frauman AG, Cocks TM: Increased expression of protease-activated receptor-2 (PAR2) and PAR4 in human coronary artery by inflammatory stimuli unveils endothelium-dependent relaxations to PAR2 and PAR4 agonists. Circ Res 2001;89:92-98.

273. Sabri A, Muske G, Zhang H, et al: Signaling properties and functions of two distinct cardiomyocyte protease-activated receptors. Circ Res 2000;86:1054-1061.

274. Shapiro MJ, Weiss EJ, Faruqi TR, et al: Protease-activated receptors 1 and 4 are shut off with distinct kinetics after activation by thrombin. J Biol Chem 2000;275:25216-25221.

275. Sabri A, Guo J, Elouardighi H, et al: Mechanisms of protease-activated receptor-4 actions in cardiomyocytes: Role of Src tyrosine kinase. J Biol Chem 2003;278:11714-11720.

276. Robertson SC, Tynan J, Donoghue DJ: RTK mutations and human syndromes: When good receptors turn bad. Trends Genet 2000;16:368.

277. Rentschler S, Zander J, Meyers K, et al: Neuregulin-1 promotes formation of the murine cardiac conduction system. Proc Natl Acad Sci U S A 2002;99:10464-10469.

278. Zhao YY, Sawyer DR, Baliga RR, et al: Neuregulins promote survival and growth of cardiac myocytes. Persistence of ErbB2 and ErbB4 expression in neonatal and adult ventricular myocytes. J Biol Chem 1998;273:10261-10269.

279. Baliga RR, Pimental DR, Zhao YY, et al: NRG-1-induced cardiomyocyte hypertrophy. Role of PI-3-kinase, p70$^{S6K}$, and MEK-MAPK-RSK. Am J Physiol 1999;277:H2026-H2037.

280. Feldman AM, Lorell BH, Reis SE Trastuzumab in the treatment of metastatic breast cancer: Anticancer therapy versus cardiotoxicity. Circulation 2000;102:272-274.

281. Bolger AP, Anker SD: Tumour necrosis factor in chronic heart failure: A peripheral view on pathogenesis, clinical manifestations and therapeutic implications. Drugs 2000;60:1245-1257.

282. Liu PP, Le J, Nian M: Nuclear factor-kappaB decoy: Infiltrating the heart of the matter in inflammatory heart disease. Circ Res 2001;89:850–852.

283. Baumgarten G, Knuefermann P, Mann DL: Cytokines as emerging targets in the treatment of heart failure. Trends Cardiovasc Med 2000;10:216–223.

284. Frangogiannis NG, Smith CW, Entman ML: The inflammatory response in myocardial infarction. Cardiovasc Res 2002;53:31–47.

285. Shi C, Zhang X, Chen Z, et al: Leukocyte integrin Mac-1 recruits toll/interleukin-1 receptor superfamily signaling intermediates to modulate NF-kappaB activity. Circ Res 2001;89:859–865.

286. Kupatt C, Habazettl H, Goedecke A, et al: Tumor necrosis factor-alpha contributes to ischemia- and reperfusion-induced endothelial activation in isolated hearts. Circ Res 1999;84:392–400.

287. Sack MN, Smith RM, Opie LH: Tumor necrosis factor in myocardial hypertrophy and ischaemia: An anti-apoptotic perspective. Cardiovasc Res 2000;45:688–695.

288. Sack M: Tumor necrosis factor-alpha in cardiovascular biology and the potential role for anti-tumor necrosis factor-alpha therapy in heart disease. Pharmacol Ther 2002;94:123–135.

289. Mann DL: Inflammatory mediators and the failing heart: past, present, and the foreseeable future. Circ Res 2002;91:988–998.

290. Meldrum DR: Tumor necrosis factor in the heart. Am J Physiol 1998;274:R577–R595.

291. Hallenbeck JM: The many faces of tumor necrosis factor in stroke. Nature Med 2002;8:1363–1368.

292. Condorelli G, Morisco C, Latronico MV, et al: TNF-alpha signal transduction in rat neonatal cardiac myocytes: Definition of pathways generating from the TNF-alpha receptor. FASEB J 2002;16:1732–1737.

293. Tracey KJ, Cerami A: Tumor necrosis factor, other cytokines and disease. Annu Rev Cell Biol 1993;9:317–343.

294. Locksley RM, Killeen N, Lenardo MJ: The TNF and TNF receptor superfamilies: Integrating mammalian biology. Cell 2001;104:487–501.

295. Idriss HT, Naismith JH: TNF alpha and the TNF receptor superfamily: Structure-function relationship(s). Microsc Res Tech 2000;50:184–195.

296. Kadokami T, Frye C, Lemster B, et al: Anti-tumor necrosis factor-alpha antibody limits heart failure in a transgenic model. Circulation 2001;104:1094–1097.

297. Kurrelmeyer KM, Michael LH, Baumgarten G, et al: Endogenous tumor necrosis factor protects the adult cardiac myocyte against ischemic-induced apoptosis in a murine model of acute myocardial infarction. Proc Natl Acad Sci USA 2000;97:5456–5461.

298. Ashkenazi A, Dixit V: Death receptors: Signaling and modulation. Science 1998;281:1305–1308.

299. Baud V, Karin M: Signal transduction by tumor necrosis factor and its relatives. Trends Cell Biol 2001;11:372–377.

300. Hsu H, Shu HB, Pan MG, et al: TRADD-TRAF2 and TRADD-FADD interactions define two distinct TNF receptor 1 signal transduction pathways. Cell 1996;84:299–308.

301. Rothe M, Wong SC, Henzel WJ, et al: A novel family of putative signal transducers associated with the cytoplasmic domain of the 75 kDa tumor necrosis factor receptor. Cell 1994;78:681–692.

302. Chinnaiyan AM, O'Rourke K, Tewari M, et al: FADD, a novel death domain-containing protein, interacts with the death domain of Fas and initiates apoptosis. Cell 1995;81:505–512.

303. Liu ZG, Hsu H, Goeddel DV, et al: Dissection of TNF receptor 1 effector functions: JNK activation is not linked to apoptosis while NF-kappaB activation prevents cell death. Cell 1996;87:565–576.

304. Stanger BZ, Leder P, Lee TH, et al: RIP: A novel protein containing a death domain that interacts with Fas/APO-1 (CD95) in yeast and causes cell death. Cell 1995;81:513–523.

305. Kelliher MA, Grimm S, Ishida Y, et al: The death domain kinase RIP mediates the TNF-induced NF-kappaB signal. Immunity 1998;8:297–303.

306. Yu PW, Huang BC, Shen M, et al: Identification of RIP3, a RIP-like kinase that activates apoptosis and NFkappaB. Curr Biol 1999;9:539–542.

307. Arch RH, Gedrich RW, Thompson CB: Tumor necrosis factor receptor-associated factors (TRAFs)–a family of adapter proteins that regulates life and death. Genes Dev 1998;12:2821–2830.

308. Rothe M, Sarma V, Dixit VM, et al: TRAF2-mediated activation of NF-kappa B by TNF receptor 2 and CD40. Science 1995;269:1424–1427.

309. Park YC, Ye H, Hsia C, et al: A novel mechanism of TRAF signaling revealed by structural and functional analyses of the TRADD-TRAF2 interaction. Cell 2000;101:777–787.

310. Lee SY, Reichlin A, Santana A, et al: TRAF2 is essential for JNK but not NF-kappaB activation and regulates lymphocyte proliferation and survival. Immunity 1997;7:703–713.

311. Devin A, Cook A, Lin Y, et al: The distinct roles of TRAF2 and RIP in IKK activation by TNF-R1: TRAF2 recruits IKK to TNF-R1 while RIP mediates IKK activation. Immunity 2000;12:419–429.

312. Medzhitov R: CpG DNA: Security code for host defense. Nat Immunol 2001;2:15–16.

313. Hashimoto C, Hudson KL, Anderson KV: The Toll gene of Drosophila, required for dorsal-ventral embryonic polarity, appears to encode a transmembrane protein. Cell 1988;52:269–279.

314. Belvin MP, Anderson KV: A conserved signaling pathway: The Drosophila toll-dorsal pathway. Annu Rev Cell Dev Biol 1996;12:393–416.

315. Lemaitre B, Nicolas E, Michaut L, et al: The dorsoventral regulatory gene cassette spatzle/Toll/cactus controls the potent antifungal response in Drosophila adults. Cell 1996;86:973–983.

316. Asea A, Kraeft SK, Kurt-Jones EA, et al: HSP70 stimulates cytokine production through a CD14-dependant pathway, demonstrating its dual role as a chaperone and cytokine. Nat Med 2000;6:435–442.

317. Ohashi K, Burkart V, Flohe S, et al: Cutting edge: heat shock protein 60 is a putative endogenous ligand of the toll-like receptor-4 complex. J Immunol 2000;164:558–561.

318. Rock FL, Hardiman G, Timans JC, et al: A family of human receptors structurally related to Drosophila Toll. Proc Natl Acad Sci USA 1998;95:588–593.

319. Wesche H, Henzel WJ, Shillinglaw W, et al: MyD88: an adapter that recruits IRAK to the IL-1 receptor complex. Immunity 1997;7:837–847.

320. Shimazu R, Akashi S, Ogata H, et al: MD-2, a molecule that confers lipopolysaccharide responsiveness on Toll-like receptor 4. J Exp Med 1999;189:1777–1782.

321. Nemoto S, Vallejo JG, Knuefermann P, et al: Escherichia coli LPS-induced LV dysfunction: Role of toll-like receptor-4 in the adult heart. Am J Physiol Heart Circ Physiol 2002;282:H2316–H2323.

322. Muzio M, Ni J, Feng P, et al: IRAK (Pelle) family member IRAK-2 and MyD88 as proximal mediators of IL-1 signaling. Science 1997;278:1612–1615.

323. Adachi O, Kawai T, Takeda K, et al: Targeted disruption of the MyD88 gene results in loss of IL-1- and IL-18-mediated function. Immunity 1998;9:143–150.

324. Kawai T, Adachi O, Ogawa T, et al: Unresponsiveness of MyD88-deficient mice to endotoxin. Immunity 1999;11:115–122.

325. Fitzgerald KA, Palsson-McDermott EM, Bowie AG, et al: Mal (MyD88-adapter-like) is required for Toll-like receptor-4 signal transduction. Nature 2001;413:78–83.

326. Horng T, Barton GM, Medzhitov R: TIRAP: An adapter molecule in the Toll signaling pathway. Nat Immunol 2001;2:835–841.

327. Cao Z, Xiong J, Takeuchi M, et al: TRAF6 is a signal transducer for interleukin-1. Nature 1996;383:443–446.

328. Cao Z, Henzel WJ, Gao X: IRAK: A kinase associated with the interleukin-1 receptor. Science 1996;271:1128–1131.

329. Li X, Commane M, Jiang Z, et al: IL-1-induced NFkappa B and c-Jun N-terminal kinase (JNK) activation diverge at IL-1 receptor-associated kinase (IRAK). Proc Natl Acad Sci U S A 2001;98:4461–4465.

330. Aravind L, Dixit VM, Koonin EV: Apoptotic molecular machinery: Vastly increased complexity in vertebrates revealed by genome comparisons. Science 2001;291:1279–1284.

331. Lomaga MA, Yeh WC, Sarosi I, et al: TRAF6 deficiency results in osteopetrosis and defective interleukin-1, CD40, and LPS signaling. Genes Dev 1999;13:1015–1024.

332. Hollinger S, Hepler JR: Cellular regulation of RGS proteins: Modulators and integrators of G protein signaling. Pharmacol Rev 2002;54:527–559.

333. Wedegaertner PB, Wilson PT, Bourne HR: Lipid modifications of trimeric G proteins. J Biol Chem 1995;270:503–506.

334. McIntire WE, MacCleery G, Garrison JC: The G protein beta subunit is a determinant in the coupling of Gs to the $\beta_1$-adrenergic and A2a adenosine receptors. J Biol Chem 2001;276:15801–15809.

335. Siffert W, Rosskopf D, Siffert G, et al: Association of a human G-protein $\beta_3$ subunit variant with hypertension. Nat Genet 1998;18:45–48.

336. Virchow S, Ansorge N, Rosskopf D, et al: The G protein beta3 subunit splice variant G$\beta_3$s causes enhanced chemotaxis of human neutrophils in response to interleukin-8. Naunyn Schmiedebergs Arch Pharmacol 1999;360:27–36.

337. Baumgart D, Naber C, Haude M, et al: G protein $\beta_3$ subunit 825T allele and enhanced coronary vasoconstriction on alpha(2)-adrenoceptor activation. Circ Res 1999;85:965–969.

338. Cook LA, Schey KL, Wilcox MD, et al: Heterogeneous processing of a G protein γsubunit at a site critical for protein and membrane interactions. Biochemistry 1998;37:12280–12286.

339. Hansen CA, Schroering AG, Robishaw JD: Subunit expression of signal transducing G proteins in cardiac tissue: Implications for phospholipase C-β regulation. J Mol Cell Cardiol 1995;27:471–484.

340. Balcueva EA, Wang Q, Hughes H, et al: Human G protein $\gamma_{11}$ and $\gamma_{14}$ subtypes define a new functional subclass. Exp Cell Res 2000; 257:310–319.

341. Ray K, Kunsch C, Bonner LM, et al: Isolation of cDNA clones encoding eight different human G protein γ subunits, including three novel forms designated the $\gamma_4$, $\gamma_{10}$, and $\gamma_{11}$ subunits. J Biol Chem 1995;270:21765–21771.

342. Wang Q, Mullah BK, Robishaw JD: Ribozyme approach identifies a functional association between the G protein $\beta_1\gamma_7$ subunits in the β-adrenergic receptor signaling pathway. J Biol Chem 1999;274:17365–17371.

343. Wang Q, Mullah B, Hanson C, et al: Ribozyme-mediated suppression of the G protein $\gamma_7$ subunit suggests a role in hormone regulation of adenylylcyclase activity. J Biol Chem 1997;272:26040–26048.

344. Robillard L, Ethier N, Lachance M, et al: Gβγ subunit combinations differentially modulate receptor and effector coupling *in vivo*. Cell Signal 2000;12:673–682.

345. Vatner SF, Vatner DE, Homcy CJ: β-Adrenergic receptor signaling: An acute compensatory adjustment-inappropriate for the chronic stress of heart failure? Insights from Gsα overexpression and other genetically engineered animal models. Circ Res 2000; 86:502–506.

346. Gu C, Ma YC, Benjamin J, et al: Apoptotic signaling through the β-adrenergic receptor: A new $G_s$ effector pathway. J Biol Chem 2000;275:20726–20733.

347. Ma YC, Huang J, Ali S, et al: Src tyrosine kinase is a novel direct effector of G proteins. Cell 2000;102:635–646.

348. Jain M, Lim CC, Nagata K, et al: Targeted inactivation of G$\alpha_i$ does not alter cardiac function or β-adrenergic sensitivity. Am J Physiol Heart Circ Physiol 2001;280:H569–H575.

349. Jiang M, Gold MS, Boulay G, et al: Multiple neurological abnormalities in mice deficient in the G protein $G_o$. Proc Natl Acad Sci USA 1998;95:3269–3274.

350. Rudolph U, Spicher K, Birnbaumer L: Adenylyl cyclase inhibition and altered G protein subunit expression and ADP-ribosylation patterns in tissues and cells from $G_{i2}\alpha$-/-mice. Proc Natl Acad Sci USA 1996;93:3209–3214.

351. Sowell MO, Ye C, Ricupero DA, et al: Targeted inactivation of $\alpha_{i2}$ or $\alpha_{i3}$ disrupts activation of the cardiac muscarinic K$^+$ channel, $I_K{}^+$Ach, in intact cells. Proc Natl Acad Sci U S A 1997;94:7921–7926.

352. Yatani A, Okabe K, Codina J, et al: Heart rate regulation by G proteins acting on the cardiac pacemaker channel. Science 1990;249:1163–1166.

353. Retondaro FC, Dos Santos Costa PC, Pedrosa RC, et al: Presence of antibodies against the third intracellular loop of the m2 muscarinic receptor in the sera of chronic chagasic patients. FASEB J 1999;13:2015–2020.

354. Redfern CH, Coward P, Degtyarev MY, et al: Conditional expression and signaling of a specifically designed Gi-coupled receptor in transgenic mice. Nat Biotechnol 1999;17:165–169.

355. Strathmann M, Simon MI: G protein diversity: A distinct class of α subunits is present in vertebrates and invertebrates. Proc Natl Acad Sci USA 1990;87:9113–9117.

356. Wilkie TM, Scherle PA, Strathmann MP, et al: Characterization of G-protein α subunits in the $G_q$ class: Expression in murine tissues and in stromal and hematopoietic cell lines. Proc Natl Acad Sci USA 1991;88:10049–10053.

357. Smrcka AV, Hepler JR, Brown KO, et al: Regulation of polyphosphoinositide-specific phospholipase C activity by purified Gq. Science 1991;251:804–807.

358. Berstein G, Blank JL, Smrcka AV, et al: Reconstitution of agonist-stimulated phosphatidylinositol 4,5-bisphosphate hydrolysis using purified m1 muscarinic receptor, $G_{q/11}$, and phospholipase C-β1. J Biol Chem 1992;267:8081–8088.

359. Venkatakrishnan G, Exton JH: Identification of determinants in the α-subunit of $G_q$ required for phospholipase C activation. J Biol Chem 1996;271:5066–5072.

360. Berstein G, Blank JL, Jhon D-Y, et al: Phospholipase C-β1 is a GTPase-activating protein for $G_{q/11}$, its physiological regulator. Cell 1992;70:411–418.

361. Conklin BR, Chabre O, Wong YH, et al: Recombinant Gqα. J Biol Chem 1992;267:31–34.

362. Qian N-X, Winitz S, Johnson GL: Epitope-tagged Gq α subunits: Expression of GTPase-deficient α subunits persistently stimulates phosphatidylinositol-specific phospholipase C but not mitogen-activated protein kinase activity regulated by the M1 muscarinic acetylcholine receptor. Proc Natl Acad Sci U S A 1993;90:4077–4081.

363. Wilson BA, Zhu X, Ho M, et al: *Pasteurella multocida* toxin activates the inositol triphosphate signaling pathway in *Xenopus* oocytes via $G_q$α-coupled Phospholipase c-β1. J Biol Chem 1997; 272:1268–1275.

364. Zywietz A, Gohla A, Schmelz M, et al: Pleiotropic effects of Pasteurella multocida toxin are mediated by Gq-dependent and -independent mechanisms: Involvement of Gq but not G11. J Biol Chem 2001;276:3840–3845.

365. Adams JW, Brown JH: G-proteins in growth and apoptosis: lessons from the heart. Oncogene 2001;20:1626–1634.

366. LaMorte VJ, Thorburn J, Absher D, et al: $G_q$- and Ras-dependent pathways mediate hypertrophy of neonatal rat ventricular myocytes following $\alpha_1$-adrenergic stimulation. J Biol Chem 1994; 269:13490–13496.

367. D'Angelo DD, Sakata Y, Lorenz JN, et al: Transgenic G$\alpha_q$ overexpression induces cardiac contractile failure in mice. Proc Natl Acad Sci USA 1997;94:8121–8126.

368. Mende U, Kagen A, Cohen A, et al: Transient cardiac expression of constitutively active G$\alpha_q$ leads to hypertrophy and dilated cardiomyopathy by calcineurin-dependent and independent pathways. Proc Natl Acad Sci USA 1998;95:13893–13898.

369. Umemori H, Inoue T, Kume S, et al: Activation of the G protein $G_{q/11}$ through tyrosine phosphorylation of the α subunit. Science 1997;276:1878–1881.

370. Rogers JH, Tamirisa P, Kovacs A, et al: RGS4 causes increased mortality and reduced cardiac hypertrophy in response to pressure overload. J Clin Invest 1999;104:567–576.

371. Offermanns S, Hashimoto K, Watanabe M, et al: Impaired motor coordination and persistent multiple climbing fiber innervation of cerebellar Purkinje cells in mice lacking Gαq. Proc Natl Acad Sci USA 1997;94:14089–14094.

372. Offermanns S, Toombs CF, Hu Y-H, et al: Defective platelet activation in G$\alpha_q$-deficient mice. Nature 1997;389:183–186.

373. Offermanns S, Zhao L-P, Gohla A, et al: Embryonic cardiomyocyte hypoplasia and craniofacial defects in G$\alpha_q$/G$\alpha_{11}$-mutant mice. EMBO J 1998;17:4304–4312.

374. Wettschureck N, Rutten H, Zywietz A, et al: Absence of pressure overload induced myocardial hypertrophy after conditional inactivation of Galphaq/Galpha11 in cardiomyocytes. Nat Med 2001;7:1236–1240.

375. Adams JW, Pagel AL, Means CK, et al: Cardiomyocyte apoptosis induced by Galphaq signaling is mediated by permeability transition pore formation and activation of the mitochondrial death pathway. Circ Res 2000;87:1180–1187.

376. Howes AL, Arthur JF, Zhang T, et al: Akt-mediated cardiomyocyte survival pathways are compromised by G$\alpha_q$-induced phosphoinositide 4,5-bisphosphate depletion. J Biol Chem 2003;278: 40343–40351.

377. Luttrell LM, van Biesen T, Hawes BE, et al: G-protein-coupled receptors and their regulation: activation of the MAP kinase signaling pathway by G-protein-coupled receptors. Adv Second Messenger Phosphoprotein Res 1997;31:263–277.

378. Pierce KL, Luttrell LM, Lefkowitz RJ: New mechanisms in heptahelical receptor signaling to mitogen activated protein kinase cascades. Oncogene 2001;20:1532–1539.

379. Thorburn A, Thorburn J, Chen S-Y, et al: H-Ras-dependent pathways can activate morphological and genetic markers of cardiac muscle cell hypertrophy. J Biol Chem 1993;268:2244–2249.

380. Chiloeches A, Paterson HF, Marais R, et al: Regulation of Ras-GTP loading and Ras-Raf association in neonatal rat ventricular

myocytes by G protein-coupled receptor agonists and phorbol ester: Activation of the extracellular signal-regulated kinase cascade by phorbol ester is mediated by Ras. J Biol Chem 1999;274:19762–19770.

381. Ramirez MT, Sah VP, Zhao X, et al: The MEKK-JNK pathway is stimulated by $\alpha_1$-adrenergic receptor and Ras activation and is associated with *in vitro* and *in vivo* cardiac hypertrophy. J Biol Chem 1997;272:14057–14061.

382. Clerk A, Pham FH, Fuller SJ, et al: Regulation of mitogen-activated protein kinases in cardiac myocytes through the small G protein Rac1. Mol Cell Biol 2001;21:1173–1184.

383. Aoki H, Richmond M, Izumo S, et al: Specific role of the extracellular signal-regulated kinase pathway in angiotensin II-induced cardiac hypertrophy in vitro. Biochem J 2000;347(Pt 1):275–284.

384. Hunter JJ, Tanaka N, Rockman HA, et al: Ventricular expression of a MLC-2/v-Ras fusion gene induces cardiac hypertrophy and selective diastolic dysfunction in transgenic mice. J Biol Chem 1995;270:23173–23178.

385. Gottshall KR, Hunter JJ, Tanaka N, et al: Ras-dependent pathways induce obstructive hypertrophy in echo-selected transgenic mice. Proc Natl Acad Sci USA 1997;94:4710–4715.

386. Kozma R, Ahmed S, Best A, et al: The Ras-related protein Cdc42Hs and bradykinin promote formation of peripheral actin microspikes and filopodia in Swiss 3T3 fibroblasts. Mol Cell Biol 1995;15:1942–1952.

387. Nobes CD, Hall A: Rho, rac and cdc42 GTPases regulate the assembly of multimolecular focal complexes associated with actin stress fibers, lamellipodia, and filopodia. Cell 1995;81:53–62.

388. Schmidt G, Aktories K: Bacterial cytotoxins target Rho GTPases. Naturwissenschaften 1998;85:253–261.

389. Sah VP, Hoshijima M, Chien KR, et al: Rho is required for $G\alpha_q$ and $\alpha_1$-adrenergic receptor signaling in cardiomyocytes: Dissociation of Ras and Rho pathways. J Biol Chem 1996;271:31185–31190.

390. Hoshijima M, Sah VP, Wang Y, et al: The low molecular weight GTPase Rho regulates myofibril formation and organization in neonatal rat ventricular myocytes: Involvement of Rho kinase. J Biol Chem 1998;273:7725–7730.

391. Aikawa R, Komuro I, Yamazaki T, et al: Rho family small G proteins play critical roles in mechanical stress-induced hypertrophic responses in cardiac myocytes. Circ Res 1999;84:458–466.

392. Thorburn J, Xu S, Thorburn A: MAP kinase- and Rho-dependent signals interact to regulate gene expression but not actin morphology in cardiac muscle cells. EMBO J 1997;16:1888–1900.

393. Laufs U, Kilter H, Konkol C, et al: Impact of HMG CoA reductase inhibition on small GTPases in the heart. Cardiovasc Res 2002;53:911–920.

394. Takemoto M, Node K, Nakagami H, et al: Statins as antioxidant therapy for preventing cardiac myocyte hypertrophy. J Clin Invest 2001;108:1429–1437.

395. Oi S, Haneda T, Osaki J, et al: Lovastatin prevents angiotensin II-induced cardiac hypertrophy in cultured neonatal rat heart cells. Eur J Pharmacol 1999;376:139–148.

396. Yamazaki M, Zhang Y, Watanabe H, et al: Interaction of the small G protein RhoA with the C terminus of human phospholipase D1. J Biol Chem 1999;274:6035–6038.

397. Chong LD, Traynor-Kaplan A, Bokoch GM, et al: The small GTP-binding protein Rho regulates a phosphatidylinositol 4-phosphate 5-kinase in mammalian cells. Cell 1994;79:507–513.

398. Oude Weernink PA, Schulte P, Guo Y, et al: Stimulation of phosphatidylinositol-4-phosphate 5-kinase by Rho-kinase. J Biol Chem 2000;275:10168–10174.

399. Chatah NE, Abrams CS: G-protein-coupled receptor activation induces the membrane translocation and activation of phosphatidylinositol-4-phosphate 5-kinase I alpha by a Rac- and Rho-dependent pathway. J Biol Chem 2001;276:34059–34065.

400. Walker SJ, Brown HA: Specificity of Rho insert-mediated activation of phospholipase D1. J Biol Chem 2002;277:26260–26267.

401. Amano M, Fukata Y, Kaibuchi K: Regulation and functions of Rho-associated kinase. Exp Cell Res 2000;261:44–51.

402. Gong MC, Fujihara H, Somlyo AV, et al: Translocation of *rhoA* associated with $Ca^{2+}$ sensitization of smooth muscle. J Biol Chem 1997;272:10704–10709.

403. Fukata Y, Amano M, Kaibuchi K: Rho-Rho-kinase pathway in smooth muscle contraction and cytoskeletal reorganization of non-muscle cells. Trends Pharmacol Sci 2001;22:32–39.

404. Uehata M, Ishizaki T, Satoh H, et al: Calcium sensitization of smooth muscle mediated by a Rho-associated protein kinase in hypertension. Nature 1997;389:990–994.

405. Kuwahara K, Saito Y, Nakagawa O, et al: The effects of the selective ROCK inhibitor, Y27632, on ET-1-induced hypertrophic response in neonatal rat cardiomyocytes: Possible involvement of Rho/ROCK pathway in cardiac muscle cell hypertrophy. FEBS Lett 1999;452:314–318.

406. Seasholtz TM, Majumdar M, Brown JH: Rho as a mediator of G protein-coupled receptor signaling. Mol Pharmacol 1999;l55:949.

407. Sah VP, Seasholtz TM, Sagi SA, et al: The role of Rho in G protein-coupled receptor signal transduction. Ann Rev Pharmacol Toxicol 2000;40:459–489.

408. Aoki H, Izumo S, Sadoshima J: Angiotensin II activates RhoA in cardiac myocytes: A critical role of RhoA in angiotensin II-induced premyofibril formation. Circ Res 1998;82:666–676.

409. Sah VP, Minamisawa S, Tam SP, et al: Cardiac-specific overexpression of RhoA results in sinus and atrioventricular nodal dysfunction and contractile failure. J Clin Invest 1999;103:1627–1634.

410. Seasholtz TM, Majumdar M, Kaplan DD, et al: Rho and Rho kinase mediate thrombin-stimulated vascular smooth muscle cell DNA synthesis and migration. Circ Res 1999;84:1186–1193.

411. Seasholtz TM, Zhang T, Morissette MR, et al: Increased expression and activity of RhoA is associated with increased DNA synthesis and reduced $p27^{Kip1}$ expression in the vasculature of hypertensive rats. Circ Res 2001;89:488–495.

412. Manser E, Leung T, Salihuddin H, et al: A brain serine/threonine protein kinase activated by Cdc42 and Rac1. Nature 1994;367:40–46.

413. Knaus UG, Morris S, Dong H-J, et al: Regulation of human leukocyte p21-activated kinases through G protein-coupled receptors. Science 1995;269:221–223.

414. Vojtek AB, Cooper JA: Rho family members: activators of MAP kinase cascades. Cell 1995;82:527–529.

415. Coso OA, Chiariello M, Yu J-C, et al: The small GTP binding proteins Rac1 and Cdc42 regulate the activity of the JNK/SAPK signaling pathway. Cell 1995;81:1137–1146.

416. Minden A, Lin A, Claret F-X, et al: Selective activation of the JNK signaling cascade and c-Jun transcriptional activity by the small GTPases Rac and Cdc42Hs. Cell 1995;81:1147–1157.

417. Qiu R-G, Chen J, Kirn D, et al: An essential role for Rac in Ras transformation. Nature 1995;374:457–459.

418. Khosravi-Far R, Solski PA, Clark GJ, et al: Activation of Rac1, RhoA, and mitogen-activated protein kinases is required for Ras transformation. Mol Cell Biol 1995;15:6443–6453.

419. Olson MF, Ashworth A, Hall A: An essential role for Rho, Rac, and Cdc42 GTPases in cell cycle progression through $G_1$. Science 1995;269:1270–1272.

420. Ridley AJ, Paterson HF, Johnston CL, et al: The small GTP-binding protein rac regulates growth factor-induced membrane ruffling. Cell 1992;70:401–410.

421. Hall A: Rho GTPases and the actin cytoskeleton. Science 1998;279:509–519.

422. Sander EE, ten Klooster JP, van Delft S, et al: Rac downregulates Rho activity: Reciprocal balance between both GTPases determines cellular morphology and migratory behavior. J Cell Biol 1999;147:1009–1021.

423. Pracyk JB, Tanaka K, Hegland DD, et al: A requirement for the rac1 GTPase in the signal transduction pathway leading to cardiac myocyte hypertrophy. J Clin Invest 1998;102:929–937.

424. Sussman MA, Welch S, Walker A, et al: Altered focal adhesion regulation correlates with cardiomyopathy in mice expressing constitutively active rac1. J Clin Invest 2000;105:875–886.

425. Clerk A, Sugden PH: Small guanine nucleotide-binding proteins and myocardial hypertrophy. Circ Res 2000;86:1019–1023.

426. Cali JJ, Parekh RS, Krupinski J: Splice variants of type VIII adenylyl cyclase. Differences in glycosylation and regulation by $Ca^{2+}$/calmodulin. J Biol Chem 1996;271:1089–1095.

427. Gu C, Sorkin A, Cooper DM: Persistent interactions between the two transmembrane clusters dictate the targeting and functional assembly of adenylyl cyclase. Curr Biol 2001;11:185–190.

428. Seebacher T, Linder JU, Schultz JE: An isoform-specific interaction of the membrane anchors affects mammalian adenylyl cyclase type V activity. Eur J Biochem 2001;268:105–110.

429. Villacres EC, Wu Z, Hua W, et al: Developmentally expressed $Ca^{2+}$-sensitive adenylyl cyclase activity is disrupted in the brains of

type I adenylyl cyclase mutant mice. J Biol Chem 1995;270: 14352–14357.

430. Abdel-Majid RM, Leong WL, Schalkwyk LC, et al: Loss of adenylyl cyclase I activity disrupts patterning of mouse somatosensory cortex. Nat Genet 1998;19:289–291.

431. Cui H, Green RD: Cell-specific properties of type V and type IX adenylyl cyclase isozymes in 293T cells and embryonic chick ventricular myocytes. Biochem Biophys Res Commun 2001;283:107–112.

432. Schwencke C, Yamamoto M, Okumura S, et al: Compartmentation of cyclic adenosine 3′, 5′-monophosphate signaling in caveolae. Mol Endocrinol 1999;13:1061–1070.

433. Lai HL, Lin TH, Kao YY, et al: The N terminus domain of type VI adenylyl cyclase mediates its inhibition by protein kinase C. Mol Pharmacol 1999;56:644–650.

434. Premont RT, Chen J, Ma HW, et al: Two members of a widely expressed subfamily of hormone-stimulated adenylyl cyclases. Proc Natl Acad Sci U S A 1992;89:9809–9813.

435. Aprigliano O, Rybin VO, Pak E, et al: $\beta_1$- and $\beta_2$-adrenergic receptors exhibit differing susceptibility to muscarinic accentuated antagonism. Am J Physiol 1997;272:H2726–H2735.

436. Puceat M, Bony C, Jaconi M, et al: Specific activation of adenylyl cyclase V by a purinergic agonist. FEBS Lett 1998;431:189–194.

437. Puceat M, Clement-Chomienne O, Terzic A, et al: Alpha 1-adrenoceptor and purinoceptor agonists modulate Na-H antiport in single cardiac cells. Am J Physiol 1993;264:H310–H319.

438. Tobise K, Ishikawa Y, Holmer SR, et al: Changes in Type VI adenylyl cyclase isoform expression correlate with a decreased capacity for cAMP generation in the aging ventricle. Circ Res 1994;74:596–603.

439. Tepe NM, Lorenz JN, Yatani A, et al: Altering the receptor-effector ratio by transgenic overexpression of type V adenylyl cyclase: Enhanced basal catalytic activity and function without increased cardiomyocyte beta-adrenergic signalling. Biochemistry 1999; 38:16706–16713.

440. Georget M, Mateo P, Vandecasteele G, et al: Augmentation of cardiac contractility with no change in L-type $Ca^{2+}$ current in transgenic mice with a cardiac-directed expression of the human adenylyl cyclase type 8 (AC8). FASEB J 2002;16:1636–1636.

441. Lipskaia L, Defer N, Esposito G, et al: Enhanced cardiac function in transgenic mice expressing a $Ca^{2+}$-stimulated adenylyl cyclase. Circ Res 2000;86:795–801.

442. Hokin MR, Hokin LE: Enzyme secretion and the incorporation of $^{32}P$ into phospholipids of pancreas slices. J Biol Chem 1953; 203:967–977.

443. Michell RH: Inositol phospholipids and cell surface receptor function. Biochim Biophys Acta 1975;415:81–147.

444. Berridge MJ: Inositol trisphosphate and diacylglycerol: Two interacting second messengers. Ann Rev Biochem 1987;56:159–193.

445. Berridge MJ, Irvine RF: Inositol trisphosphate, a novel second messenger in cellular signal transduction. Nature 1984;312:315–321.

446. Streb H, Irvine RF, Berridge MJ, et al: Release of $Ca^{2+}$ from a nonmitochondrial intracellular store in pancreatic acinar cells by inositol-1,4,5 trisphosphate. Nature 1983;306:67–69.

447. Rhee SG: Inositol phospholipids-specific phospholipase C: Interaction of the gamma 1 isoform with tyrosine kinase. Trends Biochem Sci 1991;16:297–301.

448. Rhee SG, Choi KD: Multiple forms of phospholipase C isozymes and their activation mechanisms. Adv Second Messenger Phosphoprotein Res 1992;26:35–61.

449. Singer WD, Brown HA, Sternweis PC: Regulation of eukaryotic phosphatidylinositol-specific phospholipase C and phospholipase D. Annu Rev Biochem 1997;66:475–509.

450. Rebecchi MJ, Pentyala SN: Structure, function, and control of phosphoinositide-specific phospholipase C. Physiol Rev 2000; 80:1291–1335.

451. Rhee SG: Regulation of phosphoinositide-specific phospholipase C. Annu Rev Biochem 2001;70:281–312.

452. Wing MR, Houston D, Kelley GG, et al: Activation of phospholipase C-epsilon by heterotrimeric G protein betagamma-subunits. J Biol Chem 2001;276:48257–48261.

453. Kelley GG, Reks SE, Ondrako JM, et al: Phospholipase C(epsilon): A novel Ras effector. EMBO J 2001;20:743–754.

454. Lopez I, Mak EC, Ding J, et al: A novel bifunctional phospholipase c that is regulated by Galpha 12 and stimulates the Ras/mitogen-activated protein kinase pathway. J Biol Chem 2001; 276:2758–2758.

455. Evellin S, Nolte J, Tysack K, et al: Stimulation of phospholipase C-epsilon by the M3 muscarinic acetylcholine receptor mediated by cyclic AMP and the GTPase Rap2B. J Biol Chem 2002;277: 16805–16813.

456. Schmidt M, Evellin S, Weernink PA, et al: A new phospholipase-C-calcium signalling pathway mediated by cyclic AMP and a Rap GTPase. Nat Cell Biol 2001;3:1020–1024.

457. Essen LO, Perisic O, Cheung R, et al: Crystal structure of a mammalian phosphoinositide-specific phospholipase C delta. Nature 1996;380:595–602.

458. Brown JH, Brown SL: Agonists differentiate muscarinic receptors that inhibit cyclic AMP formation from those that stimulate phosphoinositide metabolism. J Biol Chem 1984;259:3777–3781.

459. Brown JH, Goldstein D: Differences in muscarinic receptor reserve for inhibition of adenylate cyclase and stimulation of phosphoinositide hydrolysis in chick heart cells. Mol Pharmacol 1986;30:566–570.

460. Brown JH, Jones LG: Phosphoinositide metabolism in the heart. In Putney TW (ed): Phosphoinositide and Receptor Mechanisms. New York, Alan R. Russ, 1986, pp 245–270.

461. Brown JH, Martinson EA: Phosphoinositide-generated second messengers in cardiac signal transduction. Trends Cardiovasc Med 1992;2:209–214.

462. Renard D, Poggioli J: Does the inositol tris/tetrakisphosphate pathway exist in rat heart? FEBS Lett 1987;217:117–123.

463. Moschella MC, Marks AR: Inositol 1,4,5-trisphosphate receptor expression in cardiac myocytes. J Cell Biol 1993;120:1137–1146.

464. Kijima Y, Saito A, Jetton TL, et al: Different intracellular localization of inositol 1,4,5-trisphosphate and ryanodine receptors in cardiomyocytes. J Biol Chem 1993;268:3499–3506.

465. Perez PJ, Ramos-Franco J, Fill M, et al: Identification and functional reconstitution of the type 2 inositol 1,4,5-trisphosphate receptor from ventricular cardiac myocytes. J Biol Chem 1997;272: 23961–23969.

466. Woodcock EA, Lambert KA, Du XJ: Ins(1,4,5)P3 during myocardial ischemia and its relationship to the development of arrhythmias. J Mol Cell Cardiol 1996;28:2129–2138.

467. Harrison SN, Autelitano DJ, Wang BH, et al: Reduced reperfusion-induced $Ins(1,4,5)P_3$ generation and arrhythmias in hearts expressing constitutively active $\alpha_{1B}$-adrenergic receptors. Circ Res 1998;83:1232–1240.

468. Matkovich SJ, Woodcock EA: $Ca^{2+}$-activated but not G protein-mediated inositol phosphate responses in rat neonatal cardiomyocytes involve inositol 1,4,5-trisphosphate generation. J Biol Chem 2000;275:10845–10850.

469. Lipp P, Laine M, Tovey SC, et al: Functional InsP3 receptors that may modulate excitation-contraction coupling in the heart. Curr Biol 2000;10:939–942.

470. Jaconi M, Bony C, Richards S, et al: Inositol 1,4,5-trisphosphate directs $Ca^{2+}$ flow between mitochondria and the endoplasmic/sarcoplasmic reticulum role in regulating cardiac autonomic $Ca^{2+}$ spiking. Mol Biol Cell 2000;11:1845–1858.

471. Jones LG, Goldstein D, Brown JH: Guanine nucleotide-dependent inositol trisphosphate formation in chick heart cells. Circ Res 1988;62:299–305.

472. Schnabel P, Gas H, Nohr T, et al: Identification and characterization of G protein-regulated phospholipase C in human myocardium. J Mol Cell Cardiol 1996;28:2419–2427.

473. Arthur JF, Matkovich SJ, Mitchell CJ, et al: Evidence for selective coupling of alpha 1-adrenergic receptors to phospholipase C-beta 1 in rat neonatal cardiomyocytes. J Biol Chem 2001; 276:37341–37346.

474. Wang S, Gebre-Medhin S, Betsholtz C, et al: Targeted disruption of the mouse phospholipase C beta3 gene results in early embryonic lethality. FEBS Lett 1998;441:261–265.

475. Xie W, Samoriski GM, McLaughlin JP, et al: Genetic alteration of phospholipase C beta3 expression modulates behavioral and cellular responses to mu opioids. Proc Natl Acad Sci USA 1999;96:10385–10390.

476. Romoser VA, Graves TK, Wu D, et al: Calcium responses to thyrotropin-releasing hormone, gonadotropin-releasing hormone and somatostatin in phospholipase css3 knockout mice. Mol Endocrinol 2001;15:125–135.

477. Jiang H, Kuang Y, Wu Y, et al: Roles of phospholipase C beta2 in chemoattractant-elicited responses. Proc Natl Acad Sci USA 1997;94:7971–7975.

478. Li Z, Jiang H, Xie W, et al: Roles of PLC-beta2 and -beta3 and PI3Kgamma in chemoattractant-mediated signal transduction. Science 2000;287:1046–1049.

479. Kim D, Jun KS, Lee SB, et al: Phospholipase C isozymes selectively couple to specific neurotransmitter receptors. Nature 1997; 389:290–293.

480. Jiang H, Lyubarsky A, Dodd R, et al: Phospholipase C beta 4 is involved in modulating the visual response in mice. Proc Natl Acad Sci U S A 1996;93:14598–14601.

481. Rameh LE, Rhee SG, Spokes K, et al: Phosphoinositide 3-kinase regulates phospholipase Cgamma-mediated calcium signaling. J Biol Chem 1998;273:23750–23757.

482. Puceat M, Vassort G: Purinergic stimulation of rat cardiomyocytes induces tyrosine phosphorylation and membrane association of phospholipase C gamma: A major mechanism for $InsP_3$ generation. Biochem J 1996;318:723–728.

483. Bony C, Roche S, Shuichi U, et al: A specific role of phosphatidylinositol 3-kinase gamma: A regulation of autonomic $Ca^{2+}$ oscillations in cardiac cells. J Cell Biol 2001;152:717–728.

484. Marrero MB, Schieffer B, Paxton WG, et al: Electroporation of pp60c-src antibodies inhibits the angiotensin II activation of phospholipase C-gamma 1 in rat aortic smooth muscle cells. J Biol Chem 1995;270:15734–15738.

485. Marrero MB, Paxton WG, Duff JL, et al: Angiotensin II stimulates tyrosine phosphorylation of phospholipase C-gamma 1 in vascular smooth muscle cells. J Biol Chem 1994;269:10935–10939.

486. Tappia PS, Padua RR, Panagia V, et al: Fibroblast growth factor-2 stimulates phospholipase C beta in adult cardiomyocytes. Biochem Cell Biol 1999;77:569–575.

487. Hong F, Moon K, Kim SS, et al: Role of phospholipase C-gamma1 in insulin-like growth factor I-induced muscle differentiation of H9c2 cardiac myoblasts. Biochem Biophys Res Commun 2001; 282:816–822.

488. Ji QS, Winnier GE, Niswender KD, et al: Essential role of the tyrosine kinase substrate phospholipase C-gamma1 in mammalian growth and development. Proc Natl Acad Sci USA 1997;94:2999–3003.

489. Williams RL, Katan M: Structural views of phosphoinositide-specific phospholipase C: Signalling the way ahead. Structure 1996; 4:1387–1394.

490. Allen V, Swigart P, Cheung R, et al: Regulation of inositol lipid-specific phospholipase cdelta by changes in $Ca^{2+}$ ion concentrations. Biochem J 1997;327(Pt 2):545–552.

491. Kim YH, Park TJ, Lee YH, et al: Phospholipase C-delta1 is activated by capacitative calcium entry that follows phospholipase C-beta activation upon bradykinin stimulation. J Biol Chem 1999; 274:26127–26134.

492. Wojcikiewicz RJH, Tobin AB, Nahorski SR: Desensitization of cell signalling mediated by phosphoinositidase C. Trends Pharmacol Sci 1993;14:279–285.

493. Homma Y, Emori Y: A dual functional signal mediator showing RhoGAP and phospholipase C-δ stimulating activities. EMBO J 1995;14:286–291.

494. Das T, Baek KJ, Gray C, et al: Evidence that the Gh protein is a signal mediator from alpha 1-adrenoceptor to a phospholipase C. II. Purification and characterization of a Gh-coupled 69-kDa phospholipase C and reconstitution of alpha 1-adrenoceptor, Gh family, and phospholipase C. J Biol Chem 1993;268:27398–27405.

495. Feng JF, Rhee SG, Im MJ: Evidence that phospholipase δ1 is the effector in the $G_h$ (transglutaminase II)-mediated signaling. J Biol Chem 1996;271:16451–16454.

496. Zhang J, Tucholski J, Lesort M, et al: Novel bimodal effects of the G-protein tissue transglutaminase on adrenoceptor signalling. Biochem J 1999;343(Pt 3):541–549.

497. Chen S, Lin F, Iismaa S, et al: $\alpha_1$-Adrenergic receptor signaling via $G_h$ is subtype specific and independent of its transglutaminase activity. J Biol Chem 1996;271:32385–32391.

498. Small K, Feng JF, Lorenz J, et al: Cardiac specific overexpression of transglutaminase II (G(h)) results in a unique hypertrophy phenotype independent of phospholipase C activation. J Biol Chem 1999;274:21291–21296.

499. Song C, Hu CD, Masago M, et al: Regulation of a novel human phospholipase C, PLCepsilon, through membrane targeting by Ras. J Biol Chem 2001;276:2752–2757.

500. Jin TG, Satoh T, Liao Y, et al: Role of the CDC25 homology domain of phospholipase Cepsilon in amplification of Rap1-dependent signaling. J Biol Chem 2001;276:30301–30307.

501. Stoyanov B, Volinia S, Hanck T, et al: Cloning and characterization of a G-protein activated human phosphoinositide-3 kinase. Science 1995;269:690–693.

502. Stephens LR, Eguinoa A, Erdjument-Bromage H, et al: The G beta gamma sensitivity of a PI3K is dependent upon a tightly associated adaptor, p101. Cell 1997;89:105–114.

503. Naga Prasad SV, Esposito G, Mao L, et al: Gbetagamma-dependent phosphoinositide 3-kinase activation in hearts with in vivo pressure overload hypertrophy. J Biol Chem 2000;275:4693–4698.

504. Sasaki T, Suzuki A, Sasaki J, et al: Phosphoinositide 3-kinases in immunity: Lessons from knockout mice. J Biochem (Tokyo) 2002; 131:495–501.

505. Shioi T, Kang PM, Douglas PS, et al: The conserved phosphoinositide 3-kinase pathway determines heart size in mice. EMBO J 2000;19:2537–2548.

506. Sam F, Sawyer DB, Xie Z, et al: Mice lacking inducible nitric oxide synthase have improved left ventricular contractile function and reduced apoptotic cell death late after myocardial infarction. Circ Res 2001;89:351–356.

507. Toker A: Protein kinases as mediators of phosphoinositide 3-kinase signaling. Mol Pharmacol 2000;57:652–658.

508. Kisseleva MV, Wilson MP, Majerus PW: The isolation and characterization of a cDNA encoding phospholipid-specific inositol polyphosphate 5-phosphatase. J Biol Chem 2000;275:20110–20116.

509. Taylor V, Wong M, Brandts C, et al: 5′ phospholipid phosphatase SHIP-2 causes protein kinase B inactivation and cell cycle arrest in glioblastoma cells. Mol Cell Biol 2000;20:6860–6871.

510. Dyson JM, O'Malley CJ, Becanovic J, et al: The SH2-containing inositol polyphosphate 5-phosphatase, SHIP-2, binds filamin and regulates submembraneous actin. J Cell Biol 2001;155:1065–1079.

511. Schwartzbauer G, Robbins J: The tumor suppressor gene pten can regulate cardiac hypertrophy and survival. J Biol Chem 2001;276:35786–35793.

512. Toker A, Newton AC: Cellular signalling: Pivoting around PDK-1. Cell 2000;103:185–188.

513. Le Good JA, Ziegler WH, Parekh DB, et al: Protein kinase C isotypes controlled by phosphoinositide 3-kinase through the protein kinase PDK1. Science 1998;281:2042–2045.

514. Toker A, Newton AC: Akt/protein kinase B is regulated by autophosphorylation at the hypothetical PDK-2 site. J Biol Chem 2000;275:8271–8274.

515. Brazil DP, Park J, Hemmings BA: PKB binding proteins: Getting in on the Akt. Cell 2002;111:293–303.

516. Testa JR, Bellacosa A: AKT plays a central role in tumorigenesis. Proc Natl Acad Sci U S A 2001;98:10983–10985.

517. Pham FH, Sugden PH, Clerk A: Regulation of protein kinase B and 4E-BP1 by oxidative stress in cardiac myocytes. Circ Res 2000;86:1252–1258.

518. Fujio Y, Nguyen T, Wencker D, et al: Akt promotes survival of cardiomyocytes in vitro and protects against ischemia-reperfusion injury in mouse heart. Circulation 2000;101:660–667.

519. Kuwahara K, Saito Y, Harada M, et al: Involvement of cardiotrophin-1 in cardiac myocyte-nonmyocyte interactions during hypertrophy of rat cardiac myocytes in vitro. Circulation 1999;100:1116–1124.

520. Hirota H, Chen J, Betz UAK, et al: Loss of a gp130 cardiac muscle cell survival pathway is a critical event in the onset of heart failure during biomechanical stress. Cell 1999;97:189–198.

521. Oh H, Fujio Y, Kunisada K, et al: Activation of phosphatidylinositol 3-kinase through glycoprotein 130 induces protein kinase B and p70 S6 kinase phosphorylation in cardiac myocytes. J Biol Chem 1998;273:9703–9710.

522. Camper-Kirby D, Welch S, Walker A, et al: Myocardial Akt activation and gender: Increased nuclear activity in females versus males. Circ Res 2001;88:1020–1027.

523. Matsui T, Li L, del Monte F, et al: Adenoviral gene transfer of activated phosphatidylinositol 3′-kinase and Akt inhibits apoptosis of hypoxic cardiomyocytes in vitro. Circulation 1999; 100:2373–2379.

524. Matsui T, Tao J, del Monte F, et al: Akt activation preserves cardiac function and prevents injury after transient cardiac ischemia in vivo. Circulation 2001;104:330–335.

525. Miao W, Luo Z, Kitsis RN, et al: Intracoronary, adenovirus-mediated Akt gene transfer in heart limits infarct size following ischemia-reperfusion injury in vivo. J Mol Cell Cardiol 2000; 32:2397–2402.

526. Taniyama Y, Walsh K: Elevated myocardial Akt signaling ameliorates doxorubicin-induced congestive heart failure and promotes heart growth. J Mol Cell Cardiol 2002;34:1241–1247.

527. Shioi T, McMullen JR, Kang PM, et al: Akt/protein kinase B promotes organ growth in transgenic mice. Mol Cell Biol 2002;22:2799–2809.

528. Matsui T, Li L, Wu JC, et al: Phenotypic spectrum caused by transgenic overexpression of activated Akt in the heart. J Biol Chem 2002;277:22896–22901.

529. Cook SA, Matsui T, Li L, et al: Transcriptional effects of chronic Akt activation in the heart. J Biol Chem 2002;277:22528–22533.

530. Condorelli G, Drusco A, Stassi G, et al: Akt induces enhanced myocardial contractility and cell size in vivo in transgenic mice. Proc Natl Acad Sci USA 2002;99:12333–12338.

531. Iaccarino G, Rockman HA, Shotwell KF, et al: Myocardial overexpression of GRK3 in transgenic mice: Evidence for in vivo selectivity of GRKs. Am J Physiol 1998;275:H1298–H1306.

532. Daaka Y, Pitcher JA, Richardson M, et al: Receptor and Gβγ isoform-specific interactions with G protein-coupled receptor kinases. Proc Natl Acad Sci USA 1997;94:2180–2185.

533. Eckhart AD, Duncan SJ, Penn RB, et al: Hybrid transgenic mice reveal in vivo specificity of G protein-coupled receptor kinases in the heart. Circ Res 2000;86:43–50.

534. Koch WJ, Inglese J, Stone WC, et al: The binding site for the βγ subunits of heterotrimeric G proteins on the β-adrenergic receptor kinase. J Biol Chem 1993;268:8256–8260.

535. Tiruppathi C, Yan W, Sandoval R, et al: G protein-coupled receptor kinase-5 regulates thrombin-activated signaling in endothelial cells. Proc Natl Acad Sci USA 2000;97:7440–7445.

536. Rockman HA, Choi DJ, Rahman NU, et al: Receptor-specific in vivo desensitization by the G protein-coupled receptor kinase-5 in transgenic mice. Proc Natl Acad Sci USA 1996;93:9954–9959.

537. Sallese M, Mariggio S, D'Urbano E, et al: Selective regulation of $G_q$ signaling by G protein-coupled receptor kinase 2: Direct interaction of kinase N terminus with activated Gαq. Mol Pharmacol 2000;57:826–831.

538. Carman CV, Parent JL, Day PW, et al: Selective regulation of $Gα_{q/11}$ by an RGS domain in the G protein-coupled receptor kinase, GRK2. J Biol Chem 1999;274:34483–34492.

539. Luttrell LM, Ferguson SS, Daaka Y, et al: β-arrestin-dependent formation of β2 adrenergic receptor-Src protein kinase complexes. Science 1999;283:655–661.

540. DeFea KA, Zalevsky J, Thoma MS, et al: β-arrestin-dependent endocytosis of proteinase-activated receptor 2 is required for intracellular targeting of activated ERK1/2. J Cell Biol 2000;148:1267–1281.

541. McDonald PH, Chow CW, Miller WE, et al: Beta-arrestin 2: A receptor-regulated MAPK scaffold for the activation of JNK3. Science 2000;290:1574–1577.

542. Lefkowitz RJ, Rockman HA, Koch WJ: Catecholamines, cardiac β-adrenergic receptors, and heart failure. Circulation 2000; 101:1634–1637.

543. Iaccarino G, Dolber PC, Lefkowitz RJ, et al: β-adrenergic receptor kinase-1 levels in catecholamine-induced myocardial hypertrophy: Regulation by β-but not α1-adrenergic stimulation. Hypertension 1999;33:396–401.

544. Winstel R, Freund S, Krasel C, et al: Protein kinase cross-talk: membrane targeting of the β-adrenergic receptor kinase by protein kinase C. Proc Natl Acad Sci U S A 1996;93:2105–2109.

545. Pronin AN, Benovic JL: Regulation of the G protein-coupled receptor kinase GRK5 by protein kinase C. J Biol Chem 1997; 272:3806–3812.

546. Lechat P, Packer M, Chalon S, et al: Clinical effects of β-adrenergic blockade in chronic heart failure: A meta-analysis of double-blind, placebo-controlled, randomized trials. Circulation 1998; 98:1184–1191.

547. Rockman HA, Chien KR, Choi DJ, et al: Expression of a beta-adrenergic receptor kinase 1 inhibitor prevents the development of myocardial failure in gene-targeted mice. Proc Natl Acad Sci USA 1998;95:7000–7005.

548. Harding VB, Jones LR, Lefkowitz RJ, et al: Cardiac beta ARK1 inhibition prolongs survival and augments beta blocker therapy in a mouse model of severe heart failure. Proc Natl Acad Sci USA 2001;98:5809–5814.

549. Shah AS, White DC, Emani S, et al: In vivo ventricular gene delivery of a beta-adrenergic receptor kinase inhibitor to the

550. Manning BS, Shotwell K, Mao L, et al: Physiological induction of a beta-adrenergic receptor kinase inhibitor transgene preserves β-adrenergic responsiveness in pressure-overload cardiac hypertrophy. Circulation 2000;102:2751–2757.

551. Choi DJ, Koch WJ, Hunter JJ, et al: Mechanism of β-adrenergic receptor desensitization in cardiac hypertrophy is increased β-adrenergic receptor kinase. J Biol Chem 1997;272:17223–17229.

552. Hayes JS, Brunton LL, Brown JH, et al: Hormonally specific expression of cardiac protein kinase activity. Proc Natl Acad Sci USA 1979;76:1570–1574.

553. Livesey SA, Kemp BE, Re CA, et al: Selective hormonal activation of cyclic AMP-dependent protein kinase isoenzymes in normal and malignant osteoblasts. J Biol Chem 1982;257:14983–14987.

554. Tortora G, Cho-Chung YS: Type II regulatory subunit of protein kinase restores cAMP-dependent transcription in a cAMP-unresponsive cell line. J Biol Chem 1990;265:18067–18070.

555. Brandon EP, Zhuo M, Huang YY, et al: Hippocampal long-term depression and depotentiation are defective in mice carrying a targeted disruption of the gene encoding the RI beta subunit of cAMP-dependent protein kinase. Proc Natl Acad Sci USA 1995;92:8851–8855.

556. Gray PC, Scott JD, Catterall WA: Regulation of ion channels by cAMP-dependent protein kinase and A-kinase anchoring proteins. Curr Opin Neurobiol 1998;8:330–334.

557. Fraser ID, Cong M, Kim J, et al: Assembly of an A kinase-anchoring protein-β2-adrenergic receptor complex facilitates receptor phosphorylation and signaling. Curr Biol 2000;10:409–412.

558. Shih M, Lin F, Scott JD, et al: Dynamic complexes of β2-adrenergic receptors with protein kinases and phosphatases and the role of gravin. J Biol Chem 1999;274:1588–1595.

559. Lin F, Wang H, Malbon CC: Gravin-mediated formation of signaling complexes in β2-adrenergic receptor desensitization and resensitization. J Biol Chem 2000;275:19025–19034.

560. Davare MA, Avdonin V, Hall DD, et al: A β2 adrenergic receptor signaling complex assembled with the $Ca^{2+}$ channel $Ca_v1.2$. Science 2001;293:98–101.

561. Gao T, Yatani A, Dell'Acqua ML, et al: cAMP-dependent regulation of cardiac L-type $Ca^{2+}$ channels requires membrane targeting of PKA and phosphorylation of channel subunits. Neuron 1997; 19:185–196.

562. Yang J, Drazba JA, Ferguson DG, et al: A-kinase anchoring protein 100 (AKAP100) is localized in multiple subcellular compartments in the adult rat heart. J Cell Biol 1998;142:511–522.

563. Dempsey EC, Newton AC, Mochly-Rosen D, et al: Protein kinase C isozymes and the regulation of diverse cell responses. Am J Physiol Lung Cell Mol Physiol 2000;279:L429–L438.

564. Ron D, Luo J, Mochly-Rosen D: C2 region-derived peptides inhibit translocation and function of beta protein kinase C in vivo. J Biol Chem 1995;270:24180–24187.

565. Csukai M, Chen CH, De Matteis MA, et al: The coatomer protein β'-COP, a selective binding protein (RACK) for protein kinase Cε. J Biol Chem 1997;272:29200–29206.

566. Rybin VO, Sabri A, Short J, et al: Cross regulation of nPKC isoform function in cardiomyocytes: Role of PKCε in activation loop phosphorylations and PKCδ in hydrophobic motif phosphorylations. J Biol Chem 2003;278:14555–14564.

567. Ishii H, Jirousek MR, Koya D, et al: Amelioration of vascular dysfunctions in diabetic rats by an oral PKC-β inhibitor. Science 1996;272:728–731.

568. Kariya K, Karns LR, Simpson PC: Expression of a constitutively activated mutant of the β-isozyme of protein kinase C in cardiac myocytes stimulates the promoter of the β-myosin heavy chain isogene. J Biol Chem 1991;266:10023–1002.

569. Wakasaki H, Koya D, Schoen FJ, et al: Targeted overexpression of protein kinase CβII isoform in myocardium causes cardiomyopathy. Proc Natl Acad Sci USA 1997;94:9320–9325.

570. Takeishi Y, Chu G, Kirkpatrick DM, et al: In vivo phosphorylation of cardiac troponin I by protein kinase CβII decreases cardiomyocyte calcium responsiveness and contractility in transgenic mouse hearts. J Clin Invest 1998;102:72–78.

571. Bowman JC, Steinberg SF, Jiang T, et al: Expression of protein kinase C-β in the heart causes hypertrophy in adult mice and sudden death in neonates. J Clin Invest 1997;100:2189–2195.

572. Jiang T, Pak E, Zhang HL, et al: Endothelin-dependent actions in cultured AT-1 cardiac myocytes: the role of the ε-isoform of protein kinase C. Circ Res 1996;78:724-736.

573. Strait JB, III, Martin JL, Bayer A, et al: Role of protein kinase Cε in hypertrophy of cultured neonatal rat ventricular myocytes. Am J Physiol Heart Circ Physiol 2001;280:H756-H766.

574. Takeishi Y, Ping P, Bolli R, et al: Transgenic overexpression of constitutively active protein kinase Cε causes concentric cardiac hypertrophy. Circ Res 2000;86:1218-1223.

575. Leitges M, Schmedt C, Guinamard R, et al: Immunodeficiency in protein kinase C-β-deficient mice. Science 1996;273:788-791.

576. Khasar SG, Lin YH, Martin A, et al: A novel nociceptor signaling pathway revealed in protein kinase Cε mutant mice. Neuron 1999;24:253-260.

577. Roman BB, Geenen DL, Leitges M, et al: PKCβ is not necessary for cardiac hypertrophy. Am J Physiol Heart Circ Physiol 2001; 280:H2264-H2270.

578. Hu K, Mochly-Rosen D, Boutjdir M: Evidence for functional role of ε PKC isozyme in the regulation of cardiac Ca²⁺ channels. Am J Physiol Heart Circ Physiol 2000;279:H2658-H2664.

579. Chen CH, Gray MO, Mochly-Rosen D: Cardioprotection from ischemia by a brief exposure to physiological levels of ethanol: Role of epsilon protein kinase C. Proc Natl Acad Sci USA 1999;96:12784-12789.

580. Dorn GW, Souroujon MC, Liron T, et al: Sustained *in vivo* cardiac protection by a rationally designed peptide that causes ε protein kinase C translocation. Proc Natl Acad Sci USA 1999;96:12798-12803.

581. Sabri A, Wilson BA, Steinberg SF: Dual actions of the Gα_q agonist Pasteurella multocida toxin to promote cardiomyocyte hypertrophy and enhance apoptosis susceptibility. Circ Res 2002;90:850-857.

582. Braun AP, Schulman H: The multifunctional calcium/calmodulin-dependent protein kinase: From form to function. Annu Rev Physiol 1995;57:417-445.

583. Nairn AC, Bhagat B, Palfrey HC: Identification of calmodulin-dependent protein kinase III and its major Mr 100,000 substrate in mammalian tissues. Proc Natl Acad Sci U S A 1985;82:7939-7943.

584. Lee JC, Edelman AM: A protein activator of Ca²⁺ calmodulin-dependent protein kinase Ia. J Biol Chem 1994;269:2158-2164.

585. Tokumitsu H, Enslen H, Soderling TR: Characterization of a Ca²⁺/calmodulin-dependent protein kinase cascade: Molecular cloning and expression of calcium/calmodulin-dependent protein kinase kinase. J Biol Chem 1995;270:19320-19324.

586. Edman CF, Schulman H: Identification and characterization of δ_B-CaM kinase and δ_C-CaM kinase from rat heart, two new multifunctional Ca²⁺/calmodulin-dependent protein kinase isoforms. Biochim Biophys Acta 1994;1221:89-101.

587. Miyano O, Kameshita I, Fujisawa H: Purification and characterization of a brain-specific multifunctional calmodulin-dependent protein kinase from cerebellum. J Biol Chem 1992;267:1198-1203.

588. Kanaseki T, Ikeuchi Y, Sugiura H, et al: Structural features of Ca²⁺/calmodulin-dependent protein kinase II revealed by electron microscopy. J Cell Biol 1991;115:1049-1060.

589. Tobimatsu T, Fujisawa H: Tissue specific expression of four types of rat calmodulin-dependent protein kinase II transcripts. J Biol Chem 1989;264:17907-17912.

590. Schworer CM, Rothblum LI, Thekkumkara TJ, et al: Identification of novel isoforms of the δ subunit of Ca²⁺/calmodulin-dependent protein kinase II. J Biol Chem 1993;268:14443-14449.

591. Mayer P, Mohlig M, Idlibe D, et al: Novel and uncommon isoforms of the calcium sensing enzyme calcium/calmodulin dependent protein kinase II in heart tissue. Basic Res Cardiol 1995;90:372-379.

592. Baltas LG, Karczewski P, Krause E-G: The cardiac sarcoplasmic reticulum phospholamban kinase is a distinct δ-CaM kinase isozyme. FEBS Lett 1995;373:71-75.

593. Srinivasan M, Edman CF, Schulman H: Alternative splicing introduces a nuclear localization signal that targets multifunctional CaM kinase to the nucleus. J Cell Biol 1994;126:839-852.

594. Ramirez MT, Zhao X, Schulman H, et al: The nuclear δ_B isoform of Ca²⁺/calmodulin-dependent protein kinase II regulates atrial natriuretic factor gene expression in ventricular myocytes. J Biol Chem 1997;272:31203-31208.

595. Witcher DR, Kovacs RJ, Schulman H, et al: Unique phosphorylation site on the cardiac ryanodine receptor regulates calcium channel activity. J Biol Chem 1991;266:11144-11152.

596. Hain J, Onoue H, Mayrleitner M, et al: Phosphorylation modulates the function of the calcium release channel of sarcoplasmic reticulum from cardiac muscle. J Biol Chem 1995;270:2074-2081.

597. Karczewski P, Kuschel M, Baltas LG, et al: Site-specific phosphorylation of a phospholamban peptide by cyclic nucleotide- and Ca²⁺/calmodulin-dependent protein kinases of cardiac sarcoplasmic reticulum. Basic Res Cardiol 1997;92(Suppl 1):37-43.

598. Bassani RA, Mattiazzi A, Bers DM: CaMKII is responsible for activity-dependent acceleration of relaxation in rat ventricular myocytes. Am J Physiol 1995;268:H703-H712.

599. Maier LS, Bers DM: Calcium, calmodulin, and calcium-calmodulin kinase II: Heartbeat to heartbeat and beyond. J Mol Cell Cardiol 2002;34:919-939.

600. Marks AR: Ryanodine receptors/calcium release channels in heart failure and sudden cardiac death. J Mol Cell Cardiol 2001;33:615-624.

601. Xiao R-P, Cheng H, Lederer WJ, et al: Dual regulation of Ca²⁺/calmodulin-dependent kinase II activity by membrane voltage and by calcium influx. Proc Natl Acad Sci USA 1994;91:9659-9663.

602. Anderson ME, Braun AP, Schulman H, et al: Multifunctional Ca²⁺/calmodulin-dependent protein kinase mediates Ca²⁺-induced enhancement of the L-type Ca²⁺ current in rabbit ventricular myocytes. Circ Res 1994;75:854-861.

603. Yuan W, Bers DM: Ca-dependent facilitation of cardiac Ca current is due to Ca-calmodulin-dependent protein kinase. Am J Physiol 1994;267:H982-H993.

604. Dzhura I, Wu Y, Colbran RJ, et al: Calmodulin kinase determines calcium-dependent facilitation of L-type calcium channels. Nat Cell Biol 2000;2:173-177.

605. Anderson ME, Braun AP, Wu Y, et al: KN-93, an inhibitor of multifunctional Ca²⁺/calmodulin-dependent protein kinase, decreases early afterdepolarizations in rabbit heart. J Pharmacol Exp Ther 1998;287:996-1006.

606. Wu Y, Roden DM, Anderson ME: Calmodulin kinase inhibition prevents development of the arrhythmogenic transient inward current. Circ Res 1999;84:906-912.

607. Wu Y, Temple J, Zhang R, et al: Calmodulin kinase II and arrhythmias in a mouse model of cardiac hypertrophy. Circulation 2002;106:1288-1293.

608. Wu Y, MacMillan LB, McNeill RB, et al: CaM kinase augments cardiac L-type Ca²⁺ current: a cellular mechanism for long Q-T arrhythmias. Am J Physiol 1999;276:H2168-H2178.

609. Gruver CL, DeMayo F, Goldstein MA, et al: Targeted developmental overexpression of calmodulin induces proliferative and hypertrophic growth of cardiomyocytes in transgenic mice. Endocrinology 1993;133:376-388.

610. Colomer JM, Means AR: Chronic elevation of calmodulin in the ventricles of transgenic mice increases the autonomous activity of calmodulin-dependent protein kinase II, which regulates atrial natriuretic factor gene expression. Mol Endocrinol 2000;14:1125-1136.

611. Passier R, Zeng H, Frey N, et al: CaM kinase signaling induces cardiac hypertrophy and activates the MEF2 transcription factor in vivo. J Clin Invest 2000;105:1395-1406.

612. Colomer JM, Mao L, Rockman HA, et al: Pressure overload selectively up-regulates Ca²⁺/calmodulin-dependent protein kinase II in vivo. Mol Endocrinol 2003;17:183-192.

613. Zhang T, Johnson EN, Gu Y, et al: The cardiac-specific nuclear δ_B isoform of Ca²⁺/calmodulin-dependent protein kinase II induces hypertrophy and dilated cardiomyopathy associated with increased protein phosphatase 2A activity. J Biol Chem 2002; 277:1261-1267.

614. Zhang T, Maier LS, Dalton ND, et al: The δ_C isoform of Ca²⁺/calmodulin-dependent protein kinase II is activated in cardiac hypertrophy and induces dilated cardiomyopathy and heart failure. Circ Res 2003;92:912-919.

615. Maier LS, Zhang T, Chen L, et al: Transgenic CaMKIIδ_C overexpression uniquely alters cardiac myocyte Ca²⁺ handling: Reduced SR Ca²⁺ load and activated SR Ca²⁺ release. Circ Res 2003;92:904-911.

616. Bers DM: Calcium fluxes involved in control of cardiac myocyte contraction. Circ Res 2000;87:275-281.

617. Hagemann D, Bohlender J, Hoch B, et al: Expression of Ca²⁺/calmodulin-dependent protein kinase II δ-subunit isoforms in rats with hypertensive cardiac hypertrophy. Mol Cell Biochem 2001;220:69-760.

618. Boknik P, Heinroth-Hoffman I, Kirchhefer U, et al: Enhanced protein phosphorylation in hypertensive hypertrophy. Cardiovasc Res 2001;51:717–728.

619. Currie S, Smith GL: Calcium/calmodulin-dependent protein kinase II activity is increased in sarcoplasmic reticulum from coronary artery ligated rabbit hearts. FEBS Lett 1999;459:244–248.

620. Netticadan T, Temsah RM, Kawabata K, et al: Sarcoplasmic reticulum Ca²⁺/calmodulin-dependent protein kinase is altered in heart failure. Circ Res 2000;86:596–605.

621. Mishra S, Sabbah HN, Jain JC, et al: Reduced Ca²⁺-calmodulin-dependent protein kinase activity and expression in LV myocardium of dogs with heart failure. Am J Physiol 2003; 284:H876–H883.

622. Kirchhefer U, Schmitz W, Scholz H, et al: Activity of cAMP-dependent protein kinase and Ca²⁺/calmodulin-dependent protein kinase in failing and nonfailing human hearts. Cardiovasc Res 1999;42:254–261.

623. Hoch B, Meyer R, Hetzer R, et al: Identification and expression of δ-isoforms of the multifunctional Ca²⁺/calmodulin dependent protein kinase in failing and nonfailing human myocardium. Circ Res 1999;84:713–721.

624. Hempel P, Hoch B, Bartel S, et al: Hypertrophic phenotype of cardias calcium\calmodulin-dependent protein kinase II is reversed by angiotensin converting enzyme inhibition. Basic Res Cardiol 2002;97:96–101.

625. Wright SC, Schellenberger U, Ji L, et al: Calmodulin-dependent protein kinase II mediates signal transduction in apoptosis. FASEB J 1997;11:843–849.

626. Fladmark KE, Brustugun OT, Mellgren G, et al: Ca²⁺/calmodulin-dependent protein kinase II is required for microcystin-induced apoptosis. J Biol Chem 2002;277:2804–2811.

627. Zhu WZ, Wang SQ, Chakir K, et al: Linkage of β₁-adrenergic stimulation to apoptotic heart cell death through protein kinase A-independent activation of Ca²⁺/calmodulin kinase II. J Clin Invest 2003;111:617–625.

628. Molkentin JD: Calcineurin and beyond: Cardiac hypertrophic signaling. Circ Res 2000;87:731–738.

629. Tian J, Karin M: Stimulation of Elk1 transcriptional activity by mitogen-activated protein kinases is negatively regulated by protein phosphatase 2B (calcineurin). J Biol Chem 1999;274:15173–15180.

630. Wang HG, Pathan N, Ethell IM, et al: Ca²⁺-induced apoptosis through calcineurin dephosphorylation of BAD. Science 1999; 284:339–343.

631. Molkentin JD: Calcineurin, mitochondrial membrane potential, and cardiomyocyte apoptosis. Circ Res 2001;88:1220–1222.

632. Matsuda S, Moriguchi T, Koyasu S, et al: T lymphocyte activation signals for interleukin-2 production involve activation of MKK6-p38 and MKK7-SAPK/JNK signaling pathways sensitive to cyclosporin A. J Biol Chem 1999;273:12378–12382.

633. Crabtree GR: Calcium, calcineurin, and the control of transcription. J Biol Chem 2001;276:2313–2316.

634. Rothermel BA, McKinsey TA, Vega RB, et al: Myocyte-enriched calcineurin-interacting protein, MCIP1, inhibits cardiac hypertrophy in vivo. Proc Natl Acad Sci USA 2001;98:3328–3333.

635. Ghosh S, May MJ, Kopp EB: NF-kappa B and Rel proteins: Evolutionarily conserved mediators of immune responses. Annu Rev Immunol 1998;16:225–260.

636. Valen G, Yan ZQ, Hansson GK: Nuclear factor kappa-B and the heart. J Am Coll Cardiol 2001;38:307–314.

637. Morishita R, Sugimoto T, Aoki M, et al: In vivo transfection of cis element "decoy" against nuclear factor-kappaB binding site prevents myocardial infarction. Nat Med 1997;3:894–899.

638. Sawa Y, Morishita R, Suzuki K, et al: A novel strategy for myocardial protection using in vivo transfection of cis element 'decoy' against NFkappaB binding site: Evidence for a role of NFkappaB in ischemia-reperfusion injury. Circulation 1997;96:II-4.

639. Purcell NH, Tang G, Yu C, et al: Activation of NF-kappa B is required for hypertrophic growth of primary rat neonatal ventricular cardiomyocytes. Proc Natl Acad Sci USA 2001;98:6668–6673.

640. Gupta S, Purcell NH, Lin A, et al: Activation of nuclear factor-kappaB is necessary for myotrophin-induced cardiac hypertrophy. J Cell Biol 2002;159:1019–1028.

641. Kukreja RC: NFkappaB activation during ischemia/reperfusion in heart: friend or foe? J Mol Cell Cardiol 2002;34:1301–1304.

642. Ghosh G, van Duyne G, Ghosh S, et al: Structure of NF-kappa B p50 homodimer bound to a kappa B site. Nature 1995;373:303–310.

643. Chen FE, Huang DB, Chen YQ, et al: Crystal structure of p50/p65 heterodimer of transcription factor NF-kappaB bound to DNA. Nature 1998;391:410–413.

644. Karin M, Ben Neriah Y: Phosphorylation meets ubiquitination: The control of NF-[kappa]B activity. Annu Rev Immunol 2000;18: 621–663.

645. Mercurio F, DiDonato JA, Rosette C, et al: p105 and p98 precursor proteins play an active role in NF-kappa B-mediated signal transduction. Genes Dev 1993;7:705–718.

646. Solan NJ, Miyoshi H, Carmona EM, et al: RelB cellular regulation and transcriptional activity are regulated by p100. J Biol Chem 2002;277:1405–1418.

647. Xiao G, Harhaj EW, Sun SC: NF-kappaB-inducing kinase regulates the processing of NF-kappaB2 p100. Mol Cell 2001;7:401–409.

648. Rothwarf DM, Karin M: The NF-κ B activation pathway: A paradigm in information transfer from membrane to nucleus. Sci STKE 1999;1999:RE1.

649. DiDonato JA, Hayakawa M, Rothwarf DM, et al: A cytokine-responsive IkappaB kinase that activates the transcription factor NF-kappaB. Nature 1997;388:548–554.

650. Yaron A, Hatzubai A, Davis M, et al: Identification of the receptor component of the IkappaBalpha-ubiquitin ligase. Nature 1998; 396:590–594.

651. Zandi E, Chen Y, Karin M: Direct phosphorylation of IkappaB by IKKalpha and IKKbeta: Discrimination between free and NF-kappaB-bound substrate. Science 1998;281:1360–1363.

652. Li Q, Van Antwerp D, Mercurio F, et al: Severe liver degeneration in mice lacking the IkappaB kinase 2 gene. Science 1999;284:321–325.

653. Tanaka M, Fuentes ME, Yamaguchi K, et al: Embryonic lethality, liver degeneration, and impaired NF-kappa B activation in IKK-beta-deficient mice. Immunity 1999;10:421–429.

654. Rudolph D, Yeh WC, Wakeham A, et al: Severe liver degeneration and lack of NF-kappaB activation in NEMO/IKKgamma-deficient mice. Genes Dev 2000;14:854–862.

655. Makris C, Godfrey VL, Krahn-Senftleben G, et al: Female mice heterozygous for IKK gamma/NEMO deficiencies develop a dermatopathy similar to the human X-linked disorder incontinentia pigmenti. Mol Cell 2000;5:969–979.

656. Schmidt-Supprian M, Bloch W, Courtois G, et al: NEMO/IKK gamma-deficient mice model incontinentia pigmenti. Mol Cell 2000;5:981–992.

657. Chu WM, Ostertag D, Li ZW, et al: JNK2 and IKKbeta are required for activating the innate response to viral infection. Immunity 1999;11:721–731.

658. Chu W, Gong X, Li Z, et al: DNA-PKcs is required for activation of innate immunity by immunostimulatory DNA. Cell 2000;103: 909–918.

659. Senftleben U, Li ZW, Baud V, et al: IKKbeta is essential for protecting T cells from TNFalpha-induced apoptosis. Immunity 2001; 14:217–230.

660. Miller BS, Zandi E: Complete reconstitution of human IkappaB kinase (IKK) complex in yeast: Assessment of its stoichiometry and the role of IKKgamma on the complex activity in the absence of stimulation. J Biol Chem 2001;276:36320–36326.

661. Yamaoka S, Courtois G, Bessia C, et al: Complementation cloning of NEMO, a component of the IkappaB kinase complex essential for NF-kappaB activation. Cell 1998;93:1231–1240.

662. Zandi E, Rothwarf DM, Delhase M, et al: The IkappaB kinase complex (IKK) contains two kinase subunits, IKKalpha and IKKbeta, necessary for IkappaB phosphorylation and NF-kappaB activation. Cell 1997;91:243–252.

663. Mercurio F, Zhu H, Murray BW, et al: IKK-1 and IKK-2: Cytokine-activated IkappaB kinases essential for NF-kappaB activation. Science 1997;278:860–866.

664. Woronicz JD, Gao X, Cao Z, et al: IkappaB kinase-beta: NF-kappaB activation and complex formation with IkappaB kinase-alpha and NIK. Science 1997;278:866–869.

665. Hu Y, Baud V, Oga T, et al: IKKalpha controls formation of the epidermis independently of NF-kappaB. Nature 2001;410:710–714.

666. May MJ, D'Acquisto F, Madge LA, et al: Selective inhibition of NF-kappaB activation by a peptide that blocks the interaction of NEMO with the IkappaB kinase complex. Science 2000;289: 1550–1554.

667. Rothwarf DM, Zandi E, Natoli G, et al: IKK-gamma is an essential regulatory subunit of the IkappaB kinase complex. Nature 1998; 395:297–300.

668. Delhase M, Hayakawa M, Chen Y, et al: Positive and negative regulation of IkappaB kinase activity through IKKbeta subunit phosphorylation. Science 1999;284:309-313.

669. Ling L, Cao Z, Goeddel DV: NF-kappaB-inducing kinase activates IKK-alpha by phosphorylation of Ser-176. Proc Natl Acad Sci USA 1998;95:3792-3797.

670. Taylor SS, Radzio-Andzelm E, Hunter T: How do protein kinases discriminate between serine/threonine and tyrosine? Structural insights from the insulin receptor protein-tyrosine kinase. FASEB J 1995;9:1255-1266.

671. Cao Y, Bonizzi G, Seagroves TN, et al: IKKalpha provides an essential link between RANK signaling and cyclin D1 expression during mammary gland development. Cell 2001;107:763-775.

672. Takeda K, Takeuchi O, Tsujimura T, et al: Limb and skin abnormalities in mice lacking IKKalpha. Science 1999;284:313-316.

673. Zhang SQ, Kovalenko A, Cantarella G, et al: Recruitment of the IKK signalosome to the p55 TNF receptor: RIP and A20 bind to NEMO (IKKgamma) upon receptor stimulation. Immunity 2000;12: 301-311.

674. Tada K, Okazaki T, Sakon S, et al: Critical roles of TRAF2 and TRAF5 in tumor necrosis factor-induced NF-kappa B activation and protection from cell death. J Biol Chem 2001;276:36530-36534.

675. Heldwein KA, Golenbock DT, Fenton MJ Recent advances in the biology of toll-like receptors. Mod Asp Immunobiol 2001;1:249-252.

676. Kovacic B, Ilic D, Damsky CH, et al: c-Src activation plays a role in endothelin-dependent hypertrophy of the cardiac myocyte. J Biol Chem 1998;273:35185-35193.

677. Puceat M, Roche S, Vassort G: Src family tyrosine kinase regulates intracellular pH in cardiomyocytes. J Cell Biol 1998;141:1637-1646.

678. Sadoshima J, Izumo S: The heterotrimeric $G_q$ protein-coupled angiotensin II receptor activates $p21^{ras}$ via the tyrosine kinase-Shc-Grb2-Sos pathway in cardiac myocytes. EMBO J 1996;15: 775-787.

679. Yue TL, Gu JL, Wang C, et al: Extracellular signal-regulated kinase plays an essential role in hypertrophic agonists, endothelin-1 and phenylephrine-induced cardiomyocyte hypertrophy. J Biol Chem 2000;275:37895-37901.

680. Eble DM, Strait JB, Govindarajan G, et al: Endothelin-induced cardiac myocyte hypertrophy: Role for focal adhesion kinase. Am J Physiol Heart Circ Physiol 2000;278:H1695-H1707.

681. Wu JY, Cohen IS: Tyrosine kinase inhibition reduces $i_f$ in rabbit sinoatrial node myocytes. Pflugers Arch 1997;434:509-514.

682. Felsch JS, Cachero TG, Peralta EG Activation of protein tyrosine kinase PYK2 by the m1 muscarinic acetylcholine receptor. Proc Natl Acad Sci USA 1998;95:5051-5056.

683. Sabri A, Govindarajan G, Griffin TM, et al: Calcium- and protein-kinase C-dependent activation of the tyrosin kinase PYK2 by angiotensin II in vascular smooth muscle. Circ Res 1998;83:841-851.

684. Widmann C, Gibson S, Jarpe MB, et al: Mitogen-activated protein kinase: Conservation of a three-kinase module from yeast to human. Physiol Rev 1999;79:143-180.

685. Kyriakis JM, Avruch J: Mammalian mitogen-activated protein kinase signal transduction pathways activated by stress and inflammation. Physiol Rev 2001;81:807-869.

686. Hagemann C, Blank JL: The ups and downs of MEK kinase interactions. Cell Signal 2001;13:863-875.

687. Bueno OF, Molkentin JD: Involvement of extracellular signal-regulated kinases 1/2 in cardiac hypertrophy and cell death. Circ Res 2002;91:776-781.

688. Glennon PE, Kaddoura S, Sale EM, et al: Depletion of mitogen-activated protein kinase using an antisense oligodeoxynucleotide approach downregulates the phenylephrine-induced hypertrophic response in rat cardiac myocytes. Circ Res 1996;78:954-961.

689. Bueno OF, De Windt LJ, Lim HW, et al: The dual-specificity phosphatase MKP-1 limits the cardiac hypertrophic response in vitro and in vivo. Circ Res 2001;88:88-96.

690. Sugden PH: Signalling pathways in cardiac myocyte hypertrophy. Ann Med 2001;33:611-622.

691. Michel MC, Li Y, Heusch G: Mitogen-activated protein kinases in the heart. Naunyn Schmiedebergs Arch Pharmacol 2001;363: 245-266.

692. Bueno OF, De Windt LJ, Tymitz KM, et al: The MEK1-ERK1/2 signaling pathway promotes compensated cardiac hypertrophy in transgenic mice. EMBO J 2000;19:6341-6350.

693. Sugden PH, Clerk A: "Stress-responsive" mitogen-activated protein kinases (c-Jun N-terminal kinases and p38 mitogen-activated protein kinases) in the myocardium. Circ Res 1998;83:345-352.

694. Force T, Pombo CM, Avruch JA, et al: Stress-activated protein kinases in cardiovascular disease. Circ Res 1996;78:947-953.

695. Feuerstein GZ, Young PR: Apoptosis in cardiac diseases: Stress- and mitogen-activated signaling pathways. Cardiovasc Res 2000;45:560-569.

696. Zechner D, Thuerauf DJ, Hanford DS, et al: A role for the p38 mitogen-activated protein kinase pathway in myocardial cell growth, sarcomeric organization, and cardiac-specific gene expression. J Cell Biol 1997;139:115-127.

697. Nemoto S, Sheng Z, Lin A: Opposing effects of Jun kinase and p38 mitogen-activated protein kinases on cardiomyocyte hypertrophy. Mol Cell Biol 1998;18:3518-3526.

698. Wang Y, Huang S, Sah VP, et al: Cardiac muscle cell hypertrophy and apoptosis induced by distinct members of the p38 mitogen-activated protein kinase family. J Biol Chem 1998;273:2161-2168.

699. Bogoyevitch MA, Ketterman AJ, Sugden PH: Cellular stresses differentially activate c-Jun N-terminal protein kinases and extracellular signal-related protein kinases in cultured ventricular myocytes. J Biol Chem 1995;270:29710-29717.

700. Laderoute KR, Webster KA: Hypoxia/reoxygenation stimulates Jun kinase activity through redox signaling in cardiac myocytes. Circ Res 1997;80:336-344.

701. Clerk A, Fuller SJ, Michael A, et al: Stimulation of "stress-regulated" mitogen-activated protein kinases (stress-activated protein kinases/c-Jun N-terminal kinases and p38-mitogen-activated protein kinases) in perfused rat hearts by oxidative and other stresses. J Biol Chem 1998;273:7228-7234.

702. Bogoyevitch MA, Gillespie-Brown J, Ketterman AJ, et al: Stimulation of the stress-activated mitogen-activated protein kinase subfamilies in perfused heart: p38/RK mitogen-activated protein kinases and c-Jun N-terminal kinases are activated by ischemia and reperfusion. Circ Res 1996;79:162-173.

703. Yin T, Sandhu G, Wolfgang CD, et al: Tissue-specific pattern of stress kinase activation in ischemic/reperfused heart and kidney. J Biol Chem 1997;272:19943-19950.

704. Aoki H, Kang PM, Hampe J, et al: Direct activation of mitochondrial apoptosis machinery by c-Jun N-terminal kinase in adult cardiac myocytes. J Biol Chem 2002;277:10244-10250.

705. Ma XL, Kumar S, Gao F, et al: Inhibition of p38 mitogen-activated protein kinase decreases cardiomyocyte apoptosis and improves cardiac function after myocardial ischemia and reperfusion. Circulation 1999;99:1685-1691.

706. Wang Y, Su B, Sah VP, et al: Cardiac hypertrophy induced by mitogen-activated protein kinase kinase 7, a specific activator for c-Jun $NH_2$-terminal kinase in ventricular muscle cells. J Biol Chem 1998; 273:5423-5426.

707. Choukroun G, Hajjar R, Fry S, et al: Regulation of cardiac hypertrophy in vivo by the stress-activated protein kinases/c-Jun $NH_2$-terminal kinases. J Clin Invest 1999;104:391-398.

708. Finn SG, Dickens M, Fuller SJ: c-Jun N-terminal kinase-interacting protein 1 inhibits gene expression in response to hypertrophic agonists in neonatal rat ventricular myocytes. Biochem J 2001; 358:489-495.

709. Sadoshima J, Montagne O, Wang Q, et al: The MEKK1-JNK pathway plays a protective role in pressure overload but does not mediate cardiac hypertrophy. J Clin Invest 2002;110:271-279.

710. Zhang D, Gaussin V, Taffet GE, et al: TAK1 is activated in the myocardium after pressure overload and is sufficient to provoke heart failure in transgenic mice. Nature Med 2000;6:556-563.

711. Hines WA, Thorburn J, Thorburn A: Cell density and contraction regulate p38 MAP kinase-dependent responses in neonatal rat cardiac myocytes. Am J Physiol 1999;277:H331-H341.

712. Aikawa R, Komuro I, Yamazaki T, et al: Oxidative stress activates extracellular signal-regulated kinases through Src and Ras in cultured cardiac myocytes of neonatal rats. J Clin Invest 1997; 100:1813-1821.

713. Zhu W, Zou Y, Aikawa R, et al: MAPK superfamily plays an important role in daunomycin-induced apoptosis of cardiac myocytes. Circulation 1999;100:2100-2107.

714. Minamino T, Yujiri T, Papst PJ, et al: MEKK1 suppresses oxidative stress-induced apoptosis of embryonic stem cell-derived cardiac myocytes. Proc Natl Acad Sci U S A 1999;96:15127-15132.

715. Andreka P, Zang J, Dougherty C, et al: Cytoprotection by Jun kinase during nitric oxide-induced cardiac myocyte apoptosis. Circ Res 2001;88:305-312.

716. Dougherty CJ, Kubasiak LA, Prentice H, et al: Activation of c-Jun N-terminal kinase promotes survival of cardiac myocytes after oxidative stress. Biochem J 2002;362:561-571.

717. Craig R, Larkin A, Mingo AM, et al: p38 MAPK and NF-kappa B collaborate to induce interleukin-6 gene expression and release. Evidence for a cytoprotective autocrine signaling pathway in a cardiac myocyte model system. J Biol Chem 2000;275:23814-23824.

## EDITOR'S CHOICE

Chien KR, Ross J, Jr, Hoshijima M: Calcium and heart failure: The cycle game. Nat Med 2003;9:508-509.
*A short review of recent experimental and clinical studies that support a pivotal role of signaling pathways that control calcium cycling in genetically based and acquired forms of heart failure.*
Coughlin SR: Protease-activated receptors in the cardiovascular system. Cold Spring Harb Symp Quant Biol 2002;67:197-208.
*The thrombin receptor has a unique pathway of activation based upon the cleavage of the receptor by this serine protease following ligand binding; a unique class of G-protein coupled receptor.*
Crackower MA, Oudit GY, Kozieradzki I, Sarao R, Sun H, Sasaki T, Hirsch E, Suzuki A, Shioi T, Irie-Sasaki J, et al: Regulation of myocardial contractility and cell size by distinct PI3K-PTEN signaling pathways. Cell 2002;110:737-749.
*Pivotal study that documents a key role of PI3 kinase in the control of in vivo cardiac contractility.*
Kioussi C, Briata P, Baek SH, Rose DW, Hamblet NS, Herman T, Ohgi KA, Lin C, Gleiberman A, Wang J, et al: Identification of a Wnt/Dvl/beta-Catenin → Pitx2 pathway mediating cell-type-specific proliferation during development. Cell 2002;111:673-685.
*A comprehensive study of signaling pathways for cardiac neural crest proliferation, with implications for congenital heart diseases.*
Li AC, Glass CK: The macrophage foam cell as a target for therapeutic intervention. Nat Med 2002;8:1235-1242.
*A timely review of recent work that links cytokine and nuclear hormone receptor signaling in monocytes as a critical pathway for atherosclerosis.*
Olson EN, Schneider MD: Sizing up the heart: Development redux in disease. Genes Dev. 2003;17:1937-1956
*Comprehensive review of cardiac myocyte signaling by leaders in the field.*
Pandur P, Lasche M, Eisenberg LM, Kuhl M: Wnt-11 activation of a non-canonical Wnt signalling pathway is required for cardiogenesis. Nature 2002;418:636-641.
*Wnts play multiple roles in cardiogenesis.*
Rockman HA, Koch WJ, Lefkowitz RJ: Seven-transmembrane-spanning receptors and heart function. Nature 2002;415:206-212.
*Studies of the beta-adrenergic receptor signaling in in vitro systems and in vivo in mouse models provide a paradigm for understanding the role of G-protein coupled receptors in the cardiovascular system and many other organ systems.*
Semenza GL: Angiogenesis in ischemic and neoplastic disorders. Annu Rev Med 2003;54:17-28.
*Oxygen sensing by the HIF transcriptional factor pathway is key in in vivo angiogenesis.*
Zhang J, Campbell RE, Ting AY, Tsien RY: (). Creating new fluorescent probes for cell biology. Nat Rev Mol Cell Biol 2002;3:906-918.
*A new generation of molecular probes allows the direct assessment of biochemical signals in specific compartments in living cells; historic work of wide impact.*

# chapter 8

# Genetic Approaches to Cardiovascular Disease

*Carl J. Vaughan*
*Craig T. Basson*

In this chapter, we describe the evolution of molecular genetics and its practical application to cardiovascular diseases. Since the early recognition that many cardiovascular diseases have a familial basis, pedigree analysis has become critical for modern practice. Advances in molecular biology coupled with elucidation of gene structure and function have further enhanced genetic approaches to cardiovascular disease. Investigation of familial monogenic diseases not only has been enlightening because of the specific genes discovered but, even more importantly, has highlighted multigene molecular and biochemical pathways in cardiovascular homeostasis whose manipulation has great therapeutic potential. Linkage analysis and positional cloning studies remain fundamentals of contemporary cardiovascular genetic analyses. Such studies have deciphered mysteries surrounding pathogenesis of several disorders such as dilated and hypertrophic cardiomyopathies, cardiac arrhythmias, cardiac tumors, dyslipoproteinemias, vasculopathies, and congenital heart malformation; they have highlighted key molecular paradigms in cardiovascular pathophysiology. For instance, study of congenital heart disease has led to seminal descriptions of transcriptional cascades that have fundamentally changed our perceptions and understanding of genes that orchestrate cardiac development. One can now appreciate that mutations in single regulatory genes that control cardiogenesis may cause solitary cardiac defects such as isolated atrial septal defects (ASDs) or ventricular septal defects (VSDs) and may also lead to complex cardiac phenotypes. Such transcriptional regulatory networks may ultimately be manipulated to modify a variety of complex pathophysiologic responses including ischemic left ventricular dysfunction, heart failure, atherosclerosis, and hypertension. Further advances are expected in the coming decades. The Human Genome Project (HGP) has provided a foundation on which to build a study of complex polygenic diseases, and the field of pharmacogenomics coupled with the advent of proteinomics and gene therapy promises more tailored and specific therapies for a wide variety of polygenic cardiovascular diseases. In addition to embracing these new genetic concepts, technologies, and approaches, physicians will need to be comfortable with the language and strategies of genetic medicine and will need to guide societal direction of the ethical dilemmas that arise along with the clinical application of modern genetics.

## PATTERNS OF INHERITANCE

In 1865, Mendel defined basic principles of inheritance of alleles at a single locus.[1] These Mendelian inheritance patterns (Figure 8-1) can be generally categorized into groups depending on the location of the relevant gene (i.e., on an autosome or sex chromosome) and the dominant or recessive effects of the allele. Thus, traits or disease can be inherited in autosomal dominant, autosomal recessive, X-linked recessive, or X-linked dominant fashions.[2,3] In addition, some traits are consequences of expression of genes in the distinct mitochondrial genome, and thus, mitochondrial disorders are inherited in a non-Mendelian fashion.

### Autosomal Dominant

Autosomal dominant disorders are the most prevalent Mendelian cardiovascular genetic disorders (Figure 8-1*A*). Examples of autosomal dominant cardiovascular disorders include hypertrophic cardiomyopathy (HCM), Marfan's syndrome (MFS), hereditary long QT syndrome (LQTS), and familial hypercholesterolemia. Any child of an affected individual has a 50% chance of being affected by the inherited disease. Because the disease gene is autosomal (i.e., not on a sex chromosome), dominant disorders occur without gender preference and with male-to-male transmission. Because only one disease allele is required for the phenotype to manifest, the disease is seen in every generation. There are exceptions to both these rules often resulting from the impact of interactions with other modifying genes. For instance, disease genes that are responsive to hormone levels may result in differences in male versus female disease manifestations, which is one form of so-called variable expressivity. In some cases, skip generations occur, that is, individuals who do not exhibit any disease manifestations but still transmit the disease to offspring and thus must carry a disease allele. This phenomenon is termed *incomplete* or *reduced* penetrance. Unaffected individuals do not carry the defective allele and do not transmit the disease to their offspring. Common examples of cardiovascular diseases that are transmitted in an autosomal dominant manner are listed in Table 8-1.

### Autosomal Recessive

In autosomal recessive disorders (Figure 8-1*B*), individuals must have two disease alleles. Thus, both parents

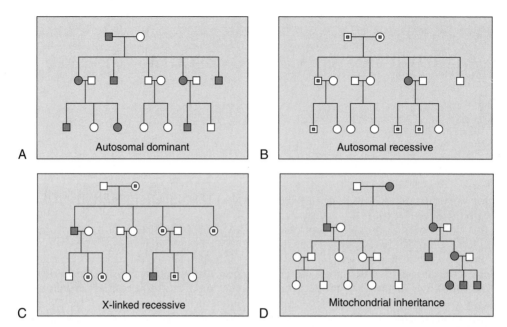

**FIGURE 8-1.** Patterns of inheritance. *A,* Autosomal dominant. *B,* Autosomal recessive. *C,* X-linked recessive. *D,* Mitochondrial inheritance. *Squares,* male; *circles,* female. Affected and unaffected individuals are represented by solid and open symbols, respectively. Symbols with central dot represent carriers.

must either be affected or unaffected heterozygotes. If both parents are affected, all children will be affected. If both parents are unaffected heterozygotes, each child has a 25% chance of being affected and a 50% chance of being an unaffected heterozygous carrier of the disorder. Therefore, one fourth of the offspring of two unaffected heterozygotes will carry two defective copies of the gene and will be affected. Half of the offspring will be heterozygous carriers of the disorder. Because heterozygotes are not affected, clinical manifestations of disease are not seen in every generation. As in autosomal dominant disorders, males and females are equally affected by autosomal recessive disorders. Inborn errors of metabolism, cystic fibrosis, and sickle cell anemia are examples of autosomal recessive disorders.

Common examples of cardiovascular diseases that are transmitted in an autosomal recessive manner include dilated cardiomyopathy, arrhythmogenic right-ventricular dysplasia, and homocysteinuria (Table 8-1).

## X-linked Inheritance

X-linked inheritance has specific features because of the presence of two X-chromosomes in the female and only one in the male. Both X-linked dominant and X-linked recessive disorders are known, but most X-linked diseases are recessive. Examples of X-linked recessive disorders with cardiovascular manifestations include Duchenne's muscular dystrophy (DMD) and fragile X syndrome. A typical X-linked recessive pedigree is

■ ■ ■

**TABLE 8-1**    EXAMPLES OF AUTOSOMAL DOMINANT, AUTOSOMAL RECESSIVE, AND X-LINKED CARDIOVASCULAR DISEASES

| Autosomal Dominant | Autosomal Recessive | X-linked Recessive |
|---|---|---|
| Hypertrophic cardiomyopathy | Dilated cardiomyopathy | Duchenne's muscular dystrophy |
| Dilated cardiomyopathy | Arrhythmogenic right ventricular | Fragile X syndrome |
| Familial hypercholesterolemia | dysplasia | |
| Hereditary long QT syndrome | Friedreich's ataxia | |
| Arrhythmogenic right | Gaucher's disease | |
| ventricular dysplasia | Ellis van Crevald's syndrome | |
| Marfan's syndrome | Homocystinuria | |
| Williams syndrome | Hereditary long QT syndrome | |
| Holt-Oram syndrome | | |
| Carney's complex | | |
| Atrial septal defect with heart block | | |
| Alagille's syndrome | | |
| Noonan's syndrome | | |
| Char's syndrome | | |

shown in Figure 8-1C. A hallmark of an X-linked recessive disorder is the absence of male-to-male transmission because a father never transmits his X-chromosome to his son. By contrast, a father transmits a copy of his X-chromosome to his daughters. Therefore, all daughters of an affected male are carriers. X-linked dominant cardiovascular disorders have not been described.

## Mitochondrial Inheritance

Mitochondrial disorders are maternally inherited because the egg, not the sperm, transmits cytoplasmic mitochondrial DNA to offspring.[4,5] Because each germ and somatic cell can contain different amounts of mitochondrial DNA, the risk of disease transmission to offspring is difficult to predict. This results in a non-Mendelian pattern of inheritance (Figure 8-1D). The severity and often highly variable expressivity of the phenotype in a mitochondrial disorder is often related to the ratio of mutant to normal mitochondrial DNA (mtDNA) in a cell. Organs with high-energy requirements (muscles, eyes, and kidneys) appear to be more susceptible to mitochondrial disorders.[6] An example of a mitochondrial disorder is MELAS syndrome (mitochondrial myopathy, encephalopathy, lactic acidosis, and stroke-like episodes), and the inheritance pattern of such mitochondrial disorders is seen in Figure 8-1D.

## Complexity in the Basic Pedigree

A common confounder in cardiovascular disease is age-related penetrance.[7] Although the genotype is fixed at conception, the disorder may not manifest until late in life. HCM is an age-related disease. For instance, HCM often does not manifest on the echocardiogram until after puberty. A more dramatic example is the subset of HCM resulting from mutations in myosin binding protein C. Individuals with this disorder frequently do not show evidence of cardiac hypertrophy until after age 50.[8] This delayed onset of disease has occasionally led to patients with this disorder being misclassified as having a hypertensive cardiomyopathy. In addition to altered penetrance, marked variable phenotypic expressivity characterizes cardiovascular disorders such as MFS,[9,10] hereditary LQTS,[11] HCM,[8,12] Holt-Oram syndrome,[13] and familial ASDs with conduction disease.[14]

## CHROMOSOMAL SYNDROMES

### Structure of Chromosomes

The normal human somatic cell has 46 chromosomes, including 2 sex chromosomes (X,Y). During interphase, the largest portion of the cell cycle, the chromosomes are not visible as individual objects under a light microscope. However, during cell division, the chromosomes become condensed and are visible as dark distinct bodies within the nuclei of cells. The chromosomes are most easily seen and identified at the metaphase stage of cell division. Chromosomes can be identified by characteristic banding patterns in karyotypes that are obtained by staining chromosomes with various dyes, such as Giemsa, that produce unique light and dark banding patterns. The bandwidth and the order of the bands are specific to each particular chromosome; a trained cytogeneticist can identify each chromosome by observing its banding pattern under a microscope. Newer methods have been developed that do not rely on Giemsa banding (G-banding). Advances in molecular cytogenetics, especially the technique of fluorescent *in situ* hybridization (FISH), have allowed more precise definition of chromosomal structures, which are difficult to identify using conventional G-banding.[15] Spectral karyotyping (SKY), a novel approach based on hybridization of 24 fluorescent-labeled chromosome painting probes was developed, which permits a simultaneous but differential high-resolution color display of all human chromosomes.[16,17]

## Gross Chromosomal Abnormalities

Numerical chromosomal abnormalities occur when the normal human chromosome complement of a cell is altered. When a cell has a balanced extra set of chromosomes in multiples of 23, it is described as polyploid. For example, when a single egg is fertilized by two sperm, the resulting cells are triploid (i.e., 69XXY, 69XXX, 69XYY). In general, triploidy and tetraploidy are lethal and result in spontaneous abortion of the fetus. Aneuploidy is a term used to describe a cell in which an individual chromosome of a chromosome pair is missing (monosomy) or an extra copy of a chromosome is present (trisomy). Trisomies are common and are found in more than 50% of chromosomally abnormal fetuses. Like trisomies, monosomies are usually lethal unless they involve the sex chromosomes. Three well-described trisomies associated with significant cardiovascular disease and are compatible with live birth are trisomy 21 (Down's syndrome),[18] trisomy 13 (Patau's syndrome),[19] and trisomy 18 (Edwards' syndrome)[20] (Table 8-2). Trisomy 21 is often associated with common atrioventricular canal, an ostium primum ASD, VSD, patent ductus arteriosus (PDA), and cleft anterior mitral valve leaflet; trisomy 13 with ASD, VSD, and PDA; and trisomy

■ ▨ ■

**TABLE 8-2**  EXAMPLES OF CARDIOVASCULAR DISEASE ASSOCIATED WITH CHROMOSOMAL ANEUPLOIDIES

| **Trisomies** | |
|---|---|
| Trisomy 13 (Patau's syndrome) | ASD, VSD, PDA, DORV, CCHD |
| Trisomy 18 (Edwards' syndrome) | VSD, PDA, polyvalvular dysplasia, CCHD |
| Trisomy 21 (Down's syndrome) | Endocardial cushion defect, VSD, cleft mitral valve, CCHD |
| **Monosomies** | |
| Monosomy X (Turner's syndrome) | Coarctation of the aorta, VSD, bicuspid aortic valve, aortic aneurysm |

ASD, atrial septal defect; CCHD, complex congenital heart disease; DORV, double-outlet right ventricle; PDA, patent ductus arteriosus; VSD, ventricular septal defect.

18 with ASD, double outlet right ventricle, VSD, and PDA. Survival in these disorders depends on the severity of the congenital defect. Monosomy and trisomy arise during either meiosis or mitosis by the process of nondisjunction, in which the two sister chromatids fail to separate during anaphase. The frequency of nondisjunction increases with increasing maternal age.

For certain autosomal genes, one allele must be inherited from the mother and one from the father. If both chromosomes come from the same parent, it is termed uniparental disomy (UPD).[21] The effects of UPD usually include growth retardation, small stature, and behavioral abnormalities. Isolated case reports have described UPD in association with congenital heart disease.[22] The need for a single copy of each chromosome (one from the father and one from the mother) is a consequence of genomic imprinting.[23] Imprinting is due to the functional differences in the expression of genes, depending on whether they are maternally or paternally derived.[24] The mechanism of imprinting is not fully understood but appears to involve methylation of cytosine residues upstream of a gene that control its rate of transcription.[24] The signal to imprint a gene occurs in the gonad and will, therefore, be different depending on whether the gene passes through the mother or the father. The concept of imprinting has become increasingly important as attempts are made to unravel contiguous gene syndromes, developmental diseases, and the role of position effects in genetic disease.[25]

In addition to anomalies of chromosome number, structural abnormalities or rearrangements of individual chromosomes may also cause disease. Such aberrations include interchromosomal and intrachromosomal translocations and inversions and variable-size chromosomal deletions and insertions. The severity of the phenotype depends on the nature and number of the genes contained in the affected chromosomal region. Large abnormalities often have complex phenotypes, reflecting the loss of a number of genes that may have wide-ranging functions in many organs including the heart. Small deletions (microdeletions) (Table 8-3) may not be detectable using standard karyotype analysis.[15,17] However, these deletions may be detected using DNA probes or FISH analysis.[15,17] Microdeletions may have more subtle phenotypes. Chromosomal rearrangements may also produce disease by altering expression of genes adjacent to but not included within a deletion or translocation/inversion breakpoint by changing the location of a gene, a so-called position effect.

Several diseases with cardiovascular phenotypes have been associated with specific chromosomal rearrangements, and these findings indicate chromosomal regions that harbor genes critical in cardiovascular disease

pathogenesis. For instance, chromosome 7 deletions have been demonstrated in patients with the complex Williams syndrome (supravalvular aortic stenosis [SVAS], hypercalcemia, precocious personality),[26] and subsequent investigation has shown that haploinsufficiency of the chromosome 7 elastin gene is responsible for SVAS.[27] Despite advances in modern genetic technology, clinically available high-resolution karyotyping and FISH studies with probes specific for gene segments known to be associated with disease still play important roles in establishing the location of gene(s) responsible for human cardiovascular disease. For example, congenital heart disease, particularly conotruncal defects in the setting of DiGeorge's or velocardiofacial syndrome, is associated with deletion of chromosome 22 band q11.[28] Conotruncal defects occur in the setting of cleft palate, unusual facies, and hyperparathyroidism.[2] The first clues pointing to this abnormal genetic locus came from cytogenetic analyses of patients with unbalanced translocations and partial monosomy of chromosome 22[28-30] and with the observation that small deletions of chromosome 22q were present in about 10% of patients with DiGeorge's syndrome. Subsequent studies have demonstrated that most syndromic patients have large rearrangements or microdeletions in chromosome 22q11, and current data suggest that about 80% to 95% of individuals with DiGeorge's/velocardiofacial syndrome (VCFS) have microdeletions.[29-31]

The observation that mutations in T-box transcription factors cause syndromic congenital heart disease (e.g., TBX5 in Holt-Oram syndrome, and TBX3 in ulnar-mammary syndrome)[32,33] prompted investigations to focus attention on the TBX1 gene often included in 22q deletions in patients with DiGeorge's syndrome. Studies in mice now suggest that TBX1 may be an important gene in the pathogenesis of DiGeorge's syndrome. Mice that are hemizygous deficient for TBX1 exhibit severe defects of aortic arch development.[34] Notably, TBX1 missense mutations have not yet been reported in humans with DiGeorge's syndrome who do not harbor a deletion at chromosome 22q11[35] or in patients with 22q deletions not encompassing TBX1. Thus, we cannot yet exclude involvement of other genes in the pathogenesis of human DiGeorge's syndrome. Interestingly, mouse models have also demonstrated that loss of the CrKl gene, whose 22q homologue is often deleted in DiGeorge's syndrome patients, results in aortic arch defects.[36]

Karyotype analysis should be considered an important opportunity to provide a global overview of chromosomal integrity, and cytogenetic studies remain an integral part of the molecular genetic evaluation of individuals with either sporadic or inherited diseases. An abnormal karyotype may highlight subchromosomal regions for

■ ■ ■

**TABLE 8-3**   EXAMPLES OF CARDIOVASCULAR DISEASE ASSOCIATED WITH CHROMOSOMAL MICRODELETIONS

| | |
|---|---|
| del(7)(q11.2) (Williams syndrome) | Supravalvular aortic stenosis |
| del (22)(q11.2) (DiGeorge's syndrome) | Conotruncal anomalies |
| del(20)(p11.2p12) (Alagille's syndrome) | Peripheral pulmonic stenosis, tetralogy of Fallot |

further molecular genetic analysis. For instance, we previously described the cytogenetic analysis of a giant invasive cardiac lipoma in a patient with a history of multiple lipomatosis (cutaneous lipoma, lipomatous gynecomastia, lipomatous hypertrophy of the interatrial septum, and dyslipidemia).[37] Cytogenetic studies of cells derived from the cardiac lipoma demonstrated a t(2;19)(p13;p13.2) chromosomal translocation.[37] The breakpoint of this translocation maps near a number of genes that regulate cardiovascular homeostasis, for example, the apolipoprotein gene cluster. This single case with an informative karyotype highlights the unique opportunity that cytogenetic investigation may afford investigators who are confronted with unusual presentations of disease. Ongoing studies of the regions of chromosomes 2 and 19 perturbed by the translocation in this unusual infiltrating cardiac lipoma will identify a gene or genes that participate in adipocyte growth and differentiation and may also provide insight into syndromes of multiple lipomatosis and dyslipidemia.

# IDENTIFYING DISEASE GENES

DNA provides the alphabet for a genetic language that encodes all proteins in a cell. The appreciation that misprints in this alphabet cause disease was a quantum leap in the understanding of disease pathogenesis and provided an impetus to discover methods to pinpoint the genes responsible for many diseases. To date, scientists' greatest successes have been in the identification of molecular causes for monogenic forms of cardiovascular disease. The search for disease genes that cause single-gene human disorders has been founded on principles of Mendelian inheritance and has exploited the occurrence of chromosomal anomalies to accelerate the arduous search for loci associated with disease.

Because there are at least 40,000 genes in the human genome,[38-41] early investigators attempting to isolate disease genes in the absence of genome sequence had a formidable task. Many of the earliest advances using linkage analysis involved genes located on the X chromosome, because X-linked diseases could be identified by inspecting family pedigrees. One example of an X-linked disease is familial cardiomyopathy resulting from DMD.[2] DMD is an X-linked recessive disorder that usually appears in early childhood with progressive muscular weakness and wasting.[2,42] Cardiac involvement is common in DMD and usually manifests as a dilated cardiomyopathy or with arrhythmias or heart block.[43] DMD is caused by mutations in the *dystrophin* gene that encodes dystrophin, a large subsarcolemmal rod-shaped protein.[44] Dystrophin is thought to stabilize the sarcomere (and hence the contractile apparatus of a cell) by linking the actin cytoskeleton to the extracellular matrix via a dystrophin-associated glycoprotein complex.

However, most genes are located on an autosome and their chromosomal location cannot be deduced by inspecting the family pedigree. The identification of these autosomal diseases, therefore, requires a different approach that relies on linking the disease trait to some

genetic marker that specifically defines a chromosomal region or locus. This process of linking a disease to a chromosomal location using genetic markers is called linkage analysis.

## Linkage Analysis to Demonstrate Genetic Causes of Disease

The initial step in a typical positional cloning-candidate strategy to identify a disease gene is to identify the chromosomal location of the gene that causes the disorder. This approach relies on classic Mendelian genetics. Inspection of the family pedigree determines the mode of inheritance: autosomal dominant, autosomal recessive, X-linked, or mitochondrial (Figure 8-1). If a family is of sufficient size to provide statistical power, then genetic linkage analysis can be used to determine the chromosomal location of the disease gene. Genetic linkage analysis has been facilitated through the discovery and mapping of numerous genetic polymorphisms used to genotype family members. These genetic markers are distributed throughout the genome. Some of the earliest linkage studies were done with ABO blood groups and HLA antigen types. Subsequently, restriction fragment length polymorphisms (RFLPs) with known map locations on each chromosome were used.[45] These polymorphisms usually arise in a population when a single base-pair change occurs that alters the cleavage site for a restriction endonuclease. When the cleavage site is altered, cutting DNA with a restriction endonuclease will generate DNA fragments of differing lengths that may be used to genotype a family. Linkage by RFLP analysis is laborious because it generally requires time-consuming Southern blot analysis of large quantities of genomic DNA. It has now been largely replaced by PCR-based analysis of DNA markers such as variable number tandem repeats (VNTRs),[46] short tandem repeats (STRs),[47] and single-nucleotide polymorphisms (SNPs). The most commonly used markers today for linkage analysis are STRs. These markers are sequences of DNA that are polymorphic within the general population[48-50]; that is, the number of repeats in each STR varies. This allows amplification of these STRs in each member of a family to provide a genotype that can be correlated with the particular phenotype under investigation.

Results from linkage analysis are expressed as a statistical expression of the likelihood that a particular genetic marker will be co-inherited with the phenotype more often than expected by chance alone.[51,52] The logarithm of the odds (LOD score) is the logarithm (base 10) of the calculated odds ratio in favor of linkage between the marker and the disease gene.[52] The higher the LOD score, the more likely it is that the marker and the disease gene associated with the phenotype are linked. Clear criteria for statistical significance of linkage have been established for monogenic diseases.[52] A LOD score =3.0 (or odds of 1000:1) derived from a random genome search is considered significant for linkage to a previously unknown locus because it is equivalent to $p = 0.05$.[52] A LOD score of =−2.0 (odds of 1:100) provides statistically significant evidence that excludes linkage to a locus. Once a statistically significant locus for a disorder has been established (LOD score =3.0, $p < 0.05$), one can ask whether families with this same disorder are linked to this same locus (so-called genetic homogeneity) or whether the disease in other families may be due to gene defects at other loci (so-called genetic heterogeneity). Because the statistical question requires fewer tests, lower LOD scores have greater statistical significance. Thus, in this case a LOD score =1.3 (odds 1:20 in favor of linkage) are sufficient to establish linkage to a know locus with $p < 0.05$. Because the magnitude of a LOD score is affected not only by proximity of the genotyped polymorphisms but also by the family size and number of informative individuals in any given analysis, it is possible to link disease in much smaller nuclear families to a known locus, although they might have insufficient power for a random genome search for an unknown locus. A common statistical genetic error that leads to false-positive linkage is to sum LOD scores derived from small families with insufficient power to achieve a LOD score =3.0 separately to achieve statistical power in a random genome search. This methodology is only acceptable if genetic homogeneity exists and heterogeneity can be excluded.

Early genetic linkage analysis was hampered by a lack of dense maps of highly polymorphic chromosomal markers. However, modern genetic maps include STR and other genetic markers spaced at approximately 1-cM intervals along the length of each chromosome.[53] Such panels of markers are commonly used to genotype families for linkage to identify loci associated with inherited diseases. Although locus identification is an investigational predecessor to disease gene identification, genotyping with genetic markers tightly linked to a disease locus can provide clinical information even without knowledge or mutational analysis of a specific disease gene.[51] Inheritance of a haplotype (a set of genotypes of several linked markers) associated with a particular phenotype in a given family can provide a molecular diagnosis for individuals in that family with unclear phenotypes. The accuracy of haplotype-based diagnosis increases as the genetic interval over which the genetic markers are spaced decreases. We have previously used haplotype analysis to predict diagnosis of a familial cardiac myxoma syndrome even before the disease gene had been identified.[54,55] Similarly, haplotype analysis has provided molecular diagnosis in MFS in which DNA sequencing is generally not feasible because of the large size of the *fibrillin-1* disease gene.[56]

## Disease Gene Identification

Identification of a disease gene at a mapped locus generally depends on a hybrid of two complimentary strategies: candidate gene approach and positional cloning. In a pure candidate gene approach, genes are selected for mutational analysis based on the encoded protein's known structure or function without consideration of the genes' map locations. In a pure positional approach, molecular biologic techniques are used to clone the mutated DNA without consideration of the gene product's function. Most often, a hybrid positional-candidate approach is used in which small regions with known genes are cloned and then genes in the cloned segments are prioritized for mutational analysis based on predictions about their function. With the availability of increasingly dense gene maps, positional cloning strategies can narrow the locus genetically and physically to prioritize a small list of candidate genes that can then be analyzed for sequence variants. For instance, we used a positional-candidate gene approach to identify mutations in the *PRKAR1α* gene as the cause of familial cardiac myxomas in the disorder Carney's complex.[57] In Carney's complex, familial cardiac myxomas are associated with spotty pigmentation of the skin (lentiginosis), blue nevi, and endocrine overactivity.[58] Once linkage analyses established a chromosomal locus for Carney's complex at chromosome 17q24,[54] evaluation of genes known to be mapped to this chromosomal region resulted in the analysis of the *PRKAR1α* gene as an attractive candidate for Carney's complex. *PRKAR1α* encodes the R1α regulatory subunit of cAMP-dependent protein kinase A (PKA).[59] Prior investigation of Peutz-Jeghers syndrome, a similar disorder associated with tumor formation and cutaneous hyperpigmentation, showed that mutations in the *STK11* serine threonine kinase gene can cause tumorigenesis and therefore suggested that kinase gene mutations might also cause Carney's complex.[60] Subsequent analyses have shown that, just as *STK11* haploinsufficiency causes Peutz-Jeghers syndrome, *PRKAR1α* haploinsufficiency causes Carney's complex.[57]

It is critical to distinguish among sequence variants, that is, between polymorphisms and mutations. Polymorphisms are sequence variants that occur at least with a moderately high frequency in a population. A mutation is a rare sequence variant that, in and of itself, causes a change in a phenotype or a disease. Criteria used to define a sequence variant as a mutation for Mendelian diseases include (1) a resultant change in protein structure, function, and/or expression; (2) absence of the variant in 100 normal unrelated chromosomes; and (3) cosegregation of the variant with the consequent disease in affected families. Criteria are less well defined for acquired sequence variants that may be somatic disease-causing mutations. Sequence variants that are polymorphisms may still affect phenotypes and disease and are of significant interest for investigators studying genetic causes of non-Mendelian complex traits such as hypertension, atherosclerosis, asthma, and diabetes.

## MOLECULAR PATHOGENESIS OF GENETIC DISEASE

### Haploinsufficient Diseases

In general, two molecular mechanisms underlie most genetic diseases: alteration of gene dose or perturbation of cellular homeostasis by an abnormal protein. Most commonly, gene dose changes reflect a dose reduction secondary to haploinsufficiency. By contrast, perturbation of cellular homeostasis occurs via a so-called dominant negative effect. The term *haploinsufficiency* describes a disease process in which the loss of a single copy of a gene produces disease. Well-described cardiovascular diseases that have been attributed to haploinsufficiency include familial heterozygous hypercholesterolemia resulting from LDL receptor gene haploinsufficiency,[61] and SVAS resulting from elastin gene haploinsufficiency.[27] In haploinsufficient diseases, the mutant allele is either one in which the disease gene is completely deleted or one in which nonsense or frameshift mutations give rise to an abnormal mRNA predicted to encode a "truncated" protein but instead undergoes nonsense-mediated decay (NMD).[62-64] Although the precise underlying molecular mechanisms are incompletely understood, NMD occurs when the cellular machinery recognizes a premature "stop" or termination codon (PTC; introduced by nonsense or frameshift mutations) before the final exon of the open reading frame.[62-64] The subsequent degradation of mutant mRNA leads to a halving of synthesis of normal protein (compared with unaffected individuals) and a pathologic phenotype. For instance, in familial heterozygous hypercholesterolemia, PTCs in the LDL receptor gene lead to NMD, a 50% reduction in LDL receptor expression, and a consequent reduction in LDL receptor-mediated endocytosis of LDL cholesterol and hypercholesterolemia (Figure 8-2). Haploinsufficiency has also been applied to non-Mendelian disorders including microdeletion syndromes such as DiGeorge's syndrome and aneuploidies such as Turner's syndrome (45,X).[65] In some cases, mRNAs with PTCs may escape NMD but result in a functional haploinsufficiency because the encoded truncated protein is no longer functional. However, if the truncated protein interferes with normal protein function, then it can have a dominant negative effect (see the following). Although missense point mutations often produce a dominant negative effect, they too can result in the production of a completely nonfunctional protein, that is, functional haploinsufficiency.

## Dominant Negative Diseases

In a dominant negative process, a gene mutation results in the translation of an abnormal protein (Figure 8-3). The abnormal protein impairs the function of a normal protein either through direct interaction with the protein encoded from a normal allele or through interactions with protein binding partners. This disease-causation mechanism has also been termed a *poison peptide theory.* For example, a dominant negative activity occurs if a mutant protein is able to bind either wild-type protein itself or the downstream targets of the wild-type protein but is incapable of generating the anticipated physiologic signals as a consequence of that binding. Examples of cardiovascular disorders resulting from a dominant negative process that are discussed in more detail in subsequent sections include some cases of HCM (Figure 8-2),[12] MFS,[10,66] and hereditary LQTS.[11] Observations in several diseases sug-

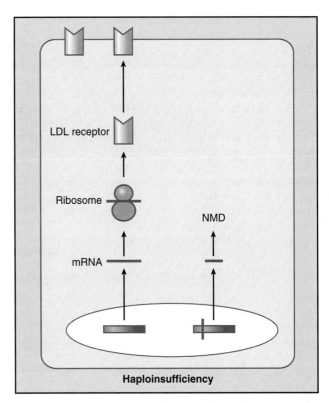

**FIGURE 8-2.** Molecular bases of haploinsufficient disease. Haploinsufficiency is a disease process in which the loss of a single coding copy of a gene produces disease. In haploinsufficient diseases, the disease allele is completely deleted or is affected by nonsense or frameshift mutations that give rise to an abnormal mRNA. Such mRNA would be predicted to encode a "truncated" protein but instead is degraded by the cell via NMD. Examples of haploinsufficient diseases include heterozygous familial hypercholesterolemia and Carney's complex due to nonsense/frameshift mutations in one allele of the LDL receptor or the *PRKAR1α* gene, respectively, and supravalvular aortic stenosis resulting from deletion of one copy of the *elastin* gene.

gest that some mutations in a given gene may lead to haploinsufficiency and others to a poison peptide. Still others may produce a mixture of haploinsufficient and dominant negative effects.

For example, in type IV Ehlers Danlos syndrome, a missense mutation in *COL3A1* leads to a deficiency in type III procollagen by impaired collagen assembly.[67,68] The type III procollagen molecule is a polymer made of three identical peptides (homotripolymer). When one allele of *COL3A1* is defective there is approximately a 1:8 chance that a homotripolymer will contain three normal peptides. Accordingly, 7/8 homotripolymers will contain at least one defective peptide. Thus, there will be overall deficiency in normally assembled type III procollagen, and this marked reduction in intact type III procollagen polymers accounts for the prominent connective tissue disease phenotypes of Ehlers Danlos syndrome IV including skin fragility, joint laxity, and rupture of large arteries. In the case of the frameshift (1832delAA, 413delC, and 555delT) and the missense 4294CT (Arg1432Ter) mutations of *COL3A1*, true haploinsufficiency of *COL3A1* occurs and produces a vascular phenotype similar to the vascular features of

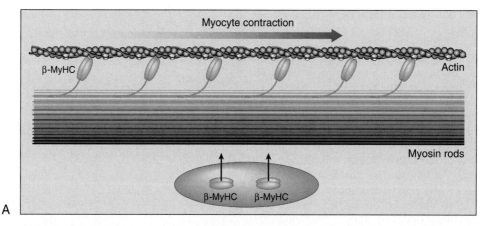

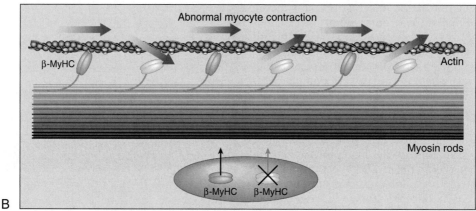

**FIGURE 8-3.** Molecular bases of dominant negative disease. A dominant negative process is one in which a gene mutation results in the translation of an abnormal protein that impedes the function of normal protein either through direct interaction with the protein encoded from the normal allele or through interactions with protein binding partners. An example of a dominant negative disease is HCM. In the normal state a uniform population of β-myosin heavy chain (β-MyHC) molecules will lead to normal actin-myosin cross-bridging and contraction. When, for example, mutations arise in the β-MyHC and abnormal population of β-MyHC molecules *(gray)* gives rise to abnormal crossbridging and myocellular contraction. This abnormal contraction at the cellular level is also thought to be ultimately responsible for the myocyte disarray, hypertrophy, and fibrosis seen in HCM.

Ehlers Danlos syndrome type IV and, therefore, calls into question the labeling of disease as purely dominant negative or haploinsufficient.[69]

## MONOGENIC PARADIGMS

The study of monogenic familial disorders has led to the identification of many disease genes that cause human cardiovascular disease. Monogenic cardiovascular disease can be categorized broadly in terms of the predominant cardiac phenotype. This is schematically represented in Figure 8-4. These categories include the cardiomyopathies, the channelopathies responsible for inherited disorders of cardiac rhythm, familial vasculopathies, and tumor syndromes that affect the heart. In addition, the appreciation that single-gene disorders may cause complex and diverse developmental cardiac defects has also led to paradigm shifts in the molecular understanding of congenital heart disease. Many of these diseases are described in detail in subsequent chapters. In this chapter, we mention certain disorders that highlight major genetic advances and that have fundamentally altered the understanding of disease causation.

## Hypertrophic Cardiomyopathy Is a Disease of the Sarcomere

The study of familial HCM is a particularly illuminating example of how molecular genetics has transformed the understanding of a perplexing cardiovascular disorder with significant morbidity and mortality. HCM is a relatively common disease with an incidence on the order of 1 in 500 that is clinically diagnosed by cardiac hypertrophy and pathologically characterized by myocyte hypertrophy disarray and myocardial fibrosis.[70] HCM is the most common cause of sudden death in the young.[71] More than 100 mutations in nine genes have been identified in HCM.[12,70,71] Most of these genes encode proteins within the sarcomeric contractile apparatus, and these observations have suggested that HCM is a disease of the sarcomere. The β-myosin heavy chain, cardiac troponin T, α-tropomyosin, and myosin binding protein-C genes are most commonly involved, together accounting for more than 60% of cases.[2,70] These genetic insights have paved the way for experimental studies showing that mutations in sarcomeric proteins cause a number of functional defects within the sarcomere including reduced ATPase activity of myosin,[72] altered cross-bridge

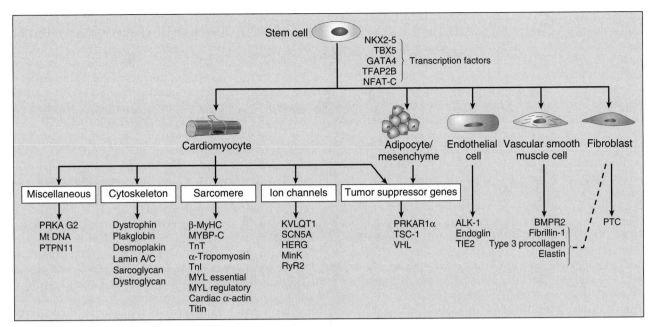

**FIGURE 8-4.** Evolving paradigms of monogenic cardiovascular disease. This schematic presents predominant cell-types and cardiovascular structures that underlie monogenic cardiovascular disorders. The disease-causing genes are listed below each cell type or compartment. This allows one to appreciate broad associations between related genes and cardiac structures that have prompted general paradigms for disease causation. For instance, HCM and familial long QT syndrome are both diseases of the cardiomyocyte but have contrasting molecular personalities. HCM is generally believed to be a disease of the sarcomere and mutations in many sarcomeric genes have been described in this condition. In contrast, ion channel gene mutations do not cause structural heart disease and are predominantly associated with the development of malignant arrhythmias. Although these pathways are represented in a hierarchical fashion, this schematic admittedly oversimplifies the true complexity of these pathways in the cardiovascular system that operate *in vivo* as a complicated web of interdependent and interacting molecules that control cardiac homeostasis. However, it also highlights exceptions that will promote new disease paradigms. This is reflected in a miscellaneous group in the figure, in which certain genes do not conform with the other compartment models. For instance, association of *PRKAG2* mutations with HCM and with Wolff-Parkinson-White syndrome suggests nonsarcomeric causes for hypertrophy and non-ion-channel causes for arrhythmias.

kinetics,[73] reduced myocyte contractility, altered calcium handling,[74] and a predisposition to arrhythmia generation.[75] It has been hypothesized that the primary abnormality in HCM is not specifically one of abnormal force generation but rather one of inefficient use of ATP.[76] The description of families with HCM and accessory pathways (pre-excitation or Wolff-Parkinson-White syndrome) with mutations in *PRKAG2*, encoding the gamma(2) subunit of AMP-activated protein kinase (AMPK) may provide some support for this hypothesis.[76,77] Because AMPK provides a central sensing mechanism that protects cells from depletion of ATP supplies, it has been proposed that myocellular energy compromise is a unifying pathogenic mechanism in all forms of HCM.[76] However, recent data suggest that AMPK mutations may not lead to true cellular hypertrophy but may lead to the same echocardiographic endpoint via abnormal cellular glycogen deposition.[78] Because abnormal glycogen storage is not a feature of classic HCM, it is unclear whether these data shed light on HCM caused by sarcomeric mutations.

## Transcription Factors Orchestrate Cardiac Development

Mutations in several transcription factors have been shown to cause congenital heart disease. Congenital structural heart disease is often estimated to occur in at least 0.5% of the general population.[79] Defects in cardiac septation including ASD, VSD, and atrioventricular canal septal defects form a major portion of congenital heart disease, and these defects occur in up to 5% of live births.[79] Major advances have been made in the understanding of the genetic orchestration of cardiac septation. Mutant genes encoding two transcription factors have been described in families with inherited ASDs and/or VSDs. Holt-Oram syndrome, also called heart-hand syndrome, is an autosomal dominant condition characterized by upper extremity abnormalities in association with ASD or VSD.[2,13] Mutation in the *TBX5* T-box transcription factor gene causes Holt-Oram syndrome.[32] Most *TBX5* mutations are truncation mutations (nonsense or frameshift) that result in *TBX5* haploinsufficiency, but missense mutations have also been identified.[32,80,81] Although *TBX5* haploinsufficiency produces severe malformation of both heart and limbs, the missense mutations thus far identified modify specific DNA binding sites and produce either severe heart or severe limb abnormalities but not both.[82] Mutations in the homeobox transcription factor gene *NKX2-5* have also been described in families with inherited structural heart disease, in particular ASDs, and progressive atrioventricular node dysfunction.[83,84] *NKX* gene family members are homologous to the *Drosophila tinman* gene that participates in specification of heart muscle progenitors.[85] At least some human *NKX2-5* mutations disrupt the homeobox encoding region of the gene and are predicted to cause disease through *NKX2.5* haploinsufficiency. Recent data shows that mutations in *GATA4* (which interacts with *TBX5* and *NKX2.5*) also cause septal defects and congenital heart disease (See Editor's Choice). PDA is a relatively common cardiac defect that occurs in approximately 1 in 2000 children.[86] PDA may occur alone or in association with complex congenital heart disease. Char's syndrome is a rare autosomal dominant syndrome that includes dysmorphic facies, abnormal fifth finger, and PDA.[87] Molecular genetic studies of families affected by Char's syndrome have identified mutations in *TFAP2B*, which encodes a neural crest-related helix-span-helix transcription factor.[88,89]

Taken together, the study of these rare syndromes has highlighted a number of key developmental pathways regulated by several important transcription factors (*TBX5*, *NKX2-5*, and *TFAP2B*) that appear to operate in a hierarchical fashion to regulate cardiogenesis (Figure 8-4). This hierarchy refers to the control of many downstream genes and developmental pathways by a number of critical upstream genes that dictate many of the steps in cardiac development. Many of these upstream genes that orchestrate heart development are transcription factors. This hierarchy helps one understand why even perturbation of single genes encoding these factors may cause a spectrum of defects as seen with mutations in *NKX2-5*. Mutation of downstream genes may also cause congenital heart disease. Alagille's syndrome is a human autosomal dominant developmental disorder characterized by liver, heart, eye, skeletal, craniofacial, and kidney abnormalities.[2,90] Alagille's syndrome is caused by mutations in the *Jagged 1 (JAG1)* gene, which encodes a ligand for Notch family receptors.[90] Most *JAG1* mutations seen in Alagille's syndrome patients are null alleles, suggesting *JAG1* haploinsufficiency as a primary cause of this disorder.

These molecular genetic studies also highlight the historic but, in retrospect, misleading characterization of congenital heart defects classified purely along anatomic lines and show that groups of conditions should more appropriately be aggregated under broad developmental categories such as diseases of septation, conotruncal defects, heterotaxy syndromes, and neural crest defects. Given that specific malformations (i.e., ASD) are found to be due to two or more different causes (i.e., mutations in *TBX5* or *NKX2-5*), this then identifies portions of the heart as fields or morphogenetic units that may undergo discrete developmental responses because of distinct genetic insults[91] (Figure 8-4).

## Familial Arrhythmias and Channelopathies

LQTS is a group of cardiac disorders that produces sudden death in otherwise healthy people. Prolongation of the QT interval is associated with lethal ventricular arrhythmias such as ventricular tachycardia and *torsades de pointes*.[11] There are at least two modes of inheritance of LQTS. The Jervell and Lange-Nielsen syndrome was described in 1957 and is inherited as an autosomal recessive trait and is associated with deafness.[92] A more common form, the Romano Ward syndrome, is not associated with deafness and is inherited as an autosomal dominant trait.[93] To define the genes involved in LQTS, familial forms of the

disorder were studied. Molecular genetic and positional cloning studies initially demonstrated linkage of LQTS to chromosome 11p15.5, and mutations in the *KVLQT1* gene were subsequently identified at this locus.[94] This discovery gave the first glimpse of the molecular pathogenesis of arrhythmia in LQTS and fueled many additional studies. Currently at least six genes are known to cause LQTS including *KVLQT1* (LQT1), *HERG* (LQT2), *SCN5A* (LQT3), *minK* (LQT5), *MiRP1* (LQT6),[95-97] and an as yet unidentified gene on chromosome 4q25-27 (LQT4).[98] The investigation of ion channel genes in other arrhythmias led to the discovery that mutations in the *SCN5A* gene also cause some cases of Brugada's syndrome (which is characterized by right bundle branch block, ST elevation in leads V1 to V3, and sudden death) and familial ventricular fibrillation.[99] Thus, such findings also highlight the pleiotropic nature of *SCN5A* mutations that may cause diverse phenotypes including LQTS, ventricular fibrillation, and atrioventricular block.

The genetic basis of a third class of arrhythmias has recently become apparent. Mutations in the cardiac ryanodine receptor RyR2 have been shown to cause familial catecholaminergic ventricular tachycardia.[100-102] The relationship between cellular mechanisms by which RyR2 mutations cause familial ventricular tachycardia in some kindreds but ARVC in others remains unclear. However, one overall unifying theme among most of these disorders is that mutations in critical proteins that form ion channels in myocardium cause arrhythmias. In LQTS, this molecular genetic data has allowed us to make broad genotype-phenotype correlations. In turn, clinicians are compelled to change the traditional way that they approach arrhythmias and have learned important lessons about potentially useful and dangerous drugs in these disorders.[103] Many drugs such as quinidine, erythromycin, cisapride, and azole antifungals have promiscuous effects on channels such as the HERG channel and may prolong the QT interval and lead to a predisposition for *torsades de pointes*. Moreover, the recognition that many cases of more common acquired LQTS are related to subtle cardiac channelopathies,[104] resulting from cardiac ion channel polymorphisms, force clinicians to carefully consider the selection of drugs used to treat common infections and allergies.[103,104]

## Kinases May Act as Tumor Suppressor Genes in the Heart

The application of molecular genetics to the study of familial disorders involving cardiac tumors has given us important insights into the pathogenesis of these neoplasms and the role of several genes that function as tumor suppressors in the heart. Primary tumors of the heart are uncommon, with an estimated incidence of 0.0017% to 0.19% in unselected patients at autopsy.[105] The most common primary cardiac tumor in adults is the myxoma. Myxomas generally develop in the atria and most commonly arise from the left side of the interatrial septum near the *fossa ovalis*.[105,106] Most cardiac myxomas are isolated sporadic lesions, but at least 7%[105] occur as components of a familial autosomal dominant syndrome that has previously been referred to as LAMB (lentigines, atrial myxoma, mucocutaneous myxoma, and blue nevi[107]) or NAME (nevi, atrial myxoma, myxoid neurofibroma, and ephelides)[108] and more recently as Carney's complex.[58] In these syndromes, familial cardiac myxomas are associated with spotty pigmentation of the skin (lentiginosis) and endocrine overactivity. Clinical and genetic linkage studies of affected families led to the identification of a statistically significant human chromosomal locus for a disease gene at chromosome 17q24.[54] Refined linkage analysis and positional cloning studies demonstrated that most familial cardiac myxomas in Carney's complex are caused by mutations in the chromosome 17q24 gene *PRKAR1α* that encodes the R1α regulatory subunit of cAMP-dependent PKA.[57]

*PRKAR1α* may act as a tumor suppressor gene within the heart via regulation of PKA activity. Haploinsufficiency of *PRKAR1α* resulting from heterozygous frameshift and nonsense mutations in the *PRKAR1α* gene causes Carney's complex.[57] Truncated R1α protein encoded by mutant *PRKAR1α* is not detectable by Western blot analysis. Although tumorigenesis may require a second somatic mutation, it is not required to occur in *PRKAR1α;* a second mutation has not been detected in the *PRKAR1α* wild-type allele and loss of *PRKAR1α* heterozygosity in most cardiac myxomas excised from patients with Carney's complex. However, we have detected a reversal of the ratio of R1α to R2β in myxomas, and this regulatory unit isoform switch may contribute to tumorigenesis.[57] The recognition that a significant portion of myxomas occur as part of a familial syndrome has important implications for family members of an affected individual.[55] Establishing a clinical or molecular diagnosis should prompt annual echocardiographic screening of individuals at risk to allow early detection and treatment of cardiac myxomas—the most serious manifestation of Carney's complex.

Causes of other cardiac tumors must be determined. The most common primary cardiac tumor in children is rhabdomyomas that are almost invariably associated with tuberous sclerosis resulting from mutations in the *TSC1, TSC2, TSC3,* and as yet unidentified genes.[2]

## Extracellular Matrix Proteins Control Vascular Homeostasis

The study of well-defined clinical syndromes such as MFS, Ehlers-Danlos syndrome type IV, and Williams syndrome (which includes SVAS) has provided a framework for the understanding of inherited structural vascular disease. MFS is due to mutation in the *fibrillin-1* gene *(FBN1)* that encodes fibrillin-1, a 350-kDa glycoprotein that is the major structural constituent of extracellular mircrofibrils.[2,109] MFS affects approximately 1 in 10,000 individuals and has protean manifestations including dislocation of the ocular lens, long bone overgrowth, and aortic aneurysm formation.[110] Numerous MFS mutations have been described, but no clear genotype-phenotype correlation has been established. Analysis of mutations in MFS indicates that virtually every family has a unique mutation.[2,111] Most mutations are missense mutations that alter a single amino acid. Nonsense mutations, small insertions and deletions, and exon splicing

errors have also been described. Although some mutations in *FBN1* are predicted to produce mutant protein and cause disease through a dominant negative effect (as described previously),[10,109] other mutations produce disease through *FBN1* mRNA NMD and haploinsufficiency.[62,112] Therefore, the original paradigm of a dominant negative process in which microfibrils containing abnormal fibrillin-1 cause defective elastic fiber assembly during development has recently been questioned. It now appears that fibrillin-1 plays a dynamic role in vascular cell handling of extracellular matrix protein homeostasis. Abnormal cellular attachments between vascular smooth muscle cells (VSMCs) and a defective microfibril scaffold leads to changes in the VSMCs that alter their phenotype and initiate pathologic remodeling of the extracellular matrix, elastolysis, and inflammation.[113]

SVAS is a condition in which the aorta just distal to the sinuses of Valsalva is narrowed.[2,26,27] SVAS may occur as an isolated trait or as part of Williams syndrome, which also comprises infantile hypercalcemia and an abnormal facies, and is a contiguous gene syndrome.[2,26,27] In SVAS, major branches of the pulmonary artery may also exhibit narrowing. As in MFS, the cause of SVAS was determined through linkage analysis and positional cloning studies. SVAS is due to mutations in the gene encoding tropoelastin *(ELN)* at chromosome 7q11.26. Mutations in *ELN* cause SVAS through haploinsufficiency in *ELN*.[27,114] This is a different paradigm than that described previously in MFS, which may be due to either dominant negative effects or haploinsufficiency. It appears that the developmental consequences of haploinsufficiency of *ELN* are distinct from the consequences of abnormal matrix homeostasis in a vessel that has already developed normally. In SVAS, elastin levels are reduced by approximately 50% during development causing a stenotic phenotype. By contrast, in MFS, elastin levels are not reduced during development, but abnormal extracellular matrix handling leads to pathologic homeostasis of elastin and other matrix proteins as described previously. The contrasting phenotypes of MFS and SVAS (both including elastin) highlight the importance of animal and functional studies in the understanding of pathophysiologic implications of fundamental genetic discoveries.

As the exploration of monogenic cardiovascular disease proceeds, investigators will continue to be challenged and excited by new and often unexpected disease models, such as the mutations in *PRKAG2* that cause familial Wolff-Parkinson-White syndrome.[77] The concept that a common phenotype may arise because of mutations in widely biologically diverse genes represents a formidable challenge for contemporary investigators. The molecular genetic analysis of arrhythmogenic right ventricular dysplasia (ARVD) exemplifies this challenge in which a similar phenotype occurs resulting from mutations in the *plakglobin* gene (that encodes a cell surface adhesion molecule)[115] and the *ryanodine receptor 2 (RyR2)* gene that encodes a sarcolemmal ion channel.[102] Moreover, recent data demonstrate the importance of acquired somatic mutations in the genesis of cardiovascular disease. Such mutations may result from environmental exposures and may affect the nuclear and mitochondrial genomes. Such genetic disorders do not affect the germ cells and are not familial. Therefore, they are not approachable through typical Mendelian trait analyses. For instance, Lerman et al.[116] have studied an adenosine-sensitive form of common right ventricular outflow tract tachycardia. Although they were not able to ascertain a family history of the disorder in their patients, they characterized the presence of missense mutation in the gene encoding G$\alpha$i2. Interestingly, this mutation was present only in DNA from myocardial biopsies taken from the electrophysiologically mapped arrhythmia focus and not from biopsies taken from remote cardiac regions. *In vitro* studies further demonstrated that the mutation did confer adenosine resistance. Thus, these studies highlight the potential contribution of acquired, nonfamilial genetic variation to cardiovascular disease.

## BENCH TO BEDSIDE

### Genetic Testing

Genetic testing for cardiovascular disease is increasingly available and increasingly sought. With identification of the genetic bases for a growing number of monogenic disorders, the clinical use of DNA-based testing to establish a molecular diagnosis is more feasible. In general, however, the use of genetic testing is still not of incremental clinical value. Most disorders are diagnosed based on well-validated clinical criteria and do not need DNA sequencing to establish the diagnosis. In many cases, disorders such as HCM are genetically heterogenous, and genetic testing is not practical because of the large number of potential genes involved and the existence of unique mutations in most families. In other diseases, the number of genes associated with a condition may be small, but their large size is prohibitive. MFS is an excellent example of such a disorder, and the size of the *FBN1* gene renders routine DNA testing impractical.[117] Moreover, even if rapid, cost-effective methods to sequence DNA were available, the sensitivity and specificity of mutational analysis of *FBN1* in MFS would not make such testing clinically attractive. Finally, the lack of clear genotype-phenotype correlation in MFS also makes the potential use of *FBN1* mutational analysis (even as a research tool) of dubious value. This array of limitations has hampered DNA-based diagnosis not only in MFS but also in conditions including HCM, LQTS, and familial dyslipidemias.

Even in families with monogenic disorders and known mutations, DNA-based genetic diagnosis may not be clinically helpful because the information derived may not predict well an individual patient's phenotype or course. For instance, in Holt-Oram syndrome in which genotype-phenotype correlations have been established in patient cohorts, variable expressivity of the disorder confounds prediction of any given patient's phenotype. Marked intrafamilial variability of Holt-Oram syndrome phenotypes is the rule, likely resulting from effects of as yet unidentified modifier genes. These difficulties in the clinical application of genetic testing are further exacerbated in polygenic disorders.

However, in some monogenic disorders and certain rare situations, DNA-based diagnosis may be very useful. If a disorder is oligogenic (i.e., caused by a few genes) and these genes are not prohibitively large, then genetic testing may be considered. This is most appropriate when such knowledge will alter either diagnostic or therapeutic approaches to a patient or a family. This must be performed by experienced clinician-scientists who are well versed in counseling patients and families regarding probable outcomes and potentially unrevealing results. Genetic testing for *PRKAR1$\alpha$* mutations among families with Carney's complex has been useful.[57] The most devastating aspect of this condition is the development of cardiac myxomas that frequently appear as a stroke in a young patient. The identification of a mutation in a family allows a preclinical diagnosis to be made in family members who are not suspected of having this disorder. This allows annual surveillance echocardiography to be initiated and can significantly affect clinical outcome by identifying myxoma formation at an early stage.

Genetic testing may be used more frequently in the future as the technology for rapid screening of candidate genes improves. In addition, increased understanding of the clinical significance of specific mutations and the effects of modifying genetic influences may make this process more rewarding in guiding both diagnostic and therapeutic practice.

### Clinical Utility of Linkage Analysis

Genetic linkage analysis and haplotype analysis may occasionally be used in the clinical evaluation of individuals in families with inherited heart disease. In general, this often occurs in the context of a research study in which family members have access to investigators with an interest in a particular disorder. Linkage analysis studies are not usually available in commercial laboratories and require a dedicated laboratory and a pedigree-oriented approach. Haplotype analysis has been used to make a molecular diagnosis in patients with a number of diseases including MFS[56] and HCM[118] and in families with dilated cardiomyopathies.[2] We have used haplotype analysis to establish molecular diagnosis of Carney's complex in the absence of clear clinical indicators.[55] Molecular prediction of increased risk for development of cardiac myxomas prompts institution of surveillance echocardiography to detect tumor development before embolic stroke. Similarly, we have employed haplotype analysis in the evaluation of families with familial aortic aneurysm (FAA) disease. FAA is an autosomal dominant disorder that is genetically heterogeneous[119] and may be caused by mutations in several genes including *fibrillin-1, fibrillin-2,* and *type III procollagen.* By systematically testing markers flanking these loci, we have been able to establish linkage between FAA and loci associated with aneurysm formation such as the FBN1 locus.[119] These studies have allowed us to identify individuals within these families with the disease haplotype. This, in turn, has prompted more intensive surveillance and the institution of preventive strategies to prevent aortic dilation.

## Preimplantation Genetic Diagnosis

Preimplantation genetic diagnosis (PGD) is a technique that allows the diagnosis of a genetic disorder in very early embryos before implantation in the uterus. PGD was initially performed using Y chromosome specific DNA amplification for couples at risk for having children with X-linked disorders.[120] Today, PGD is most commonly applied to single-gene disorders in which the mutation in a family has already been characterized.[121,122] The approach involves IVF and requires several embryos for diagnosis to choose an unaffected embryo or embryos for implantation. The technique involves removal of one or two cells from the 8- or 16-cell embryos. DNA is amplified using PCR and sequenced to determine whether the specific mutation in the parent is present. Thus, embryos that do not contain the mutation are identified for implantation. PGD has been applied to a number of diseases including sickle cell anemia,[123] cystic fibrosis,[121] and MFS.[122] In the future, PGD may offer many families the opportunity of avoiding devastating diseases. PGD has now been applied successfully to individuals with Holt-Oram syndrome (see Editor's Choice). Many ethical issues confound this evolving technology, and great societal care, attention, and discussion will be needed to address concerns about appropriate application of these technologies.

## GENETIC ADVANCES IN THE NEW MILLENIUM

### The Human Genome Project

The previous century established the cellular basis of hereditary heart diseases and defined the molecular role of DNA in this process.[124] The latter half of the century saw an exponential growth in the understanding of the cellular machinery that processes and reads DNA and converts this code into functioning protein. The last 25 years have seen a dramatic increase in the understanding of genes and their role in normal physiology and in disease. The task of linking genes to disease has, for the most part, only occurred in the last decade. The latter stages of this process converged with the delineation of the human genome sequence by the HGP Public Consortium and the Celera private effort.[38,39] The outcome of the HGP represents not only the completion of a project but also a new beginning. Just as DNA has been likened to a genetic alphabet, the genome sequence may be considered a dictionary of related and unrelated genetic words (genes). The challenge that lies ahead is to convert these words into a comprehensible language and to relate this new lexicon to human disease.

Controversy still surrounds current estimates of the number of genes in the human genome. It is now estimated that the genome contains between 35,000 and 50,000 genes.[38,39] It was initially anticipated that the number of genes would reach approximately 100,000. A smaller number of genes in the human genome may still provide remarkable biologic complexity because of alternatively splicing gene transcripts. However, it remains possible that the number of genes is still greater than 35,000 and may yet reach a much higher estimate. Contemporary bioinformatic analyses may underestimate the true number of genes by recognizing only those genes that closely resemble already known genes.[40,41] Investigators who are currently performing biologic studies *in vitro* and in animal models rather than purely human genomic studies continue to identify novel transcripts that cannot be solely accounted for on the basis of alternative splicing. Moreover, comparative genomic studies that are only at their early stages but that are progressing rapidly with the increasing availability of complete genome sequences from multiple mammalian and nonmammalian species may also foster identification of novel genes not predicted by bioinformatic analysis of genome sequences from a single or limited number of species.

Contemporary gene prediction software and algorithms may significantly underestimate the number of transcripts in the human genome. A comparison of the predicted transcript sequences from the Celera and HGP sequencing efforts indicates that novel genes predicted by both groups are largely nonoverlapping.[40] This lack of overlap may reflect differences in the algorithms used to predict putative genes and highlights the need for a more comprehensive approach to gene identification in the future. Regardless, about 10,000 genes have been cataloged in the online *Mendelian Inheritance in Man* (OMIM)[2] that documents all inherited diseases and their causal gene mutations. Thus, considerable work remains in translating gene sequence to gene function. Physician-scientists in the coming decades must integrate the genes that have been named, cataloged, and enumerated by the HGP with the accumulating delineation of cellular and organismal regulatory pathways responsible for homeostatic and pathologic processes.

Nonetheless, gene sequence has already had an impact. It has led to the expedited discovery of disease genes by enhancing positional cloning strategies and allowing investigators to identify new candidates at previously described loci. More than 30 genes were positionally cloned using just the early draft sequence from the HGP.[38] Examples of cardiovascular disease genes that were identified using the partial sequence from the HGP include the *CCM1* gene that causes cerebral arteriovenous malformations,[125] the *PRKAR1a* gene that causes Carney's complex and familial cardiac myxomas,[57] and the *EVC* gene that causes Ellis Van Creveld's syndrome.[126]

### Single-Nucleotide Polymorphisms

The HGP sequencing effort has cataloged and mapped more than 1.42 million SNPs.[38,127] These represent sites-of-variation and are single-base changes that form the basis for genetic variation. The HGP has fully integrated these SNPs with the sequence, physical, and genetic maps of the genome.[38] A comprehensive study of such SNPs will be fundamental to understanding many diseases. The SNP map will be used to study human genetics from many different perspectives including population genetics, evolution, and human disease gene identification.

A SNP map will also form the template for genome-wide association studies between genetic polymorphisms and human disease. These polymorphisms may separately and in combination confer risk for common human disorders in the appropriate environment without causing the disease itself in a Mendelian fashion. Although current efforts have facilitated detection and analysis of SNPs that occur in coding regions of genes and in known regulatory regions (intronic and exonic), these SNPs likely reflect just a small fraction of the variants that modify human phenotypes. Comparative genomic studies (see later) and targeted investigation of specific biologic processes in cellular proliferation and differentiation and organismal morphogenesis are likely to identify currently unsuspected novel intronic motifs that are critical for regulation of gene expression. These genomic segments will certainly be high-priority targets for future studies. Deciphering the relationship between genetic variation and physiology on a genomic scale is expected to provide fundamental new insights into the mechanism of human disease.

The promise that SNP analysis will allow genes that underlie complex diseases such as CAD, hypertension, diabetes, and stroke to be identified is a powerful incentive to establish the technology for large-scale analysis of SNPs. Ongoing development of new genotyping strategies are establishing high-throughput, accurate, inexpensive technologies that need to be coupled with powerful computational databases to process and analyze the data. Such experimental and computational approaches provide tools to analyze this data in a combinatorial fashion. It is unlikely that individual SNPs confer significant risk but rather that collections of SNPs within genes and among different genes set the clinical stage for disease. We have already had glimpses of novel strategies that may allow mapping of haplotypes on a chromosome-wide scale and perhaps ultimately on a genome-wide level. Patil et al.[128] have developed a novel, efficient, high-density oligonucleotide array strategy to define allele haplotypes, composed of blocks of SNPs in close proximity for all of chromosome 21. Several scientists have proposed that even though the number of SNPs is high, there are only a limited number of haplotypes in a given population. Thus, genotyping of only a small portion of the genome's SNPs may predict a critical disease-predisposing haplotype. This hypothesis has led to the somewhat controversial proposal of generating a haplotype map of the genome rather than a high-density SNP map for analysis of complex traits.

## Polygenic Disease

Genetically complex diseases, such as diabetes, hypertension, cancer, and coronary heart disease, are common disorders in most populations and usually are a consequence of the interactions between multiple predisposing genetic factors (as well as environmental influences). The study of these multifactorial diseases has been difficult because simple Mendelian patterns of inheritance are not applicable. The understanding of the genetic basis of these polygenic disorders is the single biggest hurdle facing investigators and the future utility of the HGP. Although the task is demanding, some attempts have already been made to unravel some critical polygenic diseases.

CAD severity is determined by both genetic and environmental factors. A family history of CAD is considered to be a major risk factor for the development of CAD. Much research has focused on evaluating the genetic background of CAD through the analysis of candidate genes, such as angiotensin-I converting enzyme (ACE) and apolipoprotein E (APOE). An association between an insertion/deletion (ID) polymorphism of the ACE gene and MI has been reported,[129] but this remains controversial.[130] Other genes are also implicated in the development of CAD including genes encoding proteins involved in lipid metabolism like apolipoprotein B,[131] CETP,[132] or lipoprotein lipase.[133]

However, most of the key genetic risk factors involved in CAD remain unknown. One approach to discover the molecular genetic basis of complex disorders has been to perform genome-wide susceptibility scans. A number of susceptibility loci have been described. One complex phenotype that has been studied is the atherogenic lipoprotein phenotype (ALP). This is characterized by increased levels of triglyceride-rich lipoproteins, reductions in HDL, and a threefold increased risk of MI. Linkage was found between the ALP and the LDL receptor locus on chromosome 19.[134,135] Linkage has also been shown between total cholesterol concentrations and the chromosome 19 locus in a genome scan in Pima Indians.[136] Studies in Finland in pedigrees with familial combined hyperlipidemia (FCHL) showed linkage with chromosome 1q21–q23.[137,138] Recently, an association between CAD and a locus on chromosome 16p13-pter has been reported in Indo-Mauritians.[139] The investigators used a genome-wide scan choosing a very extreme phenotype in an isolated population to attempt to reduce the genetic complexity.[140] Small, inbred populations such as the Pima Indians and other populations in Finland have provided unique opportunities to use linkage disequilibrium to study the small but additive effects of predisposing genetic variations. Similarly, the study of monogenic diseases such as Tangier's disease[141] and sitosterolemia[142] have highlighted new genes and pathways that may play a prominent role in the pathophysiology of complex diseases such as atherosclerosis and dyslipidemias. These studies represent a bridge between the present and the future—a bridge that has been assembled mainly by the genome sequencing programs. These studies also underscore the complexity of the task that lies ahead and the need for new strategies to tackle complex diseases.

## Comparative Genomics

Comparative genomic studies using the human genome sequence and genome sequences of other species will shed important light on human disease. Human and murine comparative sequence studies at the apolipoprotein gene cluster at human chromosome 11q23 have already led to the identification of a new apolipoprotein gene *APOAV* that appears to be a major determinant of plasma triglyceride levels.[143] In humans, polymorphisms in the *APOAV* gene are significantly correlated with plasma triglyceride levels.[143]

It will be particularly intriguing to learn how common genetic polymorphisms impact prevalent cardiovascular diseases such as hypertension, diabetes, dyslipidemias, and atherosclerosis. However, many pitfalls and controversies will arise. Studies have already reported the association of a variety of SNPs and hypertension, dyslipidemia, and thrombotic cardiovascular disease. Investigators have observed the statistical association of CAD and a number of SNPs in important genes, including platelet glycoprotein IIb/IIIa receptor,[144] factor V Leiden (R506Q),[145] prothrombin G20210A,[145] and P-selectin (T715P).[146] However, the durability of this strategy is being questioned by a recent case-control study using high-throughput genomic technology to examine the role of a large number of candidate genes in premature CAD.[147] Although this study describes an association between SNPs in thrombospondin genes and CAD, it could not detect an association between premature CAD and previously described polymorphisms.

Clearly, to yield results of biologic and clinical importance the approaches to SNP analysis must evolve further. Large, population-based DNA repositories are needed. For maximum impact, these repositories must be married to large clinical databases. SNP and haplotype analyses must be high-throughput, systematic, prospective, ethnically diverse, and genome-wide. This approach will not only be informative in terms of the relationships between SNPs and disease but also will allow determination of the relationship between genetic variants and health. All information gathered in such large association studies should be regarded not as conclusions but rather as hypotheses to be prospectively evaluated in large clinical outcome and intervention trials.

## Pharmacogenomics

Unique individual responses to drug therapy are significant confounders of therapeutic protocols for cardiovascular disease. Patient-specific drug responsiveness may be mediated through heritable factors. Pharmacogenomics focuses on (1) the identification of specific genes as targets for novel drug therapies and (2) delineation of genetic variation that affects a patient's response to drugs. Investigation in this arena has already had significant payoffs for individuals with some cancers by providing targets for genetically targeted therapy in diseases like chronic myelogenous leukemia and by helping to stratify patient candidacy for certain toxic chemotherapies. For patients with cardiovascular disease, pharmacogenomics is on the horizon. Inevitably, genome-wide scans will identify new genes and novel genetic pathways that will be a target for future drug development for the treatment of cardiovascular diseases such as hypertension, atherosclerosis, and diabetes. Individuals with certain genotypes may need different pharmacologic approaches tailored to the particular genetic nuances of their disease. For instance, one individual may be predisposed to MI because of a prothrombotic state driven primarily by variations in platelet receptors or clotting factors. Conversely, another individual may develop MI because of progressive obstructive CAD resulting from a heritable genotype associated with abnormalities of lipid metabolism or antioxidant defenses. Many individuals will have mixtures of both. In the future, genotype-tailored therapy in such individuals might vary the role of combination antiplatelet drugs or anticoagulants versus lipid-modifying drugs.

Pharmacogenomics has already contributed to analyses of the effects of genetic variation on cardiovascular drug efficacy and safety.[104] Polymorphisms in many genes, including those encoding receptors, enzymes, drug transporters, and signaling pathways, may be important determinants of clinical response. The most immediately applicable variants are SNPs in genes whose products are involved in drug metabolism. Functional SNPs (i.e., those polymorphisms that change the structure of the encoded protein) in genes controlling any aspect of metabolism can lead to an exaggerated or reduced clinical response to a cardiac drug. SNPs have been identified in more than 20 human drug-metabolizing enzymes, and these SNPs show marked ethnic diversity. Important examples include SNPs in members of the cytochrome P450 enzyme system (CYP450).[104] The CYP450 system is a multigene family of enzymes found mainly in the liver that is responsible for metabolizing many drugs.[148] In slow metabolizers, the genes encoding certain members of the CYP450 system contain SNPs that reduce the efficacy of the enzyme leading to enhanced drug effect. For example, SNPs in CYP2C9, which metabolizes warfarin, has a profound effect on the dose requirement and bleeding risk.[149] Similarly, SNPs in CYP2D6 (which is highly polymorphic and is inactive in 6% of the white population) may have important pharmacologic consequences in patients who are prescribed flecainide, amiodarone, or propranolol.[148,150]

LQTS is an archetype of how modern molecular genetics contributes both to individual therapy and to drug safety. The use of genotype-phenotype correlation has identified sets of clinical triggers of differing significance for each genotype.[97] Events in LQT1 patients almost always occur during conditions associated with increased sympathetic activity (e.g., exercise). LQT2 events largely occur during increased emotion or while at rest, and arrhythmias are associated with auditory stimuli, such as those produced by telephone calls or alarm clocks. By contrast, LQT3 events usually happen at rest or asleep without arousal. These genotype-phenotype correlates have prompted gene-specific therapy. They suggest that β-blockers are safe and effective in patients with LQT1 and that flecainide (a sodium channel blocking drug) may be more effective in LQT3 (which is due to mutations the sodium channel gene *SCN5A*).[151]

Pharmacogenomic and molecular genetic studies in the acquired form of LQTS also suggest a role for more widespread DNA testing. Genetic testing may be able to predict individuals at risk for *torsades de pointes* resulting from commonly prescribed drugs. Drugs associated with acquired LQTS include terfenadine, erythromycin, phenothiazines, and tricyclic antidepressants.

Most of these medications block HERG channels, leading to reduced repolarizing potassium currents.[152] Increased susceptibility of the HERG channel to these compounds is intriguing and appears to be due to the unique structural features of the HERG ion channel.[152] The inner cavity of the HERG channel is larger than that of other ion channels and can accommodate and bind to drugs. In addition, recent studies have demonstrated that drug-induced arrhythmias can be due to sporadic mutations and common SNPs in MiRP1.[153] MiRP1 is a subunit of the cardiac potassium channel I(Kr) that has been associated with inherited LQTS. It is also likely that mutations and SNPs in other ion channels also mediate clinically significant arrhythmias.

In the short term, pharmacogenomics may be applied to prevent common drug interactions and to assess patient suitability for drugs with narrow therapeutic margin. Pharmacogenomics DNA-based testing may also be useful to screen patients for potential drug induced arrhythmias or acquired LQTS. In the future, however, genotype-specific therapy will likely be employed to develop personalized therapy in a variety of cardiovascular diseases.

## Gene Therapy for Cardiovascular Disease

Gene therapy may be defined as the genetic modification of cells to produce a therapeutic effect.[154] Most studies to date have involved attempts to replace a single abnormal gene with a normal copy. Examples include restoration of the cystic fibrosis transmembrane regulator in patients with cystic fibrosis,[155] replacement of dystrophin in DMD,[156] and restoration of the LDL receptor in familial homozygous hypercholesterolemia.[157] Success in single-gene disorders has been quite limited, and the search for ideal vectors to deliver gene therapy and maintain the transgene has been frustrating. Gene therapy has also been applied to patients in an attempt to produce a therapeutic effect. Cytostatic therapies to limit restenosis after angioplasty have been attempted using the retinoblastoma gene targeted to VSMCs.[158] Angiogenic genes such as vascular endothelial growth factor (VEGF) have been delivered to the myocardium in patients with ischemic cardiomyopathies in an attempt to revascularize ischemic regions.[159,160] These strategies have met with some success in preliminary trials but have not yet translated into clinical practice. At its conception, gene therapy promised much, but there are still considerable technical obstacles to overcome before gene therapy becomes an established standard of care. Careful and meticulous study of gene therapy both at the bench and at the bedside will likely foster new approaches to cardiovascular disease in the future.

## CONCLUSION

The molecular genetic study of human cardiovascular disease has been rewarding and has fundamentally changed the way that clinicians view most disorders of the heart and circulation. This field was founded on Mendelian principles and evolved rapidly in tandem with the discovery of DNA and the discovery of gene structure and function. The development of linkage analysis, PCR, and more powerful computers allowed advances to take place rapidly. Prototypical models of many cardiovascular diseases that will form a scaffold for future more complex investigations were established in the previous decade. The next era will be centered on the HGP and will define new biologic and bioinformatic models to study complex polygenic diseases. The understanding of inherited predisposition to disease and the discovery of genetic abnormalities that individuals may acquire over a lifetime of toxic exposures will be united. Developments will embrace many diverse disciplines including genomics, proteinomics, pharmacogenetics, and gene therapy. The integration of these modalities into research, and ultimately clinical practice, will transform molecular genetics and the way that cardiology and medicine are practiced.

## REFERENCES

1. Olby RC: Origins of Mendelism. London, Constable and Co Ltd, 1966.
2. Online Mendelian Inheritance in Man, OMIM (TM): McKusick-Nathans Institute for Genetic Medicine, Johns Hopkins University (Baltimore, MD) and National Center for Biotechnology Information, National Library of Medicine (Bethesda, MD), 2000. World Wide Web URL: http://www.ncbi.nlm.nih.gov/omim/
3. Becker KL: Pedigree analysis. I. Dominance, recessiveness and sex-linkage. Postgrad Med 1966;40:6-12.
4. Suomalainen A: Mitochondrial DNA and disease. Ann Med 1997;29:235-246.
5. Wallace DC, Brown MD, Lott MT: Mitochondrial genetics. In Rimoin DL, Conner JM, Pyeritz RE (eds): Principles and Practice of Medical Genetics, 3rd ed. New York, Churchill Livingstone, 1997, p 277-332.
6. Hayakawa M, Sugiyama S, Hattori K, et al: Age-associated damage in mitochondrial DNA in human hearts. Mol Cell Biochem 1993;119:95-103.
7. Becker KL: Pedigree analysis. II. Clinical discrepancies and limitations. Postgrad Med 1966;40:171-174.
8. Niimura H, Bachinski LL, Sangwatanaroj S, et al: Mutations in the gene for cardiac myosin-binding protein C and late-onset familial hypertrophic cardiomyopathy. N Engl J Med 1998;338:1248-1257.
9. Milewicz DM, Chen H, Park ES, et al: Reduced penetrance and variable expressivity of familial thoracic aortic aneurysms/dissections. Am J Cardiol 1998;82:474-479.
10. Robinson PN, Godfrey M: The molecular genetics of Marfan syndrome and related microfibrillopathies. J Med Genet 2000;37:9-25.
11. Vincent GM: Long QT syndrome. Cardiol Clin 2000;18:309-325.
12. Spirito P, Seidman CE, McKenna WJ, Maron BJ: The management of hypertrophic cardiomyopathy. N Engl J Med 1997;336:775-785.
13. Basson CT, Cowley GS, Solomon SD, et al: The clinical and genetic spectrum of the Holt-Oram syndrome (heart-hand syndrome). N Engl J Med 1994;330:885-891.
14. Benson DW, Sharkey A, Fatkin D, et al: Reduced penetrance, variable expressivity, and genetic heterogeneity of familial atrial septal defects. Circulation 1998;97:2043-2048.
15. Shaffer LG: Diagnosis of microdeletion syndromes by fluorescence in situ hybridization (FISH). In Dracapoli NC, Haines J, Korf BR, et al. (eds): Current Protocols in Human Genetics. New York, John Wiley and Sons, 1997, pp 8.10.1-8.10.14.
16. Schrock E, du Manoir S, Veldman T, et al: Multicolor spectral karyotyping of human chromosomes. Science 1996;273:494-497.
17. Lee C, Lemyre E, Miron PM, Morton CC: Multicolor fluorescence in situ hybridization in clinical cytogenetic diagnostics. Curr Opin Pediatr 2001;13:550-555.

18. Perloff JK: Atrial septal defect: Simple and complex. In Perloff JK (ed): Clinical Recognition of Congenital Heart Disease, 4th ed. Philadelphia, WB Saunders, 1994, p 354.

19. Perloff JK: Atrial septal defect: Simple and complex. In Perloff JK (ed): Clinical Recognition of Congenital Heart Disease, 4th ed. Philadelphia, WB Saunders, 1994. p 305.

20. Perloff JK: Double outlet ventricle. In Perloff JK (ed): Clinical Recognition of Congenital Heart Disease, 4th ed. Philadelphia, WB Saunders, 1994, p 488.

21. Knoll JH, Nicholls RD, Magenis RE, et al: Angelman and Prader-Willi syndromes share a common chromosome 15 deletion but differ in parental origin of the deletion. Am J Med Genet 1989;32:285-290.

22. O'Riordan S, Greenough A, Moore GE, et al: Case report: Uniparental disomy 16 in association with congenital heart disease. Prenat Diagn 1996;16:963-965.

23. Hall JG: Genomic imprinting: Review and relevance to human disease. Am J Med Genet 1990;46:857-873.

24. Pfeifer K: Mechanisms of genomic imprinting. Am J Hum Genet 2000;67:777-787.

25. Cleary MA, van Raamsdonk CD, Levorse J, et al: Disruption of an imprinted gene cluster by a targeted chromosomal translocation in mice. Nat Genet 2001;29:78-82.

26. Curran ME, Atkinson DL, Ewart AK, et al: The elastin gene is disrupted by a translocation associated with supravalvular aortic stenosis. Cell 1993;73:159-168.

27. Ewart AK, Morris CA, Atkinson D, et al: Hemizygosity at the elastin locus in a developmental disorder, Williams syndrome. Nat Genet 1993;5:11-16.

28. de la Chapelle AR, Herva R, Koivisto M, Aula O: A deletion in chromosome 22 can cause DiGeorge syndrome. Hum Genet 1981;57:253-256.

29. Driscoll DA, Budarf ML, Emanuel BS: A genetic etiology for DiGeorge syndrome: Consistent deletions and microdeletions of 22q11. Am J Hum Genet 1992;50:924-933.

30. Driscoll DA, Salvin J, Sellinger B, et al: Prevalence of 22q11 microdeletions in DiGeorge and velocardiofacial syndromes: Implications for genetic counselling and prenatal diagnosis. J Med Genet 1993;30:813-817.

31. Goldmuntz E, Clark BJ, Mitchell LE, et al: Frequency of 22q11 deletions in patients with conotruncal defects. J Am Coll Cardiol 1998;32:492-498.

32. Basson CT, Bachinsky DR, Lin RC, et al: Mutations in human TBX5 cause limb and cardiac malformation in Holt-Oram syndrome. Nat Genet 1997;15:30-35.

33. Bamshad M, Lin RC, Law DJ, et al: Mutations in human TBX3 alter limb, apocrine and genital development in ulnar-mammary syndrome. Nat Genet 1997;16:311-315.

34. Merscher S, Funke B, Epstein JA, et al: TBX1 is responsible for cardiovascular defects in velo-cardio-facial/DiGeorge syndrome. Cell 2001;104:619-629.

35. Lindsay EA, Vitelli F, Su H, et al: Tbx1 haploinsufficiency in the DiGeorge syndrome region causes aortic arch defects in mice. Nature 2001;410:97-101.

36. Guris DL, Fantes J, Tara D, et al: Mice lacking the homologue of the human 22q11.2 gene CRKL phenocopy neurocristopathies of DiGeorge syndrome. Nat Genet 2001;27:293-298.

37. Vaughan CJ, Weremowicz S, Goldstein MM, et al: A t(2;19) (p13;p13.2) in a giant invasive cardiac lipoma from a patient with multiple lipomatosis. Genes Chromosomes Cancer 2000;28:133-137.

38. International Human Genome Sequencing Consortium: Initial sequencing and analysis of the human genome. Nature 2001;409:860-921.

39. Venter JC, Adams MD, Myers EW, et al: The sequence of the human genome. Science 2001;291:1304-1351.

40. Hogenesch JB, Ching KA, Batalov S, et al: A comparison of the Celera and Ensembl predicted gene sets reveals little overlap in novel genes. Cell 2001;106:413-415.

41. Zhuo D, Zhao WD, Wright FA, et al: Assembly, annotation, and integration of UNIGENE clusters into the human genome draft. Genome Res 2001;11:904-918.

42. Towbin JA, Bowles NE: The failing heart. Nature 2002; 415:227-233.

43. Nigro G, Comi LI, Politano L, Bain RJ: The incidence and evolution of cardiomyopathy in Duchenne muscular dystrophy. Int J Cardiol 1990;26:271-277.

44. Muntoni F, Cau M, Ganau A, et al: Brief report: Deletion of the dystrophin muscle-promoter region associated with X-linked dilated cardiomyopathy. N Engl J Med 1993;23;329:921-925.

45. Ruddle FH: A new era in mammalian gene mapping: Somatic cell genetics and recombinant DNA methodologies. Nature 1981;294:115-120.

46. Nakamura Y, Leppert M, O'Connell P, et al: Variable number of tandem repeat (VNTR) markers for human gene mapping. Science 1987;235:1616-1622.

47. Jeffreys AJ, Wilson V, Thein SL: Individual-specific 'fingerprints' of human DNA. Nature 1985;316:76-79.

48. Dib C, Faure S, Fizames C, et al: A comprehensive genetic map of the human genome based on 5,264 microsatellites. Nature 1996;380:152-154.

49. The BAC Resource Consortium: Integration of cytogenetic landmarks into the draft sequence of the human genome. Nature 2001;409:953-958.

50. Broman KW, Murray JC, Sheffield VC, et al: Comprehensive human genetic maps: Individual and sex-specific variation in recombination. Am J Hum Genet 1998;63:861-869.

51. Lathrop GM, Lalouel JM, Julier C, et al: Strategies for multilocus linkage analysis in humans. Proc Natl Acad Sci USA 1984; 81:3443-3446.

52. Ott J: Analysis of Human Genetic Linkage. Baltimore, Johns Hopkins University Press, 1991.

53. UCSC Human Genome Project Working Draft 22 December 2001 assembly (hg10): Available at http://genome.cse.ucsc.edu/

54. Casey M, Mah C, Merliss AD, et al: Identification of a novel genetic locus for familial cardiac myxomas and Carney complex. Circulation 1998;98:2560-2566.

55. Goldstein MM, Casey M, Carney JA, Basson CT: Molecular genetic diagnosis of the familial myxoma syndrome (Carney complex). Am J Med Genet 1999;86:62-65.

56. Judge DP, Biery NJ, Dietz HC: Characterization of microsatellite markers flanking FBN1: Utility in the diagnostic evaluation for Marfan syndrome. Am J Med Genet 2001;99:39-47.

57. Casey M, Vaughan CJ, He J, et al: Mutations in the protein kinase A R1alpha regulatory subunit cause familial cardiac myxomas and Carney complex. J Clin Invest 2000;106:R31-R38.

58. Carney JA, Gordon H, Carpenter PC, et al: The complex of myxomas, spotty pigmentation, and endocrine overactivity. Medicine 1985;64:270-283.

59. Brandon EP, Idzerda RL, McKnight GS: PKA isoforms, neural pathways, and behaviour: Making the connection. Curr Opin Neurobiol 1997;7:397-403.

60. Jenne DE, Reimann H, Nezu J, et al: Peutz-Jeghers syndrome is caused by mutations in a novel serine threonine kinase. Nat Genet 1998;18:38-43.

61. Goldstein JL, Brown MS, Stone NJ: Genetics of the LDL receptor: Evidence that the mutations affecting binding and internalization are allelic. Cell 1977;12:629-41.

62. Frischmeyer PA, Dietz HC: Nonsense-mediated mRNA decay in health and disease. Hum Mol Genet 1999;8:1893-1900.

63. Hentze MW, Kulozik AE: A perfect message: RNA surveillance and nonsense-mediated decay. Cell 1999;96:307-310.

64. Mendell JT, Dietz HC: When the message goes awry: Disease-producing mutations that influence mRNA content and performance. Cell 2001;107:411-414.

65. Zinn AR, Ross JL: Turner syndrome and haploinsufficiency. Curr Opin Genet Dev 1998;8:322-327.

66. Liu W, Qian C, Comeau K, et al: Mutant fibrillin-1 monomers lacking EGF-like domains disrupt microfibril assembly and cause severe Marfan syndrome. Hum Mol Genet 1996;5:1581-1587.

67. Pyeritz RE: Ehlers-Danlos syndrome. N Engl J Med. 2000;342:730-732.

68. Pepin M, Schwarze U, Superti-Furga A, Byers PH: Clinical and genetic features of Ehlers-Danlos syndrome type IV, the vascular type. N Engl J Med. 2000;342:673-680.

69. Schwarze U, Schievink WI, Petty E, et al: Haploinsufficiency for one COL3A1 allele of type III procollagen results in a phenotype similar to the vascular form of Ehlers-Danlos syndrome, Ehlers-Danlos syndrome type IV. Am J Hum Genet 2001;69:989-1001.

70. Marian AJ, Roberts R: The molecular genetic basis for hypertrophic cardiomyopathy. J Mol Cell Cardiol 2001;33:655-670.

71. Maron BJ, Shirani J, Poliac LC, et al: Sudden death in young competitive athletes: Clinical, demographic, and pathological profiles. JAMA 1996;276:199-204.

72. Sweeney HL, Straceski AJ, Leinwand LA, et al: Heterologous expression of a cardiomyopathic myosin that is defective in its actin interaction. J Biol Chem 1994;269:1603-5.

73. Kim SJ, Iizuka K, Kelly RA, et al: An alpha-cardiac myosin heavy chain gene mutation impairs contraction and relaxation function of cardiac myocytes. Am J Physiol 1999;276:H1780-787.

74. Fatkin D, McConnell BK, Mudd JO, et al: An abnormal Ca(2+) response in mutant sarcomere protein-mediated familial hypertrophic cardiomyopathy. J Clin Invest 2000;106:1351-1359.

75. Berul CI, McConnell BK, Wakimoto H, et al: Ventricular arrhythmia vulnerability in cardiomyopathic mice with homozygous mutant myosin-binding protein C gene. Circulation 2001;104:2734-2739.

76. Blair E, Redwood C, Ashrafian H, et al: Mutations in the gamma(2) subunit of AMP-activated protein kinase cause familial hypertrophic cardiomyopathy: Evidence for the central role of energy compromise in disease pathogenesis. Hum Mol Genet 2001;10:1215-1220.

77. Gollob MH, Green MS, Tang AS, et al: Identification of a gene responsible for familial Wolff-Parkinson-White syndrome. N Engl J Med 2001;344:1823-1831.

78. Arad M, Benson DW, Perez-Atayde AR, et al: Constitutively active AMP kinase mutations cause glycogen storage disease mimicking hypertrophic cardiomyopathy. J Clin Invest 2002;109:357-362.

79. Roguin N, Du ZD, Barak M, et al: High prevalence of muscular ventricular septal defect in neonates. J Am Coll Cardiol 1995;26:1545-1548.

80. Yang J, Hu D, Xia J, et al: Three novel TBX5 mutations in Chinese patients with Holt-Oram syndrome. Am J Med Genet 2000;92:237-240.

81. Ghosh TK, Packham EA, Bonser AJ, et al: Characterization of the TBX5 binding site and analysis of mutations that cause Holt-Oram syndrome. Hum Mol Genet 2001;10:1983-1994.

82. Basson CT, Huang T, Lin RC, et al: Different TBX5 interactions in heart and limb defined by Holt-Oram syndrome mutations. Proc Natl Acad Sci USA 1999;96:2919-2924.

83. Schott JJ, Benson DW, Basson CT, et al: Congenital heart disease caused by mutations in the transcription factor NKX2-5. Science 1998;281:108-111.

84. Benson DW, Silberbach GM, Kavanaugh-McHugh A, et al: Mutations in the cardiac transcription factor NKX2.5 affect diverse cardiac developmental pathways. J Clin Invest 1999;104:1567-1573.

85. Bodmer R: The gene tinman is required for specification of the heart and visceral muscles in Drosophila. Development 1993;118:719-729.

86. Mullins CE, Pagotto L: Patent ductus arteriosus. In Garson AJ, Bricker JT, Fisher DJ, Neish SR (eds): The Science and Practice of Pediatric Cardiology. Baltimore, William & Wilkins, 1998, pp 1181-1197.

87. Char F: Peculiar facies with short philtrum, duck-bill lips, ptosis and low-set ears: A new syndrome? Birth Defects 1978; 14:303-305.

88. Satoda M, Pierpont ME, Diaz GA, et al: Char syndrome, an inherited disorder with patent ductus arteriosus, maps to chromosome 6p12-p21. Circulation 1999;99:3036-3042.

89. Satoda M, Zhao F, Diaz GA, et al: Mutations in TFAP2B cause Char syndrome, a familial form of patent ductus arteriosus. Nat Genet 2000;25:42-46.

90. Li L, Krantz ID, Deng Y, et al: Alagille syndrome is caused by mutations in human Jagged1, which encodes a ligand for Notch 1. Nat Genet 1997;16:243-251.

91. Opitz JM, Clark EB: Heart development: An introduction. Am J Med Genet 2000;97:238-247.

92. Jervell A, Lange-Nielsen F: Congenital deaf-mutism, functional heart disease with prolongation of the QT interval, and sudden death. Am Heart J 1957;54:59-68.

93. Ward O: A new familial cardiac syndrome in children. J Ir Med Assoc 1964;54:103-106.

94. Wang Q, Curran ME, Splawski I, et al: Positional cloning of a novel potassium channel gene: KVLQT1 mutations cause cardiac arrhythmias. Nat Genet 1996;12:17-23.

95. Keating MT, Sanguinetti MC: Molecular and cellular mechanisms of cardiac arrhythmias. Cell 2001;104:569-580.

96. Schwartz PJ, Priori SG, Spazzolini C, et al: Genotype-phenotype correlation in the long-QT syndrome: Gene-specific triggers for life-threatening arrhythmias. Circulation 2001;103:89-95.

97. Splawski I, Shen J, Timothy KW, et al: Spectrum of mutations in long-QT syndrome genes. KVLQT1, HERG, SCN5A, KCNE1, and KCNE2. Circulation 2000;102:1178-1185.

98. Schott JJ, Charpentier F, Peltier S, et al: Mapping of a gene for long QT syndrome to chromosome 4q25-27. Am J Hum Genet 1995;57:1114-1122.

99. Chen Q, Kirsch GE, Zhang D, et al: Genetic basis and molecular mechanism for idiopathic ventricular fibrillation. Nature 1998;392:293-296.

100. Laitinen PJ, Brown KM, Piippo K, et al: Mutations of the cardiac ryanodine receptor (RyR2) gene in familial polymorphic ventricular tachycardia. Circulation 2001;103:485-490.

101. Tiso N, Stephan DA, Nava A, et al: Identification of mutations in the cardiac ryanodine receptor gene in families affected with arrhythmogenic right ventricular cardiomyopathy type 2 (ARVD2). Hum Mol Genet 2001;10:189-194.

102. Priori SG, Napolitano C, Tiso N, et al: Mutations in the cardiac ryanodine receptor gene (hRyR2) underlie catecholaminergic polymorphic ventricular tachycardia. Circulation 2001;103:196-200.

103. Roden DM: Pharmacogenetics and drug-induced arrhythmias. Cardiovasc Res 2001;50:224-231.

104. Abbott GW, Sesti F, Splawski I, et al: MiRP1 forms IKr potassium channels with HERG and is associated with cardiac arrhythmia. Cell. 1999;97:175-187.

105. Reynen K: Cardiac myxomas. N Engl J Med 1995;333:1610-1617.

106. Burke AP, Virmani R: Atlas of Tumor Pathology. Third Series Fascicle 16. Tumors of the Heart and Great Vessels. Washington DC, Armed Forces Institute of Pathology, 1996.

107. Rhodes AR, Silverman RA, Harrist TJ, Perez-Atayde AR: Mucocutaneous lentigines, cardiocutaneous myxomas, and multiple blue nevi: The "LAMB" syndrome. J Am Acad Dermatol 1984;10:72-82.

108. Atherton DJ, Pitcher DW, Wells RS, MacDonald DM: A syndrome of various cutaneous pigmented lesions, myxoid neurofibromata and atrial myxoma: The NAME syndrome. Br J Dermatol 1980;103:421-429.

109. Dietz HC, Cutting GR, Pyeritz RE, et al: Marfan syndrome caused by a recurrent de novo missense mutation in the fibrillin gene. Nature 1991;352:337-339.

110. De Paepe A, Devereux RB, Dietz HC, et al: Revised diagnostic criteria for the Marfan syndrome. Am J Med Genet 1996;62:417-426.

111. Pereira L, Levran O, Ramirez F, et al: A molecular approach to the stratification of cardiovascular risk in families with Marfan's syndrome. N Engl J Med 1994;331:148-153.

112. Dietz HC, Mecham RP: Mouse models of genetic diseases resulting from mutations in elastic fiber proteins. Matrix Biol 2000;19:481-488.

113. Bunton TE, Biery NJ, Myers L, et al: Phenotypic alteration of vascular smooth muscle cells precedes elastolysis in a mouse model of Marfan syndrome. Circ Res 2001;88:37-43.

114. Ewart AK, Morris CA, Ensing GJ, et al: A human vascular disorder, supravalvular aortic stenosis, maps to chromosome 7. Proc Natl Acad Sci USA 1993;90:3226-3230.

115. McKoy G, Protonotarios N, Crosby A, et al: Identification of a deletion in plakoglobin in arrhythmogenic right ventricular cardiomyopathy with palmoplantar keratoderma and woolly hair (Naxos disease). Lancet 2000;355:2119-2124.

116. Lerman BB, Dong B, Stein KM, et al: Right ventricular outflow tract tachycardia due to somatic mutation in a G protein subunit alpha12. J Clin Invest 1998;101:2862-2868.

117. Biery NJ, Eldadah ZA, Moore CS, et al: Revised genomic organization of FBN1 and significance for regulated gene expression. Genomics 1999;56:70-77.

118. Dausse E, Komajda M, Fetler L, et al: Familial hypertrophic cardiomyopathy: Microsatellite haplotyping and identification of a hot spot for mutations in the beta-myosin heavy chain gene. J Clin Invest 1993;92:2807-2813.

119. Vaughan CJ, Casey M, He J, et al: Identification of a chromosome 11q23.2-q24 locus for familial aortic aneurysm disease, a genetically heterogeneous disorder. Circulation 2001;103: 2469-2475.

120. Handyside AH, Kontogianni EH, Hardy K, Winston RM: Pregnancies from biopsied human preimplantation embryos sexed by Y-specific DNA amplification. Nature 1990;344:768-770.

121. Goossens V, Sermon K, Lissens W, et al: Clinical application of preimplantation genetic diagnosis for cystic fibrosis. Prenat Diagn 2000;20:571-581.

122. Blaszczyk A, Tang YX, Dietz HC, et al: Preimplantation genetic diagnosis of human embryos for Marfan's syndrome. J Assist Reprod Genet 1998;15:281-284.

123. Xu K, Shi ZM, Veeck LL, et al: First unaffected pregnancy using preimplantation genetic diagnosis for sickle cell anemia. JAMA 1999;281:1701-1706.

124. Watson JD, Crick FHC: Molecular structure of nucleic acids: A structure for deoxyribose nucleic acid. Nature 1953; 171:737-738.

125. Laberge-le Couteulx S, Jung HH, et al: Truncating mutations in CCM1, encoding KRIT1, cause hereditary cavernous angiomas. Nat Genet 1999;23:189-193.

126. Ruiz-Perez VL, Ide SE, Strom TM, et al: Mutations in a new gene in Ellis-van Creveld syndrome and Weyers acrodental dysostosis. Nat Genet 2000;24:283-286.

127. Sachidanandam R, Weissman D, Schmidt SC, et al: A map of human genome sequence variation containing 1.42 million single nucleotide polymorphisms. Nature 2001;409:928-933.

128. Patil N, Berno AJ, Hinds DA, et al: Blocks of limited haplotype diversity revealed by high-resolution scanning of human chromosome 21. Science 2001;294:1719-1723.

129. Cambien F, Poirier O, Lecerf L, et al: Deletion polymorphism in the gene for angiotensin-converting enzyme is a potent risk factor for myocardial infarction. Nature 1992;359:641-644.

130. Agerholm-Larsen B, Nordestgaard BG, Tybjaerg-Hansen A: ACE gene polymorphism in cardiovascular disease: Meta-analyses of small and large studies in whites. Arterioscler Thromb Vasc Biol 2000;20:484-492.

131. Tybjaerg-Hansen A, Steffensen R, Meinertz H, et al: Association of mutations in the apolipoprotein B gene with hypercholesterolemia and the risk of ischemic heart disease. N Engl J Med 1998;338:1577-1584.

132. Kuivenhoven JA, Jukema JW, Zwinderman AH, et al: The role of a common variant of the cholesteryl ester transfer protein gene in the progression of coronary atherosclerosis: The Regression Growth Evaluation Statin Study Group. N Engl J Med 1988;338:86-93.

133. Wittrup HH, Tybjaerg-Hansen A, Abildgaard S, et al: A common substitution (Asn291Ser) in lipoprotein lipase is associated with increased risk of ischemic heart disease. J Clin Invest 1997;99:1606-1613.

134. Nishina PM, Johnson JP, Naggert JK, Krauss RM: Linkage of atherogenic lipoprotein phenotype to the low density lipoprotein receptor locus on the short arm of chromosome 19. Proc Natl Acad Sci USA 1992;89:708-712.

135. Rotter JI, Bu X, Cantor RM, et al: Multilocus genetic determinants of LDL particle size in coronary artery disease families. Am J Hum Genet 1996;58:585-594.

136. Imperatore G, Knowler WC, Pettitt DJ, et al: A locus influencing total serum cholesterol on chromosome 19p: Results from an autosomal genomic scan of serum lipid concentrations in Pima Indians. Arterioscler Thromb Vasc Biol 2000;20: 2651-2656.

137. Pajukanta P, Nuotio I, Terwilliger JD, et al: Linkage of familial combined hyperlipidaemia to chromosome 1q21-q23. Nat Genet 1998;18:369-373.

138. Pei W, Baron H, Muller-Myhsok B, et al: Support for linkage of familial combined hyperlipidemia to chromosome 1q21-q23 in Chinese and German families. Clin Genet 2000;57:29-34.

139. Francke S, Manraj M, Lacquemant C, et al: A genome-wide scan for coronary heart disease suggests in Indo-Mauritians a susceptibility locus on chromosome 16p13 and replicates linkage with the metabolic syndrome on 3q27. Hum Mol Genet 2001; 10:2751-2765.

140. Lander ES, Schork NJ: Genetic dissection of complex traits. Science 1994;265:2037-2048.

141. Bodzioch M, Orso E, Klucken J, et al: The gene encoding ATP-binding cassette transporter 1 is mutated in Tangier disease. Nat Genet 1999;22:347-351.

142. Lee MH, Lu K, Hazard S, et al: Identification of a gene, ABCG5, important in the regulation of dietary cholesterol absorption. Nat Genet 2001;27:79-83.

143. Pennacchio LA, Olivier M, Hubacek JA, et al: An apolipoprotein influencing triglycerides in humans and mice revealed by comparative sequencing. Science 2001;294:169-173.

144. Ridker PM, Hennekens CH, Lindpaintner K, et al: Mutation in the gene coding for coagulation factor V and the risk of myocardial infarction, stroke, and venous thrombosis in apparently healthy men. N Engl J Med 1995;332:912-917.

145. De Stefano V, Martinelli I, Mannucci PM, et al: The risk of recurrent deep venous thrombosis among heterozygous carriers of both factor V Leiden and the G20210A prothrombin mutation. N Engl J Med 1999;341:801-806.

146. Kee F, Morrison C, Evans AE, et al: Polymorphisms of the P-selectin gene and risk of myocardial infarction in men and women in the ECTIM extension study: Etude cas-temoin de l'infarctus myocarde. Heart 2000;84:548-552.

147. Topol EJ, McCarthy J, Gabriel S, et al: Single nucleotide polymorphisms in multiple novel thrombospondin genes may be associated with familial premature myocardial infarction. Circulation 2001;104:2641-2644.

148. Hiratsuka M, Mizugaki M: Genetic polymorphisms in drug-metabolizing enzymes and drug targets. Mol Genet Metab 2001;73:298-305.

149. Aithal GP, Day CP, Kesteven PJ, Daly AK: Association of polymorphisms in the cytochrome P450 CYP2C9 with warfarin dose requirement and risk of bleeding complications. Lancet 1999;353:717-719.

150. Wolf CR, Smith G, Smith RL: Pharmacogenetics. Br Med J 2000;320:987-990.

151. Benhorin J, Taub R, Goldmit M, et al: Effects of flecainide in patients with new SCN5A mutation: Mutation-specific therapy for long-QT syndrome? Circulation 2000;101:1698-1706.

152. Mitcheson JS, Chen J, Lin M, et al: A structural basis for drug-induced long QT syndrome. Proc Natl Acad Sci USA 2000;97:12329-12333.

153. Sesti F, Abbott GW, Wei J, et al: A common polymorphism associated with antibiotic-induced cardiac arrhythmia. Proc Natl Acad Sci USA 2000;97:10613-10618.

154. Kaji EH, Leiden JM: Gene and stem cell therapies. JAMA 2001;285:545-550.

155. Knowles MR, Hohneker KW, Zhou Z, et al: A controlled study of adenoviral-vector-mediated gene transfer in the nasal epithelium of patients with cystic fibrosis. N Engl J Med 1995;333:823-831.

156. Morgan JE: Cell and gene therapy in Duchenne muscular dystrophy. Hum Gene Ther 1994;5:165-173.

157. Grossman M, Raper SE, Kozarsky K, et al: Successful ex vivo gene therapy directed to liver in a patient with familial hypercholesterolaemia. Nat Genet 1994;6:335-341.

158. Chang MW, Barr E, Seltzer J, et al: Cytostatic gene therapy for vascular proliferative disorders with a constitutively active form of the retinoblastoma gene product. Science 1995;267:518-522.

159. Losordo DW, Vale PR, Symes JF, et al: Gene therapy for myocardial angiogenesis: Initial clinical results with direct myocardial injection of phVEGF165 as sole therapy for myocardial ischemia. Circulation 1998;98:2800-2804.

160. Isner JM, Losordo DW: Therapeutic angiogenesis for heart failure. Nat Med 1999;5:491-492.

## EDITOR'S CHOICE

Garg V, Kathiriya IS, Barnes R, et al: GATA4 mutations cause human congenital heart defects and reveal an interaction with TBX5. Nature 2003;424:443-447.

*Study of patients with congenital heart disease extends previous work in the mouse that implicated GATA4 in critical steps of cardiogenesis; underscores the importance of combing mouse and human based genetic approaches.*

Gerull B, Gramlich M, Atherton J, et al: Mutations of TTN, encoding the giant muscle filament titin, cause familial dilated cardiomyopathy. Nat Genet 2002;30:201-204.

*Human mutations in titin lead to human heart failure; forms mechanistic connection with other work in mouse and human systems that implicates titin as part of the stretch sensor machinery of heart muscle.*

He J, McDermott DA, Song Y, et al: Preimplantation genetic diagnosis of Holt-Oram syndrome and congenital heart disease. Am J Med Genet 2003; in press.

*Reports the first application of preimplantation molecular genetic diagnosis of congenital heart disease and demonstrates feasability of this technology for families with inherited heart defects.*

Hobbs HH, Graf GA, Yu L, et al: Genetic defenses against hypercholesterolemia. Cold Spring Harb Symp Quant Biol 2002;67:499–505.

*New pathways for cholesterol regulation uncovered by studies of rare forms of human monogenic disorders.*

Lifton RP, Wilson FH, Choate KA, Geller DS: Salt and blood pressure: New insight from human genetic studies. Cold Spring Harb Symp Quant Biol 2002;67:445–450.

*Leader in the field describes seminal work in uncovering new genes and pathways for monogenic forms of human hypertension; establishing links to common forms of hypertension appears to be the next step.*

Mohler PJ, Schott JJ, Gramolini AO, et al: Ankyrin-B mutation causes type 4 long-QT cardiac arrhythmia and sudden cardiac death. Nature 2003;421:634–639.

*Important study that elucidates the first nonchannel gene defect to be linked to long QT; mouse models appear warranted to explore the potential mechanistic link with channels that are already genetically linked to this syndrome.*

Schmitt JP, Kamisago M, Asahi M, et al: Dilated cardiomyopathy and heart failure caused by a mutation in phospholamban. Science 2003;299:1410–1413.

*A new class of human dilated cardiomyopathy mutation is established in a nonsarcomeric, noncytoskeletal gene; supports the concept that enhanced activity of phospholamban is the critical step in heart failure progression in both genetic and acquired forms of human heart failure.*

Splawski I, Timothy KW, Tateyama M, et al: Variant of SCN5A sodium channel implicated in risk of cardiac arrhythmia. Science 2002; 297:1333–1336.

*A functional variant of a long QT related channel gene is an important genetic risk factor for arrythmogenesis; documents that studies of rare genetic disorders can provide candidate genes that may be responsible for disease susceptibility in large populations.*

# chapter 9

# Gene Transfer Approaches for Cardiovascular Disease

*Elizabeth G. Nabel*

## GENE TRANSFER APPROACHES FOR CARDIOVASCULAR DISEASE

Since the 1980s, molecular genetic approaches have fundamentally changed the understanding of normal cardiovascular function and the pathophysiologic basis of cardiovascular disease in humans. The cloning of many genes important for the development and function of the cardiovascular system has profoundly increased the understanding of cardiac physiology and has also provided powerful new tools for assessing susceptibility to cardiovascular disease. More recently, this revolution in molecular cardiology has generated enthusiasm for the development of novel gene and gene therapy approaches for the treatment of a variety of cardiovascular disorders, including hyperlipidemia, atherosclerosis, restenosis, and congestive heart failure (CHF).

Somatic gene therapy can be defined as the ability to introduce genetic material (RNA) into an appropriate cell type or tissue *in vivo* in such a way that it alters the cell's pattern of gene expression to produce a therapeutic effect. The genetic material used in these approaches includes eukaryotic and prokaryotic genes (with associated transcriptional regulatory elements) and RNA molecules encoding intracellular, cell surface, and secreted polypeptides and synthetic oligonucleotides and ribozymes. Since 1990, there has been remarkable progress in this field built largely on a solid foundation of basic scientific advances in the areas of viral genetics, eukaryotic gene expression, and the cloning of human disease-related genes.[1,2] In addition, public concerns about the safety of gene therapy have led to the establishment of national agencies, such as the Recombinant Advisory Committee (RAC), that oversee gene therapy trials in humans. These agencies have served to stimulate public debate about the ethical issues involved in this novel type of genetic therapy.

Gene therapy in humans became a reality in the early 1990s when several clinical trials for single-gene replacement in inherited disorders and cancer were begun.[3,4] Since then, the field has expanded dramatically; there are currently more than 500 trials of gene therapy under way worldwide.[5] These trials, which have enrolled more than 2500 patients, have demonstrated the safety of current gene transfer technologies; published reports have described low-level morbidity and no treatment-related mortality.[6] The notable exception is a gene therapy related death in a patient with preexisting liver disease who received an intrahepatic artery infusion of high-titer adenoviral vectors.[7] Despite this tragic death, there has been a favorable safety profile to date and beginning evidence of therapeutic efficacy of gene therapy in humans.[8,9] This relative lack of success largely reflects (1) the embryonic nature of the field as a whole, (2) the choices of challenging disease targets for initial gene therapy trials in humans, and (3) the difficulties involved with gene delivery and the stability of gene expression in humans.[10] However, gene transfer experiments in both animals and humans have provided a wealth of new information about normal mammalian biology and cardiovascular pathophysiology. In particular, the ability to stably program recombinant gene expression in a variety of cell types *in vivo* has allowed direct testing of the role of specific gene products in cardiovascular disease. In many ways these basic scientific advances represent the most important legacy to date.

This chapter summarizes the current understanding of the utility of gene therapy for the treatment of acquired and inherited cardiovascular diseases; it is recognized that, in many ways, this is truly a field in evolution. Any successful gene therapy approach requires a therapeutic gene, a vector for delivering that gene to the appropriate cell, and in many cases a method for delivering this vector to a localized site of the organism or patient *in vivo*. Each of these components must be carefully tailored to the disease being treated. For example, a disease such as restenosis may require only transient transgene expression in vascular smooth muscle cells (VSMCs) localized to the site of a balloon angioplasty. In contrast, gene therapy for a disease such as familial hypercholesterolemia would likely require long-term transgene expression in large numbers of hepatocytes, and gene therapy for CHF might require transgene expression in cardiac myocytes throughout the ventricular myocardium. These profoundly different spatial, temporal, and cellular requirements would almost certainly necessitate the use of different transgenes, vectors, and catheter delivery systems in the treatment of these three diseases.

Accordingly, this discussion of cardiovascular gene therapy (1) reviews the different vector and catheter systems currently available for delivering therapeutic genes to cells of the cardiovascular system, (2) describes possible disease targets and appropriate potential therapeutic genes for these cardiovascular disorders, and in particular (3) emphasizes the hurdles that must be overcome en route to successful gene therapy for specific cardiovascular diseases in humans. In addition, we have attempted to illustrate some of the novel insights into cardiovascular biology that have been derived from early gene transfer experiments. Because of the large number of publications in this area, it has been impossible to include all citations. We apologize for any inadvertent omissions of specific references. The reader is also referred to additional reviews in the areas of vector development,[11-13] clinical trials,[14] and cardiovascular gene therapy.[15-17]

## VECTORS FOR CARDIOVASCULAR GENE THERAPY

In the early days of gene therapy, many workers were searching for the ideal vector: one that would allow efficient transduction and long-term stable transgene expression in many different cell types *in vivo,* while demonstrating little or no risk of persistent infection, immunogenicity, host cell mutagenesis, or patient-to-patient transmission. It is now clear that such a vector does not exist and is unlikely to be constructed. Instead, a number of different vectors have been developed, each with unique properties that recommend their use for specific cell types and diseases. None of these vectors has been fully optimized. This process of optimization will ultimately determine the utility of gene therapy for specific diseases in humans. There are several considerations that are important in evaluating the potential of any vector for gene therapy in humans: (1) its efficiency of transduction of different cell types *in vitro* and *in vivo,* (2) the size and type of genetic material that it can transduce, (3) the ability to target its genetic material to specific cell compartments, (4) the intracellular stability of its genetic material, (5) its ability to produce stable transcription and translation of component transgenes, (6) its immunogenicity *in vivo,* (7) its cytotoxicity, and (8) its potential for disseminated infection of the host or host-to-host transmission. This information is summarized in Figure 9-1 and Table 9-1.

## Viral Vectors

Over millions of years, mammalian viruses have evolved efficient mechanisms for transducing a wide variety of cells *in vivo.* Thus, in many ways vectors derived from these viruses are ideally suited for introducing therapeutic transgenes into a wide variety of human tissues. On the other hand, humans have co-evolved efficient host defense mechanisms (inflammation and immunity) to eliminate viral pathogens. Thus, the major challenge in using viral vectors for gene therapy is retaining their highly efficient transduction mechanisms while providing a means for evading host immune and inflammatory responses. This problem has not been entirely solved, but recent work has suggested that genetic engineering of viral genomes in combination with transient immunosuppressive regimens may eventually provide solutions that will allow these modified vectors to be used successfully for gene therapy in humans.

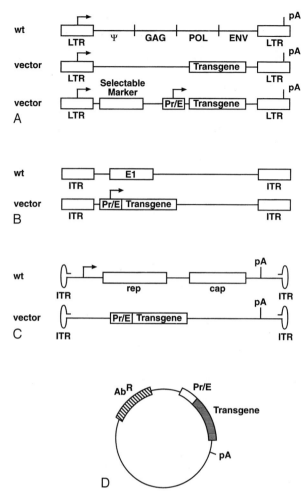

**FIGURE 9-1.** Schematic illustrations of viral and plasmid vectors for gene transfer. *A,* Structure of wild-type and replication-defective retroviral vectors. The structure of a wild-type (wt) retrovirus is shown in the top panel and is based on the structure of the Maloney murine leukemia virus. These viruses contain three genes (*gag, pol, and env*) flanked by LTRs. The packaging sequence (ψ) is located at the left end of the genome. The start of viral transcription is shown by an arrow; the pA site is located in the 3′ LTR. Two different retroviral vectors are shown in the bottom two panels. In the first, expression of the transgene is driven from the LTR promoter (*middle panel*). The second vector contains a selectable marker gene driven from the LTR promoter and a second transgene driven from an internal promoter-enhancer (Pr/E) (*bottom panel*). *B,* The structure of the wt and replication-defective adenovirus vectors. The wt vector contains an intact E1 region (E1). In the first-generation replication-defective vector shown in the bottom panel, the E1 region has been replaced with a transgene driven by an internal promoter-enhancer (Pr/E). The virus is flanked by ITRs. *C,* The structure of wt and replication-defective AAV vectors. The wt AAV vector shown in the top panel contains the rep and cap viral genes flanked by ITRs. The viral promoter (*arrow*) is at the left end of the genome. In the replication-defective AAV vector (*bottom panel*), the rep and cap genes have been deleted and replace with a foreign transgene driven from an internal Pr/E. *D,* A typical plasmid DNA vector used for gene transfer. The vector contains a foreign transgene driven by a viral or cellular Pr/E and a pA. The vector also contains an AbR gene for selection and propagation in bacteria.

### Retroviral Vectors

Retroviruses have been the most widely used vector system for gene therapy experimentation in both animals and humans.[18-21] Their popularity derives from the simplicity of their genome, which can be easily manipulated

**TABLE 9-1    ADVANTAGES AND DISADVANTAGES OF DIFFERENT VECTORS FOR CARDIOVASCULAR GENE THERAPY**

| Vector/Transgene | Advantages | Disadvantages |
|---|---|---|
| Retroviruses | Stably integrate into host genome<br>Easily manipulated viral genome<br>No viral gene products; relatively nonimmunogenic<br>Highly efficient transduction of many cell types | Low titers<br>Capacity for insertional mutagenesis<br>*In vitro* instability<br>Transcriptional shut-off *in vivo*<br>Require cell proliferation for infection |
| Lentiviruses | Efficient transduction of replicating and nonreplicating cells<br>Stably integrate into host genome<br>Wide tropism in mammalian cells<br>Relatively nonimmunogenic | *In vivo* stability in the cardiovascular system is unknown<br>Capacity for insertional mutagenesis |
| Adenoviruses | Maintained as an episome<br>Highly efficient transduction of replicating and nonreplicating cells<br>Stable *in vivo* in absence of immune response<br>High-level transgene expression *in vivo*<br>Relatively nonpathogenic<br>High titers | Evoke potent host inflammatory and immune responses that eliminate transgene expression and preclude repeated administration<br>Difficult to target to specific cell types<br>Relatively difficult to manipulate viral genome |
| Adeno-associated virus | Infects replicating and nonreplicating cells<br>Potential for site-specific integration<br>Relatively nonimmunogenic<br>High titers<br>Nonpathogenic in humans | Can accept only small transgenes<br>Difficult to produce in large quantities<br>Does not appear to stably transduce all cell types *in vivo*<br>Potential for insertional mutagenesis |
| Plasmid DNA | Easy to manipulate and produce in large quantities<br>Nonpathogenic<br>Relatively nonimmunogenic<br>Does not require an infectious vector<br>Maintained as an episome<br>Can program long-term gene expression in postmitotic cells *in vivo* | Very low transduction efficiency |
| Synthetic oligonucleotides | Easy to synthesize in large quantities<br>Relatively high transduction efficiencies if delivered with viral liposomes | Can only reduce or ablate gene expression<br>Large number of nonspecific and nonreproducible biologic effects<br>Cannot target specific cell types<br>Relatively short halflife *in vivo* |
| Ribozymes | Can specifically and effectively target mRNAs | Can only reduce or ablate gene expression<br>Difficult to deliver to cells *in vivo*<br>Stability *in vitro* unclear |

genetically to accept transgenes of up to 10,000 base-pairs (bp); from their ability to infect many mammalian cell types (at least *in vitro*); and from their capacity to stably and precisely integrate their genome into the host chromosome, thereby theoretically providing long-term transgene expression in both the initially infected cell and all of its progeny. In their wild-type form, retroviruses are single-stranded enveloped RNA viruses that encode a relatively small number of viral proteins necessary for infection. Most retroviral gene therapy vectors have been based on the murine leukemia viruses, whose genomic structure is shown in Figure 9-1. The wild-type leukemia virus genome is flanked by long terminal repeats (LTRs), each of which is composed of unique 3′ (U3) and 5′ (U5) sequences. The 5′ LTR contains a single promoter, which is used to transcribe all of the viral genes. Simple retroviruses contain only three genes: *gag*, which encodes the structural proteins involved in making the virus core; *pol*, which encodes the viral reverse transcriptase, integrase, and protease; and *env*, which encodes the viral envelope glycoproteins. Other important sequence elements include the packaging sequence (Ψ), which is required for packaging the genome into viral particles, and the polyadenylation sequence (pA), which is located in the 3′ UTR.

One of the major advantages of retroviral vectors is the ability to remove all of the viral genes and replace them with transgene sequences and transcriptional regulatory elements. The viral gene products necessary to generate infectious particles can then be supplied in *trans* by a packaging cell line. Practically speaking, the genetically modified retroviral genome in the form of a cDNA cloned into a plasmid containing the LTRs, the packaging sequence, the transgenes (with or without their own promoters), and the pA is transfected into a packaging cell line that has been engineered previously to constitutively express the *gag*, *pol*, and *env* gene products. The resulting transfectants produce high-titer retroviral particles, which can be harvested and used directly for gene transfer experiments. Such gene therapy vectors are capable of infecting a wide range of host cells but lack the genes necessary to produce further infectious virus; thus, the risk of systemic infection and/or patient-to-patient transmission of the vector is minimized. A second attractive feature of these vectors is that their host range is determined by the envelope glycoprotein expressed by the packaging cell line. Therefore, it is possible to produce ecotropic retroviruses that will infect only murine cells or amphotropic vectors that will infect a wide variety of species (including humans) by transfecting the same vector into packaging cell lines expressing different envelope genes.

After infection of a mammalian cell *in vitro* or *in vivo*, the RNA genome of the typical replication-defective retroviral vector undergoes reverse transcription to yield a double-stranded DNA copy. This retroviral cDNA is then randomly integrated into the host genome, a process mediated by the terminal attachment sites and the viral integrase. Typically, infection results in the integration of 1 to 10 copies of the viral genome per cell. After integration into the host genome, the viral genome is transcribed either from the endogenous pro-moter in the 5′ LTR or from an internal promoter that has been engineered into the vector. The integrated viral genome is replicated with the host chromosome and is, therefore, passed on to all of the progeny of the infected cell.

Despite their relative advantages, the use of retroviral vectors has been greatly limited by several important technical and biologic problems. First, it has been difficult to produce high-titer stocks of these viruses. The typical retroviral vector cannot be produced at titers of much more than $10^6$ plaque-forming units (pfu, or infectious units) per milliliter, which is insufficient for most *in vivo* gene therapy experiments in humans. (In contrast, both adenoviral and adeno-associated viral vectors can be produced at titers of more than $10^{10}$ pfu/mL). Second, classical retroviral vectors require cell proliferation for efficient infection and intetration.[22,23] Although this is not a problem for *ex vivo* infection of cultured cells, it has greatly limited the use of these vectors for *in vivo* gene transfer, because most primary cells do not actively proliferate *in vivo*. This is particularly problematic for cardiovascular gene therapy because, as described later, cardiac myocytes are postmitotic, and vascular smooth muscle and endothelial cells rarely proliferate. Third, despite the fact that retroviral vectors are stably expressed in cultured cells *in vitro,* the transcription of many of these vectors is extinguished in primary cells *in vivo* after relatively short periods of time.[22] The mechanism underlying this transcriptional shut-off remains unclear. Fourth, the random integration of retroviral vectors poses the risk of insertional mutagenesis and, in particular, neoplastic transformation if the virus integrates into or near an oncogene or a tumor suppressor gene. Although this risk does not appear to be high in experiments involving stocks of highly purified replication-defective vectors, some studies have suggested that many stocks of retroviral vectors are contaminated with low levels of replication-competent virus (RCV), which is produced by recombination after transfection of the packaging cell line.[24] The use of such contaminated preparations in monkeys has been associated with lethal tumors caused by the widespread integration of the RCV.[25]

Despite these problems several studies have rekindled the hope that retrovirus vectors may eventually find some utility in gene therapy in humans. For example, it has been reported that retroviral vectors based on human immunodeficiency virus (HIV) genome are capable of efficiently transducing nonreplicating cells *in vivo*.[26] Similarly, it is now possible to produce pseudo-typed retroviral particles containing the envelope glyco-protein from the vesicular stomatitis virus.[27] Such pseudotyped viruses can be prepared at much higher titers (at least $10^9$ pfu/mL) than traditional amphotropic viruses. It has also been possible to target retroviral vectors to specific cell lineages by modifying the envelope protein to contain peptide recognition sites for lineage-specific cell-surface receptors.[28] Finally, it has been suggested that transcriptional shut-off of retroviral vectors can be prevented by replacing the retroviral LTR promoters with highly active cellular promoters and enhancers.[22]

In summary, retroviral vectors have several unique advantages that make them attractive vectors for gene therapy in humans. However, to date, their use, particularly in cardiovascular gene therapy, has been limited by several difficult technical and biologic problems. Research advances have suggested that it may now be possible to overcome some of these problems, and, therefore, the use of appropriately modified retroviral vectors in animal models of cardiovascular gene therapy may be re-explored.

### Lentiviral Vectors

Recent progress has been made in the development of lentiviral vectors for gene therapy. These vectors are based on the lentivirus genus of retroviruses that includes HIV.[29] Lentiviral vectors infect both dividing and nondividing cells because of the ability of the preintegration complex, or viral shell, to penetrate intact membranes of the target cell nucleus. In addition, lentiviral vectors can stably integrate into chromosomes resulting in stable gene expression for at least 6 months. These vectors have a wide tropism, infecting many mammalian cells including neurons, macrophages, hematopoietic stem cells, retinal photoreceptors, muscle, and liver cells.[30] In the cardiovascular system, there have been recent reports of gene transfer using lentiviral vectors to characterize gene expression *in vivo*. A lentiviral vector encoding a green fluorescent protein has been employed to monitor gene expression by magnetic resonance imaging using catheter-based gene transfer.[31] Lentiviral vectors may also be useful in the treatment of AIDS because these viruses have evolved to infect and express viral genes in human T cells and monocytes/macrophages.[30] Although lentiviral vectors offer advantages over retroviral vectors for human gene therapy purposes, concerns regarding their safety with regard to HIV has slowed application to clinical trials.

### Adenoviral Vectors

Since 1990, replication-defective adenovirus (RDAd) vectors have been widely used for gene therapy experimentation in both animals and humans. Adenoviruses are double-stranded linear DNA viruses that in their wild-type form cause self-limited respiratory tract infections in humans.[32] The wild-type adenovirus genome is a 36-kDa molecule that is divided into 100 map units (see Figure 9-1). A number of properties make adenoviral vectors ideally suited for cardiovascular gene therapy in humans.[33-35] First, unlike retroviral vectors, adenoviruses infect a wide variety of replicating and nonreplicating cell types both *in vitro* and *in vivo*. In particular, these vectors have been shown to efficiently infect cardiac myocytes *in vivo* after either intramyocardial injection[36,37] or intracoronary artery infusion.[38] They also have been used to efficiently transduce vascular endothelial and smooth muscle cells both *in vitro* and after catheter-mediated delivery *in vivo*.[38-41] Finally, these vectors can be used to efficiently transduce both hepatocytes[42,43] and skeletal myocytes[44-47] *in vivo*, which makes them potentially useful vectors for gene

therapy approaches designed to produce transgene-encoded serum proteins. Adenovirus vectors can be produced at very high titers (up to $10^{12}$ pfu/mL), thereby allowing efficient gene transfer *in vivo* with small volumes of virus. This is a significant advantage of being able to accept large promoter/transgene cassettes (up to 6 kilobases in first-generation vectors and more than 20 kilobases in recently modified vectors). Finally, adenoviruses display a relatively favorable safety profile; they do not integrate into the host genome, and have not been associated with malignancies in humans. Moreover, wild-type adenoviruses have been used to safely vaccinate large numbers of military recruits.[48]

Most adenoviral vectors used in previous gene therapy experiments are derived from adenovirus serotypes 2 and 5, both of which are minimally pathogenic in humans. First-generation adenovirus vectors were rendered replication-defective by removal of the E1 region (map units 1 to 9) of the genome that normally encodes two transcriptional regulatory proteins (E1A and E1B) that are required for the expression of late viral genes and for the induction of the lytic cycle of the virus.[49,50] This region of the genome is then replaced by a transgene under the transcriptional control of appropriate promoter and enhancer elements (see Figure 9-1). Because the E1 deletion renders them replication-incompetent, adenovirus vectors must be propagated on a permissive cell clone such as 293[51] or 911[52] that stably express the E1 gene products in *trans*. After administration *in vivo,* these vectors are capable of efficiently transducing a large number of rodent, canine, simian, and human cell types. However, because they lack E1 genes, they are incapable of regenerating infectious progeny, thereby preventing generalized infection or patient-to-patient transmission of the vector.

Despite their numerous advantages for *in vivo* gene transfer into cells of the cardiovascular system, the use of first-generation adenovirus vectors has thus far been limited by host inflammatory and immune responses that severely shorten the duration of gene expression *in vivo* and that preclude repeated administration of these vectors.[53-60] Whereas infection of immunocompromised animals, such as mice with severe combined immunodeficiency (SCID), or of neonatal rodents (in which tolerance to foreign antigens can be induced easily) produces life-long transgene expression in multiple organs (including the liver and skeletal and cardiac muscle), infection of immunocompetent animals results in transgene expression that peaks at 5 to 7 days and is undetectable in most cases by 20 to 30 days after infection. Work from several groups has demonstrated that this transient gene expression is caused by complex immune responses involving non–antigen-specific inflammation caused by viral infection and cell death and humoral and cellular immune responses directed against both viral and foreign transgene proteins.[53,56-59] For example, cytotoxic T cells directed against viral and transgene proteins have been shown to eliminate virus-infected cells, antibody responses against secreted foreign transgene proteins have been demonstrated to neutralize the physiologic effects of these proteins,[53,58] and neutralizing antibodies produced against the viral capsids prevent reinfection with the virus.[59] In addition, cytokine responses may play a role in eliminating the viral genome from infected cells.

Despite these problems, the finding that infection of immunocompromised hosts with these same vectors produces life-long high-level transgene expression with minimal organ pathology strongly suggests that it may be possible to alter host immune responses in such a way that these vectors are useful for cardiovascular gene therapy in humans. Several reports have suggested novel approaches to this problem. These approaches fall into two categories: modifications of the viral genome and transient immunosuppression of the infected host. It has been shown that the use of self transgenes at least in skeletal muscle appears to significantly reduce host immune responses and prolongs transgene expression in immunocompetent mice for as long as 2 years.[58,61] Similarly, the construction of second- and third-generation vectors containing deletions in the E2 and E4 genes, which are also required for late viral gene expression, has been shown to prolong transgene expression in immunocompetent animals.[60,62,63] Finally, it has been possible to produce "gutted" adenovirus vectors, in which all of the viral genes have been replaced with transgene sequences.[64] Such vectors may also prolong transgene expression, but they have not yet been tested extensively *in vivo*.

A second approach to this problem involves transient immunosuppression of the host around the time of virus infection. Transient immunosuppression with a variety of agents, including α-CD4 and α-CD40 monoclonal antibodies,[65,66] CTLA4-Ig (a competitive antagonist of the CD28 second signal in T cell activation),[67] cyclophosphamide, and cyclosporine, has been shown to prolong transgene expression in rodents. Moreover, treatment with α-CD4 monoclonal antibodies (mAbs) has been shown in some cases to abrogate the neutralizing antibody response, thereby allowing readministration of the virus. Finally, it should be emphasized that although long-term transgene expression is clearly desirable in diseases such as the inherited hyperlipidemias and CHF, transient transgene expression as seen with first-generation adenovirus vectors may actually be preferable in diseases such as restenosis after balloon angioplasty, in which short-term modifications of VSMC gene expression are sufficient to inhibit formation of the restenotic lesion.

In summary, RDAd vectors are in many ways ideally suited for *in vivo* cardiovascular gene therapy in the heart, blood vessels, liver, and skeletal muscle. To date, their use for many diseases has been limited by host inflammatory and immune responses directed against both viral and transgene proteins. Modifications of the viral genome and transient immunosuppressive regimens hold promise for significantly enhancing the utility of these vectors for cardiovascular gene therapy.

### Adeno-Associated Viral Vectors

Adeno-associated virus (AAV) is a defective human parvovirus that displays several properties that make it potentially attractive as a vector for gene therapy in humans.[68-70] The virus can be prepared at high titers

($>10^{10}$ pfu/mL), is normally nonpathogenic in humans, and is able to infect a broad range of cell types *in vitro*. In the absence of concomitant adenovirus infection, wild-type AAV also displays the interesting property of becoming integrated in a site-specific manner into a single 7-kilobase region on human chromosome 19.[71] The AAV genome is a single-stranded, linear, 5-kilobase DNA molecule (see Figure 9-1).[69] The genome is flanked by 145-bp inverted terminal repeats (ITRs) that contain the sequences necessary for packaging and for DNA replication and integration. The coding region contains two open reading frames (ORFs). The left ORF encodes at least four replication (Rep) proteins that are involved in DNA replication, whereas the right ORF encodes the viral capsid (Cap) proteins (VP1, VP2, and VP3). Either the right or both ORFs can be deleted and replaced with one or more transgenes in conjunction with transcriptional regulatory elements to produce AAV-based gene therapy vectors. As a result of packaging constraints, even vectors containing a complete deletion of both ORFS can accept transgene cassettes of only 4 to 5 kilobases, which thereby limits the types of transgenes that can be used with this vector system. Propagation of such internally deleted AAV vectors requires both the AAV Rep and Cap proteins and five adenoviral proteins: E1A, E1B, E2A, E4, and VA. Because of these complex packaging requirements, it has not been possible to produce a convenient helper cell line for the packaging of AAV vectors. Instead, the vectors are currently propagated by cotransfection of cells with the AAV vector and a nonpackageable plasmid to provide AAV Rep and Cap proteins, followed by infection of the transfected cells with wild-type or mutant helper adenovirus.[72] AAV prepared by this protocol can be separated from contaminating adenovirus by both heat treatment (AAV is relatively resistant to heating) and by equilibrium density gradient centrifugation. Although AAV infects a wide variety of cells *in vitro,* it is not yet clear which cell types can be stably transduced with AAV *in vivo*. Efficient transduction of both skeletal myocytes and CNS neurons has been demonstrated after direct injection of AAV into rodents.[73,74] In these experiments, transgene expression was stable for periods of months, and there were few signs of local inflammation. Interestingly, however, AAV does not seem to produce high-level stable transgene expression in the liver. Whether it has the ability to transduce cardiac myocytes and vascular endothelial and smooth muscle cells remains unknown and will be an important determinant of the usefulness of this vector for cardiovascular gene therapy.[75]

As with both retroviral and adenoviral vectors, there are a number of problems associated with the use of AAV vectors that will need to be solved before they are used in gene therapy in humans.[72] First, the lack of a packaging cell line and the need for co-infection with adenovirus make it difficult to prepare large quantities of pure AAV vectors. Second, deletion of internal sequences appears to reduce the titer of the resulting vectors from 10- to 10,000-fold. Of equal importance, deletion of the viral genes during vector construction abrogates the ability of the vectors to become integrated in a site-specific manner into the human genome, thereby raising the possibility of insertional mutagenesis and neoplastic transformation. Thus, although AAV is a potentially attractive vector for cardiovascular gene therapy in humans, better methods are needed for the production of large amounts of purified vector, and much more must be learned about its biology *in vivo* before its usefulness can be accurately assessed.

## Nonviral Vectors

### DNA and RNA Vectors

To date, RNA has been difficult to use as a gene therapy vector *in vivo* because of its instability and sensitivity to RNAases. Despite this problem, ribozymes that can specifically eliminate the expression of individual genes are attractive candidates for altering cardiovascular gene expression *in vivo*. Thus far, most work with ribozymes has been performed in cultured cells. However, some attempts have focused on the expression of ribozymes from adenovirus or plasmid DNA vectors *in vivo*. The reader is referred to several reviews for a more detailed discussion of ribozyme-mediated gene therapy.[76-78]

In 1990, Wolff et al.[79] made the surprising observation that plasmid DN injected directly into skeletal muscle is taken up and expressed for long periods of time by a small percentage of skeletal myocytes in the area of injection. Subsequently, it was shown that cardiac myocytes (but not most other cell types) can also be transduced with foreign genes after direct DNA injection into the myocardium.[80-82] The molecular basis of this remarkable property of skeletal and cardiac muscle remains unknown. However, this technique has been used to program the expression of a variety of genes in rodent and canine cardiac and skeletal cardiac myocytes *in vivo*.[79-83] It has also proved useful as a technique for the molecular dissection of cellular promoters and enhancers *in vivo* without the need to make transgenic mice.[82,84] It has been reported that naked DNA can also be used to transduce cells in the vessel wall after introduction on a hydrophilic gel-coated catheter, albeit with very low efficiency.[85]

Plasmid DNA has a number of advantages as a gene therapy vector. Plasmids are easy to construct and can be inexpensively produced in large quantities as homogeneous chemical solutions. The use of plasmid vectors obviates the need for an infectious agent and thereby eliminates the possibilities of generalized infection of the host and patient-to-patient transmission of the vector. The injection of pure plasmid DNA does not cause significant inflammation and the use of plasmid vectors encoding self transgenes (and in some cases even foreign transgenes) has resulted in long-term transgene expression *in vivo* and has not generally been associated with immune responses either to the DNA or to the transgene product[79-83,86] This has made it possible to readminister plasmid vectors to produce increased levels of transgene expression. Despite these advantages, the use of plasmid DNA vectors has thus far been limited by the relatively low efficiencies of transduction *in vivo*.[79-82] At best, 1% of cells in a relatively small area surrounding the site of plasmid administration have been shown to be transduced. This low transduction efficiency probably reflects both the lack of receptor-mediated endocytosis of plasmid DNA and its extensive degradation and relatively poor nuclear translocation after incorporation into the lysosomal compartment after cellular uptake. Despite attempts by many groups, it has thus far been impossible to significantly increase this relatively low transduction efficiency.

In summary, the simplicity and flexibility of plasmid DNA vectors make them attractive gene therapy vehicles. However, their more widespread use in most gene therapy applications in humans will await the development of more efficient *in vivo* delivery systems. Perhaps lessons learned from viruses that have evolved efficient mechanisms for entering cells and evading lysosomal degradation can be used to construct hybrid synthetic vectors that allow efficient *in vivo* gene delivery with the use of plasmid DNAs.

### Synthetic Oligonucleotides

Antisense oligonucleotides (ASOs) are short (10 to 30 bp) chemically synthesized DNA molecules that are designed to be complementary to the coding sequence of an RNA of interest.[87] Chemical modifications such as the substitution of sulfur for one of the nonbridging oxygen atoms of the phosphate backbone (to produce so-called phosphorothiorates) can be used to render ASOs more stable to nuclease degradation and to enhance their stability in serum and in cells. Such ASOs can be introduced into cells by simple diffusion or by liposome-mediated transfer, the efficiency of which can be further enhanced by the inclusion of fusogenic viruses such as hemagglutinating virus of Japan (HVJ).[88] Once inside the cell, single-stranded ASOs are thought to form double-stranded complexes with their complementary RNA and to decrease its translational efficiency either by steric hindrance or, more likely, by activating RNAase H-mediated degradation of the double-stranded RNA complex.[87] Thus, ASOs can theoretically be used to specifically reduce or ablate the expression of one of more genes in a wide variety of cell types. In addition, double-stranded synthetic oligonucleotides containing binding sites for specific transcription factors can be used as decoys to ablate the transcription of genes that require those factors for expression.[89]

Because they can be chemically synthesized in large quantities and do not require an infectious agent for cell transduction, ASOs are potentially attractive targets for *in vivo* gene therapy. However, in view of their short half-life *in vivo* and their ability to only ablate (as opposed to program and enhance gene expression), they will probably be useful only in the treatment of diseases necessitating transient reductions in gene expression. As described later, ASOs have been used both *in vitro* and *in vivo* to modulate cardiovascular gene expression. In particular, ASOs complementary to cell cycle regulatory proteins such as c-myc,[90,91] c-myb,[92] proliferating cell nuclear antigen (PCNA),[93,94] cdc2,[95] and double-stranded oligonucleotide decoys for the transcription factor E2F[96] have been used to inhibit VSMC proliferation *in vitro* and to reduce restenosis after balloon angioplasty *in vivo*.

Despite initial enthusiasm about the use of ASOs in gene therapy in humans, important concerns have been raised about both the specificity and reproducibility of ASO-mediated biologic effects.[87] At least three nonspecific effects have been shown to account for many of the previously observed biologic activities of ASOs. First, both the oligonucleotides themselves and chemical contaminants of individual batches of ASOs can have nonspecific cytotoxic effects, including effects mediated by their binding to specific intracellular and cell surface proteins. These effects can vary from batch to batch of ASOs. Second, some oligonucleotides affect the expression of multiple genes in addition to that of the gene against which they were originally designed. This effect is sequence specific (and presumably mediated by base pairing with additional RNAs) and, therefore, cannot be controlled with the use of scrambled or mutant oligonucleotides. Finally, ASOs containing CpG dinucleotides have been shown to produce non–antigen-specific polyclonal activation of the humoral immune system in rodents.[97] In summary, despite initially encouraging results, the utility of ASOs for cardiovascular gene therapy will be limited by their relatively short half-life, by the fact that they can be used only to decrease gene expression, and, most importantly, by their ratio of specific to nonspecific biologic effects.

### Liposomes

One method for potentially increasing the efficiency of DNA and ASO transduction is to complex the DNA with lipids.[98,99] Such DNA-lipid complexes both potentially increase the stability of the DNA and facilitate cellular entry by promoting fusion with the plasma membrane. DNA liposome complexes are typically made by mixing DNA (or RNA) with various cationic and neutral lipids. Liposome-mediated gene transfer is potentially attractive because it does not require an infectious vector and can be used to deliver a wide variety of easily constructed DNA vectors to many different cell types. In addition, liposome DNA complexes can theoretically be targeted to specific cell lineages by the incorporation of lineage-specific receptor-binding proteins. Several reports have demonstrated that the efficiency of liposome-mediated gene transfer can be increased both by changes in lipid structure[100] and by incorporating adenoviral or fusogenic viral proteins into the complexes.[88] A variety of liposomes have proved remarkably useful for increasing the efficiency of gene transfer into many cell types in vitro.[100-106] However, to date they have been less successful in vivo. This difference may reflect their relative instability in serum, nonspecific uptake by cells of the reticuloendothelial system, and/or fundamental differences between their ability to transduce proliferating cells in culture and primary $G_0$ cells in vivo. Thus, although they are potentially attractive gene therapy vehicles, it will be necessary to increase the in vivo efficiency of liposomes by at least 10- to 1000-fold before they will demonstrate general utility for gene therapy of most cardiovascular disorders in humans.

## CELL TRANSPLANTATION

The ability to transplant normal or genetically engineered cells represents an alternative approach to in vivo gene therapy that might prove useful for the treatment of some cardiovascular diseases. For example, previous studies have shown that it is possible to transplant primary murine skeletal myoblasts into adult mouse skeletal muscle by simple intramuscular injection.[107-112] Such transplanted cells fuse both with each other and with endogenous myocytes to become stably incorporated into the muscle for periods of months to years. Despite efficient myoblast transplantation in rodents, this approach has to date not proved successful in humans with Duchenne's muscular dystrophy.[113] This difference may reflect the fact that the recipient muscle in such patients is inflamed and fibrotic, that immune responses directed against the transplanted myoblasts were not syngeneic with the patients' muscle, or that there are fundamental differences in the ability to colonize murine and human muscle with transplanted cells. Soonpaa et al[114] reported that embryonic cardiac myocytes and genetically modified skeletal myoblasts can be transplanted into mouse myocardium in vivo by direct injection. Such transplanted cardiac myocytes were shown to survive for at least several weeks and to form intercalated disks with the endogenous cardiac myocytes. In addition, injection of genetically modified skeletal myoblasts expressing transforming growth factor $\beta^1$ into the myocardium resulted in the formation of stable intracardiac grafts that promoted neovascularization of the surrounding myocardium.[115] Finally, several groups have shown that it is possible to transplant normal or genetically modified endothelial cells onto denuded vessels and for these cells to obtain at least short-term survival.[116]

Although each of these cellular transplantation approaches has potential for human therapy, they are all plagued by the need to culture cells from each patient to be treated or to provide long-term immunosuppression to prevent the rejection of transplanted autologous cells. In addition, many diseases (such as inherited skeletal and cardiac myopathies) would require the transplantation of large numbers of cells and their delivery to large areas of cardiac and skeletal muscle. However, the recent interest in stem cell biology has now reopened the issue of cellular implants as a therapeutic approach for cardiovascular diseases in humans. It is possible that in the future, gene therapy will be combined with stem cell biology to develop potential therapies.[117]

## CELLULAR TARGETS FOR CARDIOVASCULAR GENE TRANSFER

Many cell types have been employed as targets for cardiovascular gene therapy. These include cells of the cardiovascular system, such as cardiac myocytes and vascular endothelial and smooth muscle cells, and noncardiovascular cells, such as hepatocytes and skeletal myocytes. This section reviews the issues involved in transducing each of these cell types in vitro and in vivo.

## *Ex Vivo* Versus *In Vivo* Gene Transfer

An appreciation of the important practical differences between *ex vivo* and *in vivo* gene transfer approaches is critical to understanding the unique hurdles associated with cardiovascular gene therapy. *Ex vivo* gene transfer involves the removal of cells from a host organism, gene transduction *in vitro,* and then transplantation of the genetically modified cells back into the host.[116] Most initial gene therapy experiments used *ex vivo* gene transfer approaches, primarily because of the lack of efficient techniques for transducing primary cells *in vivo.* However, despite the relative ease of *ex vivo* gene transfer, in most cases it is not practical for the treatment of large numbers of patients because it requires isolating and culturing primary cells from each patient to be treated. More importantly, *ex vivo* gene transfer is not therapeutically feasible for most cardiovascular diseases because it is difficult to culture, transduce, and efficiently reimplant most cardiovascular cell types, including cardiac myocytes and VSMCs. Thus, in many ways the field of cardiovascular gene therapy was predicated on the development of novel and efficient methods for transducing these cells directly *in vivo.* As described in more detail later, this involved the simultaneous development of novel vectors and catheters that could be used to deliver genes to the appropriate cardiovascular cell typed *in vivo.*

## Cardiac Myocytes

Cardiac myocytes represent an attractive but particularly difficult target for gene therapy. These cells are terminally differentiated and become postmitotic (i.e., permanently withdrawn from the cell cycle) within the first few weeks of life. Therefore, *ex vivo* gene transfer techniques that require culturing and transducing cardiomyocytes *in vitro* before transplanting them back into a host organism are not feasible. Instead, it has been necessary to develop direct gene transfer techniques that are capable of transducing these quiescent cells *in vivo.* As described later, at least three such techniques have now been developed: (1) direct injection of plasmid DNA into the left ventricular myocardium,[80-82] (2) intramyocardial infection of RDAds,[36,37] and (3) intracoronary infusion of RDAds or synthetic oligonucleotides.[38] The relative advantages and disadvantages of each of these approaches are summarized in Table 9-1. Briefly, direct DNA injection can produce long-term recombinant gene expression *in vivo,* but this is limited to a small area surrounding the site of injection and is extremely inefficient, resulting in transduction of less than 1% of the cells surrounding the injection site.[80-82] In contrast, RDAds injected into the myocardium or infused into the coronary arteries provide highly efficient gene transduction (into as many as 80% of cardiac myocytes) but produce only transient recombinant gene expression *in vivo* because of host immune responses directed against both viral and foreign transgene proteins.[36-38] Moreover, these vectors cannot be readministered, because of potent neutralizing antibody responses generated after an initial infection. Finally, synthetic oligonu-

cleotides have been used as antisense reagents, and their duration of action and specificity remain unclear.

## Vascular Smooth Muscle Cells

VSMCs are important for maintaining normal vessel homeostasis. However, they have also been implicated in the pathogenesis of atherosclerosis and other vascular proliferative disorders, including restenosis after percutaneous revascularization procedures.[118] Thus, the ability to program recombinant gene expression in these cells *in vivo* should yield important new insights into normal and pathophysiologic vessel function. It has been demonstrated that VSMCs can be transduced with relatively high efficiency *in vivo* by catheter-mediated delivery of RDAd.[39,119,120] In addition, perivascular application of synthetic oligonucleotides in pluronic gels has also been reported to yield efficient VSMC gene transduction *in vivo.*[92] Because the endothelium presents a barrier to intraluminal gene delivery to VSMCs, it is necessary to remove or disrupt it before endoluminal catheter-mediated gene transfer to VSMCs. Although this is not a problem in gene therapy approaches designed to treat restenosis after balloon angioplasty, it may complicate the interpretation of experiments in which catheter-mediated gene transfer is used to probe normal vascular function. The advantages and disadvantages of each of the vector systems used to transduce VSMCs *in vivo* are summarized in Table 9-1.

## Endothelial Cells

Endothelial cells are important regulators of vascular function *in vivo.* Initial studies demonstrated that it is possible to transduce cultured endothelial cells *in vitro* by using retroviruses or DNA-liposome complexes and to reimplant these genetically modified cells onto denuded arteries *in vivo.*[116] Subsequent studies demonstrated efficient transduction of vascular endothelial cells *in vivo* through the use of catheter-mediated delivery of RDAd vectors.[38,41] Low levels of gene transfer into endothelial cells have also been reported after *in vivo* infection with replication-defective retroviral vectors[101] and with DNA-liposome complexes.[102,105,106] Gene transfer into endothelial cells represents a potentially attractive approach for local vascular gene therapy and, in addition, has been used to produce recombinant hormones and cytokines that are secreted into the blood to provide systemic effects.[110]

## Hepatocytes and Skeletal Myocytes

Hepatocytes represent the major site of synthesis of many plasma proteins, including lipoproteins and clotting factors. The liver also serves as the major site of LDL metabolism. Therefore, there has been interest in developing efficient systems for programming transgene expression in hepatocytes *in vivo.* Initial experiments used an *ex vivo* approach in which primary hepatocytes isolated after partial hepatectomy were transduced by infection with replication-defective retroviral vectors encoding recombinant proteins and then reimplanted into the host by portal vein infusion.[121,122] The usefulness of this method was limited by the relatively small numbers of hepatocytes that could be transduced *ex vivo*. In rabbits, approximately 2% of hepatocytes displayed transgene expression,[121] whereas in humans less than 1% of hepatocytes demonstrated transgene expression after infusion of genetically modified hepatocytes.[122] These observations, combined with the tragic gene therapy death in an intrahepatic artery trial,[7] have dampened enthusiasm for both *ex vivo* and *in vivo* approaches to hepatic gene therapy for metabolic diseases.

Skeletal myocytes are another potential source for gene therapy applications. Several groups have demonstrated that genetically modified skeletal myocytes could be used to stably deliver physiologic levels of recombinant proteins such as growth hormone to the systemic circulation of mice.[108,109] This finding was somewhat surprising because it had not been appreciated that skeletal myocytes had a secretory potential. In the initial experiments, skeletal muscle stem cells (myoblasts) were transduced with retroviral or plasmid vectors encoding human growth hormone *in vitro,* and these genetically modified cells were then injected intramuscularly into syngeneic mice. The injected myoblasts were shown to fuse both with themselves and with the endogenous myocytes to become stably incorporated into the muscle. Moreover, they continued to secrete physiologic levels of growth hormone into the systemic circulation of the injected mice for at least 3 months. These *ex vivo* gene transfer studies represented important proof of principal experiments concerning the use of genetically modified skeletal muscle, but the findings were not practical for the long-term therapy of inherited or acquired human serum protein deficiencies.

*In vivo* gene transfer approaches using skeletal muscle have demonstrated the potential for therapy in humans. A single intramuscular injection into mice with $10^9$ pfu of a RDAd vector encoding murine erythropoietin (Epo) produced physiologically significant increases in Epo that were stable for more than 2 years.[58,61] As long as mice were injected with RDAd encoding a self protein to which they were tolerant (e.g., murine Epo), immune responses did not eliminate transgene expression. Thus, it appears that, in skeletal muscle, immune responses to the adenoviral proteins are not as problematic as they are after intravenous injection of the same vectors.

Intramuscular injection of plasmid DNA represents a second viable approach to the treatment of serum protein deficiencies. One report demonstrated that a single intramuscular injection of as little as 10 µg of a plasmid DNA vector encoding Epo can be used to program physiologically significant levels of Epo in the systemic circulation of mice.[86] The levels of Epo expression obtained in these experiments were proportional to the dose of DNA administered and were stable for at least 90 days. The intramuscular injection of plasmid DNA has several advantages as compared with intramuscular injection of RDAd. First, it is simple to construct and prepare large quantities of homogeneously pure plasmid DNA vectors. Second, immune responses are much less of a problem with DNA vectors than with adenovirus vectors, thus making it possible to readminister DNA vectors—a pos-

sibility that has not proved feasible after an initial infection with RDAd, at least in rodents and rabbits. Finally, because intramuscular injection of naked DNA does not require an infectious vector, there is no risk of persistent or systemic infection or of patient-to-patient transmission. Despite these advantages, intramuscular injection of plasmid DNA is not nearly as efficient as the injection of RDAd. Therefore, although it may be therapeutically useful for the delivery of potent cytokines such as Epo, it does not yet represent a feasible delivery system for serum proteins such as clotting factors or lipoproteins, which are required at much higher therapeutic concentrations in serum.

## CATHETER DELIVERY SYSTEMS

Delivering therapeutic vectors to the appropriate site *in vivo* represents one of the major challenges to many gene therapy approaches for cardiovascular disease. As discussed earlier, intravenous injection of adenovirus vectors successfully targets the liver, whereas intramuscular injection of both DNA and plasmid vectors can be used to localize recombinant gene expression to skeletal muscle. In contrast, more sophisticated systems are required to deliver therapeutic vectors to specific sites in the vasculature for the treatment of atherosclerosis or restenosis or to the myocardium for the treatment of cardiomyopathies or arrhythmias. Several catheters have been tested as vector delivery systems in animals and humans (Figure 9-2). This section reviews the usefulness of these catheters for the delivery of specific types of vectors to the heart and vasculature.

### Double-Balloon Catheters

Double-balloon catheters contain two balloons (proximal and distal) tandemly arrayed on a single infusion catheter (see Figure 9-2). The area of the catheter between the two balloons contains one or more pores

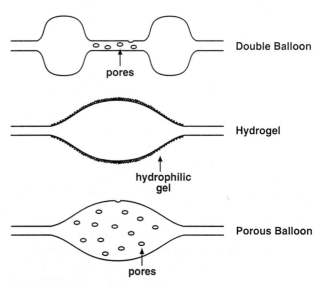

**FIGURE 9-2.** Catheters for cardiovascular gene therapy.

through which gene therapy vectors (or drugs) can be infused or removed. After the catheter is positioned in the vessel, the simultaneous low-pressure inflation of both balloons creates a sealed potential space in the vessel lumen from which blood can be evacuated and that can be filled with an aqueous solution containing an appropriate gene therapy vector. The vector solution can be left in contact with the vessel wall for variable periods of time and then flushed from the vessel before both balloons are deflated, thereby minimizing the extent of systemic dispersion of the vector. The advantages of these catheters are their simplicity, their ability to localize vector delivery, and the relative lack of vascular disruption produced by the low-pressure balloons. Because peripheral arteries have relatively few side branches, the double-balloon catheter represents an effective means of producing stable localized vector delivery in these vessels. However, because the coronary arteries have frequent side branches (occurring every 2 to 4 mm), this type of catheter is unlikely to be useful in its present form for vector delivery to sites of coronary angioplasty, because much of the vector will be "lost" down these side branches.

## Porous and Microporous Infusion Catheters

A variety of porous and microporous infusion catheters have been used to deliver vectors into the arterial wall (see Figure 9-2). Although the details of their construction differ significantly, they are all based on the principle of a balloon that can be inflated against the arterial wall and that contains pores of various sizes for the infusion of vector-containing solutions. Large pore sizes tend to enable efficient intra-arterial delivery but often at the cost of significant mechanical injury to the vessel as a result of high-velocity jetting of solution into the vessel wall. Smaller pores entail less injury but may not deliver vectors as efficiently into the vessel. These types of catheters, particularly microporous catheters, may prove more useful for coronary artery delivery than the double-balloon catheters, because their use should not be adversely affected by frequent coronary artery side branches.[123]

## Hydrogel Catheters

Hydrogel catheters (see Figure 9-2) contain a balloon coated with a hydrophilic gel that forms a sponge-like surface that can be impregnated with different aqueous solutions. The balloon can be dipped in solutions of vector, which can then be dried on the gel and covered with a removable sheath that is used to introduce the catheter into the appropriate intravascular site. After removal of the sheath, the balloon is inflated against the arterial wall, and the vector is delivered into the arterial wall at the site of balloon inflation. Because most viral vectors do not survive drying, this type of catheter is probably most useful for delivery of plasmid DNA vectors. Moreover, because naked DNA does not efficiently transduce VSMCs *in vivo,* the most promising uses of this catheter delivery system involve the intra-arterial delivery of plasmid DNA vectors encoding potent secreted

cytokines, such as vascular endothelial growth factor (VEGF)[85] and nitric oxide synthase (NOS).[124] In such cases, low-level production of recombinant proteins by relatively few cells has been reported to have demonstrable biologic effects.

## Other Delivery Devices

Several additional devices hold some promise for cardiovascular gene therapy but have not yet been tested extensively. As described earlier, plasmid DNA injected into the myocardium is taken up and stably expressed in cardiac myocytes surrounding the site of injection.[80-82] Although most initial experiments used injection under direct visualization via hypodermic needles, several catheters have been designed to permit a catheter-based subendocardial DNA injection technique.[125] These catheters, which can be introduced by arterial or venous access into the right or left ventricular cavity, contain a sheathed needle on one end that can be inserted through the endocardial surface into the myocardium under fluoroscopic guidance and used for the intramyocardial injection of plasmid DNA solutions. Such a catheter may prove useful for programming localized transgene expression at specific sites in the myocardium. Iontophoretic catheters that allow electrophoresis of vectors into localized sites in the vessel wall have also been developed. Finally, drug coated stents are now FDA approved[126,127]; however, the next generation of coated stents will likely deliver plasmid DNA vectors to VSMCs in the coronary and peripheral arteries. Combined stent and gene therapy will prove useful for preventing the VSMC proliferation that results in in-stent restenosis.

## CARDIOVASCULAR DISEASE TARGETS FOR GENE THERAPY

A large number of cardiovascular diseases are potential targets for gene therapy. Although early efforts focused on using gene transfer as correction therapy for single-gene recessive disorders, investigators now recognize that gene transfer holds promise for common acquired cardiovascular diseases, such as myocardial and peripheral ischemia, restenosis, and heart failure. As shown in Figure 9-3, gene therapy approaches may be useful throughout the progression of coronary artery disease, from strategies designed to modify cardiac risk factors to the treatment of vascular proliferative syndromes to novel therapies for myocardial ischemia and infarction, heart failure, and malignant arrhythmias. Most experimentation in cardiovascular gene therapy in animals and humans has focused on angiogenesis, vascular proliferative disorders, cardiomyopathies, arrhythmias, and hyperlipidemias. Accordingly, the following discussion focuses on these areas; it is recognized that other cardiovascular diseases may also eventually prove to be attractive targets for gene therapy. At the onset, it is important to realize as well that successful cardiovascular gene therapy requires the coordination of three components: vector, device, and therapeutic gene (Figure 9-4). Each

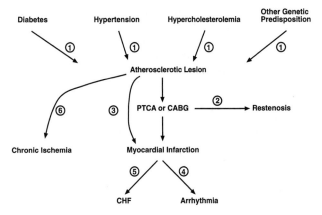

**FIGURE 9-3.** Potential targets for intervention in the progression of atherosclerotic vascular disease. Potential targets include risk factor modification (*1*), treatment of vascular proliferative disorders such as restenosis after PTCA or CABG (*2*), stabilization of atherosclerotic plaque for the prevention of vascular occlusive syndromes such as myocardial infarction (*3*), treatment of cardiac arrhythmias (*4*), treatment of myocardial dysfunction following myocardial infarction or in association with other cardiomyopathies (*5*), and ability to program angiogenesis in skeletal and cardiac muscle in patients with chronic ischemic syndrome (*6*).

leg of this three-legged stool is critical; failure to optimize one component will likely lead to failure of the entire experiment.

## Angiogenesis

Despite dramatic advances in the medical, catheter-based, and surgical therapies of coronary and peripheral atherosclerosis, chronic cardiac and limb ischemia remain major public health problems. The purification and characterization of a series of polypeptide angiogenic growth factors have raised the possibility of programming small vessel neovascularization in ischemic tissues as a therapy for severe chronic cardiac and limb

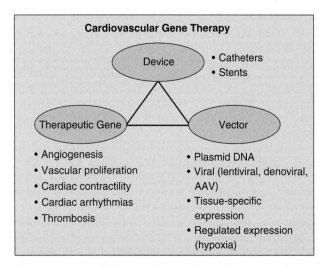

**FIGURE 9-4.** Components of cardiovascular gene therapy. Successful gene therapy into blood vessels and the heart requires the coordination of three components: vectors, devices, and therapeutic genes. Examples of each of the components are provided.

ischemia. The concept of "therapeutic angiogenesis" dates back 30 years to the work of Judah Folkman on neovascularization.[128] Angiogenesis (development of endothelial tubes) and vasculogenesis (development of intact arteries) lead to vascular formation in the embryo. Recent evidence suggests that these processes lead to neovascularization in the adult in normal and pathologic conditions.[129] Although many growth factors and cytokines have angiogenic activity, the two growth factors most widely studied in preclinical and clinical gene transfer studies are VEGF and basic fibroblast growth factor (bFGF).

Early animal model studies using intramuscular injection of bFGF into rabbits with surgically induced syndromes of hind limb ischemia demonstrated increased capillary densities and evidence of augmented collateral blood flow in the treated animals.[129,130] The intra-arterial administration of bFGF protein enhanced collateral blood flow and preserved left ventricular function in an animal model of chronic myocardial ischemia.[131] Takeshita et al[132] extended these initial protein studies to gene transfer. In an initial series of experiments in rabbits with surgically induced hind limb ischemia, they showed that hydrogel catheter-mediated intra-arterial gene transfer of 400 μg of a plasmid DNA vector encoding the angiogenic peptide VEGF caused increased capillary density and increased distal blood flow in the ischemic limb. These findings suggested that small quantities (nanograms to micrograms) of VEGF secretion were required to program neovascularization in severe limb ischemia.

Based on these preclinical experiments, several phase I studies have evaluated the safety and toxicity of plasmid DNA and adenoviral vectors encoding VEGF or bFGF for coronary and peripheral ischemia. A trial of intra-arterial gene transfer of plasmid DNA encoding human VEGF$_{165}$, coded onto an angioplasty balloon, reported the safe delivery of the vector and gene and indirect angiographic evidence of angiogenesis in the peripheral circulation.[133] In this study, plasmid DNA was coated onto an angioplasty balloon, and the DNA was mechanically delivered to a focal atherosclerotic lesion in the superficial femoral artery. The intent was to induce collateral formation distal to the angioplasty site. This delivery method is not optimal because the site of growth factor activity is distal to the site of transduction, and there is no documentation of recombinant VEGF activity in the distal circulation. Demonstration of efficacy awaits phase II and III trials. A more practical approach is the direct injection of vectors into peripheral skeletal muscle near the site of the arterial lesion. This approach has been tested in two trials of VEGF gene therapy. In a phase I study, 400 μg of plasmid DNA encoding VEGF$_{165}$ was injected intramuscularly in patients with peripheral vascular disease.[134] Adverse events related to the vector or gene were not observed. Indices of clinical efficacy were not adequately tested in this phase I protocol. The investigators noted increased pain-free walking time and increased ankle-brachial index in some patients, an indirect measure of improved circulation. Subsequent clinical trials of VEGF to stimulate angiogenesis in peripheral vascular disease in patients with rest pain or ischemic foot ulcers have noted some lower extremity edema in one third of patients and indirect evidence of clinical improvement in 60% to 70% of patients.[135] These phase I studies provide the safety basis for proceeding with phase II and III dose escalation and efficacy trials, but they should not be interpreted as demonstrating clinical efficacy. More recently, a phase I study of $VEGF_{121}$, delivered by adenoviral vectors into peripheral skeletal muscle, reported improvement of endothelial cell function in treated patients, suggesting a benefit to peripheral arterial circulation.[136]

To stimulate angiogenesis in the coronary circulation, preclinical animal studies and phase I human studies have been conducted. The intracoronary delivery of a recombinant adenovirus that directs the expression of FGF-5 can induce therapeutic angiogenesis and restoration of ischemia-inhibited function in an experimental pig model of chronic coronary arterial stenosis.[137] Vectors encoding VEGF have been delivered by a transepicardial approach at the time of bypass surgery[138] or directly into the left ventricle or transendocardially by a catheter.[139] Other phase I studies have been conducted in patients not suitable for revascularization (percutaneous transluminal angioplasty of coronary arteries [PTCA] or CABG).[140] Plasmid $VEGF_{165}$ was administered by direct injection via a limited anterior thoracotomy into the myocardium of patients with inoperable coronary artery disease. The safety of this approach was demonstrated and some measures of improved symptoms (an increase in exercise time and reduced ischemia on myocardial perfusion scanning) were obtained. Adenoviral vectors encoding $VEGF_{121}$ were directly injected into the myocardium of patients undergoing coronary artery bypass surgery.[138] The adenoviral vectors were well tolerated. Symptoms and exercise duration improved, whereas myocardial perfusion studies were not changed in this phase I study. In a small pilot phase I study of plasmid VEGF2 delivered percutaneously by a left ventricular injection catheter, the plasmid DNA was delivered safely,[141] and on the basis of these results a phase II/III study has been initiated.

In summary, these preclinical animal studies and phase I human studies of angiogenesis in the peripheral and coronary circulation have demonstrated that delivery of plasmid or adenoviral vectors encoding VEGF by direct injection or through a catheter have been safe and well tolerated. Indirect measures of improved perfusion and a reduction in symptoms in this small number of patients are encouraging and provide the impetus for phase II/III studies that will be required to determine optimal dosing and clinical efficacy.

## Vascular Proliferative Disorders

Gene transfer has been a useful tool to probe the regulatory pathways involved in VSMC proliferation. Arterial lesions in cardiovascular diseases are characterized by the proliferation of VSMCs and the deposition of connective tissue matrix.[118] Mitogens that stimulate VSMC growth have been well described; however, the proteins that limit intimal hyperplasia are not as well understood. Animal gene transfer models have been created to overexpress growth regulator proteins, and these models have served two purposes: to investigate the molecular pathways that regulate smooth muscle cell growth and to develop potential therapeutic approaches to treating vascular diseases characterized by excessive VSMC proliferation.

VSMCs are normally quiescent and proliferate at low indices. When stimulated to divide by mitogens, cells enter $G_0/G_1$ phase of the cell cycle. Progression through $G_1$ is regulated by the assembly and phosphorylation of cyclin/cyclin-dependent kinase (CDK) complexes, cyclin D-Cdk4, Cdk6, and cyclin E-Cdk2.[142] The cyclin-dependent kinase inhibitors (CKIs) are cellular proteins that inhibit cyclin-CDK activity and prevent phosphorylation of the retinoblastoma gene product (Rb), resulting in $G_1$ arrest (Figure 9-5). CKIs directly implicated in mitogen-dependent CDK regulation are p21,[Cip1] p27,[Kip1] and p16.[Ink4] In the vasculature, p21[Cip1] and p27[Kip1] are endogenous inhibitors of VSMC proliferation through their effects on cyclin E-Cdk2.[143]

Several approaches have been devised to overexpress the CKIs in the vasculature to inhibit vascular proliferation. Studies have examined the role of CKIs, including p21,[Cip1] p27,[Kip1] and p16[Ink4] to inhibit the kinase activities of cyclin-CDK complexes. For example, p21[Cip1] was known to inhibit cell cycle progression in fibroblasts and to protect cells from DNA damage, but the regulation of vascular growth during vascular remodeling by this or other CKIs was unclear. Expression of human p21[Cip1] in rat and pig VSMCs inhibited growth factor stimulation of cell proliferation and arrested cells in $G_1$ phase of the cell cycle.[144,145] Growth arrest of these cells was associated with inhibition of Rb phosphorylation. Likewise, p27[Kip1] is an important regulator of VSMC proliferation in vitro and in vivo.[146] Expression of p27[Kip1] inhibits vascular proliferation and intimal formation through disruption of cyclin E-cdk2 complexes, making this CKI a molecular target for restenosis and other vascular proliferative diseases.

Other gene transfer approaches have been employed to study growth regulation of vascular cells, particularly proliferation of smooth muscle cells and macrophages within atherosclerotic plaques. A prodrug approach, with the herpes simplex virus *thymidine kinase* gene *(HSV-tk)* and the nucleoside analog ganciclovir, has been examined in several animal models of restenosis, including atherosclerotic vessels.[119,147,148] *HSV-tk,* when expressed in mammalian cells, encodes the enzyme thymidine kinase, which phosphorylates ganciclovir. Incorporation of phosphorylated ganciclovir into replicating DNA in dividing cells leads to DNA chain termination, resulting in cell death. Metabolites of the enzymatic reaction are diffusible into adjacent cells (presumably via gap junctions), where they disrupt DNA replication and promote cell killing in dividing cells (the so-called bystander effect). There are several advantages to this approach. Specificity for replicating cells is achievable because cell killing occurs only in dividing cells, and nondividing cells are not affected. The timing of cell death can be regulated by administration of the

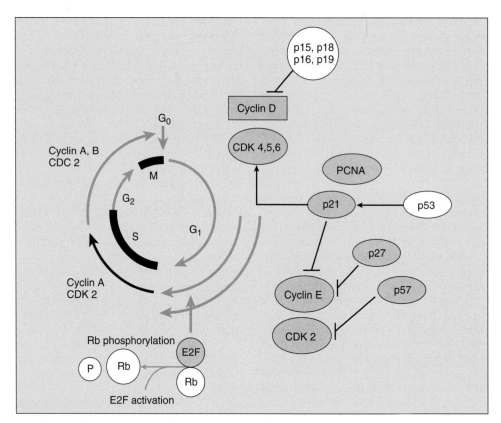

**FIGURE 9-5.** Regulation of the cell cycle. Progression of the cell-cycle $G_1$/S checkpoint is regulated by the assembly and activation of cyclins and CDKs that phosphorylate and inactivate the retinoblastoma gene product (Rb). CKIs complex with cyclin-CDKs to promote G1 arrest. *(Modified with permission from Boehm M, Nabel EG: Cell cycle and cell migration: New pieces to the puzzle. Circulation 2001;103:2879–2881.)*

drug. The bystander effect allows a greater number of cells to be eliminated than if the toxic metabolite remained intracellular; thus, gene transfer efficiency is less critical. Finally, local gene transfer can achieve high local concentrations without systemic toxic effects. The effectiveness of *HSV-tk* gene transfer and ganciclovir treatment has been examined in three animal models of gene transfer: balloon-injured pig and rat arteries and balloon-injured, atherosclerotic rabbit arteries. Adenoviral gene transfer of *HSV-tk* and ganciclovir treatment was associated with significant reductions in smooth muscle cell proliferation and intimal hyperplasia in balloon-injured pig iliofemoral,[119] hyperlipidemic rabbit,[148] and rat carotid[147] arteries.

ASOs represent another strategy to suppress the function of specific gene products in vascular cells, although this approach has not been as effective *in vivo* as adenoviral gene transfer. C-myb ASOs were delivered by Simons et al[92] to the adventitia of injured rat carotid arteries with a pluronic gel; a reduction in *c-myb* RNA was observed, which was associated with a decrease in neointimal formation. Antisense c-myc[90] oligonucleotides were also embedded in a pluronic gel and wrapped around the outer surface of injured rat carotid arteries, on which similar reductions in intimal hyperplasia were observed. A single, local intraluminal administration of antisense cdc2 kinase and PCNA oligonucleotides with HVJ liposomes resulted in prolonged (6-week) suppression of intimal thickening in

balloon-injured rat arteries.[93] Morishita et al[95] demonstrated similar results with antisense to cdk2 kinase as well.

An interesting application of this technology is treatment of bypass vein hyperplasia. Veins, when placed in an arterial position to bypass a stenosis, become "arterialized" when subjected to hemodynamic pressures and shear stress from the arterial circulation. Normally, veins have several layers of smooth muscle cells in the media. After exposure to arterial pressures, intimal hyperplasia develops, presumably as a result of mitogen stimulation of smooth muscle cells from the altered hemodynamic forces. This process has been studied in a rabbit model in which internal jugular veins are interposed in a carotid artery. Treatment of veins with cdc2 and PCNA ASOs before insertion in an arterial position resulted in a reduction in intimal hyperplasia, in comparison with veins treated with control oligonucleotides.[149] This concept has served as the basis for a clinical trial in which patients undergoing peripheral bypass surgery have veins harvested from the lower extremity, incubated with double-stranded oligonucleotide decoys to the transcription factor E2F, and then placed in a bypass position.[150] Patients were randomized to one of three groups: placebo, E2F decoys, and scrambled oligonucleotides. There were no perioperative deaths, and the number of postoperative complications was similar across the three groups. A statistically significant decrease in time to primary graft failure was observed in the E2F decoy group.

Phase III studies will be required to validate these results.

Although the cell cycle has been a major focus of gene therapy efforts to treat vascular proliferative diseases, other cellular targets have also been investigated. Heme oxygenases (HOs) are the rate-limiting enzymes in heme degradation, catalyzing the cleavage of the heme ring to form ferrous iron, carbon monoxide, and biliverdin. Three distinct isoforms of HO have been cloned. Heme oxygenase-1 (HO-1) is an inducible protein activated in systemic inflammatory conditions by oxidant stress. Vascular injury is also characterized by a local reparative process with inflammatory components, and, hence, it is likely that HO-1 plays an important role in vascular remodeling. Indeed, HO-1 has broad protective effects on the vasculature. HO-1 induces vasodilation in blood vessels and protects against pathologic vasoconstriction.[151] In addition, HO-1 has antiproliferative properties through the upregulation of p21[Cip1]. HO-1 also protects against vascular thrombosis through antioxidant mechanisms in the vessel wall.[152] HO-1 has become an exciting molecular target for local treatments of vascular diseases using drug-coated stents and gene transfer.

NO is a potent vasodilator involved in the regulation of vascular tone in many circulatory beds. NO is synthesized from L-arginine by NOSs, and there are two classes of NOSs: constitutive and inducible.[153,154] the constitutive enzymes are calcium and calmodulin dependent and were initially identified in brain (NOS I) and endothelial (NOS III, or ecNOS) cells. The inducible NOS isoform (NOS II, or iNOS) is typically expressed in cells only after exposure to cytokines and is calcium independent. In VSMCs and in platelets, NO activates soluble guanylate cyclase, which increases intracellular guanosine $3',5'$-cyclic monophosphate (cGMP), thereby inducing vasorelaxation and inhibiting platelet aggregation. NO is also an important modulator of VSMCs as a result of its antiproliferative actions. The vascular biology of NOS has been studied in several animal models with the use of NOS vectors. Transfection of ecNOS vectors with HVJ liposomes into injured rat carotid arteries was associated with local NO generation and a reduction in intimal hyperplasia.[124] The functions of other vasoactive molecules have been studied in situ through gene transfer methods, including angiotensin-converting enzyme (ACE)[155] and endothelin-1 (EI-1).[156]

Cell proliferation is a prominent feature of in-stent restenosis. Drug-coated stents are currently being tested as primary therapies for in-stent restenosis.[126,127] In the future, it is likely that DNA- or vector-coated stents will be developed, encoding one or more genes that have antiproliferative, anti-inflammatory, and antithrombotic actions.

## Thrombosis

The development of transgenic mice has been a powerful tool for the analysis of coagulation factors and their role in the development of atherosclerosis and other vascular diseases. Murine models for a number of defects in the fibrinolytic system have been constructed, including mice deficient in fibrinogen,[157] plasminogen,[158] plasminogen activator inhibitor-1 (PA1-1),[159] urokinase plasminogen activator (uPA) and tissue plasminogen activator (TPA),[160] factor V,[161] tissue factor,[162] a thrombin receptor,[163] and thrombomodulin.[164] These studies have produced important and surprising results. For example, deficiency in a thrombin receptor[163] and factor Va[161] in mice is embryonic lethal, which suggests that thrombin activation proceeds through a factor V pathway, and factor V is an essential component of the prothrombinase complex. Interestingly, only approximately 50% of the mice deficient in factor V and thrombin receptor die during embryogenesis. Although the mechanism is not unknown, the findings suggest a role for thrombin in the development of placental blood vessels.

These animal models are also being used to explore the genetic contributions to complex traits, such as atherosclerosis, and to dissect the pathophysiology of vascular diseases, such as the role of protease inhibitors of cell migration and proliferation. Adenoviral vectors have been constructed to express fibrinolytic proteins, and these vectors have been infused into mice deficient in coagulation proteins to "rescue" a phenotype. For example, mice deficient in PAI-1 demonstrate accelerated neointimal formation after vascular injury, in comparison with mice with normal levels of PAI-1. Mice deficient in uPA appear "protected" and exhibit reduced intimal lesions after injury. Adenoviral-mediated gene transfer of PAI-1 to mice deficient in PAI-1 reverses the phenotype, that is, neointimal formation is reduced.[165] The utility of these gene transfer approaches to the treatment of thrombotic diseases in humans has not been completely tested. It will be interesting to compare the efficacy of genetic therapies with that of protein therapies for local thrombotic lesions as the genetic approaches are further refined and carried from preclinical stages to clinical trials in humans.

## Plaque Rupture and Transplant Atherosclerosis

Two other vascular diseases, not previously discussed, account for significant cardiovascular morbidity and mortality and may be targets for genetic therapy in the future. Plaque rupture is the major cause of unstable coronary syndromes and is the result of ongoing inflammation, thrombosis, and matrix degradation within an atherosclerotic plaque. This syndrome has been difficult to study because of a lack of an appropriate small or large animal model. Furthermore, many cytokine, growth factor, coagulation, and protease genes contribute to the pathophysiology of the disease process, and hence it is difficult to elucidate the role of a single gene or protein, in view of the interplay and redundancy of multiple factors. Nonetheless, this is a disease for which further understanding and improved treatment are urgently needed, and genetic approaches are likely to make important contributions in the future.

The major cause of death from cardiac transplantation is progressive coronary atherosclerosis, which is characterized as a diffuse, intimal thickening throughout the coronary circulation. The cause of this type of atherosclerosis is different from that of standard atherosclerosis in that ongoing inflammation contributes significantly to the development of atherosclerotic lesions. Transplant atherosclerosis has also been difficult to study because of a lack of relevant animal models. Several models of pig transplantation, however, have been developed to mimic the disease in humans and have been useful tools for testing novel forms of therapy. Transplantation atherosclerosis is another vascular proliferative disease in which patients may benefit from genetic therapy, but further investigation is awaited.

## Hyperlipidemias

Several acquired and inherited lipid disorders are independent risk factors for the development of atherosclerotic vascular disease, myocardial infarction, and stroke. These include the hypercholesterolemia states (mostly associated with increased LDL-cholesterol [LDL-C]), syndromes of decreased HDL, and inherited elevations in lipoprotein A (Lp[a]). Although drug therapy with bile acid-binding resins and 3-hydroxy-3-methylglutaryl-coenzyme A (HMG CoA) reductase inhibitors have significantly reduced the risk of cardiovascular morbidity and mortality in many hypercholesterolemia patients, large numbers of patients have lipid disorders that are not fully responsive to standard pharmacologic therapy. These disorders include heterozygous and homozygous FH caused by inherited defects in the $LDL_R$. The lack of effective pharmacologic therapy for these patients has stimulated efforts to develop novel gene therapy approaches for these disorders.

The development of gene transfer approaches for the hyperlipidemias has been greatly facilitated by the generation of mouse models that closely mimic the pathophysiology of the hyperlipidemias in humans. Wild-type mice do not represent a good model system of the lipid disorders in humans. In mice, HDL rather than LDL is the major circulating lipoprotein, and mice are remarkably resistant to atherosclerosis even after prolonged feeding with a high-fat diet. Gene targeting approaches have been used to produce mice that lack either apo E.[164] Apo E-deficient mice have marked elevations in plasma cholesterol with a dramatic shift in the distribution of their cholesterol from HDL to very low density lipoprotein (VLDL) and chylomicron remnants. Of more importance, atherosclerosis develops spontaneously in these mice, even when they are maintained on a regular chow diet. These mice have for provided excellent small animal models for gene therapy and have also facilitated the use of *in vivo* gene transfer approaches to test hypotheses concerning the role of specific lipoproteins and lipid-modifying enzymes in regulating lipid metabolism and atherogenesis.

Apo E is a 36-kDa apolipoprotein that plays a critical role in the uptake of multiple lipoproteins by hepatic LDL and LDL remnant receptors.[166] There are three human alleles of the apo E gene (apo Ew, apo E3, and apo E4) that display different affinities for the lipoprotein receptors. Patients with inherited apo E deficiency or who are homozygous for the apo E2 allele that displays decreased affinity for the lipoprotein receptors have elevated plasma cholesterol-rich VLDL and chylomicron remnants. Of more importance, premature atherosclerotic vascular disease develops in these patients. Like their human counterparts, the apo E-deficient mice demonstrate marked hypercholesterolemia with elevated VLDL and chylomicron remnants.[167] They also exhibit spontaneous atherosclerosis even when maintained on a normal chow diet. Adenovirus-mediated gene transfer of the human apo E3 cDNA into hepatocytes of apo E-deficient mice by intravenous injection resulted in the complete correction of the dyslipidemia in these mice and, more important, in markedly reduced atherosclerosis in these animals.[168] These findings suggest that similar gene therapy approaches could be used for the treatment of patients with apo E disorders. However, gene therapy of the apo E disorders in humans awaits the development of a vector system that can program efficient and stable transgene expression in hepatocytes *in vivo*.

## Myocardial Diseases

Heart failure is one of the most common causes of cardiovascular morbidity and mortality, afflicting more than 4 million Americans and representing the leading cause of hospitalization in patients older than 65 years. Although improvements in pharmacologic therapy have both decreased mortality and improved the quality of life for patients with heart failure, it remains a devastating disease with 1-year mortality rates of approximately 10% to 50% for medially treated patients with New York Heart Association (NYHA) classes II to IV CHF.[169] Advances in the ability to program recombinant gene expression in cardiac myocytes *in vivo* have generated enthusiasm for developing novel gene- and cell-based therapies for this disorder. Several different gene therapy approaches might be useful for the treatment of heart failure.

### Gene Therapy to Enhance Myocardial Contractility

Since the 1980s, a great deal has been learned about the molecular pathways that regulate cardiac myocyte contractility. The β-adrenergic receptor (β-AR) system is a powerful regulator of the inotropic state of the normal myocardium and derangements in this system have been demonstrated to contribute in important ways to impaired myocardial function in patients with heart failure. In a set of pioneering studies, Milano et al[170] produced transgenic mice that overexpress the $β_2$-AR under the control of the cardiac α-MHC promoter. These mice, which express 200-fold increased levels of β-AR, displayed significantly increased heart rates and markedly enhanced contractility in the absence of exogenous β-agonists. The findings suggest that overexpression of positive regulators of the β-adrenergic pathway might be an effective method of increasing the myocardial contractility in the failing heart. However, whether such an approach can be used to increase the contractility of failing myocytes remains unclear, as do the long-term effects of β-adrenergic stimulation. This is particularly important because previous clinical trials have demonstrated increased mortality in patients with heart failure treated with positive inotropic drugs.[171]

## Gene Transfer to Program Replication of Cardiac Myocytes or Conversion of Fibroblasts to Myocytes

Cardiac myocytes are terminally differentiated postmitotic cells. The inability of adult cardiac myocytes to proliferate accounts for the failure of myocardial regeneration after myocardial injury. The molecular pathways that regulate cell cycle progression have been identified[172]; thus, in the future it may be possible to introduce genes into cardiac myocytes to regenerate their proliferative capacity, thereby allowing replacement of dead or damaged myocytes. An alternative approach to cardiomyocyte replacement involves transferring appropriate lineage-determining genes into cardiac fibroblasts to convert them into cardiomyocytes. Although to date such cardiomyocyte determining genes have not yet been identified, experiments with skeletal muscle determining genes such as *MyoD* support the validity of this approach. These studies have shown that infection of cardiac fibroblasts *in vivo* with a replication-defective retrovirus encoding the skeletal muscle determining gene *MyoD* can permanently convert these cells into skeletal myocytes that express contractile proteins.[173] Although these approaches are conceptually promising, the feasibility of both requires the identification of the appropriate cell cycle regulatory and lineage determining genes and the development of gene delivery systems that can program stable transgene expression in large numbers of cardiac myocytes and fibroblasts *in vivo*.

## Myocyte Transplantation

Organ transplantation is an effective, albeit costly, therapy for patients with end-stage CHF. However, the limited availability of donor hearts has severely limited the numbers of patients who can be treated by cardiac transplantation. Pioneering work by Soonpaa et al[114] has suggested that cellular transplantation may represent a viable alternative to whole-organ transplantation in these patients. Specifically, they showed that fetal cardiac myocytes and skeletal myoblasts injected directly into the left ventricular myocardium are capable of forming stable intracardiac grafts. The ability to use skeletal myoblasts to repopulate the myocardium would be especially attractive because syngeneic myoblasts could be easily (and repeatedly) isolated from each patient to be treated. Unfortunately, thus far, injected skeletal myoblasts have not been shown to form electrical junctions with endogenous cardiomyocytes; therefore it is less likely that they could be entrained to contract synchronously with the myocardium.[114] In contrast, engrafted fetal cardiac myocytes were shown to form intercalated disks with the endogenous cardiomyocytes.[174] However, from a practical standpoint, there is currently no readily available source of syngeneic fetal cardiac myocytes that could be used to treat large numbers of patients with heart failure. In addition, there is currently no available method that would allow the implantation of large numbers of skeletal or cardiac myocytes throughout the myocardium. Thus, although cellular transplantation is a theoretically attractive therapy for heart failure, a number of hurdles, including a source of cells and the development of a system for delivering these cells diffusely throughout the myocardium, must be overcome before this therapy is feasible for the treatment of heart failure in humans.

## Myocardial Signaling Pathways

A new major area of emphasis is signaling pathways that cause myocyte development, differentiation, and hypertrophy. Major decisions of a cell, whether to divide, differentiate, or die, are influenced by signals from the environment. These signals, received by membrane receptors, culminate in the nucleus with the activation and repression of specific sets of genes. Intracellular calcium is a common currency among many of the signaling pathways that control cell fate. Recent studies have identified calcium-sensing molecules and transcription factors that govern these signaling pathways in myocytes. On the basis of this research, molecular targets are being identified for translational research and development of new gene- and protein-based therapies.

Myocyte enhancer factor-2 (MEF-2) is one transcriptional effector of diverse calcium signaling pathways.[175] MEF-2 binds directly to the promoters or enhancers of most muscle-specific genes and interacts with members of the MyoD family of basic helix-loop-helix (bHLH) proteins to activate the skeletal muscle differentiation program. Loss of function mutations of the murine MEF2C gene have demonstrated an essential role for MEF2 in myogenesis of muscle cells, and MEF2 factors have also been implicated in myocyte hypertrophy and VSMC proliferation and differentiation.[176,177] Calcineurin is a serine/threonine phosphatase that is activated by the binding of calcium and calmodulin, and MEF2 factors are downstream targets of calmodulin and calcineurin signaling. Modulation of calcineurin may prevent cardiac hypertrophy.[178] Furthermore, the histone deacetylases (HDACs) act as transcriptional repressors of MEF2; calcium signaling through the calcium/calmodulin-dependent protein kinase (CaMK) activates MEF2 by disrupting MEF2-HDAC interactions.[179] Hence, modulation of the HDAC proteins may be an another approach to suppress cardiac hypertrophy.

An important calcium signaling pathway in cardiac contractility is calcium release from stores in the sarcoplasmic reticulum (SR) through a calcium release channel, the ryanodine receptor. Cardiac relaxation, in return, is mediated by the reuptake of calcium by the SR calcium pump, $Ca^{2+}$-ATPase, which maintains SR calcium stores for subsequent cardiac contraction. The β-adrenergic pathway controls this system through activated of the cyclic AMP-dependent protein kinase A, which phosphorylates phospholamban, an endogenous inhibitor of the calcium pump. Phosphorylation of phospholamban prevents its inhibitory effect on $Ca^{2+}$-ATPase, leading to augmentation of pump function and cardiac contractility and relaxation. A pivotal role for SR calcium cycling the progression of heart failure has been discovered.[180] Inhibition of phospholamban by gene ablation can completely prevent the onset of heart failure in mice with a cardiomyopathic muscle LIM protein (MLP) mutation.[180] Furthermore, gene transfer of the $Ca^{2+}$-ATPase gene into the myocardium prevents the onset of heart failure in animal models of the disease.[181] Therapeutic strategies to activate calcium cycling without augmenting cAMP may prevent the increases in cardiac cAMP levels that are toxic and lead to myocyte death and arrhythmogenesis.

## Cardiac Arrhythmias

In the United States, more than 400,000 people die from sudden cardiac death and lethal arrhythmias each year. High-risk individuals are difficult to identify, and, aside from implantable defibrillators, therapeutic options are limited. Genetic alterations of various ion channels produce heritable cardiac arrhythmias that predispose affected individuals to sudden death. Investigations of these channelopathies provide the basis for new strategies of treatment, including gene therapy.[182] One example is the Kv channel-interacting protein 2 (KChIP2). A defect in KChIP2 leads to a loss of the transient outward potassium current and susceptibility to ventricular tachycardia.[183] A second approach is to investigate pathways that account for acquired forms of the disease. For example, because the cells of the electrical conduction system arise from cardiac muscle precursors, defects in the pathways that guide the differentiation between ventricular myocyte and Purkinje cell lineages could cause susceptibility to cardiac-associated sudden death. Evidence for this comes from studies of HF-1b, an SP-1 related transcription factor that is preferentially expressed in ventricular and conduction system lineages.[184] These studies have demonstrated that cardiac associated sudden death can occur from defects in the transition between ventricular and conduction system cell lineages.[184] A recent approach is to use gene transfer to target SERCA1 and Kir2.1 that disrupts ventricular excitability without altering cardiac contractility.[185] Modulation of the pathways leading to sudden cardiac death through gene transfer may prove to be a useful therapeutic strategy.

## CONCLUSIONS AND FUTURE DIRECTIONS

Since the 1980s, remarkable progress has been made in the field of somatic gene therapy. The development and improvement of multiple vector systems and the cloning of a wide variety of human disease-related genes have dramatically expanded the numbers of diseases that can be approached through the use of gene transfer technology. The use of transgenic- and gene-targeting approaches has created important new animal models of human diseases that will be invaluable in developing and testing new gene therapy approaches. Such experiments in animals have already provided important proof of principal data concerning the potential efficacy of gene therapy for the treatment of a wide variety of cardiovascular diseases, including angiogenesis, vascular diseases, heart failure, and arrhythmias. Importantly, gene transfer experiments in animals have revealed a great deal about normal biology, including host responses to viral pathogens, the molecular pathways involved in VSMC proliferation, and the roles of multiple proteins in regulating lipid metabolism *in vivo*.

Despite this extraordinary progress, many important hurdles remain before these advances can be translated into highly effective gene therapies for common cardiovascular diseases. There is clearly a need for better vectors that can efficiently program transgene expression in different cardiovascular cell types without evoking host immune responses to either vector-encoded or transgene proteins. As such efficient vectors are developed researchers will need to envision ways to target these vectors to specific cardiovascular cell types *in vivo*. Improved catheters are also needed for delivering these vectors to the myocardium, vasculature, and peripheral organs. Finally, a better understanding of the normal and pathophysiologic pathways that regulate cardiovascular function in health and disease is needed. Such knowledge will be immensely helpful in designing rational gene therapies for cardiovascular diseases. If history is an accurate predicator of future progress, gene therapy should play an increasingly important role in cardiovascular therapeutics in the future.

## REFERENCES

1. Pfeifer A, Verma IM: Gene therapy: Promises and problems. Annu Rev Genomics Hum Genet 2001;2:177–211.
2. Leiden JM: Human gene therapy: The good, the bad, and the ugly. Circ Res 2000;86:923–925.
3. Blaese RM, Culver KW, Miller AD, et al: T lymphocyte-directed gene therapy for ADA-SCID: Initial trial results after 4 years. Science 1995;270:475–480.
4. Nabel GJ, Nabel EG, Yang Z, et al: Direct gene transfer with DNA-liposome complexes in melanoma: Expression, biologic activity, and lack of toxicity in humans. Proc Natl Acad Sci USA 1993;90:11307–11311.
5. Anderson WF: Excitement in gene therapy! Hum Gene Ther 2001;12:1483–484.
6. Ferber D: Gene therapy: Safer and virus-free? Science 2001; 294:1638–1642.
7. Raper SE, Yudkoff M, Chirmule N, et al: A pilot study of in vivo liver-directed gene transfer with an adenoviral vector in partial ornithine transcarbamylase deficiency. Hum Gene Ther 2002;13:163–175.
8. Cavazzana-Calvo M, Hacein-Bey S, de Saint Basile G, et al: Gene therapy of human severe combined immunodeficiency (SCID)-XI disease. Science 2000;288:669–672.
9. Kay MA, Manno CS, Ragni MV, et al: Evidence for gene transfer and expression of factor IX in haemophilia B patients treated with an AAV vector. Nat Genet 2000;24:257–261.
10. Leiden JM: Gene therapy: Promise, pitfalls, and prognosis. N Engl J Med 1995;333:871–873.
11. Galimi F, Verma IM: Opportunities for the use of lentiviral vectors in human gene therapy. Curr Top Microbiol Immunol 2002; 261:245–254.
12. Mizuguchi H, Kay MA, Hayakawa T: Approaches for generating recombinant adenovirus vectors. Adv Drug Deliv Rev 2001; 52:165–176.

13. Kay MA, Gloriosc JC, Naldini L: Viral vectors for gene therapy: The art of turning infectious agents into vehicles of therapeutics. Nat Med 2001;7:33-740.
14. Baumgartner I, Isner JM: Somatic gene therapy in the cardiovascular system. Annu Rev Physiol 2001;63:427-450.
15. Duckers HJ, Nabel EG: Prospects for genetic therapy of cardiovascular disease. Med Clin North Am 2000;84:199-213.
16. Yla-Herttuala S, Martin JF: Cardiovascular gene therapy. Lancet 2000;355:213-222.
17. Pislaru S, Janssesn SP, Gersh BJ, et al: Defining gene transfer before expecting gene therapy. Circulation 2002;106:631-636.
18. Miller A: Retroviral vectors. Curr Top Microbiol Immunol 1992;158:1-24.
19. Boris L, Temin H: Recent advances in retrovirus vector technology. Curr Opin Genet Dev 1993;3:102-109.
20. Kotani H, Newton PB III, Zhang S, et al: Improved methods of retroviral vector transduction and production for gene therapy. Hum Gene Ther 1994;5:19-28.
21. Friedmann T: A brief history of gene therapy. Nat Genet 1992;2:93-98.
22. Miller D, Adam M, Miller A: Gene transfer by retrovirus vectors occurs only in cells that are actively replicating at the time of infection. Mol Cell Biol 1990;10:4239-4242.
23. Roe T, Reynolds T, Uy G, Brown P: Integration of murine leukemia virus DNA depends on mitosis. EMBO J 1993;12:2099-2108.
24. Otto E. Jones-Trower A, Vanin EF, et al: Characterization of a replication-competent retrovirus resulting from recombination of packaging and vector sequences. Hum Gene Ther 1994;5:567-575.
25. Vanin EF, Kaloss M, Broscius C, Nienhuis AW: Characterization of replication-competent retroviruses from nonhuman primates with virus-induced T-cell lymphomas and observations regarding the mechanism of oncogenesis. J Virol 1994;68:4241-4250.
26. Naldini L, Blomer U, Gallay P, et al: In vivo gene delivery and stable transduction of nondividing cells by lentiviral vector. Science 1996;272:263-267.
27. Burns J, Friedmann T, Driever W, et al: Vesicular stomatitis virus G glycoprotein pseudotyped retroviral vectors: Concentration to very high titer and efficient gene transfer into mammalian and nonmammalian cells. Proc Natl Acad Sci USA 1994;90:8033-8037.
28. Kashara N, Dozy AM, Kan YW: Tissue-specific targeting of retroviral vectors through ligand-receptor interactions. Science 1994;266:1373-1376.
29. Buchschachter GL, Wong Staal F: Development of lentiviral vectors for gene therapy for human diseases. Blood 2000;95:2499-2504.
30. Amado RG, Chen ISY: Lentiviral vectors: The promise of gene therapy within reach? Science 1999;285:674-676.
31. Yang X, Atalar E, Li D, et al: Magnetic resonance imaging permits in vivo monitoring of catheter-based vascular gene delivery. Circulation 2001;104:1588-1590.
32. Horwitz M: The adenoviruses. In Fields B, Knipe D (eds): Virology. New York, Raven Press, 1990, pp 1723-1742.
33. Bergner KL: Development of adenovirus vectors for the expression of heterologous genes. Biotechniques 1989;6:616-629.
34. Berkner K: Expression of heterologous sequences in adenoviral vectors. Curr Top Microbiol Immunol 1992;158:39-66.
35. Wilson JM: Adenoviruses as gene-delivery vehicles. N Engl J Med 1996;334:1185-1187.
36. Kass-Eisler A, Falck-Pedersen E, Alvira M, et al: Quantitative determination of adenovirus-mediated gene delivery to rat cardiac myocytes in vitro and in vivo. Proc Natl Acad Sci USA 1993;90:11498-11502.
37. Guzman RJ, Lemarchand P, Crystal RG, et al: Efficient gene transfer in myocardium by direct injection of adenovirus vectors. Circ Res 1993;88:1202-1207.
38. Barr E, Carroll J, Kalynych A, et al: Efficient catheter-mediated gene transfer into the heart using replication-defective adenovirus. Gene Ther 1994;1:51-58.
39. Guzman R, Lemarchand P, Crystal R, et al: Efficient and selective adenovirus-mediated gene transfer into vascular neointima. Circulation 1993;88:2838-2848.
40. Lee S, Trapnell B, Rade J, et al: In vivo adenoviral vector-mediated gene transfer into balloon-injured rat carotid arteries. Circ Res 1993;73:797-807.
41. Lemarchand P, Jones M, Yamada I, Crystal R: In vivo gene transfer and expression in normal uninjured blood vessels using replication-deficient recombinant adenovirus vectors. Circ Res 1993;72:1132-1138.
42. Herz J, Gerard RD: Adenovirus-mediated transfer of low density lipoprotein receptor gene acutely accelerates cholesterol clearance in normal mice. Proc Natl Acad Sci USA 1993;90:2812-2816.
43. Jaffe HA, Danel C, Longenecker G, et al: Adenovirus-mediated in vivo gene transfer and expression in normal rat liver. Nat Genet 1992;1:372-378.
44. Stratford-Perricaudet LD, Makeh I, Perricaudet M, Briand P: Widespread long-term gene transfer to mouse skeletal muscles and heart. J Clin Invest 1992;90:626-630.
45. Quantin B, Perricaudet LD, Tajbakhsh S, Mandel JL: Adenovirus as an expression vector in muscle cells in vivo. Proc Natl Acad Sci USA 1992;89:2581-2584.
46. Ragot T, Vincent N, Chafey P, et al: Efficient adenovirus-mediated transfer of a human minidystrophin gene to skeletal muscle of mdx mice. Nature 1993;361:647-650.
47. Tripathy S, Goldwasser E, Barr E, Leiden J: Stable delivery of physiologic levels of recombinant erythropoietin to the systemic circulation by intramuscular injection of replication-defective adenovirus. Proc Natl Acad Sci USA 1994;91:11557-11561.
48. Gurwith MJ, Horwith GS, Impellizzeri CA, et al: Current use and future directions of adenovirus vaccine. Semin Respir Infect 1989;4:299-303.
49. Haj-Ahmad Y, Graham FL: Development of a helper-independent human adenovirus vector and its use in the transfer of the herpes simplex virus thymidine kinase gene. J Virol 1986;57:267-274.
50. Karlsson S, Doren KV, Schweiger SG, et al: Stable gene transfer and tissue specific expression of a human globin gene using adenoviral vectors. EMBO J 1986;5:2377-2385.
51. Graham FL, Smiley J, Russel WC, Nairn R: Characteristics of a human cell line transformed by DNA from human adenovirus type 5. J Gen Virol 1977;36:59-72.
52. Fallaux FJ, Kranenburg O, Cramer SJ, et al: Characterization of 911: A new helper cell line for the titration and propagation of early region 1-deleted adenoviral vectors. Hum Gene Ther 1996;7:215-222.
53. Dai Y: Cellular and humoral immune responses to adenoviral vectors containing factor IX gene: Tolerization of factor IX and vector antigens allows for long-term expression. Proc Natl Acad Sci USA 1995;92:1401-1405.
54. Smith TAG: Adenovirus mediated expression of therapeutic plasma levels of human factor IX in mice. Nat Genet 1993;5:397-402.
55. Rosenfeld MA: In vivo transfer of the human cystic fibrosis transmembrane conductance regulator gene to the airway epithelium. Cell 1992;68:143-155.
56. Yang Y, Ertl J, Wilson JM: MHC class 1-restricted cytoxic T lymphocytes to viral antigens destroy hepatocytes in mice infected with E1-deleted recombinant adenoviruses. Immunity 1994;1:433-442.
57. Yang Y, Li Q, Ertl HC, Wilson JM: Cellular immunity to viral antigens limits E1-deleted adenoviruses for gene therapy. Proc Natl Acad Sci USA 1994;91:4407-4411.
58. Tripathy SK, Black HB, Goldwasser E, Leiden JM: Immune responses to transgene-encoded proteins limit the stability of gene expression after injection of replication-defective adenovirus vectors. Nat Med 1996;2:545-550.
59. Yang Y, Li Q, Ertl HC, Wilson JM: Cellular and humoral immune response to viral antigens create barriers to lung-directed gene therapy with recombinant adenoviruses. J Virol 1995;69:2004-2015.
60. Yang Y, Nunes FA, Berencsi K, et al: Inactivation of E2a in recombinant adenoviruses improves the prospect for gene therapy for cystic fibrosis. Nat Genet 1994;7:362-369.
61. Svensson EC, Black HB, Dugger DL, et al: Long term erythropoietin expression in rodents and non-human primates following intramuscular injection of a replication-defective adenoviral vector. Hum Gen Ther 1997;8:1797-1806.

62. Yeh P, Dedieu JF, Orsini C, et al: Efficient dual transcomplementation of adenovirus E1 and E4 regions from a 293-derived cell line expressing a minimal E4 functional unit. J Virol 1996;70: 559–565.

63. Wang Q, Finer MH: Second-generation adenovirus vectors. Nat Med 1996;2:714–716.

64. Kochanek S, Clemens PR, Mitani K, et al: A new adenoviral vector: Replacement of all viral coding sequences with 28 kb of DNA independently expressing both full-length dystrophin and beta-galactosidase. Pro Natl Acad Sci USA 1996;93:5731–5736.

65. DeMatteo RP, Markmann JF, Kozarsky KF, et al: Prolongation of adenoviral transgene expression in mouse liver by T lymphocyte subset depletion. Gene Ther 1996;11:191–196.

66. Yang Y, Su Q, Grewal IS, et al: Transient subversion of CD40 ligand function diminishes immune responses to adenovirus vectors in mouse liver and lung tissues. J Virol 1996;70:6370–6377.

67. Kay M: Long-term hepatic adenovirus-mediated gene expression in mice following CTLA4lg administration. Nat Genet 1995;11:191–196.

68. Kremer EJ, Perricaudet M: Adenovirus and adeno-associated virus mediated gene transfer. [Review.] Br Med Bull 1995;51:31–44.

69. Berns K: Parvovirus replication. Microbiol Rev 1990;50:316–329.

70. Nahreini P, Larsen P, Srivastava A: Cloning and integration of DNA fragments in human cells via the inverted terminal repeats of the adeno-associated virus 2 genome. Gene 1992;119:265–272.

71. Kotin R, Linden R, Berns K: Characterization of a preferred site on human chromosome 19q for integration of adeno-associated virus DNA by nonhomologous recombination. EMBO J 1992;11: 5071–5078.

72. Rolling F, Samulski RJ: AAV as a viral vector for human gene therapy. Generation of recombinant virus. Mol Biotechnol 1995;3:9–15.

73. Kaplitt MB, Leone P, Samulski RJ, et al: Long-term gene expression and phenotypic correction using adeno-associated virus vectors in the mammalian brain. Nat Genet 1994;8:148–154.

74. Kessler PD, Podsakoff GM, Chen X, et al: Gene delivery to skeletal muscle results in sustained expression and systemic delivery of a therapeutic protein. Proc Natl Acad Sci USA 1996;93: 14082–14087.

75. Lynch CM, Hara PS, Leonard JC, et al: Adeno-associated virus vectors for vascular gene delivery. Circ Res 1997;80:497–505.

76. Barinaga M: Ribozymes: Killing the messenger by destroying RNA that carries the message of the disease: Ribozymes, RNA molecules that act as enzymes, are on the verge of leaving the lab for the clinic. Science 1993;262:1512–1514.

77. Cech TR: Ribozymes and their medical implications. JAMA 1998;260:3030–3034.

78. Castanotto D, Rossi JJ, Sarver N: Antisense catalytic RNAs as therapeutic agents. Adv Pharmacol 1994;25:289–317.

79. Wolff J, Malone R, Williams P, et al: Direct gene transfer into mouse muscle in vivo. Science 1990;247:1465–1468.

80. Lin H, Pramacek MS, Morle G: Expression of recombinant genes in myocardium in vivo after direct injection of DNA. Circulation 1990;82:2217–2221.

81. Acsadi G, Jiao S, Jani A: Direct gene transfer and expression into rat heart in vivo. New Biol 1990;3:71–81.

82. Kitsis R, Buttrick P, McNally E: Hormonal modulation of a gene injected into rat heart in vivo. Proc Natl Acad Sci USA 1991;88:4138–4142.

83. Harsford RV, Schott R, Shen Y, et al: Gene injection into canine myocardium as a useful model for studying gene expression in the heart of large mammals. Circ Res 1993;2:688–695.

84. Parmacek MS, Vora AJ, Shen T: Identification and characterization of a cardiac-specific transcriptional regulatory element in the slow/cardiac troponin C gene. Mol Cell Biol 1992;12: 1967–1976.

85. Riessen R, Rahimizadeh H, Blessing E, et al: Arterial gene transfer using pure DNA applied directly to a hydrogel-coated angioplasty balloon. Hum Gene Ther 1993;4:749–758.

86. Tripathy SK, Svensson EC, Black HB, et al: Long-term expression of erythropoietin in the systemic circulation of mice after intramuscular injection of plasmid DNA vector. Proc Natl Acad Sci USA 1996;93:10876–10880.

87. Stein CA, Cheng YC: Antisense oligonucleotides as therapeutic agents: Is the bullet really magical? Science 1993;262:1004–1012.

88. Morishita R, Higaki J, Aoki M, et al: Novel strategy of gene therapy in cardiovascular disease with HVJ-liposome method. Contrib Nephrol 1996;118:254–264.

89. Bielinska A, Shivdasani RA, Zhang LQ, Nabel GJ: Regulation of gene expression with double-stranded phosphorothioate oligonucleotides. Science 1990;250:997–1000.

90. Bennett M, Anglin S, McEwan J, et al: Inhibition of vascular smooth muscle cell proliferation in vitro and in vivo by c-myc antisense oligonucleotides. J Clin Invest 1994;93:820–828.

91. Shi Y, Fard A, Galeo A, et al: Transcatheter delivery of c-myb antisense oligomers reduces neointimal formation in a porcine model of coronary artery balloon injury. Circulation 1994;90: 944–951.

92. Simons M, Edleman ER, DeKeyser JL, et al: Anti-sense c-myb oligonucleotides inhibit intimal arterial smooth muscle cell accumulation in vivo. Nature 1992;359:67–70.

93. Morishita R, Gibbons G, Ellison K, et al: Single intraluminal delivery of antisense cdc2 kinase and proliferating-cell nuclear antigen oligonucleotides results in chronic inhibition of neointimal hyperplasia. Proc Natl Acad Sci USA 1993;90:8474–8478.

94. Simons M, Edelman E, Rosenberg R: Antisense proliferating cell nuclear antigen oligodeoxynucleotide targeting the messenger RNA encoding proliferating cell nuclear antigen. Circulation 1992;86:538–547.

95. Morishita R, Gibbons GH, Horiuchi M, et al: Intimal hyperplasia after vascular injury is inhibited by antisense cdk 2 kinase oligonucleotides. J Clin Invest 1994;1458:1464–1469.

96. Morishita R, Gibbons GH, Horiuchi M, et al: A gene therapy strategy using a transcription factor decoy of the E2F binding site inhibits smooth muscle proliferation in vivo. Proc Natl Acad Sci USA 1995;92:5855–5859.

97. Krieg AM, Yi Ak, Matson S, et al: CpG motifs in bacterial DNA trigger direct B-cell activation. Nature 1995;374:546–549.

98. Felgner P, Gadek T, Holm M, et al: Lipofection: A highly efficient, lipid-mediated DNA transfection procedure. Proc Natl Acad Sci USA 1987;84:7413–7417.

99. Lasic DD, Papahadjopoulos D: Liposomes revisited. Sciences 1995;267:1275–1276.

100. San H, Yang Z, Pompili V, et al: Safety and short-term toxicity of a novel cationic lipid formulation for human gene therapy. Hum Gene Ther 1993;4:781–788.

101. Nabel E, Plautz G, Nabel G: Site-specific gene expression in vivo by direct gene transfer into the arterial wall. Science 1990;249:1285–1288.

102. Nabel E, Plautz G, Nabel G: Transduction of a foreign histocompatibility gene into the arterial wall induces vasculitis. Proc Natl Acad Sci USA 1992;89:5157–5161.

103. Leclerc G, Gal D, Takeshita S, et al: Percutaneous arterial gene transfer in a rabbit model: Efficiency in normal and balloon-dilated atherosclerotic arteries. J Clin Invest 1992;90:936–944.

104. Chapman G, Lim C, Gammon R, et al: Gene transfer into coronary arteries of intact animals with a percutaneous balloon catheter. Circ Res 1992;71:27–33.

105. Nabel E, Yang Z, Liptay S, et al: Recombinant fibroblast growth factor B gene expression in porcine arteries induces intimal hyperplasia in vivo. J Clin Invest 1993;91:1822–1829.

106. Nabel EG, Yang ZY, Plautz G, et al: Recombinant fibroblast growth factor-1 promotes intimal hyperplasia and angiogenesis in arteries in vivo. Nature 1993;362:844–846.

107. Rando TA, Balu HM: Primary mouse myoblast purification, characterization, and transplantation for cell-mediated gene therapy. J Cell Biol 1994;125:1275–1287.

108. Barr E, Leiden JM: Systemic delivery of recombinant proteins by genetically modified myoblasts. Science 1991;245: 1507–1509.

109. Dhawan J, Pabn L, Pavlath G, et al: Systemic delivery of human growth hormone by injection of genetically engineered myoblasts. Science 1991;254:1509–1512.

110. Osborne WR, Ramesh N, Lau S, et al: Gene therapy for long-term expression of erythropoietin in rats. Proc Natl Acad Sci USA 1995;92:8055–8058.

111. Dai Y, Roman M, Naviaux RK, Verma IM: Gene therapy via primary myoblasts: Long-term expression of factor IX protein following transplantation in vivo. Proc Natl Acad Sci USA 1992;89: 10892–10895.

112. Yao S, Kurachi K: Expression of human factor IX in mice after injection of genetically modified myoblasts. Proc Natl Acad Sci USA 1992;89:3357–3361.

113. Mendell JR: Myoblast transfer in the treatment of Duchenne's muscular dystrophy. N Engl J Med 1995;333:832–838.

114. Soonpaa MH, Koh GY, Klulg MG, et al: Formation of nascent intercalated disks between grafted fetal cardiomyocytes and host myocardium. Science 1994;264:98–101.

115. Koh GY, Kim S-J, Klug MG, et al: Targeted expression of transforming growth factor-B1 in intracardiac grafts promotes vascular endothelial cell DNA Synthesis. J Clin Invest 1995;95:114–121.

116. Nabel EG, Plautz FM, Stanley JC, et al: Recombinant gene expression in vivo within endothelial cells. Science 1989;244:1344–1346.

117. Nabel EG: Stem cells combined with gene transfer for therapeutic vasculogenesis. Circulation 2002;105:672–674.

118. Ross R: The pathogenesis of atherosclerosis: A perspective for the 1990s. Nature 1993;362:801–809.

119. Ohno T, Gordon D, San H, et al: Gene therapy for vascular smooth muscle cell proliferation after arterial injury. Science 1994;265:781–784.

120. Chang MW, Barr E, Seltzer J, et al: Cytostatic gene therapy for vascular proliferative disorders using a constitutively active form of retinoblastoma gene product. Science 1994;267:518–522.

121. Chowdhury J, Grossman M, Gupta S, et al: Long-term improvement of hypercholesterolemia after ex vivo gene therapy in LDL$_R$-deficient rabbits. Science 1991;254:1802–1805.

122. Grossman M, Raper SE, Kozarsky K, et al: Successful ex vivo gene therapy directed to liver in patients with familial hypercholesterolemia. Nat Genet 1994;6:335–341.

123. Vareene O, Pislaru S, Gillijns H, et al: Local adenovirus-mediated transfer of human endothelial nitric oxide synthase reduces luminal narrowing after coronary angioplasty in pigs. Circulation 1998;98:919–926.

124. von der Leyen HE, Gibbons GH, Morishita R, et al: Gene therapy inhibiting neointimal vascular lesion: In vivo transfer of endothelial cell nitric oxide synthase gene. Proc Natl Acad Sci USA 1995;92:1137–1141.

125. Bao J, Naimark W, Palasis M, et al: Intramyocardial delivery of FGF2 in combination with radio frequency transmyocardial revascularization. Catheter Cardiovasc Interv 2001;53:429–434.

126. Sousa JE, Costa MA, Abizaid AC, et al: Sustained suppression of neointimal proliferation by sirolimus-eluting stents: One-year angiographic and intravascular ultrasound follow-up. Circulation 2001;104:1996–1998.

127. Helman AW, Cheng L, Jenkins GM, et al: Paclitaxel stent coating inhibits neointimal hyperplasia at 4 weeks in a porcine model of coronary restenosis. Circulation 2002;103:2289–2295.

128. Folkman J: Tumor angiogenesis: Therapeutic implications. N Engl J Med 1971;285:1182–1186.

129. Carmeliet P, Jain RK: Angiogenesis in cancer and other diseases. Nature 2000;407:249–257.

130. Pu LQ, Sniderman AD, Brassard R, et al: Enhanced revascularization of the ischemic limb by means of angiogenic therapy. Circulation 1993;88:208–215.

131. Harada K, Grossman W, Friedman M, et al: Basic fibroblast growth factor improves myocardial function in chronically ischemic porcine hearts. J Clin Invest 1994;94:623–630.

132. Takeshita S, Weir L, Chen D, et al: Therapeutic angiogenesis following arterial gene transfer of vascular endothelial growth factor in a rabbit model of hindlimb ischemia. Biochem Biophys Res Commun 1996;227:628–635.

133. Isner JM, Pieczek A, Schainfeld R, et al: Clinical evidence of angiogenesis following arterial gene transfer of phVEGF$_{165}$. Lancet 1996;248:370–374.

134. Baumgartner I, Pieczek A, Manor O, et al: Constitutive expression of phVEGF165 following intramuscular gene transfer promotes collateral vessel development in patients with critical limb ischemia. Circulation 1998;97:1114–1123.

135. Baumgartner I, Rauh G, Pieczek A, el al: Lower-extremity edema associated with gene transfer of naked DNA vascular endothelial growth factor. Ann Int Med 2000;132:880–884.

136. Rajagopalan S, Shah M, Luciano A, et al: Adenovirus-mediated gene transfer of VEGF(121) improves lower-extremity endothelial function and flow reserve. Circulation 2001;104:753–755.

137. Giordano FJ, Ping P, McKirnan MD, et al: Intracoronary gene transfer of fibroblast growth factor-5 increases blood flow and contractile function in an ischemic region of the heart. Nat Med 1996;2:534–539.

138. Rosengart TK, Lee LY, Patel SR, et al: Six-month assessment of a phase I trial of angiogenic gene therapy for the treatment of coronary artery disease using direct intramyocardial administration of an adenovirus vector expressing the VEGF$_{121}$ cDNA. Ann Surg 1999;230:466–472.

139. Vale PR, Losordo DW, Milliken CE, et al: Randomized, single-blind, placebo-controlled pilot study of catheter-based myocardial gene transfer for therapeutic angiogenesis utilizing LV electromechanical mapping in patients with chronic myocardial ischemia. Circulation 2001;103:2138–2143.

140. Losorodo DW, Vale PR, Symes J, et al: Gene therapy for myocardial angiogenesis: Initial clinical results with direct myocardial injection of phVEGF$_{165}$ as sole therapy for myocardial ischemia. Circulation 1998;98:2800–2804.

141. Vale PR, Losordo DW, Milliken CE, et al: Randomized, single-blind, placebo-controlled pilot study of catheter-based myocardial gene transfer for therapeutic angiogenesis using left ventricular electromechanical mapping in patients with chronic myocardial ischemia. Circulation 2001;103:2138–2143.

142. Sherr CJ, Roberts JM: Inhibitors of mammalian G1 cyclin-dependent kinases. Genes Dev 1995;9:1149–1163.

143. Tanner FC, Yang Z-Y, Duckers E, et al: Expression of cyclin-dependent kinase inhibitors in vascular disease. Circ Res 1998;82:396–403.

144. Chang MW, Barr E, Lu M, et al: Adenovirus-mediated overexpression of the cyclin/cyclin-dependent kinase inhibitor p21 inhibits vascular smooth muscle cell proliferation and neointima formation in the rat carotid artery model of balloon angioplasty. J Clin Invest 1995;96:2260–2268.

145. Yang Z, Simari R, Perkins N, et al: Role of the p21 cyclin-dependent kinase inhibitor in limiting intimal cell proliferation in response to arterial injury. Proc Natl Acad Sci USA 1996;93:1905–1910.

146. Tanner FC, Akyurek L, San H, et al: Differential effects of cyclin-dependent kinase inhibitors on vascular smooth muscle cell proliferation. Circulation 2000;101:2022–2025.

147. Chang MW, Ohno T, Gordon D, et al: Adenovirus-mediated transfer of the herpes simplex virus thymidine kinase gene inhibits vascular smooth muscle cell proliferation and neointima formation following balloon angioplasty. Mol Med 1995;1:172–181.

148. Simari R, San H, Rekhter M, et al: Regulation of cellular proliferation and intimal formation following balloon injury in atherosclerotic rabbit arteries. J Clin Invest 1996;98:225–235.

149. Mann MJ, Gibbons GH, Kernoff RS, et al: Genetic engineering of vein grafts resistant to atherosclerosis. Proc Natl Acad Sci USA 1995;92:4502–4506.

150. Mann MJ, Whittemore AD, Donaldson MC, et al: Ex-vivo gene therapy of human vascular bypass grafts with E2F decoys: The PREVENT single-centre, randomized, controlled trial. Lancet 1999;354:1493–1498.

151. Duckers HJ, Boehm M, True A, et al: Heme oxygenase-1 protects against vascular constriction and proliferation. Nat Med 2001;7:693–698.

152. True AL, San H, Kesselheim J, et al: Deletion of heme oxygenase-1 accelerates arterial thrombus formation. Arter Thromb Vas Biol 2001;21:704.

153. Kelly RA, Ballignard JL, Smith TW: Nitric oxide and cardiac function. Circ Res 1996;79:363–380.

154. Jia L, Bonaventura C, Bonaventura J: A dynamic activity of blood involved in vascular control. Nature 1996;380:221–226.

155. Morishita R, Gibbons GH, Ellison KE, et al: Evidence for direct local effect of angiotensin in vascular hypertrophy: In vivo gene transfer of angiotensin converting enzyme. J Clin Invest 1994;94:978–984.

156. Schott E, Tostes RCA, San H, et al: Expression of a recombinant pre-proendpthelin-1 gene in arteries stimulates vascular contractility by increased sensitivity to angiotensin 1. Am J Physiol 1997;272:H2385–2393.

157. Suh TT, Holback K, Jensen NJ, et al: Resolution of spontaneous bleeding events but failure of pregnancy in fibrinogen-deficient mice. Genes Dev 1995;9:2020–2023.

158. Polplis VA, Carmeliet P, Vazirzadeh S, et al: Effects of disruption of the plasminogen gene on thrombosis, growth, and health in mice. Circulation 1992;92:2585–2593.

159. Carmeliet P, Stassen JM, Schoonjans L, et al: Plasminogen activator inhibito-1 gene deficient mice. I. Generation by homologous recombination and characterization. J Clin Invest 1993;92:2746–2755.

160. Carmeliet P, Schoonjans L, Kieckens L, et al: Physiological consequences of loss of plasminogen activator gene function in mice. Nature 1994;368:419–424.

161. Cui J, O'Shea S, Purkayastha A, et al: Fatal haemmorrhage and incomplete block to embryogenesis in mice lacking coagulation factor V. Nature 1996;384:66–68.

162. Carmeliet P, Mackman N, Moons L, et al: Role of tissue factor in embryonic blood vessels development. Nature 1996;383:73–75.

163. Connolly AJ, Ishihara H, Kahn ML, et al: Role of the thrombin receptor in development and evidence for a second receptor. Nature 1996;381:516–519.

164. Healy AM, Rayburn HB, Rosenberg RD, Weiler H: Absence of the blood-clotting regulator thrombomodulin causes embryonic lethality in mice before development of a functional cardiovascular system. Proc Natl Acad Sci USA 1995;92:850–854.

165. Carmeliet P, Moons L, Lignen R, et al: Inhibitory role of plasminogen activator inhibitor-1 in arterial wound healing and neointima formation: A gene targeting and gene transfer study in mice. Circulation 1997;96:3180–3191.

166. Mahley RW: Apolipoprotein E: Cholesterol transport protein with expanding role in cell biology. Science 1988;240:622–630.

167. Plump AS, Smith JD, Aalto-Setala TH, et al: Severe hypercholesterolemia and atherosclerosis in apolipoprotein E-deficient mice created by homologous recombinants in ES cells. Cell 1992;1992:343–353.

168. Kashyap VS, Santamarina-Fojo S, Brown DR, et al: Apolipoprotein E deficiency in mice: Gene replacement and prevention of atherosclerosis using adenovirus vectors. J Clin Invest 1995;96:1612–1620.

169. Pfeffer M, Braunwald E, Moye LA, et al: Effect of captopril on mortality and morbidity in patients with left ventricular dysfunction after myocardial infarction: Results of the survival and ventricular enlargement trial. N Engl J Med 1992;327:669–677.

170. Milano CA, Allen LF, Rockman HA, et al: Enhanced myocardial function in transgenic mice overexpressing beta 2-adrenergic receptor. Science 1994;264:582–586.

171. Packer M, Carver JR, Rodeheffer RJ, Group PSR: Effect of oral milrinone on mortality in severe chronic heart failure. N Engl J Med 1991;325:1468–1475.

172. Sherr CJ, Roberts JM: CDK inhibitors: Positive and negative regulators of G1-phase progression. Genes Dev 1999;13:1501–1512.

173. Black BL, Olson EN: Transcriptional control of muscle development by myocyte enhancer factor-2 (MEF2) proteins. Annu Rev Cell Dev Biol 1998;14:167–196.

174. McKinsey TA, Zhang CL, Olson EN, et al: MEF2: A calcium-dependent regulator of cell division, differentiation and death. Trends Biochem Sci 2002;27:40–47.

175. Passier R, Zeng H, Frey N, et al: CaM kinase signaling induces cardiac hypertrophy and activates the MEF2 transcription factor in vivo. J Clin Invest 2000;105:1395–1406.

176. Kolodziejczyk SM, Wang L, Balazsi K, et al: MEF2 is upregulated during cardiac hypertrophy and its required for normal post-natal growth of the myocardium. Curr Biol 1999;9:1203–1206.

177. Lin Q, Lu J, Yanagisawa H, et al: Requirement of the MADS-box transcription factor MEF2C for vascular development. Development 1998;125:4565–4574.

178. Semsarian C, Giewat M, Georgakopoulos D, et al: The L-type calcium-channel inhibitor diltiazem prevents cardiomyopathy in a mouse model. J Clin Invest 2002;109:1013–1020.

179. Lu J, McKinsey TA, Nicol RL, et al: Signal-dependent activation of the MEF2 transcription factor by dissociation from histone deacetylases. Proc Natl Acad Sci USA 2000;97:4070–4075.

180. Minamisawa S, Hoshijima M, Chu GM, et al: Chronic phospholamban-sarcoplasmic reticulum calcium ATPase interaction is the critical calcium cycling defect in dilated cardiomyopathy. Cell 1999;99:313–322.

181. Miyamoto MI, del Monte F, Schmidt U, et al: Adenoviral gene transfer of SERCA2a improves left ventricular function in aortic-banded rats in transition to heart failure. Proc Natl Acad Sci USA 2000;97:793–798.

182. Marban E: Cardiac channelopathies. Nature 2002;415:213–218.

183. Kuo HC, Cheng CF, Clark RB, et al: A defect in the Kv channel-interacting protein 2 (KchIP2) gene leads to a complete loss of Ito and confers susceptibility to ventricular tachycardia. Cell 2001;107:801–813.

184. Nyuyen-Tran VT, Kubalak SW, Minamisawa S, et al: A novel genetic pathway for cardiac sudden death via defects in the transition between ventricular and conduction system cell lineages. Cell 2000;102:671–682.

185. Ennis IL, Li RA, Murphy AM, et al: Dual gene therapy with SERCA1 and Kir2.1 abbreviates excitation without suppressing contractility. J Clin Invest 2002;109:393–400.

## EDITOR'S CHOICE

Fraites TJ, Jr., Schleissing MR, Shanely RA, et al: Correction of the enzymatic and functional deficits in a model of Pompe disease using adeno-associated virus vectors. Mol Ther 2002;5:571–578.
*AAV shows efficacy for long-term gene replacement in a mouse model of Pompe's disease, human studies on the horizon.*

Hacein-Bey-Abina S, von Kalle C, Schmidt M, et al: A serious adverse event after successful gene therapy for X-linked severe combined immunodeficiency. N Engl J Med 2003;348:255–256.
*Follow-up studies of patients receiving retroviral gene therapy indicate an incidence of tumors, which may reflect insertion of the viral vector into a critical gene; clinical studies continued but additional caution and monitoring are required.*

Hood JD, Bednarski M, Frausto R, et al: Tumor regression by targeted gene delivery to the neovasculature. Science 2002;296:2404–2407.
*Novel approach to deliver genes to targeted cell types via a nonviral delivery system that uses an integrin receptor based mechanism.*

Hoshijima M, Ikeda Y, Iwanaga Y, et al: Chronic suppression of heart-failure progression by a pseudophosphorylated mutant of phospholamban via in vivo cardiac rAAV gene delivery. Nat Med 2002;8:864–871.
*Toward heart gene therapy for end-stage heart failure with AAV-based systems to promote calcium cycling via the inhibition of phospholamban, the endogenous muscle specific SERCA inhibitory peptide.*

Kaspar BK, Vissel B, Bengoechea T, et al: Adeno-associated virus effectively mediates conditional gene modification in the brain. Proc Natl Acad Sci USA 2002;99:2320–2325.
*AAV may prove useful for the activation of conditional mutations in the brain and elsewhere via the in vivo delivery of cre recombinase.*

Kootstra NA, Verma IM: Gene therapy with viral vectors. Annu Rev Pharmacol Toxicol 2003;43:413–439.
*Leader in the field outlines the progress to date and the problems ahead with viral vectors for gene therapy; refreshing intellectual honesty of a very challenging but important problem.*

Nakai H, Montini E, Fuess S, et al: AAV serotype 2 vectors preferentially integrate into active genes in mice. Nat Genet 2003;34:297–302.
*AAV vectors integrate into the host genome, but not with the same frequency as retroviral vectors.*

Song S, Morgan M, Ellis T, et al: Sustained secretion of human alpha-1-antitrypsin from murine muscle transduced with adeno-associated virus vectors. Proc Natl Acad Sci USA 1998;95:14384–14388.
*Human AAV-mediated gene therapy for alpha-1 antitrypsin deficiency is on the horizon.*

Tiscornia G, Singer O, Ikawa M, Verma IM: A general method for gene knockdown in mice by using lentiviral vectors expressing small interfering RNA. Proc Natl Acad Sci USA 2003;100:1844–1848.
*Lentiviruses become powerful tools for expressing RNAi that will allow the knockdown of specific genes in living cells in the mouse; could become alternative to knockouts with further technologic improvements.*

■ ■ ■ chapter **1 0**

# Cardiac Development and Congenital Heart Disease

*Deepak Srivastava*
*Eric N. Olson*

Although impressive advances have been made in the diagnosis and treatment of congenital heart disease (CHD), it remains the leading noninfectious cause of death in infants. CHD occurs in nearly 1% of live births and is estimated to be the cause of 10% of spontaneous abortions.[1] Surgical palliation for many congenital heart defects has resulted in an increasing population of adults surviving with complex CHD and has spawned a new subspecialty within adult cardiology. In addition, some forms of adult-onset heart disease have their origin in cardiac developmental defects. The most notable of these is aortic valve stenosis, which is most commonly associated with a congenitally bicuspid aortic valve, present in 1% of the general population.

Although the cause of CHD remains poorly understood, it is clear that the complex process of heart development involves a combination of hemodynamic forces and morphogenetic events that are exquisitely sensitive to mild perturbations. Infants born with CHD typically have isolated cardiovascular defects affecting only one chamber, septum, or valve of the heart. These findings suggest that relatively independent molecular developmental programs might exist for each specific region of the heart. In recent years, the study of numerous genes involved in cardiogenesis (using human and animal models) has provided insight into the genetic pathogenesis of CHD. Here, we review aspects of cardiac morphogenesis that are relevant to CHD, describe animal model systems used to study heart development, and provide examples of genes that have regionally restricted effects on the cardiovascular system.

## MORPHOGENESIS OF THE CARDIOVASCULAR SYSTEM

A functioning cardiovascular system is essential by the middle of the third week of gestation to satisfy the nutritional requirements of the developing human embryo. Beginning soon after gastrulation, cardiac progenitor cells within the anterior lateral plate mesoderm become committed to a cardiogenic fate in response to an inducing signal that emanates from the adjacent endoderm.[2] The specific signaling molecules responsible for this commitment are unknown, but members of the TGF-β family are necessary for this step.[3] In addition, recent studies have shown that inhibition of a signaling molecule, Wnt, in the anterior lateral mesoderm is necessary for cardiogenesis.[4,5] The bilaterally symmetric heart primordia migrate to the midline and fuse to form a single beating heart tube (Fig. 10-1). The straight heart tube has an outer myocardium and an inner endocardium that is separated by an extracellular matrix (ECM) called the cardiac jelly. The linear heart tube is organized along an anterior-posterior (AP) axis to form the future regions of the four-chambered heart. Rightward looping of the heart tube converts the AP polarity to a left-right (L-R) polarity. The ventricular chambers mature by ballooning from the outer curvature of the looped heart, and the inner curvature undergoes extensive remodeling to align the inflow and outflow portions of the heart with the appropriate ventricular chambers. Further septation and remodeling eventually leads to the four-chambered heart.

Another major cell type that contributes to the development of the heart is a population of migratory neural crest cells known as the cardiac neural crest (see Fig. 10-1). These neural crest cells populate the aortic sac, where they are necessary for the proper septation of the truncus arteriosus into the aorta and pulmonary artery and for formation of the semilunar valves and superior portion of the ventricular septum. Cardiac neural crest cells also populate the bilaterally symmetric aortic arch arteries, where they are necessary for proper remodeling of the aortic arch arteries into a left aortic arch with normal branching of the head and neck vessels. Each aortic arch artery contributes to a specific segment of the mature arch as indicated in Figure 10-1.

Over the last decade, heart development has emerged as a paradigm for organogenesis based on molecular and genetic studies in model organisms. Cardiac genetic pathways are highly conserved across diverse species,

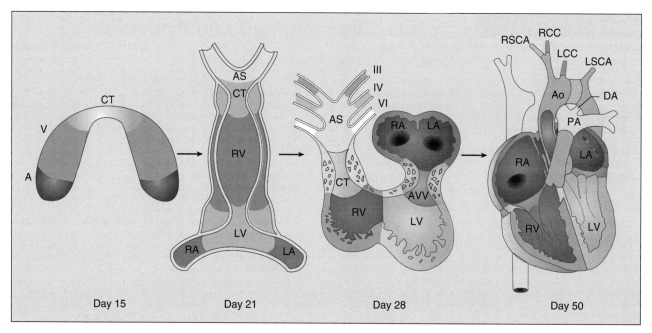

**FIGURE 10-1.** Schematic of cardiac morphogenesis. Cardiac development seen from a ventral view. Cardiogenic precursors form a crescent *(left-most panel)* that is specified to form specific segments of the linear heart tube, which is patterned along the AP axis to form the various regions and chambers of the looped and mature heart. Each cardiac chamber balloons from the outer curvature of the looped heart tube in a segmental fashion. Neural crest cells populate the bilaterally symmetric aortic arch arteries (III, IV, and VI) and aortic sac (AS) that together contribute to specific segments of the mature aortic arch. Mesenchymal cells form the cardiac valves from the conotruncal (CT) and atrioventricular valve (AVV) segments. Corresponding days of human embryonic development are indicated. Ao, aorta; DA, ductus arteriosus; LA, left atrium; LCC, left common carotid; LSCA, left subclavian artery LV, left ventricle; PA, pulmonary artery; RA, right atrium; RCC, right common carotid; RSCA, right subclavian artery; RV, right ventricle. *(From Srivastava D, Olson EN: A genetic blueprint for cardiac development. Nature 2000;407:221–226.)*

from flies to humans, and thus have allowed the use of multiple model systems to explain the molecular mechanisms involved in CHD. At a cellular level, the essential genes for cardiomyocyte formation are similar in humans and in the fruit fly, *Drosophila,* which has a primitive linear heart tube known as a dorsal vessel. *Drosophila* has the advantages of having a rapid breeding time and a simple genome. Most importantly, its DNA can be chemically mutated in a random fashion. Subsequently, by searching for flies with abnormal hearts and identifying the responsible mutations (reverse genetics), genes that are associated with specific developmental defects can be identified. However, the form and function of the vertebrate heart are not similar to those of the fruit fly. Vertebrates share many organotypic features, and there is a conservation of genetic pathways that govern higher order structures such as chambers. Zebrafish can be studied using chemical mutagenesis, phenotype analysis, and reverse genetics, similar to flies, and have the advantage of being vertebrates with two-chambered hearts. In addition, a functioning circulatory system is not necessary until late stages of zebrafish development, allowing visualization of defects while the fish are still alive. To study four-chambered hearts, efforts have focused on chick and mouse model systems. The chick has easily accessible embryos that make it useful for surgical and molecular manipulation. However, the chick system is limited because true genetic studies are not possible. Mice, which have a cardiovascular system nearly identical to that of humans, are mammals and allow *in vivo* genetic manipulation. Using direct gene targeting, mouse

models for some types of CHD have been generated. Each model system has unique advantages, and each has provided important insights into the development of the human heart.

Most cardiac phenotypes in model systems occur in the presence of homozygous mutations of critical cardiac developmental genes and result in embryonic death. In contrast, infants born with CHD likely have heterozygous mutations of one or more critical genes that predispose to the observed phenotype. In the next few sections, we provide examples of genes that are expressed and function in specific regions of the heart and that may contribute to CHD.

## DEFECTS OF ATRIAL AND VENTRICULAR DEVELOPMENT

Infants born with CHD provide evidence for chamber-specific molecular programs. For example, in hypoplastic right ventricle conditions, only the right ventricle does not develop properly, whereas the left ventricle and atria have normal structure and function. Several transcription factors have been shown to be expressed in a chamber-specific pattern. Two members of the basic helix-loop-helix family of transcription factors, dHAND and eHAND (deciduum/extraembryonic membrane, heart, autonomic nervous system, neural crest-derived tissues), are predominantly expressed in the right and left ventricles, respectively.[6,7] Deletion of the *dHAND* gene in mice results in hypoplasia of the right ventricle, providing evidence that mutation of a single gene can ablate an entire chamber.[7] The *dHAND* gene appears to regulate survival of ventricular cells, although the downstream targets of *dHAND* that regulate right ventricular survival remain to be identified.

Myocyte enhancer binding factor-2 (MEF2) is another transcription factor that plays a critical role in ventricular development. Initially studied in *Drosophila*, MEF2 has four orthologs in mammals that are expressed in precursors of the cardiac, skeletal, and smooth muscle lineages in vertebrates.[8-10] Targeted deletion of one of these, MEF2C, in mice results in hypoplasia of the right and left ventricles but not of the atria.[11] The chamber-specific role of MEF2C, despite its homogenous expression in the heart, suggests that MEF2C is a necessary cofactor for other ventricular-restricted regulatory proteins.

The ECM also plays a critical role in ventricular development, because two ECM proteins are necessary for proper right ventricular development. Versican, a chondroitin sulfate proteoglycan, and hyaluronan synthase-2 (Has2) are expressed in the endocardial cushions and in the ventricular myocardium. When *versican* or *Has2* is disrupted in mice, the right ventricle is hypoplastic, and the left ventricle is less affected.[12,13] The mechanism by which perturbation of ECM proteins results in right ventricular hypoplasia is being explored.

Defects of the atrial or ventricular septum are the most common types of CHD. Genetic linkage analyses of families with autosomal dominant inheritance of CHD have revealed a critical role for two transcription factors in the genesis of septal defects. In humans, point mutations of *NKX2.5* cause familial atrial septal defects and conduction abnormalities in addition to sporadic cases of a variety of other types of CHD such as tetralogy of Fallot and Ebstein's anomaly.[14,15] *Nkx2.5* is a homeodomain protein whose ortholog in *Drosophila*, *tinman*, is necessary for formation of the dorsal vessel.[16] In mice, targeted disruption of *Nkx2.5* results in the arrest of heart formation after the straight tube stage in homozygous-null embryos,[17,18] and careful analysis of heterozygotes has identified abnormalities of the atrial septum and the conduction system.[19] Analysis of the mutated human gene products revealed important structure-function relationships of the *Nkx2.5* protein,[20] but the mechanism for how *NKX2.5* mutations result in CHD remains unknown.

Tbx5 is a transcription factor that is mutated in individuals with the Holt-Oram syndrome, characterized by ventricular and atrial septal defects along with limb anomalies.[21] *Tbx5* is expressed highly in the septum and future left ventricular segment during mouse embryogenesis.[22] Targeted deletion of *Tbx5* in mice results in embryonic death in the homozygous state, whereas heterozygous mice have atrial and ventricular septal defects and limb anomalies.[23] Further studies in mice will likely elucidate how *Tbx5* regulates ventricular and septal formation.

## DEFECTS IN CONOTRUNCAL AND AORTIC ARCH DEVELOPMENT

Defects of the cardiac outflow tract (e.g., tetralogy of Fallot, persistent truncus arteriosus, double-outlet right ventricle) or aortic arch (e.g., coarctation, interrupted aortic arch, patent ductus arteriosus) account for 20% to 30% of all CHD.[24] The 22q11 deletion syndrome (del22q11) has provided an entry point to study the molecular pathways critical for the generation of these defects. This deletion syndrome is the most common human gene deletion syndrome and is the second most common genetic cause of CHD after trisomy 21.[25] Of individuals with del22q11, 75% have defects of the conotruncus and/or aortic arch, both of which are derived from the cardiac neural crest, in addition to pharyngeal arch defects that include cleft palate, dysmorphic facial features, thymic hypoplasia, and hypoparathyroidism.[26-29] Of patients with this syndrome, 85% to 90% have a monoallelic microdeletion of chromosome 22q11 spanning approximately 3 Mb that contains nearly 30 genes.[30] Extensive human genetic analyses have failed to identify the critical genes for del22q11. In an effort to identify the important genes in this locus, mouse models were generated that deleted syntenic portions of the commonly deleted region on 22q11.[31-33] Using such approaches, Tbx1, a transcription factor that is expressed in the pharyngeal arches,[34] appears to be one likely candidate gene because heterozygous mice have fourth aortic arch artery anomalies, including interrupted aortic arch type B and anomalous right subclavian artery,[33,35,36] although other features of the syndrome have not been reproduced in mice. *Tbx1* is regulated by the signaling molecule sonic hedgehog (*Shh*) in the developing pharyngeal arches,[37] and accordingly mice harboring mutation in *Shh* have aortic arch defects similar to those observed in *Tbx1* mutants.[38] Transcription factors of the forkhead (Fox) class mediate the *Shh* signal and directly activate Tbx1 transcription in the pharyngeal endoderm (Foxa2) and head mesenchyme (Foxc1 and Foxc2).[38] Interestingly, Foxc1 or Foxc2 mutant mice have aortic arch defects similar to Tbx1 mutants. Further understanding of *Tbx1* gene regulation may provide diagnostic and preventive approaches in the future.

Additional genes in the 22q11 region may contribute to other aspects of the del22q11 phenotype. A patient with the del22q11 phenotype has been described with a small deletion encompassing a gene involved in a ubiquitin-dependent pathway (*UFD1*) and the cell cycle regulator (*CDC45*),[39] although the roles of these genes in development remain unclear. In addition, homozygous deletion of *Crkl*, a gene in the 22q11 locus encoding for a signaling adaptor protein, results in a phenotype similar to the *Tbx1* homozygous null mouse and displays many features of del22q11. How the genes in this locus function independently or combinatorially will be the subject of future studies.

Numerous other genes involved in conotruncal and craniofacial development have been identified by targeted disruption studies in mice. Mice lacking endothelin-1 (ET-1) or its receptor $ET_A$ have postmigratory neural crest defects reminiscent of del22q11.[40,41] In ET-1 and $ET_A$-deficient mice, dHAND and eHAND are downregulated in neural crest-derived tissues, suggesting that the HAND transcription factors function downstream of this signaling cascade.[42] Recent studies have identified a neural crest-specific enhancer for *dHAND* which is a target for activation by the ET-1 signaling pathway.[43] Targeted deletion of *dHAND* results in programmed cell death of the postmigratory neural crest cells, suggesting that dHAND is necessary for survival of these neural crest-derived cells. Neuropilin-1, a downstream target of dHAND, is expressed in neural crest-derived tissues, and targeted deletion of it in mice also results in a phenotype similar to del22q11.[44,45] Similarly, mutations in Pax3 cause persistent truncus arteriosus in mice. Dissection of these and other molecular pathways in mice represents a promising approach to elucidate the bases for cardiovascular developmental defects.

The zebrafish mutant *gridlock* has no circulation to the posterior trunk and tail because of a blockage in the dorsal aorta where the bilateral aortae fuse.[46] This phenotype is similar to aortic coarctation in humans. Positional cloning revealed mutations in a gene encoding a hairy-related transcription factor similar to the mammalian *HRT2/Hey2* gene. Aortic coarctation is known to have a high familial recurrence rate, and it will be interesting to determine if mutations of *gridlock* are present in a subset of these affected patients.

Human genetic studies have identified the gene responsible for Alagille syndrome, characterized by biliary atresia and conotruncal defects. Mutations were identified in *Jagged-1*, a membrane-bound ligand that was originally identified in *Drosophila*.[47,48] *Jagged-1* mutations have since been identified in patients with isolated pulmonary stenosis or tetralogy of Fallot.[49] Jagged-1 is a ligand for the transmembrane receptor Notch, which is involved in embryonic patterning and cellular differentiation.

The ductus arteriosus is derived from the sixth aortic arch artery, and lack of ductal closure after birth results in patent ductus arteriosus, which is the third most common form of CHD. Pedigree analysis of individuals with familial patent ductus arteriosus identified heterozygous mutations of the transcription factor TFAP2B.[50] This suggests a critical role for TFAP2B or its downstream targets in the normal closure of the ductus arteriosus after birth.

## DEFECTS IN VALVE DEVELOPMENT

Congenital abnormalities of the cardiac valves are commonly seen in infants and children. The cardiac valves develop from regional swellings of ECM, known as the cardiac cushions. Reciprocal signaling between the endocardial and myocardial cell layers induces a transformation of endocardial cells into mesenchymal cells. Migration of these cells into the cushions and differentiation into the fibrous tissue of the valves then occurs. These cells are also responsible for the septation of the common atrioventricular (AV) canal into separate right- and left-sided orifices. Trisomy 21, or Down's syndrome, is commonly associated with incomplete septation of the AV valves. A mouse model of trisomy 21 has been generated, but to date the responsible gene(s) on chromosome 21 remain unknown.

Nuclear factor of activated T cells-c (NF-ATc) is a transcription factor that is needed for cytokine gene expression in activated lymphocytes; it is controlled by calcineurin, a calcium-regulated phosphatase. In the heart, NF-ATc expression is restricted to the endocardium. By gene targeting in mice, NF-ATc was found to be necessary for formation of the semilunar valves and, to some extent, the AV valves.[51,52]

Although lack of cardiac valve leaflets is a rare cardiac anomaly, thickened valve leaflets that result in stenotic valves are a common form of CHD. The Smad proteins are intracellular transcriptional mediators of signaling initiated by TGF-β ligands. Smad6 is specifically expressed in the AV cushions and outflow tract during cardiogenesis and is a negative regulator of TGF-β signaling. Targeted disruption of *Smad6* in mice results in thickened and gelatinous AV and semilunar valves, similar to those observed in human disease.[53] In addition to *Smad6*, there are likely other genes in the TGF-β signaling pathway that, when mutated, result in the formation of stenotic and hyperplastic valves. Inhibition of such pathologic processes holds promise as a therapeutic strategy in recurrent valvar stenosis refractory to valvuloplasty.

## DEFECTS OF CARDIAC LOOPING AND LEFT-RIGHT ASSYMETRY

Abnormal cardiac looping underlies a variety of CHD. Proper folding of the straight heart tube aligns the atrial chambers with their appropriate ventricles and the right and left ventricles with the pulmonary artery and aorta, respectively. The atrioventricular septum (AVS), which divides the common AV canal into a right and left AV orifice, moves to the right to position the AVS over the ventricular septum. Simultaneously, the conotruncus septates into the aorta and pulmonary artery and moves to the left so that the conotruncal septum is positioned over the ventricular septum (Fig. 10-2). This movement converts the two-chambered heart to a four-chambered heart.

Arrest or incomplete movement of the AVS or conotruncus may result in malalignment of the inflow and outflow tracts (see Fig. 10-2). When the AVS fails to shift to the right, it results in both AV orifices emptying into the left ventricle (double-inlet left ventricle), whereas failure of the conotruncus to shift to the left results in both the aorta and pulmonary artery arising from the right ventricle (double-outlet right ventricle). *Fog-2* is a zinc-finger protein that may play a role in this process. Deletion of *Fog-2* in mice results in embryos that have a single AV valve that empties into the left ventricle in addition to pulmonic valve stenosis and absence of the coronary vasculature.[54,55] The morphologic defects in *Fog-2* mutants are likely secondary to improper folding of the heart tube resulting in malalignment of the inflow and outflow tracts. Such defects in folding may be secondary to failure of myocardialization, a process in which myocardial cells evacuate the inner curvature of the heart and migrate into the cushions.

Abnormalities in the process of cardiac looping described previously are often observed in the setting of randomized L-R patterning of the heart, lungs, and

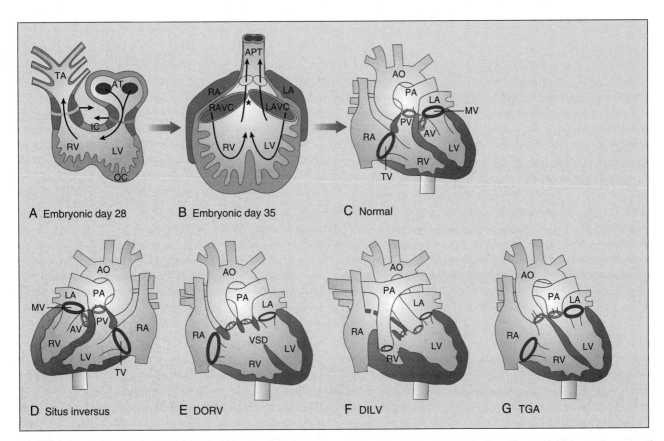

**FIGURE 10-2.** Normal and abnormal cardiac morphogenesis associated with left-right signaling. *A,* As the linear heart tube loops rightward with inner curvature (IC) remodeling and outer curvature (OC) proliferation, the endocardial cushions of the inflow and outflow tracts become adjacent to one another. Subsequently, the AVS shifts to the right, while the aortopulmonary trunk (APT) shifts to the left. *B,* The inflow tract is divided into the right atrioventricular canal (RAVC) and left atrioventricular canal (LAVC) by the AVS (∗). The outflow tract, known as the truncus arteriosus (TA), becomes the aortopulmonary trunk (APT) on septation. *C,* Ultimately, the left (LA) and right atrium (RA) are aligned with the left ventricle (LV) and right ventricle (RV), respectively. The lv and rv become aligned with the aorta (AO) and pulmonary artery (PA), respectively, after 180-degree rotation of the great vessels. *D,* If the determinants of the left-right axis are coordinately reversed, then a condition known as situs inversus results. *E,* If the apt fails to shift to the left, then a condition known as double-outlet right ventricle (DORV) results, in which the right ventricle is aligned with both the aorta and pulmonary artery. *F,* Likewise, if the AVS fails to shift to the right, both atria communicate with the left ventricle in a condition known as double-inlet left ventricle (DILV). *G,* Transposition of the great arteries (TGA) results if the apt fails to twist resulting in communication of the rv with ao and lv with pa. *(Reproduced with permission from Kathiriya IS, Srivastava D: Left-right asymmetry and cardiac looping: Implications for cardiac development and congenital heart disease. Am J Med Genet 2001;97:271–279.)*

visceral organs. The heart is the first organ to visibly break the bilateral symmetry present in the early embryo. A cascade of signaling molecules that regulates L-R asymmetry has been identified and provides a framework in which to consider human L-R defects. Asymmetric expression of Shh leads to expression of the TGF-β members (nodal and lefty) in the left lateral plate mesoderm.[56] The left-sided expression of nodal induces rightward looping of the straight heart tube. In the right lateral mesoderm, Shh and nodal are inhibited by an activin-receptor mediated pathway. Conversely, the snail-related zinc finger transcription factor is expressed in the right lateral mesoderm and is repressed by Shh on the left.[57] Ultimately, the activin and nodal-dependent pathways result in expression of the transcription factor Pitx2 on the left side of visceral organs.[58] The asymmetric expression of Pitx2 is sufficient for the establishment of L-R asymmetry in the heart, lungs, and gut.

Recent studies have revealed how the initial asymmetry of molecules such as Shh might be established. Henson's node contains ciliary processes that beat in a vortical fashion creating a leftward movement of morphogens around the node.[59] In mice homozygous for the *inversus viscerum (iv)* mutation, L-R orientation of the heart and viscera is randomized.[60] The *iv* gene encodes for L-R dynein that might act as a force generating component in cilia that are present in the node.[61,62] Mice with situs inversus totalis *(inv)* have complete reversal of L-R asymmetry, but the function of the *inv* gene remains unknown. These findings may provide the mechanism for situs inversus in Kartagener's syndrome, also known as immotile cilia syndrome.

Patients with heterotaxy syndromes display randomization of the cardiac, pulmonary, and gastrointestinal situs, and patients with situs inversus totalis have a well-coordinated reversal of L-R asymmetry. Disruption of the signaling cascades on the left or right side of the embryo results in randomization of cardiac looping and often leads to bilateral right (asplenia syndrome) or left (polysplenia syndrome) sidedness, respectively. In humans, point mutations of several genes involved in the L-R signaling cascade have been identified including ZIC3, a zinc finger transcription factor; activin receptor IIB; and cryptic, a cofactor of nodal.[63]

## CARDIOMYOCYTE SPECIFICATION AND DIFFERENTIATION

In contrast to the dramatic progress in identifying genes that control cardiac morphogenesis, relatively little is known of initial steps in heart formation that involve commitment of mesodermal cells to the cardiac lineage and the subsequent differentiation to form contractile cardiomyocytes. This facet of cardiac development has been difficult to dissect, in part because of apparent functional redundancy among the genes that control these early processes in vertebrates. For example, although tinman is required for heart formation in Drosophila, there are several tinman orthologs in vertebrates that are coexpressed in the developing heart.[64] As discussed earlier, the best characterized of these genes, NKX2.5, is expressed at the right time and place in vertebrate embryos to fulfill a role analogous to that of tinman in flies, and gene replacement studies have shown that the mouse NKX2.5 gene can substitute for some of the functions of tinman when introduced into Drosophila embryos.[65,66] However, the initial steps in cardiac development occur normally in mice lacking NKX2.5,[18] which suggests that other members of this family of homeobox genes may share common functions with NKX2.5. The finding that abnormalities in cardiac morphogenesis are not manifested until later in development of mice (and humans) harboring NKX2.5 mutations suggests that the cardiac-expressed Nk-type homeobox genes exhibit unique functions at later developmental stages or, more likely, that subtle cardiac abnormalities become more apparent as the heart begins to function under a hemodynamic load. Further evidence that NKX2.5 may share common early functions with other members of this multigene family has come from the observation that forced expression of dominant negative versions of NKX2.5 in frog or fish embryos results in severe early effects on the heart that are not seen with single-gene mutations.[67,68]

Another barrier to the identification of genes that act nonredundantly to control the initial steps in cardiogenesis is the fact that loss of function mutations in such genes are likely to result in early embryonic death. Thus, identification of such genes is more likely to come from approaches other than human or mouse genetics. Thus, the wealth of DNA sequence information provided by recent genome projects represents a valuable untapped resource.

As an example of such an approach, a powerful cardiac transcription factor named myocardin was recently identified using a bioinformatics-based approach to identify novel genes present only as unknown cDNA sequences from cardiac cDNA libraries.[69] During mouse embryogenesis, myocardin is expressed in the earliest cardiac precursor cells within the cardiac crescent, and its expression is maintained in the heart until adulthood. Myocardin activates cardiac genes by interacting with serum response factor (SRF), a ubiquitous transcription factor that binds the promoters of numerous cardiac genes. Frog embryos injected with a dominant negative mutant of myocardin fail to form a heart or to activate cardiac gene expression. Because myocardin belongs to a family of related genes with similar functions, it is unlikely that it would have been identified by genetic studies because of functional redundancy. Whether myocardin plays roles in later stages of heart development remains to be determined, but its expression throughout the heart from embryogenesis to adulthood underscores its potential importance at multiple developmental stages.

The identification of early cardiac control genes like myocardin not only promises to yield insights into the molecular mechanisms for heart formation but also provides opportunities for cardiac regeneration through the ectopic expression of such genes in noncardiac cells. Although such approaches are still largely conceptual, it is easy to imagine that genes that specify cardiac cell identity may soon be harnessed as a means of repairing abnormalities resulting from CHD and from cardiac disease in adults.

## SUMMARY

The early findings described here have identified some of the genes and molecular mechanisms involved in heart development, but the etiology of CHD is complex and likely results from a combination of genetic and environmental influences. By using multiple animal systems, numerous new genes have been identified that are critical for cardiac development.[70] Genetic analyses in humans with CHD have revealed point mutations in some of these critical genes. The identification of mutated genes in affected individuals will only be the first step, because it is becoming increasingly clear that similar genetic abnormalities result in a spectrum of phenotypes in humans. These differences are likely due to other genetic and environmental influences. Over the next decade, the challenge will be to identify environmental and epigenetic factors that result in CHD in the setting of appropriate genetic susceptibility. Thus, genetic identification and subsequent environmental alteration could result in the prevention of some forms of CHD.

### Acknowledgments

D.S. Is supported by grants from the NHLBI/NIH, March of Dimes Birth Defects Foundation and Smile Train Inc. E.N.O. is supported by grants from the NHLBI/NIH and Donald W. Reynolds Foundation.

# REFERENCES

1. Hoffman JI: Incidence of congenital heart disease: II. Prenatal incidence. Pediatr Cardiol 1995;16:155-165.
2. Schultheiss TM, Xydas S, Lassar AB: Induction of avian cardiac myogenesis by anterior endoderm. Development 1995;121:4203-4214.
3. Schultheiss TM, Burch JB, Lassar AB: A role for bone morphogenetic proteins in the induction of cardiac myogenesis. Genes Dev 1997;11:451-462.
4. Schneider VA, Mercola M: Wnt antagonism initiates cardiogenesis in Xenopus laevis. Genes Dev 2001;15:304-315.
5. Marvin MJ, Di Rocco G, Gardiner A, et al: Inhibition of Wnt activity induces heart formation from posterior mesoderm. Genes Dev 2001;15:316-327.
6. Srivastava D, Cserjesi P, Olson EN: A subclass of bHLH proteins required for cardiac morphogenesis. Science 1995;270:1995-1999.
7. Srivastava D, Thomas T, Lin Q, et al: Regulation of cardiac mesodermal and neural crest development by the bHLH transcription factor, dHAND. Nat Genet 1997;16:154-160.
8. Nguyen HT, Bodmer R, Abmayr SM, et al: D-mef2: A Drosophila mesoderm-specific MADS box-containing gene with a biphasic expression profile during embryogenesis. Proc Natl Acad Sci USA 1994;91:7520-7524.
9. Lilly B, Zhao B, Ranganayakulu G, et al: Requirement of MADS domain transcription factor D-MEF2 for muscle formation in Drosophila. Science 1995;267:688-693.
10. Black BL, Olson EN: Transcriptional control of muscle development by myocyte enhancer factor-2 (MEF2) proteins. Annu Rev Cell Dev Biol 1998;14:167-196.
11. Lin Q, Schwarz J, Bucana C, et al: Control of mouse cardiac morphogenesis and myogenesis by transcription factor MEF2C. Science 1997;276:1404-1407.
12. Yamamura H, Zhang M, Markwald RR, et al: A heart segmental defect in the anterior-posterior axis of a transgenic mutant mouse. Dev Biol 1997;186:58-72.
13. Camenisch TD, Spicer AP, Brehm-Gibson T, et al: Disruption of hyaluronan synthase-2 abrogates normal cardiac morphogenesis and hyaluronan-mediated transformation of epithelium to mesenchyme. J Clin Invest 2000;106:349-360.
14. Schott JJ, Benson DW, Basson CT, et al: Congenital heart disease caused by mutations in the transcription factor NKX2-5. Science 1998;281:108-111.
15. Benson DW, Silberbach GM, Kavanaugh-McHugh A, et al: Mutations in the cardiac transcription factor NKX2.5 affect diverse cardiac developmental pathways. J Clin Invest 1999;104:1567-1573.
16. Bodmer R: The gene tinman is required for specification of the heart and visceral muscles in Drosophila. Development 1993;118:719-729.
17. Tanaka M, Chen Z, Bartunkova S, et al: The cardiac homeobox gene Csx/Nkx2.5 lies genetically upstream of multiple genes essential for heart development. Development 1999;126:1269-1280.
18. Lyons I, Parsons LM, Hartley L, et al: Myogenic and morphogenetic defects in the heart tubes of murine embryos lacking the homeo box gene Nkx2-5. Genes Dev 1995;9:1654-1666.
19. Biben C, Weber R, Kesteven S, et al: Cardiac septal and valvular dysmorphogenesis in mice heterozygous for mutations in the homeobox gene Nkx2-5. Circ Res 2000;87:888-895.
20. Kasahara H, Lee B, Schott JJ, et al: Loss of function and inhibitory effects of human CSX/NKX2.5 homeoprotein mutations associated with congenital heart disease. J Clin Invest 2000;106:299-308.
21. Basson CT, Bachinsky DR, Lin RC, et al: Mutations in human TBX5 cause limb and cardiac malformation in Holt-Oram syndrome. Nat Genet 1997;15:30-35.
22. Bruneau BG, Logan M, Davis N, et al: Chamber-specific cardiac expression of Tbx5 and heart defects in Holt-Oram syndrome. Dev Biol 1999;211:100-108.
23. Bruneau BG, Nemer G, Schmitt JP, et al: A murine model of Holt-Oram syndrome defines roles of the T-Box transcription factor Tbx5 in cardiogenesis and disease. Cell 2001;106:709-721.

24. Fyler DC: Trends. In Fyler DC (ed): Nadas' Pediatric Cardiology. Philadelphia, Hanley & Belfus, 1992, pp 273-280.
25. Scambler PJ: The 22q11 deletion syndromes. Hum Mol Genet 2000;9:2421-2426.
26. Ryan AK, Goodship JA, Wilson DI, et al: Spectrum of clinical features associated with interstitial chromosome 22q11 deletions: A European collaborative study. J Med Genet 1997;34:798-804.
27. DiGeorge AM: Discussion on a new concept of the cellular basis of immunology. J Pediatr 1965;67:907.
28. Shprintzen RJ, Goldberg RB, Lewin ML, et al: A new syndrome involving cleft palate, cardiac anomalies, typical facial facies, and learning disabilities: Velo-cardio-facial syndrome. Cleft Palate Craniofac J 1998;15:56-62.
29. Kinouchi A, Mori K, Ando M, et al: Facial appearance of patients with conotruncal anomalies. Pediatrics (Japan) 1976;17:84-87.
30. Driscoll DA, Budarf ML, Emanuel BS: A genetic etiology for DiGeorge syndrome: Consistent deletions and microdeletions of 22q11. Am J Hum Genet 1992;50:924-933.
31. Puech A, Saint-Jore B, Merscher S, et al: Normal cardiovascular development in mice deficient for 16 genes in 550 kb of the velocardiofacial/DiGeorge syndrome region. Proc Natl Acad Sci USA 2000;97:10090-10095.
32. Lindsay EA, Botta A, Jurecic V, et al: Congenital heart disease in mice deficient for the DiGeorge syndrome region. Nature 1999;401:379-383.
33. Merscher S, Funke B, Epstein JA, et al: TBX1 is responsible for cardiovascular defects in velo-cardio-facial/DiGeorge syndrome. Cell 2001;104:619-629.
34. Chapman DL, Garvey N, Hancock S, et al: Expression of the T-box family genes, Tbx1-Tbx5, during early mouse development. Dev Dyn 1996;206:379-390.
35. Lindsay EA, Vitelli F, Su H, et al: Tbx1 haploinsufficiency in the DiGeorge syndrome region causes aortic arch defects in mice. Nature 2001;410:97-101.
36. Jerome LA, Papaioannou VE: DiGeorge syndrome phenotype in mice mutant for the T-box gene, Tbx1. Nat Genet 2001;27:286-291.
37. Garg V, Yamagishi C, Hu T, et al: Tbx1, a DiGeorge syndrome candidate gene is regulated by Sonic Hedgehog during pharyngeal arch development. Dev Biol 2001;235:62-73.
38. Yamagishi H, Maeda J, Hu T, et al: Tbx1 is regulated by tissue-specific forkhead proteins through a common sonic hedgehog-responsive enhancer. Genes Dev 2003;17:269-281.
39. Yamagishi H, Garg V, Matsuoka R, et al: A molecular pathway revealing a genetic basis for human cardiac and craniofacial defects. Science 1999;283:1158-1161.
40. Kurihara Y, Kurihara H, Oda H, et al: Aortic arch malformations and ventricular septal defect in mice deficient in endothelin-1. J Clin Invest 1995;96:293-300.
41. Clouthier DE, Hosoda K, Richardson JA, et al: Cranial and cardiac neural crest defects in endothelin-A receptor-deficient mice. Development 1998;125:813-824.
42. Thomas T, Kurihara H, Yamagishi H, et al: A signaling cascade involving endothelin-1, dHAND and msx1 regulates development of neural-crest-derived branchial arch mesenchyme. Development 1998;125:3005-3014.
43. Charité J, McFadden DG, Merlo G, et al: Role of Dlx-6 in regulation of an endothelin-1 dependent, dHAND branchial arch enhancer. Genes Dev 2001;15:3039-3049.
44. Kawasaki T, Kitsukawa T, Bekku Y, et al: A requirement for neuropilin-1 in embryonic vessel formation. Development 1999;126:4895-4902.
45. Yamagishi H, Olson EN, Srivastava D: The basic helix-loop-helix transcription factor, dHAND, is required for vascular development. J Clin Invest 2000;105:261-270.
46. Zhong TP, Rosenberg M, Mohideen MP, et al: Gridlock, an HLH gene required for assembly of the aorta in zebrafish. Science 2000;287:1820-1824.
47. Li L, Krantz ID, Deng Y, et al: Alagille syndrome is caused by mutations in human Jagged1, which encodes a ligand for Notch1. Nat Genet 1997;16:243-251.
48. Oda T, Elkahloun AG, Pike BL, et al: Mutations in the human Jagged1 gene are responsible for Alagille syndrome. Nat Genet 1997;16:235-242.

49. Krantz ID, Smith R, Colliton RP, et al: Jagged1 mutations in patients ascertained with isolated congenital heart defects. Am J Med Genet 1999;84:56–60.

50. Satoda M, Zhao F, Diaz GA, et al: Mutations in TFAP2B cause Char syndrome, a familial form of patent ductus arteriosus. Nat Genet 2000;25:42–46.

51. Ranger AM, Grusby MJ, Hodge MR, et al: The transcription factor NF-ATc is essential for cardiac valve formation. Nature 1998;392:186–190.

52. de la Pompa JL, Timmerman LA, Takimoto H, et al: Role of the NF-ATc transcription factor in morphogenesis of cardiac valves and septum. Nature 1998;392:182–6.

53. Galvin KM, Donovan MJ, Lynch CA, et al: A role for Smad6 in development and homeostasis of the cardiovascular system. Nat Genet 2000;24:171–174.

54. Svensson EC, Huggins GS, Lin H, et al: A syndrome of tricuspid atresia in mice with a targeted mutation of the gene encoding Fog-2. Nat Genet 2000;25:353–356.

55. Tevosian SG, Deconinck AE, Tanaka M, et al: FOG-2, a cofactor for GATA transcription factors, is essential for heart morphogenesis and development of coronary vessels from epicardium. Cell 2000;101:729–739.

56. Levin M, Johnson RL, Stern CD, et al: A molecular pathway determining left-right asymmetry in chick embryogenesis. Cell 1995;82:803–814.

57. Isaac A, Sargent MG, Cooke J: Control of vertebrate left-right asymmetry by a snail-related zinc finger gene. Science 1997;275:1301–1304.

58. Piedra ME, Icardo JM, Albajar M, et al: Pitx2 participates in the late phase of the pathway controlling left-right asymmetry. Cell 1998;94:319–324.

59. Nonaka S, Tanaka Y, Okada Y, et al: Randomization of left-right asymmetry due to loss of nodal cilia generating leftward flow of extraembryonic fluid in mice lacking KIF3B motor protein. Cell 1998;95:829–837.

60. Brueckner M, D'Eustachio P, Horwich AL: Linkage mapping of a mouse gene, iv, that controls left-right asymmetry of the heart and viscera. Proc Natl Acad Sci USA 1989;86:5035–5038.

61. Supp DM, Witte DP, Potter SS, et al: Mutation of an axonemal dynein affects left-right asymmetry in inversus viscerum mice. Nature 1997;389:963–966.

62. Supp DM, Brueckner M, Kuehn MR, et al: Targeted deletion of the ATP binding domain of left-right dynein confirms its role in specifying development of left-right asymmetries. Development 1999;126:5495–5504.

63. Kathiriya IS, Srivastava D: Left-Right asymmetry and cardiac looping: Implications for cardiac development and congenital heart disease. Am J Med Genet 2001;97:271–279.

64. Harvey RP: NK-2 homeobox genes and heart development. Dev Biol 1996;178:203–216.

65. Ranganayakulu G, Elliott D, Harvey R, et al: Divergent roles for NK-2 class homeobox genes in cardiogenesis in flies and mice. Development 1998;125:3037–3048.

66. Park M, Lewis C, Turbay D, et al: Differential rescue of visceral and cardiac defects in Drosophila by vertebrate tinman-related genes. Proc Natl Acad Sci USA 1998;95:9366–9371.

67. Fu Y, Yan W, Mohun TJ, et al: Vertebrate tinman homologues XNkx2-3 and XNkx2-5 are required for heart formation in a functionally redundant manner. Development 1998;125:4439–4449.

68. Grow MW, Kreig PA: Tinman function is essential for vertebrate heart development: Elimination of cardiac differentiation by dominant inhibitory mutants of the tinman-related genes, XNks2-3 and XNkx2-5. Dev Biol 1998;204:187–196.

69. Wang D-Z, Chang P, Wang Z, et al: Activation of cardiac gene expression by myocardin, a transcriptional cofactor for serum response factor. Cell 2001;105:851–862.

70. Srivastava D, Olson EN: A genetic blueprint for cardiac development. Nature 2000;407:221–226.

## EDITOR'S CHOICE

Bao ZZ, Bruneau BG, Seidman JG, et al: Regulation of chamber-specific gene expression in the developing heart by Irx4. Science 1999;283:1161–1164.
*Irx gene family joins a growing list of genes that control cardiac morphgenesis and cardiac chamber development.*

Bisgrove BW, Morelli SH, Yost HJ: Genetics of Human Laterality Disorders: Insights from Vertebrate Model Systems. Annu Rev Genomics Hum Genet. 2003.
*Summary of advances in understanding genetic pathways that control laterality in the heart and other organ systems.*

Chen F, Kook H, Milewski R, et al: Hop is an unusual homeobox gene that modulates cardiac development. Cell 2002;110:713–723.
*New facet of the Nkx2.5 pathway that regulates cardiogenesis*

Clevers H: Inflating cell numbers by Wnt. Mol Cell 2002;10:1260–1261.
*Leader in Wnt signaling highlights work that is relevant to the development of the heart and many other systems.*

Garg V, Kathiriya IS, Barnes R, et al. GATA4 mutations cause human congenital heart defects and reveal an interaction with TBX5. Nature 2003;424:443–447.
*GATA-4 joins Nkx2.5, TBX5 as a monogenic cause of congenital heart disease.*

Gibson-Brown JJ: T-box time in England. Dev Cell 2002;3:625–630.
*Tbx family reunion; multiple roles in multiple organs, but a recurring theme can be found that ties the family together.*

Hamblet NS, Lijam N, Ruiz-Lozano P, et al: Dishevelled 2 is essential for cardiac outflow tract development, somite segmentation and neural tube closure. Development 2002;129:5827–5838.
*Converging pathways for outflow tract defects; companion paper to the PTX story.*

Harvey RP: Patterning the vertebrate heart. Nat Rev Genet 2002;3:544–556.
*Excellent review with lucid illustrations on a complex topic.*

Kelly RG, Brown NA, Buckingham ME: The arterial pole of the mouse heart forms from Fgf10-expressing cells in pharyngeal mesoderm. Dev Cell 2001;1:435–440.
*Traces of the secondary heart field; molecular markers should facilitate further understanding of its role in cardiac morphogenesis.*

Marvin MJ, Di Rocco G, Gardiner A, et al: Inhibition of Wnt activity induces heart formation from posterior mesoderm. Genes Dev 2001;15:316–327.
*Negative regulation is critical to allow the onset of cardiogenesis*

Pandur P, Lasche M, Eisenberg LM, Kuhl M: Wnt-11 activation of a non-canonical Wnt signalling pathway is required for cardiogenesis. Nature 2002;418:636–641.
*Wnts come in many forms and trigger diverse steps of cardiogenesis.*

Schneider VA, Mercola M: Wnt antagonism initiates cardiogenesis in Xenopus laevis. Genes Dev 2001;15:304–315.
*Companion paper to Marvin et al.*

Shin CH, Liu ZP, Passier R, et al: Modulation of cardiac growth and development by HOP, an unusual homeodomain protein. Cell 2002;110:725–735.
*Companion paper to Chen et al.*

Stainier DY, Beis D, Jungblut B, Bartman T: Endocardial cushion formation in zebrafish. Cold Spring Harb Symp Quant Biol 2002;67:49–56.
*Zebrafish models provide deeper mechanistic insight into valvular morphogenesis.*

Sucov HM: Molecular insights into cardiac development. Annu Rev Physiol 1998;60:287–308.
*Highlights role of retinoids in cardiac development.*

Tevosian SG, Deconinck AE, Tanaka M, et al: FOG-2, a cofactor for GATA transcription factors, is essential for heart morphogenesis and development of coronary vessels from epicardium. Cell 2000;101:729–739.
*Epicardial-myocardial crosstalk is critical for coronary arteriogenesis; key role of Gata-4 and its co-factors in this cell-cell interaction.*

# chapter 11

# Development of Cardiac Pacemaking and Conduction System Lineages

*Robert G. Gourdie*
*Steven W. Kubalak*
*Terence X. O'Brien*
*Kenneth R. Chien*
*Takashi Mikawa*

According to legend, Galileo Galilei used his own pulse to time the swing of a cathedral lamp as he pondered the mathematical laws governing its oscillation. Although Galileo and others subsequently developed more objective timepieces, the heartbeat remains a natural marvel—an exemplar for regularity and consistency. During the lifetime of an average person the heart undergoes more than two and a half billion contraction cycles. Although modulated by neural input, the autonomous rhythm of the heart has it origins in a multicomponent set of specialized muscle tissues collectively referred to as the pacemaking and conduction system (PCS) (Fig. 11-1). The components of this system include a pacemaker (the sinuatrial node), an electrical impulse delay generator for separating the contraction of the atrial and ventricular chambers of the heart (the atrioventricular [AV] node), and a wiring harness (the His-Purkinje system) for fast and coordinate conduction of impulse within the ventricles.

The anatomy, histology, electrophysiology, and cellular properties of PCS tissues have long been the subject of experimentation and characterization. However, with the advent of modern biologic tools, there is fresh impetus in unraveling the molecular and cellular processes that regulate the genesis and integration of these specialized sets of cardiac tissue during development. In addition to increasing our basic knowledge, these novel mechanistic insights are of significance to clinicians. Because of its decisive function in initiating and coordinating the heartbeat, dysfunction of the PCS is a direct cause of pathologic disturbances to impulse conduction and arrhythmia. Growing understanding of the developmental biology of these specialized tissues is providing insight into the molecular cause of cardiac pathology in adults and children. Such insight, in conjunction with technologies such as stem cell manipulation, could eventually yield paths to the treatment or replacement of PCS tissues damaged by disease or congenital malformation.

## THE FUNCTIONAL EMERGENCE OF PACEMAKING AND CONDUCTION SYSTEM COMPONENTS

### Pacemaking Activity

A cellular focus of dominant pacemaking activity or automaticity (Fig. 11-2) is the first element of the PCS that is functionally recognizable during heart development. This dominant automaticity arises within the "flared" inflow region located at the posterior end of the embryonic tubular heart.[17-20] Electrical excitation initiated at pacemaker cells spreads anteriorly via gap junctions between myocytes toward the outflow region of the single-chambered organ. The rhythmic sequence of posterior-anterior excitation spread induces the concordant propagation of waves of slow, peristaltic contraction along the heart.[21,22] In the chick embryo, first establishment of lead pacemaker activity occurs at around 25 to 35 hours of development[20]—a developmental stage corresponding approximately to 3 weeks of embryonic age in humans. At this early stage of morphogenesis, the tube heart has a simple histologic organization consisting of a few concentric layers—a thin outer layer of epithelioid myocytes, an intermediate stratum of acellular matrix, and an inner lining of endocardial cells.[23-25] Initially, the pacemaker focus at the inflow pole is left sided.[17,26] As development proceeds, dominant automaticity shifts to cells in the right-hand side of the inflow region.

Although myocytes along the length the tube heart elicit action potentials (APs), the electrogenic mechanisms that underlie differentiation of spontaneous beating and dominant automaticity are not well understood. There is a distinct posterior-to-anterior distribution of pacemaking dominance along the early heart.[19] Studies of I(f) and hyperpolarization-activated cyclic nuclide gated (HCN) membrane channels have implicated these currents in spontaneous beating, and HCN1 has a specific role in the formation of SA node pacemaker

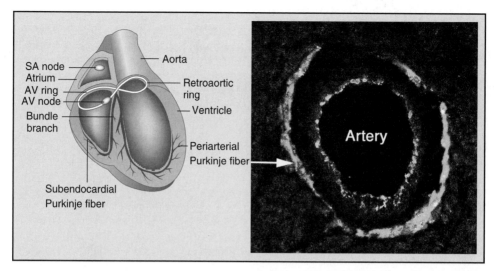

**FIGURE 11-1.** Basic structural and functional organization of the embryonic pacemaking and conduction system (PCS). The heartbeat is set by the ***sinuatrial (SA) node***. From this focus of pacemaking activity, propagating action potential spreads through atrial muscle, eventually focusing into the ***atrioventricular (AV) node*** where it is delayed briefly before ventricular activation. Following exit from the node, the propagating action potential accelerates along the His bundle and ***bundle branches,*** finally activating working ventricular muscle via a network of ***Purkinje fiber*** conduction cells. The model shown in the right hand panel is based on the embryonic chick heart. In the chick, the terminalmost component of the conduction system penetrates into the ventricular muscle in intimate association with coronary arteries. The ***periarterial Purkinje fiber*** shown in the left hand panel has been simultaneously labeled for three markers of conduction lineage: a gap junction protein Cx40 (yellow in color insert), a myosin heavy chain (green in color insert), and Nkx2.5 (red in color insert), a transcription factor. The endothelial cells lining the artery also contain Cx40 gap junctions. See the following references for further reading on the discovery of structure and function of the developing and mature PCS, including classics by Purkinje,[1] His,[2] Tawara,[3] Wenckebach,[4] Hering,[5] and Keith and Flack.[6] Also see references 1 to 16. (See color plate.)

currents.[27,28] Gene targeting in different animal models have also indicated roles for ion channels in pacemaker dominance. Mutations of an Ih channel are associated with slowed intrinsic heart rate in zebrafish.[29] More recently, knockout of the $Na^+$-$Ca^{2+}$ exchanger gene in mice was reported to result in the development of a looped, tubular heart that did not beat spontaneously.[30]

## Atrioventricular Delay

The development of a segment of AV canal myocardium in the looping, tube heart marks the first emergence of a specialized component that acts to delay impulse propagation (see Fig. 11-2).[22,31,35] In the chick embryo, an AV junctional delay is evident from around 42 hours of development, a timing that corresponds to around 8 and 25 days of embryonic age in mice and humans, respectively. The AV canal is one of three segments (including the inflow and outflow segments of the looping tube heart) that display peristaltic electromechanical properties analogous to those in the unlooped tube heart.[22] These phenotypically "primitive" segments flank the early atrial and ventricular chambers and appear to function as sphincter-like valves, probably serving to increase the pumping efficiency of the embryonic heart. Similar to the APs of the tubular heart, AV canal myocytes display a gradual depolarization phase consistent with a predominance of slow, voltage-gated $Ca^{2+}$ channels.[33,34] Concomitantly, atrial and ventricular segments develop more rapid and powerful contractions—a change associated with increases in the velocity of excitation propagation and the evolution of APs that incorporate a

high-amplitude, fast-rising depolarization.[22,31,35] Studies in mice indicate that intercellular coupling in the tubular heart, and later in the AV canal, is dominated by connexin45[36]—a gap junction channel displaying high voltage sensitivity and low conductance. Interestingly, Cx45 is also a pre-eminent connexin within the SA node and the AV node and ring system of the mouse and other mammalian species.[37-40] Thus, the mechanism of AV delay in the developing and mature heart is probably not simply a function of the characteristics of specific populations of membrane ion channels. A significant contribution may also be made by intercellular coupling properties within specialized myocardial compartments such as the embryonic AV canal and nodes of the adult heart.

## Rapid Impulse Conduction in the Ventricles

The final major component of the PCS to differentiate functionally is a network of fast conducting cells responsible for synchronizing and coordinating the contraction of the increasingly bulky ventricles. In the adult heart of higher vertebrates such as birds and mammals, this network corresponds to the His-Purkinje system of specialized conduction cardiomyocytes. This fast-conducting network is identified by a topologic shift in the sequence of ventricular activation (see Fig. 11-2).[41] Before the shift, electrical excitation initially spreads from the AV junction toward the tip or apex of the ventricle. Following the shift, the progressive course of activation undergoes an apparent reversal, such that the entire ventricle is depolarized in a rapid apex-to-base sequence. In the

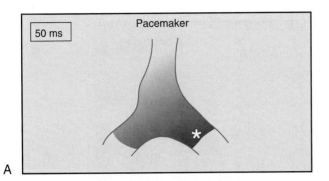

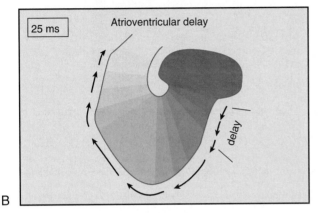

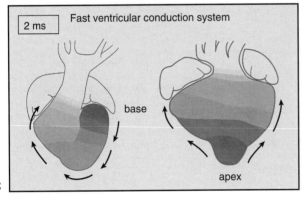

**FIGURE 11-2.** Functional emergence of the three major components of the PCS in the chick. *A,* A ***dominant pacemaker*** (i.e., SA node-like) emerges initially in the left inflow region (star) of the tube heart (Hamburger and Hamilton (HH) developmental stage 10 to 11). *B,* AV impulse delay (i.e., an ***AV nodelike function***) develops first at the junction of the atria and ventricles in the looped tube heart (e.g., ~HH 15 to 17). *C,* A shift in the sequence of activation spread as observed from the ventricular epicardium marks differentiation of a ***His-Purkinje-like function*** of fast ventricular conduction. The right-hand HH 28 heart retains the more primitive sequence, initiating activation from the left-ventricular base. Later in the HH 31 heart, activation spreads first from the apex of the ventricle. Note that the entire tubular heart (e.g., in A) is approximately 0.5 mm in length—less than one tenth of the ventricular base-apex distance of the HH 31 heart. The arrows indicate course of activation spread. Isochrones are in milliseconds in the right-hand corner of each box. (See color plate.) *(B and C from Reckova M, Rosengarten C, deAlmeida A, et al: Hemodynamics is a key epigenetic factor in development of the cardiac conduction system. Circ Res 2003;93:77-85.)*

chick embryo, this topologic shift appears to be correlated with completion of ventricular septation at around 7 to 8 days of embryonic development,[41,42] although some workers have reported activation of the apex at slightly earlier stages.[22] In the mouse embryo, ventricular

activation from the apex has been reported to be initiated from around 10.5 days of embryonic development, a timing that precedes the completion of ventricular septation.[43] Although no specific data exists for humans, the studies in chick and mouse suggest that apex-to-base activation in humans may emerge between the sixth and eighth week of embryogenesis.

At present, the structural basis of the topologic shift in the embryonic ventricle is not well understood. One interpretation is that it reflects a developmental linkage event between two specialized myocardial compartments (i.e., the AV node and the His-Purkinje system) that occurs at or around ventricular septation. One line of support for this interpretation comes from retroviral lineage tracing studies that indicate that the peripheral conduction cells differentiate independent of central or proximal elements of the PCS in the chick heart.[15,44] Studies of markers (including HNK-1) in the embryonic chick and human heart have also revealed apparent breaks and linkages in expression pattern between specialized myocardial compartments that may reflect the occurrence of a discontinuous process necessary for establishment of electrical continuity along the mature PCS.[42,45]

## PHENOTYPIC HETEROGENEITY OF PACEMAKING AND CONDUCTION SYSTEM LINEAGES

The previous section demonstrated that certain PCS characteristics are labile and that some undergo definite shifts in topology. Upcoming sections of this review discuss new questions that are currently debated by PCS researchers. Before this discussion, however, it is important that the electrophysiologic and gene expression characteristics of the heterogeneous (but uniformly cardiomyocyte) tissues of the PCS should be briefly addressed (Fig. 11-3). This topic has been given more extensive coverage by us[15,16] and others[9,10,14,46,47] in earlier articles.

### Nodal Phenotypes

Cells composing nodal tissues show characteristics similar to myocardial cells in the embryonic tubular heart.[9,14,46] Parallels drawn between embryonal and nodal myocytes include resemblance in electrophysiology—AP morphologies and conduction velocities are similar; histology—the myocytes are similarly small in size and have more irregular shapes than other myocardial lineages; ultrastructure—both have poorly developed myofibrils and sarcoplasmic reticulum and a low frequency of intercellular junctions; and gene expression—embryonal and nodal myocytes often share expression of embryonic isoforms of contractile and cytoskeletal proteins and intercellular junctional proteins. However, care must be taken that this parallel is not pushed too far. The evidence is that mature nodal cells have a functional phenotype as specialized as any part of the PCS. Reports of such specialization include increases in levels of specific membrane channels,

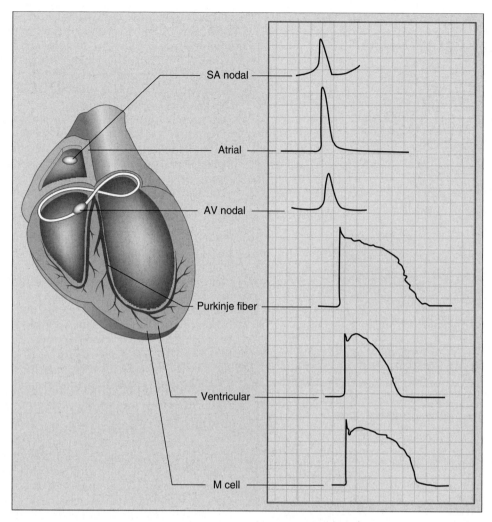

**FIGURE 11-3.** Cardiomyocyte electrophysiologic phenotypes. Each of the six APs shown are representative of different cardiomyocyte types present in the sinu-ventricular conduction pathway. All APs are drawn to the same scale. Horizontal lines on Aps (X-axis) show 0 potential level. Each of these lines is ~400 ms in duration. Position of the cellular AP along the X-axis indicates approximate order of the activation sequence. The maximum diastolic potential (Y-axis) of the SA node AP is ~50 millivolts. (See color plate.)

receptors, and signal transduction proteins[48-50] and downregulation of a protein involved in $Ca^{2+}$ regulation.[51] Also, with respect to integration of pacemaker function in the adult, studies in mammals indicate significant heterogeneity in terms of cell morphology, pacemaker activity, AP, densities of various ionic currents, and gap junctional connexins within the SA node.[52] Studies of connexin localization in the rodent AV node also reveal myocytes displaying heterotypic characteristics within this tissue.[37] Cellular heterogeneity in connexin distribution appears to be particularly complex at the interface between the nodes and adjacent myocardial compartments (Fig. 11-4).

## Conduction System Phenotypes

The network of ventricular conduction tissues specialized for rapid propagation of impulse in the mature vertebrate heart also demonstrate complex and heterogeneous phenotypes.[9,10,13-16] In apparent consistency with a fast wiring function and classical cable theory, conduction cells are often described as having a larger

diameter than working myocytes. However, although increased cellular size and other histologic characteristics such as decreased sarcomeric organization and increased glycogen storage granules are features of Purkinje fibers in many mammalian species,[9] Purkinje fibers in rodent and chicken hearts are often difficult to distinguish from ventricular myocytes by histologic criteria. It should also be noted that the anatomic distribution of conduction cells in avian species demonstrates unique features.[7,8,13,53,54] These include an intramural component that codistributes with coronary arteries and a network of conduction-like cells within the atria that display phenotypic characteristics similar to those in the ventricle. However, consistent phenotypic differences do exist between working myocytes and cells of the conduction system.[9,13-16,55-57] One self-evident difference is more rapid longitudinal spread of electrical excitation. Compared with working myocytes, conduction cells are also typically characterized electrophysiologically by faster AP upstroke, prolonged AP duration, higher membrane diastolic potential, and greater electrical restitution properties (see Fig. 11-3). In terms of molecular

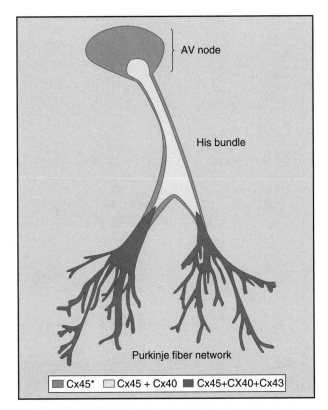

**FIGURE 11-4.** Connexin distribution patterns in the mouse AV conduction system (see references 37 and 39). Connexins define distinct compartments of cardiomyocytes along the axis of AV conduction. Note that the domain of Cx45 expressing tissue encompasses the entire AV conduction system and is always slightly broader than those domains coexpressing other connexins. Cx40 expression occurs within a coaxial core of cells found mainly in the His-Purkinje system. (See color plate.)

phenotype, a number of working myocyte-specific genes are typically not expressed or expressed at considerably lower levels by conduction cells.[58-60] Genes usually associated with neural tissues or skeletal muscle, including neurofilaments, CNS-associated glycoproteins, and myofiber contractile apparatus proteins, are often found localized to subpopulations of conduction cells in different species.[14-16,46,61-70] Conduction cells also possess distinct sets of ion channels,[71-73] channel-associated proteins,[74,75] and gap junctional connexins.[39,40,76-82] Because the gap junction is the organelle of most pertinence to cell-to-cell conductance of excitation, the intercellular coupling properties of these specialized tissues deserve special attention.

Cx40 was first identified as the predominant isoform of the His-Purkinje system in the chick.[77] In all higher vertebrates thus far examined, Cx40 is also the major connexin isoform of the His-Purkinje system.[39,40,78-81] Nonetheless, studies in various species, including humans, indicate that variations in levels and isoforms of other connexins can occur within the developing and mature conduction system (e.g., for mouse in Fig. 11-4). Indeed, studies in rodents suggest that complex patterns of coexpression of Cx40, Cx43, and Cx45 occur between conduction cells (see Fig. 11-4).[37,40,78-82] At present, the reason for such cell-to-cell variation in gene expression

pattern is not understood, although it may relate to electrical integration at Purkinje-myocyte junctions.

## CELLULAR ONTOGENESIS OF PACEMAKING AND CONDUCTION SYSTEM LINEAGES

The lineage of pacemaking and conduction cells is currently attracting much interest and some debate. This discussion is somewhat puzzling because the term *cell lineage* is used in slightly varying ways. Our thinking on this topic can be explained by an analogy. Several of us authors have what are termed *foreign accents*—a common occurrence in the United States. Sometimes we are asked "Where are you from?" Another consequence of having an accent is that we occasionally embarrass our children in front of their school friends because "we speak funny." It is a fascinating truism that given a tape recording of virtually any youngster of immigrant parents raised in the United States, most of us would hear an American dialect indistinguishable from that spoken by their school classmates. Indeed, it can be a tricky business using spoken accent to guess "where a person is from." Researchers using the phenotypic characteristics of cells as a guide to the embryonic origins of those cells are faced with a related problem. For example, because embryonic pacemaker myocytes and mature SA nodal cells share similar anatomic locations at the cardiac inflow, AP morphologies and unique genes in common do not necessarily imply a lineage relationship between these cells. One can never actually be sure of the convergence of function and phenotype. The only way to reliably establish the origins of cells within a given mature tissue is to tag the antecedents of those cells earlier using a stable marker of cell lineage that can only be transmitted vertically to the descendants of the initially tagged cells. To continue the previous analogy, a guess as to the origins of an American youngster would be improved by examining a family heirloom, passed down from his or her parents and grandparents.

### Lineage Tracing Studies

To date, direct lineage studies of nodal tissues have not been undertaken, although Burch et al.[83] have used the Cre-lox system in the mouse to provide insight into the origin of cells in the AV canal that probably include AV nodal progenitors. There is now a growing body of information on the lineage of conduction cells in the chick embryonic heart.[15,16,44] This work has relied on the use of defective retroviruses, modified so that they cannot produce further infectious virions but still retain the ability to integrate into and be replicated with the genomic DNA of the host cell. In a sense, the strategy takes advantage of a native characteristic of this unique class of animal pathogen. Although the modified retrovirus can no longer reproduce horizontally by infecting other cells, it can vertically propagate by making itself an involuntary "heirloom" of the particular cell lineage it has infected. One interesting feature of this method is that its power to generate information improves at lower levels of discernible retroviral infection; to assist detection, a marker such as LacZ is incorporated into the virus. This occurs because at lower titrations of infectious particles, virally defined clones generated by the division of an infected cell can be more readily resolved. As a result, in addition to lineage derivation, questions of phenotype diversification, changes in clonal composition over time, and, to a lesser extent, cell division behaviors can be addressed by analyses of these clonal groups of cells.

One of the initial fruits of this approach was a fresh perspective of the organization of ventricular muscle in the chick embryo, revealing that it had a compound organization based around facets of lineage-related myocytes.[84-86] Subsequent findings have related to the individual fate of myocytes within these facets and, in particular, the unequivocal origin of conduction tissues from cardiomyogenic rather than from neurogenic cells.[44,85] The timing of neural crest (NC) migration to the heart and expression of neuronal markers by conduction cells in various species led to the hypothesis that conduction cells were transdifferentiated from neurally derived lineages.[87] However, direct retroviral lineage tracing of NC progenitors in chick embryos revealed that a significant contribution by neural populations to the conduction system was unlikely.[85,88] Evidence from two groups, based on the use of Cre-lox technology to mark presumptive NC derivatives in the mouse embryo, also argued against a neurogenic contribution to the conduction system.[89,90] By contrast, microinjection of defective retrovirus into the embryonic chick heart before the arrival of migrating cell populations, such as the NC, resulted in frequent incorporation of lineage marker within cells of the conduction system.[44,85]

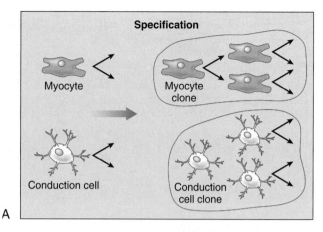

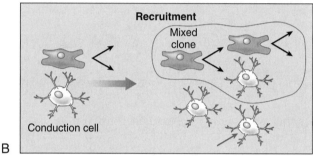

**FIGURE 11-5.** Outgrowth versus recruitment. Two models of conduction cell differentiation. The composition of cardiomyocyte clones gives clues as to how the specialized conduction network elaborates. It is predicted from an "outgrowth" model of conduction system differentiation (top panel) that individual cardiomyocyte clones will consist of only one cell type proliferating either from differentiated working myocyte or from conduction cell progenitors. Conversely, if "recruitment" of multipotent cardiomyogenic cells to the conduction system occurs (bottom panel), then it is predicted that clones will contain multiple cardiomyocyte phenotypes. Retroviral clonal analysis in the chick embryo supports a recruitment model (see Fig. 11-6).

## "Outgrowth" or "Recruitment" of a Cardiomyogenic Lineage within the Embryonic Heart

Although retroviral lineage tracing data has localized the progenitors of the developing conduction network to cardiomyogenic cells in the embryonic heart, there are different schools of thought as to how such cells give rise to this system of specialized tissues (Fig. 11-5). It has been proposed that the cellular constituents of conduction tissues are derived from the division of previously differentiated (specified) conduction cells—the *outgrowth* model. Alternately, it has been proposed that conduction cells are recruited from a pool of multipotent cardiomyogenic cells that have not yet differentiated a specialized phenotype—the *recruitment* model. Based on the first of these hypothetical options, the network of conduction tissue could be conceived as increasing in complexity by proliferative outgrowth from an original pool of conduction cells—rather like the roots of a tree growing into the ground. One difficulty for the outgrowth model is that commitment to non-DNA synthesis, and thus significantly reduced proliferation, is one of the earliest emerging characteristics of cells differentiating

into a conduction lineage.[85,91,92] This property appears to be a consistent feature of both avian and mammalian species. Thus, one must question how the mature conduction network would grow if it could only be derived from a specific pool of nondividing or very slowly dividing cells present in the millimeter-long heart of all vertebrate embryos. Presumably, if this were a conserved mechanism for elaboration of the conduction system, the dilemma would be more acute for whales than hummingbirds.

The phenotypes of myocytes composing retroviral clones in the developing chick ventricle poses a second problem for the outgrowth model, at least in this avian species. Retroviral targeting of cells in the looped, tubular heart has been found to result in the subsequent generation of virally defined clones that contained both working myocytes and conduction cells. This heterocellular motif was found within clones incorporating central conduction fascicles, such as the His bundle, and in the subendocardial and periarterial network of cells composing the peripheral conduction system[44,85] (Fig. 11-6). A clone containing working myocytes and conduction cells logically cannot occur if the only source of conduction cells is other conduction cells. Putting it

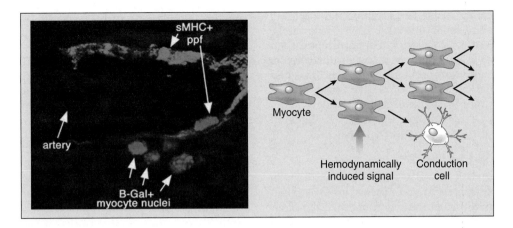

**FIGURE 11-6.** Induction of periarterial Purkinje fiber conduction cells. The right hand panel shows a cluster of red nuclei delineating a clone of LacZ expressing cells infected with a defective retrovirus. The clone contains both working myocytes and an sMHC+ (green in color insert) Purkinje fiber—a pattern consistent with the occurrence of localized recruitment of a multipotent progenitor cell to specialized myocardial lineages in the avian heart (e.g., Fig. 11-5). The left hand panel shows a model in which hemodynamically sensitive factors (e.g., the endothelin-1 signaling pathway) from arterial tissues locally mediate this divergence into either working myocytes or Purkinje fiber conduction cells within a cardiomyogenic lineage. (See color plate.)

another way, if only prespecified conduction progenitors gave rise to conduction cells, then one would expect to find myocardial clones composed only of these specialized cells. Thus, retroviral lineage analyses have lent support to a recruitment model of conduction system development in the chick. This model proposes that there is a pool of multipotent cardiomyogenic cells present in the embryonic heart and that the conduction system elaborates over development by a process of localized and progressive recruitment from this pool. Although birthdating analyses indicate that the conscription of cells to the central conduction system (e.g., the AV and retroaortic rings, His bundle, and bundle branches) ceases after the completion of ventricular septation, elaboration of the peripheral network of conduction cells by inductive recruitment appears to continue almost until hatching.[44,85]

Whether these findings in the chick embryo can be extended to other species is not known. There is a wealth of inferential morphologic, physiologic, and gene expression data in mammalian species, including humans, that would support the idea that the entire conduction system derives from the outgrowth of specific domains present within the early embryonic heart.[14,93] One of the most persuasive of these is a study by Rentschler et al.[43] who studied transgenic mice expressing LacZ under the control of a regulatory enhancer sequence derived from the engrailed-2 (En2) gene. The study reported that LacZ expression in one of the transgenic lines studied delineated the entire developing and mature cardiac conduction system extending proximally from the SA node to the most peripheral Purkinje fibers in the ventricles. Optical mapping was used to confirm that the LacZ expressing tissues demonstrated activation patterns consistent with the function of specialized conduction tissues. Significant LacZ expression also occurred in nonconduction system cells in this mouse, particularly in the atria. A subsequent study has indicated that a

neuregulin-induced expansion of the LacZ expressing domain in the heart of this transgenic may occur by conversion (i.e., recruitment) of non-LacZ expressing cells without recourse to increased proliferation.[94] Definitive answers as to whether the murine conduction system during normal development elaborates by proliferative outgrowth of specified progenitors or recruitment of noncommitted multipotent cells will probably require lineage and clonal analysis approaches analogous to those used in studies of the chick embryo.

## CELLULAR AND MOLECULAR FACTORS INVOLVED IN DIFFERENTIATION OF CONDUCTION OF LINEAGES

As described previously, the periarterial Purkinje fibers (see Fig. 11-1)—conduction cells that penetrate deep into the ventricles in association with the coronary arterial bed—are a unique feature of the chick heart. The study of these cells, which compose the most peripheral part of the conductive network in the chick, has helped shape ideas about the factors involved in the inductive recruitment of specialized cardiac lineages. To understand the evolution of these ideas, one must first understand the development of the coronary arterial bed.

The tissues that give rise to the arterial plumbing of the heart are not generated by outgrowth from the aorta as once thought but migrate into the tubular heart from the proepicardial organ (PEO)—a source of extracardiac mesenchyme.[95-102] In the chick embryo, after making contact with the looped, tubular heart at the AV canal (around embryonic day 3), cells from the PEO migrate over the myocardium, first forming the epicardium and subsequently initiating migration into the heart proper. Concurrent with the ingrowth of PEO cells, discontinuous endothelial channels form, anastomose, and eventually fuse with the aortic sinus initiating perfusion of the coronary bed around embryonic day 7.[103,104] Coronary arteries continue to elaborate, establishing a closed vascular bed around embryonic day 14.[105] Importantly, the upregulation of early markers of specialization such as Cx40 in Purkinje fibers in just a few myocyte layers around arteries begins around embryonic day 10,[77] correlating with the emergence of a functional arterial plexus.

## Is There a Link Between the Plumbing and the Wiring of the Heart?

Retroviral clonal analysis has revealed that cardiomyogenic cells are recruited to the conduction system in close association with the branching of coronary arteries.[44] If a functional arterial bed was involved in mediating localized patterns of recruitment to the peripheral conduction system, then it might be predicted that alterations to arterial branching would lead to concerted changes in Purkinje fiber distribution. Two complementary strategies involving either inhibition or activation of coronary arterial branching in chick embryos have been used to test this hypothesis.[106] Ablation of the cardiac NC results in a 3D derangement of the coronary vascular plexus[107] and dramatic reductions in the density of intramural arteries.[106] Concomitant with this suppression of coronary arterial development, it was found that differentiation of periarterial Purkinje fibers was significantly inhibited. No Purkinje fibers differentiated in NC-ablated hearts except those that occurred in association with the infrequent vascular structures that managed to persist; thus, arteries are necessary in the differentiation of the intramural component of the conduction system. In the second set of experiments, retroviral-mediated overexpression of FGF was used to promote localized zones of myocardial hypervascularization. Ectopic Purkinje fibers developed subepicardially (i.e., at a location at which Purkinje fibers do not normally differentiate) adjacent to vessels within these hypervascularized sectors, leading to the conclusion that these experimentally induced arterial branches were sufficient for the localized induction of Purkinje fibers.

The cell type that mediates this inductive process is unknown. As discussed subsequently there is evidence that endothelial cells may have a role—coronary arterial and endocardial endothelia in the cases of periarterial and subendocardial Purkinje fibers, respectively.[16] Certain extracardiac cell populations, including the cardiac NC[85,88] and epicardially derived cells,[102] also show intimate patterns of association with certain elements of the developing PCS. However, whether the interaction of these migratory cell populations with the PCS serve functions in the differentiation and/or maturation of cardiac specialized tissues remains to be determined.

## Molecular Induction and Patterning of Conduction Tissues

A noteworthy feature in relation to arterial development is that localized differentiation of periarterial Purkinje fibers correlates with initiation of significant perfusive

function in this part of the vascular bed; interestingly, Purkinje fibers never differentiate adjacent to veins. This observation has led to the hypothesis that paracrine signaling by arterial tissues, particularly those signals elicited by hemodynamic changes, might have a role in the molecular induction and patterning of conduction cells. Support for this idea has come from experiments in which cultured embryonic myocytes were exposed to endothelin-1 (ET-1), a shear-stress sensitive cytokine prominent in the endocardium and coronary arterial bed.[108-111] Treatment of embryonic myocytes with ET-1 was found to increase expression of some markers of Purkinje fiber cells.[58] Further experimental evidence of the ability of ET-1 to promote differentiation of Purkinje fibers *in vivo* has been provided by a strategy involving overlapping domains of viral-mediated expression of endothelin converting enzyme (ECE-1) and prepro ET-1 (a secreted but inactive precursor of ET-1).[59] Modification of preproET-1 to active ET-1 is a two-step process, first involving proteolytic cleavage to Big-ET-1 followed by a highly specific conversion of Big-ET-1 to ET-1 by the ECE-1 protease.[112,113] Exogenous coexpression of ECE-1 and preproET-1 in the embryonic chick heart resulted in the ectopic and precocious differentiation of Purkinje fibers.[59] In addition, the pattern of localized activation of secreted forms of the ET-1 ligand by exogenously expressed converting enzyme suggested that there is a mechanism that regulates the timing and location of endogenous Purkinje fiber differentiation (Fig. 11-7). Localized ET-dependent induction of embryonic myocytes *in vivo* may be explained by the distribution of endogenous ECE-1. This theory is supported by *in situ* hybridization analyses of ECE-1 mRNA distributions in the chick embryo,[59] which have revealed a time course of expression at the endocardium and coronary arteries consistent with the patterns of localized recruit-

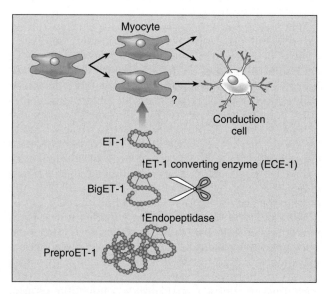

**FIGURE 11-7.** A model for the molecular induction of Purkinje fiber conduction cells. The site of specific cleavage of Big-ET-1 by ECE-1 may be a mechanism by which localized induction of conduction cells occurs.

ment of cardiomyogenic cells to the peripheral conduction system.[85]

Preliminary evidence indicates that ECE-1 expression may be subject to modulation by hemodynamics. Increasing load on the chick embryonic ventricle (by banding the outflow tract) leads to upregulated ECE-1 expression in the ventricular subendocardium[114] and precocious differentiation of His-Purkinje function.[115] Thus, the initial inference that coronary hemodynamics is an epigenetic determinant of selection of periarterial Purkinje fiber fate may be more generally applicable in the induction and patterning of the PCS (see Fig. 11-3). The interplay between biophysical factors and paracrine signaling in the embryonic heart may provide new avenues for exploring the origins of plasticity leading to congenital abnormalities in cardiac structure and function.

## Transcriptional Regulation of Conduction Lineage Differentiation

Presently, the understanding of the transcriptional control of conduction cell differentiation is at an early stage. In the chick embryo, expression of Msx-2, a homeodomain transcription factor, has been described as delineating progenitors of the central conduction system in a ring of tissue between the undivided ventricles of the early embryonic heart.[116] Although Msx-2 is also present in a subset of central conduction tissues at later developmental stages, it is never expressed in peripheral subendocardial and periarterial conduction cells. Recently, it has been shown that another transcription factor Csx/Nkx2.5 is present at elevated levels in the central[117] and peripheral[60,117] conduction systems of the developing chick heart. Pertinently, this tissue-restricted expression of Nkx2.5 is transient and correlates with the timing of cell recruitment to the central and peripheral conduction systems as characterized by retroviral lineage tracing studies.[85] Interestingly, Wnt11 appears to demonstrate a similar transient and differential pattern of expression in central elements of the developing chick peripheral conduction system similar to that described for Msx-2 and Nkx2.5.[118] Two other transcription factors, GATA4 and myoD, are also upregulated in the differentiating conduction cells of the chick embryo.[60] Although less is known about the detailed spatiotemporal pattern of expression of these latter two factors, myoD has been shown to be upregulated subsequent to induction of Purkinje fiber-like phenotype *in vitro* by ET-1. Although myoD is a well-characterized component of the transcriptional machinery regulating skeletal muscle differentiation,[119] other transcription factors present in this pathway have not been detected in either conduction cells *in vivo* or Purkinje-fiber-like cells promoted by ET-1 treatment.[60] Therefore, it seems likely that regulation of conduction cell differentiation in the chick is controlled by a transcriptional program distinct from those involved in the development of either working myocytes or skeletal muscle cells.

## DOES INSIGHT INTO CONDUCTION SYSTEM LINEAGE DIVERSIFICATION AFFECT UNDERSTANDING OF THE ORIGINS OF CARDIAC DISEASE IN HUMANS?

As in the chick embryo, Nkx2.5 is elevated in cells of the developing conduction system of humans and mice.[117] Consistent with a potential role in conduction cell differentiation, multiple and specific classes of heterozygous mutations in the Nkx2.5 locus have been shown to be associated with functional and structural defects of AV conduction in humans.[120,121] The mechanistic consequences of the specific genetic defects causing disruption of AV conduction in humans are beginning to be characterized in animal models. Recent studies in the avian embryo suggest that, although Nkx2.5 upregulation is necessary for the early stages of differentiation of specialized phenotype, continued overexpression of Nkx2.5 results in suppression of genes associated with the development of mature conduction cells.[122] Progressive AV conduction defects and heart failure have been reported in transgenic mice expressing one of the mutant forms of Nkx2.5 identified from studies of humans.[123] Interestingly, increases in Nkx2.5 expression have also been found in animal models of adult cardiac hypertrophy.[124] Thus, elevated levels of Nkx2.5 may also be part of an adaptive response of working myocardial tissues to certain disease states.

Holt-Oram syndrome, a rare human genetic disease characterized by limb and cardiac defects including conduction abnormalities, is associated with mutations in the T-box gene *Tbx5*.[125] Tbx5 expression has been reported in the human AV node,[126] and haploinsufficiency of this gene in mice leads to downregulation of the atrial and conduction system associated genes *ANF* and *connexin40*.[127] Similar to the phenotype observed in the connexin40 knockout,[79] mice with a single Tbx5 allele display abnormalities in ventricular activation including AV block.

The HF1b knockout mouse is a transgenic model that may provide a link between conduction tissue differentiation and cardiac disease.[75] Mice deficient in HF-1b survive to term but develop defects to ventricular activation and often die suddenly and unexpectedly from spontaneous ventricular arrhythmias. Single-cell analyses in these mice have revealed that markers distinguishing ventricular and conduction lineages were disrupted, with increased heterogeneity of APs measured from cardiomyocytes isolated from the ventricle. One hypothesis posed to account for the observed phenotype was that knockout of the *HF1b* gene may affect the mechanisms responsible for transition between myocyte and conduction cell fates during embryogenesis.

The growing body of evidence for diversification of myocyte phenotype (other than a simple division between ventricular myocytes and Purkinje fibers) may be important in understanding the developmental origins of cardiac disease. A distinct transitional population of myocytes (M cells; see Fig. 11-3), distributed subepicardially and intramurally, has been described as eliciting AP forms in a spectra intermediate between those of working myocytes and Purkinje fibers.[128,129] At present, the developmental biology of AP heterogeneity within the mammalian ventricular wall remains largely uninvestigated. This lack of information is cause for concern because recent data suggests that these nonuniformities in myocyte electrophysiology have clinical relevance in predisposing the heart to arrhythmia.[130,131] As outlined in this review, there is a growing understanding of the molecular and cellular mechanisms involved in the induction and patterning of specialized conduction cells in the embryonic chick ventricle. Whether this information will provide insight into developmental origins of other heterogeneities within atrial, ventricular, and conduction cell lineages in humans awaits further work.

## Acknowledgments

We would like to thank David Sedmera, Jacqui Bond, and Brett Harris for their critical reading of this manuscript. The assistance of Jane Jourdan in preparation of the manuscript references and proofreading is much appreciated. We also thank David Sedmera for conceiving and drafting Figure 11-2, and Tanya Rittman for her input on artwork.

## REFERENCES

1. Purkinje JE: Mikroscopisch-neurologische Beobachtungen. Arch Anat Physiol Swiss Med 1845;12:281-295.
2. His W: Die Tätigkeit des embryonalen Herzens und deren Bedeutung für die Lehre von der Herzbewegung beim Erwachsenen. Arb Med Klini Leipzig 1893;14-49.
3. Tawara S: Das Reizleitungssystem des Säugetierherzens—Eine anatomisch-pathlogische Studie über das Atrioventrikularbündel und die Purkinjeschen Fäden. Jena, Verlag von Gustav Fischer, 1906.
4. Wenckebach KF: Beiträge zur Kenntnis der menschlichen Herztätigkeit. (Contributions to the knowledge of human cardiac activity). Arch Anat Physiol 1906;297-354.
5. Hering HE: Nachweis, dass das His'sche Übergangsbündel Vorhof und Kammer des Säugethierherzens functionell verbindet. Pflügers Arch ges Physiol 1905;180:267-208.
6. Keith A, Flack MW: The form and nature of the muscular connections between the primary division of the vertebrate heart. J Anat Physiol 1907;41:172-189.
7. Davies F: The conducting system of the bird's heart. J Anat 1930;64:129-146.
8. James TN, Sherf L: Specialized tissues and preferential conduction in the atria of the heart. Am J Cardiol 1971;28:414-427.
9. Virágh S, Challice CE: The impulse generation and conduction system of the heart. In Challice CE, Virágh S (eds): Ultrastructure of the Mammalian Heart. New York, London, Academic Press, 1973, pp 43-89.
10. Viragh S, Challice CE: The development of the early atrioventricular conduction system in the embryonic heart. Can J Physiol Pharmacol 1983;61:775-792.
11. Davies MJ, Anderson RH, Becker AE: The Conduction System of the Heart. London, Butterworths, 1983.
12. Anderson RH, Ho SY: The architecture of the sinus node, the atrioventricular conduction axis, and the internodal atrial myocardium. J Cardiovasc Electrophysiol 1998;9:1233-1248.
13. Lamers WH, de Jong F, de Groot IJM, et al: The development of the avian conduction system. Eur J Morphol 1991;29:233-253.
14. Moorman AFN, de Jong F, Denyn MMFJ, et al: Development of the cardiac conduction system. Circ Res 1998;82:629-644.
15. Gourdie RG, Kubalak S, Mikawa T: Conducting the embryonic heart: Orchestrating development of specialized cardiac tissues. Trends Cardiovasc Med 1999;9:17-25.
16. Mikawa T, Gourdie RG, Hyer J, et al: Cardiac conduction system development. In Tomanek R, Runyan R (eds): Formation of the Heart and Its Regulation. Birkhauser, Boston, 2001, pp 121-135.
17. Kamino K, Hirota A, Fujii S: Localization of pacemaking activity in early embryonic heart monitored using voltage-sensitive dye. Nature 1981;290:595-597.
18. Yada T, Sakai T, Komuro H, et al: Development of electrical rhythmic activity in early embryonic cultured chick double-heart monitored optically with a voltage-sensitive dye. Dev Biol 1985;110:455-466.
19. Satin J, Fujii S, de Haan RL: Development of cardiac heartbeat in early chick embryos is regulated by regional cues. Dev Biol 1988;129:103-113.
20. Kamino K: Optical approaches to ontogeny of electrical activity and related functional organization during early heart development. Physiol Rev 1991;71:53-91.
21. Patten BM, Kramer TC: The initiation of contraction in the embryonic chicken heart. Am J Anat 1933;53:349-375.
22. de Jong F, Opthof T, Wilde AAM, et al: Persisting zones of slow impulse conduction in developing chicken hearts. Circ Res 1992;71:240-250.
23. Manasek FJ: Embryonic development of the heart. I. A light and electron microscopic study of myocardial development in the early chick embryo. J Morphol 1968;125:329-365.
24. Fishman MC, Chien KR: Fashioning the vertebrate heart: Earliest embryonic decisions. Development 1997;124:2099-2117.
25. Markwald RR, Wessels A: Overview of heart development. In Tomanek R, Runyan R (eds): Formation of the Heart and Its Regulation. Birkhauser, Boston, 2001, pp 1-22.
26. Goss CM: The physiology of the embryonic mammalian heart before circulation. Am J Physiol 1942;137:146-152.
27. Yasui K, Liu W, Opthof T, et al: I(f) current and spontaneous activity in mouse embryonic ventricular myocytes. Circ Res 2001;88:536-542.
28. Kaupp UB, Seifert R: Molecular diversity of pacemaker ion channels. Annu Rev Physiol 2001;63:235-257.
29. Baker K, Warren KS, Yellen G, et al: Defective "pacemaker" current (Ih) in a zebrafish mutant with a slow heart rate. Proc Natl Acad Sci USA 1997;94:4554-4559.
30. Koushik SV, Wang J, Rogers R, et al: Targeted inactivation of the sodium-calcium exchanger (Ncx1) results in the lack of a heartbeat and abnormal myofibrillar organization. FASEB J 2001;7:1209-1211.
31. Lieberman M, Paes de Carvalho A: The electrophysiological organization of the embryonic chick heart. J Gen Physiol 1965;49:351-363.
32. Lieberman M, Paes de Carvalho A: The spread of excitation in the embryonic chick heart. J Gen Physiol 1965;49:365-379.
33. Galper JB, Catterall WA: Developmental changes in the sensitivity of embryonic heart cells to tetrodotoxin and D600. Dev Biol 1978;65:216-227.
34. Sperelakis N: Electrophysiology of calcium antagonists. J Mol Cell Cardiol 1987;19:19-47.
35. Arguello C, Alanis J, Pantoja O, et al: Electrophysiological and ultrastructural study of the atrioventricular canal during the development of the chick embryo. J Mol Cell Cardiol 1986;18:499-510.
36. Alcolea S, Theveniau-Ruissy M, Jarry-Guichard T, et al: Downregulation of connexin 45 gene products during mouse heart development. Circ Res 1999;841:365-379.
37. Coppen SR, Severs NJ, Gourdie RG: Cx45 expression delineates an extended conduction system in the embryonic and adult rodent heart. Dev Genet 1999;9:82-91.
38. Coppen SR, Kodama I, Boyett MR, et al: Connexin45, a major connexin of the rabbit sinoatrial node, is co-expressed with connexin43 in a restricted zone at the nodal-crista terminalis border. J Histochem Cytochem 1999;47:907-918.
39. Gourdie RG, Lo CW: Cx43 gap junctions in cardiac development and disease. In Perrachia C (ed): Current Topics in Membranes, vol 49, Gap Junctions. Academic Press, San Diego, 2000, pp 581-602.

40. Severs NJ, Rothery S, Dupont E, et al: Immunocytochemical analysis of connexin expression in the healthy and diseased cardiovascular system. Microsc Res Tech 2001;3:301-322.

41. Chuck ET, Freeman DM, Watanabe M, et al: Changing activation sequence in the embryonic chick heart: Implications for development of the cardiac conduction system of the chick. Circ Res 1997;81:470-476.

42. Chuck ET, Watanabe M: Differential expression of PSA-NCAM and HNK-1 epitopes in the developing cardiac conduction system of the chick. Dev Dyn 1997;209:182-195.

43. Rentschler S, Vaidya DM, Tamaddon H, et al: Visualization and functional characterization of the developing murine cardiac conduction system. Development 2001;128:1785-1792.

44. Gourdie RG, Mima T, Thompson RP, et al: Terminal diversification of the myocyte lineage generates Purkinje fibers of the cardiac conduction system. Development 1995;121:1423-1431.

45. Blom NA, Gittenberger-de Groot AC, DeRuiter MC, et al: Development of the cardiac conduction tissue in human embryos using HNK-1 antigen expression: Possible relevance for understanding of abnormal atrial automaticity. Circulation 1999;99:800-806.

46. Schiaffino S: Protean patterns of gene expression in the heart conduction system. Circ Res 1997;80:749-750.

47. Franco D, Icardo JM: Molecular characterization of the ventricular conduction system in the developing mouse heart: Topographical correlation in normal and congenitally malformed hearts. Cardiovasc Res 2001;49:417-429.

48. Zahler R, Brines M, Kashgarian M, et al: The cardiac conduction system in the rat expresses the 2 and 3 isoforms of the Na+,K+-ATPase. Proc Natl Acad Sci USA 1992;89:99-103.

49. Gorza L, Schiaffino S, Volpe P: Inositol 1,4,5-triphosphate receptor in heart: Evidence for its concentration in Purkinje myocytes of the conduction system. J Cell Biol 1993;121:345-353.

50. Eschenhagen T, Laufs U, Schmitz W et al: Enrichment of G protein alpha-subunit mRNAS in the AV-conducting system of the mammalian heart. J Mol Cell Cardiol 1995;27:2249-2263.

51. Nakamura K, Robertson M, Liu G, et al: Complete heart block and sudden death in mice overexpressing calreticulin. J Clin Invest 2001;10:1245-1253.

52. Boyett MR, Honjo H, Kodama I: The sinoatrial node, a heterogeneous pacemaker structure. Cardiovasc Res 2000;47:658-687.

53. Vassall-Adams PR: The development of the atrioventricular bundle and its branches in the avian heart. J Anat 1982;134:169-183.

54. Lu Y, James TN, Yamamoto S, Terasaki F: Cardiac conduction system in the chicken: Gross anatomy plus light and electron microscopy. Anat Rec 1993;236:493-510.

55. Hoffman BF, Cranefield PF: Electrophysiology of the Heart. New York, Future Publishing Co, 1976.

56. Robinson RB, Boyden PA, Hoffman BF, et al: Electrical restitution process in dispersed canine cardiac Purkinje and ventricular cells. Am J Physiol 1987;253:H1018-1025.

57. Dangman KH, Danilo P Jr, Hordof AJ, et al: Electrophysiologic characteristics of human ventricular and Purkinje fibers. Circulation 1982;65:362-368.

58. Gourdie RG, Wei Y, Klatt SK, et al: Endothelin-induced conversion of heart muscle cells into impulse conducting Purkinje fibers. Proc Natl Acad Sci U S A 1998;95:6815-6818.

59. Takebayashi-Suzuki K, Yanagisawa M, Gourdie RG, et al: Induction of cardiac Purkinje fiber differentiation by co-expression of preproendothelin-1 and endothelin converting enzyme-1. Development 2000;127:3523-3532.

60. Takebayashi-Suzuki K, Pauliks LB, Eltsefon Y, et al: Purkinje fibers of the avian heart express a myogenic transcription factor program distinct from cardiac and skeletal muscle. Dev Biol 2001;234:390-401.

61. Sartore S, Pierobon-Bormioli S, Schiaffino S: immunohistochemical evidence for myosin polymorphism in the chicken heart. Nature 1978;274:82-83.

62. Wessels A, Vermeulen JL, Verbeek FJ, et al: Spatial distribution of "tissue-specific" antigens in the developing human heart and skeletal muscle. III. An immunohistochemical analysis of the distribution of the neural tissue antigen G1N2 in the embryonic heart; implications for the development of the atrioventricular conduction system. Anat Rec 1992;232:97-111.

63. Watanabe M, Timm M, Fallah-Najmabadi H: Cardiac expression of polysialylated NCAM in the chicken embryo: Correlation with the ventricular conduction system. Dev Dyn 1992;194:128-141.

64. Gorza L, Vitadello M: Distribution of conduction system fibers in the developing and adult rabbit heart revealed by an antineurofilament antibody. Circ Res 1989;65:360-369.

65. McCabe CF, Gourdie RG, Cole CJ, et al: Spatiotemporal distribution of the developmentally regulated protein EAP-300 during cardiac development. Dev Dyn 1995;203:51-60.

66. Alyonycheva T, Cohen-Gould L, Siewert C et al: Skeletal muscle-specific myosin binding protein-H is expressed in Purkinje fibers of the cardiac conduction system. Circ Res 1997;80:665-672.

67. González-Sánchez A, Bader D: Characterization of a myosin heavy chain in the conductive system of the adult and developing chicken heart. J Cell Biol 1989;100:270-275.

68. Vitadello M, Vettore S, Lamar E, et al: Neurofilament M mRNA is expressed in conduction system myocytes of the developing and adult rabbit heart. J Mol Cell Cardiol 1998;128:1833-1844.

69. Gorza L, Vettore S, Vitadello M: Molecular and cellular diversity of heart system myocytes. Trends Cardiovasc Med 1994;4:153-159.

70. Thornell LE, Price MG: The cytoskeleton in muscle cells in relation to function. Biochem Soc Trans 1991;19:1116-1120.

71. Callewaert G, Vereecke J, Carmeliet E: Existence of a calcium-dependent potassium channel in the membrane of cow cardiac Purkinje cells. Pflugers Arch 1986;406:424-426.

72. Light PE, Cordeiro JM, French RJ: Identification and properties of ATP-sensitive potassium channels in myocytes from rabbit Purkinje fibres. Cardiovasc Res 1999;44:356-369.

73. Han W, Wang Z, Nattel S: A comparison of transient outward currents in canine cardiac Purkinje cells and ventricular myocytes. Am J Physiol Heart Circ Physiol 2000;279:H466-H474.

74. Kupershmidt S, Yang T, Anderson ME, et al: Replacement by homologous recombination of the minK gene with lacZ reveals restriction of minK expression to the mouse cardiac conduction system. Circ Res 1998;84:146-152.

75. Nguyen-Tran VTB, Minamisawa S, Kubalak SW, et al: A novel genetic pathway for sudden cardiac death via defects in the transition between ventricular and conduction system cell lineages. Cell 2000;102:671-682.

76. Saffitz JE, Davis LM, Darrow BJ, et al: The molecular basis of anisotropy: Role of gap junctions. J Cardiovasc Electrophysiol 1995;6:498-510.

77. Gourdie RG, Green CR, Severs NJ, et al: Evidence for a distinct gap-junctional phenotype in conduction tissues of the developing and mature avian heart. Circ Res 1993;72:278-289.

78. Gros DB, Jongsma HJ: Connexins in mammalian heart function. Bioessays 1996;18:719-730.

79. Jalife J, Morley GE, Vaidya D: Connexins and impulse propagation in the mouse heart. J Cardiovasc Electrophysiol 1999;10:1649-1663.

80. Gourdie RG, Severs NJ, Green CR, et al: The spatial distribution and relative abundance of gap-junctional connexin40 and connexin43 correlate to functional properties of components of the cardiac atrioventricular conduction system. J Cell Sci 1993;105:985-991.

81. Gros D, Jarry-Guichard T, Ten Velde I, et al: Restricted distribution of connexin40, a gap junctional protein, in mammalian heart. Circ Res 1994;74:839-851.

82. Coppen SR, Dupont E, Rothery S, et al: Connexin45 expression is preferentially associated with the ventricular conduction system in mouse and rat heart. Circ Res 1998;82:232-243.

83. Davis DL, Edwards AV, Juraszek AL, et al: A GATA-6 gene heart-region-specific enhancer provides a novel means to mark and probe a discrete component of the mouse cardiac conduction system. Mech Dev 2001;108:105-119.

84. Mikawa T, Fischman DA: The polyclonal origin of myocyte lineages. Annu Rev Physiol 1996;58:509-521.

85. Cheng G, Litchenberg WH, Mikawa T, et al: Development of the conduction system involves recruitment within a multipotent cardiomyogenic lineage. Development 1999;126:5041-5049.

86. Mikawa T, Borisov A, Brown AMC, et al: Clonal analysis of cardiac morphogenesis in the chicken embryo using a replication-defective retrovirus. I. Formation of the ventricular myocardium. Dev Dyn 1992;193:11-23.

87. Gorza L, Schiaffino S, Vitadello M: Heart conduction system: A neural crest derivative? Brain Res 1988;457:360–366.

88. Poelmann RE, Gittenberger-de Groot AC: A subpopulation of apoptosis-prone cardiac neural crest cells targets to the venous pole: Multiple functions in heart development? Dev Biol 1999;207: 271–286.

89. Jiang X, Rowitch DH, Soriano P, et al: Fate of the mammalian cardiac neural crest. Development 2000;127:1607–1616.

90. Epstein JA, Li J, Lang D, Chen F, et al: Migration of cardiac neural crest cells in Splotch embryos. Development 2000;127: 1869–1878.

91. Thompson RP, Kanai T, Gourdie RG, et al: Organization and function of early specialized myocardium. In Clark EB, Markwald RR, Takao A (eds): Developmental Mechanisms of Congenital Heart Disease. Armonk, NY, Futura Publishing Co, 1995, pp 269–279.

92. Rumiantsev PP: DNA synthesis and mitotic division of myocytes of the ventricles, atria and conduction system of the heart during the myocardial development in mammals. Tsitologiia 1978;20: 132–141.

93. Wenink AC: Development of atrio-ventricular conduction pathways. Bull Assoc Anat (Nancy) 1976;60:623–629.

94. Rentschler S, Zander J, Meyers K, et al: Neuregulin-1 promotes formation of the murine cardiac conduction system. Proc Natl Acad Sci U S A 2002;99:10464–10469.

95. Poelmann RE, Gittenberger-de Groot AC, Mentink MM, et al: Development of the cardiac coronary vascular endothelium, studied with antiendothelial antibodies, in chicken-quail chimeras. Circ Res 1993;73:559–568.

96. Mikawa T, Gourdie RG: Pericardial mesoderm generates a population of coronary smooth muscle cells migrating into the heart along with ingrowth of the epicardial organ. Dev Biol 1996;174:221–232.

97. Dettman RW, Denetclaw W Jr, Ordahl CP, et al: Common epicardial origin of coronary vascular smooth muscle, perivascular fibroblasts, and intermyocardial fibroblasts in the avian heart. Dev Biol 1998;193:169–181.

98. Manner J, Perez-Pomares JM, Macias D, et al: The origin, formation and developmental significance of the epicardium: A review. Cells Tissues Organs 2001;169:89–103.

99. Ho E, Shimada Y: Formation of the epicardium studied with the scanning electron microscope. Develop Biol. 1978; 66:579–85.

100. Hiruma T, Hirakow R: Epicardial formation in embryonic chick heart: Computer-aided reconstruction, scanning, and transmission electron microscopic studies. Am J Anat 1989;184:129–138.

101. Manner J: Experimental study on the formation of the epicardium in chick embryos. Anat Embryol (Berl) 1993;187:281–289.

102. Gittenberger-de Groot AC, Vrancken Peeters MP, Mentink MM, et al: Epicardium-derived cells contribute a novel population to the myocardial wall and the atrioventricular cushions. Circ Res 1998;82:1043–1052.

103. Bogers AJ, Gittenberger-de Groot AC, Poelmann RE, et al: Development of the origin of the coronary arteries, a matter of ingrowth or outgrowth? Anat Embryol (Berl) 1989;180:437–441.

104. Waldo KL, Willner W, Kirby ML: Origin of the proximal coronary artery stems and a review of ventricular vascularization in the chick embryo. Am J Anat 1990;188:109–120.

105. Rychter Z, Ostadal B: Mechanism of the development of coronary arteries in chick embryo. Folia Morphol (Praha) 1972;19: 113–124.

106. Hyer J, Johansen M, Prasad A, et al: Induction of Purkinje fiber differentiation by coronary arterialization. Proc Natl Acad Sci U S A 1999;19:13214–13218.

107. Hood LC, Rosenquist TH: Coronary artery development in the chick: Origin and deployment of smooth muscle cells, and the effects of neural crest ablation. Anat Rec 1992;234:291–300.

108. Yanagisawa M, Kurihara H, Kimura S, et al: A novel potent vasoconstrictor peptide produced by vascular endothelial cells. Nature 1988;332:411–415.

109. Masaki T, Kimura S, Yanagisawa M, et al: Molecular and cellular mechanism of endothelin regulation: Implications for vascular function. Circulation 1991;84:1457–1468.

110. Yoshizumi M, Kurihara H, Sugiyama T, et al: Hemodynamic shear stress stimulates endothelin production by cultured endothelial cells. Biochem Biophys Res Commun 1989;161:859–864.

111. Yoshisue H, Suzuki K, Kawabata A, et al: Large scale isolation of non-uniform shear stress-responsive genes from cultured human endothelial cells through the preparation of a subtracted cDNA library. Atherosclerosis 2002;162:323–334.

112. Emoto N, Yanagisawa M: Endothelin-converting enzyme-2 is a membrane-bound, phosphoramidon-sensitive metalloprotease with acidic pH optimum. J Biol Chem 1995;270:15262–15268.

113. Xu D, Emoto N, Giaid A, et al: ECE-1: A membrane-bound metalloprotease that catalyzes the proteolytic activation of big endothelin-1. Cell 1994;78:473–485.

114. Mikawa T, Gourdie RG, Poma CP, et al: Induction and patterning of the impulse conducting Purkinje fiber network. In Clark, EB, Takao A, Nakazawa M (eds): Etiology and Morphogenesis of Congenital Heart Disease. Armonk, NY, Futura Publishing Co, 2000.

115. Reckova M, Rosengarten C, deAlmeida A, et al: Hemodynamics is a key epigenetic factor in development of the cardiac conduction system. Circ Res 2003;93:77–85.

116. Chan-Thomas PS, Thompson RP, Robert B, et al: Expression of homeobox genes Msx-1 (Hox-7) and Msx-2 (Hox-8) during cardiac development in the chick. Dev Dyn 1993;197:203–216.

117. Thomas PS, Kasahara H, Edmonson AM, et al: Elevated expression of Nkx-2.5 in developing myocardial conduction cells. Anat Rec 2001;263:307–313.

118. Bond J, Sedmera D, Jourdan J, et al: Wnt11 and Wnt7a are up-regulated in association with differentiation of cardiac conduction cells in vitro and in vivo. Dev Dyn 2003;227:536–543.

119. Olson EN, Srivastava D: Molecular pathways controlling heart development. Science 1996;272:671–676.

120. Schott JJ, Benson DW, Basson CT, et al: Congenital heart disease caused by mutations in the transcription factor NKX2-5. Science 1998;281:108–111.

121. Benson DW, Silberbach GM, Kavanaugh-McHugh A, et al: Mutations in the cardiac transcription factor NKX2.5 affect diverse cardiac developmental pathways. J Clin Invest 1999;104: 1567–1573.

122. O'Brien TX, Edmonson AM, Rackley MS, et al: Role of the cardiac transcription factor Nkx2.5 in the cardiac conduction system. Circulation 2001;14:II-288.

123. Kasahara H, Wakimoto H, Liu M, et al: Progressive atrioventricular conduction defects and heart failure in mice expressing a mutant Csx/Nkx2.5 homeoprotein. J Clin Invest 2001;108:189–201.

124. Thompson JT, Rackley MS, O'Brien TX: Upregulation of the cardiac homeobox gene Nkx2-5 (CSX) in feline right ventricular pressure overload. Am J Physiol 1998;274:H1569–573.

125. Basson CT, Bachinsky DR, Lin RC, et al: Mutations in human TBX5 cause limb and cardiac malformation in Holt-Oram syndrome. Nat Genet 1997;15:30–35.

126. Hatcher CJ, Goldstein MM, Mah CS, et al: Identification and localization of TBX5 transcription factor during human cardiac morphogenesis. Dev Dyn 2000;219:90–95.

127. Bruneau BG, Nemer G, Schmitt JP, et al: A murine model of Holt-Oram syndrome defines roles of the T-box transcription factor Tbx5 in cardiogenesis and disease. Cell 2001;106:709–721.

128. Antzelevitch C, Sicouri S: Clinical relevance of cardiac arrhythmias generated by afterdepolarizations: Role of M cells in the generation of U waves, triggered activity and torsade de pointes. J Am Coll Cardiol 1994;23:259–277.

129. Antzelevitch C, Shimizu W, Yan GX, et al: The M cell: Its contribution to the ECG and to normal and abnormal electrical function of the heart. J Cardiovasc Electrophysiol 1999;10:1297–1299.

130. Shimizu W, Antzelevitch C: Cellular basis for long QT, transmural dispersion of repolarization, and torsade de pointes in the long QT syndrome. J Electrocardiol 1999;32:177–184.

131. Anyukhovsky EP, Sosunov EA, Gainullin RZ, Rosen MR: The controversial M cell. J Cardiovasc Electrophysiol 1999;10:244–260.

## EDITOR'S CHOICE

Arad M, Moskowitz IP, Patel VV, et al: Transgenic mice overexpressing mutant PRKAG2 define the cause of Wolff-Parkinson-White syndrome in glycogen storage cardiomyopathy. Circulation 2003;107:2850–2856.

*A mutation that was initially associated with cardiomyopathy also leads to WPW; surprising finding that defects in glycogen storage can lead to both muscle and conduction system phenotypes via a type of storage disorder and secondary myocyte injury.*

Bruneau BG, Nemer G, Schmitt JP, et al: A murine model of Holt-Oram syndrome defines roles of the T-box transcription factor Tbx5 in cardiogenesis and disease. Cell 2001;106:709-721.

*Important paper that utilizes a genetically engineered mouse model to outline TBX5 pathways that are responsible for congenital heart disease and the onset of conduction system disease.*

Cheng CF, Kuo HC, Chien KR: Genetic modifiers of cardiac arrhythmias. Trends Mol Med 2003;9:59-66.

*A review that summarizes recent studies in experimental model systems that have uncovered new genetic pathways for arrythmogenesis that extend beyond the well-characterized list of channelopathies.*

Chien KR, Olson EN: Converging pathways and principles in heart development and disease: CV@CSH. Cell 2002;110:153-162.

*Summarizes new relationships between developmental studies and disease pathways; highlights of important Cold Spring Harbor Meeting.*

Harvey RP, Lai D, Elliott D, et al: Homeodomain factor Nkx2-5 in heart development and disease. Cold Spring Harb Symp Quant Biol 2002;67:107-114.

*One of the pioneers in the molecular analysis of cardiovascular developmental biology summarizes pivotal work of the most conserved and celebrated cardiac regulatory genes, Nkx2.5.*

Kanzawa N, Poma CP, Takebayashi-Suzuki K, et al: Competency of embryonic cardiomyocytes to undergo Purkinje fiber differentiation is regulated by endothelin receptor expression. Development 2002;129:3185-3194.

*Uncovering developmental pathways for conduction system formation: key role of endothelial signaling.*

Kondo RP, Anderson RH, Kupershmidt S, et al: Development of the cardiac conduction system as delineated by minK-lacZ. J Cardiovasc Electrophysiol 2003;14:383-391.

*Tracing the conduction system with genetically engineered mice.*

Ludwig A, Budde T, Stieber J, et al: Absence epilepsy and sinus dysrhythmia in mice lacking the pacemaker channel HCN2. Embo J 2003;22:216-224.

*Pacmaker channel KO mice link heart and brain dysfunction.*

Nguyen-Tran VT, Kubalak SW, Minamisawa S, et al: A novel genetic pathway for sudden cardiac death via defects in the transition between ventricular and conduction system cell lineages. Cell 2000;102:671-682.

*New pathway for cardiac arrythmogenesis and sudden death via defects in the developmental control of conduction system formation.*

Rentschler S, Morley GE, Fishman GI: Molecular and functional maturation of the murine cardiac conduction system. Cold Spring Harb Symp Quant Biol 2002;67:353-361.

*Leader in the field of cardiac conduction system development summarizes progress to date.*

Rentschler S, Zander J, Meyers K, et al: Neuregulin-1 promotes formation of the murine cardiac conduction system. Proc Natl Acad Sci USA 2002;99:10464-10469.

*Further convincing evidence of a critical role of endothelial signals in conduction system development.*

Robinson RB, Siegelbaum SA: Hyperpolarization-activated cation currents: From molecules to physiological function. Annu Rev Physiol 2003;65:453-480.

*One of the co-discoverers of the HCN pacemaker channel gene family highlights recent work in the field.*

Tanaka M, Berul CI, Ishii M, et al: A mouse model of congenital heart disease: Cardiac arrhythmias and atrial septal defect caused by haploinsufficiency of the cardiac transcription factor Csx/Nkx2.5. Cold Spring Harb Symp Quant Biol 2002;67:317-325.

*Links between Nkx2.5 and conduction system development and disease.*

Wang J, Chen S, Nolan MF, Siegelbaum SA: Activity-dependent regulation of HCN pacemaker channels by cyclic AMP: Signaling through dynamic allosteric coupling. Neuron 2002;36:451-461.

*Studies of the pacemaker channel penetrate to single molecule level; the amazing breakthroughs in understanding the structural basis of ion channel function by Rod Mackinnon are likely to have a major impact on cardiovascular biology and medicine in the coming decade.*

# chapter 12

# Cardiac Laterality and Congenital Heart Disease

*Pilar Ruiz-Lozano*
*Angel Raya*
*Kenneth R. Chien*
*Juan Carlos Izpisua-Belmonte*

## INTRODUCTION AND CLINICAL CONSIDERATIONS

The vertebrate body plan exhibits bilateral symmetry. However, the internal organs are asymmetrically located relative to the left and right sides of the midline. The position of the heart and viscera is strictly regulated and highly conserved throughout evolution. The normal left-right (L-R) anatomic position is called *situs solitus.* Laterality defects can occur in the form of isomerism, heterotaxia, or *situs inversus* (Fig. 12-1). Isomerisms result from a failure to achieve L-R asymmetry at the level of individual organs. Examples of isomerism include midline liver, same pulmonary lobation in both sides of the lung (pulmonary isomerism), and identical atrial structures in both sides of the heart (atrial isomerism). In contrast, heterotaxia describes a situation in which one or more of the individual organ systems develop with reversed L-R polarity (e.g., right-sided stomach, left-sided liver, or intestinal malrotation), because of a failure to properly coordinate the asymmetric development of multiple organ systems. The failure to properly align the L-R axis with the other two body axes, which is characterized by a complete inversion of the global L-R axis in the absence of additional clinical manifestations,[1,2] produces a condition known as *situs inversus.* Rough estimations place the incidence of L-R malformations in humans at 1 in 5000 births, with cases divided equally between *situs inversus* and *situs ambiguous* (heterotaxia).[3,4] This figure may underestimate the actual incidence of each. Complete reversal *(situs inversus)* may escape detection because it poses no detriment to the individual, and cases of *situs ambiguous* with normal hearts or with clinically silent cardiac malformations may not come to medical attention. For example, in an analysis of 18 patients with intestinal malrotation, 7 were found to have polysplenia, and 6 of them displayed either double or interrupted vena cava[5] (for a review see reference 6).

Except for the complete mirror-reversal of the heart, however, most cases of incorrect laterality lead to severe cardiac malfunction.[7] Certain congenital heart defects, such as arterial inversion, atrioventricular discordance, or ventriculoatrial discordance, can be considered as het-erotaxia or segmental defects of *situs. Situs* defects that do not involve the heart are more rare and include polysplenia, abnormal lung lobation, anomalies in the major vessels, and anomalies in gastrointestinal mesenteric attachment.

The discordance between organ *situs* observed in individuals with heterotaxia suggests that the pathways determining *situs* for individual organs are separable. However, certain laterality defects in different organs seem to be associated, suggesting coincidental specification of their primordia. Left atrial isomerism is associated with left bronchial isomerism, bilateral anterior caval veins, and ambiguous atrioventricular junction but a relatively normal ventriculoarterial junction.[8] In certain congenital syndromes, such as Kartagener's syndrome, abnormalities in organ *situs* are associated with defects in the development of cilia[9] and respiratory and fertility dysfunction.

## EVOLUTIONARY PERSPECTIVE

Asymmetries in the positioning of the internal organs are characteristic of vertebrates. However, invertebrate organisms show subtle but strictly conserved asymmetric patterns. For example, the gut of the fruit fly *(Drosophila melanogaster)* rotates in a very conserved and genetically regulated manner.[10] From an evolutionary perspective, the progression from bilateral symmetry to global, handed asymmetry requires important changes on at least three distinct levels of organization. These could have arisen in three sequential steps. The first step—the evolution of individual organ asymmetries—would have provided an initial level of complexity over the ancestral state of simple bilateral symmetry. The next step—the development of globally coordinated asymmetry—would have required the evolution of an additional level of regulation to ensure that all of the developing organ systems adopted consistent L-R orientations relative to each other. The final stage—characterized by global, *handed* asymmetry—would have required the innovation of an initial biasing mechanism to consistently orient the L-R axis with reference to the other two primary axes of the body.

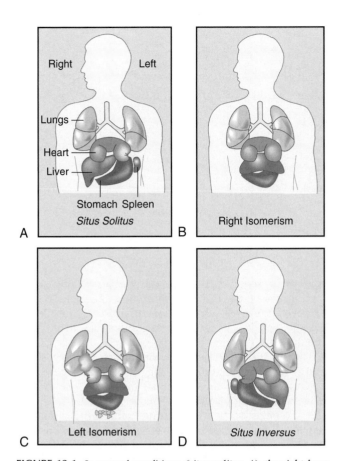

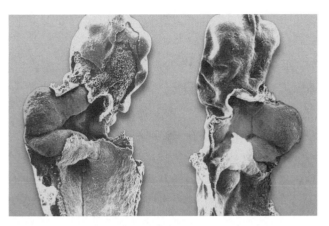

**FIGURE 12-2.** Developing heart (in red in color plate) in chick embryos shows the importance of retinoic acid on the correct heart asymmetry. Exposure to normal retinoic acid concentrations results in a heart that loops properly *(left image)*. After exposure to elevated levels of retinoic acid, however, the heart loops in the opposite direction *(right image)*. (See color plate.) *(Modified from Izpisua Belmonte JC: How the body tells left from right. Sci Am 1999;280[6]:46–51.)*

**FIGURE 12-1.** In normal conditions *(situs solitus, A)*, the right lung has three lobes, whereas the left lung has two. In addition, the apex of the heart points to the left side, the liver is on the right side, and the stomach and spleen are on the left side. Although not shown in the figure, the gut coils counterclockwise in the abdominal cavity. In the condition known as right isomerism *(B)*, also called asplenia syndrome, the heart and lungs are double-right (as indicated by the structure of the heart chambers and by both lungs having three lobes), as is the liver, which is generally found in a midline position. The stomach may be located on either side or in the midline, and the spleen is absent. In left isomerism *(C)*, also called polysplenia syndrome, the heart and lungs are double-left; the liver may be double-left, located in a midline position, or normal; and the stomach is usually found in a midline position. There is always more than one spleen (termed splenules), although multilobulated single spleens may also occur. *Situs inversus* refers to the complete mirror-image reversal of organ asymmetry *(D)*. Because laterality defects are highly variable, the figure depicts simplified cases, and is not intended to portray accurately the whole range of possible defects. The terms *situs inversus* and right or left isomerism can also be used to describe laterality defects in individual organs, even if they are not included in specific syndromes. (See color plate.) *(Modified from Izpisua Belmonte JC: How the body tells left from right. Sci Am 1999;280[6]:46–51.)*

## GENETICS OF THE LATERALITY SYNDROMES

The existence of inherited human syndromes with laterality defects (Figs. 12-1 and 12-2), together with the description of mouse and zebrafish mutants strongly suggests that the process of L-R determination is under genetic control.[11-15] This expectation has been confirmed by the recent identification of several genes that display striking, side-specific patterns of expression in

the early embryo. Recent studies in *Xenopus,* chicks, and mice have led to the description of a cascade of gene expression that regulates organ position in vertebrates.[8,12,13,16-21] Also, surgical manipulations in chick and frog embryos have further helped define the roles that specific embryonic structures play during the process of L-R determination. This experimental data suggest that the positions of internal organs are genetically controlled at four main levels: (1) the initial breaking of symmetry, which leads to the establishment of specific patterns of gene expression in and around the embryonic organizer; (2) the relay of L-R positional information from the organizer to the lateral plate mesoderm (LPM); (3) the stabilization of broad domains of side-specific gene expression in the LPM; and (4) the transfer of L-R information to the organ primordia and the elaboration of specific programs of asymmetric morphogenesis.

## The Initial Breaking of Symmetry

The embryo must integrate information concerning the relative orientations of the anteroposterior (AP) and dorsoventral (DV) axes, which are established at an earlier stage in development, and use this information to produce an initial difference or "bias" between cells on either side (left or right) of the embryonic midline.

Recent studies in the mouse[22-24] and the mouse node[25] have provided the first experimentally deduced model of L-R axis determination from any class of vertebrate (Figs. 12-3 and 12-4). The term *node* in mammals defines a structure that is equivalent to the early embryonic organizer region identified through classical transplantation studies in frogs (Spemann's organizer) and in birds (Hensen's node). The node induces the axial specification of the body plan, and it is the source of the axial mesoderm, head primordia, endoderm lining the foregut, notochord, and axial mesoderm responsible for patterning the neural tube and somites.[26,27] The involvement of the mouse node in L-R specification may come from the

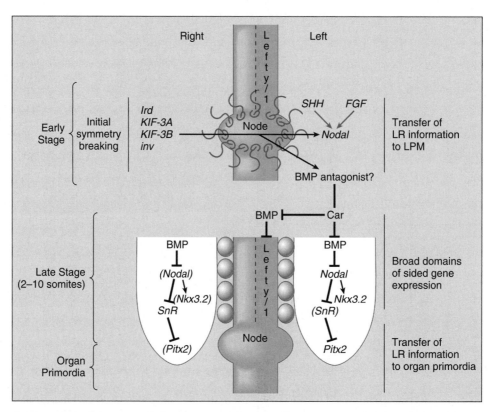

**FIGURE 12-3.** In the early mouse embryo, it is postulated that a leftward nodal flow activates left-specific gene expression, represented by asymmetric expression of Nodal in and around the node. Several components of the molecular motors in the cilia have been shown to be necessary for this initial breaking of symmetry (lrd, KIF-3A, KIF-3B). The product of the *inv* gene is also necessary for this step, although its exact function is still unclear. The transfer of asymmetric information from the node to the LPM is carried out in the chick by means of the protein Caronte. Car protein on the left side antagonizes the repression of *Nodal* transcription by BMPs. In turn, Nodal represses SnR, which is itself a repressor of Pitx2, so that SnR is expressed on the right and Pitx2 in the left LPM. At the midline, the Lefty-1 protein might act as a barrier, thus preventing ectopic expression of left-specific genes in the right side of the embryo. *(Model modified from Capdevila J, Vogan KJ, Tabin CJ, Izpisua Belmonte JC: Mechanisms of left-right determination in vertebrates. Cell 2000:101:9–21.)*

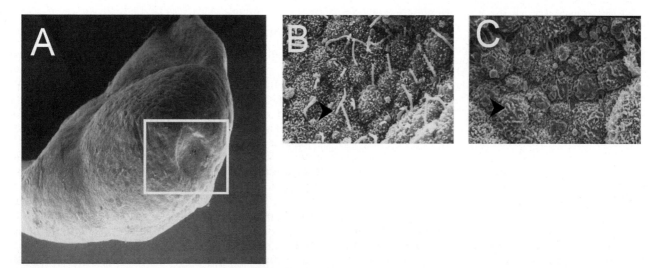

**FIGURE 12-4.** Scanning electron microscopy of mouse embryonic day 8. *A,* Localization and structure of the normal mouse node. *B,* High magnification of the embryonic node showing monociliated cells in wild-type embryos. *C,* Ciliary deficiency in *Kif3A*-mutant mice. Nodal cilia may mediate the initial breakage of bilateral symmetry in vertebrates. *(Image provided by Marszalek J, Goldstein L, UCSD, San Diego, CA.)*

activity of a cluster of monociliated cells that are located in the ventral portion of the node. These nodal monocilia, which project into the extraembryonic space surrounding the egg cylinder, exhibit a vortical motion that generates a leftward flow of extraembryonic fluid in the node region. This so-called nodal flow has been proposed to function as the initiating event in the formation of the L-R axis by causing an initial L-R difference in the relative distribution of one or more secreted factors, thus triggering the activation of distinct signaling pathways on the left and right sides of the embryo (reviewed in reference 15). Alternatively, activation of the nodal cilia itself may be the signal that triggers the first asymmetry.[28]

Strong support for the cilia model has come from studies of the *inversus viscerum (iv)*[29] and *(inv)*[30] mice, classical mutant strains characterized by a high incidence of *situs inversus.* Half of the *iv* mutant mice display *situs inversus,* suggesting that the function of the *iv* gene is to regulate the handed development of L-R asymmetries, because in its absence asymmetries develop randomly.[31,32] The product of the *iv* locus, called left-right dynein (Lrd),[33] has been identified as an axonemal-type dynein heavy chain molecule expressed specifically in monociliated cells of the node from late gastrulation through early neurulation.[21,34] In contrast to the randomized *situs* in the *iv* mutation, all *inv* homozygous mutants display *situs inversus.* The product of the inv mutation has also recently been characterized.[35] The *inv* gene product encodes an ankyrin-repeat protein.[35] To achieve its function inversin does not need to be expressed in a tissue-restricted manner (because ubiquitous expression of inversin rescues the *inv* phenotype), but perhaps it is required for providing cell polarity in certain structures.[35] In keeping with the presumed function of Lrd as a critical force-generating component of the ciliary machinery, nodal cilia in the *iv* mutant mice are completely immotile and fail to produce any discernible nodal flow.[23] Nodal flow in the *inv* mutants is also affected (slower),[23] and recent studies point to the existence of two populations of monicilia in the node: motil cilia (Lrd positive), and immotile cilia (polycystin-2 positive) that sense calcium signaling in the left margin at the node.[28] These findings support studies of human populations, in which a correlation between *situs* abnormalities and ciliary dysfunction has long been noted.[9] The development of complex *situs* defects in mice deficient for either KIF3A[24,36] or KIF3B,[22] two kinesin molecules required for the assembly of nodal cilia, lends further support to the hypothesis that nodal cilia in the mouse are critical for proper establishment of the L-R axis. In addition, genetic mapping in humans has led to the discovery of the gene *DNAH5,* which encodes for a protein expressed in the node and other ciliary structures. Mutations in *DNAH5* result in ciliary defects and *situs inversus* in 50% of the patients with ciliary dysfunction,[37] demonstrating that mutations in human *DNAH5* randomize the position of internal organs.

The suggestion that the node is the site where symmetry is first broken is also supported by a series of observations made in chicks, in which a transient morphologic asymmetry is apparent at the early chick node.[38]

In the avian model the morphologic asymmetry is paralleled with asymmetrical gene expression in the node. Likewise, a number of genes are expressed asymmetrically at the chick node, including left-side expression of *Sonic hedgehog (Shh),*[38] and right-restricted expression of *Fgf-8.*[39] The fact that these early asymmetries in the chick are all centered at the node strongly implies that this is the site where L-R patterning information first originates in the chick and argues that the underlying mechanism of symmetry-breaking might be similar between birds and mammals. If the activity of monocilia does represent a universal mechanism for specifying the L-R axis in vertebrates, one would expect to find cilia and other components of the ciliary machinery (including homologues of Lrd) present in the organizer region of other vertebrate model systems. In fact, recent studies have demonstrated the existence of conserved nodal cilia in a broad spectrum of species, which include chick, Xenopus and zebrafish.[40] Thus, although it remains to be seen how general this newly postulated mechanism of symmetry-breaking truly is, it has produced a number of testable hypotheses and remains the only model of L-R axis determination currently supported by empirical studies.

## Transmission of Left-Right Information from the Node to the Lateral Plate

Accordingly to the current model, the earliest molecular asymmetries in the mouse occur after the establishment of the nodal flow. Regardless of how L-R orientation is established in different species, the intermediate part of the determination process converges on Nodal expression on the left side of the embryo, and on bone morphogenetic protein (BMP) signaling on the right side of the embryo (Figs. 12-3 and 12-5).[12,41] Once the orientation of L-R asymmetry relative to the A-P and D-V body axis is established, asymmetric cascades of gene expression (distinct left- and right-sided cascades) reinforce and transmit this information to the tissues that form asymmetric organs.[12,41] Small domains of asymmetric gene expression can be detected at the perinodal region with the appearance of the TGF-β family members *Nodal and Lefty-1.* The transmission of the L-R positional information from the organizer to broader domains of the LPM can be monitored at the molecular level by the establishment of a second, broader domain of left-sided *Nodal* expression in the LPM.[42-44] Significantly, left-specific expression of *Nodal* within the LPM has been observed in all vertebrates examined to date, and aberrant patterns of *Nodal* expression in the LPM are closely correlated with *situs* abnormalities in a variety of mutants and experimental situations.[14,42-48] Moreover, misexpression of *Nodal* on the right side of the embryo is sufficient to randomize *situs* determination in multiple organ systems,[47,49]suggesting that *Nodal* plays a critical role in coordinating development of the global L-R axis.[11]

The relay of L-R positional information from the node to the lateral plate is marked by the interaction of several TGF-β family members. Induction of *Nodal* within the

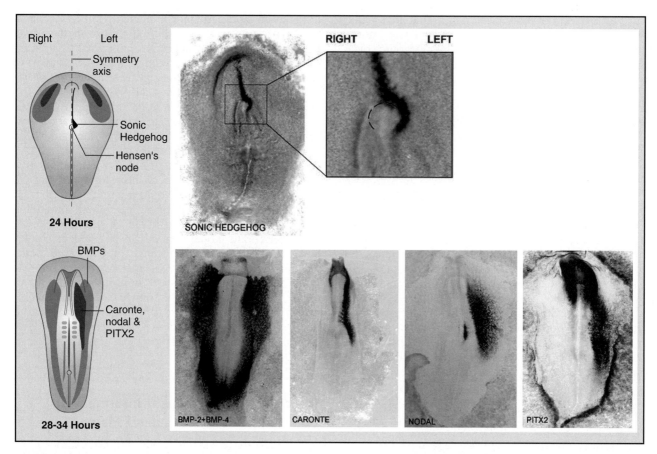

**FIGURE 12-5.** Genes that are active on one side of the embryo, such as in this early chick, establish the normal L-R asymmetry of internal organs. The gene encoding Sonic Hedgehog (dark blue in top images, in color plate) is one of the first to become active, on the left side of the embryo above the Hensen's node. Ten hours later, Sonic Hedgehog is no longer active, and its activity has been replaced by that of *Nodal* and *Pitx2* (dark blue in the lower images). The transfer of asymmetric information is carried out by the protein Caronte (in dark blue in middle images), whose left-sided expression is induced by Sonic Hedgehog. Caronte allows the expression of Nodal on the left side of the embryo, by inhibiting BMPs activity (in green in middle images), which, in turn, represses Nodal expression on the right side. (See color plate.) *(Modified from Izpisua Belmonte JC: How the body tells left from right. Sci Am 1999;280[6]:46–51.)*.

left LPM represents a key step in the establishment of the L-R axis and *Shh* is necessary and sufficient for inducing *Nodal* expression in the left LPM.[42,49] Recent studies suggest that a number of different molecules may participate in this inductive process, acting in a cooperative manner to achieve the rapid spread of *Nodal* signaling throughout the entire lateral plate. A class of TGF-β related ligands known as BMPs suppress *Nodal* expression in the right side.[50] Similarly, suppression of the available BMPs in the left side of the embryo (chicken) is required for *Nodal* expression in the left side, both adjacent to the node and in the LPM. In the avian embryos, suppression of BPM signaling in the left side is achieved the *Cerberus*-related gene *Caronte (Car)*.[51-53] *Car* functions, in part, by binding BMP. *Car* expression is initially bilaterally symmetrical, but it later becomes restricted to a small patch of cells in the left side, adjacent to the *Shh*-expressing cells of the node, and subsequently spread throughout the entire left LPM. Consistent with its putative role as a key intermediate signal between *Shh* and *Nodal*, *Car* expression is dependent on *Shh* signaling, and misexpression of *Car* is sufficient to induce *Nodal* expression. These results support a model in which BMP signaling functions to repress *Nodal* expression bilater-

ally within the LPM; the antagonistic activity of *Car* operates, in turn, to relieve the repressive effects of BMPs on the left side of the embryo, leading to the activation of *Nodal* transcription in the left LPM.

Although no homologues of *Car* have been identified so far in other vertebrates, several lines of evidence suggest that the regulation of *Nodal* expression by BMP-mediated repression may be a conserved feature of the vertebrate L-R cascade. In the mouse, for example, a deficiency in *Smad-5*, a gene that encodes an intracellular mediator of BMP signaling, results in bilateral expression of *Nodal* in the LPM.[54] This suggests that BMPs, which are also expressed bilaterally in the LPM in the mouse,[55] might actively repress *Nodal* through a pathway involving *Smad-5*. Similarly, in *Xenopus*, it has been recently shown that a BMP-dependent pathway, signaling through the ALK2 receptor, functions to repress *Nodal* on the right side of the embryo.[20,56-58] However, in zebrafish, unlike in other vertebrates, *BMP4* is expressed asymmetrically in the heart field, and it appears to be exclusively involved in the determination of heart *situs*. Whether any other BMP in the zebrafish embryo acts in the LPM by repressing *Nodal* transcription remains to be determined.

BMP antagonism may not be the only factor regulating *Nodal* expression. Indeed, there is evidence to suggest that *Nodal* maintains its own expression within the left LPM. This hypothesis is based on the observation that mice deficient for the EGF-CFC gene *Cryptic,* which encodes an essential, extracellular cofactor for *Nodal,* fail to express *Nodal* in the left LPM, despite the fact that the earlier asymmetric expression of *Nodal* in the perinodal region develops normally in these mice.[59,60] These observations imply that the medial asymmetric domain of *Nodal* may participate directly in the induction of the second, broad domain of *Nodal* within the LPM, or alternatively, that *Nodal* signaling may be required for the maintenance of its own transcription within the left LPM, operating via a classical positive feedback loop. The finding that *Nodal* can activate transcription from its own promoter supports both hypotheses.

In summary, the transfer of L-R information from the node to the periphery, and the subsequent amplification and spread of signals within the lateral plate, is achieved by the combinatorial action of a number of factors, all of which appear to converge on the regulation of *Nodal* transcription. In particular, the antagonism of BMP-mediated repression of *Nodal* on the left side appears to be an important feature of the vertebrate L-R cascade, which is shared by several vertebrates and represents an essential step in the initial establishment of *Nodal* expression within the left LPM. Other positively acting factors, including *Nodal* itself, may likewise participate in this initial inductive process and may also contribute to achieving the rapid spread of *Car* and *Nodal* expression throughout the entire left lateral plate. Researchers are now faced with the challenge of establishing the various roles that these inductive factors (and others to be discovered) play in the process and of determining the degree to which specific molecular players, such as *Car,* have been conserved over the course of evolution.

## Stabilization of Side-Specific Gene Expression in the LPM

The failure to maintain distinct domains of side-specific gene expression can result in a wide range of laterality defects. Therefore, vertebrate embryos have adopted a number of regulatory strategies to prevent the contralateral spread of asymmetric signaling cascades.

A first level of regulation is provided by members of the FGF family, as shown by experiments in chicken embryos. *Fgf-4* and *Fgf-8* are both expressed exclusively in the right side of the node beginning at stage 5, in a pattern that can be considered complementary to *Shh.*[39,61] Significantly, application of FGF protein to the left side of the node blocks induction of normal left-sided genes, including *Car*[51,52] and *Nodal.*[39] These observations suggest that FGFs may function to prevent the inappropriate activation of the *Shh*-dependent, left-sided pathway in cells to the right of the node, ensuring that the fidelity of the initial L-R decision is maintained during subsequent stages of development.

A second level of regulatory control that is common to all vertebrates occurs at the level of the embryonic mid-line. In particular, it has been noted that mouse and zebrafish mutants with defects in axial midline structures often display L-R patterning defects in conjunction with altered expression of left-specific genes.[45,62-66] Likewise, studies of laterality defects in conjoined twins have implied that long-range L-R patterning signals do exist and can travel substantial distances *in utero* but are prevented from crossing the embryonic midline. Together, these and other observations have led to the proposal that a "midline barrier" (physical, biochemical, or both) exists that prevents the activation of left-specific genes in the right side of the embryo, presumably by preventing long-range signals from crossing over from the left to the right side.[49,67]

The analysis of *lefty-1*-deficient mice has provided valuable insights into the barrier problem. In the mouse, *lefty-1* is expressed in the left half of the floor plate,[68] and its inactivation results in expression of left-specific genes in the right side of the embryo,[67] demonstrating that *lefty-1* activity is required for midline barrier function. Because Lefty proteins are members of the TGF-β superfamily, it has been suggested that *lefty-1* might function at the midline by binding to *Car,* the presumed long-range signal that relays L-R information from the node to the left LPM, thereby preventing *Car* from interfering with the BMP-mediated repression of *Nodal* on the right side.[51,52] However, the possibility that Car and Lefty proteins interact physically still remains to be determined. Interestingly, in the chick, *Car* appears to act as the endogenous inducer of *lefty-1* expression in the midline (probably by antagonizing a local BMP activity), thus establishing a negative regulatory loop that could ensure that *Car* activity is completely restricted to the left side of the embryo.[51,52] In the mouse, *lefty-1* expression in the left side of the floor plate is mediated by a combination of bilateral enhancers and a right side-specific silencer.[69] Thus, it is conceivable that this right-specific silencer element may be responding to some BMP-dependent factor in the right side of the midline, whereas in the left side, the BMP-dependent pathway is antagonized by *Car* or some other BMP antagonist, leading to activation of *lefty-1* transcription.

These results also permit interpretation of the phenotype of *Shh*-deficient mice in the light of a requirement for *Shh* in maintaining the integrity of the midline barrier. Indeed, although the initial description of the phenotype of *Shh*-deficient mice did not report any laterality defects, a closer examination of the phenotype of these mice has revealed a number of distinct *situs* abnormalities, including left pulmonary isomerism and randomization of axial turning.[70,71] Like *lefty-1*-deficient mice, *Shh* mutant embryos also show ectopic expression of left-specific genes on the right side. These patterning defects can all be explained by the fact that *Shh*-deficient mice lack a discernible floor plate and fail to express *lefty-1,*[70,71] and thus are unable to restrict the contralateral spread of long-range signals originating from the left side.

One additional mechanism that appears to restrict the range of *Nodal* signaling is the putative negative feedback role of *lefty-2,* a second *lefty* gene expressed in the left LPM.[67] The antagonism of Nodal signaling by Lefty proteins, which appears to be highly conserved among vertebrates,[72-74] involves a direct competition between Nodal and Lefty proteins for common receptor binding sites, fine-tuning the amount of Nodal signal effectively received by cells. Because the *lefty-2* gene also appears to be a transcriptional target of Nodal signaling, it is thought that Lefty-2 functions as a feedback inhibitor of Nodal signaling, restricting its range of action. In light of these findings, it is possible that the presence of Lefty-1 in the midline might also serve to limit the contralateral spread of Nodal signaling by reducing the effective concentration of Nodal in regions further away from the source of Nodal production.

Altogether, a complex regulatory cascade of negative interactions plays a major role in stabilizing side-specific gene expression within the left LPM. Moreover, and although not identical, it appears that the basic pathway that stabilizes gene expression in the LPM is conserved among vertebrates and that the *lefty* genes play a crucial role, being at the crossroads of several key regulatory interactions.

## Asymmetric Organ Development

The establishment and stabilization of side-specific gene expression in the LPM is the strategy that the embryo uses to direct asymmetric development of organs. Thus, all the complex mechanisms outlined previously are aimed at providing a specific, consistent bias to the organogenetic processes, such that organ primordia develop by performing a stereotyped choreography of loops and turns that result in the normal disposition of organs.

An important factor acting downstream of *Nodal* in the left LPM is the bicoid-type homeobox gene *Pitx2*.[67,72,75-87] Unlike other left-specific genes, *Pitx2* is also expressed at subsequent stages in the left side of several LPM-derived organ primordia, including the heart, gut, and stomach, which makes it a good candidate to mediate the transfer of L-R information from the LPM to the developing organs. Recently, it has been shown that *Pitx2c,* which encodes one of the isoforms of the *Pitx2* gene, induces its own transcription, which could act as a maintenance mechanism after *Nodal* expression fades in the left LPM. Ectopic *Pitx2* has been shown to cause laterality defects in a variety of vertebrates, and *Pitx2*-deficient mice display laterality defects that include right pulmonary isomerism, which is consistent with a role for *Pitx2* as a left determinant.[77,78,80,88] However, the direction of heart looping is normal in *Pitx2*-deficient mice, which clearly indicates that factors in addition to *Pitx2* contribute to the asymmetric development of the heart. Thus, the identification of additional targets of *Nodal* or *Pitx2* expressed in organ primordia may provide further insights into the mechanisms that control asymmetric development of individual organs within the context of the development of the general L-R axis of the embryo.

Other genes shown to be downstream of *Nodal* in the LPM, such as *cSnail-related (SnR)* (in the right[89]) and the homeobox gene *Nkx3.2* (in the left),[90] may also be involved in directing asymmetric organ development.

The chick *SnR* gene,[89] which encodes a zinc-finger protein conserved in the mouse, is initially expressed bilaterally in the presumptive anterior cardiac mesoderm. As development proceeds, expression becomes stronger in the right LPM, and bilateral expression in the lateral edges of the somites is also detected. In the chick, *Nodal* acts as a repressor of *SnR* and as an activator of *Nkx3.2,* and treatment of embryos with antisense oligonucleotides specific for *SnR* results in randomization of L-R development, accompanied by ectopic expression of *Pitx2* in the right LPM. This observation suggests that *SnR* represses *Pitx2* expression and that *Nodal* activates *Pitx2* in the left LPM through repression of *SnR,* thus providing an additional level of regulatory complexity. Unexpectedly, the mouse *Nkx3.2* gene is also expressed in the right LPM, in contrast to the chick and *Xenopus Nkx3.2,* which are expressed on the left side.[90] However, the potential involvement of this gene in directing L-R development has not yet been characterized. Conceivably, other genes that are expressed in the right LPM and continue to be expressed in the right side of organ primordia might also exist, performing functions similar to the ones mediated by *Pitx2* on the left side.

A few specific targets for *Pitx2, SnR,* or *Nkx3.2* have been identified so far, and very little is known about how asymmetric organ development is controlled at the cellular level. However, there are several other known genes that display side-specific expression patterns in the heart, gut, or stomach primordia. For example, the extracellular matrix proteins Flectin[91] and hLAMP[91] are expressed in the left side of the heart tube in the chick, whereas *Fibrillin-2* is expressed in the right side. In zebrafish (but not in the mouse[55]), *Bmp-4* is expressed predominantly in the left side of the heart tube, and its function has been shown to be required for normal L-R development of the heart.[92] Also in zebrafish, *rtk2,* a gene encoding an Eph receptor, is expressed on the right side of the gut primordia, and the adhesion protein DM-GRASP is expressed in the right side in the hepatic diverticulum.[92] In the case of the digestive system, it is known that the left side of the stomach primordia has an increased growth rate that results in the so-called greater curvature of the stomach and, secondarily, in the precise positioning of the spleen in the left upper side of the abdominal cavity. Similarly, the asymmetric development of the intestine appears to depend on increased growth rates in two specific places: the duodenum and the central part of the primitive loop. Thus, local processes involving differential control of cell proliferation and/or cell death are likely to be involved in directing asymmetric development of organs, but clear links between particular gene activities and specific morphogenetic or proliferative functions in organ primordia are still missing.

The L-R cascade not only controls asymmetry of visceral organs but also controls two other processes: body axis rotation and body wall closure. The rotation of the body axis, or axial turning, follows the rightward looping of the heart tube in revealing the emergence of morphologic laterality in vertebrate embryos. In mice, rats, and other mammals, rotation of the embryo from a dorsally flexed to a ventrally flexed position always occurs in the same direction and results in several asymmetries, as revealed by the placement of chorioallantoic placenta, tail, and umbilical vessels to the right side, and vitelline vessels to the left side of the embryo. In chick embryos, a similar body rotation occurs between stages 11 and 20. It is thought that asymmetric cell proliferation in the embryonic body and extraembryonic membrane directs body rotation, and *Pitx2* may be involved in this process through its activities in the body wall mesoderm and amnion. In the mouse, *Pitx2* is expressed in both the left and right distal ends of the lateral body wall mesoderm at E-.5, with a stronger expression in the left side similar to the pattern observed in the chick. In *Pitx2*-deficient embryos, the body wall fails to close and abdominal and thoracic organs are extruded toward the left side, which could be due to the failure of the left lateral body wall to turn inward to meet the right lateral body wall in *Pitx2*-deficient embryos. Lack of *Pitx2* also appears to thicken the mesoderm and the amnion on the left side of the embryo through an increase in cell proliferation, creating a physical constraint that disrupts the movement of the left body wall and the rotation of the posterior part of the embryo.

It may appear intuitive that alterations in *situs* of abdominal organs always follow alterations of *situs* of thoracic organs; however, a perfect correlation between abdominal and thoracic *situs* is only observed in wild-type embryos and in the *inv* mouse, which exhibits a complete reversal of organ *situs*, presumably caused by a reversal of the whole system of L-R determination from the very early stages of development.[30] Instead, there are many situations in which thoracic and abdominal *situs* are uncoupled. In *lefty-1*-deficient mice, for example, laterality defects are restricted to thoracic organs, whereas *situs* of abdominal organs is completely normal.[67] This may be due to the fact that ectopic expression of *Nodal*, *lefty-2* and *Pitx2* is restricted to the anterior part of the LPM in these mutants. In some rare human syndromes, by contrast, normal thoracic *situs* is accompanied by abdominal *situs inversus* or *situs ambiguus*, which would suggest some alteration of L-R development that specifically affects abdominal organs, probably involving alterations of gene expression in the posterior LPM of the developing embryo. Taking this argument to the extreme, it follows that very specific organ *situs* defects may conceivably result from very localized alterations at different levels of the L-R cascade. Interestingly, the study of the regulatory sequences of the mouse *lefty-2* gene has revealed that the left-specific enhancer of *lefty-2* is actually composed of two separable elements: one for the anterior left LPM and another for the posterior left LPM.[69] This finding supports the notion that the expression of key regulators of L-R development may be controlled independently in the thorax and abdomen (reviewed in reference 12).

## HUMAN GENETICS OF LATERALITY

Autosomal dominant, autosomal recessive, and X-linked inheritance patterns have been described for syndromic human *situs* abnormalities. However, knowledge of these defects is largely limited to the clinical evaluation of familial cases. Several known genes in the L-R signaling cascade have been cloned in humans, often as a result of mapping candidate genes for diverse syndromes. Herein we briefly summarize the involvement of the recently described genes in the L-R cascade in human syndromes.

Primary ciliary dyskinesia (PCDS, MIM 242650) is characterized by recurrent infections of the respiratory tract resulting from reduced mucociliary clearance and by sperm immobility. In addition, one half of the affected individuals have *situs inversus* (Kartagener's syndrome), which results from randomization of the L-R asymmetry. Recently, it has been localized to chromosome 5p, a PDC locus containing the gene *DNAH5*. The *DNAH5* gene is an excellent candidate gene for Kartagener's syndrome because it is expressed in the embryonic organizer (together with lung; kidney; and to a minor extent heart, brain, and testis), its mutations manifest in an autosomal recessive inheritance, and 50% of the analyzed human samples display *situs inversus*. The described mutations in *DNAH5* result in deficient cilia characterized by an absence of the out dynein arm on all peripheral doublets. Mutations in rodents for other genes that alter ciliary function also result in *situs inversus (lrd, Kif3A, Kif3B)* but have severe developmental defects resulting in early embryonic death, suggesting that other functions may also account for the randomization of L-R asymmetry in these mutants. Together, the phenotype resulting from mutations in *DNAH5, lrd,* and the *Kif3A* and *Kif3B* genes support a role for nodal cilia in the regulation of L-R asymmetry in humans. However, the precise mechanism of its regulation is currently unknown.

*Lefty* mutations may be associated with human L-R axis malformations. Two lefty homologues, lefty A and lefty B, have been described in humans.[93] FISH analysis has localized the two *lefty* genes to 1q42, a region synthenic to the mouse 1H5, in which mouse lefty has been localized.[68] Lefty A is identical to ebaf, a cDNA previously identified in a search for genes expressed in human endometrium.[94] The deduced amino acid sequences of Lefty A and Lefty B are more similar to each other than to lefty-1 or lefty-2. Analysis of 126 human cases of L-R axis malformations showed one nonsense and one missense mutation in lefty A. Both mutations lie in the cysteine-knot region of the protein. Affected individuals show left pulmonary isomerism, cardiac malformations (atrioventricular canal defect, hypoplastic left ventricle, and interrupted inferior vena cava), polysplenia, and right-sided stomach.[95] With the exception of the spleen defects, this phenotype is reminiscent of the left thoracic isomerism displayed by the lefty-1 mutant mouse.

Mutation in the human X-linked *ZIC3* gene results in *situs ambiguous* with complex heart malformations; asplenia or polysplenia; and other midline abnormalities, including symmetric liver, abnormal lung lobation, and intestinal malrotation. These abnormalities result from the inability of the embryo to establish normal L-R asymmetry during development.[96] However, ciliary structure and function are normal. Human *ZIC3* is 91% identical to the previously identified mouse *Zic3* gene and is related to the *Drosophila* pair-rule gene *odd paired (opa)*. Interestingly, the fly *opa* is required for the appropriate expression of *wingless*, a segment polarity gene that interacts with *hedgehog* to maintain parasegmental identity.[97,98] These results suggest that the *ZIC3* gene product may interact with *Shh* to maintain the integrity of the midline barrier.

Heterozygous mutations of *Nodal* in humans may be associated with human *situs* abnormalities as shown by the *situs ambiguus* resulting from an arginine-to-glutamine amino acid substitution in the prodomain of Nodal. Because of its essential role in gastrulation,[99-101] mutations in human *Nodal* are extremely rare and suggest that the arg183gln mutation corresponds to a mild loss-of-function version of the *Nodal* gene.

The *ACVR2B* gene maps to 3p22-p21.3.[93,102] Mutations in the type IIB activin receptor gene are associated with low frequency to some cases of L-R axis malformations in humans.[103] Among 112 sporadic and 14 familial cases of L-R axis malformations, 2 missense substitutions in *ACVR2B* were detected.[103]

In humans, *Shh* and *Pitx2* map in 7q36 and 4q25-q26, respectively. *Shh* is a candidate gene for the autosomal dominant holoprosencephaly type 3[104] and for basal cell carcinoma (BCC). Mutations in the *Pitx2* homeodomain[84] and reduction of *Pitx2* expression have been correlated with Reiger's syndrome. However, laterality defects resulting from mutations in the human *Shh* or *Pitx2* loci have not been detected so far, probably because of the deleterious nature of these mutations if they occur in a homozygous state.

## GENES AND ENVIRONMENT

Environmental factors are risk factors in the development of malformations in the L-R axis. For instance, exposure to high doses of retinoic acid can induce laterality defects in a variety of vertebrates, including humans. Retinoid acid exposure in the embryo has the same consequences as mutations in *lefty-1* gene.[67] Retinoic acid exposure decreases the expression of *lefty-1*, thus disrupting the definition of the embryonic midline.[71,105]

An increased risk of L-R malformations have also been observed in the offspring of mothers with nongestational diabetes mellitus,[106] and the risk seems to be dependent on genetic background.[107] In a line of nonobese diabetic (NOD) mice,[107] a high incidence of L-R abnormalities has been observed if the dam was hyperglycemic early in gestation. The incidence is higher (65%) if the sire is from the NOD strain, decreases if the sire is from strain ICR (from which NOD is derived), and decreases to background levels with C57Bl sires. These results suggest that the genetic background of the embryo lowers the threshold for malformations induced by environmental agents (reviewed in reference 6).

## CONCLUSION

Recently, significant progress has been made in identifying the individual molecular components necessary for determining L-R patterning decisions and their position within the signaling cascade hierarchy. In the chick, an activin or activin-related molecule appears to be critical for initiation of asymmetric gene expression in the vicinity of the node. In mice, nodal flow breaks the initial bilateral symmetry and signals the onset of a molecular cascade of asymmetric gene expression. In all vertebrates, *Nodal* and *Lefty* and their downstream target, *Pitx2*, are essential components of a left-sided signaling cascade. Any disturbance of their normal expression pattern in the left LPM is associated with alterations in organ *situs*.

The availability of gene knockout for specific mouse genes and the positional cloning of human genes responsible for familial situs abnormalities will allow the complete delineation of the intracellular events that translate and maintain positional information to the developing organs.

## REFERENCES

1. Merklin RL, Varano NR: Situs inversus and cardiac defects: A study of 111 cases of reversed asymmetry. J Thorac Cardiovasc Surg 1995;44:1-110.
2. Togersen J: Genetic factors in visceral asymmetry in the development of pathological changes of the lungs, heart and abdominal organs. Arch Pathol 1949;47:556-593.
3. Afzelius BA: Situs inversus and ciliary abnormalities: What is the connection? Int J Dev Biol 1995;39:839-844.
4. Ferencz C, Boughman JA: Congenital heart disease in adolescents and adults: Teratology, genetics, and recurrence risks. Cardiol Clin 1993;11:557-567.
5. Zissin R, Rathaus V, Oscadchy A, et al: Intestinal malrotation as an incidental finding on CT in adults. Abdom Imaging 1999;24:550-555.
6. Casey B: Genetics of human situs abnormalities. Am J Med Genet 2001;101:356-358.
7. Burn J, Goodship J: Developmental genetics of the heart. Curr Opin Genet Dev 1996;6:322-325.
8. Lander A, King T, Brown NA: Left-right development: Mammalian phenotypes and conceptual models. Cell Dev Biol 1998;9:35-41.
9. Gershoni-Baruch R, Gottfried E, Pery M, et al: Immotile cilia syndrome including polysplenia, situs inversus, and extrahepatic biliary atresia. Am J Med Genet 1989;33:390-393.
10. Ligoxygakis P, Strigini M, Averof M: Specification of left-right asymmetry in the embryonic gut of Drosophila. Development 2001;128:1171-1174.
11. Capdevila I, Belmonte JC: Knowing left from right: The molecular basis of laterality defects. Mol Med Today 2000;6(3):112-118.
12. Capdevila J, Vogan KJ, Tabin CJ, Izpisua Belmonte JC: Mechanisms of left-right determination in vertebrates. Cell 2000:101:9-21.
13. Harvey RP: Links in the left/right axial pathway. Cell 1998;94:273-276.
14. Levin M: Left-right asymmetry in vertebrate embryogenesis. Bioessays 1997;19:287-296.
15. Ruiz-Lozano P, Ryan AK, Izpisua-Belmonte JC: Left-right determination. Trends Cardiovasc Med 2000;10:258-262.
16. Cooke J, Isaac A: A cascade of gene action controlling heart asymmetry and torsion in embryonic development. Trends Cardiovasc Med 1998;8:215-220.
17. Harvey RP: Cardiac looping—an uneasy deal with laterality. Semin Cell Dev Biol 1998;9:101-108.
18. Olson EN, Srivastava D: Molecular pathways controlling heart development. Science 1996;272:671-676.
19. Overbeek PA: Right and left go dhand and ehand. Nat Genet 1997;16:119-121.
20. Ramsdell AF, Yost HJ: Molecular mechanisms of vertebrate left-right development. Trends Genet 1998;14:459-465.
21. Supp DM, Brueckner M, Potter SS: Handed asymmetry in the mouse: Understanding how things go right (or left) by studying how they go wrong. Semin Cell Dev Biol 1998;9:77-87.

22. Nonaka S, Tanaka Y, Okada Y, et al: Randomization of left-right asymmetry due to loss of nodal cilia generating leftward flow of extraembryonic fluid in mice lacking kif3b motor protein [published erratum appears in Cell 1999;99:117]. Cell 1998;95: 829–837.

23. Okada Y, Nonaka S, Tanaka Y, et al: Abnormal nodal flow precedes situs inversus in iv and inv mice [in process citation]. Mol Cell, 1999;4:459–468.

24. Takeda S, Yonekawa Y, Tanaka Y, et al: Left-right asymmetry and kinesin superfamily protein kif3a: New insights in determination of laterality and mesoderm induction by kif3a-/-mice analysis. J Cell Biol 1999;145:825–836.

25. Sulik K, Dehart DB, Iangaki T, et al: Morphogenesis of the murine node and notochordal plate. Dev Dyn 1994;201:260–278.

26. Halpern ME, Ho RK, Walker C, Kimmel CB: Induction of muscle pioneers and floor plate is distinguished by the zebrafish no tail mutation. Cell 1993;75:99–111.

27. Placzek M, Tessier-Lavigne M, Yamada T, et al: Mesodermal control of neural cell identity: Floor plate induction by the notochord. Science 1990;250:985–988.

28. McGrath J, Somlo S, Makora S, Tranx, Breuckner M: Two populations of node monocilia initiate left-right asymmetry in the mouse. Cell 003;114:61–73.

29. Hummel KP, Chapman DB: Visceral inversion and associated anomalies in the mouse. J Hered 1959;50:9–13.

30. Yokoyama T, Copeland NG, Jenkins NA, et al: Reversal of left-right asymmetry: A situs inversus mutation [see comments]. Science 1993;260:679–682.

31. Icardo JM, Sanchez de Vega MJ: Spectrum of heart malformations in mice with situs solitus, situs inversus, and associated visceral heterotaxy. Circulation 1991;84:2547–2558.

32. Layton WM Jr: Random determination of a developmental process: Reversal of normal visceral asymmetry in the mouse. J Hered 1976;67:336–338.

33. Brueckner M, D'Eustachio P, Horwich AL: Linkage mapping of a mouse gene, iv, that controls left-right asymmetry of the heart and viscera. Proc Natl Acad Sci USA 1989;86:5035–5038.

34. Supp DM, Witte DP, Potter SS: Mutation of an axonemal dynein affects left-right asymmetry in inversus viscerum mice. Nature 1997;389:963–66.

35. Morgan D, Turnpenny L, Goodship J, et al: Inversin, a novel gene in the vertebrate left-right axis pathway, is partially deleted in the inv mouse [published erratum appears in Nat Genet 1998;20:312]. Nat Genet 1998;20:149–156.

36. Marszalek JR, Ruiz-Lozano P, Roberts E, et al: Situs inversus and embryonic ciliary morphogenesis defects in mouse mutants lacking the kif3a subunit of kinesin-ii. Proc Natl Acad Sci USA 1999;96: 5043–5048.

37. Olbrich H, Haffner K, Kispert A, et al: Mutations in dnah5 cause primary ciliary dyskinesia and randomization of left-right asymmetry. Nat Genet 2002;30:143–144.

38. Cooke J: Vertebrate embryo handedness [letter]. Nature 1995;374: 681.

39. Boettger T, Wittler L, Kessel M: Fgf8 functions in the specification of the right body side of the chick. Curr Biol 1999;9:277–280.

40. Essner JJ, Vogan KJ, Wagner MK, Tabin CJ, Yost HJ, Brueckner M: Conserved function of embryonic nodal cilia. Nature 2002;418: 37–38.

41. Mercola M, Levin M: Left-right asymmetry determination in vertebrates. Annu Rev Cell Dev Biol 2001;17:779–805.

42. Collignon J, Varlet I, Robertson EJ: Relationship between asymmetric nodal expression and the direction of embryonic turning. Nature 1996;381:155–18.

43. Levin M, Johnson RL, Stern CD: A molecular pathway determining left-right asymmetry in chick embryogenesis. Cell 1995;82: 803–814.

44. Lowe LA, Supp DM, Sampath K, et al: Conserved left-right asymmetry of nodal expression and alterations in murine situs inversus [see comments]. Nature 1996;381:158–161.

45. Lohr JL, Danos MC, Yost HJ: Left-right asymmetry of a nodal-related gene is regulated by dorsoanterior midline structures during xenopus development. Development 1997;124:1465–1472.

46. Rebagliati MR, Toyama R, Fricke C, et al: Zebrafish nodal-related genes are implicated in axial patterning and establishing left-right asymmetry. Dev Biol 1998;199:261–272.

47. Sampath K, Cheng AM, Frisch A, Wright CV: Functional differences among Xenopus nodal-related genes in left-right axis determination. Development 1997;124:3293–3302.

48. Sampath K, Rubinstein AL, Cheng AM, et al: Induction of the zebrafish ventral brain and floorplate requires cyclops/nodal signalling. Nature 1998;395:185–189.

49. Levin M, Pagan S, Roberts DJ, et al: Left/right patterning signals and the independent regulation of different aspects of situs in the chick embryo. Dev Biol 1997;189:57–67.

50. Hsu DR, Economides AN, Wang X, et al: The Xenopus dorsalizing factor gremlin identifies a novel family of secreted proteins that antagonize bmp activities. Mol Cell 1998;1:673–683.

51. Rodriguez Esteban C, Capdevila J, Economides AN, et al: The novel cer-like protein caronte mediates the establishment of embryonic left-right asymmetry [see comments]. Nature 1999;401:243–251.

52. Yokouchi Y, Vogan KJ, Pearse RV 2nd, Tabin CJ: Antagonistic signaling by caronte, a novel cerberus-related gene, establishes left-right asymmetric gene expression. Cell 1999;98:573–583.

53. Zhu L, Marvin MJ, Gardiner A, et al: Cerberus regulates left-right asymmetry of the embryonic head and heart. Curr Biol 1999;9:931–938.

54. Chang H, Huylebroeck D, Verschueren K, et al: Smad5 knockout mice die at mid-gestation due to multiple embryonic and extraembryonic defects. Development 1999;126:1631–1642.

55. Winnier G, Blessing M, Labosky PA, Hogan BL: Bone morphogenetic protein-4 is required for mesoderm formation and patterning in the mouse. Genes Dev 1995;9:2105–2116.

56. Hyatt BA, Yost HJ: The left-right coordinator: The role of vg1 in organizing left-right axis formation. Cell 1998;93:37–46.

57. Yost HJ: The genetics of midline and cardiac laterality defects. Curr Opin Cardiol 1998;13:185–189.

58. Yost HJ: Diverse initiation in a conserved left-right pathway? Curr Opin Genet Dev 1999;9:422–426.

59. Gaio U, Schweickert A, Fischer A, et al: A role of the cryptic gene in the correct establishment of the left-right axis. Curr Biol 1999;9:1339–1342.

60. Yan YT, Gritsman K, Ding J, et al: Conserved requirement for egf-cfc genes in vertebrate left-right axis formation. Genes Dev 1999;13:2527–2537.

61. Shamim H, Mason I: Expression of fgf4 during early development of the chick embryo. Mech Dev 1999;85:189–92.

62. Danos MC, Yost HJ: Role of notochord in specification of cardiac left-right orientation in zebrafish and Xenopus. Dev Biol 1996;177:96–103.

63. Dufort D, Schwartz L, Harpal K, Rossant J: The transcription factor hnf3beta is required in visceral endoderm for normal primitive streak morphogenesis. Development 1998;125:3015–3025.

64. Izraeli S, Lowe LA, Bertness VL, et al: The sil gene is required for mouse embryonic axial development and left-right specification. Nature 1999;399:691–694.

65. King T, Brown NA: Developmental biology: Antagonists on the left flank [news; comment]. Nature 1999;401:222–223.

66. Melloy PG, Ewart JL, Cohen MF, et al: No turning, a mouse mutation causing left-right and axial patterning defects. Dev Biol 1998;193:77–89.

67. Meno C, Shimono A, Saijoh Y, et al: Lefty-1 is required for left-right determination as a regulator of lefty-2 and nodal. Cell 1998;94: 287–297.

68. Meno C, Ito Y, Saijoh Y, et al: Two closely-related left-right asymmetrically expressed genes, lefty-1 and lefty-2: Their distinct expression domains, chromosomal linkage and direct neuralizing activity in Xenopus embryos. Genes Cells 1997;2:513–524.

69. Saijoh Y, Adachi H, Mochida K, et al: Distinct transcriptional regulatory mechanisms underlie left-right asymmetric expression of lefty-1 and lefty-2. Genes Dev 1999;13:259–269.

70. Chiang C, Litingtung Y, Lee E, et al: Cyclopia and defective axial patterning in mice lacking sonic hedgehog gene function. Nature 1996;383:407–413.

71. Tsukui T, Capdevila J, Tamura K, et al: Multiple left-right asymmetry defects in shh(-/-) mutant mice unveil a convergence of the shh and retinoic acid pathways in the control of lefty-1. Proc Natl Acad Sci U S A 1999;96:11376–11381.

72. Bisgrove BW, Essner JJ, Yost HJ: Regulation of midline development by antagonism of lefty and nodal signaling. Development 1999;126:3253–3262.

73. Meno C, Gritsman K, Ohishi S, et al: Mouse lefty2 and zebrafish antivin are feedback inhibitors of nodal signaling during vertebrate gastrulation. Mol Cell 1999;4:287–298.

74. Thisse C, Thisse B: Antivin, a novel and divergent member of the tgfbeta superfamily, negatively regulates mesoderm induction. Development 1999;126:229–240.

75. Blum M, Steinbeisser H, Campione M, Schweickert A: Vertebrate left-right asymmetry: Old studies and new insights. Cell Mol Biol (Noisy-le-grand) 1999;45:505–16.

76. Campione M, Ros MA, Icardo JM, et al: Pitx2 expression defines a left cardiac lineage of cells: Evidence for atrial and ventricular molecular isomerism in the iv/iv mice. Dev Biol 2001;231:252–264.

77. Kitamura K, Miura H, Miyagawa-Tomita S, et al: Mouse pitx2 deficiency leads to anomalies of the ventral body wall, heart, extra- and periocular-mesoderm and right pulmonary isomerism [in process citation]. Development 1999;126:5749–5758.

78. Lin CR, Kioussi C, O'Connell S, et al: Pitx2 regulates lung asymmetry, cardiac positioning and pituitary and tooth morphogenesis. Nature 1999;401:279–282.

79. Logan M, Pagan-Westphal SM, Smith DM, et al: The transcription factor pitx2 mediates situs-specific morphogenesis in response to left-right asymmetric signals. Cell 1998;94:307–317.

80. Lu MF, Pressman C, Dyer R, et al: Function of Rieger syndrome gene in left-right asymmetry and craniofacial development. Nature 1999;401:276–278.

81. Piedra ME, Icardo JM, Albajar M, et al: Pitx2 participates in the late phase of the pathway controlling left-right asymmetry. Cell 1998;94:319–324.

82. Ryan AK, Blumberg B, Rodriguez-Esteban C, et al: Pitx2 determines left-right asymmetry of internal organs in vertebrates. Nature 1998;394:545–551.

83. Schweickert A, Campione M, Steinbeisser H, Blum M: Pitx2 isoforms: Involvement of pitx2c but not pitx2a or pitx2b in vertebrate left-right asymmetry. Mech Dev 2000;90:41–51.

84. Semina EV, Reiter RS, Murray JC: Isolation of a new homeobox gene belonging to the pitx/rieg family: Expression during lens development and mapping to the aphakia region on mouse chromosome 19. Hum Mol Genet 1997;6:2109–2116.

85. St Amand TR, Ra J, Zhang Y, et al: Cloning and expression pattern of chicken pitx2: A new component in the shh signaling pathway controlling embryonic heart looping. Biochem Biophys Res Commun 1998;247:100–105.

86. St Amand TR, Zhang Y, Semina EV, et al: Antagonistic signals between bmp4 and fgf8 define the expression of pitx1 and pitx2 in mouse tooth-forming anlage. Dev Biol 2000;217:323–332.

87. Yoshioka H, Meno C, Koshiba K, et al: Pitx2, a bicoid-type homeobox gene, is involved in a lefty-signaling pathway in determination of left-right asymmetry. Cell 1998;94:299–305.

88. Gage PJ, Suh H, Camper SA: Dosage requirement of pitx2 for development of multiple organs. Development 1999;126:4643–4651.

89. Isaac A, Sargent MG, Cooke J: Control of vertebrate left-right asymmetry by a snail-related zinc finger gene [see comments]. Science 1997;275:1301–1304.

90. Schneider A, Mijalski T, Schlange T, et al: The homeobox gene it nkx3.2 is a target of left-right signalling and is expressed on opposite sides in chick and mouse embryos. Curr Biol 1999;9:911–914.

91. Smith SM, Dickman ED, Thompson RP, et al: Retinoic acid directs cardiac laterality and the expression of early markers of precardiac asymmetry. Dev Biol 1997;182:162–171.

92. Schilling TF, Concordet JP, Ingham PW: Regulation of left-right asymmetries in the zebrafish by shh and bmp4. Dev Biol 1999;210:277–287.

93. Kosaki R, Gebbia M, Kosaki K, et al: Left-right axis malformations associated with mutations in acvr2b, the gene for human activin receptor type iib. Am J Med Genet 1999;82:70–76.

94. Kothapalli R, Buyuksal I, Wu SQ, et al: Detection of ebaf, a novel human gene of the transforming growth factor beta superfamily association of gene expression with endometrial bleeding. J Clin Invest 1997;99:2342–2350.

95. Kosaki K, Curry CJ, Roeder E, Jones KL: Ritscher-schinzel (3c) syndrome: Documentation of the phenotype. Am J Med Genet 1997;68:421–427.

96. Gebbia M, Ferrero GB, Pilia G, et al: X-linked situs abnormalities result from mutations in zic3 [see comments]. Nat Genet 1997;17:305–308.

97. Benedyk MJ, Mullen JR, DiNardo S: Odd-paired: A zinc finger pair-rule protein required for the timely activation of engrailed and wingless in Drosophila embryos. Genes Dev 1994;8:105–117.

98. Cimbora DM, Sakonju S: Drosophila midgut morphogenesis requires the function of the segmentation gene odd-paired. Dev Biol 1995;169:580–595.

99. Conlon FL, Lyons KM, Takaesu N, et al: A primary requirement for nodal in the formation and maintenance of the primitive streak in the mouse. Development 1994;120:1919–1928.

100. Jones CM, Kuehn MR, Hogan BL, et al: Nodal-related signals induce axial mesoderm and dorsalize mesoderm during gastrulation. Development 1995;121:3651–3662.

101. Zhou X, Sasaki H, Lowe L, et al: Nodal is a novel tgf-beta-like gene expressed in the mouse node during gastrulation. Nature 1993;361:543–547.

102. Ishikawa S, Kai M, Murata Y, et al: Genomic organization and mapping of the human activin receptor type iib (hactr-iib) gene. J Hum Genet 1998;43:132–134.

103. Kosaki K, Casey B: Genetics of human left-right axis malformations. Semin Cell Dev Biol 1998;9:89–99.

104. Belloni E, Muenke M, Roessler E, et al: Identification of sonic hedgehog as a candidate gene responsible for holoprosencephaly. Nat Genet 1996;14:353–356.

105. Chazaud C, Chambon P, Dolle P: Retinoic acid is required in the mouse embryo for left-right asymmetry determination and heart morphogenesis. Development 1999;126:2589–2596.

106. Splitt M, Wright C, Sen D, Goodship J: Left-isomerism sequence and maternal type-1 diabetes. Lancet 1999;354:305–306.

107. Morishima M, Ando M, Takao A: Visceroatrial heterotaxy syndrome in the nod mouse with special reference to atrial situs. Teratology 1991;44:91–100.

## EDITOR'S CHOICE

Essner JJ, Vogan KJ, Wagner MK, et al: Conserved function for embryonic nodal cilia. Nature 2002;418:37–38.

*Unifying finding that links the onset of left-right asymmetry in the heart and other organs to an early role of cilia in a specialed region of the early embryo.*

Kramer KL, Barnette JE, Yost HJ: PKCgamma regulates syndecan-2 inside-out signaling during xenopus left-right development. Cell 2002;111:981–990.

*Multiple signals control laterality in the embryo, suggesting that the onset of laterality defects will be quite complex.*

Kramer KL, Yost HJ: Cardiac left-right development: Are the early steps conserved? Cold Spring Harb Symp Quant Biol 2002;67:37–43.

*Excellent review that ties many separate pieces of the puzzle together.*

Levin M, Thorlin T, Robinson KR, et al: Asymmetries in H+/K+-ATPase and cell membrane potentials comprise a very early step in left-right patterning. Cell 2002;111:77–89.

*Unsuspectedly, even ion transporters can play regulatory roles in early steps of cardiac morphogenesis.*

McGrath J, Brueckner M: Cilia are at the heart of vertebrate left-right asymmetry. Curr Opin Genet Dev 2003;13:385–392.

*Nice review on the role of cilia in laterality from a leading pediatric cardiologist.*

McGrath J, Somlo S, Makova S, et al: Two populations of node monocilia initiate left-right asymmetry in the mouse. Cell 2003;114:61–73.

*Most recent chapter on the cilia story and left-right asymmetry using mouse models to dissect pathways.*

Raya, A, Kawakami Y, Rodriguez-Esteban C, et al: Notch activity induces Nodal expression and mediates the establishment of left-right asymmetry in vertebrate embryos. Genes Dev 2003;17:1213–1218.

*Notch signals are critical players in the laterality pathway.*

# chapter 13

# Pharyngeal Apparatus and Cardiac Neural Crest Defects

*Antonio Baldini*

Classic tissue ablation experiments in chicks have demonstrated the importance of neural crest cells in cardiovascular development.[1,2] Cardiac neural crest cells constitute a subpopulation of neuroectodermal cells that migrates from the hindbrain (rhombomeres 6 to 8), undergoes ectomesenchymal transformation, and populates the pharyngeal arches and the outflow tract of the heart. Once at their place of destination, these cells differentiate to form the skeletal and connective tissues of the arches and the vascular smooth muscle cells of the pharyngeal arch arteries (PAAs).[3-6] Physical elimination of these cells by microsurgery causes a number of developmental defects affecting the outflow tract of the heart, aortic arch, and some of the pharyngeal arch and pouch derivatives.[7-10] This chapter reviews the cardiac neural crest in the broader context of pharyngeal arch and pouch development and aims to dissect their interactions with other cellular components of the embryonic pharyngeal apparatus (endoderm, mesoderm, and ectoderm) and to identify the gene networks that control these interactions.[11,12]

The pharyngeal apparatus develops as a unit and determines, among other things, the proper connection of the heart to the systemic and pulmonary circulation. Some of the most common birth defects, including approximately 30% of congenital heart defects, are attributable to maldevelopment of the pharyngeal apparatus. Genetics is the most powerful tool available to dissect this developmental process, and most of the current knowledge about this system derives from molecular embryology and analysis of genetically defined models.

## CARDIAC NEURAL CREST AND THE DEVELOPMENT OF THE PHARYNGEAL APPARATUS

The term *pharyngeal apparatus* is used here to indicate the transient, vertebrate-specific embryonic structures called pharyngeal arches and pharyngeal pouches. The pharyngeal apparatus develops in a cranial-caudal direction with growth and segmental folding of the endodermal lining. The apparatus receives cellular contributions from all three germ layers—endoderm, mesoderm, and ectoderm (Fig. 13-1). Embryonic endoderm lines the digestive and respiratory tubes. These two tubes share a common chamber in the anterior region of the embryo—the pharynx. The pharyngeal endoderm directly contributes to the development of the thyroid,

parathyroids, and thymus, and it is thought to be a rich source of signaling molecules with inductive abilities directed toward the underlying mesenchyme.[11,12] The pharyngeal arches are populated by mesodermal cells and migratory cells of neural crest origin. As they form, each arch includes a blood vessel (PAA) that connects the heart, via the aortic sac, to the dorsal aortae (Figs. 13-1*D* and 13-2). During development the PAAs undergo extensive and asymmetric remodeling that causes growth of some arteries and regression of others (Fig. 13-2), a process that leads to the formation of the mature aortic arch and to connections with the great arteries.

Physical ablation of the neural crest that contributes to the pharyngeal arches has underlined the importance of the migrating neural crest-derived cells for the development of the pharyngeal apparatus.[10] However, these experiments have also shown that they are not required for segmentation of the pharynx (i.e., the process of formation of the multiple "arch-pouch" modules), which is thought to be an intrinsic function of the endoderm.[11] Ablation experiments have also shown that neural crest cells are not required for the formation of the PAAs but that they are important for their growth and maintenance.[8] Perhaps the closest phenotypic approximations of the ablation model is DiGeorge syndrome (DGS) in humans and *Pax3* mutations in mice. The role of neural crest cells in the pathogenesis of DGS, which is discussed later in this chapter, is questionable. *Pax3*-mutant mice develop a complex cardiovascular and noncardiovascular phenotype, including persistent truncus arteriosus (PTA) and thymus and parathyroid defects. These defects are thought to be due to a severe reduction in the number of neural crest-derived cells that populate the pharyngeal arches and outflow tract of the heart.[6,13-15] Interestingly, *Pax3* heterozygous and homozygous mutations in humans cause Waardenburg syndrome (OMIM 193500[16]), which is not associated with cardiovascular defects, casting doubts on the significance of this particular model for human congenital heart disease.

## PHARYNGEAL ARCH ARTERY REMODELING, MATURE GREAT ARTERY PATTERNING, AND THE AORTIC ARCH

The PAAs in mammals develop as five paired and symmetrical vessels (named first, second, third, fourth, and sixth, like the pharyngeal arches within which they are

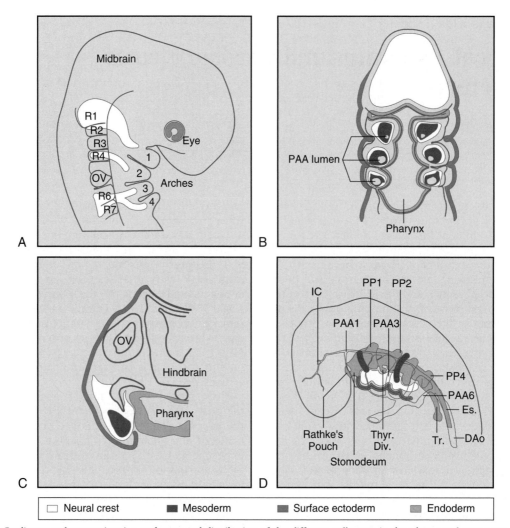

**FIGURE 13-1.** Cardiac neural crest migration pathways and distribution of the different cell types in the pharyngeal apparatus. *A,* Lateral view showing the three major streams directed to arches 1, 2, and 3-4. *B,* Coronal section showing the segmental organization of the embryonic pharynx. *C,* Transverse section at the level of the otic vesicle (OV) through the second pharyngeal arch. *D,* Pharyngeal endoderm-lined pouches and how they relate to vessels. DAo, dorsal aorta; Es, esophagus; PAA, pharyngeal arch arteries; PP, pharyngeal pouch; TD, thyroid diverticulum; Tr, trachea. (See color plate.) *(A–C modified from Graham A, Smith A: Patterning the pharyngeal arches. Bioessays 2001;23:54–61. D, modified from Carlson BM: Patten's Foundations of Embryology. New York, McGraw-Hill, 1996.)*

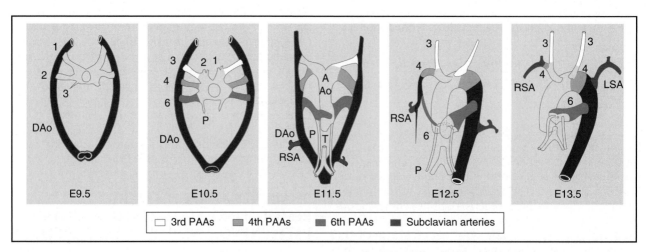

**FIGURE 13-2.** PAA remodeling during development, stages refers to mouse embryonic day. The arrangement at E13.5 is essentially the same as that in embryos at term. *Arrow* on E11.5 panel indicates the origin of the aorticopulmonary septum. DAo, dorsal aorta; LSA, left subclavian artery; P, pulmonary artery; RSA, right subclavian artery; T, trachea. Numbers refer to PAAs. (See color plate.) *(Modified from Kaufman MH: The Atlas of Mouse Development. San Diego, Academic Press, 1992.)*

located), which form progressively in a cranial-caudal order (Fig. 13-2). The formation of all these arteries is complete by approximately embryonic day (E) 10.5 in the mouse. The first and second PAAs regress early. The third PAA participates in the formation of the mature common carotid arteries. The left fourth PAA contributes to the aortic arch, and the right fourth becomes a small segment connecting the right common carotid with the right subclavian artery. The right sixth PAA regresses, and the left sixth becomes the ductus arteriosus. The remodeling of the PAAs proceeds in concert with the remodeling of the dorsal aortae, which in the early embryo are two large symmetrical vessels connected to the outflow tract of the heart via the PAAs. The left dorsal aorta becomes the mature descending and dorsal aorta, whereas the right dorsal aorta regresses (Figs. 13-2 and 13-3).

During a relatively narrow time window (24 to 36 hours in mice), the developing PAAs have a limited capacity to adapt to possible defects and rearrange themselves, presumably following hemodynamic cues, to keep the heart and great arteries connected. For example, the right fourth PAA ensures the connection of the right subclavian artery to the right common carotid artery. If the right fourth PAA fails, the right subclavian artery most commonly connects to the descending aorta because of the persistence of the right dorsal aorta, which normally regresses. Figure 13-3 illustrates some of the abnormalities that may

derive from a failure of formation, growth, or remodeling of the fourth PAAs. The finding of any such abnormality in human patients or mouse mutants is diagnostic of fourth PAA failure but does not provide any information as to when and where in the fourth PAA development -the problem occurred. It is important to note that some of the abnormalities shown in Figure 13-3 (e.g., aberrant origin of the right subclavian artery) may be clinically silent, whereas others (e.g., interruption of the aortic arch type B [IAA-B]) are very severe. These defects are embryologically and genetically closely related. Familial recurrence of these clinically silent abnormalities may be the sign of an underlying genetic defect that in some family members may manifest itself in a much more dramatic phenotype.

Although the genetics of PAA development is far from understood, a number of genes are known to play a role in this process. Neuropilin-1, a semaphorin-3 receptor that also binds an isoform of VEGF, is required for the development of the fourth and sixth PAAs.[17] Heterozygous mutation of *Tbx1*, a candidate gene for DGS (see in the following), affects early growth and remodeling of the fourth PAAs (Fig. 13-4), whereas its homozygous mutation prevents the formation of the third, fourth, and sixth PAAs.[18-20] Endothelin-1, its receptor $ET_A$, and the endothelin converting enzyme I *(EceI)*, are required for the development of the third and fourth PAAs; more specifically, loss of function of any of these

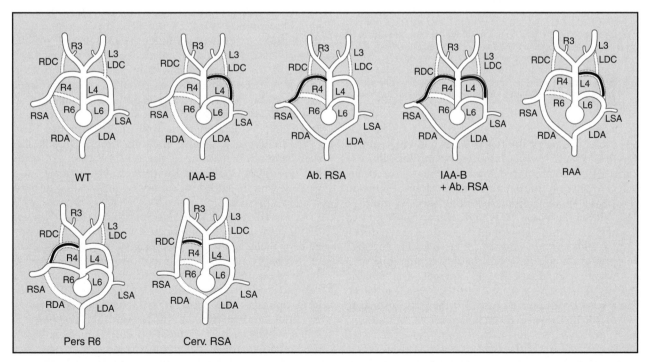

**FIGURE 13-3.** The different types of great vessel abnormalities derived from the developmental failure of one or both fourth PAA. The solid black line indicates the failed fourth PAA. *Dotted* lines indicate the normally regressing vessels. L3, 4, 6; R3, 4, 6, left and right third, fourth, and sixth PAAs. Ab. RSA, aberrant origin of the RSA resulting from failure of R4 and persistence of RDA. Because the RDA lies dorsal to the trachea and esophagus, this abnormality is also known as retroesophageal RSA. Cerv. RSA, cervical RSA, resulting from failure of R4 and persistence of RDC. LDA, left dorsal aorta. LDC, left ductus caroticus. LSA, left subclavian artery. Pers. R6, abnormal persistence of the right sixth PAA connecting the right subclavian artery with the pulmonary trunk. This is secondary to R4 failure. RAA, right aortic arch, resulting from L4 failure combined with RDA persistence. RDA, right dorsal aorta. Only the LDA persists in embryos at term. RDC, right ductus caroticus; the most cranial segments of the embryonic dorsal aortae, destined to regress. RSA, right subclavian artery. WT, normal arrangement. IAA-B, interruption of the aortic arch type B, resulting from L4 failure.

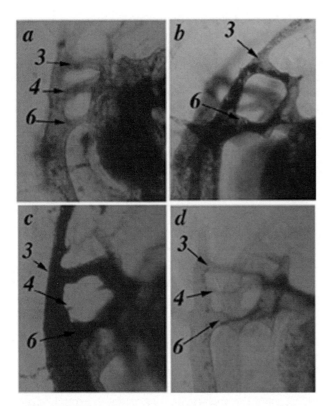

**FIGURE 13-4.** Diagnosis of fourth PAA abnormalities using intracardiac India ink injection. Lateral view of cleared E10.5 mouse embryos. *A,* Wild-type embryo showing the normal pattern, third, fourth, and sixth PAAs are clearly visible. *B, C,* and *D,* Show the same test on *Df1/+* embryos, which are heterozygously deleted for a chromosomal region homologous to the DGS deleted region on 22q11.2. *B,* The left fourth PAA is missing, whereas the right fourth PAA (visible in the background) is normal. *C,* The fourth PAA is greatly reduced in size and partially nonpatent to ink. *D,* The fourth PAA is present but very reduced in size. (See color plate.) *(From Lindsay EA, Baldini A: Recovery from arterial growth delay reduces penetrance of cardiovascular defects in mice deleted for the DiGeorge syndrome region. Hum Mol Genet 2001;10: 997-1002.)*

genes causes failure of the fourth PAAs and enlargement of the third PAAs.[21-24] *Foxc1* and *Foxc2* and *Semaphorin 3C* and *Tgfβ2* are required for late remodeling of the fourth PAA.[25-28] A preliminary conclusion of current data is that PAA development is controlled by multiple genetic networks; some of which overlap with known pathways of vessel development (e.g., *Neuropilin1*). However, most genes known to be relevant for PAA development do not have an obvious connection with the known vasculogenesis and angiogenesis genetic pathways. It is interesting to note that genes involved in the formation and early growth of the PAAs appear to be distinct from those involved in late vessel remodeling. This is perhaps not surprising given the specialized and different nature of the two processes. Developmental expression analyses of genes involved in PAA development reveal that they may be expressed in the neural crest–derived and non–neural crest–derived mesenchyme of the arches, paraxial mesoderm, pharyngeal endoderm, or endothelium, suggesting that interactions between all tissue components of the pharyngeal apparatus are critical for cardiovascular development.

## OUTFLOW TRACT DEVELOPMENT

During evolution, the outflow tract of the heart has acquired a complex septation process to allow separation of the systemic and pulmonary circulations. Septation errors, including malrotation of the septum, account for a large proportion of congenital cardiovascular defects. These include tetralogy of Fallot (TOF) (a combination of pulmonary stenosis with ventricular septal defect [VSD], overriding aorta, and right ventricular hypertrophy), PTA, double-outlet right ventricle (DORV), transposition of great arteries (TGA), and perimembranous VSDs. There are three distinct components of the outflow septum: the aorticopulmonary septum (the most dorsal component, originating from the aortic sac; see arrow in Fig. 13-2); the truncal septum, originating from the truncal cushions and separating the aorta and pulmonary valves; and the conal septum, the most ventral portion, important for the closure of the ventricular septum (Fig. 13-5).

The outflow tract (specifically the portion proximal to the aortic sac, i.e., the conus and truncus) is initially a conduit formed by an external myocardial layer and an internal endothelial layer (Fig. 13-5*A*). As the embryos develops, two mesenchymal swellings form between the two layers, named the truncus and the conus ridges (Fig. 13-5*B* and *C*). These swellings are populated by neural crest–derived cells and later fuse to divide the lumen of the outflow into two vessels (aorta and pulmonary trunk) (Fig. 13-5*E*). The ridges undergo a characteristic rotation so that the final septum has a spiral morphology (Fig. 13-5*D*). The myocardial wall of the outflow tract is contributed by muscle cell precursors migrating from a so-called secondary heart field, which is distinct from that contributing to the heart tube.[29-31] These observations provide an embryologic rationale for understanding genetic abnormalities of the outflow tract of the heart, which is distinct from and rarely associated with abnormalities of the heart itself. In contrast, mouse mutants or human diseases that have abnormalities of the outflow tract are often but not always associated with PAA abnormalities, suggesting genetic and developmental links with the pharyngeal apparatus.

As for PAA development, current genetic knowledge of the outflow tract implicates a number of different genes (Table 13-1). The TGFβ signaling pathway is one of the pathways involved in conotruncal development. TGFβ2 is required for normal development of the truncal and conal septa. *TGFβ2–/–* mice have PTA,[28] perimembranous VSD, and DORV, which are defects of septation and alignment of the outflow, respectively. BMPs, which are part of the TGFβ superfamily, also play a role in conotruncal development. Mice that have lost both *Bmp6* and *Bmp7* have PTA.[41] *Bmp4* is strongly expressed in the muscle wall of the conotruncus, but unfortunately the early lethality of the homozygous mutation does not allow the study of its role in outflow development in mice. Tissue-specific mutation of *Bmp4* will probably clarify this issue. The retinoid signaling pathway also plays a role in the conotruncus because homozygous mutation of the retinoic acid receptor gene

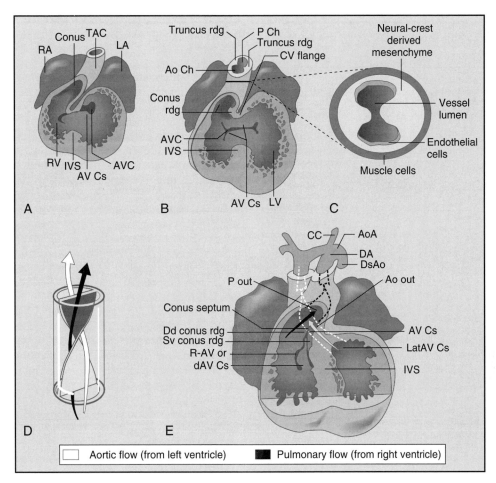

**FIGURE 13-5.** Development and septation of the outflow tract of the mammalian heart. *A*, Early morphology, the conotruncus is a simple tube, the conus and truncus arteriosus communis (TAC). *B*, Prongs of mesenchymal tissue or ridges (rdg) appear and start defining two communicating channels in the conus and truncus for the aortic (Ao Ch) and pulmonary (P Ch) blood flows. *C*, Magnified section through the truncus showing the location of cells of different origin that contribute to the development of the outflow. *D*, The spiral septum of the conotruncus. *E*, The aorta and pulmonary trunk are completely separated by the truncal septum. Below the valvular plane, the conal ridges are responsible for the closure of the ventricular septum by contributing to its perimembranous section. AoA, aortic arch; AoOut, aortic outflow; AVC, atrioventricular canal; AV Cs, atrioventricular canal cushion; CC, common carotid artery; CV, flange, conoventricular flange; DA, dorsal aorta; Dd conus rdg, dextrodorsal conus ridge; DsAo, descending aorta; IVS, interventricular septum; LA, left atrium; LatAV Cs, lateral atrioventricular canal cushion; LV, left ventricle; P out pulmonary outflow; RA, right atrium; R-AV, right atrioventricular orifice; RV, right ventricle; Sv conus rdg, sinistroventral conus ridge. *(Modified from Carlson BM: Patten's Foundations of Embryology. New York, McGraw-Hill, 1996.)*

*Rxrα* causes PTA in mice. A reduction in number of cardiac neural crest cells has been proposed to be the basis of PTA in a number of mouse mutants, including *Pax3* and *Semaphorin3C* mutants.[6,15,27]

## PHARYNGEAL APPARATUS AND HUMAN CONGENITAL HEART DISEASE

Results obtained with genetically modified models predict that human cardiovascular defects secondary to pharyngeal arch and pouch maldevelopment should be associated with a complex yet characteristic clinical picture. This may include craniofacial abnormalities, especially of the mid and lower face; palatal defects; and parathyroid and thymic abnormalities. Cardiovascular defects should include conotruncal and/or aortic arch defects. The explanation for this phenotypic association

is intuitive, if one considers the concerted development of these structures (thymus, parathyroid, aortic arch, face, and palate) from essentially a single embryonic apparatus. Table 13-2 lists some of the genes known to cause phenotypic complexes attributable to maldevelopment of the pharyngeal apparatus.

The concept of a developmental field defect[48-50] has been proposed to describe the characteristic phenotypic association. The DGS phenotype (described in the following) is the most typical example of a disorder of the pharyngeal apparatus associated with congenital heart disease. This syndrome, however, is remarkably homogeneous from a genetic standpoint because most patients have the same genetic defect (i.e., a small deletion of chromosome 22). This may be due to one or more of the following reasons: (1) the chromosomal deletion is frequent, (2) there are very few gene mutations that can cause this phenotypic

■ ■ ■

**TABLE 13-1** GENES KNOWN TO BE INVOLVED IN AORTIC ARCH OR CONOTRUNCAL DEVELOPMENT

| | MOUSE MUTATION | | HUMAN MUTATION | | |
|---|---|---|---|---|---|
| Gene | Het | Hom | Het | Hom | References |
| Pax3 | n/c | PTA, Arch | n/c | n/c | 32 |
| Foxc1 | n/c | Arch | n/c | n/a | 26 |
| Foxc2 | n/c | Arch | VSD, ToF (uncommon) | n/a | 25 |
| RXRα | n/c | PTA, DORV | n/a | n/a | 33 |
| RARs Compound mutants | n/c | Arch, PTA, VSD, DORV | n/a | n/a | 34 |
| Tbx1 | Arch, VSD | PTA, Arch, VSD | *Del22q11 Arch, PTA, ToF, VSD | n/a | 18–20 |
| Neurofibromin1 | n/c | DORV, valve defects | PS, Arch (uncommon) | n/a | 35–37 |
| TGFβ2 | n/c | PTA, DORV | n/a | n/a | 28 |
| Jagged1 | n/c | Vascular abnormalities? | ToF | n/a | 38,39 |
| Neurotrophin3 | n/c | VSD, ToF | n/a | n/a | 40 |
| Neuropilin1 | n/c | Vascular abnormalities PTA, Arch | n/a | n/a | 17 |
| Sema3C | n/c | PTA, Arch | n/a | n/a | 27 |
| Endothelin1 | n/c | Arch | n/a | n/a | 21 |
| ETa | n/c | Arch | n/a | n/a | 23 |
| ECE1 | n/c | Arch | n/a | n/a | 24 |
| Bmp6/Bmp7 Double mutants | n/c | PTA | n/a | n/a | 41 |
| Sox4 | n/c | PTA, DORV | n/a | n/a | 42 |
| Crkol | n/c | Arch | *Del22q11 Arch, PTA, ToF | n/a | 43 |
| c-Jun | n/c | PTA, Arch | n/a | n/a | 44 |
| Rae28 | n/c | VSD, OAo, PS | n/a | n/a | 45 |
| Fog2 | n/c | ToF, Abn. coronary A | n/a | n/a | 46 |
| Cited2 | n/c | Arch, VSD, OAo, DORV | n/a | n/a | 47 |

*Single gene mutations not identified yet.

?, cardiac morphology data were not reported; Abn. coronary a., abnormal coronary artery; Arch, defects of the aortic arch patterning; DORV, double-outlet right ventricle; Het, heterozygous; Hom, homozygous; n/a, not available; n/c, no cardiovascular abnormalities reported; OAo, aortic diameter; PS, infundibular or valvular pulmonary stenosis; PTA, persistent truncus arteriosus; ToF, tetralogy of Fallot; VSD, perimembranous ventricular septal defects.

association, and (3) the DGS cases without deletion are etiologically heterogeneous and may be caused by the mutation of several genes or by teratogens. Although the first reason is unquestionably true, the second reason is highly speculative and is in apparent contrast with data from mouse models that indicate the genetic complexity of the development of the pharyngeal apparatus. However, a complete DGS phenotype can only be caused by genes functioning early and extensively enough to affect virtually all the derivatives of

the pharyngeal apparatus. The phenotype of mice lacking Tbx1, a DGS candidate gene, is perhaps the most severe and extensive pharyngeal apparatus defect described so far, resulting in lack of formation or abnormalities of all the arches and pouches.[18,19] In contrast, most of the other reported mutant phenotypes affect these structures only partially. Consistent with this observation is the fact that most human disorders relevant to this chapter exhibit a partial phenotype (e.g., isolated conotruncal defects).

■ ■ ■

**TABLE 13-2** MUTATION THAT CAUSES ABNORMALITIES OF THE CONOTRUNCUS AND/OR AORTIC ARCH AND OF THE DERIVATIVES OF THE PHARYNGEAL APPARATUS

| Gene | Aortic Arch | Conotruncus | Thymus | Parathyroids | Craniofacial | References |
|---|---|---|---|---|---|---|
| Pax3 | x | x | x | x | x | 32 |
| ETA | x | x | x | x | x | 23 |
| Endothelin1 | x | x | x | x | x | 21 |
| ECE1 | x | x | x | x | x | 24 |
| Tbx1 | x | x | x | x | x | 18–20 |
| RARs Compound mutants | x | x | x | x | x | 34 |
| Rae28 | | x | x | x | x | 45 |
| Crkol | x | | x | | x | 43 |
| Foxc1 | x | | | | x | 26 |
| Foxc2 | x | | | | x | 25 |

x, presence of abnormalities in mutants.

The disorders that are described in the following were selected because they exhibit abnormalities of aortic arch patterning, outflow septation, and perimembranous ventricular septation. Teratogenic disorders were selected among those that have known or presumed connections with known genetic pathways. For virtually all of the disorders discussed in this chapter, the pathogenesis is not well understood, which underlines the need for further research in this field because it is relevant to a large number of birth defects in general and to congenital heart disease in particular.

## GENETIC DISORDERS

### DiGeorge Syndrome/Velocardiofacial Syndrome/Conotruncal Anomaly Face/del22q11 Syndromes

DGS[51] (OMIM 188400), also known as velocardiofacial syndrome or conotruncal anomaly face, is the most characteristic and frequent disorder of the pharyngeal apparatus (1 in 4000 live births). It is characterized by craniofacial anomalies, aortic arch patterning defects (mainly IAA-B), conotruncal heart defects (mainly PTA, TOF, and VSD), and thymus and parathyroid aplasia and hypoplasia.[52] Most of the derivatives of the pharyngeal arches and pouches are affected. The disorder is usually caused by a heterozygous chromosomal deletion of chromosome 22q11.2 (del22q11). Investigators have been studying this syndrome intensely because the gene(s) responsible for this phenotype must be a major player in the development of the pharyngeal apparatus. The chromosomal deletion associated with this syndrome, del22q11, includes approximately 30 genes, and the findings of rare patients with nonoverlapping deletions have confused efforts to localize the gene.[52] Investigators turned to mouse modeling using a recently developed technology to generate precisely engineered chromosomal deficiencies.[53] Mice carrying a 1-Mb chromosomal deletion that includes most of the genes homologous to those deleted in DGS (Df1/+ mice) exhibited cardiovascular defects similar to those observed in del22q11 patients, secondary to defective development of the fourth PAAs[54] (Fig. 13-4) including aberrant origin of right subclavian artery and IAA-B. Some mice also showed VSD and overriding of the aorta. In addition, the Df1/+ mouse model was later shown to have parathyroid and thymus developmental anomalies[55] and a behavioral phenotype reminiscent of del22q11 syndrome.[56] The fourth PAA abnormality was characterized as an early growth defect following normal formation of the artery. The vessel growth defect is associated with delayed or absent formation of a smooth muscle wall around the artery. Smooth muscle cells surrounding the fourth PAAs are thought to be derived from neural crest cells; however, no neural crest migration defect could be identified in these mutants, suggesting a defect of differentiation or recruitment of smooth muscle cells.[57] Interestingly, many embryos were able to overcome this initial arterial growth defect. This phenomenon, not previously reported in congenital heart disease

models, causes incomplete penetrance of arch defects at birth,[57] and it is strongly affected by the genetic background of the mice.[55] These findings provide a genetic framework for future studies into penetrance of heart defects and possibly even their prevention.

The gene responsible for the Df1/+ cardiovascular phenotype has been identified as Tbx1, a putative transcription factor.[18-20] Homozygous mutation of Tbx1 prevents the formation of PAAs 3, 4, and 6; arches 3, 4, and 6; and pouches 2, 3, and 4 and causes severe hypoplasia of the second arch.[18,19] Striking in these mutants is the severe hypoplasia of the pharynx and lack of the characteristic segmentation of the pharyngeal apparatus, leading to a hypothesis that the primary role of Tbx1 is in endoderm segmentation.[19,52] Consistent with this hypothesis is the strong expression of Tbx1 in the endoderm of the pharyngeal pouches. Along with PAA defects, Tbx1−/− mice exhibit PTA, absent thymus and parathyroids, and craniofacial abnormalities.[18] Perhaps surprisingly, homozygous mutation of Tbx1 does not cause embryonic lethality. However, Tbx1−/− pups die soon after birth, presumably because of cardiovascular defects.[18]

Whether Tbx1 is the only gene involved in the pathogenesis of DGS is not known. Although this gene is consistently deleted in patients with DGS, patients with mutation of only Tbx1 have not been identified, suggesting that these mutations are very rare, are located outside the coding region of the gene, or are not sufficient to cause a phenotype that clinically appears as DGS.

Interestingly, another gene, Crkol, has been identified in the del22q11 region; Crkol mutations cause aortic arch defects.[43] This gene is not haploinsufficient in mice and is not deleted in some del22q11 syndrome patients. Nevertheless, it could contribute to the DGS phenotype.

### Alagille Syndrome, JAGGED1, and the NOTCH pathway

Alagille's syndrome (AS) (OMIM 118450) is an autosomal dominant condition caused by mutation of JAGGED1, a Notch ligand.[38,39] Congenital heart disease is present in 95% of AS patients; TOF is the most common finding. Mutations of JAGGED1 have been associated with familial and sporadic TOF, in which patients have mild extracardiac findings that are thought to be insufficient for a clinical diagnosis of AS.[58,59] Therefore, a fraction of TOF cases without a syndromic diagnosis may be due to JAGGED1 mutations.

Interestingly, other connections have been proposed between the Notch signaling pathway and cardiovascular development.[26] Homozygous mutation of the forkhead transcription factors Foxc1 and Foxc2 causes aortic arch patterning abnormalities, most likely resulting from defects in late remodeling of the PAAs.[25,60] These two genes are important for the development of the ocular, cardiovascular, and genitourinary systems. Foxc1−/−; Foxc2−/− double mutants exhibit generalized vascular defects. The two genes are expressed in both endothelial cells and vascular smooth muscle cells, although they are not required for the differentiation of the two cell types.[26] Heterozygous mutations of FOXC1 cause primary congenital glaucoma in human patients[61] (OMIM 601090) but no heart defects. A similar defect has been described in *Foxc1+/−* mice. *FOXC2* heterozygous mutations cause the lymphedema-distichiasis syndrome[62] (OMIM 602402). Congenital heart defects (VSD and TOF) have been reported in these patients, but they are uncommon.

## Noonan Syndrome

Noonan syndrome[63] (OMIM 163950) is an autosomal dominant condition characterized by craniofacial dysmorphisms, short stature, motor delay, deafness, and cardiovascular abnormalities. The most common cardiovascular findings are pulmonary valvular stenosis, hypertrophic cardiomyopathy, and atrial septal defects. Because of its relatively frequent incidence, Noonan syndrome is an important genetic cause of pulmonary stenosis. The causative gene had been located in the chromosomal region 12q24. The protein-tyrosine-phosphatase *SHP2* gene is localized within the critical region, and recently, mutations within this gene have been identified in Noonan syndrome patients.[64] Shp2 is a required signal-enhancing component of EGFR signal transduction.[65] A mouse knockout of *Shp2* has been reported; *Shp2+/−* mice are normal but, because of early lethality, the cardiovascular phenotype of *Shp2−/−* animals could not be analyzed. However, mice double heterozygous *Egfr+/−*; *Shp2+/−* exhibit semilunar (aortic and pulmonary) valve thickening, which results in stenosis and myocardial hypertrophy.[66]

## CHARGE Syndrome

Previously referred to as CHARGE association, CHARGE is currently referred to as a syndrome because of its recognizable pattern of malformations (OMIM 214800). The acronym[67] stands for coloboma, heart anomaly, choanal atresia, retardation, and genital and ear anomalies. Congenital heart disease occurs in 85% of the patients, and the most common abnormality is TOF. The genetic defect causing this syndrome is unknown.

## Opitz Syndrome

Opitz syndrome[68] (OMIM 300000) is characterized by midline abnormalities including cleft lip, laryngeal cleft, hypospadias, agenesis of the corpus callosum, and congenital heart disease. The cardiovascular phenotype includes arch abnormalities and conotruncal defects.[69] Opitz's syndrome is genetically heterogeneous; two loci have been identified, one X-linked (Xp22) and one autosomic (22q11.2).[70] The gene mutated in the X-linked locus has been identified as *MID1*.[71] The MID1 protein belongs to the B-box family of proteins and is found associated with microtubules.[72] Mutations causing Opitz syndrome impair the ability of this protein to bind microtubules.[72] MID1 has a E3 ubiquitin ligase activity that targets the catalytic subunit of protein phosphatase 2A (PP2Ac). Mutation of *MID1* leads to accumulation of PP2Ac, and it has been proposed that this may be the pathogenetic basis of Opitz syndrome.[73] How MID1 mutation causes cardiovascular defects remains to be elucidated. The Opitz syndrome gene localized at 22q11.2 remains to be identified, and some patients have been reported to carry a chromosomal deletion in the same region as DGS *(del22q11)*.[74]

## Chromosomal Abnormalities

Chromosomal abnormalities are the most common known cause of congenital heart disease. The multigenic nature of these rearrangements makes the genetic dissection of these disorders, and eventually the identification of the critical genes, extremely difficult with the current methods of investigation. Only recently, sophisticated chromosomal manipulation technologies in mice have opened up new possibilities for functional studies of these disorders.[52,53]

Among the chromosomal abnormalities associated with conotruncal heart defects, I briefly discuss two that are recurrent. The recombinant chromosome 8 syndrome[75,76] (OMIM 179613) exhibits mental retardation, facial abnormalities, seizures, and cardiovascular abnormalities. Cardiovascular abnormalities are important components of the syndrome and include TOF and other conotruncal abnormalities.[77] Cytogenetically, the rearrangement Rec8 is defined as rec(8)dup(8q) inv(8)(p23.1q22.1), and it derives from a parental pericentric inversion of chromosome 8, inv(8)(p23.1q22.1). This pericentric inversion, which is not associated with an abnormal phenotype, is thought to result from aberrant recombination between repetitive DNA sequences that are located at the chromosomal breakpoints of the inversion.[78] Progeny of carriers of the inversion have a 6% chance of having a Rec8 rearrangement.

Aortic arch defects, pulmonary stenosis, and VSD may be associated with heterozygous chromosomal deletions of the short arm of chromosome 8, band 8p23. *GATA4*, a transcription factor that regulates cardiomyocyte transcription program and that is required for cardiovascular development,[79,80] is localized in this region. Therefore, it was considered to be a candidate for the cardiovascular abnormalities associated with this deletion syndrome.[81] However, it has been shown that in at least some of the patients, *GATA4* is not deleted, making it an unlikely candidate.[82]

### Isolated Conotruncal and Arch Defects

Most cardiovascular abnormalities affecting structures derived from PAAs and conotruncus occur without association with apparent extracardiac developmental defects (OMIM 217095). Among the most common defects are PTA, TOF, perimembranous VSDs, and aortic arch abnormalities. The cause of isolated defects is unknown (with the few exceptions discussed previously). Simple Mendelian inheritance in some familial cases suggested transmission as a single gene trait,[83,84] but most cases are sporadic. Perhaps genetic or nongenetic insults leading to these defects act at a late developmental stage (e.g., affecting the maintenance or late remodeling of great arteries) or interfere specifically with development of the cardiovascular structures. The identification of genes involved in these defects will be important but extraordinarily challenging, especially for the sporadic cases.

## DISORDERS INDUCED BY TERATOGENS

### Retinoic Acid-Related Disorders

Retinoic acid is the active metabolite of vitamin A (retinol). Deficiency or excess of retinoic acid causes considerable problems to embryonic development in general and to cardiovascular development in particular. Vitamin A deficiency during pregnancy can cause aortic arch and conotruncal anomalies in human embryos and in animal models. The use of drugs containing vitamin A or retinoic acid analogs may cause the so-called retinoic acid embryopathy, or isotretinoin embryopathy (OMIM 243440). Isotretinoin is a vitamin A analog used for treatment of acne. Physical findings in patients include craniofacial and ear anomalies and conotruncal and aortic arch defects.[85-88]

Retinoic acid is produced by a two-step process: (1) retinol is oxidized into retinaldehyde by an alcohol dehydrogenase or alcohol dehydrogenase/reductase and (2) retinaldehyde is then converted into retinoic acid by retinaldehyde dehydrogenases (RALDH), of which RALDH2 is thought to be the main source of retinoic acid production in early mouse embryogenesis.[89] Biologic activity of retinoic acid is mediated by interactions with two classes of receptors: RARs ($\alpha$, $\beta$, and $\gamma$) and RXRs ($\alpha$, $\beta$, and $\gamma$). To dissect the retinoid signaling pathway, genetic experiments have aimed at the targeted mutation of genes coding for RALDH2 or retinoic acid receptors in mice. RALDH2-deficient mouse embryos die at E10.5 with severe developmental defects, including cardiovascular abnormalities.[90] Most of the cardiovascular defects can be rescued by administration of retinoic acid to the pregnant mother.[91] *Rxr*$\alpha$−/− animals exhibit PTA and DORV. Individual mutation of RARs did not cause cardiovascular or other vitamin A deficiency phenotypes, possibly because of functional redundancy. However, phenotypic abnormalities were revealed in compound mutants.[34] The cardiovascular defects included abnormalities of the aortic arch patterning and PTA.

### Fetal Alcohol Syndrome

Consumption of alcohol during pregnancy can lead to cardiovascular abnormalities, including VSDs, aortic arch defects,[92,93] and abnormalities resembling DGS.[94] Similar results have been described in animal models.[95] The phenotypic picture associated with alcohol consumption is reminiscent of the vitamin A deficiency, and it has been proposed that ethanol induces inhibition of alcohol dehydrogenase-catalyzed synthesis of retinoic acid.[96,97] This could effectively reduce the amount of available retinoic acid during embryonic development, hence establishing a link between fetal alcohol syndrome and retinoic acid function.

## CONCLUSIONS

Although conotruncal and aortic arch defects can be categorized into a limited number of anatomic types, the genetic failures leading to those defects are much more diverse. As developmental genetics tools become increasingly sophisticated, substantial differences in the pathogenesis of cardiovascular malformations in genetically defined mouse models are becoming apparent. For example, *Tbx1* mutations affect the early growth and remodeling or formation of the PAAs, whereas *Foxc1*, *Foxc2*, *Sema3C*, or *Tgfβ2* mutations affect late remodeling. However, the outcome of these mutations in term embryos may be the same, namely interruption of the aortic arch. Hence, the first conclusion from this brief review is that the cause of a given anatomic defect may be genetically heterogeneous. Conversely, a given gene mutation can generate different anatomic defects in different individuals, even if the individuals are genetically identical (mice of inbred strains or human monozygotic twins). A corollary of the latter conclusion is that clinically benign anomalies (e.g., aberrant origin of the right subclavian artery) may be a sign of an underlying genetic mutation.

Although many genes have been shown to be important for outflow and aortic arch development in mice, only a few have been proven to be relevant to human congenital heart disease. The most trivial explanation for this apparent discrepancy is that most of these mouse genes have not been tested for mutations in human patients. Testing requires a large effort and considerable resources, at least until low-cost high-throughput technologies are available for mutation searches. Hence, understanding the genetics of sporadic congenital heart disease cases remains a major challenge. Gene mutation in model systems is still, and will remain for the foreseeable future, the most effective strategy to identify genes relevant to cardiovascular development. Further investigation of the human genetics of congenital heart disease will require a synthesis between model system data and mutational analysis technology. The process will require two advances: (1) development of a catalog of genes important for pharyngeal arch and pouch development, as determined by model systems and human genetics data, and (2) development of large-scale, low-cost technologies for rapid sequencing of a large number of genes in congenital heart disease patients.

Current knowledge indicates that the genetics of pharyngeal arch and pouch development is complex and dependent on multiple genes, mainly encoding for transcription factors and signaling and signal transduction molecules. Despite early studies emphasizing the importance of neural crest-derived cells, it is becoming clear that the concerted development of, and tissue interactions between, the different components of the pharyngeal apparatus are key issues in pharyngeal-dependent cardiovascular development. In particular, the importance of the pharyngeal endoderm as a source of inductive signals is being carefully considered.[12,37,98,99] Critical issue are to understand how the different tissue components communicate with each other, what signaling molecules are involved, and how their activities and the transcription of their genes is controlled. For example, if the endoderm drives the development of the pharyngeal apparatus, how does it signal to the neural crest-derived mesenchyme, and what are the critical genes that respond to these signals. Candidate signaling systems, especially fibroblast growth factor, TGFβ, and hedgehog signaling, should be tested in this context.

Finally, one should consider that most known genetic syndromes associated with conotruncal and aortic arch defects are caused by gene haploinsufficiency and have incomplete penetrance and variable expressivity. Hence, gene dosage is critical, and the threshold between sufficiency and insufficiency of a given gene product may be affected by the structure or level of expression of the remaining allele, other genetic loci, and/or nongenetic factors. For example, the penetrance of cardiovascular defects in the *Df1/+* mouse model of DGS does not depend on the remaining allele; instead, it is strongly affected by other genetic loci and by nongenetic factors.[55] In addition to the obvious biologic importance of identifying modifier genes, one should also consider the possibility of artificially tipping the balance between insufficiency and sufficiency of a gene product using pharmacologic agents to boost the expression of the normal copy of the gene. This may form the basis for prevention of congenital heart disease in the future.

## REFERENCES

1. Kirby ML: Contribution of neural crest to heart and vessel morphology. In Harvey RP, Rosenthal N (eds): Heart Development. New York, Academic Press, 1999, pp 179–190.
2. Creazzo TL, Godt RE, Leatherbury L, et al: Role of cardiac neural crest cells in cardiovascular development. Annu Rev Physiol 1998;60:267–286.
3. Noden DM: The embryonic origins of avian cephalic and cervical muscles and associated connective tissues. Am J Anat 1983;168:257–276.
4. Couly GF, Coltey PM, Le Douarin NM: The triple origin of skull in higher vertebrates: A study in quail-chick chimeras. Development 1993;117:409–429.
5. Jiang X, Rowitch DH, Soriano P, et al: Fate of the mammalian cardiac neural crest. Development 2000;127:1607–1616.
6. Epstein JA, Li J, Lang D, et al: Migration of cardiac neural crest cells in Splotch embryos. Development 2000;127:1869–1878.
7. Kirby ML, Bockman DE: Neural crest and normal development: A new perspective. Anat Rec 1984;209:1–6.
8. Bockman DE, Redmond ME, Waldo K, et al: Effect of neural crest ablation on development of the heart and arch arteries in the chick. Am J Anat 1987;180:332–341.
9. Bockman DE, Redmond ME, Kirby ML: Alteration of early vascular development after ablation of cranial neural crest. Anat Rec 1989;225:209–217.
10. Kirby ML, Waldo KL: Neural crest and cardiovascular patterning. Circ Res 1995;77:211–215.
11. Veitch E, Begbie J, Schilling TF, et al: Pharyngeal arch patterning in the absence of neural crest. Curr Biol 1999;9:1481–1484.
12. Graham A, Smith A: Patterning the pharyngeal arches. Bioessays 2001;23:54–61.
13. Franz T: The Splotch (Sp1H) and Splotch-delayed (Spd) alleles: Differential phenotypic effects on neural crest and limb musculature. Anat Embryol (Berl) 1993;187:371–377.
14. Conway SJ, Henderson DJ, Kirby ML, et al: Development of a lethal congenital heart defect in the splotch (Pax3) mutant mouse. Cardiovasc Res 1997;36:163–173.
15. Conway SJ, Bundy J, Chen J, et al: Decreased neural crest stem cell expansion is responsible for the conotruncal heart defects within

the splotch (Sp(2H))/Pax3 mouse mutant. Cardiovasc Res 2000;47:314–328.
16. McKusick V: Online mendelian inheritance in man. www.ncbi.nlm.nih.gov/Omim/, 2001.
17. Kawasaki T, Kitsukawa, T, Bekku Y, et al: A requirement for neuropilin-1 in embryonic vessel formation. Development 1999;126:4895–4902.
18. Jerome LA, Papaioannou VE: DiGeorge syndrome phenotype in mice mutant for the T-box gene, Tbx1. Nat Genet 2001;27:286–291.
19. Lindsay EA, Vitelli F, Su H, et al: Tbx1 haploinsufficieny in the DiGeorge syndrome region causes aortic arch defects in mice. Nature 2001;410:97–101.
20. Merscher S, Funke B, Epstein JA, et al: TBX1 is responsible for cardiovascular defects in velo-cardio-facial/DiGeorge syndrome. Cell 2001;104:619–629.
21. Kurihara H, Kurihara Y, Maemura K, Yazaki Y: The role of endothelin-1 in cardiovascular development. Ann NY Acad Sci 1997;811:168–176; discussion 176–177.
22. Yanagisawa H, Hammer RA, Richardson JA, et al: Role of endothelin-1/endothelin-A receptor-mediated signaling pathway in the aortic arch patterning in mice. J Clin Invest 1998;102:22–33.
23. Clouthier DE, Hosoda K, Richardson JA, et al: Cranial and cardiac neural crest defects in endothelin-A receptor-deficient mice. Development 1998;125:813–824.
24. Yanagisawa H, Yanagisawa M, Kapur, RP, et al: Dual genetic pathways of endothelin-mediated intercellular signaling revealed by targeted disruption of endothelin converting enzyme-1 gene. Development 1998;125:825–836.
25. Iida K, Koseki H, Kakinuma H, et al: Essential roles of the winged helix transcription factor MFH-1 in aortic arch patterning and skeletogenesis. Development 1997;124:4627–4638.
26. Kume T, Jiang H, Topczewska JM, Hogan BL: The murine winged helix transcription factors, Foxc1 and Foxc2, are both required for cardiovascular development and somitogenesis. Genes Dev 2001;15:2470–2482.
27. Feiner L, Webber AL, Brown CB, et al: Targeted disruption of semaphorin 3C leads to persistent truncus arteriosus and aortic arch interruption. Development 2001;128:3061–3070.
28. Bartram U, Molin DS, Wissel J, et al: Double-outlet right ventricle and overriding tricuspid valve reflect disturbances of looping, myocardialization, endocardial cushion differentiation, and apoptosis in TGFβ(2)-knockout mice. Circulation 2001;103:2745–2752.
29. Kelly RG, Brown NA, Buckingham ME: The arterial pole of the mouse heart forms from Fgf10-expressing cells in pharyngeal mesoderm. Dev Cell 302;1:435–440.
30. Mjaatvedt CH, Nakaoka T, Moreno Radriquez R, et al: The outflow tract of the heart is recruited from a novel heart-forming field. Dev Biol 2001;238:97–109.
31. Waldo KL, Kumiski DH, Wallis KT, et al: Conotruncal myocardium arises from a secondary heart field. Development 2001;128:3179–3188.
32. Franz T: Persistent truncus arteriosus in the Splotch mutant mouse. Anat Embryol 1989;180:457–464.
33. Gruber PJ, Kubalak SW, Pexieder T, et al: RXR alpha deficiency confers genetic susceptibility for aortic sac, conotruncal, atrioventricular cushion, and ventricular muscle defects in mice. J Clin Invest 1996;98:1332–1343.
34. Mendelsohn C, Lohnes D, Decimo D, et al: Function of the retinoic acid receptors (RARs) during development. II. Multiple abnormalities at various stages of organogenesis in RAR double mutants. Development 1994;120:2749–2771.
35. Brannan CI, Perkins AS, Vogel KS, et al: Targeted disruption of the neurofibromatosis type-1 gene leads to developmental abnormalities in heart and various neural crest-derived tissues [published erratum appears in Genes Dev 1994;8:2792]. Genes Dev 1994;8:1019–1029.
36. Jacks T, Shih TS, Schmitt EM, et al: Tumour predisposition in mice heterozygous for a targeted mutation in Nf1. Nat Genet 1994;7:353–361.
37. Lakkis MM, Epstein JA: Neurofibromin modulation of ras activity is required for normal endocardial-mesenchymal transformation in the developing heart. Development 1998;125:4359–4367.

38. Oda T, Elkahloun AG, Pike BL, et al: Mutations in the human Jagged1 gene are responsible for Alagille syndrome [see comments]. Nat Genet 1997;16: 235-242.

39. Li L, Krantz ID, Deng Y, et al: Alagille syndrome is caused by mutations in human Jagged1, which encodes a ligand for Notch1 [see comments]. Nat Genet 1997;16:243-251.

40. Donovan MJ, Hahn R, Tessarollo L, Hempstead BL: Identification of an essential nonneuronal function of neurotrophin 3 in mammalian cardiac development. Nat Genet 1996;14:210-213.

41. Kim RY, Robertson EJ, Solloway MJ: Bmp6 and Bmp7 are required for cushion formation and septation in the developing mouse heart. Dev Biol 2001;235:449-466.

42. Ya J, Schilhan MW, DeBoer PA, et al: Sox4-deficiency syndrome in mice is an animal model for common trunk. Circ Res 1998;83:986-994.

43. Guris DL, Fantes J, Tara D, et al: Mice lacking the homologue of the human 22q11.2 gene CRKL phenocopy neurocristopathies of DiGeorge syndrome. Nat Genet 2001;27:293-298.

44. Eferl R, Sibilia M, Hilberg F, et al: Functions of c-Jun in liver and heart development. J Cell Biol 1999;145:1049-1061.

45. Takihara Y, Tomotsone D, Shirai M, et al: Targeted disruption of the mouse homologue of the Drosophila polyhomeotic gene leads to altered anteroposterior patterning and neural crest defects. Development 1997;124: 3673-3682.

46. Tevosian SG, Deconinck AE, Taraka H, et al: FOG-2, a cofactor for GATA transcription factors, is essential for heart morphogenesis and development of coronary vessels from epicardium. Cell 2000;101: 729-739.

47. Bamforth SD, Braganca J, Eloranta JJ, et al: [46_AU30]Cardiac malformations, adrenal agenesis, neural crest defects and exencephaly in mice lacking Cited2, a new Tfap2 co-activator. Nat Genet 2001;29:469-474.

48. Lammer EJ, Opitz JM: The DiGeorge anomaly as a developmental field defect. Am J Med Genet Suppl 1986;2:113-127.

49. Opitz JM, Lewin SO: The developmental field concept in pediatric pathology-especially with respect to fibular a/hypoplasia and the DiGeorge anomaly. Birth Defects Orig Artic Ser 1987;23:277-292.

50. Thomas RA, Landing BH, Wells TR: Embryologic and other developmental considerations of thirty-eight possible variants of the DiGeorge anomaly. Am J Med Genet Suppl 1987;3:43-66.

51. DiGeorge AM: A new concept of the cellular basis of immunity. J Pediatr 1965;67:907-908.

52. Lindsay EA: Chromosomal microdeletions: Dissecting del22q11 syndrome. Nat Rev Genet 2001;2:858-868.

53. Yu Y, Bradley A: Mouse genomic technologies engineering chromosomal rearrangements in mice. Nat Rev Genet 2001;2: 780-790.

54. Lindsay EA, Botta A, Jorecic V, et al: Congenital heart disease in mice deficient for the DiGeorge syndrome region. Nature 1999;401:379-383.

55. Taddei I, Morishima M, Huynh T, Lindsay EA: Genetic factors are major determinants of phenotypic variability in a mouse model of the DiGeorge/del22q11 syndromes. Proc Natl Acad Sci USA 2001;98:11428-11431.

56. Paylor R, McIlwain KL, McAninch R, et al: Mice deleted for the DiGeorge/velocardiofacial syndrome region show abnormal sensorimotor gating and learning and memory impairments. Hum Mol Genet 2001;10:2645-2650.

57. Lindsay EA, Baldini A: Recovery from arterial growth delay reduces penetrance of cardiovascular defects in mice deleted for the DiGeorge syndrome region. Hum Mol Genet 2001;10: 997-1002.

58. Krantz ID, Smith R, Colliton RP, et al: Jagged1 mutations in patients ascertained with isolated congenital heart defects. Am J Med Genet 1999;84: 56-60.

59. Eldadah ZA, Hamosh A, Biery NJ, et al: Familial tetralogy of Fallot caused by mutation in the jagged1 gene. Hum Mol Genet 2001;10: 163-169.

60. Winnier GE, Kume T, Deng K, et al: Roles for the winged helix transcription factors MF1 and MFH1 in cardiovascular development revealed by nonallelic noncomplementation of null alleles. Dev Biol 1999;213: 418-431.

61. Nishimura DY, Swiderski RE, Alward WL, et al: The forkhead transcription factor gene FKHL7 is responsible for glaucoma phenotypes which map to 6p25. Nat Genet 2998;19:140-147.

62. Fang J, Dagenais SL, Erikson RR, et al: Mutations in FOXC2 (MFH-1), a forkhead family transcription factor, are responsible for the hereditary lymphedema-distichiasis syndrome. Am J Hum Genet 2000;67: 1382-1388.

63. Noonan JA: Hypertelorism with Turner phenotype. A new syndrome with associated congenital heart disease. Am J Dis Child 1968;116:373-380.

64. Tartaglia M, Mehler EL, Goldberg R, et al: Mutations in PTPN11, encoding the protein tyrosine phosphatase SHP-2, cause Noonan syndrome. Nat Genet 2001;29:465-468.

65. Van Vactor D, O'Reilly AM, Neel BG: Genetic analysis of protein tyrosine phosphatases. Curr Opin Genet Dev 1998;8:112-126.

66. Chen B, Bronson RT, Klaman LD, et al: Mice mutant for Egfr and Shp2 have defective cardiac semilunar valvulogenesis. Nat Genet 2000;24:296-299.

67. Pagon RA, Graham JM Jr, Zonana J, Yong SL: Coloboma, congenital heart disease, and choanal atresia with multiple anomalies: CHARGE association. J Pediatr 1981;99:223-227.

68. Opitz JM: G syndrome (hypertelorism with esophageal abnormality and hypospadias, or hypospadias-dysphagia, or "Opitz-Frias" or "Opitz-G" syndrome)-perspective in 1987 and bibliography. Am J Med Genet 1987;28:275-285.

69. Jacobson Z, Glickstein J, Hensle T, Marion RW: Further delineation of the Opitz G/BBB syndrome: Report of an infant with complex congenital heart disease and bladder exstrophy, and review of the literature. Am J Med Genet 1998;78:294-299.

70. Robin NH, Feldman GJ, Aronson AL, et al: Opitz syndrome is genetically heterogeneous, with one locus on Xp22, and a second locus on 22q11.2. Nat Genet 1995;11:459-461.

71. Quaderi NA, Schweiger S, Gaudenz K, et al: Opitz G/BBB syndrome, a defect of midline development, is due to mutations in a new RING finger gene on Xp22. Nat Genet 1997;17:285-291.

72. Cainarca S, Messali S, Ballabio A, Meroni G: Functional characterization of the Opitz syndrome gene product (midin): Evidence for homodimerization and association with microtubules throughout the cell cycle. Hum Mol Genet 1999;8:1387-1396.

73. Trockenbacher A, Suckow V, Foerster J, et al: MID1, mutated in Opitz syndrome, encodes an ubiquitin ligase that targets phosphatase 2A for degradation. Nat Genet 2001;29:287-294.

74. McDonald-McGinn DM, Driscoll DA, Bason L, et al: Autosomal dominant "Opitz" GBBB syndrome due to a 22q11.2 deletion [see comments]. Am J Med Genet 1995;59:103-113.

75. Fujimoto A, Wilson MG, Towner JW: Familial inversion of chromosome No. 8: An affected child and a carrier fetus. Humangenetik 1975;27:67-73.

76. Sujansky E, Smith AC, Prescott KE, et al: Natural history of the recombinant (8) syndrome. Am J Med Genet 1993;47:512-525.

77. Gelb BD, Towbin JA, McCabe ER, Sujansky E: San Luis Valley recombinant chromosome 8 and tetralogy of Fallot: A review of chromosome 8 anomalies and congenital heart disease. Am J Med Genet 1991;40:471-476.

78. Graw SL, Sample T, Bleskan J, et al: Cloning, sequencing, and analysis of inv8 chromosome breakpoints associated with recombinant 8 syndrome. Am J Hum Genet 2000;66:1138-1144.

79. Kuo CT, Morrisey EE, Anandappa R, et al: GATA4 transcription factor is required for ventral morphogenesis and heart tube formation. Genes Dev 1997;11: 1048-1060.

80. Molkentin JD, Lin Q, Duncan SA, Olson EN: Requirement of the transcription factor GATA4 for heart tube formation and ventral morphogenesis. Genes Dev 1997;11:1061-1072.

81. Pehlivan T, Pober BR, Brueckner M, et al: GATA4 haploinsufficiency in patients with interstitial deletion of chromosome region 8p23.1 and congenital heart disease. Am J Med Genet 1999;83: 201-206.

82. Giglio S, Graw SL, Gimelli G, et al: Deletion of a 5-cM region at chromosome 8p23 is associated with a spectrum of congenital heart defects. Circulation 2000;102:432-437.

83. Pierpont ME, Gobel JW, Moller JH, Edwards JE: Cardiac malformations in relatives of children with truncus arteriosus or interruption of the aortic arch. Am J Cardiol 1988;61:423-427.

84. Rein AJ, Dollberg S, Gale R: Genetics of conotruncal malformations: Review of the literature and report of a consanguineous kindred with various conotruncal malformations. Am J Med Genet 1990;36:353-355.

85. Benke PJ: The isotretinoin teratogen syndrome. JAMA 1984;251:3 267-269.

86. Braun JT, Franciosi RA, Mastri AR, et al: Isotretinoin dysmorphic syndrome. Lancet 1984;1:506-507.

87. Lott IT, Bocian M, Pribram HW, Leitner M: Fetal hydrocephalus and ear anomalies associated with maternal use of isotretinoin. J Pediatr 1984;105:597-600.

88. Lammer EJ, Chen DT, Hoar RM, et al: Retinoic acid embryopathy. N Engl J Med 1985;313:837-841.

89. Niederreither K, McCaffery P, Drager UC, et al: Restricted expression and retinoic acid-induced downregulation of the retinaldehyde dehydrogenase type 2 (RALDH-2) gene during mouse development. Mech Dev 1997;62:67-78.

90. Niederreither K, Vermot J, Dolle P, Chambon P: Embryonic retinoic acid synthesis is essential for early mouse post-implantation development. Nat Genet 1999;21:444-448.

91. Niederreither K, Vermot J, Messaddeq N, et al: Embryonic retinoic acid synthesis is essential for heart morphogenesis in the mouse. Development 2001;128:1019-1031.

92. Jones KL, Smith DW: The fetal alcohol syndrome. Teratology 1975;12:1-10.

93. Steeg CN, Woolf P: Cardiovascular malformations in the fetal alcohol syndrome. Am Heart J 1979;98:635-637.

94. Ammann AJ, Wara DW, Cowan MJ, et al: The DiGeorge syndrome and the fetal alcohol syndrome. Am J Dis Child 1982;136:906-908.

95. Daft PA, Johnston MC, Sulik KK: Abnormal heart and great vessel development following acute ethanol exposure in mice. Teratology 1986;33:93-104.

96. Deltour L, Ang HL, Duester G: Ethanol inhibition of retinoic acid synthesis as a potential mechanism for fetal alcohol syndrome. FASEB J 1996;10:1050-1057.

97. Zachman RD, Grummer MA: The interaction of ethanol and vitamin A as a potential mechanism for the pathogenesis of fetal alcohol syndrome. Alcohol Clin Exp Res 1998;22:1544-1556.

98. Piotrowski T, Nusslein-Volhard C: The endoderm plays an important role in patterning the segmented pharyngeal region in zebrafish (Danio rerio). Dev Biol 2000;225:339-356.

99. van den Hoff MJ, Moorman AF: Cardiac neural crest: The holy grail of cardiac abnormalities? Cardiovasc Res 2000;47:212-216.

## EDITOR'S CHOICE

Abu-Issa R, Smyth G, Smoak I, et al: Fgf8 is required for pharyngeal arch and cardiovascular development in the mouse. Development 2002;129:4613-4625.

*One of a trio of papers (See Franke et al and below) indicating the FGF 8 pathways may play a critical role in the onset of outflow tract defects in the setting of Digeorge Syndrome and related cardiac neural crest defects.*

Frank DU, Fotheringham LK, Brewer JA, et al: Moon AM: An Fgf8 mouse mutant phenocopies human 22q11 deletion syndrome. Development 2002;129:4591-4603.

*One of the trio of papers identifying a potential role of FGF 8 in Digeorge; see Abu-Issa et al above.*

Gitler AD, Brown CB, Kochilas L, et al: Neural crest migration and mouse models of congenital heart disease. Cold Spring Harb Symp Quant Biol 2002;67:57-62.

*Excellent review of mouse models of congenital heart disease.*

Gitler AD, Zhu Y, Ismat FA, et al: Nf1 has an essential role in endothelial cells. Nat Genet 2003;33:75-79.

*Systematic, rigorous conditional mutagenesis in multiple cell types indicates a key role for the endothelial cell lineages in outflow tract development.*

Hamblet NS, Lijam N, Ruiz-Lozano P, et al: Dishevelled 2 is essential for cardiac outflow tract development, somite segmentation and neural tube closure. Development 2002;129:5827-5838.

*Wnt/DVL pathways play a key role in cardiac outflow tract developmentn and are likely to have a similar important role in pathways for congenital heart disease.*

Jiang X, Rowitch DH, Soriano P, et al: Fate of the mammalian cardiac neural crest. Development 2000;127:1607-1616.

Kioussi C, Briata P, Baek SH, et al: Identification of a Wnt/Dvl/beta-Catenin -> Pitx2 pathway mediating cell-type-specific proliferation during development. Cell 2002;111:673-685.

*Wnt/DVL pathway (see Hamblet et al. above) connects with Pitx2 pathways for outflow tract development related to control of the proliferative capacity of cardiac neural crest cells.*

Kioussi C, Briata P, Baek SH, et al: Pitx genes during cardiovascular development. Cold Spring Harb Symp Quant Biol 2002;67:81-87.

*Fascinating story of Pitx2 in cardiac development.*

Stalmans I, Lambrechts D, De Smet F, et al: VEGF: a modifier of the del22q11 (DiGeorge) syndrome? Nat Med 2003;9:173-182.

*A link between angiogenesis and DiGeorge, most likely via endothelial related pathways.*

Yamagishi H, Maeda J, Hu T, et al: Tbx1 is regulated by tissue-specific forkhead proteins through a common Sonic hedgehog-responsive enhancer. Genes Dev 2003;17:269-281.

*Elegant molecular analysis of the mechanisms that control the expression of TBX1, a key player in the DiGeorge phenotype.*

# chapter 14

# Monogenic Causes of Congenital Heart Disease

*Joachim P. Schmitt*
*Christine E. Seidman*

Cardiac development is a critical and complex embryologic process that requires the integration of cell commitment, growth, looping, septation, and chamber specification. Usually these processes proceed with precision, but every year 32,000 infants in the United States and about 1 million worldwide are born with a defect in normal cardiac development. Epidemiologic and pathologic investigations of human congenital heart malformations have identified multiple teratogens, infectious agents, and factors in the maternal environment that are important causes for some cardiac defects. However, in most cases the cause remains unknown. In a posthumous publication, Dr. Helen Taussig[1] speculated that because "common cardiac malformations occur in otherwise 'normal' individuals. These malformations must be genetic in origin (and) neither exposure to toxic substances nor the parents can be held accountable for the occurrence of (most) congenital abnormalities." Recent molecular studies indicate the prophetic nature of her observations. Multiple congenital heart defects have been identified that are produced by gene mutations, which are transmitted as Mendelian traits and inherited in a dominant or recessive, X-linked, or autosomal fashion.

The incidence of congenital cardiovascular malformation approaches 1 per 100 in live births,[2-4] and these malformations occur in approximately 10% of stillborn infants. Almost one third of congenital heart abnormalities are ventricular septal defects (VSDs), but atrial septal defects (ASDs), pulmonary valve stenosis, and combined defects of atrial and ventricular septa and the tetralogy of Fallot are not uncommon. Each of these disorders accounts for 7% to 10% of cardiac malformations found in newborns. Table 14-1 reviews the 20 most common diagnostic groups identified from the Baltimore-Washington Infant Study on 906,626 live births.[5] Importantly, all of the defects listed severely disturb normal blood and/or oxygen supply of organs and often demand immediate surgical corrections. Epidemiologic data also indicates considerable variation in the precise congenital defects exhibited by related, affected individuals. For example the Baltimore-Washington Infant Heart Study[5] demonstrated an increased incidence of tetralogy of Fallot, transposition of the great arteries, and truncus arteriosus in family members of individuals with VSDs. Such findings suggest that developmental pathways are shared by unrelated structures that participate in different aspects of cardiac functions. A corollary to this observation might be that

clinically distinct malformations arising from a single genetic cause tend to hinder recognition of the heritable nature of human congenital heart disease (CHD).

To appreciate the mechanisms underpinning structural malformations of the heart requires an understanding of normal cardiac development. The heart begins to form during the third week of human embryonic life with establishment of a primitive vascular system. Although the earliest molecular mechanisms that specify cells to adopt a cardiac fate are largely unknown, cell migration early in gastrulation indicates commencement of cardiac embryogenesis. Populations of mesodermal cells migrate bilaterally away from the primitive streak and toward the anterior endoderm where they coalesce to form a horseshoe-shaped plexus, often called the cardiac crescent (Fig. 14-1A). As the embryo folds cephalocaudally the lateral regions of the crescent merge, except at their most caudal ends, to shape a linear heart tube (Fig. 14-1B). Cells within the linear heart have specified myocyte programs: caudal and central cells are fated to become atrial and ventricular myocytes, respectively, and more cranial cells form the constituents of the outflow tract. The linear heart tube is an active heart that pumps blood from the caudal to cephalic poles into the first aortic arch and dorsal aorta.

During the fourth week of embryonic life the growing linear heart tube undergoes looping (Fig. 14-1C): cranial portions of the tube shift in a ventrocaudal direction and to the right, and the caudal portion bends in a dorsocranial direction and to the left. The resultant bend repositions individual cardiac chambers into an adult anatomic position (Fig. 14-1D).

Throughout cardiac looping the myocardium is also remodeled. Expansion of cells results in ventricular trabeculation. Proliferation of ridge-like protrusions produce cardiac cushions within the atrioventricular canal; these swellings approach each other and fuse, dividing atria from ventricles. With remodeling, these structures become mitral and tricuspid valves. Atrial septation occurs by sequential growth of the septum primum and secundum, while an interatrial foramen is maintained to allow blood to traverse from the right to the left atrium. Establishment of the interventricular septum depends on division of the right from left ventricles and juxtaposition of the developing aortic and pulmonary trunks, processes that integrate growth, extensive remodeling of the inner curvature of the myocardium, and migration of neural crest-derived cells (Fig. 14-2).

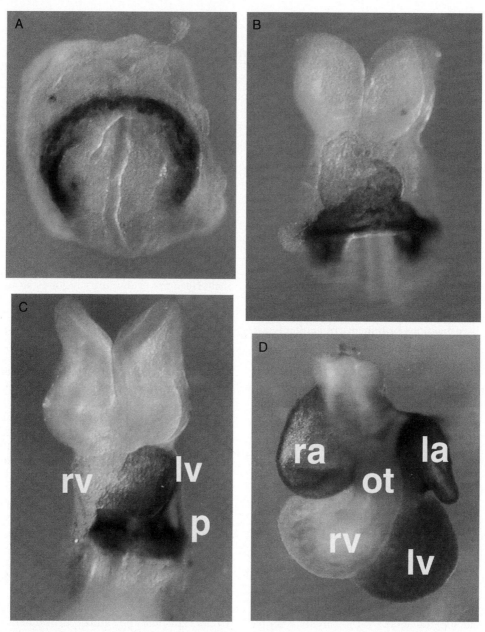

**FIGURE 14-1.** Developmental structures of the mammalian heart illuminated by *in situ* hybridization of *Tbx5*. Primitive myocardial cells initially form a cardiac crescent *(A)*, the first morphologic structure of the developing heart. The crescent coalesces to form a midline, beating linear heart tube *(B)* that undergoes looping *(C)*, growth, and remodeling to become the mature four-chambered heart *(D)*. LA, left atrium; LV, left ventricle; P, pericardium; OT, outflow tract; RA, right atria; RV, right ventricle. *(Modified from Bruneau BG, Logan M, Davis N, et al: Chamber-specific cardiac expression of Tbx5 and heart defects in Holt-Oram syndrome. Dev Biol 1999;211:100–108, with permission.)*

A wealth of insights into some of the many molecular signals responsible for cardiac embryogenesis has come from studies of model organisms, and specific genes have been defined that are critical to direct the complex developmental processes outlined previously.[6] Several transcription factors, initially identified in *Drosophila* (tinman) and mice (Nkx2.5 or Csx, MEF2, Gata) are important for cardiac cell differentiation.[7,8] From studies in chicks, the roles of sonic hedgehog, activin receptor IIa, and CNR1 have been recognized for establishment of axis, a necessary step for subsequent cardiac looping. In mice, *iv* and *inv* genes are involved in left-right asymmetry at later stages in cardiac development.[7,9,10] TGFβ

family members and BMP have been implicated in vertebrate atrioventricular valve formation and conotruncus development.[7,11] Tbx5 participates in early maturation of the atria and primitive left-ventricular and later functions in cardiac septation. Tbx1 and neural crest cells are essential for vertebrate atrioventricular valve formation and maturation of the outflow tract.

Discovery of these molecular signals is relevant to understanding congenital heart disorders. Spacing model systems in which the genes noted previously have been genetically mutated have produced a myriad of structural heart malformations, presumably because of the consequences that dysregulation of one gene has on down-

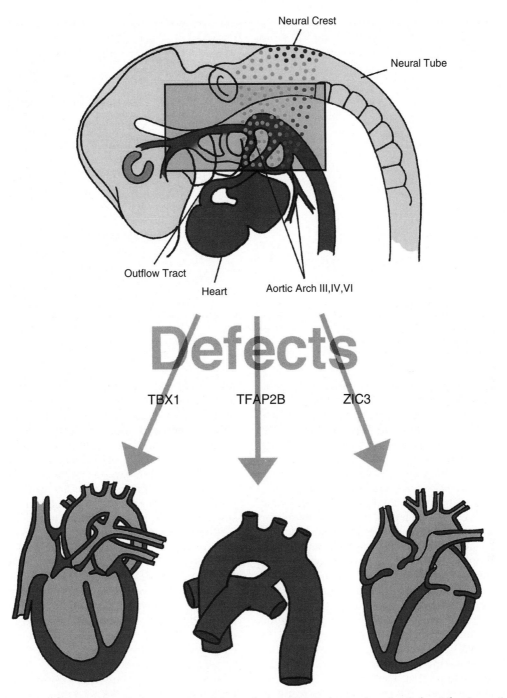

**FIGURE 14-2.** Neural crest cells in cardiac development. Migrating neural crest cells populate aortic arches 3, 4, and 6 and contribute to the cardiac outflow tract and vascular development of the great arteries. Neural crest cells (light gray) expressing *ZIC3* (black) and *TFAP2B* (dark gray) migrate through tissues expressing *TBX1* (box). Defects in these transcription factors can cause congenital heart defects including tetralogy of Fallot *(left)*, PDA *(center)*, and dextrocardia with normally related great arteries *(right)*.

stream molecular targets. Although currently only a few genes identified in model systems have been directly implicated in human heart malformations, the single-gene defects that have been defined (Table 14-1) collectively indicate an important paradigm: CHD occurs when the molecular blueprint for development is disturbed. Except for *Jag1*, which encodes a ligand to a transmembrane receptor, human CHD genes encode transcription factors that directly or indirectly activate the expression

of other genes and in so doing regulate cell fate decisions, orchestrate migration, and program development.

## ATRIAL AND VENTRICULAR SEPTAL DEFECTS

Defects in cardiac septation arise as isolated findings, in the context of other structural malformations of

■ ■ ■

**TABLE 14-1** SINGLE-GENE DEFECTS IN HUMAN HEART MALFORMATIONS

| Malformation | Prevalence* | Gene Defect† |
|---|---|---|
| VSD, membranous | 9.87 | *TBX5, TBX1, NKX2.5* |
| VSD, muscular | 4.73 | *TBX5, TBX1, NKX2.5* |
| Pulmonic stenosis | 3.78 | *JAG1,* chromosomes 12q2, 17q11.2 |
| Atrioventricular septal defect | 3.53 | *TBX5, NKX2.5* |
| Tetralogy of Fallot | 3.26 | *NKX2.5, JAG1, TBX,* chromosome *22q* (TBX1) |
| Atrial septal defect | 3.21 | *TBX5, NKX2.5* |
| Transposition of great arteries | 2.64 | |
| Hypoplastic left heart | 1.78 | *NKX2.5* |
| Laterality/looping | 1.44 | *ZIC3, LEFTA* |
| Coarctation of aorta | 1.39 | |
| Patent arterial duct | 0.88 | *TFAP2B* |
| Aortic valve stenosis | 0.81 | |
| Bicuspid aortic valve | 0.74 | |
| Total anomalous pulmonary venous return | 0.66 | Chromosome 4 |
| Pulmonary atresia | 0.59 | |
| Interrupted aortic arch | 0.58 | |
| Common arterial trunk | 0.49 | |
| Ebstein anomaly | 0.47 | *NKX2.5* |
| Tricuspid atresia | 0.36 | |
| Double-outlet right ventricle without TGA | 0.33 | |

*Prevalence per 10,000, based on the Baltimore-Washington Infant Study: 1981-1989.[5]
†Gene mutations and loci demonstrated to cause malformations. In most instances, mutations in these genes have been associated with inherited congenital defects. Note that mutations in the same gene can produce quite different malformations.

the heart, and as components of multisystem syndromic disorders. Using linkage strategies, the location of three gene mutations that produce cardiac septation defects have been located on chromosomes 5p, 5q35, and 12q24. Each disease locus results in autosomal dominant transmission with variable expression of ASD and VSD.

The congenital heart gene encoded at 5p remains unknown. Affected individuals exhibit cardiac disease only, most commonly an isolated ASD, but in some instances atrial septal aneurysm, aortic stenosis, or persistent left superior vena cava are also observed. The 5p locus is characterized by incomplete penetrance. A disease haplotype has been identified in clinically unaffected parents of children who had an affected haplotype and structural heart disease. Whether spontaneous closure of an unrecognized ASD or VSD contributes to variable penetrance of this disease gene is unknown.

The disease genes encoded on chromosomes 5q35 and 12q24 are *NKX2-5* and *TBX5,* respectively. Both genes encode transcription factors that are strongly expressed by the time that the cardiac crescent is formed (Fig. 14-1*A*). Mutations in either gene result in autosomal dominant inheritance of ASDs, VSDs, and a wide spectrum of other cardiac structural malformations that are often associated with defects in normal cardiac electrophysiology.

## *NKX2-5*

The *Drosophila tinman* gene is so named because gene deletion in flies results in the absence of the dorsal vessel, which is the insect equivalent of the vertebrate heart. *NKX2-5,* also known as *CSX,* is the human homolog of *tinman* and encodes a homeobox transcription factor that is expressed from the earliest stage of cardiac development, throughout embryogenesis, and in the adult atria and ventricles.[12-14] However, *Nkx2-5* transcripts are

not found in derivatives of the endocardial cushion including the tricuspid valve and atrioventricular bundles or in the vasculature and the epicardium.[14]

Experiments in mice that were genetically engineered to lack functional *Nkx2-5* alleles have indicated the importance of this transcription factor in mammalian cardiac development. Homozygous mutants are embryonic lethal and exhibit defects in myocardial growth and differentiation[15,16]; the atrioventricular canal remains open and the single ventricle is connected to a poorly developed outflow tract. Ventricular maturation is also abnormal; trabeculae were poorly developed and endocardial cushion formation was deficient in homozygous *Nkx2.5*-null mice. Attenuated expression of transcripts encoding proteins important for ventricular development and growth, including low levels of myosin light chain (MLC)-2v, ANF, BNP, and SM22a, are found in *Nkx2-5* deficient mice, and *eHand* expression is abolished.[15-17] Thus, *Nkx2-5* appears to be an essential transcription factor for the ventricular-specific developmental program.

Remarkably, the phenotypes observed in humans who carry a heterozygous *NKX2-5* mutation are strikingly different from phenotypes seen in mice that lack this transcription factor. Human defects are compatible with life, although a range of congenital structural malformations have been reported, most prominently secundum ASDs but also VSDs, tetralogy of Fallot, subvalvular aortic stenosis, ventricular hypertrophy, pulmonary atresia, and mitral valve malformations.[18,19] Human studies have also uncovered an unrecognized role for *NKX2-5* in normal cardiac electrophysiology: conduction delays in the atrioventricular node are found in almost all individuals with congenital heart defects caused by *NKX2-5* gene mutations. In some, these electrophysiologic abnormalities were the sole clinical manifestation of a mutation. Electrophysiologic deficits are usually progressive, and worsening atrioventricular block frequently has necessitated pacemaker implantation in affected individuals. Unrecognized electrophysiologic abnormalities may account for sudden death that occurs many years after uncomplicated surgical repair of an ASD in individuals with *NKX2-5* defects.

Human *NKX2-5* mutations encode both missense amino acid residues and premature termination of the transcription factor. However the consequences of these different defects may be the same. Biochemical analyses of mutant *NKX2-5* constructs, engineered to contain human missense defects, indicate that these impair DNA binding and/or disrupt homodimerization,[20] a consequence that would render mutant peptides inactive. *NKX2-5* mutations that produce either haploinsufficiency or a functional null allele would reduce by half the physiologic levels of this transcription factor. Given the congenital heart anomalies associated with reduced levels of NKX2-5, one can conclude that physiologic concentrations of this molecule during cardiac embryogenesis is critically important.

The phenotypes associated with human *NKX2-5* haploinsufficiency prompted reevaluation of the impact of *Nkx2-5* gene dosage in mice. Although initially believed to be normal, mice that are heterozygous for the *Nkx2-5* deletion have recently been demonstrated to have defects in atrial septal formation, atrioventricular block, and, occasionally, bicuspid aortic valves.[16,21] Further evidence for the importance of physiologic levels of Nkx2-5 comes from an analysis of chimeric mice derived from *Nkx2-5*-deficient ES cell lines.[16] Embryos with more than 30% to 40% contribution of *Nkx2-5*-deficient cells to the heart showed a phenotype comparable to homozygous *Nkx2-5* null embryos. Milder cardiac phenotypes were observed in embryos with less contribution of *Nkx2-5*-deficient cells to the heart. Normal cardiac morphogenesis may therefore be predicated on appropriate expression of *Nkx2.5* in an adequate number of cardiac myocytes.

## TBX5

Members of the T-box gene family encode transcription factors that share a common DNA binding motif termed the T-box, which consists of 180 amino acid residues involved in DNA binding and dimerization.[22] There are 12 T-box genes encoded in the human genome, which are phylogenetically related to transcription factors[23-28] that pattern the development of a variety of tissues in diverse species. Human mutations in two T-box genes *TBX5* and *TBX1* result in CHD.

*TBX5* is encoded on chromosome 12q24. *TBX5* mutations cause Holt-Oram syndrome (HOS),[29-31] a rare autosomal dominant heart and hand disorder with an estimated prevalence of 0.95 per 100,000 total births. Approximately 85% of Holt-Oram cases are attributed to new mutations.[32] Although clinical manifestations of this disorder vary widely,[33,34] abnormalities in the upper limb preaxial radial rays are always present. These malformations may be unilateral or bilateral and range from carpal bone abnormalities that are only evident by radiographic study to more severe phenotypes that include triphalangeal or absent thumbs and phocomelia. Cardiac anomalies occur in about 85% of HOS patients. Septation

defects (ASDs and VSDs) and cardiac conduction defects, such as progressive atrioventricular block and atrial fibrillation, are common. Electrophysiologic abnormalities can occur even in the absence of septal defects.[30,33] ASDs are usually of the secundum type and can produce a common atrium syndrome with or without anomalous pulmonary venous return. VSDs often develop in the muscular trabeculated septum and may be multiple, producing a "Swiss cheese" septum. Abnormalities of cardiac isomerism are also seen.

The pattern of *Tbx5* expression during murine cardiogenesis has helped to explain the cardiac phenotypes observed in HOS. Tbx5 is found in the developing heart, eye, and forelimbs[35,36]; patterns of cardiac expression are conserved in mice and chicks[37] and presumably in other vertebrates, including humans. *Tbx5* transcripts are ubiquitous in the cardiac crescent (Fig. 14-1*A*), but, with formation of the linear heart tube, expression is strongest in the most posterior segments, regions that are destined to become right and left atrium and sinus venosus. As the heart undergoes looping, *Tbx5* expression expands anteriorly to encompass the entire future left ventricle. During chamber maturation and septation left-ventricular expression remains strong but is limited to the trabeculae of the right ventricle. This restricted expression pattern demarcates the developing right ventricular outflow tract from the trabeculated part of the right ventricle. *Tbx5* expression within the interventricular septum is also strikingly left sided and implies a developmental model in which right ventricular portions of the septum evolve from derivatives of the bulbus cordis, which exclude *Tbx5* expression.[38] Tbx5 is also detected in the developing atrioventricular valves, with higher levels on the atrial side of the valve leaflets,[31,37] suggesting that this transcription factor participates in valvulogenesis. Expression of *Tbx5* has been found in both the left and right superior vena cava and in the inferior vena cava.

Of the many different *TBX5* mutations identified in HOS patients,[29,31,39] most produce null alleles. A dominant disease phenotype, therefore, appears to reflect transcription factor haploinsufficiency. Although a 50% reduction in TBX5 levels causes severe birth defects in both the limb and the heart, the few missense mutations identified to date produce more divergent clinical findings: a predominance of either cardiac or limb malformations.[30,39] Insight into this observation has come from the three-dimensional crystal structure of a T-box protein encoded by *Xenopus laevis*. T-box motifs contain at least two DNA binding domains; residues located at the amino terminus interact with the major groove of target DNA, and residues at the carboxyl terminus interact with the minor groove of target DNA.[22] Holt-Oram missense mutations appear to affect one of these two binding domains. Distinct interactions with partner proteins that are critical for limb or heart development may explain why human *TBX5* missense mutations that perturb either 5' or 3' T-box sequences cause a preponderance of cardiac or skeletal malformations.[30]

Individuals with chromosome 12q duplications also show features of HOS, thereby suggesting a more generalized effect of *TBX5* dosage on phenotype; both underexpression and overexpression may cause disease.[40-42] This data supports the idea that normal cardiac embryogenesis requires precise regulation of the dose of transcription factors (TBX5, NKX2.5, and others) throughout development.

Lessons about the importance of *Tbx5* dosage have also come from genetically engineered models. Homozygous mice with deletions of both *Tbx5* alleles die early *in utero* and fail to develop posterior sinoatrial structures, resulting in a common atrium, hypoplastic left ventricle, and distorted right ventricle. A variety of genes known to participate in cardiogenesis are misexpressed, including *Anf, cx40, Irx4, Mlc2v, Gata4, Nkx2-5*, and *Hey2*. Overexpression of *Tbx5* in mouse[43] and chick[44] models also results in cardiac developmental anomalies. Murine haploinsufficiency of *Tbx5* (*Tbx5*[+/−]) closely resembles human HOS with forelimb, wrist, and digit malformations and cardiac septation defects with atrioventricular conduction block.[45] This model has helped in the discovery of mechanisms by which a 50% reduction in this transcription factor produces some of the developmental anomalies observed in HOS. *Anf* and *cx40* have been identified as downstream target genes of Tbx5; expression of both is diminished in *Tbx5*[+/−] mice. Promoter sequences in *Anf* and *cx40* contain binding sites for Nkx2-5 and Tbx5, and synergistic interactions between these transcription factors have been demonstrated to affect *Anf* and *cx40* expression.[45,46] This is a particularly intriguing result given the extensive overlap in human cardiac phenotypes (septation defects and atrioventricular block) that are produced by mutations in either of these transcription factor genes. Perhaps mutations that disrupt NKX2-5-TBX5 interactions alter downstream genes that are common to both transcription factors and produce common clinical phenotypes.

Striking variation in phenotype is observed among heterozygous *Tbx5*[+/−] mice bred into different genetic backgrounds. *Tbx5*[+/−] in an outbred background displays consistently mild skeletal abnormalities and cardiac malformations that are compatible with life (ASDs), whereas mice heterozygous for a null allele on an inbred background produces complex cardiac malformations and intrauterine death. These observations indicate a strong influence of modifier genes in phenotype expression. Modifier genes may also account for the considerable variation in the type and severity of limb and cardiac malformations in human HOS, even among individuals with identical *TBX5* mutations.

## DEFECTS IN STRUCTURES POPULATED BY NEURAL CREST CELLS

Neural crest cells derived from the dorsal neural tube migrate into pharyngeal arches 3, 4, and 6 early in embryonic development (Fig. 14-2). These cells contribute to the vascular development of the great arteries and to the outflow tract of the heart. Neural crest cells differentiate into the smooth muscle of the aortic arch, the ductus arteriosus, and the carotid arteries and become incorporated into the aorticopulmonary septum and the conotruncal cushions of the heart. In addition to cardiovascular tissues, these cells also contribute to the development of the thymus and thyroid and parathyroid glands.[47-49] The migration of neural crest cells is a highly orchestrated process that follows defined pathways. Cells migrate along a scaffold of fibronectin, laminin-1, vitronectin, collagens, and other extracellular matrix proteins. Proper neural crest migration and differentiation requires integration of intracellular and extracellular signals. Adhesion molecules, such as integrins, are involved in the interaction of neural crest cells with the extracellular matrix, and cadherins may allow neural crest cells to interact with each other during migration. Presently only some of critical molecular signals involved in these processes have been defined. Pax3 appears to be important for proliferation of neural crest precursors, and connexin43-mediated gap junction communication may affect migration rates. Endothelin and related receptors are required for normal postmigratory differentiation. Platelet-derived growth factor and retinoic acid have roles in neural crest migration and differentiation.[50]

Mice that have been genetically engineered to misexpress genes important for neural crest migration and development (e.g., *N-cadherin, Pax3/Splotch, connexin 43, MHF-1, endothelin-1, Patch, neurotrophin 3*, and *retinoic acid receptor* genes) exhibit an array of phenotypes. Abnormalities include defective left-right axis development; severe congenital malformations of the heart and great vessels; and malformations of the craniofacial structures, thymus, eyes, respiratory tract, and urogenital system. Similar cardiovascular phenotypes were reported with neural crest ablation in chicks.[51-54] To date only a limited number of genes that have been identified as critical for neural crest migration and function in lower vertebrate species have been implicated in human disease. Phenotypes observed in humans with mutations in *TFAP2B, TBX1*, and *ZIC3* genes include malformations of the great vessels and cardiac outflow tract and laterality defects.

## MALFORMATIONS OF THE OUTFLOW TRACT

Mutations in at least three genes, *TFAP2B, TBX1*, and *JAG-1*, are known to cause congenital cardiovascular disorders that particularly affect the cardiac outflow tract, although intracardiac malformations have also been observed with mutations in these genes. *TFAP2B* encodes a transcription factor that is expressed in neural crest cells. *TBX1* transcripts are also found in the tissue fields that become populated by neural crest cells.

### TFAP2B

The ductus arteriosus connects the pulmonary artery to the descending aorta and shunts blood away from the lungs during intrauterine life (Fig. 14-2). Normally, the ductus arteriosus closes shortly after birth, but failure of closure results in a PDA with left-to-right shunting of blood. PDA is a relatively common congenital cardiac defect (Table 14-1) that affects approximately 1 in 2000 children and may occur alone or in association with complex cardiovascular malformations.

Although a PDA may arise when one of several developmental processes go awry,[55] the occurrence rate among siblings of individuals with isolated PDA is approximately 3%, implying a strong genetic effect. Study of Char's syndrome has further advanced an appreciation of molecular genetic events that contribute to PDA. Linkage analyses in two families with Char's syndrome, an autosomal dominant disorder characterized by PDA, dysmorphic facial features, and malformed fifth digits of the hands,[56] mapped the disease locus to chromosome 6p12-p21.[57] Subsequent positional cloning and mutation analyses demonstrated missense mutations in the TFAP2B gene. TFAP2B encodes transcription factor AP-2 β (activating enhancer-binding protein 2 β), which is expressed in neural crest cells.[58] The identified missense defects perturb highly evolutionarily conserved residues at positions 264 and 289. Biochemical analyses of the functional consequences of these missense mutations indicate that heterodimers of mutant transcription factors were unable to bind target DNA sequence.[58] Mutant TFAP2B proteins also had a reduced ability to transactivate gene expression in eukaryotic cells, implying that human mutations encode functionally null alleles. Presumably the consequence of TFAP2B haploinsufficiency on neural crest development accounts for the resultant cardiovascular defects.

Like HOS, Char's syndrome causes CHD and hand anomalies (heart-hand syndromes). Coexistence of defects in these very distinct tissues has led to the hypothesis that there are shared features in cardiogenesis and limb development. Wilson[59] has proposed a cardiomelic developmental field, a region in the early embryo that gives rise to the heart and limb primordia and has suggested that qualitative or quantitative abnormalities of morphogens in this field account for both heart and hand defects. Whether this mechanism accounts for the range of genes with overlapping patterns of expression during cardiogenesis and upper limb development remains unknown.

## TBX 1

DiGeorge's syndrome is a common congenital disorder (1 out of 4000 life births) characterized by cardiac outflow tract abnormalities, usually mild facial dysmorphology, velopharyngeal insufficiency, submucous cleft palate, and thymic and parathyroid gland hypoplasia or aplasia.[60-62] Historically the dysgenesis of such diverse structures affected by DiGeorge's syndrome has been attributed to an unknown abnormality affecting the cranial neural crest cells that populate these structures. Whether DiGeorge's syndrome mutations directly perturbed a gene that is critical for neural crest cells maturation or a gene in cells that interacts with neural crest cells along their migratory pathways[63] is unclear. Most patients with DiGeorge's syndrome are hemizygous for a deletion of human chromosome 22 that can be large (3-Mb region on HSA22q11) or small (1.5-Mb nested deletion[61]). These observations indicate that haploinsufficiency of one or more genes on human chromosome 22 accounts for DiGeorge's syndrome.

Molecular genetic data has recently implicated TBX1 as the critical gene deleted in DiGeorge's syndrome.[64,65] Genetically engineered mice that are heterozygous for a Tbx1 null allele develop a high incidence of cardiac outflow tract anomalies similar to those observed in DiGeorge's syndrome patients. Homozygous null mice exhibit an even broader range of developmental anomalies that encompass most of the common human clinical features of this disorder. Mice engineered to carry a large (1.5-Mb) deletion on 22q11 also had conotruncal and parathyroid defects[64] and perinatal lethality. Importantly, these conotruncal defects could be partially rescued by a human BAC containing the TBX1 gene,[65] further evidencing the substantial role of this T-box transcription factor in DiGeorge's syndrome. Overexpression of Tbx1 in mice, like Tbx5, also causes cardiovascular defects, suggesting that too much or too little of these transcription factors disrupts important developmental pathways.

Expressed in the pharyngeal arches during early stages and mid stages of embryonic development, TBX1 is certainly required for normal maturation of these tissues, but whether this transcription factor participates in migration and other developmental functions of neural crest cells remains unknown. Whether mutation or deficiency of TBX1 alone is sufficient to cause DiGeorge's syndrome remains somewhat unresolved, because to date no human mutation has been reported that selectively disrupts this gene. Although the mouse data clearly indicates the importance of TBX1 in DiGeorge's syndrome, it is also possible that the human phenotype reflects a contiguous gene defect (decreased expression or function of several adjacent genes) or the cumulative effect of several mutated genes within the deleted chromosome 22q11 region.[66]

Abnormal neural crest migration may also cause tetralogy of Fallot, the most common form of complex CHD occurring in 1 in 3000 live births (Fig. 14-2). The cardinal malformations of the Fallot tetrad are a VSD, obstruction to right ventricular outflow, aortic dextroposition, and right ventricular hypertrophy. Recurrence rate within families (estimated risk in siblings is 1%[67]) and clinical reports of multiple affected individuals in some kindreds (who exhibit all or a subset of the malformations of the tetrad) has been interpreted to indicate that single-gene mutations can cause tetralogy of Fallot. Although both autosomal dominant and recessive modes of inheritance have been suggested, multifactorial inheritance is postulated for most cases.

Disruption of other genes in the mouse has also been reported to cause tetralogy of Fallot. Friend of Gata (Fog-2) is a transcription factor that interacts with Gata factors, a family of molecules involved in cardiogenesis. Genetic disruption of Fog-2 in mice results in tetralogy of Fallot and abnormal coronary artery development.[68] Tetralogy of Fallot has also been observed in neurotrophin 3-deficient mice. Neurotrophin 3 is one of several molecules implicated in the regulation of neural crest cell migration and survival that interacts with the tyrosine kinase receptor TrkC.[69]

Although tetralogy of Fallot can arise from microdeletion in chromosome 22q11, as one manifestation of DiGeorge's syndrome, most often this complex congenital heart lesion occurs in isolation without associated developmental abnormalities in other tissues that characterize DiGeorge's syndrome. Human mutations in *NKX2.5* (detailed previously) and in *JAG1* (see following) are known to produce isolated tetralogy of Fallot, but, given the high incidence (Table 14-1) of this congenital malformation, there are likely to be other genetic causes. The human homologs of *Fog-2* and *neurotrophin 3* and related molecules appear to be excellent candidates for tetralogy of Fallot mutations.

## JAG1

A gene with 26 exons extending over 36 kb, *JAG1* is a ligand for Notch receptors. The Notch gene family encodes transmembrane receptors and ligands that are critical for cell fate decisions made during development of both invertebrates and vertebrates.[70] Mutations in Notch genes have been implicated in a human hematologic malignancy and a neurodegenerative disorder. A chromosomal translocation t(7;9) that interrupts Notch1 *(TAN1)* encoded at 9q34 causes T-cell leukemia,[71] and *NOTCH3* mutations cause cerebral autosomal dominant arteriopathy with subcortical infarcts and leukoencephalopathy (CADASIL).[72] It is somewhat surprising, therefore, that a striking cardiovascular phenotype arises when the Notch ligand JAG1 is mutated. Missense and null mutations in *JAG1* have been identified as the cause of Alagille's syndrome,[73,74] a complex disorder that occurs in 1 per 70,000 live births. Alagille's syndrome is transmitted as an autosomal trait and produces developmental anomalies of the heart, liver, eye, skeleton, and kidney. Much of the premature morbidity associated with Alagille's syndrome reflects congenital heart malformations and chronic cholestatic liver disease.

More than 95% of Alagille's syndrome patients have congenital heart defects that vary in type and severity. Clinical examination usually reveals a cardiac murmur that reflects underlying peripheral pulmonic stenosis[75] in most patients (67%). Lesions involving the pulmonary valve or outflow tract and/or pulmonary stenosis or atresia in combination with other structural abnormalities are commonly found. Cardiac structural defects occur in 25% of patients and include ASDs and/or VSDs. Although right-sided cardiac abnormalities are more common in Alagille's syndrome, defects in the left-sided circulation (aortic stenosis, aortic coarctation, and dysplastic atrioventricular valves) also occur. *JAG1* mutations have also been identified in children with tetralogy of Fallot who lack other features of Alagille's syndrome.[76]

Expression of *JAG1* in the developing heart and associated vascular structures correlates with the congenital cardiovascular defects observed in Alagille's syndrome. *JAG1* transcripts are found in the first pharyngeal arch early in development and thereafter in pharyngeal arches 2, 3, 4, and 6. The sixth pharyngeal arch gives rise to the pulmonary artery. Strong *JAG1* expression in the developing pulmonary valve and outflow tract correlate with the predominance of right-sided heart lesions (especially pulmonary valve lesions) that are seen in Alagille's syndrome patients. *JAG1* is also expressed throughout the endocardium, myocardium, and epicardium of the atrium, whereas in the ventricle, expression is restricted to the endocardium and epicardium and absent from the myocardium. In the ductus arteriosus, *JAG1* expression accounts for the PDA that is observed in some cases of Alagille's syndrome (Fig. 14-2). The consequences of disrupted or abnormal Notch signaling caused by *JAG1* mutations remains largely unknown, but clearly this pathway establishes important processes on which late stages of mammalian cardiovascular development are predicated.

## MALFORMATIONS OF LEFT-RIGHT ASYMMETRY

Unpaired organs such as the heart, stomach, liver, or spleen are asymmetrically distributed along the left-right body axis in vertebrates. Aberrant left-right axis development can lead to random *(situs ambiguous)* or mirror-image reversed organ positioning *(situs inversus)*. *Situs inversus* occurs in 1 in 10,000 live births and by itself causes no harm to the individual. *Situs ambiguous* occurs with a frequency similar to that of *situs inversus* but is much more deleterious and is usually associated with severe and often fatal heart malformations.

Both genes and environment can contribute to the development of left-right axis malformations. For example, retinoic acid exposure may induce laterality defects in various vertebrates, including human. Furthermore, maternal (nongestational) diabetes mellitus has been shown to increase the risk of left-right malformations. Several genes (such as *Nodal, Ebaf, Pitx2,* and *cryptic*) have been implicated in left-right organ positioning in model organisms. In humans, relatively few genes have been associated with a small percentage of human *situs* defects. These include *ZIC3, LEFTB,* and *ACVR2B*.

## ZIC3

Zinc-finger in cerebellum (ZIC3) is a transcription factor encoded at Xq24 that harbors homology to proteins involved in left-right axis formation. Mutations in *ZIC3* have been identified among sporadic and familial cases of defects in laterality.[77] *ZIC3* mutations caused either mild or no consequences in women, whereas affected hemizygous men have severe complex heart malformations, including *situs ambiguous* and midline abnormalities that frequently resulted in neonatal lethality. In one family, some females heterozygous for a *ZIC3* mutation were diagnosed with *situs inversus,* whereas the affected males had *situs ambiguous*. Megarbane et al.[78] described a family harboring a *ZIC3* mutation in which affected males show a transposition of the great vessels and midline anomalies but no obvious left-right malformations. In addition, one male family member with the mutation had anatomically normal organs, thereby indicating incomplete penetrance of some *ZIC3* mutations.

Klootwijk et al.[79] generated *Zic3*-deficient mice. All *Zic3*-null mice that survived intrauterine development were found to have a kinked tail, and approximately 10% manifested other malformations, particularly neural tube defects, heart anomalies, altered lobation of the lungs, and malrotation of the gut, all characteristic of abnormal left-right specification.

Overexpression of *Zic3* resulted in hyperplastic neural and neural crest-derived tissue[80] and induction of proneural genes. Because *Zic3* is expressed in the neural plate at the earliest embryonic stages, this data is consistent with the hypothesis that this transcription factor has an important role in the induction of neuroectoderm and neural crest cells.

*LeftyA* and *LeftyB,* which are members of the TGF family, are expressed exclusively on the left side of the mouse embryo by 8.0 days post coitum.[81,82] Mice homozygous for a *LeftyA* null allele manifest left-right malformations and misexpressed *LeftyB.*[83] Analysis of the human homolog of *LeftyA* in 126 patients with left-right axis malformations showed one nonsense and one missense mutation in *LEFTYA.*[84]

Targeted disruption of the mouse activin receptor type IIB gene *(Acvr2b)* also produced abnormalities in left-right axis development.[85] Cardiopulmonary malformations included right-sided morphology of the left atrium and left lung and ASDs and VSDs. Screening for *ACVR2B* mutations in humans with either familial or sporadic axis malformations has revealed two missense mutations. Both mutations were absent from control samples, and one mutation was found in two unrelated individuals,[86] further substantiating that these *ACVR2B* defects have functional consequences.

## CLINICAL PROSPECTS

During the past decade, studies to elucidate critical pathways for normal and abnormal development of the heart have advanced significantly. The availability of complete genome sequences has simplified the mapping and identification of disease-causing gene mutations, and accelerated progress in these arenas is expected. Better understanding of the molecular causes of CHD provides opportunity for novel and visionary approaches in diagnosis and therapy.

For decades, therapy of CHD has been—and remains—surgical correction. Since the first ligation of a PDA by Robert Gross of Boston in 1938, better appreciation of anatomy and pathophysiology of congenital malformations, improved diagnostics, and the advent of cardiopulmonary bypass and deep hypothermic circulatory arrest have allowed the open repair of many lesions. Further advances in preoperative, intraoperative, and postoperative management have resulted in greatly improved survival for even the most complex congenital defects. For simple lesions, catheter interventions have become feasible; these allow correction not only in younger patients but even in neonates with CHD. However, many survivors are still at increased risk for insidious deterioration of cardiac function and chronic heart disease.

Contemporary approaches to CHD require prenatal risk assessment, ultrasonic definition of anatomy, prognostic data, and an informed management plan for termination or continuance of pregnancies with CHD. For these issues to be adequately addressed a multidisciplinary team of perinatologists, neonatologists, pediatric cardiologists, pediatric cardiac surgeons, and geneticists is required. Enhanced understanding of the genetic causes of CHD will increasingly assign a central role to the geneticist to foster earlier and accurate diagnosis, assist in an assessment of prognosis, and provide genetic counseling. Although gene therapy remains a distant prospect, one might predict that the rapid pace of developmental genetics may provide opportunities for early intervention that could modify the degree of aberrant cardiac development or avoid malformation.

Because many types of complex CHD arise from a single-gene defect there is also the possibility that corrected expression of only a single molecule may dissipate heterogeneous expressions of disease. Furthermore, the recognition of significant phenotypic heterogeneity produced by identical mutations in a single gene clearly suggests a potent role for environmental factors and/or modifier genes in influencing disease expression. Identification and targeted modification of these cofactors promises hope for affected families in the pregene therapy era. Continued application of molecular genetics in concert with growing avenues for molecular medicine should augment the clinical advances in CHD and foster exciting new treatments that may mitigate the substantial morbidity and mortality of these human disorders.

## REFERENCES

1. Taussig HB: Evolutionary origin of cardiac malformations. J Am Coll Cardiol 1988;12:1079–1086.
2. Ferencz C, Boughman JA: Congenital heart disease in adolescents and adults: Teratology, genetics, and recurrence risks. Cardiol Clin 1993;11:557–567.
3. Grabitz RG, Joffres MR, Collins-Nakai RL: Congenital heart disease: Incidence in the first year of life: The Alberta Heritage Pediatric Cardiology Program. Am J Epidemiol 1988;128:381–388.
4. Fixler DE, Pastor P, Chamberlin M, et al: Trends in congenital heart disease in Dallas County births. 197-984. Circulation 1990;81:137–142.
5. Ferencz C, Rubin JD, Loffredo CA, et al: Epidemiology of Congenital Heart Disease: The Baltimore-Washington Infant Study, 198–989. Mt. Kisko, NY, Futura Publishing Co, 1993.
6. Srivastava D, Olson EN: A genetic blueprint for cardiac development. Nature 2000;407:221–226.
7. Olson EN, Srivastava D: Molecular pathways controlling heart development. Science 1996;272:671–676.
8. Park M, Wu X, Golden K, et al: The wingless signaling pathway is directly involved in Drosophila heart development. Dev Biol 1996;177:104–116.
9. Levin M, Johnson RL, Stern CD, et al: A molecular pathway determining left-right asymmetry in chick embryogenesis. Cell 1995;82:803–814.
10. Rossant J: Mouse mutants and cardiac development: New molecular insights into cardiogenesis. Circ Res 1996;78:349–353.
11. Huang JX, Potts JD, Vincent EB, et al: Mechanisms of cell transformation in the embryonic heart. Ann NY Acad Sci 1995;752:317–330.
12. Komuro I, Izumo S: Csx: A murine homeobox-containing gene specifically expressed in the developing heart. Proc Natl Acad Sci USA 1993;90:8145–8149.
13. Lints TJ, Parsons LM, Hartley L, et al: Nkx-2.5: A novel murine homeobox gene expressed in early heart progenitor cells and their myogenic descendants. Development 1993;119:419–431.

14. Kasahara H, Bartunkova S, Schinke M, et al: Cardiac and extracardiac expression of Csx/Nkx2.5 homeodomain protein. Circ Res 1998;82:936–946.

15. Lyons I, Parsons LM, Hartley L, et al: Myogenic and morphogenetic defects in the heart tubes of murine embryos lacking the homeo box gene Nkx2-5. Genes Dev 1995;9:1654–1666.

16. Tanaka M, Chen Z, Bartunkova S, et al: The cardiac homeobox gene Csx/Nkx2.5 lies genetically upstream of multiple genes essential for heart development. Development 1999;126:1269–1280.

17. Biben C, Harvey RP: Homeodomain factor Nkx2-5 controls left/right asymmetric expression of bHLH gene eHand during murine heart development. Genes Dev 1997;11:1357–1369.

18. Schott JJ, Benson DW, Basson CT, et al: Congenital heart disease caused by mutations in the transcription factor NKX2-5. Science 1998;281:108–111.

19. Benson DW, Silberbach GM, Kavanaugh-McHugh A, et al: Mutations in the cardiac transcription factor NKX2.5 affect diverse cardiac developmental pathways. J Clin Invest 1999;104:1567–1573.

20. Kasahara H, Lee B, Schott JJ, et al: Loss of function and inhibitory effects of human CSX/NKX2.5 homeoprotein mutations associated with congenital heart disease. J Clin Invest 2000;106:299–308.

21. Biben C, Weber R, Kesteven S, et al: Cardiac septal and valvular dysmorphogenesis in mice heterozygous for mutations in the homeobox gene Nkx2-5. Circ Res 2000;87:888–895.

22. Muller CW, Herrmann BG: Crystallographic structure of the T domain-DNA complex of the Brachyury transcription factor. Nature 1997;389:884–888.

23. Agulnik SI, Papaioannou VE, Silver LM: Cloning, mapping, and expression analysis of TBX15, a new member of the T-Box gene family. Genomics 1998;51:68–75.

24. Law DJ, Garvey N, Agulnik SI, et al: TBX10, a member of the Tbx1-subfamily of conserved developmental genes, is located at human chromosome 11q13 and proximal mouse chromosome 19. Mamm Genome 1998;9:397–399.

25. Papaioannou VE, Silver LM: The T-box gene family. Bioessays 1998;20:9–19.

26. Papapetrou C, Putt W, Fox M, et al: The human TBX6 gene: Cloning and assignment to chromosome 16p11.2. Genomics 1999;55:238–241.

27. Wattler S, Russ A, Evans M, et al: A combined analysis of genomic and primary protein structure defines the phylogenetic relationship of new members if the T-box family. Genomics 1998;48:24–33.

28. Yi CH, Terrett JA, Li QY, et al: Identification, mapping, and phylogenomic analysis of four new human members of the T-box gene family: EOMES, TBX6, TBX18, and TBX19. Genomics 1999;55:10–20.

29. Basson CT, Bachinsky DR, Lin RC, et al: Mutations in human TBX5 [corrected] cause limb and cardiac malformation in Holt-Oram syndrome. Nat Genet 1997;15:30–35.

30. Basson CT, Huang T, Lin RC, et al: Different TBX5 interactions in heart and limb defined by Holt-Oram syndrome mutations. Proc Natl Acad Sci USA 1999;96:2919–2924.

31. Li QY, Newbury-Ecob RA, Terrett JA, et al: Holt-Oram syndrome is caused by mutations in TBX5, a member of the Brachyury (T) gene family. Nat Genet 1997;15:21–29.

32. Elek C, Vitez M, Czeizel E: Holt-Oram syndrome. Orv Hetil 1991;132:73–74, 77–78.

33. Basson CT, Cowley GS, Solomon SD, et al: The clinical and genetic spectrum of the Holt-Oram syndrome (heart-hand syndrome). N Engl J Med 1994;330:885–891.

34. Newbury-Ecob RA, Leanage R, Raeburn JA, et al: Holt-Oram syndrome: A clinical genetic study. J Med Genet 1996;33:300–307.

35. Chapman DL, Garvey N, Hancock S, et al: Expression of the T-box family genes, Tbx1-Tbx5, during early mouse development. Dev Dyn 1996;206:379–390.

36. Gibson-Brown JJ, Agulnik SI, Chapman DL, et al: Evidence of a role for T-box genes in the evolution of limb morphogenesis and the specification of forelimb/hindlimb identity. Mech Dev 1996;56:93–101.

37. Bruneau BG, Logan M, Davis N, et al: Chamber-specific cardiac expression of Tbx5 and heart defects in Holt-Oram syndrome. Dev Biol 1999;211:100–108.

38. Netter FH, Van Mierop LHS: Embryology. In The CIBA Collection of Medical Illustrations, Vol 5, Heart, Section III. Summit, NJ, CIBA Pharmaceutical Co, 1969.

39. Cross SJ, Ching YH, Li QY, et al: The mutation spectrum in Holt-Oram syndrome. J Med Genet 2000;37:785–787.

40. Melnyk AR, Weiss L, Van Dyke DL, et al: Malformation syndrome of duplication 12q24.1 leads to qter. Am J Med Genet 1981;10:357–365.

41. McCorquodale MM, Rolf J, Ruppert ES, et al: Duplication (12q) syndrome in female cousins, resulting from maternal (11;12)(p15.5;q24.2) translocations. Am J Med Genet 1986;24:613–622.

42. Dixon JW, Costa T, Teshima IE: Mosaicism for duplication 12q (12q13→q24.2) in a dysmorphic male infant. J Med Genet 1993;30:70–72.

43. Liberatore CM, Searcy-Schrick RD, Yutzey KE: Ventricular expression of tbx5 inhibits normal heart chamber development. Dev Biol 2000;223:169–180.

44. Hatcher CJ, Kim MS, Mah CS, et al: TBX5 transcription factor regulates cell proliferation during cardiogenesis. Dev Biol 2001;230:177–188.

45. Bruneau BG, Nemer G, Schmitt JP, et al: A murine model of Holt-Oram syndrome defines roles of the T-box transcription factor Tbx5 in cardiogenesis and disease. Cell 2001;106:709–721.

46. Hiroi Y, Kudoh S, Monzen K, et al: Tbx5 associates with Nkx2-5 and synergistically promotes cardiomyocyte differentiation. Nat Genet 2001;28:276–280.

47. Phillips MT, Kirby ML, Forbes G: Analysis of cranial neural crest distribution in the developing heart using quail-chick chimeras. Circ Res 1987;60:27–30.

48. Epstein JA, Li J, Lang D, et al: Migration of cardiac neural crest cells in Splotch embryos. Development 2000;127:1869–1878.

49. Jiang X, Rowitch DH, Soriano P, et al: Fate of the mammalian cardiac neural crest. Development 2000;127:1607–1616.

50. Maschhoff KL, Baldwin HS: Molecular determinants of neural crest migration. Am J Med Genet 2000;97:280–288.

51. Kirby ML, Stewart DE: Neural crest origin of cardiac ganglion cells in the chick embryo: Identification and extirpation. Dev Biol 1983;97:433–443.

52. Bockman DE, Kirby ML: Dependence of thymus development on derivatives of the neural crest. Science 1984;223:498–500.

53. Bockman DE, Redmond ME, Waldo K, et al: Effect of neural crest ablation on development of the heart and arch arteries in the chick. Am J Anat 1987;180:332–341.

54. Kirby ML, Waldo KL: Role of neural crest in congenital heart disease. Circulation 1990;82:332–340.

55. Nora JJ, Nora AH: Update on counseling the family with a first-degree relative with a congenital heart defect. Am J Med Genet 1988;29:137–142.

56. Char F: Peculiar facies with short philtrum, duck-bill lips, ptosis, and low-set ears: A new syndrome? Birth Defects Orig Arctic Ser 1978;14:303–305.

57. Satoda M, Pierpont ME, Diaz GA, et al: Char syndrome, an inherited disorder with patent ductus arteriosus, maps to chromosome 6p12-p21. Circulation 1999;99:3036–3042.

58. Satoda M, Zhao F, Diaz GA, et al: Mutations in TFAP2B cause Char syndrome, a familial form of patent ductus arteriosus. Nat Genet 2000;25:42–46.

59. Wilson GN: Correlated heart/limb anomalies in Mendelian syndromes provide evidence for a cardiomelic developmental field. Am J Med Genet 1998;76:297–305.

60. DiGeorge AM, Harley RD: The association of aniridia, Wilms' tumor, and genital abnormalities. Trans Am Ophthalmol Soc 1965;63:64–69.

61. Shprintzen RJ, Goldberg RB, Lewin ML, et al: A new syndrome involving cleft palate, cardiac anomalies, typical facies, and learning disabilities: Velo-cardio-facial syndrome. Cleft Palate J 1978;15:56–62.

62. Goldberg R, Motzkin B, Marion R, et al: Velo-cardio-facial syndrome: A review of 120 patients. Am J Med Genet 1993;45:313–319.

63. Van Mierop LH, Kutsche LM: Cardiovascular anomalies in DiGeorge syndrome and importance of neural crest as a possible pathogenetic factor. Am J Cardiol 1986;58:133–137.

64. Lindsay, EA, Vitelli F, Su H, et al: Tbx1 haploinsufficiency in the DiGeorge syndrome region causes aortic arch defects in mice. Nature 2001;410:97–101.

65. Merscher S, Funke B, Epstein JA, et al: TBX1 is responsible for cardiovascular defects in velo-cardio-facial/DiGeorge syndrome. Cell 2001;104:619–629.

66. Epstein JA: Developing models of DiGeorge syndrome. Trends Genet 2001;17:S13–17.

67. Boon AR, Farmer MB, Roberts DF: A family study of Fallot's tetralogy. J Med Genet 1972;9:179–192.

68. Tevosian SG, Deconinck AE, Tanaka M, et al: FOG-2, a cofactor for GATA transcription factors, is essential for heart morphogenesis and development of coronary vessels from epicardium. Cell 2000;101:729–739.

69. Donovan MJ, Lin MI, Wiegn P, et al: Brain derived neurotrophic factor is an endothelial cell survival factor required for intramyocardial vessel stabilization. Development 2000;127:4531–4540.

70. Artavanis-Tsakonas S, Matsuno K, Fortini ME: Notch signaling. Science 1995;268:225–232.

71. Ellisen LW, Bird J, West DC, et al: TAN-1, the human homolog of the Drosophila notch gene, is broken by chromosomal translocations in T lymphoblastic neoplasms. Cell 1991;66:649–661.

72. Joutel A, Corpechot C, Ducros A, et al: Notch3 mutations in CADASIL, an hereditary adult-onset condition causing stroke and dementia. Nature 1996;383:707–710.

73. Li L, Krantz ID, Deng Y, et al: Alagille syndrome is caused by mutations in human Jagged1, which encodes a ligand for Notch1. Nat Genet 1997;16:243–251.

74. Oda T, Elkahloun AG, Pike BL, et al: Mutations in the human Jagged1 gene are responsible for Alagille syndrome. Nat Genet 1997;16:235–242.

75. Emerick KM, Rand EB, Goldmuntz E, et al: Features of Alagille syndrome in 92 patients: Frequency and relation to prognosis. Hepatology 1999;29:822–829.

76. Krantz ID, Smith R, Colliton RP, et al: Jagged1 mutations in patients ascertained with isolated congenital heart defects. Am J Med Genet 1999;84:56–60.

77. Gebbia M, Ferrero GB, Pilia G, et al: X-linked situs abnormalities result from mutations in ZIC3. Nat Genet 1997;17:305–308.

78. Megarbane A, Salem N, Stephan E, et al: X-linked transposition of the great arteries and incomplete penetrance among males with a nonsense mutation in ZIC3. Eur J Hum Genet 2000;8:704–708.

79. Klootwijk R, Franke B, van der Zee CE, et al: A deletion encompassing Zic3 in bent tail, a mouse model for X-linked neural tube defects. Hum Mol Genet 2000;9:1615–1622.

80. Nakata K, Nagai T, Aruga J, et al: Xenopus Zic3, a primary regulator both in neural and neural crest development. Proc Natl Acad Sci USA 1997;94:11980–11985.

81. Meno C, Saijoh Y, Fujii H, et al: Left-right asymmetric expression of the TGF beta-family member lefty in mouse embryos. Nature 1996;381:151–155.

82. Meno C, Ito Y, Saijoh Y, Matsuda Y, et al: Two closely-related left-right asymmetrically expressed genes, lefty-1 and lefty-2: Their distinct expression domains, chromosomal linkage and direct neuralizing activity in Xenopus embryos. Genes Cells 1997;2:513–524.

83. Meno C, Shimono A, Saijoh Y, et al: Lefty-1 is required for left-right determination as a regulator of lefty-2 and nodal. Cell 1998;94:287–297.

84. Kosaki K, Bassi MT, Kosaki R, et al: Characterization and mutation analysis of human LEFTY A and LEFTY B, homologues of murine genes implicated in left-right axis development. Am J Hum Genet 1999;64:712–721.

85. Oh SP, Li E: The signaling pathway mediated by the type IIB activin receptor controls axial patterning and lateral asymmetry in the mouse. Genes Dev 1997;11:1812–1826.

86. Kosaki R, Gebbia M, Kosaki K et al: Left-right axis malformations associated with mutations in ACVR2B, the gene for human activin receptor type IIB. Am J Med Genet 1999;82:70–76.

## EDITOR'S CHOICE

Elliott DA, Kirk EP, Yeoh T, et al: Cardiac homeobox gene NKX2-5 mutations and congenital heart disease: Associations with atrial septal defect and hypoplastic left heart syndrome. J Am Coll Cardiol 2003;41:2072–2076.

*Mutations in the NKX 2.5 gene can cause a very diverse set of morphogenic defects beyond atrial septal defects, including hypoplastic left heart syndrome.*

Garg V, Kathiriya IS, Barnes R, et al: GATA4 mutations cause human congenital heart defects and reveal an interaction with TBX5. Nature 2003;424:443–447.

*GATA-4 mutations are associated with human congenital heart disease; a finding consistent with earlier studies documenting a critical importance in fetal development in the mouse. Supports the concept that studies in mouse models can be predictive of monogenic causes of CHD in humans.*

Lipshultz SE, Sleeper LA, Towbin JA, et al: The incidence of pediatric cardiomyopathy in two regions of the United States. N Engl J Med 2003;348:1647–1655.

*Cardiomyopathy is an important, often neglected genetic cause of congenital heart disease; many mutations have been shown to be related to defects in the cardiac cytoskeletal components.*

Mani A, Meraji SM, Houshyar R, et al: Finding genetic contributions to sporadic disease: A recessive locus at 12q24 commonly contributes to patent ductus arteriosus. Proc Natl Acad Sci USA 2002;99:15054–15059.

*Patent ductus arteriosus can have genetic origins.*

■ ▨ ■ c h a p t e r 1 5

# Molecular Pathways for Cardiac Hypertrophy and Heart Failure Progression

Masahiko Hoshijima
Susumu Minamisawa
Hideo Yasukawa
Kenneth R. Chien

Heart failure is emerging as a leading cause of human morbidity and mortality and is predicted to reach epidemic proportions in the early 21st century.[1] Unfortunately, current therapy for heart failure is largely based on a complex regimen of drugs that are primarily targeted at symptoms of the disease rather than the fundamental processes that drive disease progression.[2-4] One of the major difficulties has been the complexity of the disease, which is chronic, progressive, and propelled by a combination of environmental stimuli and genetic susceptibility.[5,6] Studies of rare familial forms of heart failure have documented a trend toward incomplete penetrance with a highly variable genotype-phenotype correlation, suggesting the presence of strong modifiers and associated genetic background effects.[7,8] At the same time, diverse environmental stimuli, including postinfarction injury, cardiotoxic side effects of chemotherapeutic agents, viral infection, and chronic exposure to volume and pressure overload can all serve to initiate and modify disease progression. Although decreases in cardiac contractility and relaxation are conserved features of many forms of heart failure, these acute physiologic end points do not always correlate with long-term mortality, again underscoring the complex nature of the heart failure phenotype. Heart failure is a growing, unmet clinical problem, representing both a major scientific opportunity and a clinical challenge for cardiovascular physicians and scientists alike. Many laboratories now view heart failure as the "cancer" of the cardiovascular system, because it is a classic, multifactorial, polygenic, and chronic disease that progresses to a terminal stage.

Intriguingly, a growing body of work now suggests another important parallel between the biology of cancer and the biology of heart failure. The massive, abnormal growth in cardiac muscle that accompanies heart failure shares several biologic principles and molecular pathways with cancer biology. The biologic precepts of cell growth, apoptosis, and cell survival are as important in the onset of heart failure as they are in tumor progression, and the molecular signals for cell proliferation and cardiac myocyte hypertrophy are highly conserved. Both diseases are inexorable and progressive in their nature, and a "multihit" hypothesis applies for both cancer and heart failure progression, largely based on the interplay between genetic susceptibility and environmental stimuli. This view, coupled with the integration of multiple experimental approaches including *in vivo* somatic gene transfer, bioinformatics, and computational biology, is beginning to provide new insights into the disease process. Insights from genetically based studies in mice and humans are now suggesting new therapeutic targets and strategies for intervening in the disease. With the completion of the human and mouse genome databases and physical mapping of annotated genes that provide a road map, great strides in unraveling the logic of heart failure progression can be made. This chapter highlights several advances in the understanding of the molecular pathways that drive the onset of cardiac hypertrophy and heart failure; these advances are forming the basis for a new wave of biologically targeted therapy.

## BIPHASIC TEMPORAL SIGNALING CASCADES DIRECTLY ACTIVATED BY MECHANICAL STRESS: POSITIVE AND NEGATIVE REGULATORS

Mechanical stress is one of the most important stimuli for triggering the initial steps toward heart failure. A diverse group of biochemical signals can be rapidly activated during *in vivo* pressure overload; many can be activated within a few minutes of exposure to dynamic or passive stretch that accompanies increases in aortic pressure or volume overload.[9-12] To date, the precise identity of the molecular machinery that initially senses cardiac mechanical stress has remained largely unknown. A series of studies have indicated that a subset of ion-channel or ion exchangers, such as a stretch-activated channel or a sodium-proton exchanger, are regulated by deformation of the plasma membrane and are found in cardiomyocytes exposed to mechanical or osmotic load.[13,14] These mechanical stress-related changes in ionic current have rarely been linked to the onset of hypertrophy in individual cardiomyocytes.[15] However, several transmembrane signaling pathways, including MAP kinases, Janus kinase (JAK)/signal transducers and activators of transcription (STAT), and phosphoinositide 3-kinase (PI3K)/Akt (protein kinase B) cascades, have been suggested to connect mechanical load to the onset of cardiac hypertrophy.[16-19] Following mechanical stretch of cultured cardiomyocytes, most of these cardiac signaling kinase cascades are activated, in part via the cell adhesion complex, which include integrins and integrin-associated proteins that are linked to the extracellular matrix (ECM).[20,21] Cardiac conditional knockout mice of the β1 integrin gene display a blunted MAP kinase activation following *in vivo* pressure overload.[22] In addition, ablation of melusin, an integrin-binding protein, has resulted in blunted response to pressure-overload stimulation to activate Akt/glycogen synthase kinase-3β (GSK3β) signaling and to induce cardiac hypertrophy.[23] However, further investigation will be necessary to determine the precise role of the ECM-integrin-cytoskeleton complex in cardiac mechanical stress sensing. In addition, hormonal stimuli, such as adrenergic agonists, angiotensin, endothelin, and gp130 cytokine receptor agonists also activate these signaling kinases, thereby triggering hypertrophic responses *in vitro* and *in vivo*.[16-19]

Many of these insights in the signaling pathways for cardiac hypertrophy have originated from studies in cultured neonatal rat cardiomyocytes *in vitro*, followed by studies of normal and genetically engineered mouse models that have been exposed to the pressure overload that accompanies *in vivo* aortic banding. The acute response to pressure-overload peaks within hours and includes the activation of ERK1/2, JNK, p38, Akt, and gp130/STAT and the induction of early stress-response genes, such as the suppressor of cytokine signaling-3 (SOCS3) (Fig. 15-1, Table 15-1). This early phase response is followed by a hypertrophic response, which starts within 48 hours after aortic banding and reaches a peak within 7 days. This later hypertrophic response is clearly marked by an increase in the left ventricle to body weight ratio and the induction of a series of embryonic gene markers such as ANF, skeletal actin, and β-myosin heavy chain.[9,31,32] Interestingly, there is a second peak of activation for many of signaling cascade kinases in this subacute hypertrophic response phase,[10,11] suggesting that there may be phasic and discrete roles for a subset of signaling pathways that respond to mechanical stress.

The double peak of early mechanical stress responses implicates the presence of inhibitory regulators that act

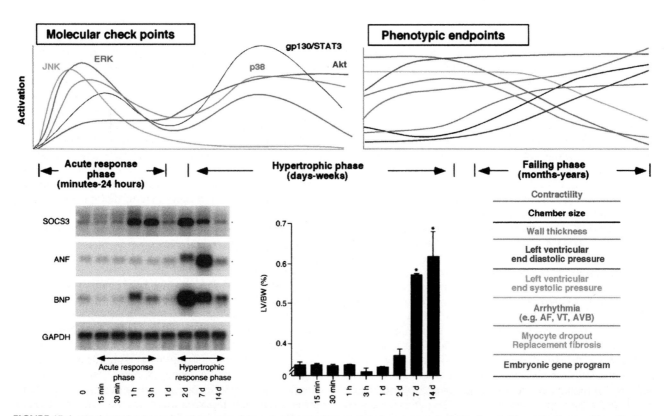

**FIGURE 15-1.** Mechanical stress-induced transmembrane signaling and integrated phenotypes of a failing heart. The activation profiles of various signaling cascades and time-dependent changes in phenotypic features of heart failure are illustrated based on our previous studies[10] and unpublished observations. Lower panels show biphasic induction of representative stress-responding marker genes and upregulation of left ventricular to body weight (LV/BW) ratio after transverse thoracic aortic constriction in normal adult mice. *(Modified from Yasukawa H, Hoshijima M, Gu Y, et al: Suppressor of cytokine signaling-e is a biomechanical stress-inducible gene that suppresses gp130-mediated cardiac myocyte hypertrophy and survival pathways. J Clin Invest 2001;108:1459–1467 and Hoshijima M, Chien KR: Mixed signals in heart failure: Cancer rules. J Clin Invest 2002;109:849–855.)*

■ ▣ ■

**TABLE 15-1** MECHANICAL STRESS-RELATED CHANGES IN GENE EXPRESSION DURING HEART FAILURE PROGRESSION IN HUMAN AND EXPERIMENTAL STUDIES

| Acute (<24 hr) Up | Hypertrophic–Failing (Days-Weeks-Years) Up | | Down |
|---|---|---|---|
| c-fos | **Secreted proteins** | **Metabolism/translational proteins** | **Cytoskeletal proteins** |
| c-jun | ANF, lipocortin I, ET-1 | Ubiquitin, pyruvate dehydrogenase α | FHL1 (failing heart) Nonsarcomeric |
| junB | HB-EGF, TGFβ1, BNP | NADH ubiquinone oxidoreductase | MLC2 |
| egr-1 | Osteoblast specific factor 2 | Creatine kinase, Myoglobin | **Ion-channels/carriers** |
| nur77 | **Cytoskeletal proteins** | Superoxide dismutase 2 | L-type Ca2+ channel |
| BNP | αMHC, βMHC | Aldose reductase, EF-1a, EF-2, IF-4AII | SERCA2 |
| SOCS3 | MLC1a/v, MLC2a | 28S, 60S ribosomal L3 | Phospholamban |
| | MLC2v, tropomyosin | **Signaling** | Kv4.2, 4.3 |
| | Troponin C, Myomesin | Gsα, βARK, adenylyl cyclase VII | Kv1.5 |
| | Smooth muscle α–actin | A-kinase, C-kinase inhibitor-1, ILK | KChIP2 |
| | Skeletal α–actin | Rap1B, SOCS3, Id-1, GATA-4 | **Signaling** |
| | α–cardiac actin | SP1/3, PGD/D2 synthase | β1-AR, type-A like Ephrin receptor |
| | FHL1(HCM), sarcosin | **Others** | **Others** |
| | Desmin, gelsolin | Heat shock 70kD proteins 1, 6, 8 | α1-Antichymotrypsin |
| | **Extracellular matrix** | Quaking protein, CARP | αB-Crystallin |
| | Fibulin, fibronectin | | Plasminogen activator inhibitor-1 |
| | Laminin, collagen | | TIM17 |
| | **Ion-channels/carriers** | | Connexin43 |
| | Na+/Ca2+ exchanger, Kv1.4 | | |
| | Voltage dependent anion channel-1 | | |

Modified from Hoshijima M, Chien KR: Mixed signals in heart failure: Cancer rules. J Clin Invest 2002;109:849–855, and references 24 to 30.

as a negative feedback loop to prevent the continuous activation of any single pathway. Naturally, there must be negative regulators of the response that leads to attenuation of the signal so that the acute response is properly terminated and an orderly compensatory hypertrophic response ensues, as opposed to unbridled reactive growth, which is often seen in mouse models of cardiac hypertrophy induced by cardiac overexpression of signaling molecules.[19] A number of studies have recently identified negative feedback regulation of these intracellular signaling pathways. SOCS3 provides an example of a biomechanical stress-inducible negative regulator, which acts to inhibit the gp130 stress-inducible pathway for myocyte survival.[10,33] Within minutes of aortic constriction, either by the action of gp130 ligands (e.g., cardiotrophin-1 and LIF) or via unknown mechanisms of direct activation, JAKs phosphorylate a transcriptional regulator STAT3 leading to the translocation of STAT3 into the nucleus, which directly activates the expression of genes that can confer myocyte hypertrophy[34,35] and survival (e.g., BCL-x),[36-38] and SOCS3.[10] SOCS3 is induced in the myocardium within 1 hour of aortic banding, peaking for several hours and suppressing JAK kinase activity by selectively binding to gp130. By inhibiting JAKs, SOCS3 negatively regulates stress-inducible gp130 activation (Fig. 15-2). It is likely that this negative regulatory circuit prevents hyperstimulation of this pathway that is induced by sustained expression of gp130-coupled cytokines, which may have independent pathologic effects on cardiac function. In this manner, the delicate balance between the activation of gp130/JAK signaling and the induction of its negative feedback regulator SOCS3 might be important in the transition between car-

diac hypertrophy and failure.[5,10] Disrupting the balance between this positive and negative regulatory loop by chronic exposure to gp130 ligands might lead to secondary effects that impair cardiac function.

A number of other novel negative regulators of cardiac signaling have recently been described. Recent studies have identified myocyte-enriched calcineurin-interacting protein-1 (MCIP1), a protein that inhibits cardiac hypertrophy by attenuating calcineurin activity.[39] The MCIP1 gene contains NFAT (nuclear factors of activated T cells) binding motifs that mediate its upregulation by calcineurin signals, thereby suggesting that MCIP1 participates in the negative feedback loop of calcineurin signaling in the myocardium.[40] A separate negative feedback regulatory system has been found for cardiac MAP kinase signaling: forced expression of MAP kinase phosphatase-1 (MKP-1) has been shown to negatively regulate the cardiac hypertrophic response by downregulating the three branches of MAP kinase cascade (p38s, JNK1/2, and ERK1/2).[41]

Given this complex temporal pattern of signaling pathways that are activated following *in vivo* pressure overload, it is not surprising that studies of the effects of the overexpression of diverse components of cardiac signaling pathways have been shown to result in cardiac hypertrophy or failure. It will become increasingly important to examine the temporal sequence of activation of these signaling pathways and to connect them to specific phenotypic features that are associated with discrete physiologic end points associated with the disease, such as defects in contractility, action potential, arrhythmogenesis, and so forth. A more meticulous gene switching in model animals[42] and high-efficiency somatic gene delivery systems have become available toward this end.[43,44]

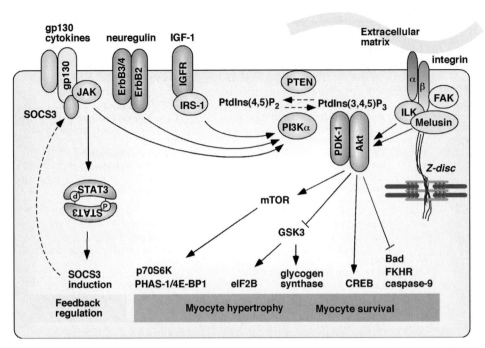

**FIGURE 15-2.** PI3K/Akt signaling in cardiomyocytes. Activation of variety of downstream molecules leads to hypertrophic and survival effects in cardiomyocytes.

# HYPERTROPHY RESPONSE: QUANTITATIVE EFFECTS OF INCREASING TRANSLATIONAL EFFICIENCY AND QUALITATIVE EFFECTS ON INDUCING AN EMBRYONIC GENE PROGRAM

## PI3K/Akt Pathway

Cardiac hypertrophy can be broken down into two central phenotypic end points: (1) quantitative effects on increasing the level of sarcomeric and other constitutive proteins and their transcripts and (2) qualitative changes in the cardiac gene program that lead to a return to the fetal phenotype. Interestingly, both of these phenotypic effects can be found during growth stimulation of diverse differentiated cell types. In this regard, insulin-like growth factor-1 (IGF-1) is a potent stimulus for both cardiac[45,46] and skeletal muscle hypertrophy[47] *in vivo*. Recent studies have clearly identified that IGF-1 increases translational efficiency of preexisting mRNAs, which underlies the hypertrophic response of skeletal muscle hypertrophy.[48–50] A number of independent approaches have convincingly shown a central role of Akt in enhancing translational efficiency by phosphorylating and thereby inhibiting GSK3.[48,49,51] Skeletal muscle atrophy leads to a decrease in the Akt/mTOR (mammalian target of rapamycin) pathway, and IGF-1 unexpectedly acts via Akt to antagonize calcineurin signaling during skeletal myotube hypertrophy. Taken together, the activation of the Akt/mTOR pathway and its downstream targets, p70S6K and PHAS-1/4E-BP1,[3,52] appear to play a central role in skeletal muscle and perhaps cardiac muscle hypertrophy and atrophy (Fig. 15-2).[53] IGF-1 activates PI3K,[54,55] thereby activating Akt and phosphoinositide-dependent

kinase 1 (PDK-1), which interact with each other and cooperatively activate downstream signaling.[52,56,57] The tumor suppressor phosphatase and tensin homolog on chromosome 10 (PTEN) antagonizes this pathway by facilitating dephosphorylation of PtdIns(3,4,5)P_3 (phosphatidylinositol-3,4,5-triphosphate).[58,59] During *in vivo* pressure overload, an increase in translational efficiency has also been documented, and myocardial Akt is particularly activated during the subacute hypertrophic response phase.[10] Taken together, a similar role for Akt signaling in heart failure-related myocardial remodeling is likely, and activation of Akt is noted in the failing human heart.[60] Transgenic mouse models of cardiac IGF-1,[61] PI3K,[62] and Akt overexpression[63–65] have been reported to induce cardiac hypertrophy and/or hyperplasia, whereas cardiac overexpression of GSK3β suppresses pressure overload or β-adrenergic stimulation-dependent hypertrophy.[53,66] In addition, *in vitro* overexpression of catalytically inactive mutant of PTEN induces cardiomyocyte hypertrophy,[67] and muscle-specific ablation of PTEN enhances *in vivo* mouse cardiac hypertrophy.[68] Taken together, PI3K/Akt and their downstream signaling appear to be an important *in vivo* determinant of cardiac size. Recently, further complexity of PI3K signaling was documented. PI3Kα is linked to receptor tyrosine kinase pathways that regulate cardiac myocyte size, and PI3Kγ, which binds to G-protein βγ subunits,[69] negatively regulates cardiomyocyte contractility through β2-adrenergic receptor/cAMP-dependent signaling.[68]

## Calcium Signaling

Numerous studies in cardiac muscle now support an important role for calcium signaling in the activation of a hypertrophic response. Earlier, activation of calmodulin

(CaM)-dependent kinase (CaMK) was reported to be involved in the regulation of a fetal gene program that is coactivated during cardiac hypertrophy.[70] CaMK activity is elevated in failing human hearts.[71] Subsequently, a series of studies using transgenic mouse models documented that cardiac overexpression of calcineurin, a calcium-CaM dependent protein phosphatase, can induce massive cardiac hypertrophy.[72] A family of transcriptional factors NFATs are located in the downstream of calcineurin signaling.[73] In addition, the cardiac overexpression of CaMKIV, a neural CaMK isotype, results in a concentric form of cardiac hypertrophy.[74] Myocyte enhancer factor-2 (MEF2), a MADS-box transcription factor highly expressed in myocytes, is a putative downstream target molecule of the CaMK pathway, and dual activation of CaMK and calcineurin-dependent pathways by calcium has been proposed to regulate cardiac hypertrophy.[19,73] In this regard, MEF2 associates with NFAT and GATA to facilitate transcriptional activation of hypertrophy-responsive genes[75] (Fig. 15-3). From studies in skeletal muscle and neural tissue, the molecular mechanism of CaMK-dependent MEF2 regulation has been proposed as follows[76]: activated CaMK phosphorylates class II histone deacetylases (HDACs) (4, 5, 7, and 9: abundant in striated muscle and brain) or perhaps MEF2-interacting transcriptional facator-2 (MITR), which is a splicing variant of HDAC and lacks the catalytic domain. Phosphorylated HDACs or MITR binds to an intracellular chaperone protein 14-3-3, and this interaction exposes a nuclear export sequence (NES) on HDACs, which leads to CRM1-dependent translocation of HDAC/14-3-3 complex to the cytoplasm. On the other hand, MITR phosphorylation leads to the redistribution of the MITR/14-3-3 complex in the nucleus

because MITR lacks the NES. The dislocation of HDACs or MITR releases MEF2-interaction-dependent suppression of muscle gene activation. However, this CaMK/HDAC/MEF2 activation sequence has not yet been proved in cardiomyocytes. Interestingly, in cardiomyocytes the CaMK phosphorylation sites of HDAC/MITR seems to be catalyzed by other kinases, because the HDAC phosphorylation activity in cardiac extracts from calcineurin-transgenic mice or mice with cardiac hypertrophy induced by pressure-overload is insensitive to chemical CaMK inhibitors and EGTA, a divalent cation chelator.[77] So far, the molecular identity of the putative cardiac HDAC kinase(s) remains unclear. On the other hand, p38 phosphorylates and directly activates MEF2.[78] It also antagonizes nuclear translocalization of NFAT.[79] In addition, GSK3 negatively regulates GATA4[80] and NFAT.[66] As described, the transcriptional factor complex, including MEF2, NFAT, and GATA, is localized in the downstream of a web of multiple kinase cascades.

Pharmacologic inhibition of calcineurin using cyclosporin A or FK506 has provided mixed results for their antihypertrophic effect in various experimental models.[81-83] However, more compelling studies, using cardiac specific expression of dominant negative forms of calcineurin[84] and endogenous calcineurin inhibitors,[32,85] have confirmed a pivotal role for the calcineurin pathway in certain *in vitro* and *in vivo* assay systems. Subsequent studies in calcineurin Aβ-deficient mice revealed that changes in heart weight to tibia length ratio are diminished following acute pressure overload or chronic angiotensin II/isoproterenol infusion.[86] Herein, the calcineurin Aβ form dominantly contributes to cardiac protein phosphatase 2B activity. In addition, targeted disruption of NFATc3, but not

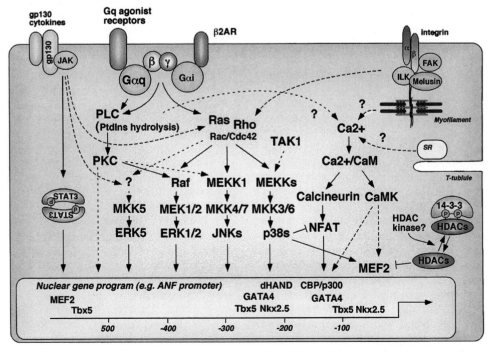

**FIGURE 15-3.** Activation of the embryonic gene program in the hypertrophic heart via diverse membrane-nucleus signaling pathways. The signaling meshwork includes Gq, small GTP-biding proteins, MAP kinases, and calcium-calcineurin/CaM. The well-characterized ANF promoter lesion is shown in the lower panel with positioning of respective transactivators, such as MEF2, Tb×5, Nk×2.5, and GATA4.

NTATc4, was shown to attenuate both pressure-overload and calcineurin–overexpression-mediated mouse cardiac hypertrophy.[87] On the other hand, calcineurin inhibition aggravated cardiac dysfunction in a hypertrophic cardiomyopathy (HCM) model carrying a point mutation of the myosin heavy chain gene,[88] which corresponds to the human inherited form of cardiomyopathy[89] and points out the need to further probe the clinical significance of calcineurin signaling in cardiac diseases.

The recent notion that the constitutive activation of CaMKIIdelta(B), the major cardiac CaMK isotype, results in a dilated form of cardiomyopathy[90] suggests another level of complexity regarding calcium-dependent signaling in the regulation of cardiac hypertrophy. The compartmental source for calcium that triggers biochemical calcium signaling has not been identified. It is uncertain whether the pool of calcium that activates components of the hypertrophic response is derived from the beat-by-beat transient increase in free cytoplasmic calcium that underlies excitation-contraction coupling[91] or whether this reflects a specific intracellular compartmentalization (such as specialized endoplasmic reticulum,[92,93] myofilaments,[94] or nuclear membrane) of calcium. Mice harboring a targeted disruption of calreticulin display embryonic cardiomyopathy, and the calreticulin-deficient myocytes show reduced NFAT translocation into the nucleus, suggesting the possibility that calcium mobilization from the distinctive cardiac cytoplasmic membrane structure where calreticulin localizes may activate calcineurin-dependent nuclear signaling.[95] Another possibility is distinctive calcium-dependent signaling pathways that dictate the particular frequency or concentration range of intracellular calcium oscillation.[96-98] The pCa of calcineurin activation is also one order of magnitude lower than that required for CaMK.[99,100] Thus, it appears that a cohesive, integrated view of the role of calcium signaling in hypertrophy is beginning to appear, although an extensive amount of work will be required. In addition, it will be of interest to determine how this calcium signaling is integrated into other calcium-independent signaling pathways for hypertrophy.

## Gq Pathways

A growing body of clinical and scientific evidence supports the viewpoint that Gq/$G_{11}$ pathways are one of the most proximal steps in the hypertrophic response.[18] By microinjection in cultured neonatal cardiomyocytes, the Gq protein was initially shown to be critical to the induction of morphologic hypertrophy and ANF expression.[101] Subsequently, studies using either *in vitro* overexpression of Gq via an adenovirus vector or *in vivo* overexpression of Gq in transgenic mice resulted in cardiomyocyte hypertrophy.[102] Excessive expression of Gq provokes cardiomyocyte apoptosis and associated cardiac dysfunction in both experimental systems. Herein, induction of a Bcl-2 family proapoptotic mitochondria-targeted protein Nix/Bni3L by Gq overexpression may play a cytopathic role via cytochrome c release and caspase-3 activation.[103] The overexpression of the inhibitory peptide for Gq suppressed *in vivo* pressure-overload-induced cardiac hypertrophy in mice,[104,105] which was confirmed by a subsequent study using mice that harbor a double cardiac-restricted ablation of both Gq and $G_{11}$.[106] The downstream signaling of Gq/$G_{11}$ activation is diverse and includes activations of small molecular GTP binding proteins, such as ras, rho, and rac; multiple MAP kinases; rho kinase; phosphatidyl inositol (PtdIns) hydrolysis; PKC; and CaMK[16-19] (Fig. 15-3). The extent of crosstalk between calcium signaling, PI3K/Akt, ECM-adhesion complex, and Gq/$G_{11}$ pathways and their differential role in triggering downstream phenotypic features of cardiac hypertrophy are currently unclear. Other membrane G-proteins, including $G_{12}$/$G_{13}$, are also involved in ligand-dependent cardiac hypertrophy.[107] A new Gq-dependent pathway has recently been uncovered, which involves the Gq-dependent transactivation of EGF receptor through cleavage of heparin-binding EGF via the extracellular metalloprotease 12 (ADAM12).[108] Further investigation will be needed to confirm that this intracellular or intercellular transactivation of tyrosine kinase receptor is indeed downstream of Gq-dependent signaling in the myocardium.

## Protein Kinase C (PKC) Signaling

PKC was originally identified in bovine brain extracts as a calcium/phospholipid-dependent protein kinase, and its diverse physiologic functions include regulation of cell proliferation, differentiation, motility, and intermediary metabolism.[109] The *in vitro* effect of activated PKC on cardiomyocyte hypertrophy was noted relatively early (using direct PKC-activating agents; e.g., phorbol esters or diacylglycerols[110]) and was later confirmed in *in vivo* cardiac overexpression studies of various isoforms of PKC in transgenic mice.[111-114] A combination of biochemical and molecular cloning strategies have now identified more than 12 members of the PKC family, which are categorized into four groups based on structural similarities: classic (cPKC), novel (nPKC), atypical (aPKC), and related genes.[115] In cardiomyocytes, cPKCα, nPKCδ, and nPKCε are relatively abundant and consistently identified; aPKCζ and aPLCλ/ι are also detectable. The presence of cPKCβ1/2 in the heart has been inconsistent between laboratories.[17,116-118] A two-step model of PKC activation has been proposed. PDK-1 accesses to the activation loop of PKCs for conformational changes associated with phosphorylation,[119] which is sufficient for the activation of aPKCs, whereas the primed cPKCs need subsequent coupling with PtdIns hydrolysis.[50,115] Gq-coupled agonists can lead to the translocation of nPKCδ and nPKCε to the cardiac membrane fraction from the cytoplasm,[120-122] and these PKC isoforms display crosstalk and partly constitute a molecular complex with MAP kinases.[123,124] Perhaps through c-Raf dependent ERK1/2 activation,[125] nPKCε has been implicated in both cardiac hypertrophy and cardioprotective effects, whereas nPKCδ is known to be proapoptotic[115] and may be linked to JNK and p38 pathways.[126] Overexpression of an nPKCε-activating peptide ψεRACK1 in mice results in mild cardiac hypertrophy,[127] whereas an nPKCε-inhibitory peptide εV1 accelerates induction of a heart failure phenotype in Gq-transgenic mice.[128] Intriguingly, nPKCε-null mice, which have normal basal cardiac function, are blunted for sphingosine-1-phosphate and ganglioside GM-1 mediated cardiac protection against ischemia-reperfusion injury.[129] The cardioprotective action of nPKCε may be related to its partial colocalization with MAP kinases near cardiac mitochondria,[130] which induces phosphorylation and inactivation of a proapoptotic protein Bad.[130,131] On the other hand, earlier immunohistologic studies using isotype-specific antibodies have documented that nPKCε can rapidly translocate from the cytosol to the Z-disc accompanied by kinase activation,[132] thereby raising the possibility that nPKCε is directly involved in remodeling of the cardiac cytoskeletal architecture or Z-disc related mechanical stress sensing machinery (see later). Two possible groups of proteins may recruit nPKCε to the Z-disc related structure: (1) β′COP, a selective binding protein (RACK) for activated nPKCε colocalizes in cardiomyocytes with cross-striation[133] and (2) some PDZ-Lim domain proteins including ENH (Enigma-homolog)[134,135] and ZASP/Cypher/Oracle[136-138] are known to interact with PKC[134,136] and colocalize at the Z-disc.[135,136]

## gp130 Signaling

The first link between gp130 signaling and cardiac hypertrophy arose via studies of a novel cytokine that was capable of activating an increase in cardiomyocyte cell size via an expression cloning approach.[34] A mouse embryonic stem cell cDNA library was screened for its activity to induce rat neonatal cardiomyocyte hypertrophy. This cytokine was named cardiotrophin-1 (CT-1) and was characterized as a member of the gp130 receptor cytokine family peptides.[34,35] Separately, an inflammatory peptide IL-6, another gp130 cytokine, was documented to induce *in vivo* and *in vitro* cardiomyocyte hypertrophy by associating with the soluble form of the sIL-6 receptor.[139] The gp130 peptide is a single transmembrane domain peptide that forms heterodimer complexes with various α subunit ligand-binding peptides. A LIF-binding subunit β (LIFR)-gp130 heterodimer was identified as CT-1 receptor on the surface of cardiomyocytes using a neutralizing antibody against LIFR.[35] Dimerized gp130 cytokine receptor activates JAKs, which then induce phosphorylation of a tyrosine residue of gp130, followed by the phosphorylation of the family of STATs. Phosphorylated and active forms of STATs result in homodimerization or heterodimerization and are translocated into the nucleus, leading to target gene expression.[140] Cardiac overexpression of STAT3 induces mild hypertrophy[141] and also promotes cardiac hypervascularization, which might be linked to VEGF induction in the myocardium.[142] Other kinase signaling cascades, including ERK1/2,[143] MEK5/ERK5,[144] and Akt,[145] have also been linked to gp130 activation. In an *in vitro* cultured rat neonatal cardiomyocyte system, CT-1/LIF-treated cardiomyocytes showed unique polymorphic features of cardiomyocyte hypertrophy,[146] which are distinct from Gq-coupling receptor agonists but often are observed in the myocytes isolated from the heart with eccentric hypertrophy. Accordingly, CT-1 induces longitudinal growth of myofilaments rather than lateral thickening of actin-myosin bundles. Protein and

RNA synthesis were also enhanced, Several characteristic markers for the embryonic gene program were reactivated: myofilaments were newly formed and cell surface area was enlarged by CT-1 treatment in cultured cardiomyocytes. The molecular mechanisms that lead to this distinct assembly of sarcomeres in series is not well understood at present but may include MEK5/ERK5 signaling[144]; Rho/Rho kinase dependent nonsarcomeric myosin light chain phosphorylation;[147] and/or formation of nascent Z-discs with segregation of α-Actinin and other associated proteins such as ALP, a Z-disc PDZ-Lim protein.[148]

## MAP Kinase Signaling

Cytoplasmic MAP kinase, MAP kinase kinase (MKK), and MKK kinase signaling cascades are activated by diverse receptor-linked membrane signaling proteins including Gq and are known to have extensive crosstalk and interaction with many of the other previously mentioned signaling cascades.[17,124] This intricate signaling meshwork includes three major nodal points, including ERK1/2, JNK1/2, and p38s (Fig. 15-3). Despite effort to determine the physiologic significance and precise downstream cardiac targets that are selectively triggered by these MAPK signaling molecules, a complete understanding of their exact role in cardiac hypertrophy and failure has been elusive because of their complexity and the inherent difficulty in distinguishing between primary and secondary effects. Endogenous activation of many of these molecules induce cardiac hypertrophy and cytoprotective effects, and enhanced activation results in toxicity with apoptotic or necrotic cell death in many cases. Synthetic small molecule kinase inhibitors are often less selective, and overexpression of dominant negative forms of kinases are uncertain for their specificity for molecular compartmentalization; however, more sophisticated genetic approaches, such as conditional gene ablation, are starting to shed light on this problem. Recent studies suggest that the MEK1/2-ERK1/2 cascade might be a central player in this kinase cascade meshwork and primarily induces a concentric form of cardiac hypertrophy and cardioprotection.[124] Cardiac-restricted MEK1 transgenic mice have mild concentric form of hypertrophy with enhanced left-ventricular contractility.[149] A significant ERK1/2 downstream nuclear target in the cardiomyocyte may be GATA4, which interacts with other cardiac specific transcriptional factors to regulate muscle gene expression[150] (see later). In contrast, cardiac p38 activation is primarily cytopathic *in vivo*,[151] which is partly due to its direct proapoptotic effects and also partly due to reduction in myofilament calcium sensitivity.[152] TAK1, a p38 upstream kinase, also promotes cardiac hypertrophy with subsequent heart failure *in vivo*.[153] JNK signaling was originally related to cardiomyocyte hypertrophy *in vitro*[154]; however, the significance of JNK signaling in *in vivo* cardiac hypertrophy was less clear in subsequent studies. MEKK1, a JNK upstream regulating kinase, was genetically ablated and has been tested in two *in vivo* mouse systems. Under conditions in which JNK activation was blunted by MEKK1 ablation, pressure-overload-induced *in vivo* hypertrophy was not affected, although there was mild induction of cytopathic changes in the myocardium.[155] On the other hand, cardiomyopathic changes in Gq transgenic mice were largely diminished by MEKK1 ablation.[156] Part of these MEKK1/JNK signaling effects have been linked to JNK-dependent phosphorylation of a gap-junction molecule, connexin43.[157] Interestingly, the significance of respective MAP kinase cascade activation has been studied in humans tissue, demonstrating the *in vivo* activation of JNK1/2 and p38. On the other hand, levels of activated ERK1/2 were found unchanged in the failing heart in these studies.[60] Although these studies in human tissue are supportive, they have inherent difficulties related to individual variability, difficulty in obtaining sufficient control specimens, and hazards in extrapolating from a one-time measurement at the end stage of the disease to the pathways that trigger the initial steps of the disease-related pathways.

## Transcriptional Regulation of Cardiac Genes

The activation of a fetal gene program is a highly conserved feature of the hypertrophic response and has been extensively studied as a means to identify pathways that might be involved in the *in vivo* response. Although the initial steps of the induction of embryonic genes are clearly reversible, chronic changes in the cardiac gene program may trigger pathologic changes in the myocardium that can be associated with irreversible dysfunction. Much of this work has focused on the inducibility of ANF gene, which is reactivated in ventricular muscle early during the hypertrophic response (Fig. 15-3). A host of cardiac transcription factors, including NKX 2.5,[158] a zinc-finger protein GATA4,[159,160] NFATs,[72] TBX5,[161,162] dHAND,[163] CBP/p300,[163,164] MEF2,[74] and another MADS box protein serum response factor (SRF),[160] work together to control the expression of ANF and a panel of downstream target genes in the embryonic gene program. The recent discovery of a new series of cardiac restricted transcriptional cofactors such as Myocardin[165] and HOP[166,167] have suggested the combinatorial control of the cardiac gene program in response to defined upstream signals. As mentioned previously, a dual enzyme system composed of histone acetyltransferases (HATs) and HDACs is associated with this transcriptional complex and serves as an epigenetic control point of the embryonic cardiac program.[76,163,164]

## PATHWAYS FOR SURROGATE FAILING HEART PHENOTYPES

### Genotype-Phenotype Relationships in Cardiomyopathy

The initial precepts that guided the understanding of human cardiomyopathies were based on the presumption that the primary determinant of the clinical phenotype is the molecular genotype. This clinical viewpoint is supported by noninvasive analyses, such as echocardiography, that can quantitatively assess differences in chamber volume, wall thickness, hypertrophy, systolic versus diastolic dysfunction, and outflow tract obstruction, leading to three clinical subtypes: HCM, dilated cardiomyopathy (DCM), and restrictive cardiomyopathy (RCM).[168,169] Genotyping of human cardiomyopathy was initiated with the surprising discovery of mutations in the β-Myosin heavy chain gene in HCM cases in large pedigrees[170]; this was subsequently expanded to include other sarcomeric gene mutations in human HCM patients, including myosin binding protein-C,[171,172] myosin light chains,[173] cardiac actin,[174] troponin-T,[171,175] troponin-I,[176] α-Tropomyosin,[171,175] and titin.[177] On the other hand, parallel analyses of candidate genes for DCM were more difficult, because of the relatively small pedigrees, incomplete penetrance, and phenotypic diversity. Eventually, studies in genetically engineered mice revealed an initial role for cytoskeletal defects in DCM via studies of mutant mice that are deficient in the cardiac Z-disc–associated cytoskeletal muscle-specific LIM protein (MLP)[178] (Fig. 15-4). Later, a missense mutation of MLP was identified in a subset of DCM patients who reside in northern Europe.[179] Different MLP mutations were also linked to familial cases of HCM.[180] Extensive links between other cytoskeletal proteins and familial forms of human DCM were subsequently established.[6,168,169]

Based on these early findings, a generalized concept was formulated that suggested that sarcomeric mutations lead to HCM, whereas cytoskeletal mutations result in DCM, thereby reflecting specific defects in the hardwiring within cardiac muscle cells that govern these two distinct phenotypes. Thus, the phenotypic diversity of familial cardiomyopathies appeared to be primarily driven by the disease genotype. However, recent experimental and clinical studies suggest a more complex genotype-phenotype relationship of cardiomyopathies[168,169] (Table 15-2). It now appears that mutations in a given sarcomeric gene can lead to a spectrum of cardiomyopathic phenotypes, often overlapping between the clinical subsets of DCM, HCM, and RCM. Although there is little doubt that the disease genotype plays a critical role in initiating the cardiomyopathic process, the ultimate clinical phenotype seems to represent the integrated effect of multiple interacting factors. This view is supported by a host of circumstantial evidence, including the poor penetrance of many cardiomyopathic genotypes; the influence of hemodynamic stress on disease progression; the secondary effects of the loss of cardiac myocyte survival and subsequent replacement fibrosis; strong modifying effects of calcium cycling and calcium signaling; and clear evidence of genetic background effects, which is also apparent in gene-targeted mouse models of cardiomyopathy.[5,204]

### Chamber Dilation: Diverse Cytoskeletal Pathways

Changes in organ size, shape, and histologic phenotype are central features of cardiomyopathy and related heart failure. Chronic increases in ventricular volume and filling pressure can lead to dilation of the cardiac chamber and subsequent thinning of the ventricular wall in the advancement of heart failure, which results in large increases in diastolic and systolic wall stress in both the

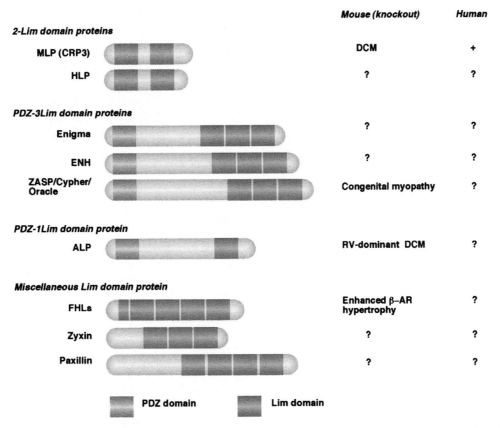

| | Mouse (knockout) | Human |
|---|---|---|
| **2-Lim domain proteins** | | |
| MLP (CRP3) | DCM | + |
| HLP | ? | ? |
| **PDZ-3Lim domain proteins** | | |
| Enigma | ? | ? |
| ENH | ? | ? |
| ZASP/Cypher/Oracle | Congenital myopathy | ? |
| **PDZ-1Lim domain protein** | | |
| ALP | RV-dominant DCM | ? |
| **Miscellaneous Lim domain protein** | | |
| FHLs | Enhanced β–AR hypertrophy | ? |
| Zyxin | ? | ? |
| Paxillin | ? | ? |

PDZ domain    Lim domain

**FIGURE 15-4.** Lim domain proteins and cardiomyopathy. Cardiac-enriched Lim domain proteins are categorized based on their domain structure. MLP-null mice were initially reported to display DCM phenotypes, followed by the identification of human MLP mutations linked to cardiomyopathy. Later, cardiomyopathic phenotypes were also noted in a series of experimental model animals in which Lim domain proteins are ablated.

■ ■ ■

## TABLE 15-2   MOLECULAR DEFECTS LINKED TO HUMAN CARDIOMYOPATHIES DEFECTS IN HUMANS

| Genomic Defects | HCM | DCM | RCM |
|---|---|---|---|
| *Sarcomere* | | | |
| Myosin heavy chain | Missense[171,181,182] | Missense[185] | |
| Myosin essential light chain | Missense[173] | | |
| Myosin regulatory light chain | Missense[173] | | |
| Cardiac actin | Missense[174] | Missense[186] | |
| Troponin-T | Missense/deletion[171,175] | Deletion[185] | |
| Troponin-I | Missense[176] | | Missense[203] |
| α-tropomyosin | Missense[171,175] | Missense[187] | |
| Myosin binding protein-C | Missense/deletion[171,172] | | |
| *Titin/titin-related protein* | | | |
| Titin | Missense[177] | Missense/deletion[188] | |
| Telethonin (T-cap) | | Missense[179] | |
| *Z-disk-associated proteins* | | | |
| MLP | | Missense[179] | |
| *Sarcolemmal cytoskeleton* | | | |
| Dystrophin | | Deletion[189-191] | |
| β-Sarcoglycan | | Deletion/duplication[192] | |
| δ-Sarcoglycan | | Missense[193] | |
| α-Dystrobrevin | | Missense[194] | |
| Metavinculin | | Deletion[195,196] | |
| *Intermediate filaments* | | | |
| Desmin | | Missense[197,198] | |
| Lamin A/C | | Missense[199] | |
| *Miscellaneous* | | | |
| Mitochondrial respiratory chain | | Missense[200] | |
| G4.5 (tafazzin) | | Nonsense[201] | |
| Phospholamban | Nonsense[183]/promoter[184] | Missense/nonsense[183-202] | |

right and left ventricular chambers. Based on the discovery of a cytoskeletal network of DCM-related genes in both experimental and clinical studies, distinct classes of cytoskeletal defects have been uncovered that include components of the macromolecular titin complex, Z-disc and intercalated disc proteins, components of the dystrophin/dystroglycan/sarcoglycan complex, and mutations in the nuclear and intermediate filaments (Table 15-2). These diverse cytoskeletal defects have been proposed to lead to chamber dilation via multiple potential mechanisms, such as abnormalities in force transmission,[178,186] force generation,[185] sarcolemmal integrity,[205] sarcomeric organization/assembly defects,[144] and intercalated disc stability.[206] In addition to these structural roles of the cardiac cytoskeleton, selective cytoskeletal mutations and associated defects may exert their effects on heart failure via specific effects on intracellular signaling pathways triggered by biomechanical or hormonal stimuli to promote cardiac remodeling.[179] MLP was demonstrated to directly bind to telethonin (T-cap), a 19-kd muscle-specific titin-interacting protein, and MLP deficiency causes T-cap dislocation from Z-disc structure. Physiologic analysis of MLP-deficient myocardium, before the gross development of DCM, has revealed a selective defect in the cardiac mechanical stress sensor, which is related to abnormalities in the titin-related complex[179] (Fig. 15-5). MLP is downregulated at the protein level in the myocardium of both sporadic DCM and ischemic cardiomyopathy patients.[207] In this manner, cardiac cytoskeletal defects in mechanical stress sensing might also trigger chamber dilation in acquired forms of heart failure, extending the observations obtained in rare forms of DCM to more common forms of heart failure.

The recent association of cytoskeletal components with distinct cardiac channels (min K)[208] and the identification of a mutation of ankyrin-B (a membrane cytoskeletal protein and an associated protein of the sarcolemmal sodium-potassium ATPase) in long QT syndrome type 4[209] have further raised the possibility of divergent roles of cytoskeletal components in the direct regulation of cardiac channels involved in the control of cardiac repolarization and/or excitation–contraction coupling. An expanding number of novel muscle-specific cytoskeletal components have been found localized in the cardiac Z-disc, thereby implying that the Z-disc may play a specialized function beyond its known role as a structural element[210] (Fig. 15-6). At the Z-disc, α-actinins are organized into a series of antiparallel dimers that crosslink polymerized actin filaments (thin filaments). The Z-disc also anchors titin, a 2- to 3-Md muscle-specific protein. Titin contains two α-actinin binding domains at its N-terminus and spans the length of each half-sarcomere, reaching to the M line in the middle of the A-band. T-cap interacts with titin at the Z-disc. As mentioned previously, a series of signaling molecules including several PKC isoforms, are known to translocate to Z-disc after activation; accordingly, Z-disc proteins with the PDZ-Lim structure including ENH[134,135] and ZASP/Cypher/Oracle[136-138] and the calcineurin-binding proteins Calsarcin/FATZ[211-213] may serve as mechanical-to-biologic signal transducers.

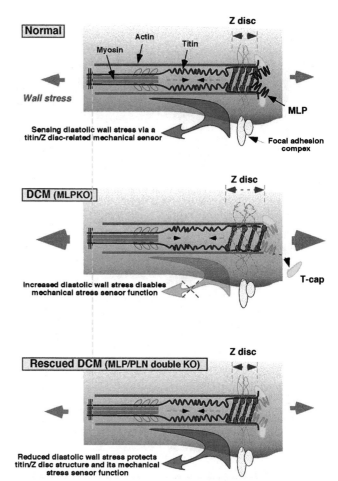

**FIGURE 15-5.** MLP/T-cap/titin complex and the cardiac stretch sensor. At peak diastole, as ventricular filling pressure rises, titin elastic segments are reshaped, generating diastolic wall stress. The change in intrinsic elasticity functions to trigger the mechanical stress sensor. In DCM (e.g., the MLP-null mouse heart), ventricular chamber dilation and wall thinning act to enhance diastolic wall stress; the increased wall stress destabilizes the function of the titin/Z-disc complex (e.g., in the MLP-null mouse heart, T-cap, which is mechanically stabilized by MLP, gradually dislocates from Z-disc); the titin/Z-disc related mechanical stress sensor fails in translating mechanical stress to the cytoplasmic signaling cascade. The diastolic wall stress reduction appears to be critical for the prevention and rescue of heart failure progression by stabilizing titin/Z-disc complex. For example, in the MLP/phospholamban double knockout (MLP/PLN double KO) mouse heart, Z-disc abnormality, which is apparent in MLP-null myocardium, is genetically rescued.[179] (*Modified from Knoll R, Hoshijima M, Hoffman HM, et al: The cardiac mechanical stretch sensor machinery involves a Z disc complex that is defective in a subset of human dilated cardiomyopathy. Cell 2002;111:943–955.*)

## Excitation-Contraction Coupling in Heart Failure Progression: A Common Pathologic Endpoint Associated with Defects in Calcium Cycling

During the course of cardiac chamber dilation, a progressive decrease in cardiac contractility and relaxation ensues, which ultimately leads to chronic heart failure. The precise link between chamber dilation and cardiac dysfunction is not completely clear, because there are numerous defects that have been associated with the

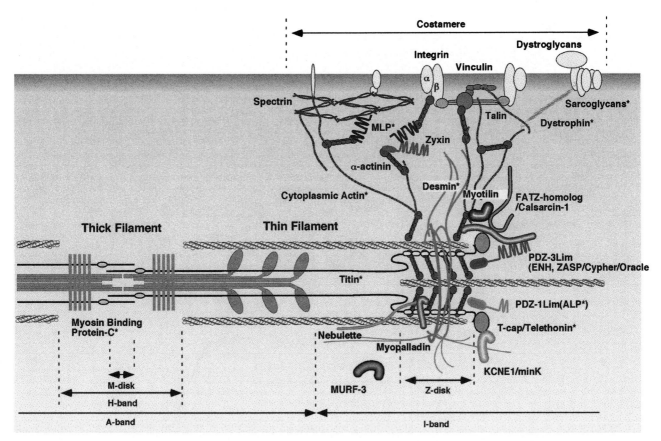

**FIGURE 15-6.** Cardiac cytoskeletal proteins and cardiomyopathy. Representative cytoskeletal proteins constituting cardiac Z-disc and connecting myofilaments to the costamere are illustrated. *(Modified from Chien KR: Genomic circuits and the integrative biology of cardiac diseases. Nature 2000;407:227–232.)*
*Proteins linked to human and experimental cardiomyopathies.

impairment of cardiac contractile function in heart failure. However, recent studies point to the central role of defects in calcium cycling in heart failure progression. These defects arise from a decrease in the activity of the SR calcium ATPase type 2 (SERCA2) that regulates diastolic and systolic function via the resequestration of calcium into the SR lumen.[214-216] During the onset of heart failure, there is a decrease in the content of SERCA2 and its activity relative to the unrestrained inhibitory effect of phospholamban (PLN), an endogenous SERCA2 inhibitory peptide.[215] In the normal heart, the inhibitory activity of PLN is under the control of the β-adrenergic receptor (β-AR)-adenylyl cyclase-cAMP dependent PKA pathway in which phosphorylation of the S16 residue of PLN leads to an inactivation of its suppressor effect on SERCA2,[217, 218] (Fig. 15-7). In human and experimental models of heart failure, PLN is hypophosphorylated,[219-221] which most likely reflects desensitization of the β-adrenergic pathway resulting from the increase in the activity of the β-adrenergic receptor kinase (βARK: GRK2) in the failing heart.[222] Recently, a PLN mutation (R9CPLN) was found in patients with familial DCM, which blocks the PKA-dependent site-specific phosphorylation in both R9CPLN and co-oligomerized wild-type PLNs.[202] Together with the experimental finding that cardiac restricted R9CPLN overexpression leads to progressive heart fail-

ure,[202] SR calcium uptake suppression appears to be a critical step in the progression of heart failure.

Although clinical and experimental studies document that simply enhancing cAMP during heart failure can lead to cardiac injury and an associated increase in mortality,[223-225] genetic complementation studies and somatic gene transfer in heart failure model animals have suggested that it is possible to markedly improve cardiac diastolic and systolic function independent of effects on cAMP levels via directly enhancing SR calcium cycling. The clear therapeutic effects of β-adrenergic receptor blockade, even at advanced stages of heart failure, suggests that any new therapy will have to be compatible with chronic β-blocker therapy.[226]

Percutaneous or intramuscular delivery of an adenovirus vector (Adeno) carrying β2-AR (Adeno/β2-AR) delivery results in enhanced contractility in normal rabbit or cardiomyopathic hamsters.[227,228] βAR kinase inhibitor peptide (βARKct)-transgenic overexpression partially rescues cardiomyopathic phenotypes of MLP-null mice[229] and R403Q mutant α-myosin heavy chain (αMHC) transgenic mice.[230] Adeno/βARKct also improves contractility and delays heart failure development in postmyocardial infarction rabbits.[231,232] Adenylyl cyclase type VI (AC-type VI) transgenic overexpression rescues the heart failure phenotype in Gq cardiomyopathic mice,[233] and percutaneous

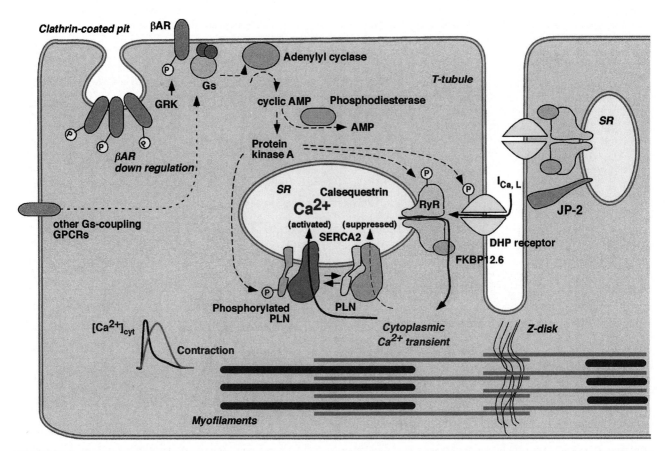

**FIGURE 15-7.** Regulatory pathways and key molecules in the control of SR calcium cycling. The G-protein coupling receptor (GPCR)/cAMP/PKA axis is the main regulating system and serves as a pharmacologic and genetic target at multiple steps in the cascade to improve cardiac contractility and relaxation in heart failure. *(Modified from Hoshijima M, Chien KR: Mixed signals in heart failure: Cancer rules. J Clin Invest 2002;109:849–855.)*

Adeno/AC-type VI delivery enhances cardiac contractility in normal pigs.[234] SERCA2 transgenic mice have enhanced cardiac function,[235] and SERCA2 transgenic overexpression partially rescues MLP-null cardiac dysfunction,[236] whereas Adeno/SERCA2 gene delivery improves cardiac contractility and prognosis of postaortic-banded rats.[237,238] PLN ablation induces a hyperkinetic phenotype in the normal mouse heart[239] and dominantly complements cardiomyopathic changes in the MLP-null animals[240] The genetic rescue effect of PLN ablation might be model-dependent, because it is not obvious in Gq transgenic mice (an apoptotic heart failure model) and homozygous myosin binding protein-C mutant animals (a neonatal-onset progressive ventricular dilation model)[241]; however, molecular intervention to target PLN-SERCA2 interaction demonstrates clear beneficial effects, which are indeed chronic.[44] Enhancement of isolated cardiomyocytes from endstage heart failure patients is also promoted by suppression of PLN expression.[242]

Diastolic leakage of calcium from SR through a SR calcium release channel (ryanodine receptor: RyR) has been linked to the PKA-dependent hyper-phosphorylation of RyR and subsequent dissociation of FKBP12.6, a stabilizing protein of RyR from the RyR/FKBP12.6 complex[243]; enhanced diastolic SR calcium leakage was later confirmed in FKBP12.6-null mice.[244] Thus, long-term beneficial effects of β-blocker therapy may be partly attributed to the stabilization of the RyR/FKBP12.6 complex.[245,246] The evidence that human RyR mutations[247-249] can lead to polymorphic ventricular tachycardia and associated sudden death[250] further supports this possibility. The *in vitro* transfection of Adeno/FKBP12.6 in cultured cardiomyocyte increases contractility,[251] suggesting that RyR stabilization may also improve cardiac contractile in the failing hearts.

## Molecular Substrates for Arrhythmogenesis in Heart Failure: Acquired Defects in Conduction Lineages, Intercellular Coupling, Repolarization, and Action Potential Duration (APD)

One of the major causes of mortality in heart failure is the onset of life-threatening malignant arrhythmias. The incidence of cardiac sudden death and associated cardiac rhythm abnormalities correlates with the severity of dysfunction, but the mechanism that serves as the substrate for this markedly increased susceptibility is unclear. In addition to the abnormal delayed inward depolarization current that is partly associated with diastolic SR calcium leak (see previous discussion), a growing body of electrophysiologic, genetic, experimental, and clinical data is supporting the concept that heterogeneity of APD throughout the myocardium of the failing heart may partly account for the arrhythmogenic substrate that creates susceptibility for reentrant ventricular tachyarrrhythmias.[252,253] Much of this insight has been gleaned from genetically based forms of arrhythmias in clinical and animal model systems. Several distinct classes of mutations have been shown to be associated with cardiac arrhythmogenesis. Studies of long QT syndrome, an autosomal dominant disease associated with an increased incidence of cardiac sudden death, have indicated that the disease is due to mutations in channel pore-forming proteins and interacting proteins of ion-transporters that can lead to prolongation of the QT interval and associated APD prolongation.[209,252] A second class of arrhythmogenic defects has recently been uncovered, which are related to abnormalities in cardiac intercellular conduction that is associated with the loss of cardiac connexins.[157,254,255] The third class of mutations associated with malfunctions in the conduction system and cardiac sudden death have been discovered in human patients and from studies using genetically engineered mouse models. The mutations occur because of defects in cardiac transcription factors that control muscle gene expression in both ventricular muscle and conduction system cell lineages.[162,256,257] Recent studies have further implicated a glycogen-storage abnormality associated with HCM that contributes to progressive conduction defects within the conduction system itself.[258-260]

Because it is unlikely that somatic mutations account for most cases of cardiac sudden death associated with progressive heart failure, the generalizable mechanisms that accompany arrhythmogenesis in this acquired form

of the disease warrant investigation. There are several conserved electrophysiologic features of human heart failure, which include elongation of APD, enhanced inward current associated with sarcolemmal sodium-calcium exchanger activity, and the loss of a transmural gradient of phase 1 $I_{to}$ potassium current.[214] The mechanisms that contribute to the loss of the $I_{to}$ gradient are unclear, and the relative importance of changes in this specific current versus the multitude of other changes in the electrophysiologic phenotype of the failing heart is unknown. Recent studies have clearly identified that the loss of $I_{to}$ can independently increase the dispersion of repolarization and confer marked susceptibility to lethal forms of ventricular tachycardia.[261] These observations are based on the discovery of a cytoplasmic accessory protein (KChIP2) that binds to the Kv4.2 and 4.3 channel proteins and that is markedly downregulated early during pressure-overload hypertrophy.[261] This negative regulation mimics the reactivation of the fetal gene program, because the KChIP2 gene is not expressed in the fetal heart until the late embryonic stage and is postnatally activated in the adult heart. Interestingly, KChIP2 quantitatively regulates the $I_{to}$ current, because heterozygotes for the mutant allele display a precise 50% decrease in current density. Mice that lack KChIP2 can display a loss of the normal $I_{to}$ current gradient across the ventricular wall and sustained polymorphic ventricular tachycardia with a single, extra stimulus in programmed stimulation studies[261] (Fig. 15-8). Because human and canine hearts express the KChIP2 gene in a gradient (epicardium greater than endocardium) that matches with the distribution of $I_{to}$ current (the Kv4.2 and 4.3 genes are uniformly expressed throughout the

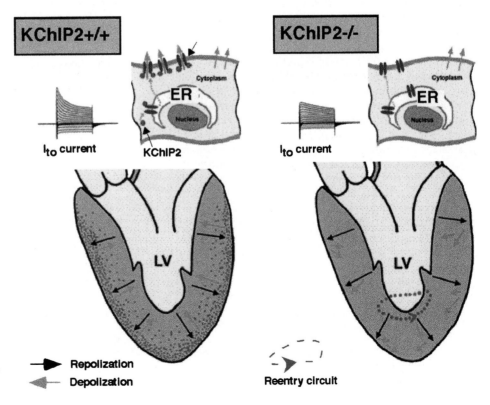

**FIGURE 15-8.** Ion transporter abnormalities and the substrate for malignant ventricular arrhythmia in KChIP2-null (KChIP-/-) myocardium. The absence of KChIP2 blocks the translocation of Kv4.2/4.3 pore-forming subunits of membrane potassium channels, leading to a loss of the cardiac $I_{to}$ current. The transmural gradient of $I_{to}$ current, which is normally high in the outer layer, is lost in the KChIP2-null myocardium, resulting in the heterogeneity of repolarization. This repolarization heterogeneity can create multiple reentry circuits with unidirectional conduction block, which provide a substrate for malignant ventricular arrhythmia. (*Modified from Kuo H, Cheng CF, Clark RB, et al: A defect in the Kv Channel-interacting protein 2 (KCHIP2) gene leads to a complete loss of I (to) and confers susceptibility to ventricular tachycardia. Cell 2001;107:801–813.*)

ventricular wall[262,263]), it is likely that the KChIP2 gene quantitatively regulates the $I_{to}$ current in the human heart. Therefore, it will be interesting to determine whether there is a downregulation of KChIP2 gene expression in the failing human heart that might account for the loss of the $I_{to}$ gradient in human heart failure. If such is the case, then defects in KChIP2 may represent a new class of genetic modifiers that can confer risk for both inheritable and acquired forms of ventricular arrhythmias. Because the expression of KChIP2 is downregulated during cardiac remodeling,[261] strategies to maintain $I_{to}$ by promoting the level of KChIP2 expression in the failing heart may represent a new therapeutic approach for combating the prevalent lethal arrhythmias associated with heart failure. The roles of other channel accessory proteins that may be important in the regulation of other cardiac currents and how they confer susceptibility to arrhythmogenesis in the setting of heart failure should be investigated.

## TOWARD NEW THERAPEUTIC PATHWAYS

Genomic databases, which provide a universal language that can be used to identify the conserved functions of cardiovascular genes in multiple species and organ systems, are ushering in a new era of integrative biology.[6] For example, numerous parallels exist between cardiac muscle and neuromuscular disorders (e.g., excitability, conduction, terminal differentiation, and innervation). Unsuspected connections between neural and cardiac developmental gene programs have been uncovered in gene-targeted mice, and conserved myocyte and neuronal cell survival factors have been discovered, which suggest the existence of other factors. Thus, major opportunities for understanding cardiac diseases may lie in working at the interface of cardiovascular science and neuroscience.

To evaluate the real clinical potential of disease pathways found in mouse models, parallel studies in larger animals will be necessary. The difficulty of germ-line gene manipulation in larger animals suggests the value of new strategies using peptide inhibitors, neutralizing antibodies, and somatic gene transfer with smart vectors that allow long-term expression. The many quantitative end points for complex *in vivo* cardiac phenotypes should empower the next frontier that lies at the boundaries of genomic databases, physiology, and human disease. We are entering a renaissance of integrative biology of the intact organism, and the heart may again play a key role in defining the circuitry for complex *in vivo* physiologic traits.

## REFERENCES

1. Cohn JN, Bristow MR, Chien KR, et al: Report of the National Heart, Lung, and Blood Institute Special Emphasis Panel on Heart Failure Research. Circulation 1997;95:766–770.
2. McMurray J, Pfeffer MA: New therapeutic options in congestive heart failure. I. Circulation 2002;105:2099–2106.
3. McMurray J, Pfeffer MA: New therapeutic options in congestive heart failure. II. Circulation 2002;105:2223–2228.
4. Angeja BG, Grossman W: Evaluation and management of diastolic heart failure. Circulation 2003;107:659–663.
5. Chien KR: Stress pathways and heart failure. Cell 1999;98:555–558.
6. Chien KR: Genomic circuits and the integrative biology of cardiac diseases. Nature 2000;407:227–232.
7. Franz WM, Muller OJ, Katus HA: Cardiomyopathies: From genetics to the prospect of treatment. Lancet 2001;358:1627–1637.
8. Charron P, Komajda M: Are we ready for pharmacogenomics in heart failure? Eur J Pharmacol 2001;417:1–9.
9. Rockman HA, Ross RS, Harris AN et al: Segregation of atrial-specific and inducible expression of an atrial natriuretic factor transgene in an in vivo murine model of cardiac hypertrophy. Proc Natl Acad Sci USA 1991;88:8277–8281.
10. Yasukawa H, Hoshijima M, Gu Y et al: Suppressor of cytokine signaling-3 is a biomechanical stress-inducible gene that suppresses gp130-mediated cardiac myocyte hypertrophy and survival pathways. J Clin Invest 2001;108:1459–1467.
11. Fischer TA, Ludwig S, Flory E et al: Activation of cardiac c-Jun NH(2)-terminal kinases and p38-mitogen-activated protein kinases with abrupt changes in hemodynamic load. Hypertension 2001;37:1222–1228.
12. http://cardiogenomics.med.harvard.edu/public-data
13. Hu H, Sachs F: Stretch-activated ion channels in the heart. J Mol Cell Cardiol 1997;29:1511–1523.
14. Ruwhof C, van der Laarse A: Mechanical stress-induced cardiac hypertrophy: Mechanisms and signal transduction pathways. Cardiovasc Res 2000;47:23–37.
15. Yamazaki T, Komuro I, Kudoh S, et al: Role of ion channels and exchangers in mechanical stretch-induced cardiomyocyte hypertrophy. Circ Res 1998;82:430–437.
16. Sadoshima J, Izumo S: The cellular and molecular response of cardiac myocytes to mechanical stress. Annu Rev Physiol 1997;59:551–571.
17. Sugden PH, Clerk A: Cellular mechanisms of cardiac hypertrophy. J Mol Med 1998;76:725–746.
18. Molkentin JD, Dorn IG 2nd: Cytoplasmic signaling pathways that regulate cardiac hypertrophy. Annu Rev Physiol 2001;63:391–426.
19. Frey N, Olson EN: Cardiac hypertrophy: The good, the bad, and the ugly. Annu Rev Physiol 2003;65:45–79.
20. Choquet D, Felsenfeld DP, Sheetz MP: Extracellular matrix rigidity causes strengthening of integrin-cytoskeleton linkages. Cell 1997;88:39–48.
21. Ross RS, Borg TK: Integrins and the myocardium. Circ Res 2001;88:1112–1119.
22. Shai SY, Harpf AE, Babbitt CJ, et al: Cardiac myocyte-specific excision of the beta1 integrin gene results in myocardial fibrosis and cardiac failure. Circ Res 2002;90:458–464.
23. Brancaccio M, Fratta L, Notte A, et al: Melusin, a muscle-specific integrin beta1-interacting protein, is required to prevent cardiac failure in response to chronic pressure overload. Nat Med 2003;9:68–75.
24. Hunter JJ, Grace A, Chien KR: Molecular and cellular biology of cardiac hypertrophy and failure. In Chien KR (ed): Molecular Basis of Cardiovascular Disease. Philadelphia, WB Saunders, 1999, pp 211–250.
25. Hwang DM, Dempsey AA, Wang RX, et al: A genome-based resource for molecular cardiovascular medicine: Toward a compendium of cardiovascular genes. Circulation 1997;96:4146–4203.
26. Yang J, Moravec CS, Sussman MA, et al: Decreased SLIM1 expression and increased gelsolin expression in failing human hearts measured by high-density oligonucleotide arrays. Circulation 2000;102:3046–3052.
27. Friddle CJ, Koga T, Rubin EM, Bristow J: Expression profiling reveals distinct sets of genes altered during induction and regression of cardiac hypertrophy. Proc Natl Acad Sci USA 2000;97:6745–6750.
28. Redfern CH, Degtyarev MY, Kwa AT, et al: Conditional expression of a Gi-coupled receptor causes ventricular conduction delay and a lethal cardiomyopathy. Proc Natl Acad Sci USA 2000;97:4826–4831.
29. Lim DS, Roberts R, Marian AJ: Expression profiling of cardiac genes in human hypertrophic cardiomyopathy: Insight into the pathogenesis of phenotypes. J Am Coll Cardiol 2001;38:1175–1180.

30. Johnatty SE, Dyck JR, Michael LH, et al: Identification of genes regulated during mechanical load-induced cardiac hypertrophy. J Mol Cell Cardiol 2000;32:805–815.

31. Chien KR, Knowlton KU, Zhu H, Chien S: Regulation of cardiac gene expression during myocardial growth and hypertrophy: Molecular studies of an adaptive physiologic response. FASEB J 1991;5:3037–5046.

32. Hunter JJ, Chien KR: Signaling pathways for cardiac hypertrophy and failure. N Engl J Med 1999;341:1276–1283.

33. Yasukawa H, Sasaki A, Yoshimura A: Negative regulation of cytokine signaling pathways. Annu Rev Immunol 2000;18: 143–164.

34. Pennica D, King KL, Shaw KJ et al: Expression cloning of cardiotrophin 1, a cytokine that induces cardiac myocyte hypertrophy. Proc Natl Acad Sci USA 1995;92:1142–1146.

35. Wollert KC, Chien KR: Cardiotrophin-1 and the role of gp130-dependent signaling pathways in cardiac growth and development. J Mol Med 1997;75:492–501.

36. Sheng Z, Pennica D, Wood WI, Chien KR: Cardiotrophin-1 displays early expression in the murine heart tube and promotes cardiac myocyte survival. Development 1996;122:419–428.

37. Fujio Y, Kunisada K, Hirota H, et al: Signals through gp130 upregulate bcl-x gene expression via STAT1-binding cis-element in cardiac myocytes. J Clin Invest 1997;99:2898–2905.

38. Yamauchi-Takihara K, Kishimoto T: A novel role for STAT3 in cardiac remodeling. Trends Cardiovasc Med 2000;10:298–303.

39. Rothermel BA, McKinsey TA, Vega RB, et al: Myocyte-enriched calcineurin-interacting protein, MCIP1, inhibits cardiac hypertrophy in vivo. Proc Natl Acad Sci USA 2001;98:3328–3333.

40. Yang J, Rothermel B, Vega RB, et al: Independent signals control expression of the calcineurin inhibitory proteins MCIP1 and MCIP2 in striated muscles. Circ Res 2000;87:E61–68.

41. Bueno OF, De Windt LJ, Lim HW, et al: The dual-specificity phosphatase MKP-1 limits the cardiac hypertrophic response in vitro and in vivo. Circ Res 2001;88:88–96.

42. Ruiz-Lozano P, Chien KR: Cre-constructing the heart. Nat Genet 2003;33:8–9.

43. Ikeda Y, Gu Y, Iwanaga Y, et al: Restoration of deficient membrane proteins in the cardiomyopathic hamster by in vivo cardiac gene transfer. Circulation 2002;105:502–508.

44. Hoshijima M, Ikeda Y, Iwanaga Y, et al: Chronic suppression of heart-failure progression by a pseudophosphorylated mutant of phospholamban via in vivo cardiac rAAV gene delivery. Nat Med 2002;8:864–871.

45. Duerr RL, Huang S, Miraliakbar HR, et al: Insulin-like growth factor-1 enhances ventricular hypertrophy and function during the onset of experimental cardiac failure. J Clin Invest 1995;95: 619–627.

46. Tanaka N, Ryoke T, Hongo M et al: Effects of growth hormone and IGF-I on cardiac hypertrophy and gene expression in mice. Am J Physiol 1998;275:H393–99.

47. Barton ER, Morris L, Musaro A, et al: Muscle-specific expression of insulin-like growth factor I counters muscle decline in mdx mice. J Cell Biol 2002;157:137–148.

48. Rommel C, Bodine SC, Clarke BA, et al: Mediation of IGF-1-induced skeletal myotube hypertrophy by PI(3)K/Akt/mTOR and PI(3)K/Akt/GSK3 pathways. Nat Cell Biol 2001;3:1009–1013.

49. Bodine SC, Stitt TN, Gonzalez M, et al: Akt/mTOR pathway is a crucial regulator of skeletal muscle hypertrophy and can prevent muscle atrophy in vivo. Nat Cell Biol 2001;3:1014–1019.

50. Glass DJ: Signalling pathways that mediate skeletal muscle hypertrophy and atrophy. Nat Cell Biol 2003;5:87–90.

51. Cohen P, Frame S: The renaissance of GSK3. Nat Rev Mol Cell Biol 2001;2:769–776.

52. Scheid MP, Woodgett JR: Pkb/akt: Functional insights from genetic models. Nat Rev Mol Cell Biol 2001;2:760–768.

53. Hardt SE, Sadoshima J: Glycogen synthase kinase-3beta: A novel regulator of cardiac hypertrophy and development. Circ Res 2002;90:1055–1063.

54. Fujio Y, Nguyen T, Wencker D, et al: Akt promotes survival of cardiomyocytes in vitro and protects against ischemia-reperfusion injury in mouse heart. Circulation 2000;101:660–667.

55. Wu W, Lee WL, Wu YY, et al: Expression of constitutively active phosphatidylinositol 3-kinase inhibits activation of caspase 3 and apoptosis of cardiac muscle cells. J Biol Chem 2000;275: 40113–40119.

56. Vanhaesebroeck B, Alessi DR: The PI3K-PDK1 connection: More than just a road to PKB. Biochem J 2000;346(Pt 3):561–576.

57. Toker A, Newton AC: Cellular signaling: Pivoting around PDK-1. Cell 2000;103:185–188.

58. Vanhaesebroeck B, Leevers SJ, Ahmadi K, et al: Synthesis and function of 3-phosphorylated inositol lipids. Annu Rev Biochem 2001;70:535–602.

59. Backman S, Stambolic V, Mak T: PTEN function in mammalian cell size regulation. Curr Opin Neurobiol 2002;12:516–522.

60. Haq S, Choukroun G, Lim H et al: Differential activation of signal transduction pathways in human hearts with hypertrophy versus advanced heart failure. Circulation 2001;103:670–677.

61. Reiss K, Cheng W, Ferber A, et al: Overexpression of insulin-like growth factor-1 in the heart is coupled with myocyte proliferation in transgenic mice. Proc Natl Acad Sci USA 1996;93:8630–8635.

62. Shioi T, Kang PM, Douglas PS et al: The conserved phosphoinositide 3-kinase pathway determines heart size in mice. EMBO J 2000;19:2537–2548.

63. Shioi T, McMullen JR, Kang PM, et al: Akt/protein kinase B promotes organ growth in transgenic mice. Mol Cell Biol 2002;22:2799–809.

64. Condorelli G, Drusco A, Stassi G et al: Akt induces enhanced myocardial contractility and cell size in vivo in transgenic mice. Proc Natl Acad Sci USA 2002;99:12333–12338.

65. Matsui T, Li L, Wu JC, et al: Phenotypic spectrum caused by transgenic overexpression of activated Akt in the heart. J Biol Chem 2002;277:22896–22901.

66. Antos CL, McKinsey TA, Frey N, et al: Activated glycogen synthase-3 beta suppresses cardiac hypertrophy in vivo. Proc Natl Acad Sci USA 2002;99:907–912.

67. Schwartzbauer G, Robbins J: The tumor suppressor gene PTEN can regulate cardiac hypertrophy and survival. J Biol Chem 2001;276:35786–35793.

68. Crackower MA, Oudit GY, Kozieradzki I, et al: Regulation of myocardial contractility and cell size by distinct PI3K-PTEN signaling pathways. Cell 2002;110:737–749.

69. Toker A, Cantley LC: Signalling through the lipid products of phosphoinositide-3-OH kinase. Nature 1997;387:673–676.

70. Ramirez MT, Zhao XL, Schulman H, Brown JH: The nuclear deltaB isoform of Ca²⁺/calmodulin-dependent protein kinase II regulates atrial natriuretic factor gene expression in ventricular myocytes. J Biol Chem 1997;272:31203–31208.

71. Kirchhefer U, Schmitz W, Scholz H, Neumann J: Activity of cAMP-dependent protein kinase and Ca²⁺/calmodulin-dependent protein kinase in failing and nonfailing human hearts. Cardiovasc Res 1999;42:254–261.

72. Molkentin JD, Lu JR, Antos CL, et al: A calcineurin-dependent transcriptional pathway for cardiac hypertrophy. Cell 1998; 93:215–228.

73. Frey N, McKinsey TA, Olson EN: Decoding calcium signals involved in cardiac growth and function. Nat Med 2000;6: 1221–1227.

74. Passier R, Zeng H, Frey N et al: CaM kinase signaling induces cardiac hypertrophy and activates the MEF2 transcription factor in vivo. J Clin Invest 2000;105:1395–1406.

75. Han J, Molkentin JD: Regulation of MEF2 by p38 MAPK and its implication in cardiomyocyte biology. Trends Cardiovasc Med 2000;10:19–22.

76. McKinsey TA, Zhang CL, Olson EN: Control of muscle development by dueling HATs and HDACs. Curr Opin Genet Dev 2001;11:497–504.

77. Zhang CL, McKinsey TA, Chang S, et al: Class II histone deacetylases act as signal-responsive repressors of cardiac hypertrophy. Cell 2002;110:479–488.

78. Zhao M, New L, Kravchenko VV, et al. Regulation of the MEF2 family of transcription factors by p38. Mol Cell Biol 1999;19: 21–30.

79. Yang TT, Xiong Q, Enslen H, et al: Phosphorylation of NFATc4 by p38 mitogen-activated protein kinases. Mol Cell Biol 2002;22: 3892–3904.

80. Morisco C, Seta K, Hardt SE et al: Glycogen synthase kinase 3beta regulates GATA4 in cardiac myocytes. J Biol Chem 2001; 276:28586–28597.

81. Olson EN, Molkentin, JD: Prevention of cardiac hypertrophy by calcineurin inhibition: Hope or hype? Circ Res 1999;84:623–632.

82. Sugden PH: Signaling in myocardial hypertrophy: Life after calcineurin? Circ Res 1999;84:633-646.

83. Wilkins BJ, Molkentin JD: Calcineurin and cardiac hypertrophy: Where have we been? Where are we going? J Physiol 2002; 541:1-8.

84. Zou Y, Hiroi Y, Uozumi H, et al: Calcineurin plays a critical role in the development of pressure overload-induced cardiac hypertrophy. Circulation 2001;104:97-101.

85. De Windt LJ, Lim HW, Bueno OF, et al: Targeted inhibition of calcineurin attenuates cardiac hypertrophy in vivo. Proc Natl Acad Sci USA 2001;98:3322-3327.

86. Bueno OF, Wilkins BJ, Tymitz KM, et al: Impaired cardiac hypertrophic response in calcineurin Abeta-deficient mice. Proc Natl Acad Sci USA 2002;99:4586-4591.

87. Wilkins BJ, De Windt LJ, Bueno OF, et al: Targeted disruption of NFATc3, but not NFATc4, reveals an intrinsic defect in calcineurin-mediated cardiac hypertrophic growth. Mol Cell Biol 2002;22:7603-7613.

88. Fatkin D, McConnell BK, Mudd JO, et al: An abnormal Ca(2+) response in mutant sarcomere protein-mediated familial hypertrophic cardiomyopathy. J Clin Invest 2000;106:1351-1359.

89. Geisterfer-Lowrance AA, Christe M, Conner DA, et al: A mouse model of familial hypertrophic cardiomyopathy. Science 1996; 272:731-734.

90. Zhang T, Johnson EN, Gu Y et al: The cardiac-specific nuclear delta(B) isoform of Ca2+/calmodulin-dependent protein kinase II induces hypertrophy and dilated cardiomyopathy associated with increased protein phosphatase 2A activity. J Biol Chem 2002; 277:1261-1267.

91. Bers DM: Cardiac excitation-contraction coupling. Nature 2002;415:198-205.

92. Mesaeli N, Nakamura K, Opas M, Michalak M: Endoplasmic reticulum in the heart, a forgotten organelle? Mol Cell Biochem 2001; 225:1-6.

93. Allen BG, Katz S: Calreticulin and calsequestrin are differentially distributed in canine heart. J Mol Cell Cardiol 2000;32: 2379-2384.

94. Semsarian C, Ahmad I, Giewat M, et al: The L-type calcium channel inhibitor diltiazem prevents cardiomyopathy in a mouse model. J Clin Invest 2002;109:1013-1020.

95. Mesaeli N, Nakamura K, Zvaritch E et al: Calreticulin is essential for cardiac development. J Cell Biol 1999;144:857-868.

96. Dolmetsch RE, Lewis RS, Goodnow CC, Healy JI: Differential activation of transcription factors induced by Ca2+ response amplitude and duration. Nature 1997;386:855-858.

97. Zhang J, Warwick PJ, Wolfrum E, et al: Saturated output of a Ge. Physical Rev A 1996;54:R4653-R4656.

98. Timmerman LA, Clipstone NA, Ho SN, et al: Rapid shuttling of NF-AT in discrimination of Ca$^{2+}$ signals and immunosuppression. Nature 1996;383:837-840.

99. Lisman J: The CaM kinase II hypothesis for the storage of synaptic memory. Trends Neurosci 194;17:406-412.

100. Bayer KU, De Koninck P, Schulman H: Alternative splicing modulates the frequency-dependent response of CaMKII to Ca(2+) oscillations. EMBO J 2002;21:3590-3597.

101. LaMorte VJ, Thorburn J, Absher D, et al: Gq- and ras-dependent pathways mediate hypertrophy of neonatal rat ventricular myocytes following alpha 1-adrenergic stimulation. J Biol Chem 1994;269:13490-13496.

102. Adams JW, Pagel AL, Means CK et al: Cardiomyocyte apoptosis induced by Galphaq signaling is mediated by permeability transition pore formation and activation of the mitochondrial death pathway. Circ Res 2000;87:1180-1187.

103. Yussman MG, Toyokawa T, Odley A, et al: Mitochondrial death protein Nix is induced in cardiac hypertrophy and triggers apoptotic cardiomyopathy. Nat Med 2002;8:725-730.

104. Akhter SA, Luttrell LM, Rockman HA, et al: Targeting the receptor-Gq interface to inhibit in vivo pressure overload myocardial hypertrophy. Science 1998;280:574-577.

105. Esposito G, Rapacciuolo A, Naga Prasad SV, et al: Genetic alterations that inhibit in vivo pressure-overload hypertrophy prevent cardiac dysfunction despite increased wall stress. Circulation 2002;105:85-92.

106. Wettschureck N, Rutten H, Zywietz A, et al: Absence of pressure overload induced myocardial hypertrophy after conditional inactivation of Galphaq/Galpha11 in cardiomyocytes. Nat Med 2001;7:1236-1240.

107. Maruyama Y, Nishida M, Sugimoto Y, et al: Galpha(12/13) mediates alpha(1)-adrenergic receptor-induced cardiac hypertrophy. Circ Res 2002;91:961-969.

108. Asakura M, Kitakaze M, Takashima S, et al: Cardiac hypertrophy is inhibited by antagonism of ADAM12 processing of HB-EGF: Metalloproteinase inhibitors as a new therapy. Nat Med 2002; 8:35-40.

109. Nishizuka Y: Intracellular signaling by hydrolysis of phospholipids and activation of protein kinase C. Science 1992;258:607-614.

110. Dunnmon PM, Iwaki K, Henderson SA, et al: Phorbol esters induce immediate-early genes and activate cardiac gene transcription in neonatal rat myocardial cells. J Mol Cell Cardiol 1990;22:901-910.

111. Bowman JC, Steinberg SF, Jiang T, et al: Expression of protein kinase C beta in the heart causes hypertrophy in adult mice and sudden death in neonates. J Clin Invest 1997;100:2189-2195.

112. Wakasaki H, Koya D, Schoen FJ, et al: Targeted overexpression of protein kinase C beta2 isoform in myocardium causes cardiomyopathy. Proc Natl Acad Sci USA 1997;94:9320-9325.

113. Takeishi Y, Ping P, Bolli R, et al: Transgenic overexpression of constitutively active protein kinase C epsilon causes concentric cardiac hypertrophy. Circ Res 2000;86:1218-1223.

114. Pass JM, Zheng Y, Wead WB, et al: PKCepsilon activation induces dichotomous cardiac phenotypes and modulates PKCepsilon-RACK interactions and RACK expression. Am J Physiol Heart Circ Physiol 2001;280:H946-55.

115. Dempsey EC, Newton AC, Mochly-Rosen D, et al: Protein kinase C isozymes and the regulation of diverse cell responses. Am J Physiol Lung Cell Mol Physiol 2000;279:L429-438.

116. Steinberg SF, Goldberg M, Rybin VO: Protein kinase C isoform diversity in the heart. J Mol Cell Cardiol 1995;27:141-153.

117. Mackay K, Mochly-Rosen D: Localization, anchoring, and functions of protein kinase C isozymes in the heart. J Mol Cell Cardiol 2001;33:1301-1307.

118. Malhotra A, Kang BP, Opawumi D, et al: Molecular biology of protein kinase C signaling in cardiac myocytes. Mol Cell Biochem 2001;225:97-107.

119. Dutil EM, Newton AC: Dual role of pseudosubstrate in the coordinated regulation of protein kinase C by phosphorylation and diacylglycerol. J Biol Chem 2000;275:10697-10701.

120. Puceat M, Hilal-Dandan R, Strulovici B, et al: Differential regulation of protein kinase C isoforms in isolated neonatal and adult rat cardiomyocytes. J Biol Chem 1994;269:16938-16944.

121. Clerk A, Bogoyevitch MA, Anderson MB, Sugden PH: Differential activation of protein kinase C isoforms by endothelin-1 and phenylephrine and subsequent stimulation of p42 and p44 mitogen-activated protein kinases in ventricular myocytes cultured from neonatal rat hearts. J Biol Chem 1994;269: 32848-32857.

122. Clerk A, Gillespie-Brown J, Fuller SJ, Sugden PH: Stimulation of phosphatidylinositol hydrolysis, protein kinase C translocation, and mitogen-activated protein kinase activity by bradykinin in rat ventricular myocytes: Dissociation from the hypertrophic response. Biochem J 1996;317(Pt 1):109-118.

123. Clerk A, Sugden PH: Untangling the Web: Specific signaling from PKC isoforms to MAPK cascades. Circ Res 2001;89:847-849.

124. Bueno OF, Molkentin JD: Involvement of extracellular signal-regulated kinases 1/2 in cardiac hypertrophy and cell death. Circ Res 2002;91:776-781.

125. Bogoyevitch MA, Marshall CJ, Sugden PH: Hypertrophic agonists stimulate the activities of the protein kinases c-Raf and A-Raf in cultured ventricular myocytes. J Biol Chem 1995;270: 26303-26310.

126. Heidkamp MC, Bayer AL, Martin JL, Samarel AM: Differential activation of mitogen-activated protein kinase cascades and apoptosis by protein kinase C epsilon and delta in neonatal rat ventricular myocytes. Circ Res 2001;89:882-890.

127. Mochly-Rosen D, Wu G, Hahn H et al: Cardiotrophic effects of protein kinase C epsilon: Analysis by in vivo modulation of PKCepsilon translocation. Circ Res 2000;86:1173-1179.

128. Wu G, Toyokawa T, Hahn H, Dorn GW 2nd: Epsilon protein kinase C in pathological myocardial hypertrophy. Analysis by combined transgenic expression of translocation modifiers and Galphaq. J Biol Chem 2000;275:29927-29930.

129. Jin ZQ, Zhou HZ, Zhu P, et al: Cardioprotection mediated by sphingosine-1-phosphate and ganglioside GM-1 in wild-type and PKC epsilon knockout mouse hearts. Am J Physiol Heart Circ Physiol 2002;282:H1970-1977.

130. Baines CP, Zhang J, Wang GW, et al: Mitochondrial PKCepsilon and MAPK form signaling modules in the murine heart: Enhanced mitochondrial PKCepsilon-MAPK interactions and differential MAPK activation in PKCepsilon-induced cardioprotection. Circ Res 2002;90:390-397.

131. Valks DM, Cook SA, Pham FH et al: Phenylephrine promotes phosphorylation of Bad in cardiac myocytes through the extracellular signal-regulated kinases 1/2 and protein kinase A. J Mol Cell Cardiol 2002;34:749-763.

132. Huang XP, Pi Y, Lokuta AJ, et al: Arachidonic acid stimulates protein kinase C-epsilon redistribution in heart cells. J Cell Sci 1997;110(Pt 14):1625-1634.

133. Csukai M, Chen CH, De Matteis MA, Mochly-Rosen D: The coatomer protein beta'-COP, a selective binding protein (RACK) for protein kinase Cepsilon. J Biol Chem 1997;272:29200-29206.

134. Kuroda S, Tokunaga C, Kiyohara Y, et al: Protein-protein interaction of zinc finger LIM domains with protein kinase C. J Biol Chem 1996;271:31029-31032.

135. Nakagawa N, Hoshijima M, Oyasu M, et al: ENH, containing PDZ and LIM domains, heart/skeletal muscle-specific protein, associates with cytoskeletal proteins through the PDZ domain. Biochem Biophys Res Commun 2000;272:505-512.

136. Zhou Q, Ruiz-Lozano P, Martone ME, Chen J: Cypher, a striated muscle-restricted PDZ and LIM domain-containing protein, binds to alpha-actinin-2 and protein kinase C. J Biol Chem 1999;274:19807-19813.

137. Faulkner G, Pallavicini A, Formentin E, et al: ZASP: A new Z-band alternatively spliced PDZ-motif protein. J Cell Biol 1999;146:465-475.

138. Passier R, Richardson JA, Olson EN: Oracle, a novel PDZ-LIM domain protein expressed in heart and skeletal muscle. Mech Dev 2000;92:277-284.

139. Hirota H, Yoshida K, Kishimoto T, Taga T: Continuous activation of gp130, a signal-transducing receptor component for interleukin 6-related cytokines, causes myocardial hypertrophy in mice. Proc Natl Acad Sci USA 1995;92:4862-4866.

140. Kishimoto T, Taga T, Akira S: Cytokine signal transduction. Cell 1994;76:253-262.

141. Kunisada K, Negoro S, Tone E, et al: Signal transducer and activator of transcription 3 in the heart transduces not only a hypertrophic signal but a protective signal against doxorubicin-induced cardiomyopathy. Proc Natl Acad Sci USA 2000;97:315-319.

142. Osugi T, Oshima Y, Fujio Y, et al: Cardiac-specific activation of signal transducer and activator of transcription 3 promotes vascular formation in the heart. J Biol Chem 2002;277:6676-6681.

143. Kodama H, Fukuda K, Pan J, et al: Significance of ERK cascade compared with JAK/STAT and PI3-K pathway in gp130-mediated cardiac hypertrophy. Am J Physiol Heart Circ Physiol 2000;279:H1635-1644.

144. Nicol RL, Frey N, Pearson G, et al: Activated MEK5 induces serial assembly of sarcomeres and eccentric cardiac hypertrophy. EMBO J 2001;20:2757-2767.

145. Oh H, Fujio Y, Kunisada K, et al: Activation of phosphatidylinositol 3-kinase through glycoprotein 130 induces protein kinase B and p70 S6 kinase phosphorylation in cardiac myocytes. J Biol Chem 1998;273:9703-9710.

146. Wollert KC, Taga T, Saito M, et al: Cardiotrophin-1 activates a distinct form of cardiac muscle cell hypertrophy: Assembly of sarcomeric units in series VIA gp130/leukemia inhibitory factor receptor-dependent pathways. J Biol Chem 1996;271:9535-9545.

147. Hoshijima M, Sah VP, Wang Y, et al: The low molecular weight GTPase Rho regulates myofibril formation and organization in neonatal rat ventricular myocytes: Involvement of Rho kinase. J Biol Chem 1998;273:7725-7730.

148. Pashmforoush M, Pomies P, Peterson KL, et al: Adult mice deficient in actinin-associated LIM-domain protein reveal a developmental pathway for right ventricular cardiomyopathy. Nat Med 2001;7:591-597.

149. Bueno OF, De Windt LJ, Tymitz KM, et al: The MEK1-ERK1/2 signaling pathway promotes compensated cardiac hypertrophy in transgenic mice. EMBO J 2000;19:6341-6350.

150. Liang Q, Wiese RJ, Bueno OF, et al: The transcription factor GATA4 is activated by extracellular signal-regulated kinase 1- and 2-mediated phosphorylation of serine 105 in cardiomyocytes. Mol Cell Biol 2001;21:7460-7469.

151. Liao P, Georgakopoulos D, Kovacs A, et al: The in vivo role of p38 MAP kinases in cardiac remodeling and restrictive cardiomyopathy. Proc Natl Acad Sci USA 2001;98:12283-12288.

152. Liao P, Wang SQ, Wang S, et al: p38 Mitogen-activated protein kinase mediates a negative inotropic effect in cardiac myocytes. Circ Res 2002;90:190-196.

153. Zhang D, Gaussin V, Taffet GE, et al: TAK1 is activated in the myocardium after pressure overload and is sufficient to provoke heart failure in transgenic mice. Nat Med 2000;6:556-563.

154. Wang Y, Su B, Sah VP, et al: Cardiac hypertrophy induced by mitogen-activated protein kinase kinase 7, a specific activator for c-Jun NH2-terminal kinase in ventricular muscle cells. J Biol Chem 1998;273:5423-5426.

155. Sadoshima J, Montagne O, Wang Q, et al: The MEKK1-JNK pathway plays a protective role in pressure overload but does not mediate cardiac hypertrophy. J Clin Invest 2002;110:271-279.

156. Minamino T, Yujiri T, Terada N, et al: MEKK1 is essential for cardiac hypertrophy and dysfunction induced by Gq. Proc Natl Acad Sci USA 2002;99:3866-3871.

157. Petrich BG, Gong X, Lerner DL, et al: c-Jun N-terminal kinase activation mediates downregulation of connexin43 in cardiomyocytes. Circ Res 2002;91:640-647.

158. Kasahara H, Usheva A, Ueyama T, et al: Characterization of homo- and heterodimerization of cardiac Csx/Nkx2.5 homeoprotein. J Biol Chem 2001;276:4570-4580.

159. Morin S, Charron F, Robitaille L, Nemer M: GATA-dependent recruitment of MEF2 proteins to target promoters. EMBO J 2000;19:2046-2055.

160. Morin S, Paradis P, Aries A, Nemer M: Serum response factor-GATA ternary complex required for nuclear signaling by a G-protein-coupled receptor. Mol Cell Biol 2001;21:1036-1044.

161. Hiroi Y, Kudoh S, Monzen K, et al: Tbx5 associates with Nkx2-5 and synergistically promotes cardiomyocyte differentiation. Nat Genet 2001;28:276-280.

162. Bruneau BG, Nemer G, Schmitt JP, et al: A murine model of Holt-Oram syndrome defines roles of the T-box transcription factor Tbx5 in cardiogenesis and disease. Cell 2001;106:709-721.

163. Dai YS, Cserjesi P, Markham BE, Molkentin JD: The transcription factors GATA4 and dHAND physically interact to synergistically activate cardiac gene expression through a p300-dependent mechanism. J Biol Chem 2002;277:24390-24398.

164. Gusterson RJ, Jazrawi E, Adcock IM, Latchman DS: The transcriptional co-activators CREB-binding protein (CBP) and p300 play a critical role in cardiac hypertrophy that is dependent on their histone acetyltransferase activity. J Biol Chem 2003;278:6838-6847.

165. Wang D, Chang PS, Wang Z, et al: Activation of cardiac gene expression by myocardin, a transcriptional cofactor for serum response factor. Cell 2001;105:851-862.

166. Shin CH, Liu ZP, Passier R, et al: Modulation of cardiac growth and development by HOP, an unusual homeodomain protein. Cell 2002;110:725-735.

167. Chen F, Kook H, Milewski R, et al: Hop is an unusual homeobox gene that modulates cardiac development. Cell 2002;110:713-723.

168. Seidman JG, Seidman C: The genetic basis for cardiomyopathy: From mutation identification to mechanistic paradigms. Cell 2001;104:557-567.

169. Towbin JA, Bowles NE: The failing heart. Nature 2002;415:227-233.

170. Seidman C, Seidman JG: Molecular genetics of inherited cardiomyopathies. In Chien KR, Breslow JL, Leiden JM, et al (eds): Molecular Basis of Cardiovascular Disease. Philadelphia, WB Saunders, 1999, pp 251-263.

171. Bonne G, Carrier L, Richard P, et al: Familial hypertrophic cardiomyopathy: From mutations to functional defects. Circ Res 1998;83:580-593.

172. Bonne G, Carrier L, Bercovici J, et al: Cardiac myosin binding protein-C gene splice acceptor site mutation is associated with familial hypertrophic cardiomyopathy. Nat Genet 1995;11:438-440.

173. Poetter K, Jiang H, Hassanzadeh S, et al: Mutations in either the essential or regulatory light chains of myosin are associated with

a rare myopathy in human heart and skeletal muscle. Nat Genet 1996;13:63-69.

174. Mogensen J, Klausen IC, Pedersen AK, et al: Alpha-cardiac actin is a novel disease gene in familial hypertrophic cardiomyopathy. J Clin Invest 1999;103:R39-43.

175. Thierfelder L, Watkins H, MacRae C, et al: Alpha-tropomyosin and cardiac troponin T mutations cause familial hypertrophic cardiomyopathy: A disease of the sarcomere. Cell 1994;77: 701-712.

176. Kimura A, Harada H, Park JE, et al: Mutations in the cardiac troponin I gene associated with hypertrophic cardiomyopathy. Nat Genet 1997;16:379-382.

177. Satoh M, Takahashi M, Sakamoto T, et al: Structural analysis of the titin gene in hypertrophic cardiomyopathy: Identification of a novel disease gene. Biochem Biophys Res Commun 1999;262: 411-417.

178. Arber S, Hunter JJ, Ross J Jr, et al: MLP-deficient mice exhibit a disruption of cardiac cytoarchitectural organization, dilated cardiomyopathy, and heart failure. Cell 1997;88:393-403.

179. Knoll R, Hoshijima M, Hoffman HM, et al: The cardiac mechanical stretch sensor machinery involves a Z disc complex that is defective in a subset of human dilated cardiomyopathy. Cell 2002; 111:943-955.

180. Geier C, Perrot A, Ozcelik C, et al. Mutations in the human muscle LIM protein gene in families with hypertrophic cardiomyopathy. Circulation 2003;107:1390-1395.

181. Tanigawa G, Jarcho JA, Kass S, et al: A molecular basis for familial hypertrophic cardiomyopathy: An alpha/beta cardiac myosin heavy chain hybrid gene. Cell 1990;62:991-998.

182. Geisterfer-Lowrance AA, Kass S, Tanigawa G, et al: A molecular basis for familial hypertrophic cardiomyopathy: A beta cardiac myosin heavy chain gene missense mutation. Cell 1990; 62:999-1006.

183. Haghighi K, Kolokathis F, Pater L, et al: Human phospholamban null results in lethal dilated cardiomyopathy revealing a critical difference between mouse and human. J Clin Invest 2003;111: 869-876.

184. Minamisawa S, Sato Y, Tatsuguchi Y, et al: Mutation of the phospholamban promoter associated with hypertrophic cardiomyopathy. Biochem Biophys Res Commun 2003;304:1-4.

185. Kamisago M, Sharma SD, DePalma SR, et al: Mutations in sarcomere protein genes as a cause of dilated cardiomyopathy. N Engl J Med 2000;343:1688-1696.

186. Olson TM, Michels VV, Thibodeau SN, et al: Actin mutations in dilated cardiomyopathy, a heritable form of heart failure. Science 1998;280:750-752.

187. Olson TM, Kishimoto NY, Whitby FG, Michels VV: Mutations that alter the surface charge of alpha-tropomyosin are associated with dilated cardiomyopathy. J Mol Cell Cardiol 2001;33:723-732.

188. Gerull B, Gramlich M, Atherton J, et al: Mutations of TTN, encoding the giant muscle filament titin, cause familial dilated cardiomyopathy. Nat Genet 2002;30:201-204.

189. Towbin JA, Hejtmancik JF, Brink P, et al: X-linked dilated cardiomyopathy. Molecular genetic evidence of linkage to the Duchenne muscular dystrophy (dystrophin) gene at the Xp21 locus. Circulation 1993;87:1854-1865.

190. Muntoni F, Cau M, Ganau A, et al: Brief report: Deletion of the dystrophin muscle-promoter region associated with X-linked dilated cardiomyopathy. N Engl J Med 1993;329:921-925.

191. Melacini P, Fanin M, Danieli GA, et al: Myocardial involvement is very frequent among patients affected with subclinical Becker's muscular dystrophy. Circulation 1996;94:3168-3175.

192. Barresi R, Di Blasi C, Negri T, et al: Disruption of heart sarcoglycan complex and severe cardiomyopathy caused by beta sarcoglycan mutations. J Med Genet 2000;37:102-107.

193. Tsubata S, Bowles KR, Vatta M, et al: Mutations in the human delta-sarcoglycan gene in familial and sporadic dilated cardiomyopathy. J Clin Invest 2000;106:655-662.

194. Ichida F, Tsubata S, Bowles KR, et al: Novel gene mutations in patients with left ventricular noncompaction or Barth syndrome. Circulation 2001;103:1256-1263.

195. Maeda M, Holder E, Lowes B, et al: Dilated cardiomyopathy associated with deficiency of the cytoskeletal protein metavinculin. Circulation 1997;95:17-20.

196. Olson TM, Illenberger S, Kishimoto NY, et al: Metavinculin mutations alter actin interaction in dilated cardiomyopathy. Circulation 2002;105:431-437.

197. Goldfarb LG, Park KY, Cervenakova L, et al: Missense mutations in desmin associated with familial cardiac and skeletal myopathy. Nat Genet 1998;19:402-403.

198. Li D, Tapscoft T, Gonzalez O, et al: Desmin mutation responsible for idiopathic dilated cardiomyopathy. Circulation 1999;100: 461-464.

199. Fatkin D, MacRae C, Sasaki T, et al: Missense mutations in the rod domain of the lamin A/C gene as causes of dilated cardiomyopathy and conduction-system disease. N Engl J Med 1999;341: 1715-1724.

200. DiMauro S, Hirano M: Mitochondria and heart disease. Curr Opin Cardiol 1998;13:190-197.

201. Bione S, D'Adamo P, Maestrini E, et al: A novel X-linked gene, G4.5. is responsible for Barth syndrome. Nat Genet 1996;12: 385-389.

202. Schmitt JP, Kamisago M, Asahi M, et al: Dilated cardiomyopathy and heart failure caused by a mutation in phospholamban. Science 2003;299:1410-1413.

203. Mogensen J, Kubo T, Duque M, et al: Idiopathic restrictive cardiomyopathy is part of the clinical expression of cardiac troponin I mutations. J Clin Invest 2003;111:209-216.

204. Hoshijima M, Chien KR: Mixed signals in heart failure: Cancer rules. J Clin Invest 2002;109:849-855.

205. Durbeej M, Campbell KP: Muscular dystrophies involving the dystrophin-glycoprotein complex: An overview of current mouse models. Curr Opin Genet Dev 2002;12:349-361.

206. Ehler E, Horowits R, Zuppinger C, et al: Alterations at the intercalated disk associated with the absence of muscle LIM protein. J Cell Biol 2001;153:763-772.

207. Zolk O, Caroni P, Bohm M: Decreased expression of the cardiac LIM domain protein MLP in chronic human heart failure. Circulation 2000;101:2674-2677.

208. Furukawa T, Ono Y, Tsuchiya H, et al: Specific interaction of the potassium channel beta-subunit minK with the sarcomeric protein T-cap suggests a T-tubule-myofibril linking system. J Mol Biol 2001;313:775-784.

209. Mohler PJ, Schott JJ, Gramolini AO, et al: Ankyrin-B mutation causes type 4 long-QT cardiac arrhythmia and sudden cardiac death. Nature 2003;421:634-639.

210. Clark KA, McElhinny AS, Beckerle MC, Gregorio CC: Striated muscle cytoarchitecture: An intricate web of form and function. Annu Rev Cell Dev Biol 2002;18:637-706.

211. Frey N, Richardson JA, Olson EN: Calsarcins, a novel family of sarcomeric calcineurin-binding proteins. Proc Natl Acad Sci USA 2000;97:14632-14637.

212. Faulkner G, Pallavicini A, Comelli A, et al: FATZ, a filamin-, actinin-, and telethonin-binding protein of the Z-disc of skeletal muscle. J Biol Chem 2000;275:41234-41242.

213. Frey N, Olson EN: Calsarcin-3, a novel skeletal muscle-specific member of the calsarcin family, interacts with multiple Z-disc proteins. J Biol Chem 2002;277:13998-4004.

214. Tomaselli GF, Marban E: Electrophysiological remodeling in hypertrophy and heart failure. Cardiovasc Res 1999;42:270-283.

215. Hasenfuss G, Pieske B: Calcium cycling in congestive heart failure. J Mol Cell Cardiol 2002;34:951-969.

216. Houser SR, Margulies KB: Is depressed myocyte contractility centrally involved in heart failure? Circ Res 2003;92:350-358.

217. Brittsan AG, Kranias EG: Phospholamban and cardiac contractile function. J Mol Cell Cardiol 2000;32:2131-2139.

218. Tada M, Toyofuku T: Molecular regulation of phospholambin function and expression. Trends in Cardiovascular medicine 1998;8:330-340.

219. Schwinger RH, Munch G, Bolck B, et al: Reduced Ca(2+)-sensitivity of SERCA 2a in failing human myocardium due to reduced serin-16 phospholamban phosphorylation. J Mol Cell Cardiol 1999;31:479-491.

220. Sande JB, Sjaastad I, Hoen IB, et al: Reduced level of serine(16) phosphorylated phospholamban in the failing rat myocardium: A major contributor to reduced SERCA2 activity. Cardiovasc Res 2002;53:382-391.

221. Frank KF, Bolck B, Brixius K, et al: Modulation of SERCA: Implications for the failing human heart. Basic Res Cardiol 2002;97(Suppl 1):172-78.

222. Rockman HA, Koch WJ, Lefkowitz RJ: Seven-transmembrane-spanning receptors and heart function. Nature 2002;415: 206-212.

223. Lohse MJ, Engelhardt S: Protein kinase a transgenes: The many faces of cAMP. Circ Res 2001;89:938-940.

224. Stevenson LW: Inotropic therapy for heart failure. N Engl J Med 1998;339:1848-1850.

225. Antos CL, Frey N, Marx SO, et al: Dilated cardiomyopathy and sudden death resulting from constitutive activation of protein kinase a. Circ Res 2001;89:997-1004.

226. Bristow MR: beta-adrenergic receptor blockade in chronic heart failure. Circulation 2000;101:558-569.

227. Shah AS, Lilly RE, Kypson AP, et al: Intracoronary adenovirus-mediated delivery and overexpression of the beta(2)-adrenergic receptor in the heart: Prospects for molecular ventricular assistance. Circulation 2000;101:408-414.

228. Tomiyasu K, Oda Y, Nomura M, et al: Direct intra-cardiomuscular transfer of beta2-adrenergic receptor gene augments cardiac output in cardiomyopathic hamsters. Gene Ther 2000;7:2087-2093.

229. Rockman HA, Chien KR, Choi DJ, et al: Expression of a beta-adrenergic receptor kinase 1 inhibitor prevents the development of myocardial failure in gene-targeted mice. Proc Natl Acad Sci USA 1998;95:7000-7005.

230. Freeman K, Lerman I, Kranias EG, et al: Alterations in cardiac adrenergic signaling and calcium cycling differentially affect the progression of cardiomyopathy. J Clin Invest 2001;107:967-974.

231. White DC, Hata JA, Shah AS, et al: Preservation of myocardial beta-adrenergic receptor signaling delays the development of heart failure after myocardial infarction. Proc Natl Acad Sci USA 2000;97:5428-5433.

232. Shah AS, White DC, Emani S, et al: In vivo ventricular gene delivery of a beta-adrenergic receptor kinase inhibitor to the failing heart reverses cardiac dysfunction. Circulation 2001;103:1311-1316.

233. Roth DM, Gao MH, Lai NC, et al: Cardiac-directed adenylyl cyclase expression improves heart function in murine cardiomyopathy. Circulation 1999;99:3099-3102.

234. Lai NC, Roth DM, Gao MH, et al: Intracoronary delivery of adenovirus encoding adenylyl cyclase VI increases left-ventricular function and cAMP-generating capacity. Circulation 2000;102:2396-2401.

235. He H, Giordano FJ, Hilal-Dandan R, et al: Overexpression of the rat sarcoplasmic reticulum Ca2+ ATPase gene in the heart of transgenic mice accelerates calcium transients and cardiac relaxation. J Clin Invest 1997;100:380-389.

236. (unpublished data by Hoshijima M, Minamisawa S, Dillmann WH, Ross J, and Chien KR)

237. Miyamoto MI, del Monte F, Schmidt U, et al: Adenoviral gene transfer of SERCA2a improves left-ventricular function in aortic-banded rats in transition to heart failure. Proc Natl Acad Sci USA 2000;97:793-798.

238. del Monte F, Williams E, Lebeche D, et al: Improvement in survival and cardiac metabolism after gene transfer of sarcoplasmic reticulum Ca(2+)-ATPase in a rat model of heart failure. Circulation 2001;104:1424-1429.

239. Kiriazis H, Kranias EG: Genetically engineered models with alterations in cardiac membrane calcium-handling proteins. Annu Rev Physiol 2000;62:321-351.

240. Minamisawa S, Hoshijima M, Chu G, et al: Chronic phospholamban-sarcoplasmic reticulum calcium ATPase interaction is the critical calcium cycling defect in dilated cardiomyopathy. Cell 1999;99:313-322.

241. Song Q, Schmidt AG, Hahn HS, et al: Rescue of cardiomyocyte dysfunction by phospholamban ablation does not prevent ventricular failure in genetic hypertrophy. J Clin Invest 2003;111:859-867.

242. del Monte F, Harding SE, Dec GW, et al: Targeting phospholamban by gene transfer in human heart failure. Circulation 2002;105:904-907.

243. Marx SO, Reiken S, Hisamatsu Y et al: PKA phosphorylation dissociates FKBP12.6 from the calcium release channel (ryanodine receptor): Defective regulation in failing hearts. Cell 2000;101:365-376.

244. Xin HB, Senbonmatsu T, Cheng DS, et al: Oestrogen protects FKBP12.6 null mice from cardiac hypertrophy. Nature 2002;416:334-338.

245. Reiken S, Gaburjakova M, Gaburjakova J, et al: Beta-adrenergic receptor blockers restore cardiac calcium release channel (ryanodine receptor) structure and function in heart failure. Circulation 2001;104:2843-2848.

246. Doi M, Yano M, Kobayashi S, et al: Propranolol prevents the development of heart failure by restoring FKBP12.6-mediated stabilization of ryanodine receptor. Circulation 2002;105:1374-1379.

247. Laitinen PJ, Brown KM, Piippo K, et al: Mutations of the cardiac ryanodine receptor (RyR2) gene in familial polymorphic ventricular tachycardia. Circulation 2001;103:485-490.

248. Priori SG, Napolitano C, Tiso N, et al: Mutations in the cardiac ryanodine receptor gene (hRyR2) underlie catecholaminergic polymorphic ventricular tachycardia. Circulation 2001;103:196-200.

249. Tiso N, Stephan DA, Nava A, et al: Identification of mutations in the cardiac ryanodine receptor gene in families affected with arrhythmogenic right ventricular cardiomyopathy type 2 (ARVD2). Hum Mol Genet 2001;10:189-194.

250. Marks AR: Ryanodine receptors/calcium release channels in heart failure and sudden cardiac death. J Mol Cell Cardiol 2001;33:615-624.

251. Prestle J, Janssen PM, Janssen AP, et al: Overexpression of FK506-binding protein FKBP12.6 in cardiomyocytes reduces ryanodine receptor-mediated Ca(2+) leak from the sarcoplasmic reticulum and increases contractility. Circ Res 2001;88:188-194.

252. Keating MT, Sanguinetti MC: Molecular and cellular mechanisms of cardiac arrhythmias. Cell 2001;104:569-580.

253. Marban E: Cardiac channelopathies. Nature 2002;415:213-218.

254. Gutstein DE, Morley GE, Tamaddon H, et al: Conduction slowing and sudden arrhythmic death in mice with cardiac-restricted inactivation of connexin43. Circ Res 2001;88:333-339.

255. Barker RJ, Gourdie, RG: JNK bond regulation: Why do mammalian hearts invest in connexin43? Circ Res 2002;91:556-558.

256. Nguyen-Tran VT, Kubalak SW, Minamisawa S, et al: A novel genetic pathway for sudden cardiac death via defects in the transition between ventricular and conduction system cell lineages. Cell 2000;102:671-682.

257. Schott JJ, Benson DW, Basson CT, et al: Congenital heart disease caused by mutations in the transcription factor NKX2-5. Science 1998;281:108-111.

258. Gollob MH, Green MS, Tang AS, et al: Identification of a gene responsible for familial Wolff-Parkinson-White syndrome. N Engl J Med 2001;344:1823-1831.

259. Blair E, Redwood C, Ashrafian H, et al: Mutations in the gamma(2) subunit of AMP-activated protein kinase cause familial hypertrophic cardiomyopathy: Evidence for the central role of energy compromise in disease pathogenesis. Hum Mol Genet 2001;10:1215-1220.

260. Arad M, Benson DW, Perez-Atayde AR, et al: Constitutively active AMP kinase mutations cause glycogen storage disease mimicking hypertrophic cardiomyopathy. J Clin Invest 2002;109:357-362.

261. Kuo HC, Cheng CF, Clark RB, et al: A defect in the Kv channel-interacting protein 2 (KChIP2) gene leads to a complete loss of I(to) and confers susceptibility to ventricular tachycardia. Cell 2001;107:801-813.

262. Rosati B, Pan Z, Lypen S, et al: Regulation of KChIP2 potassium channel beta subunit gene expression underlies the gradient of transient outward current in canine and human ventricle. J Physiol 2001;533:119-125.

263. Rosati B, Grau F, Rodriguez S, et al: Concordant expression of KChIP2 mRNA, protein and transient outward current throughout the canine ventricle. J Physiol 2003;548:815-822.

## EDITOR'S CHOICE

Intravenous nesiritide vs nitroglycerin for treatment of decompensated congestive heart failure: A randomized controlled trial. Jama 2002;287:1531-1540.

*BNP finds a home as a therapy for acute, decompensated heart failure.*

Chien KR, Ross J Jr, Hoshijima M: Calcium and heart failure: The cycle game. Nat Med 2003;9:508-509.

*Promoting calcium cycling via phospholamban inhibition is new therapeutic target to halt heart failure progression.*

del Monte F, Hajjar RJ: Targeting calcium cycling proteins in heart failure through gene transfer. J Physiol 2003;546:49-61.

*Overview of gene therapy strategies for heart failure via promting calcium cycling.*

Haghighi K, Kolokathis F, Pater L, et al: Human phospholamban null results in lethal dilated cardiomyopathy revealing a critical difference between mouse and human. J Clin Invest 2003;111:869–876.

*Human mutation results in a truncated phospholamban peptide and is associated with genetically base dilated cardiomyopathy, contains cytoplasmic inhibitory domain but also is unstable, may represent a mixed genetic effect of poison peptide and hypomorphic allele.*

Hajjar RJ, MacRae CA: Adrenergic-receptor polymorphisms and heart failure. N Engl J Med 2002;347:1196–1199.

*Nice review of the association of human variants of the beta-adrenergic receptor and heart failure.*

MacLennan DH, Kranias EG: Phospholamban: A crucial regulator of cardiac contractility. Nat Rev Mol Cell Biol 2003;4:566–577.

*Excellent review of emerging topic of clinical importance.*

Maisel AS, Krishnaswamy P, Nowak RM, et al: Rapid measurement of B-type natriuretic peptide in the emergency diagnosis of heart failure. N Engl J Med 2002;347:161–167.

*BNP as a biomarker for heart failure; rapidly finding a place as standard diagnostic test in the ER and elsewhere.*

Olson EN, Schneider MD: Sizing up the heart: Development redux in disease. Genes Dev 2003;17:1937–1956.

*Thought leaders provide excellent overview of complex field.*

Prasad SV, Perrino C, Rockman HA: Role of phosphoinositide 3-kinase in cardiac function and heart failure. Trends Cardiovasc Med 2003;13:206–212.

*PI-3 pathways may represent a new signaling pathway to regulate cardiac contractility.*

Schmitt JP, Kamisago M, Asahi M, et al: Dilated cardiomyopathy and heart failure caused by a mutation in phospholamban. Science 2003;299:1410–1413.

*Seminal paper provides first clear genetic evidence that the augmentation of phospholamban inhibitory activity is sufficient by itself to cause human dilated cardiomyopathy and heart failure; human validation of earlier studies in mice that suggested that phospholamban is a valid therapeutic target for heart failure.*

Small KM, Wagoner LE, Levin AM, et al: Synergistic polymorphisms of beta1-and alpha2C-adrenergic receptors and the risk of congestive heart failure. N Engl J Med 2002;347:1135–1142.

*Genetic susceptibility to heart failure based on variants of adrenergic receptors.*

Wehrens XH, Marks AR: Myocardial disease in failing hearts: Defective excitation-contraction coupling. Cold Spring Harb Symp Quant Biol 2002;67:533–541.

*Leader in the molecular biology of ryanodine receptors provides nice overview of large body of work.*

Wencker D, Chandra M, Nguyen K, et al: A mechanistic role for cardiac myocyte apoptosis in heart failure. J Clin Invest 2003;111:1497–1504.

*Makes the case for a pivotal role of apoptosis in heart failure progression.*

Yussman MG, Toyokawa T, Odley A, et al: Mitochondrial death protein Nix is induced in cardiac hypertrophy and triggers apoptotic cardiomyopathy. Nat Med 2002;8:725–730.

*New pathway for cell death in heart muscle cells could play important role in heart failure progression during chronic stimulation of receptors linked to Gq pathways.*

# chapter 16

# Molecular Genetics of Inherited Cardiomyopathies

*Christopher Semsarian*
*J. G. Seidman*
*Christine E. Seidman*

Cardiomyopathies are generally defined as heart muscle disorders of unknown etiology. These disorders occur as primary pathologic conditions that uniquely alter myocardial structure and function or as cardiac manifestations of systemic disease. Primary cardiomyopathies can be sporadic and nonfamilial or heritable disorders that are usually transmitted as monogenic traits. Over the past decade, there has been substantial progress in discovering the genetic basis of inherited primary cardiomyopathies,[1] a success that has largely occurred through substantial advances in molecular genetics.[2,3] Application of linkage analyses that define the chromosome location of disease-causing loci, tissue profiling to define patterns of gene expression, positional cloning techniques, and a wealth of information provided from comprehensive genome sequences derived from multiple organisms[4] have fostered identification of disease genes and human mutations.

Genetic studies of cardiomyopathies have expanded and refined traditional morphologic classifications of hypertrophic, dilated, and restrictive disease phenotypes. For example, the genetics of hypertrophic cardiomyopathy indicate that autosomal dominant gene defects typically cause clinical manifestations late in adolescence and adulthood. Autosomal recessive gene defects cause cardiomyopathy of childhood. X-linked dilated cardiomyopathies are clinically important early in men but also may appear later in life in women. Dilated cardiomyopathy transmitted on autosomes equally affects men and women but can be subclassified according to extracardiac manifestations or associated conduction system disease. Mitochondrial mutations account for matrilinear transmission of cardiomyopathies.

Progress in defining the molecular basis for each morphologic subtype of cardiomyopathy has been variable. Genetic studies of hypertrophic cardiomyopathy have been especially productive, and multiple disease genes and mutations have been defined over the last decade. As a result, hypertrophic cardiomyopathy provides a paradigm for the study of a genetic cardiac disorder and its sequelae—heart failure and sudden death. Over the past several years the chromosome locations of multiple inherited dilated cardiomyopathy loci and disease genes have also been identified. However, the chromosome

locations and causal genes that cause restrictive cardiomyopathy have not been identified. Given the rapid pace of molecular genetic research and substantive efforts in these areas, however, the genetic causes for these rare inherited cardiomyopathies will likely be discovered.

Do inherited gene mutations have relevance for the more prevalent, nonfamilial cardiomyopathies? Undoubtedly, the answer is yes but not always. Some gene defects that cause familial hypertrophic cardiomyopathy have also been demonstrated to cause sporadic disease; hence, common genetic causes account for heritable cases and some isolated cases of cardiomyopathy. There are also likely to be many distinct genetic and environmental stimuli that cause nonfamilial disease. However, despite the probable multiplicity of triggering events that remodel the myocardium, the repertoire of responses is predominantly limited to a hypertrophic, dilated, or restricted morphology. Hence, the study of inherited cardiomyopathies can also provide insights into signaling pathways that are important in familial and nonheritable disease. How does a mutation in a gene ultimately result in the clinical phenotype, and why is it that two individuals within the same family and, therefore, carrying the same gene mutation can have disparate clinical presentations, ranging from absence of symptoms to early sudden death? Genetic engineering of cell and animal models that express cardiomyopathy gene mutations provides a novel approach for defining the cellular mechanisms that ultimately perturb cardiac structure and function. Furthermore, such models provide an opportunity to identify potential modifying factors, either genetic or environmental, which may modulate expression of the mutant gene and explain, at least in part, the clinical heterogeneity that is seen. Understanding the cascade of myocyte responses to inherited gene defects should, therefore, provide an important foundation for defining the fundamental molecular basis of cardiomyopathies.

This chapter reviews genetics studies of inherited hypertrophic, dilated, and restrictive cardiomyopathies that result from mutations in nuclear genes. Molecular causes that have been discovered for inherited multisystem disorders accompanied by cardiomyopathy are briefly reviewed.

# FAMILIAL HYPERTROPHIC CARDIOMYOPATHY

## Clinical Background

Hypertrophic cardiomyopathy (Fig. 16-1A and B) is a primary disorder of the myocardium characterized by hypertrophy that most prominently affects the left ventricle in the absence of other loading conditions such as hypertension or aortic valve stenosis. There is marked diversity in the morphologic features and clinical manifestations of the disorder.[5] Clinical diagnosis is based on unexplained cardiac hypertrophy that can be subtle or massive. The hypertrophy is classically asymmetric with particular involvement of the interventricular septum, but it can also be concentric, diffuse, or focal. Asymmetric septal hypertrophy causes a resting or provocative left-ventricular outflow tract obstruction in approximately 30% of affected individuals. Although unexplained cardiac hypertrophy is an important pathologic hallmark of disease, altered cardiac morphology is an age-dependent phenotype that is often lacking in children.[6,7] Histopathologic features include disorganized myocyte architecture, such as disarray of myocyte fibers, intertwined hypertrophied myocytes with bizarre-shaped nuclei, and focal or widespread interstitial fibrosis.

The clinical management of hypertrophic cardiomyopathy is complex,[8] in part because of the heterogeneous symptoms exhibited by affected individuals and the marked variability in the natural history of this disease. Hypertrophic cardiomyopathy can occur without symptoms, but most individuals experience some dyspnea, angina, and palpitations. The natural history of the disease is usually a gradual progression of symptoms, but, in some, sudden death or severe heart failure is superimposed. Cardiac death in hypertrophic cardiomyopathy is often unexpected and occurs at any stage of life,[9] even in asymptomatic individuals. Hypertrophic cardiomyopathy remains the commonest cause of sudden cardiac death in individuals younger than 35 years who are involved in competitive athletics.[10] Considerable data indicates that ventricular arrhythmias significantly contribute to the incidence of sudden death,[11] but clinical tests are often inaccurate in assessing risk.[12] Atrial arrhythmias, embolic events, and congestive heart failure also contribute to the premature morbidity and mortality of this disorder.[9]

Family studies have demonstrated that hypertrophic cardiomyopathy occurs as a heritable disorder and is transmitted as an autosomal dominant trait or as a sporadic disease. There is neither a racial nor an ethnic predisposition to the condition. Hypertrophic cardiomyopathy is not a rare disorder; recent noninvasive studies of more than 7000 young adults demonstrated echocardiographic criteria for disease in 1 in 500 persons.[13] Whether this value reflects an accurate incidence of familial disease is unknown.

## Genetic Studies

Genetic studies in familial hypertrophic cardiomyopathy have demonstrated disease loci on chromosomes 1q31,[14] 2q31,[15] 3p,[16] 11p13-q13,[17] 12q2,[16] 14q1,[18] 15q2,[19] 15q14,[20] and 19q13.[21] Contractile protein genes (cardiac troponin T, titin, ventricular regulatory light chain, cardiac myosin binding protein-C, essential light chain, β cardiac myosin heavy chain, α tropomyosin, actin, and cardiac troponin I) have been identified at each locus. This genetic data demonstrates that hypertrophic cardiomyopathy is a disease of the sarcomere (Fig. 16-2).

Some of the clinical heterogeneity of hypertrophic cardiomyopathy can be accounted for by the substantial diversity of gene defects that cause the condition. Approximately 35% of hypertrophic cardiomyopathy results from β cardiac myosin heavy chain gene missense mutations.[22,23] More than 50 unique mutations have been reported that alter one amino acid residue in the globular head or head-rod junction of the β cardiac myosin heavy chain. These mutations are expressed with a high degree of penetrance, and most affected individuals exhibit significant myocardial hypertrophy on two-dimensional echocardiography studies. A mean maximal left-ventricular wall thickness equal to 23.7 ±7.7 mm was found in affected individuals from families with different myosin mutations.[24] Despite nearly complete disease penetrance and significant hypertrophy, survival in hypertrophic cardiomyopathy caused by a β cardiac myosin heavy chain mutation varies considerably and is, in part, mutation-specific.[22,25] For example, individuals with the Arg403Gln mutation have markedly shortened life expectancies (average age of death is 45 years), whereas survival is near normal in individuals carrying the Val606Met mutation (Fig. 16-3). The change of amino acid charge appears to influence outcome in hypertrophic cardiomyopathy, and conservative muta-

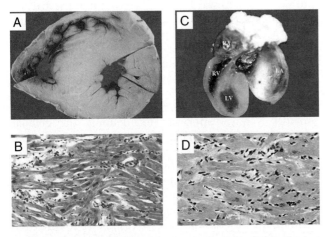

**FIGURE 16-1.** Hypertrophic cardiomyopathy in humans and mice. *A,* Postmortem examination of the heart from an Arg403Gln β cardiac myosin heavy chain mutation demonstrates massive concentric hypertrophy. *B,* Histologic findings (myocyte hypertrophy, disarray, and replacement fibrosis) of hypertrophic cardiomyopathy resulting from α tropomyosin mutation Asp175Asn are comparable to that seen in other sarcomere gene defects. *C,* A murine model of hypertrophic cardiomyopathy (based on the human Arg403Gln mutation[38]) causes sudden death following vigorous exercise. Note marked left-ventricular hypertrophy, left atrial enlargement, and an organized thrombus. *D,* Murine hypertrophic cardiomyopathy histopathology is comparable to that observed in human disease.

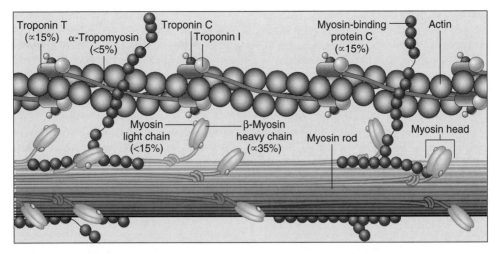

**FIGURE 16-2.** Sarcomere proteins are mutated in hypertrophic cardiomyopathy. Mutations in thick filament components (β cardiac myosin heavy chain, ventricular regulatory and essential light chains, and cardiac myosin binding protein-C) and thin filament components (cardiac troponin T, α tropomyosin) cause hypertrophic cardiomyopathy. *(Reproduced with permission from Spirito P, Seidman CE, McKenna WJ, et al: Management of hypertrophic cardiomyopathy. N Engl J Med 1997;336:775-785.)*

tions appear to be associated with a better prognosis than nonconservative mutations. Although more data is required to provide a complete profile of the phenotypes associated with each myosin mutation, preliminary data clearly indicates that genotype may assist in risk stratification for premature death in hypertrophic cardiomyopathy.

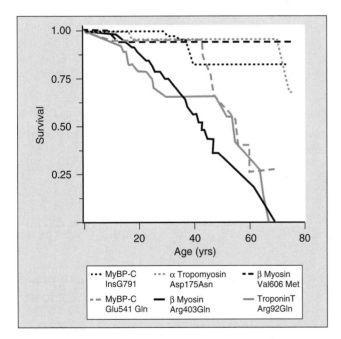

**FIGURE 16-3.** Survival in hypertrophic cardiomyopathy caused by different gene defects. Kaplan-Meier survival curves were constructed as described.[14,17,21,24] Normal life expectancy is found in patients with hypertrophic cardiomyopathy resulting from β cardiac myosin heavy chain (myosin) mutation Val606Met, α tropomyosin mutation Asp175Asn, or cardiac myosin binding protein-C (MyBP-C) mutation InsG791. Survival is markedly reduced in hypertrophic cardiomyopathy caused by β cardiac myosin heavy chain mutation Arg403Gln or cardiac troponin T mutation Arg92Gln.

A variety of cardiac troponin T gene defects (missense mutations, small deletions, and mutations in splice signals) cause approximately 15% of all hypertrophic cardiomyopathy.[23,26] The cardiac phenotype produced by these gene defects is characterized by substantially less hypertrophy than that observed with myosin mutations. The mean maximal left-ventricular wall thickness resulting from six different cardiac troponin T mutations was 16.7 ±5.5 mm, and some adults with these mutations had normal cardiac wall thickness.[26] Despite this reduced penetrance, most but not all[27] reported cardiac troponin T mutations are associated with markedly reduced survival (Fig. 16-3). Genetic diagnosis may, therefore, be particularly important in identifying individuals at risk for sudden death in hypertrophic cardiomyopathy caused by cardiac troponin T defects.

Studies of cardiac myosin binding protein-C,[28-31] a 137-kd polypeptide with structural and regulatory functions in the sarcomere, have demonstrated mutations that cause hypertrophic cardiomyopathy. During cardiac embryogenesis, cardiac myosin binding protein-C may participate in the alignment of thick filaments,[32] whereas, in the adult myocardium, phosphorylation of cardiac myosin binding protein-C by a catecholamine-sensitive pathway[33] may provide dynamic regulation of cardiac contraction in response to adrenergic stimuli. Whether these or other unknown functions are perturbed by mutations that cause hypertrophic cardiomyopathy remains unknown. A broad range of gene defects, including missense and splice signal mutations, insertions, and deletions, in cardiac myosin binding protein-C can cause hypertrophic cardiomyopathy. As in cardiac troponin T defects, penetrance is often incomplete[28-31] and is strikingly age-dependent. Cardiac myosin binding protein-C mutations may be clinically quiescent until late in adult life, with cardiac hypertrophy manifest only after the fourth and fifth decades of life.[31] This has implications for clinical screening programs that consider the absence of hypertrophy by age 20 as indicative of an unaffected individual. Clearly, individuals can develop disease much later in life and, thus, need regular clinical screening well into their 40s and 50s. In general, the prognosis associated with these mutations is markedly better than that associated with cardiac troponin T defects (detailed previously), although the risk of sudden death is increased in at least one cardiac myosin binding protein-C mutation (Fig. 16-3). Early estimates based on linkage studies[17,26] suggested that 15% of hypertrophic cardiomyopathy was caused by mutations in cardiac myosin binding protein-C. However, the findings of reduced disease penetrance associated with these gene defects, combined with good survival, may have diminished accurate estimates of the true incidence of these mutations in hypertrophic cardiomyopathy. Continued definition of cardiac myosin binding protein-C mutations may help to delineate the relationship between gene defects and late-onset hypertrophic cardiomyopathy.

Mutations in the α tropomyosin gene account for less than 5% of hypertrophic cardiomyopathy.[26] Unlike defects in other sarcomere genes, the spectrum of mutations in α tropomyosin that cause hypertrophic cardiomyopathy appears to be limited. Few disease-causing missense mutations have been identified. The Asp175Asn defect may reflect a mutational hot spot within the gene,[34] because it has arisen independently in multiple families. Intriguingly, the hypertrophic response to the α tropomyosin mutation Asp175Asn varies considerably between different families, suggesting that modifying genes and/or environment influence this cardiac phenotype. Despite this, survival is near normal in hypertrophic cardiomyopathy caused by α tropomyosin mutation Asp175Asn (Fig. 16-3).

Mutations in myosin regulatory or essential light chains rarely cause hypertrophic cardiomyopathy,[16] although the limited number of families reported with these gene defects has hindered correlation of genotype and phenotype. Distinctive cardiac morphologies have, however, been reported with some mutations (ventricular regulatory myosin Ala13Thr and Glu22Lys and myosin essential light chain Met149Vla), including predominance of midventricular hypertrophy that results in a systolic midcavity obliteration (hour-glass morphology). More typical asymmetric hypertrophy also occurs from mutations in these disease genes.[35] Further study is necessary to ascertain to what extent unusual hypertrophic cardiomyopathy phenotypes are genetically programmed.

Mutations in troponin I[21] have been considered rare causes of hypertrophic cardiomyopathy, although, with increasing sequence analyses,[23,36-38] this initial impression bears reinterpretation. Unusual patterns of hypertrophy, including a predominant apical involvement,[21,37] have also been reported with some troponin I defects.[36,38] Based on this morphologic pattern of disease, troponin I mutations may be prevalent in populations with a high incidence of apical hypertrophic cardiomyopathy, as has been reported in Japan.[39]

Mutations in cardiac actin[20,40] and titin[15] are other rare causes of hypertrophic cardiomyopathy and collectively account for less than 1% of reported cases. Little is known about the clinical correlates of these disease genes.

Genetic data on hypertrophic cardiomyopathy of the elderly implicates sarcomere protein gene mutations as a cause of this poorly understood disorder.[41] The distribution of mutations that produce hypertrophy late in life is, however, substantially different from that of familial, early-onset hypertrophic cardiomyopathy. Whereas defects in β cardiac myosin heavy chain, cardiac troponin T, and α tropomyosin account for more than 45% of familial hypertrophic cardiomyopathy, mutations in these were not identified in one study of elderly onset disease. Instead, mutations in cardiac myosin binding protein-C, troponin I, and α cardiac myosin heavy chain have been defined as causes of elderly onset hypertrophic cardiomyopathy.

A disease locus on chromosome 7q3, previously thought to cause hypertrophic cardiomyopathy,[42] has recently been reclassified as a glycogen storage disease of the heart. Affected individuals exhibit cardiac hypertrophy and electrophysiologic abnormalities (Fig. 16-4A) including Wolff-Parkinson-White syndrome,[42-45] atrial fibrillation, and progressive atrioventricular block. Cardiac histopathology also distinguishes this disorder from hypertrophic cardiomyopathy in that myocyte and myofiber disarray is absent, and intracytoplasmic vac-

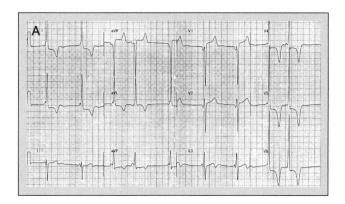

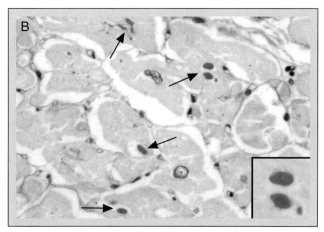

FIGURE 16-4. Clinical features discriminate *PRKAG2* mutations from hypertrophic cardiomyopathy caused by sarcomere protein gene mutations. *A,* Wolff-Parkinson-White syndrome in a 12-year-old with cardiac hypertrophy. *B,* Cardiac histopathology is notable for the absence of myocyte disarray and the presence of homogenous inclusions within vacuoles (*arrows* and *inset*) that stain with periodic acid Schiff. (*B, From J Clin Invest*)

uoles are found in myocytes. These vacuoles contain densely packed fine granular and fibrillar electron dense material, with staining properties consistent with polyglucan and amylopectin (Fig. 16-4B), a nonsoluble product of glycogen metabolism.[45] Mutations in the *PRKAG2* gene encoding the gamma-2 subunit of AMP-activated protein kinase, a molecule involved in energy metabolism and glucose utilization, have been identified in multiple families.[43-45] Given the distinctive histopathology, electrophysiologic features, and absence of involvement of the mutation in sarcomere function, cardiac hypertrophy resulting from *PRKAG2* mutations are more appropriately considered to cause a polysaccharide storage disorder of the myocardium rather than hypertrophic cardiomyopathy.

## Insights from Genetic Studies

Although hypertrophic cardiomyopathy most often occurs as a familial disease, identification of disease-causing genes has fostered genetic analyses of isolated cases of cardiac hypertrophy. Results indicate that sporadic hypertrophic cardiomyopathy, in which an affected individual's parents are clinically well, can occur from either genetic mosaicism or *de novo* mutation.[46,47] Maternal germline mosaicism accounted for transmission of a hypertrophic cardiomyopathy mutation and clinical disease to two offspring, although the defect was absent from DNA from blood samples of the clinically unaffected mother.[48] *De novo* mutation arising in germ cells can also result in transmission of disease to the offspring of unaffected parents. Collectively this data indicates that sporadic and familial hypertrophic cardiomyopathy represents a continuum of disease. Risk stratification based on insights derived from the study of familial disease and genetic counseling is also relevant to isolated cases of hypertrophic cardiomyopathy.

As the number of defined genetic defects that cause hypertrophic cardiomyopathy grow, increasing numbers of individuals are identified who bear these mutations but lack clinical manifestations of disease.[7,30,31,49] Often these genotype-positive, phenotype-negative individuals are children who can be expected to develop signs and symptoms of the disorder with age. Although there is no clear data regarding appropriate management of these individuals,[8] it would seem prudent to use genotype information for assessing risk of sudden death, whether or not cardiac hypertrophy is evident. In the future, gene-based identification and early intervention in at-risk children may improve survival in hypertrophic cardiomyopathy.

The demonstration that hypertrophic cardiomyopathy results from sarcomere gene defects (Fig. 16-2) has raised many questions about the cell biology of cardiac muscle. What is the mechanism by which a cardiac-specific phenotype results from mutations in sarcomere genes? What intracellular signaling pathways are triggered by expression of these gene defects? Is the hypertrophic response compensatory or pathologic? What factors, either genetic or environmental, modify the expression of the mutant gene? Answers to these questions may provide insights into how and why mutated contractile proteins predispose affected individuals to sudden death.

Addressing these questions in humans is limited because of the unavailability of cardiac tissue, and, in cases in which tissue is available, methods of maintaining human heart tissue in cell culture systems are inadequate. One avenue that has advanced this research has been analyses in hypertrophic cardiomyopathy mutations in skeletal muscle cells. Although β cardiac myosin heavy chains are abundant in the myocardium, they are also found in lower levels in slow-twitch skeletal muscles. Abnormal contractile properties of muscle fibers expressing a β cardiac myosin heavy chain mutation[50] and histologic evidence of central core disease[51] have been demonstrated. The clinical relevance of dysfunction detected *ex vivo* remains unclear because skeletal myopathy is a rare clinical manifestation of hypertrophic cardiomyopathy even in cases caused by α tropomyosin mutations, which are widely expressed in skeletal and cardiac muscle. The mechanism by which mutations in this peptide produce a cardiac-specific phenotype may relate to interactions with partner proteins. Hypertrophic cardiomyopathy mutations in α tropomyosin occur in regions that interact with troponin T, which is expressed as a tissue-specific isoform. Interactions with cardiac troponin T but not skeletal muscle troponin T may be perturbed, thereby restricting dysfunction to the myocardium. Alternatively some α tropomyosin mutations may alter a unique or critical function of cardiac myocytes. By analogy, essential and regulatory light chain mutations may also produce a predominantly cardiac phenotype by particularly impairing function of cardiac myosin heavy chains.

To overcome the limitations of studies in humans with hypertrophic cardiomyopathy, a variety of biochemical, cell, and animal models have been engineered to more fully examine the consequences of human sarcomere mutations on muscle structure and function. Human myosin mutations, located[23] on the three-dimensional structure of the chicken skeletal muscle myosin,[52] are widely dispersed throughout the molecule, implying that no one function of myosin (e.g., actin binding, ATP hydrolysis, force transmission, or propagation) accounts for disease. The consequences of mutations have also been assayed in reconstituted thick filaments[53] and following stable expression into[54] cells, and results generally indicate that mutant myosins have diminished motor activity without changes in enzymatic activity. Comparable biochemical studies of mutant cardiac troponin T peptides also show adverse effects of hypertrophic mutations on sarcomere filament function,[55] but responses vary depending on calcium concentrations and on whether mixtures of mutant and wild-type peptides are present,[56] as would occur in humans who carry heterozygous mutations. Such data underscores the need to assess the consequences of hypertrophic cardiomyopathy mutations in the context of cardiac muscle and whole organ physiology.

Genetically engineered mice and rabbits that express human hypertrophic cardiomyopathy have helped to address these issues. Transgenic models that overexpress mutant myosin heavy chains,[57,58] mutant cardiac troponin T,[59,60] mutant myosin binding protein-C,[61] or cardiac troponin I[62] and a model that physiologically expresses the myosin (Arg403Gln) mutation (produced by homologous recombination)[63] have been studied. All models exhibit histopathology comparable to that observed in human hypertrophic cardiomyopathy including myocyte disarray, hypertrophy, and injury with replacement fibrosis (Fig. 16-1C and D); these findings indicate that cardiac disease is not the consequence of haploinsufficiency but that it occurs from the dominant effects of mutant proteins on sarcomere function. In transgenic models, levels of mutant sarcomere protein expressed within the heart shows some correlation with the severity of myocyte dysfunction.[61] Analyses of the mechanics of Arg403Gln myosin[64] derived from heart muscle indicate enhanced actin-activated ATPase activity, increased generated force, and accelerated actin filament sliding. Taken together with data derived from *in vitro* systems, these findings collectively indicate that hypertrophic cardiomyopathy myosin mutations produce a gain of function. Although such defects might actually improve motor performance of individual molecules, inhomogeneity of mutant and wild-type peptides within the sarcomere should uncouple mechanical coordination. Increased energy consumption from enhanced ATPase activity and demands of the hypertrophic heart would further diminish any benefit from mutations causing a gain of function.

In addition to explaining the mechanisms that underlie the pathologic conditions of hypertrophic cardiomyopathy, these models provide insights with important clinical ramifications. For example, although little is known about the natural history of human troponin I mutations, transgenic mice expressing an Arg145Gly missense mutation often suffer sudden death,[62] implying that careful monitoring and intervention may be warranted in individuals with the comparable mutation. Longitudinal studies of murine models have also demonstrated that hemodynamic dysfunction precedes histopathology, suggesting that the hypertrophic phenotype occurs as a compensatory response to sarcomere mutation.[63] Discovery of intracellular signals that trigger myocyte growth and death may, therefore, provide novel avenues for intervention and prevention. One study indicated that abnormal $Ca^{2+}$ responses exhibited by mutant myocytes are early and important signaling events,[65] and research aimed at tweaking the $Ca^{2+}$ response to hypertrophic cardiomyopathy mutation is underway using mouse models. The mechanisms by which sarcomere defects increase cardiac interstitial fibrosis have also been probed; losartan blockade of angiotensin II in mutant mice has shown salutary effects by attenuating profibrotic effects and reducing collagen deposits.[66] Using murine models to define these and other signaling pathways that trigger sarcomere protein gene mutations has great promise for defining novel targets for therapeutic interventions in human hypertrophic cardiomyopathy.

The utility of these animal models has been substantially increased by miniaturization of many diagnostic procedures that are used to evaluate cardiac function in humans. For example, the role of vigorous exercise in sudden death and hypertrophic cardiomyopathy can be evaluated in exercise protocols and provocative electrophysiologic testing in mice. Profound exertion in mice with myosin mutation (Arg403Gln) appears to recapitulated sudden death events in some athletes (Fig. 16-1C), and provocative electrophysiologic testing[66] has demonstrated marked increases in arrhythmogenicity in mutant mice as compared with wild-type mice. M-mode and two-dimensional echocardiography in mice has also enabled accurate assessment of left-ventricular hypertrophy, changes in cardiac dimensions, and systolic function (fractional shortening).[61,62,65] More recently application of MRI has enabled detailed assessment of heart structure and even congenital malformations (e.g., atrial and ventricular septal defects[67]) in mice. Murine models of human cardiac disease, therefore, appear to be valuable for delineating the mechanisms of disease, for analyses of complex events such as sudden death, and as important tools for evaluating pharmacologic therapies and devices.

## DILATED CARDIOMYOPATHY

### Clinical Background

Dilated cardiomyopathy is clinically defined as cardiac chamber dilation accompanied by contractile dysfunction. This heterogeneous group of pathologic conditions is an important cause of heart failure and the most common diagnosis necessitating cardiac transplantation. Dilated cardiomyopathy is diagnosed in 36.5 per 100,000 people[68] and occurs secondary to toxic, metabolic, or infectious agents or as a primary disorder of the myocardium.

Despite recognition of the diverse causes of dilated cardiomyopathy, pathologic findings in this disorder are often nonspecific. Cardiac mass is usually increased, although there is often only modest ventricular hypertrophy but often marked ventricular and atrial chamber distention. Biopsy and postmortem histopathologic examination (Fig. 16-5A and B) typically reveals myocyte hypertrophy and death with variable degrees of replacement fibrosis and involvement of the conduction system.[69] Unlike hypertrophic cardiomyopathy, substantial distortion of cell architecture or myocyte disarray are *not* typical features of dilated cardiomyopathy. Extracellular matrix components[70] are similarly nonselectively increased and consist of fibronectin; laminin; and collagen types I, III, and IV. Although the absence of inflammatory cells is often used to discriminate dilated cardiomyopathy from myocarditis,[71] interstitial T cells and activated endothelial cells, when detected in dilated cardiomyopathy, indicate that chronic inflammation can contribute to this condition.

Individuals with dilated cardiomyopathy often initially have vague, nonspecific symptoms. With progression of disease, affected individuals develop symptoms of fatigue, exertional dyspnea, and palpitations. These symptoms worsen in parallel with deterioration in left-ventricular contractile function and/or the onset of atrial and ventricular arrhythmias, leading to overt heart failure[71] and premature death. Diagnosis is based on the

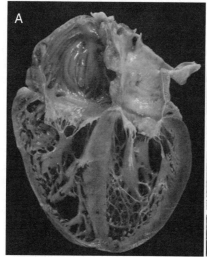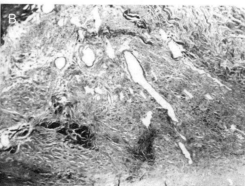

**FIGURE 16-5.** The morphologic features of dilated cardiomyopathy include (A) four-chamber dilation and normal wall thickness. Histopathologic findings (B) in familial dilated cardiomyopathy associated with conduction system disease[52] demonstrate necrosis of atrioventricular nodal cell and replacement fibrosis.

echocardiographic findings of increased systolic and diastolic cardiac dimensions associated with a reduction in contractile (systolic) function. When an underlying cause for dilated cardiomyopathy such as coronary artery disease, alcohol abuse, thyroid disease, or viral infection is excluded, a diagnosis of "idiopathic" dilated cardiomyopathy is made. It now appears that between 25% to 30% of cases of idiopathic dilated cardiomyopathy is caused by an inherited gene mutation.[68,72]

## Genetic Studies

Over the last 5 years the understanding of genetic causes of dilated cardiomyopathy has increased. Multiple disease genes and more than 15 disease loci have now been identified (Table 16-1). Although genetic insights into dilated cardiomyopathy initially lagged behind those of hypertrophic heart disease, improved therapies that have altered survival[71] and better tools for analyzing small families[2] have made genome-wide linkage studies possible. Despite these important advances, the premature mortality of affected individuals and the incidence of incomplete penetrance (absence of phenotype in genetically affected individuals) remain challenges for studying these disorders. Familial dilated cardiomyopathy can be transmitted as an autosomal recessive, X-linked, or matrilinear (mitochondrial) trait, although autosomal dominant transmission occurs most often.[2,71,72]

Identification of several disease-causing mutations in a variety of genes coupled with a clinical diversity of both cardiac and extracardiac features illustrate that dilated cardiomyopathy is both a genetically and clinically heterogeneous disease. Table 16-1 summarizes the known causative genes in human dilated cardiomyopathy and the disease loci identified in families in whom the gene has not yet been defined. Although a common cardiac phenotype is produced by each of these mutations, a variety of other clinical features ranging from skeletal myopathies to sensorineural hearing loss[2,72] can sometimes distinguish different genetic causes. Some extracardiac features can precede the onset of dilated cardiomyopathy (e.g., a form of sensorineural hearing

loss that precedes by several decades the onset of heart failure).[73]

The first autosomal dominant dilated cardiomyopathy mutation was identified by candidate gene analyses of cardiac actin on chromosome 15q14.[74] Affected individuals demonstrate no extracardiac features. More recently, linkage studies in large pedigrees have extended these findings to indicate that other sarcomere gene mutations[75-78] cause dilated cardiomyopathy. Although approximately 10% of individuals with hypertrophic cardiomyopathy ultimately "burn out" to develop a dilated phenotype, some sarcomere mutations cause dilated cardiomyopathy without an antecedent hypertrophic

■ ■ ■

## TABLE 16-1   GENETIC AND CLINICAL HETEROGENEITY OF HUMAN DILATED CARDIOMYOPATHY

| Locus | Disease Gene | Additional Phenotype |
|---|---|---|
| 1q32 | Cardiac troponin T | None |
| 14q11 | Cardiac β-myosin heavy chain | None |
| 15q2 | α-Tropomyosin | None |
| 15q14 | Cardiac actin | None |
| 1p1-q21 | Lamin A/C | Conduction disease |
| 2q35 | Desmin | Skeletal myopathy |
| Xp21 | Dystrophin | Skeletal myopathy |
| Xq28 | Tafazzin | Short stature and neutropenia |
| | δ-Sarcoglycan | None |
| 1q32 | ? | None |
| 2q14-q22 | ? | Conduction disease |
| 2q31 | Titin | None |
| 3q22-q25 | ? | Conduction disease |
| 6q23 | ? | Skeletal myopathy |
| 6q23-q24 | ? | Sensorineural hearing loss |
| 9q13-q22 | ? | None |
| 10q21-q23 | ? | Mitral valve prolapse |

phase. Indeed, onset of heart failure from sarcomere protein genes can be quite early, and several studies indicated that dilated cardiomyopathy occurs in young children.[74,75] Whether the biophysical consequences of sarcomere protein defects or the signaling pathways triggered by these mutations account for the initiation of either a dilated or a hypertrophic phenotype remains an area of active investigation.

Mutations on chromosome 1p1-1q21 and 3q22-q25 have been identified as causes of dilated cardiomyopathy in association with conduction system disease.[79,80] Affected individuals typically exhibit progressive prolongation of the normal delay in electrical activation of the atrial and ventricular chambers, and, after many years of conduction system disease, they develop cardiac chamber dilation and heart failure. Defects in the gene encoding lamin isoforms A and C have been identified in several families.[81-83] Lamin proteins are intermediate filaments that are associated with the nucleoplasmic surface of the inner nuclear envelope and are thought to provide structural integrity to the nuclear envelope and contribute mechanical support for the nucleus.[84] Although the mechanism by which lamin mutations lead to dilated cardiomyopathies remains to be discovered, an interesting piece in the puzzle has been the finding that lamin mutations can also cause autosomal dominant Emery Dreifuss muscular dystrophy (limb girdle muscular dystrophy[85]) and familial partial lipodystrophy (Dunnigan's type[86]). The location of mutations may influence disease expression because defects clustered at the extreme carboxyl terminus of the gene produce lipodystrophy. However, neither the site nor the type of lamin gene mutation appears to distinguish mutations that cause Emery Dreifuss muscular dystrophy from mutations that cause dilated cardiomyopathy and conduction system disease. Perhaps proteins that interact with lamin may help to explain the predominance of organ-specific disease expression of different mutations.

Proteins involved in maintaining the structural integrity of the other organelles have been analyzed as candidates for cardiomyopathy mutations. Proteins that stabilize myofibrils and link the contractile apparatus to the cytoskeleton have been studied, and mutations in the desmin[87] and metavinculin[88] have been found to cause autosomal dominant dilated cardiomyopathy. These mutations are also often associated with skeletal myopathy.

Structural protein mutations also account for familial dilated cardiomyopathy that is transmitted as an X-linked trait. Mutations in the dystrophin gene are well recognized as causes of either Duchenne's or Becker's muscular dystrophy,[89] but deletions in the 5′ muscle promoter of the dystrophin gene have been reported to cause a predominant cardiac phenotype.[90,91] Skeletal muscle biopsies of individuals with X-linked dilated cardiomyopathy resulting from dystrophin deletions also demonstrate classical histopathologies of Duchenne's or Becker's dystrophies, but the skeletal manifestations can be subclinical. The dystrophin-associated protein complex has also become a target for the identification of genes that cause dilated cardiomyopathy. Mutations in the δ-sarcoglycan gene, a member of this complex, has

been identified to cause autosomal dominant dilated cardiomyopathy in one family and two sporadic cases.[92]

Barth's syndrome[93] is a poorly understood disorder characterized by congenital dilated cardiomyopathy, short stature, and neutropenia. Mutations in the tafazzin gene, which encodes a protein of unknown function, cause this X-linked dilated cardiomyopathy. Affected individuals usually die early in childhood. Alternative splicing of the gene encoding tafazzins in different tissues may account for the variable end organ expression resulting from these mutations.

The expanding list of mutations defined as genetic causes of dilated cardiomyopathy appear to indicate that abnormalities in almost any participant in myocyte biology can produce this condition. Undoubtedly the continued application of high-throughput gene-screening methods will uncover other causal gene defects. Although a unified mechanism for ventricular dilation and dysfunction may never evolve, continued progress in defining genetic cause of dilated cardiomyopathy may further delineate subtypes that improve diagnosis and provide information that is relevant for management of these important cause of heart failure. The development of animal models of dilated cardiomyopathy has begun to provide a platform for such issues.

## Animal Models of Dilated Cardiomyopathy

An important question raised by defined genetic causes of dilated cardiomyopathy is how do these mutations result in cardiac remodeling and a dilated phenotype. Numerous mechanisms have been proposed including deficits in force transmission, disruption of force generation, and inadequate energy production. To address these issues, various animal models of dilated cardiomyopathy have been recently developed.

Many of the morphologic and hemodynamic features of dilated cardiomyopathy are recapitulated in animal models of this human disease. Genetic models of dilated cardiomyopathy that arose from spontaneous mutations (e.g., the naturally occurring sarcoglycan mutation in cardiomyopathic hamster Bio14.6) have been extensively studied[93] with important potential signaling mechanisms identified. More recently, animal models have been produced through the introduction of germline mutations using transgenic or recombinatorial strategies. These latter models have helped establish the consequences of mutations and have provided insights into the downstream signals triggered by inciting events. Gene mutations in mice that alter the muscle LIM protein,[94] desmin,[95] and δ-sarcoglycan[93,96] confirm that cytoskeletal dysfunction is one cause of dilated cardiomyopathy. Deficits in myocyte energy and metabolism have been modeled in mice by ablation of genes directing mitochondrial biology.[97] Animals deficient in lamin A/C[98] also develop dilated cardiomyopathy, although the signaling pathways triggered by these events remain unclear.

These animal models illustrate the complexity and multiplicity of signaling pathways by which gene mutations can remodel the heart. These studies also identify potential roles for genes that have not become evident from human studies. An example of this is seen with the δ-sarcoglycan mutations. Although humans and murine δ-sarcoglycan mutations cause dilated cardiomyopathy, the responses to these gene defects appear to be quite different. Mice lacking δ-sarcoglycan develop coronary artery spasm, which results in myocardial ischemia, necrosis, and ultimately dilated cardiomyopathy.[93,96] Administration of the calcium channel antagonist verapamil improves cardiac function and reduces coronary artery ischemia. An important role for δ-sarcoglycan in the biology of human coronary arteries has not previously been recognized. Although human mutations in this gene have been reported to cause dilated cardiomyopathy, studies of the coronary arteries from affected individuals do not indicate an ischemic mechanism.[92] Instead, human mutations appear to alter heart function through dominant negative influences on the dystrophin-sarcoglycan complex, analogous to the mechanism by which these cause skeletal muscle dystrophy. Whether disparity in clinical findings of δ-sarcoglycan mutations from these species reflect distinct properties of the different mutations studied or unique functions of δ-sarcoglycan in human versus murine hearts remains unclear.

Important insights from animal models have also come from cross-breeding strategies aimed at complementing dilated cardiomyopathy deficits by genetic manipulation of models of disease. For example, ablation of the muscle LIM protein (MLP[94]) in mice causes neonatal dilated cardiomyopathy. However, if these mutant mice are bred with mice deficient in the phospholamban gene,[99] normal cardiac function is preserved. Phospholamban is a small regulatory protein that functions as a physiologic inhibitor of SERCA2a, an ATPase-dependent pump that allows cytosolic calcium to enter the sarcoplasmic reticulum. Genetic ablation of phospholamban would, therefore, result in unregulated SERCA2a pump function, thereby enhancing calcium reuptake by the sarcoplasmic reticulum. Functional improvement of hearts that are genetically predisposed to dilated cardiomyopathy by abrogation of phospholamban function implicates that calcium is a fundamental mediator of some of the pathophysiologic components of heart failure.

These animal studies allow study of pathophysiologic mechanisms involved in the development of dilated cardiomyopathy and define potentially molecular targets for pharmacologic intervention. For example, the LIM-phospholamban studies would suggest that the pharmacologic inhibition of phospholamban might enhance heart function in dilated cardiomyopathy. It is likely that many more animal models of dilated cardiomyopathy will be developed in the future to test these hypotheses.

## RESTRICTIVE CARDIOMYOPATHY

The restrictive cardiomyopathies are probably the least well understood myocardial disorders. These unusual disorders are characterized by abnormalities of ventricular filling in the absence of abnormal cardiac morphology.[100] Most studies of the characteristic hemodynamic profiles of restrictive cardiomyopathy are based on secondary pathologic findings such as that observed with chronic hypereosinophilic syndromes (endomyocardial fibrosis[101]), amyloidosis,[102] and chloroquine toxicity.[103] Myocardial degeneration and replacement fibrosis in hypereosinophilic syndromes occur secondary to infiltration with eosinophil granule proteins; recent evidence suggests that toxic effects may be mediated through interleukin-5 production.[104] Myocardial damage occurs in familial amyloidosis, an autosomal dominant condition resulting from a mutation in transthyretin, but is unusual in secondary amyloidosis. Long-term chloroquine therapy rarely results in a cardiomyopathy characterized by endomyocardial accumulation of vacuoles and lysosomes containing dense lamellar structures.

Familial restricted cardiomyopathies are exceedingly rare. At least two reports[105,106] of familial disease suggest that the disorder can be transmitted as an autosomal dominant trait. The natural history in one five-generation kindred[106] demonstrates symptomatic disease that develops after the third decade of life, with an insidious course. Individuals who survive into the fifth decade develop a progressive nonwasting skeletal myopathy. In another four-generation kindred,[107] a desmin-associated restrictive cardiomyopathy was identified, with a highly variable age of onset, severity, and rate of progression of disease.

The cardiac phenotype of familial restrictive cardiomyopathy is similar to the phenotype that occurs with secondary disease. Biventricular size and systolic function is normal, and both familial and secondary cases have biatrial enlargement. Diastolic filling pressures are increased, and ventricular filling patterns exhibit a "dip and plateau" morphology. Nonspecific electrocardiographic findings occur, including biatrial enlargement and atrioventricular and bundle branch block. Histopathology exhibits nonspecific features of patchy fibrosis and notably absence of eosinophilia and amyloid. The chromosome location(s) and disease gene(s) responsible for familial restrictive cardiomyopathy remain to be identified.

## INHERITED SYNDROMES WITH CARDIAC PHENOTYPES

Cardiomyopathies can occur as part of several inherited syndromes. Knowledge of the molecular defects that cause these multisystem disorders are important tools for cardiovascular research (i.e., although primary causes underlying alcoholic cardiomyopathy and idiopathic dilated cardiomyopathy or hypertensive heart disease and hypertrophic cardiomyopathy are quite different, the commonality of final phenotype suggests that the myocardium responds with a limited repertoire of cellular pathways). Insights gleaned from the study of cardiomyopathies that occur in the context of another organ dysfunction may, therefore, have relevance to cardiac-specific conditions. Molecular genetic studies of cardiomyopathies that result from mitochondria gene mutations and nuclear genes involved in fatty acid β-oxidation are discussed elsewhere. Genetic studies that have discovered the causal gene of cardiomyopathies that occur in the setting of other systemic disorders are discussed in this chapter.

Mutations in emerin, a novel protein of unknown function, cause Emery-Dreifuss muscular dystrophy,[108] a disorder characterized by progressive skeletal muscle dysfunction, contractures, and cardiomyopathy typically in association with atrioventricular conduction abnormalities. Atrial paralysis, atrial fibrillation, and atrial flutter are common; symptoms often result from infranodal conduction with slow junctional rhythms and atrioventricular block. Emery-Dreifuss muscular dystrophy is transmitted as an X-linked disorder, and genetic linkage studies have demonstrated that the disease gene (and the clinical phenotypes) is genetically distinct from Duchenne's and Becker's muscular dystrophies.

Friedreich's ataxia, a neuromuscular disorder transmitted as a dominant trait, results from mutations in frataxin, a novel gene encoded on chromosome 9q of unknown function.[109] Myocardial hypertrophy is the typical clinical cardiac manifestation of Friedreich's ataxia,[110] and pathologic findings include cardiomyocyte hypertrophy, fatty degeneration with diffuse interstitial fibrosis, and eosinophil and lymphocytic infiltrates.

Hemochromatosis, a common recessive disorder affecting 1 in 400 people of Northern European ancestry, is characterized by increased iron absorption and iron deposition in parenchymal tissues. Appropriate detection and treatment results in normal survival, but untreated hemochromatosis is characterized by cardiac, liver, and pancreatic failure. An inactivating mutation (C282Y) in HLA-H, a gene related to the major histocompatibility complex class I family, has been demonstrated in 85% of patients with familial hemochromatosis.[111,112] Although the mechanism by which this molecule regulates iron metabolism is unknown, sequences (termed betaGAP for beta-globin analogous promoter) within the major histocompatibility complex have homology to the promoter sequences in the β globin gene. Major histocompatibility complex genes controlled by betaGAP may, therefore, like β globin, have a role in iron metabolism. This hypothesis has been confirmed by engineering a mouse lacking β$_2$-microglobulin.[113] The resultant phenotype was systemic iron overload, although no details on cardiac physiology have been reported.

Atrial myxomas are a rare condition that can be inherited as part of Carney's complex (cardiac and mucocutaneous myxoma, lentiginosis, and endocrine dysfunction[114]). These cardiac tumors are often multicentric, rarely metastasize, and are amenable to surgical resection. Genetic linkage studies in families with autosomal dominant transmission of this disorder have demonstrated that the disorder is genetically heterogeneous[115] and mutations in the gene encoding the R1α regulatory subunit of cAMP-dependent protein kinase A (PRKAR1α) located on chromosome 17q24 have recently been identified as one cause of familial cardiac myxomas and Carney's complex.[116,117] The disease gene encoded at a second locus on chromosome 2p16 is unknown.[115]

## CONCLUSIONS

An exponential growth in the knowledge of gene defects that cause inherited cardiomyopathies will undoubtedly continue. Molecular genetic causes provide a solid basis for a classifying and understanding many heretofore idiopathic cardiac disorders. Integration of molecular insights into clinical practice has potential advantages to the patients afflicted by these intriguing disorders and to the physicians who care for them. Identification of human mutations allows early and accurate diagnosis, enabling nonspecific strategies (i.e., avoidance of competitive athletics) and early therapeutics that can reduce the serious morbidity and mortality associated with these disorders. Continued study and development of animal models of disease should further enable studies of the integrative physiology of multiple organ systems involved in the development of cardiomyopathies. Discovery of signaling events leading from mutant protein to clinical phenotype and the identification of genetic and environmental factors that modify the response to mutations may provide new insights that can enhance the fundamental understanding of the pathogenesis of inherited cardiomyopathies and improve therapeutic intervention.

## REFERENCES

1. Seidman JG, Seidman CE: The genetic basis for cardiomyopathy: From mutation identification to mechanistic paradigms. Cell 2001;104:557-567.
2. Risch NJ: Searching for genetic determinants in the new millennium. Nature 2000;405:847-56.
3. Lockhart DJ, Winzeler EA: Genomics, gene expression and DNA arrays. Nature 2000;405:827-836.
4. See the following web sites: genomes@ncbi.nlm.nih.gov and www.tigr.org
5. Wynne J, Braunwald E: The cardiomyopathies and myocarditides: Toxic, chemical, and physical damage to the heart. In Braunwald, E (ed): Heart Disease: A Textbook of Cardiovascular Medicine, 4th ed. Philadelphia, WB Saunders, 1991, p 139.
6. Maron BJ, Spirito P, Wesley Y, et al: Development and progression of left ventricular hypertrophy in children with hypertrophic cardiomyopathy. N Engl J Med 1986;315:610-614.
7. Rosenzweig A, Watkins H, Hwang D-S, et al: Preclinical diagnosis of familial hypertrophic cardiomyopathy by genetic analysis of blood lymphocytes. N Engl J Med 1991;325:1753-1760.
8. Spirito P, Seidman CE, McKenna WJ, et al: Management of hypertrophic cardiomyopathy. N Engl J Med 1997;336:775-785.
9. Maron B, Olivotto I, Spirito P, et al: Epidemiology of hypertrophic cardiomyopathy—related death: Revisited in a large non-referral-based patient population. Circulation 2000;102:858-864.
10. Maron, B, Shirani J, Poliac LC, et al: Sudden death in young competitive athletes: Clinical, demographic, and pathological profiles. JAMA 1996;276:199-204.
11. Maron BJ, Shen W-K, Link MS, et al: Efficacy of the implantable cardioverter-defibrillator for the prevention of sudden death in hypertrophic cardiomyopathy. N Engl J Med 2000;342:365-373.
12. Fananapazir L, Chang AC, Epstein SE, McAreavey D: Prognostic determinants in hypertrophic cardiomyopathy: Prognostic evaluation of a therapeutic strategy based on clinical, Holter, hemodynamic and electrophysiological findings. Circulation 1992;86:730-740.
13. Maron BJ, Gardin JM, Flack JM, et al:. Prevalence of hypertrophic cardiomyopathy in a general population of young adults: Echocardiographic analysis of 4111 subjects in the CARDIA study. Circulation 1995;92:785-789.

14. Watkins H, MacRae CA, Thierfelder L, et al: A disease locus for familial hypertrophic cardiomyopathy maps to chromosome 1q3. Nat Genet 1993;3:333-337.

15. Satoh M, Takahashi M, Sakamoto T, et al: Structural analysis of the titin gene in hypertrophic cardiomyopathy: Identification of a novel disease gene. Biochem Biophys Res Commun 1999;262: 411-417.

16. Poetter K, Jiang H, Hassanzadeh S, et al: Mutations in either the essential or regulatory light chains of myosin are associated with a rare myopathy in human heart and skeletal muscle. Nat Genet 1996;13:63-69.

17. Carrier L, Hengstemberg C, Beckmann JS, et al: Mapping of a novel gene for familial hypertrophic cardiomyopathy to chromosome 11. Nat Genet 1993;4:311-313.

18. Jarcho JA, McKenna WJ, Pare JAP, et al: Mapping a gene for familial hypertrophic cardiomyopathy to chromosome 14q1. N Engl J Med 1989;321:1372-1378.

19. Thierfelder L, MacRae CA, Watkins H, et al: A familial hypertrophic cardiomyopathy locus maps to chromosome 15q2. Proc Natl Acad Sci 1993;90:6270-6274.

20. Mogensen J, Klausen IC, Pedersen AK, et al: α-Cardiac actin is a novel gene in familial hypertrophic cardiomyopathy. J Clin Inves 1999;103:39R-43R.

21. Kimura A, Harada H, Park J-E, et al: Mutations in the cardiac troponin I gene associated with hypertrophic cardiomyopathy. Nat Genet 1997;16:379-382.

22. Watkins H, Rosenzweig A, Hwang D-S, et al: Characteristics and prognostic implications of myosin missense mutations in familial hypertrophic cardiomyopathy. N Engl J Med 1992;326:1108-1114.

23. See the following web site: http://genetics.med.harvard.edu/~sei dman/cg3/

24. Solomon SD, Wolff S, Watkins H, et al: Left ventricular hypertrophy and morphology in familial hypertrophic cardiomyopathy associated with mutations in the β myosin heavy chain gene. J Am Coll Cardiol 1993;22:498-505.

25. Fananapazir L, Epstein ND: Genotype-phenotype correlations in hypertrophic cardiomyopathy. Circulation 1994;89:22-32.

26. Watkins H, McKenna WJ, Thierfelder L, et al: The role of cardiac troponin T and α tropomyosin mutations in hypertrophic cardiomyopathy. N Engl J Med 1995;332:1058-1064.

27. Anan R, Shono H, Kisanuki A, et al: Patients with familial hypertrophic cardiomyopathy caused by a Phe110Ile missense mutation in the cardiac troponin T gene have variable cardiac morphologies and a favorable prognosis. Circulation 1998; 98:391-397.

28. Watkins H, Conner D, Thierfelder L, et al: Mutations in the cardiac myosin binding protein-C gene on chromosome 11 cause familial hypertrophic cardiomyopathy. Nat Genet 1995;11:434-437.

29. Bonne G, Carrier L, Bercovici J, et al: Cardiac myosin binding protein-C gene splice acceptor site mutation is associated with familial hypertrophic cardiomyopathy. Nat Genet 1995;11:438-440.

30. Carrier L, Bonne G, Bahrend E, et al: Organization and sequence of human cardiac myosin binding protein C (MYBP3) and identification of mutations predicted to produce truncated proteins in familial hypertrophic cardiomyopathy. Circ Res 1997;80:427-434.

31. Niimua H, Bachinski LL, Sangwatanaroj S, et al: Mutations in the gene for cardiac myosin-binding protein C and late-onset familial hypertrophic cardiomyopathy. N Engl J Med 1998;338: 1248-1257.

32. Gilbert R, Kelly MG, Mikawa T, et al: The carboxyl terminus of myosin binding protein C (MyBP-C, C-protein) specifies incorporation into the A-band of striated muscle. J Cell Science 1996; 109:101-111.

33. Gautel M, Zuffardi O, Freiburg A, et al: Phosphorylation switches specific for the cardiac isoform of myosin binding protein-C: A modulator of cardiac contraction? EMBO J 1995;14:1952-1960.

34. Coviello DA, Maron BJ, Spirito P, et al: Clinical features of hypertrophic cardiomyopathy caused by mutation of a "hot spot" in the α tropomyosin gene. JACC 1996;199:635-640.

35. Lee W-H, Hwang TH, Kimura A, et al: Different expressivity of a ventricular essential myosin light chain gene Ala57Gly mutation in familial hypertrophic cardiomyopathy. Am Heart J 2001;141: 184-189.

36. Kokado H, Shimizu, M, Hirouki Y, et al: Clinical features of hypertrophic cardiomyopathy caused by a Lys183 deletion mutation in the cardiac troponin I gene. Circulation 2000;102:663-669.

37. Woo A, Rakowski H, Liew J, et al: Hypertrophic cardiomyopathy: Genotypic and phenotypic heterogeneity. Circulation 2000;102: II 178.

38. Pascale R, Charron P, Carrier L, et al: Distribution of disease gene in 102 genotyped families with hypertrophic cardiomyopathy. Circulation 2001;104:II521.

39. Yamaguchi H, Ishimura T, Nishiyama S, et al: Hypertrophic nonobstructive cardiomyopathy with giant negative T waves (apical hypertrophy): Ventriculographic echocardiographic features in 30 patients. Am J Cardiol 1979;44:401-412.

40. Oson TM, Doan TP, Kishimoto NY, et al: Inherited and de novo mutations in the cardiac actin gene cause hypertrophic cardiomyopathy. J Mol Cell Cardiol 2000;32:1687-1694.

41. Niimura H, Patton K, McKenna, W, et al: Sarcomere protein gene mutations in hypertrophic cardiomyopathy of the elderly. Circulation 2002;105:446-451.

42. MacRae CA, Ghaisas N, Kass S, et al: Familial hypertrophic cardiomyopathy with Wolff-Parkinson-White syndrome maps to a locus on chromosome 7q3. J Clin Invest 1995;96:1216-1220.

43. Gollob MH, Green MS, Tang AS, et al: Identification of a gene responsible for Wolff-Parkinson-White syndrome. N Engl J Med 2001;344:1823-1831.

44. Blair E, Redwood C, Ashrafian H, et al: Mutations in the gamma(2) subunit of AMP-activated protein kinase cause familial hypertrophic cardiomyopathy: Evidence for the central role of energy compromise in disease pathogenesis. Hum Molec Genet 2001; 10:1215-1220.

45. Arad M, Benson W, Perez-Atayde AR, et al: Constitutively active AMP kinase mutations cause glycogen storage disease mimicking hypertrophic cardiomyopathy. J Clin Invest 2002;109: 357-362.

46. Watkins H, Thierfelder L, Anan R, et al: Independent origin of identical β myosin heavy chain gene mutations in hypertrophic cardiomyopathy. Am J Hum Genet 1993;53: 1180-1185.

47. Watkins H, Anan R, Coviello DA, et al: A de novo mutation in α tropomyosin that causes hypertrophic cardiomyopathy. Circulation 1995;91:2302-2305.

48. Forissier J-F, Pascale R, Briault S, et al: First germline mosaicism in familial hypertrophic cardiomyopathy. J Med Genet 2000;37: 132-134.

49. Al-Mahdawi S, Chamberlain S, Cleland J, et al: Identification of a mutation in the β cardiac myosin heavy chain gene in a family with hypertrophic cardiomyopathy. Br Heart J 1993;69: 136-141.

50. Lankdord EB, Epstein ND, Fananapazir L, et al: Abnormal contractile properties of muscle fibers expression β-myosin chain mutations in patients with hypertrophic cardiomyopathy. J Clin Invest 1995;95:1409-1414.

51. Fananapazir L, Dalakis MC, Cyran F, et al: Missense mutations in the β-myosin heavy chain cause central core disease in hypertrophic cardiomyopathy. Proc Natl Acad Sci USA 1993;90: 3993-3997.

52. Rayment I, Holden HM, Sellers JR, et al: Structural interpretation of the mutations in the β-cardiac myosin that have been implicated in familial hypertrophic cardiomyopathy. Proc Natl Acad Sci USA 1995;92:3894-3868.

53. Sweeney HL, Straceski AJ, Leinwand LA, et al: Heterologous expression of a cardiomyopathic myosin that is defective in its actin interaction. J Biol Chem 1994;269:1603-1605.

54. Sata M, Ikebe M: Functional analysis of the mutations in the human cardiac β-myosin that are responsible for familial hypertrophic cardiomyopathy. J Clin Invest 1996;98: 2866-2873.

55. Lin D, Bobkova A, Homsher E, et al: Altered cardiac troponin T in vitro function in the presence of a mutation implicated in familial hypertrophic cardiomyopathy. J Clin Invest 1996;97: 2842-2848.

56. Watkins H, Seidman CE, Seidman JG, et al: Expression and functional assessment of a truncated cardiac troponin T that cause hypertrophic cardiomyopathy: Evidence for a dominant negative action. J Clin Invest 1996;11:2456-2461.

57. Vikstrom KL, Factor SM, Leinwand LA: A murine model of hypertrophic cardiomyopathy. Zeitschrift fur Kardiologie 1995;84: 49-54.

58. Marian AJ, Wu Y, McCluggage M, et al: A transgenic rabbit model for human hypertrophic cardiomyopathy. J Clin Invest 1999;104: 1683-1692.

59. Oberst L, Zhao G, Park JT, et al: Dominant-negative effect of a mutant cardiac troponin T on cardiac structure and function in transgenic mice. J Clin Invest 1998;102:1498-1505.

60. Tardiff JC, Factor SM, Tompkins BD, et al: A truncated cardiac troponin T molecule in transgenic mice suggests multiple cellular mechanisms for familial hypertrophic cardiomyopathy. J Clin Invest 1998;101:2800-2811.

61. Yang Q, Sanbe A, Osinka H, et al: A mouse model of myosin binding protein C human familial hypertrophic cardiomyopathy. J Clin Invest 1998;102:1292-1300.

62. James J, Zhang Y, Osinska H, et al: Transgenic modeling of a cardiac troponin I mutation linked to familial hypertrophic cardiomyopathy. Circ Res 2000;87:805-811.

63. Geisterfer-Lowrance AAT, Christe M, Conner DA, et al: A murine model of familial hypertrophic cardiomyopathy. Science 1996; 272:731-734.

64. Tyska MJ, Hayes E, Giewat M, et al: Single molecule mechanics of R403Q cardiac myosin isolated from the mouse model of familial hypertrophic cardiomyopathy. Circ Res 2000;86:737-744.

65. Fatkin D, McConnell BK, Mudd JO, et al: An abnormal $Ca^{2+}$ response in mutant sarcomere protein-mediated familial hypertrophic cardiomyopathy. J Clin Invest 2000;106:1351-1359.

66. Berul C, Christie M, Aronovitz MJ, et al: Electrophysiological abnormalities and arrhythmias in α MHC mutant familial hypertrophic cardiomyopathy mice. J Clin Invest 1997;99: 570-576.

67. Bruneau, BG, Nemer G, Schmitt J-P, et al: Murine model of Holt-Oram syndrome defines roles of the T-box transcription facto Tbx5 in cardiogenesis and disease. Cell 2001;106:709-722.

68. Grunig E, Tasman JA, Kucherer H, et al: Frequency and phenotypes of familial dilated cardiomyopathy. J Am Coll Cardiol 1998;31:186-194.

69. Bharati S, Surawicz B, Vidaillet HJ, et al: Familial congenital sinus rhythm anomalies: Clinical and pathological correlations. PACE 1992;15:1720-1927.

70. Nogami K, Kusachi S, Nunoyama H, et al: Extracellular matrix components in dilated cardiomyopathy: Immunohistochemical study of endomyocardial biopsy specimens. Jpn Heart J 1996;37: 483-494.

71. Cohn JN, Bristow MR, Chien KR, et al: Report of the National Heart, Lung and Blood Institute special emphasis panel on heart failure research. Circulation 1997;95:766-770.

72. Mestroni L, Rocco C, Gregori D, et al: Familial dilated cardiomyopathy: Evidence for genetic and phenotypic heterogeneity. Heart Muscle Disease Study Group. J Am Coll Cardiol 1999; 34:181-190.

73. Schonberger J, Levy H, Grunig E, et al: Dilated cardiomyopathy and sensorineural hearing loss: A heritable syndrome that maps to 6q23-24. Circulation 2000;101:1812-1818.

74. Olson TM, Michels VV, Thibodeau SN, et al: Actin mutations in dilated cardiomyopathy, a heritable form of heart failure. Science 1998;280:750-752.

75. Kamisago M, Sharma SD, DePalma SR, et al: Sarcomere protein gene mutations cause dilated cardiomyopathy. N Engl J Med 2000;343:1688-1695.

76. Li, D, Czernuszewicz G, Gonzalez O, et al: Novel cardiac troponin T mutation as a cause of familial dilated cardiomyopathy. Circulation 2001;104:2188-2193.

77. Olson T, Kishimoto N, Whitby F, et al: Mutations that alter the surface charge of α tropomyosin are associated with dilated cardiomyopathy. J Moll Cell Cardiol 2001;33:723-732.

78. Gerull B, Gramlich M, Atherton J, et al: Mutations of TTN, encoding the giant muscle filament titin, causes familial dilated cardiomyopathy. Nat Genet 2002;30:201-204.

79. Kass S, MacRae CA, Graber HL, et al: A gene defect that causes conduction system disease and dilated cardiomyopathy maps to chromosome 1cen. Nat Genet 1994;7:546-551.

80. Olson TM, Keating MT: Mapping a cardiomyopathy locus to chromosome 3p22-p25. J Clin Invest 1996;97:528-532.

81. Fatkin D, MacRae C, Sasaki T, et al: Missense mutations in the lamin A/C rod cause dilated cardiomyopathy and conduction system disease. N Engl J Med 1999;34:1715-1724.

82. Brodsky GL, Mutoni F, Miocic S, et al: Lamin A/C gene mutation associated with dilated cardiomyopathy with variable skeletal muscle involvement. Circulation 2000;101:473-476.

83. Jakobs PM, Hanson EL, Crispell KA, et al: Novel lamin A/C mutations in two families with dilated cardiomyopathy and conduction system disease. J Cardiac Failure 2001;7:249-256.

84. Stuurman N, Heins S, Aebi U: Nuclear lamins: Their structure, assembly, and interactions. J Struct Biol 1998;122:42-66.

85. Bonne G, Di Barletta MR, Varnous S, et al: Mutations in the gene encoding lamin A/C cause autosomal dominant Emery-Dreifuss muscular dystrophy. Nat Genet 1999;21:285-288.

86. Shackleton S, Lloyd DJ, Jackson SN, et al: LMNA, encoding lamin A/C, is mutated in partial lipodystrophy. Nat Genet 2000;24: 153-156.

87. Li D, Tapscoft T, Gonzalez O, et al: Desmin mutation responsible for idiopathic dilated cardiomyopathy. Circulation 1999;100:461-464

88. Olson T, Illenberger S, Kishimoto N, et al: Metavinculin mutation salter actin interaction in dilated cardiomyopathy. Circulation 2002;105:431-437.

89. Online Mendelian Inheritance in Man, OMIM (TM). Johns Hopkins University, Baltimore MD. Available at: http://www3/ncbi.nlm.nih.gov/omin/

90. Mutoni F, Wilson L, Marrosu G, et al: A mutation in the dystrophin gene selectively affecting dystrophin expression in the heart. J Clin Invest 1995;96:693-699.

91. Cox GR, Kunkel LM: Dystrophies and heart disease. Curr Opin Cardiol 1997;12:329-343.

92. Tsubata S, Bowles KR, Vatta M, et al: Mutations in the human delta-sarcoglycan gene in familial and sporadic dilated cardiomyopathy. J Clin Invest 2000;106:655-662.

93. Nigro V, Okazaki Y, Belsito A, et al: Identification of the Syrian hamster cardiomyopathy gene. Hum Molec Genet 1997;6:601-607.

94. Arber S, Hunter JJ, Ross J Jr, et al: MLP-deficient mice exhibit a disruption of cardiac cytoarchitectural organization, dilated cardiomyopathy and heart failure. Cell 1997;88:393-403.

95. Milner DJ, Weitze G, Tran D, et al: Disruption of muscle architecture and myocardial degeneration in mice lacking desmin. J Cell Bio 1996;134:1255-1270.

96. Ikeda Y, Gu Y, Iwanaga Y, et al: Restoration of deficient membrane proteins in the cardiomyopathic hamster by in vivo cardiac gene transfer. Circulation 2002;105:502-508.

97. Wallace DC: Mitochondrial diseases in man and mouse. Science 1999;283:1482-1488.

98. Sullivan T, Escalante-Alcalde D, Bhatt H, et al: Loss of A-type lamin expression compromises nuclear envelope integrity leading to muscular dystrophy. J Cell Biol 1999;147:913-920.

99. Minamisawa S, Hoshijima M, Chu G, et al: Chronic phospholamban-sarcoplasmic reticulum calcium ATPase interaction is the critical calcium cycling defect in dilated cardiomyopathy. Cell 1999;99:313-322.

100. Kushwaha SS, Fallon JT, Fuster V: Restrictive cardiomyopathy. N Engl J Med 1997;336:267-276.

101. Take M, Sekiguchi M, Hiroe M, et al: Clinical spectrum and endomyocardial biopsy findings in eosinophilic heart disease. Heart Vessels Suppl 1985;1:243-249.

102. Hesse A, Altland K, Linke RP, et al: Cardiac amyloidosis: A review and report of a new transthyretin (prealbumin) variant. Br Heart J 1993;70:111-115.

103. Verny C, deGennes C, Sebastien P, et al: Troubles de la conduction cardiaque au cours d'un traitment prolonge par chloroquine: Deux nouvelles observations. Presse Medicale 1992;21:800-804.

104. Desreumaux P, Janin A, Dubucquoi S, et al: Synthesis of interleukin-5 by activated eosinophils in patients with eosinophilic heart diseases. Blood 1993;82:1553-1560.

105. Aroney C, Bett N, Radford D: Familial restrictive cardiomyopathy. Aust N Z J Med 1988;18:877-878.

106. Fitzpatrick AP, Shapiro LM, Rickards AF, et al: Familial restrictive cardiomyopathy with atrioventricular block and skeletal myopathy. Br Heart J 1990;63:114-118.

107. Zhang J, Kumar A, Stalker HJ, et al: Clinical and moleculear studies of a large family with desmin-associated restrictive cardiomyopathy. Clin Genet 2001;59:248-256.

108. Bione S, Maestrini E, Rivella S, et al: Identification of a novel X-linked gene responsible for Emery-Dreifuss muscular dystrophy. Nat Genet 1994;8:323-327.

109. Campuzano V, Montermini L, Molto MD, et al: Friedreich's ataxia: Autosomal recessive disease caused by an intronic GAA triplet repeat expansion. Science 1996;271:1423-1427.

110. Gunal N, Saraclar M, Ozkutlu S, et al: Heart disease in Friedreich's ataxia: A clinical echocardiographic study. Acta Paediatrica Japonica 1996;38:308-311.

111. Feder JN, Gnirke A, Thomas W, et al: A novel MHC class I-like gene is mutated in patients with hereditary haemochromatosis. Nat Genet 1996;13:399-408.

112. Mahon NG, Coonar AS, Coccolo JS, et al: Haemochromatosis gene mutations in idiopathic dilated cardiomyopathy. Heart 2000;84: 541-547.

113. Rothenberg BE, Voland JR: $\beta$-2 Knockout mice develop parenchymal iron overload: A putative role for class I genes of the major histocompatibility complex in iron metabolism. Proc Natl Acad Sci USA 1996;93:1529-1534.

114. Basson CT, MacRae CA, Korf B, et al: A genetic heterogeneity of familial atrial myxoma syndromes (Carney complex). Am J Cardiol 1997;79:994-995.

115. Stratakis CA, Carney JA, Lin JP, et al: Carney complex, a familial multiple neoplasia and lentiginosis syndrome: Analysis of 11 kindreds and linkage to the short arm of chromosome 2. J Clin Invest 1996;97:699-705.

116. Casey M, Vaughan CJ, He J, et al: Mutations in the R1 $\alpha$ regulatory subunit of protein kinase A cause familial cardiac myxomas and Carney complex. J Clin Invest 2000;219:90-95.

117. Kirschner LS, Carney JA, Pack SD, et al: Mutations of the gene encoding the protein kinase A type 1-$\alpha$ regulatory subunit in patients with Carney complex. Nat Genet 2000;26:89-92.

## EDITOR'S CHOICE

Arad M, Moskowitz IP, Patel VV, et al: Transgenic mice overexpressing mutant PRKAG2 define the cause of Wolff-Parkinson-White syndrome in glycogen storage cardiomyopathy. Circulation 2003;107: 2850-2856.
*WPW due to a glycogen storage disease is associated with familial cardiomyopathy.*

Ashrafian H, Redwood C, Blair E, Watkins H: Hypertrophic cardiomyopathy: A paradigm for myocardial energy depletion. Trends Genet 2003;19:263-268.
*A different viewpoint of the mechanisms that link PRKAG2 mutations with cardiomyopathy.*

Chien KR: Genotype, phenotype: Upstairs, downstairs in the family of cardiomyopathies. J Clin Invest 2003;111:175-178.
*Improved phenotyping may be the critical to the future of the genetics of cardiomyopathies.*

Finck BN, Han X, Courtois M, et al: A critical role for PPARalpha-mediated lipotoxicity in the pathogenesis of diabetic cardiomyopathy: Modulation by dietary fat content. Proc Natl Acad Sci USA 2003;100:1226-1231.
*Nuclear hormone receptor pathways may be directly linked to diabetic cardiomyopathy.*

Gerull B, Gramlich M, Atherton J, et al: Mutations of TTN, encoding the giant muscle filament titin, cause familial dilated cardiomyopathy. Nat Genet 2002;30:201-204.
*Mutations in titin are a cause of human cardiomyopathies.*

Itoh-Satoh M, Hayashi T, Nishi H, et al: Titin mutations as the molecular basis for dilated cardiomyopathy. Biochem Biophys Res Commun 2002;291:385-393.
*Companion paper to Gerull et al makes the same case in zebrafish models; validates the zebrafish model as a tool to identify candidate genes for human cardiomyopathies.*

Morita H, DePalma SR, Arad M, et al: Molecular epidemiology of hypertrophic cardiomyopathy. Cold Spring Harb Symp Quant Biol 2002;67:383-388.
*Leaders in the genetics of human cardiac diseases highlight over a decade of advances in the field.*

Richard P, Charron P, Carrier L, et al: Hypertrophic cardiomyopathy: Distribution of disease genes, spectrum of mutations, and implications for a molecular diagnosis strategy. Circulation 2003;107: 2227-2232.
*A review of elegant genetic studies emanating from European patient populations with cardiomyopathy.*

# chapter 17

# Molecular Pathways for Dilated Cardiomyopathy

*Ronald D. Cohn*
*Kevin P. Campbell*

## THE DYSTROPHIN-GLYCOPROTEIN COMPLEX AND ITS ROLE IN THE PATHOGENESIS OF CARDIOMYOPATHY

The dystrophin-glycoprotein complex (DGC)[1-3] is a multisubunit complex comprised of peripheral and integral membrane proteins that form a structural linkage between the F-actin cytoskeleton and the extracellular matrix in striated muscle (Fig. 17-1). The proteins that comprise the DGC are structurally organized into three distinct subcomplexes. These are the cytoskeletal proteins, dystrophin and $\alpha/\beta$-syntrophins; the sarcolemmal-localized dystroglycan complex ($\alpha$ and $\beta$ subunits); and sarcoglycans ($\alpha$, $\beta$, $\gamma$, and $\delta$ subunits), sarcospan complex, DGC-associated proteins, neuronal nitric oxide synthase, and dystrobrevin.[4-6] Several forms of muscular dystrophy arise from primary mutations in genes encoding components of this complex.[4-6] Interactions between subcomplexes are evidently important for targeting to the sarcolemma and for membrane stabilization.[7] An important role of the DGC for muscle function and stability is to provide mechanical support to the plasma membrane during myofiber contraction.[8,9] In various forms of muscular dystrophy, the development of cardiomyopathy as a major complication (often associated with sudden cardiac death) has been clinically appreciated for many decades. However, within the past decade, research efforts from around the world have shed light on the pathogenetic pathways involved in the development of muscular dystrophy associated cardiomyopathy (cardiomyopathy resulting from mutations within the DGC and from other genetic forms of muscular dystrophy). This chapter highlights the current understanding of molecular pathways that are responsible for cardiomyopathies associated with structural and functional alterations of the DGC.

## DYSTROPHINOPATHIES

Dystrophin, a 427-kd protein that is absent or reduced in Duchenne's and Becker's muscular dystrophies (DMD/BMD), is located on chromosome Xp21.[10] It has been shown that the N-terminus of dystrophin interacts directly with F-actin in an extended, lateral fashion, similar to many actin side-binding proteins.[11,12] Dystrophin interacts with other DGC subcomplexes through its C-terminal domain, which directly binds to the C-terminus of $\beta$-dystroglycan, an integral membrane protein with a single transmembrane helix.[13] $\beta$-Dystroglycan binds to $\alpha$-dystroglycan, anchoring it to the extracellular surface of the sarcolemma. In turn, $\alpha$-dystroglycan serves as a laminin-2 receptor, thereby completing the structural connection between the actin cytoskeleton and the extracellular matrix.[14]

Numerous studies in DMD/BMD patients, which used ECG and functionally evaluated cardiac muscle by echocardiography, have demonstrated a steady decline of left-ventricular function that, in DMD patients, may correlate with the rate of deterioration of skeletal muscle function.[15,16] Often, the combination of respiratory failure and suppression of cardiac function causes death in DMD patients. However, it is interesting to note that autopsy studies performed in patients with DMD about 20 years ago showed macroscopic and microscopic evidence of cardiac muscle fibrosis, which was not necessarily detected by functional ECG or echocardiographic studies. Thus, today when technical advancements have improved the detection of subtle cardiac functional abnormalities, it is essential to evaluate any DMD/BMD patient even in the absence of overt clinical signs of heart failure and/or exercise intolerance. In addition to using more technically sophisticated tools, serum levels of troponin I in patients with DMD/BMD should be monitored because they may be beneficial as an early indicator of cardiac muscle damage. As recent studies in animal models have shown, troponin I can serve as an excellent heart muscle specific marker for subtle cardiac damage for DMD and limb-girdle muscular dystrophin[17] even in the presence of extensive muscle regeneration that may lead to false elevation of creatine kinase MB fractions and troponin T levels (Fig. 17-2).

Another form of cardiomyopathy caused by mutations in the dystrophin gene is allelic to DMD/BMD and has been classified as X-linked dilated cardiomyopathy (XLDC).[18] In contrast to DMD and BMD, the only apparent clinical symptom in patients with XLDC is related to the cardiac phenotype, and skeletal muscle symptoms usually are nonexistent or not prominent despite an invariable elevation of serum creatine kinase levels associated with mild histologic changes of myopathy.[19] Because of the heterogeneity of dystrophin mutations

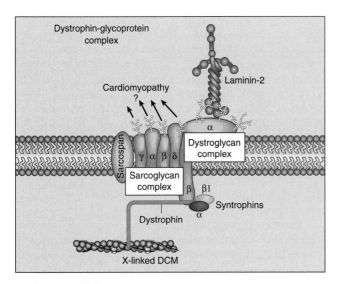

Dystrophin-glycoprotein complex

Laminin-2

Cardiomyopathy
?

Dystroglycan complex

Sarcoglycan complex

Syntrophins

Dystrophin

X-linked DCM

**FIGURE 17-1.** The DGC and cardiomyopathies associated with mutations within the DGC. (See color plate.)

identified so far, the pathogenesis underlying the selective cardiac muscle impairment in the XLDC families represents a fascinating scientific challenge. Two main regions of the dystrophin gene appeared to be most commonly involved in XLDC: the 5' end of the gene and the central hot-spot region, centered around exons 48-49 (spectrin-like).[20] From a clinical point of view the severity of cardiac involvement can be variable, ranging from an early-onset and fatal cardiomyopathy to a milder form compatible with a better prognosis. Interestingly, patients with a severe clinical phenotype almost invariably have mutations in the 5' end of the gene, whereas the less severe phenotype is associated with mutations in the spectrin-like domain.[20] Several different mutations within the 5' end of the dystrophin gene have been described in patients with XLDC. Rearrangements in the muscle promotor (M) and adjacent intron 1 have been described in three unrelated families.[21,22] In addition, a single point muta-

tion at the first exon-intron boundary, inactivating the universally conserved 5' splice site consensus sequence of the first intron has also been described.[23] In general, these mutations lead to the loss of full-length M isoform expression in the heart.[24-27] Another type of mutations within the 5' end of the dystrophin gene consists of a duplication involving exon 2-7.[28] Interestingly, these patients have a normal number of dystrophin transcripts in the cardiac and skeletal muscle, but there is a complete lack of syntrophin protein expression in the heart, indicating that the mutations breakpoints might involve regulatory regions within the 5' end of the dystrophin gene. The absence of syntrophin expression could have caused down-regulation of the dystrophin transcription in the heart alone.[28] A rather unusual type of mutation caused by an Alu-like mobile element insertion in intron 11 of the dystrophin gene was described by Ferlini et al. in 1999.[20] The described rearrangement affected the canonical splicing of exons 11 and 12 in the heart, eliminating the normal transcript and subsequent dystrophin expression in cardiac muscle only, whereas dystrophin expression in skeletal muscle was only mildly affected.[20] Another interesting splicing mutation was reported by Franz et al. in 1995.[29] A nonsense mutation in exon 29 caused exon 29 skipping in both skeletal and cardiac muscle, resulting in complete absence of the mid-rod dystrophin region in cardiac muscle. Interestingly, the mutation caused disruption of the sarcoglycan complex in cardiac muscle but not in skeletal muscle, suggesting that conformational changes in exon 29-deleted dystrophin may cause abnormal assembly of the sarcoglycan complex in cardiac muscle.[30]

Frame deletions of the spectrin-like region of the dystrophin gene usually give rise to BMD; however, a few patients with XLDC have been reported to carry in-frame deletions of exons 49-51,[31] 48-49,[31] and 48.[32] However, the pathogenesis of the isolated cardiac phenotype of patients with mutations in the spectrin-like domain is not entirely clear. It has been hypothesized that loss of intron sequences with potential regulating capacities could play a role in the development of XLDC; however, further scientific effort is needed to prove this hypothesis.

Many other studies have tried to analyze the pathogenetic mechanism from a functional and structural point of view. In cardiac muscle, dystrophin has been shown to localize as a continuous sheet at the sarcolemma with concentrated bands corresponding to the vinculin-rich costameres; unlike its localization in skeletal muscle cells, dystrophin is also found along intracellular T-tubules.[33-35] Immunohistologic and ultrastructural studies in human heart samples have shown that cardiomyocyte hypertrophy is associated with maintenance of sarcolemmal dystrophin labeling and intracellular dystrophin in parallel with more extensive T-tubular development.[33] Moreover, the sarcolemmal organization of dystrophin is lost in degenerating cells of the failing left ventricle. The association with T-tubules in cardiomyocytes suggests a functional diversity for dystrophin within the heart, because T-tubules play a role in excitation-contraction coupling

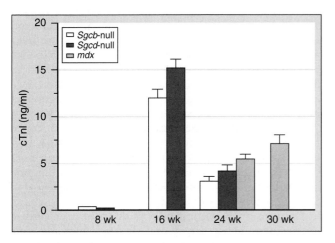

**FIGURE 17-2.** Elevation of cardiac troponin I in *Sgcb*-null, *Sgcd*-null, and *mdx* mice.

and do not serve in the transmission of contractile forces. Thus, mechanisms other than membrane fragility (such as defects in calcium handling) should be considered as pathogenetic causes of myocyte degeneration in cardiomyopathies that result from mutations within the dystrophin gene.

Functional *in vivo* studies have shown that dystrophin-deficient myocardium is specifically vulnerable to pressure overload. Abdominal aortic banding in dystrophin-deficient *mdx* mice resulted in severe myocardial cell damage followed by fibrosis.[36] Moreover, it has been shown that calcineurin and stress-activated protein kinase/p38-mitogen activated protein kinase are activated in hearts of mice deficient for dystrophin and utrophin.[37] These findings might be of particular interest because of their implication for supportive pharmacologic therapy aimed at afterload reduction in patients with DMD/BMD. In addition, no mutations within the laminin alpha 2 gene and the dystroglycan gene, two major components of the DGC, have been identified and/or associated with human or mouse models of cardiomyopathy. Thus, a combination of genetic, structural, and functional research efforts are needed to define the pathogenetic mechanism leading to heart disease in dystrophin-deficient cardiac muscle to develop strategies to treat and/or prevent heart failure in this group of disorders.

## SARCOGLYCANOPATHIES

Within the DGC, a group of single-pass transmembrane glycoproteins form a tetrameric unit consisting of α-, β-, γ-, and δ-sarcoglycan. In limb-girdle muscular dystrophy type 2 (LGMD2) four distinct subtypes are caused by mutations in sarcoglycan glycoproteins[4]: LGMD2D (α-sarcoglycan), LGMD2E (β-sarcoglycan), LGMD2C (γ-sarcoglycan), and LGMD2F (δ-sarcoglycan). During the past few years it has become increasingly clear that sarcoglycanopathies can also be associated with cardiomyopathies, in particular with β-, γ-, and δ-sarcoglycan.[38-40] Interestingly, mutations in the human δ-sarcoglycan gene have been characterized in patients with familiar and sporadic cases of dilated cardiomyopathy without significant involvement of the skeletal muscle.[40] The current focus of interest in the field is directed toward the characterization of genotype-phenotype correlations in patients with limb-girdle muscular dystrophy caused by mutations within the sarcoglycan genes. However, analysis of genetically engineered mouse models for sarcoglycanopathies have revealed some insights into the pathogenetic mechanism that might potentially lead to cardiac involvement in patients with sarcoglycan gene mutations.

By studying the different tissue distribution of the sarcoglycan-sarcospan complex (SG-SSPN), a new avenue of research was opened that revealed new insights into the pathogenesis of sarcoglycanopathies. In skeletal and cardiac muscle, the SG-SSPN complex is composed of α-, β-, γ-, and δ-sarcoglycan and sarcospan.[4] ε-Sarcoglycan, a transmembrane glycoprotein showing 43% amino acid identity with α-sarcoglycan has a broad tissue distribution, whereas α-sarcoglycan expression is restricted to skeletal and cardiac muscle.[41,42] Biochemical fractionation studies demonstrated that ε-sarcoglycan replaces α-sarcoglycan in smooth muscle as an integral component of a unique SG-SSPN complex composed of ε-, β-, and δ-sarcoglycan and sarcospan.[43] More recently, it has been demonstrated that γ-sarcoglycan is also expressed in smooth muscle and is an integral part of the smooth muscle sarcoglycan-sarcospan complex.[44] Analyzing animal models with various targeted deletions of sarcoglycan genes has shown the pathogenetic significance of the characterization of this unique sarcoglycan-sarcospan complex in smooth muscle (Fig. 17-3).

Targeted disruption of α-sarcoglycan (expressed only in skeletal and cardiac muscle) leads to progressive muscular dystrophy and to a concomitant deficiency of β-, γ-, and δ-sarcoglycan along with sarcospan in skeletal and cardiac muscle.[45] Interestingly, ε-sarcoglycan expression was still preserved in skeletal and cardiac muscle of these mice. Although the SG-SSPN complex was absent in cardiac muscle, α-sarcoglycan deficient mice do not develop cardiomyopathy. In contrast, mice with targeted disruption of β- or δ-sarcoglycan (animal models for LGMD 2E and 2F) developed severe muscular dystrophy associated with cardiomyopathy.[46,47] These mice showed the histologic hallmark of focal areas of necrosis in skeletal and cardiac muscle.[46,47] Immunohistochemical and biochemical studies of vascular smooth muscle and other smooth muscle types revealed disruption of the SG-SSPN complex in β- or δ-sarcoglycan deficient mice.[46,47] In contrast, smooth muscle expression of the SG-SSPN complex in α-sarcoglycan deficient mice was not affected. Further analysis of vascular smooth muscle in β- and δ-sarcoglycan deficient mice demonstrated that the absence of the SG-SSPN complex perturbed vascular function as demonstrated by multiple microvascular constrictions in arteries of the heart, diaphragm, and kidney.[46,47] The data indicates that vascular dysfunction initiates the cardiomyopathy and most likely exacerbates muscular dystrophy phenotype.[46,47] PET studies in several sarcoglycan-deficient patients (one patient with a known mutation in the β-sarcoglycan gene) revealed blunted coronary vasodilator reserve, suggesting dysfunction of coronary artery smooth muscle.[48] Interestingly, no abnormalities in vascular perfusion of these same tissues (including the diaphragm) were observed in mice deficient for α-sarcoglycan, ruling out the possibility that alterations within the muscle itself lead to secondary perturbation of vascular function. Mice deficient for γ-sarcoglycan also exhibit cardiomyopathy in addition to a dystrophic phenotype observed in skeletal muscle,[49] and it is believed that vascular disturbances observed in these mice are a secondary phenomenon rather than the initiating factor. The discrepancy of these results must still be explained.

The presumed pathogenetic mechanism for cardiac involvement caused by β-and/or δ-sarcoglycan mutations can be summarized as follows: disruption of the SG-SSPN complex in vascular smooth muscle leads to

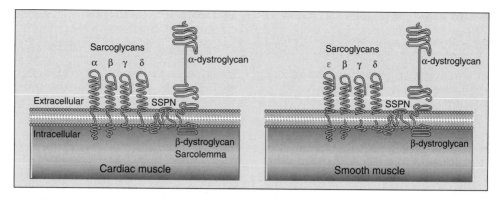

**FIGURE 17-3.** Composition of the sarcoglycan-sarcospan complex in cardiac and smooth muscle.

perturbation of vascular function as demonstrated by multiple vascular constrictions. In addition, loss of the SG-SSPN complex in cardiomyocytes causes the cardiac muscle to be prone to intermittent ischemic-like events, which eventually leads to focal myocardial necrosis and cardiomyopathy. The rationale of these findings has led to pharmacologic approaches to interfere with vascular tone to prevent cardiac injury in these mouse models.[17,46] Thus, it has been shown that short-term administration of nicorandil, a potassium channel agonist, leads to dilation of the coronary vasculature and prevents acute treadmill exercise induced heart damage in δ-sarcoglycan deficient mice.[46] Moreover, long-term treatment with verapamil, an L-type calcium channel blocker with vasodilator properties and clinical relevance, abolishes vascular constrictions and effectively prevents the development of severe cardiomyopathy in β- and δ-sarcoglycan deficient mice.[17]

The clinical relevance of the previously mentioned studies and the accuracy of extrapolating these findings to disease conditions and pathophysiology in humans will need further research. Currently, most of the clinical research is focused on identifying patients with sarcoglycanopathies who have cardiac defects, no matter how subtle. This is of particular importance because preventive therapeutic options will have to be implemented before overt clinical signs of heart failure are present. Continuous investment in the full spectrum of clinical and genetic research, from identification of human mutations to analyses of mechanism, will lead to further advances in scientific understanding and the development of therapeutic options for cardiomyopathies caused by mutations of the DGC and for cardiomyopathies in general.

## REFERENCES

1. Campbell KP, Kahl SD: Association of dystrophin and an integral membrane glycoprotein. Nature 1989;338:259-262.
2. Ervasti JM, Campbell KP: Membrane organization of the dystrophin-glycoprotein complex. Cell 1991;66:1121-1131.
3. Yoshida M, Mizuno Y, Nonaka I, Ozawa E: A dystrophin-associated glycoprotein, A3a (one of 43DAG doublets), is retained in Duchenne muscular dystrophy muscle. J Biochem (Tokyo) 1993;114:634-639.
4. Cohn RD, Campbell KP: The molecular basis of muscular dystrophy. Muscle Nerve 2000;23:1456-1471.
5. Burton EA, Davies KE: Muscular dystrophy–reason for optimism? Cell 2002;108:5-8.
6. O'Brien KF, Kunkel LM: Dystrophin and muscular dystrophy: Past, present, and future. Mol Genet Metab 2001;74:75-88.
7. Crosbie RH, Lebakken CS, Holt KH, et al: Membrane targeting and stabilization of sarcospan is mediated by the sarcoglycan subcomplex J Cell Biol 1999;145:153-165.
8. Petrof BJ, Shrager JB, Stedman HH, et al: Dystrophin protects the sarcolemma from stresses developed during muscle contraction. Proc Natl Acad Sci USA 1993;90:3710-3714.
9. Weller B, Karpati G, Carpenter S: Dystrophin-deficient mdx muscle fibers are preferentially vulnerable to necrosis induced by experimental lengthening contractions. J Neurol Sci 1990;100:9-13.
10. Koenig M, Monaco AP, Kunkel L: The complete sequence of dystrophin predicts a rod-shaped cytoskeletal protein. Cell 1988;53:219-226.
11. Rybakova IN, Amann KJ, Ervasti JM: A new model for the interaction of dystrophin with F-actin. J Cell Biol 1996;135:661-672.
12. Rybakova IN, Ervasti JM: Dystrophin-glycoprotein complex is monomeric and stabilizes actin filaments in vitro through a lateral association. J Biol Chem 1997;272:28771-28778.
13. Jung D, Yang B, Meyer J, et al: Identification and characterization of the dystrophin anchoring site on beta-dystroglycan. J Biol Chem 1995;270:27305-27310.
14. Ervasti JM, Campbell KP: A role for the dystrophin-glycoprotein complex as a transmembrane linker between laminin and actin. J Cell Biol 1993;122:809-823.
15. Utsunomiya T, Mori H, Shibuya N, et al: Long-term observation of cardiac function in Duchenne's muscular dystrophy: Evaluation using systolic time intervals and echocardiography. Jpn Heart J 1990;31:585-597.
16. Goldberg SJ, Stern LZ, Feldman L, et al: Serial two-dimensional echocardiography in Duchenne muscular dystrophy. Neurology 1982;32:1101-1105.
17. Cohn RD, Durbeej M, Moore SA, et al: Prevention of cardiomyopathy in mouse models lacking the smooth muscle sarcoglycan-sarcospan complex. J Clin Invest 2001;107:R1-7.
18. Towbin JA, Hejtmancik JF, Brink P, et al: X-linked dilated cardiomyopathy: Molecular genetic evidence of linkage to the Duchenne muscular dystrophy (dystrophin) gene at the Xp21 locus. Circulation 1993;87:1854-1865.
19. Mestroni L, Giacca M: Molecular genetics of dilated cardiomyopathy. Curr Opin Cardiol 1997;12:303-309.
20. Ferlini A, Sewry C, Melis MA, et al: X-linked dilated cardiomyopathy and the dystrophin gene. Neuromuscul Disord 1999;9:339-346.
21. Muntoni F, Cau M, Ganau A, et al: Brief report: Deletion of the dystrophin muscle-promoter region associated with X-linked dilated cardiomyopathy. N Engl J Med 1993;329:921-925.
22. Yoshida K, Nakamura A, Yazaki M, et al: Insertional mutation by transposable element, L1, in the DMD gene results in X-linked dilated cardiomyopathy. Hum Mol Genet 1998;7:1129-1132.
23. Milasin J, Muntoni F, Severini GM, et al: A point mutation in the 5′ splice site of the dystrophin gene first intron responsible for X-linked dilated cardiomyopathy. Hum Mol Genet 1996;5:73-79.
24. Muntoni F, Melis MA, Ganau A, Dubowitz V: Transcription of the dystrophin gene in normal tissues and in skeletal muscle of

a family with X-linked dilated cardiomyopathy. Am J Hum Genet 1995;56:151-157.

25. Muntoni F, Wilson L, Marrosu G, et al: A mutation in the dystrophin gene selectively affecting dystrophin expression in the heart. J Clin Invest 1995;96:693-699.

26. Nakamura A, Ikeda S, Yazaki M, et al: Up-regulation of the brain and Purkinje-cell forms of dystrophin transcripts, in Becker muscular dystrophy. Am J Hum Genet 1997;60:1555-1558.

27. Nudel U, Zuk D, Einat P, et al: Duchenne muscular dystrophy gene product is not identical in muscle and brain. Nature 1989; 337:76-78.

28. Bies RD, Maeda M, Roberds SL, et al: A 5′ dystrophin duplication mutation causes membrane deficiency of alpha-dystroglycan in a family with X-linked cardiomyopathy. J Mol Cell Cardiol 1997;29:3175-3188.

29. Franz WM, Cremer M, Herrmann R, et al: X-linked dilated cardiomyopathy: Novel mutation of the dystrophin gene. Ann N Y Acad Sci 1995;752:470-491.

30. Franz WM, Muller M, Muller OJ, et al: Association of nonsense mutation of dystrophin gene with disruption of sarcoglycan complex in X-linked dilated cardiomyopathy. Lancet 2000;355: 1781-1785.

31. Muntoni F, Di Lenarda A, Porcu M, et al: Dystrophin gene abnormalities in two patients with idiopathic dilated cardiomyopathy. Heart 1997;78:608-612.

32. Melis MA, Muntoni F, Cau M, et al: Novel nonsense mutation (C→A nt 10512) in exon 72 of dystrophin gene leading to exon skipping in a patient with a mild dystrophinopathy. Hum Mutat 1998;12(Suppl 1):S137-138.

33. Kaprielian RR, Stevenson S, Rothery SM, et al: Distinct patterns of dystrophin organization in myocyte sarcolemma and transverse tubules of normal and diseased human myocardium. Circulation 2000;101:2586-2594.

34. Klietsch R, Ervasti JM, Arnold W, et al: Dystrophin-glycoprotein complex and laminin colocalize to the sarcolemma and transverse tubules of cardiac muscle. Circ Res 1993;72:349-360.

35. Stevenson S, Rothery S, Cullen MJ, Severs NJ: Dystrophin is not a specific component of the cardiac costamere. Circ Res 1997;80:269-280.

36. Kamogawa Y, Biro S, Maeda M, et al: Dystrophin-deficient myocardium is vulnerable to pressure overload in vivo. Cardiovasc Res 2001;50:509-515.

37. Nakamura A, Harrod GV, Davies KE: Activation of calcineurin and stress activated protein kinase/p38-mitogen activated protein kinase in hearts of utrophin-dystrophin knockout mice. Neuromusc Disord 2001;11:251-259.

38. van der Kooi AJ, de Voogt WG, Barth PG, et al: The heart in limb girdle muscular dystrophy. Heart 1998;79:73-77.

39. Barresi R, Di Blasi C, Negri T, et al: Disruption of heart sarcoglycan complex and severe cardiomyopathy caused by beta sarcoglycan mutations. J Med Genet 2000;37:102-107.

40. Tsubata S, Bowles KR, Vatta M, et al: Mutations in the human delta-sarcoglycan gene in familial and sporadic dilated cardiomyopathy. J Clin Invest 2000;106:655-662.

41. Ettinger AJ, Feng G, Sanes JR: Epsilon-sarcoglycan, a broadly expressed homologue of the gene mutated in limb-girdle muscular dystrophy 2D. J Biol Chem 1997;272:32534-32538.

42. McNally EM, Ly CT, Kunkel LM: Human epsilon-sarcoglycan is highly related to alpha-sarcoglycan (adhalin), the limb girdle muscular dystrophy 2D gene. FEBS Lett 1998;422:27-32.

43. Straub V, Ettinger AJ, Durbeej M, et al: Epsilon-sarcoglycan replaces alpha-sarcoglycan in smooth muscle to form a unique dystrophin-glycoprotein complex. J Biol Chem 1999; 274: 27989-27996.

44. Barresi R, Moore SA, Stolle CA, et al: Expression of γ-sarcoglycan in smooth muscle and its interaction with the sarcoglycan-sarcospan complex. J Biol Chem 2000;275:38554-38560.

45. Duclos F, Straub V, Moore SA, et al: Progressive muscular dystrophy in alpha-sarcoglycan-deficient mice. J Cell Biol 1998;142: 1461-1471.

46. Coral-Vazquez R, Cohn RD, Moore SA, et al: Disruption of the sarcoglycan-sarcospan complex in vascular smooth muscle: A novel mechanism for cardiomyopathy and muscular dystrophy. Cell 1999;98:465-474.

47. Durbeej M, Cohn RD, Moore SA, et al: Disruption of the β-sarcoglycan gene reveals a complex pathogenetic mechanism for LGMD 2E. Mol Cell 2000;5:141-151.

48. Gnecchi-Ruscone T, Taylor J, Mercuri E, et al: Cardiomyopathy in Duchenne, Becker and sarcoglycanopathies: A role for coronary dysfunction? Muscle Nerve 1999;22:1549-1556.

49. Hack AA, Ly CT, Jiang F, et al: Gamma-sarcoglycan deficiency leads to muscle membrane defects and apoptosis independent of dystrophin. J Cell Biol 1998;142:1279-1287.

## EDITOR'S CHOICE

Badorff C, Lee GH, Lamphear BJ, et al: Enteroviral protease 2A cleaves dystrophin: Evidence of cytoskeletal disruption in an acquired cardiomyopathy. Nat Med 1999; 5:320-326.
*Links acquired forms of viral induced cardiomyopathy with genetically based forms of the disease.*

Barton ER, Morris L, Musaro A, et al: Muscle-specific expression of insulin-like growth factor I counters muscle decline in mdx mice. J Cell Biol 2002;157:137-148.
*Raises the concept of growth factor therapy for myopathies.*

Cahill KS, Toma C, Pittenger MF, et al: Cell therapy in the heart: Cell production, transplantation, and applications. Methods Mol Biol 2003;219:73-81.
*Discusses technical issues and challenges regarding cell based therapy in cardiac diseases that include myopathies.*

DelloRusso C, Scott JM, Hartigan-O'Connor D, et al: Functional correction of adult mdx mouse muscle using gutted adenoviral vectors expressing full-length dystrophin. Proc Natl Acad Sci USA 2002;99:12979-12984.
*New, less immunogenic version of adenoviral vectors shows promise for long-term expression, scalability and ease of production remain key issues.*

Helbling-Leclerc A, Bonne G, Schwartz K: Emery-Dreifuss muscular dystrophy. Eur J Hum Genet 2002;10:157-161.
*A wide variety of myopathy and other clinical phenotypes can arise from mutations in a single gene.*

Hoshijima M, Ikeda Y, Iwanaga Y, et al: Chronic suppression of heart-failure progression by a pseudophosphorylated mutant of phospholamban via in vivo cardiac rAAV gene delivery. Nat Med 2002;8:864-871.
*Makes the case for a pivotal role of calcium cycling in heart failure progression and provides pre-clinical validation for AAV mediated delivery of a phospholamban inhibitory peptide as a new therapeutic agent in advanced heart failure.*

Ikeda Y, Gu Y, Iwanaga Y, et al: Restoration of deficient membrane proteins in the cardiomyopathic hamster by in vivo cardiac gene transfer. Circulation 2002;105:502-508.
*Transcoronary high efficiency cardiac gene delivery is feasible in small experimental animals.*

Kawada T, Nakazawa M, Nakauchi S, et al: Rescue of hereditary form of dilated cardiomyopathy by rAAV-mediated somatic gene therapy: Amelioration of morphological findings, sarcolemmal permeability, cardiac performances, and the prognosis of TO-2 hamsters. Proc Natl Acad Sci USA 2002;99:901-906.
*AAV delivery of delta sarcoglycan in small animal model has beneficial effects.*

Wheeler MT, Allikian MJ, Heydemann A, McNally EM: The sarcoglycan complex in striated and vascular smooth muscle. Cold Spring Harb Symp Quant Biol 2002;6:389-397.
*The sarcoglycan complex is expressed in both heart and vascular smooth muscle; the loss of expression heart muscle and associated vasospasm may be key in driving disease progression.*

Xiong D, Lee GH, Badorff C, et al: Dystrophin deficiency markedly increases enterovirus-induced cardiomyopathy: A genetic predisposition to viral heart disease. Nat Med 2002;8:872-877.
*Genetic susceptibility to viral induced heart disease based on deficiency in dystrophin; raises the prospect that a subset of patients with cardiomyopathy and Duchenne's may have coincident viral induced etiology of progressive heart failure.*

# Excitability and Conduction

*Michael J. Ackerman*
*David E. Clapham*

The heart is composed of specialized cell types ranging from sinoatrial nodal pacing cells with few contractile elements to paced ventricular cells packed with contractile muscle protein. The heart must contract continually from the moment the fetal circulatory system is intact (approximately 5 weeks' gestation) until death usually some 70 to 80 years later. Remarkably, the heart accomplishes this feat of providing some 3 billion beats with minimal cell replacement after childhood. The filling and subsequent contraction of atria and ventricle are precisely timed to most efficiently pump blood to the periphery and to respond to increasing or decreasing demands for blood supply. The intrinsic timing devices and distribution network of the heart synchronize this pumping activity. Ion channels comprise a class of proteins ultimately responsible for the generation and orchestration of the electrical signals traversing the beating heart.

Unlike skeletal muscle cells that fuse to produce an electrical syncytium, cardiac cells make electrical continuity via low-resistance intercellular gap junctions. Each individual cell is a small battery with −50 to −90 mV across its plasma membrane (measured from the intracellular space with respect to the bathing solution ground). Depolarization is defined as a change in membrane potential to more positive voltages, whereas hyperpolarization (repolarization) refers to any change to more negative potentials. Rapid voltage changes of large tissue masses in the heart are detected as millivolt size changes in the surface electrocardiogram. P, QRS, and T waves represent atrial depolarization, ventricular depolarization, and ventricular repolarization, respectively. Transmembrane cardiac action potentials form the cellular basis for pacemaker activity, impulse spread, and control of cardiac excitation-contraction coupling. Arising in the SA node and transmitted sequentially throughout the atria, AV node, His-Purkinje system, and the ventricles, the cardiac action potential is a summation of precisely orchestrated openings and closings of distinct populations of ion channels. The molecular blueprints for most of these macromolecular pores that choreograph the heart's rhythm are now known. Cardiac channelopathies are perturbations in ion channel function and/or structural malformations that underlie heritable arrhythmia syndromes.[1-3]

This chapter reviews the current understanding of excitability and conduction as it pertains to the human cardiac action potential. Following a brief overview of basic membrane biology, the ionic currents responsible for nodal and ventricular cell action potentials are detailed. The molecular architecture of ion channels underlying these action potentials is described next. Finally, the key second-messenger-modulated ion channels of the cardiac action potential are summarized.

## THE MEMBRANE POTENTIAL

Cardiocytes are enclosed by an approximately 40-Å-thick bimolecular lipid membrane. This lipid bilayer functions as an excellent electrical insulator, permitting passage of only 1 in 1 trillion ions by simple diffusion through a square centimeter of lipid bilayer. Messages are communicated across the lipid membrane via ion channels, pumps, exchanger proteins, and receptors. The predominant cation inside the cell is $K^+$; $Na^+$ is the predominant cation outside the cell (Fig. 18-1A). Free intracellular $Ca^{2+}$ ($[Ca^{2+}]_i$) is tightly controlled to concentrations of 50 to 100 nM, roughly 20,000-fold less than the concentration in the serum. Chloride anions are 4 to 20 times higher outside the cell than inside the cell. Thus, the extracellular solution is principally NaCl, and the intracellular solution is largely KCl. Transmembrane concentration gradients are maintained by energy-requiring ion pumps and exchangers. The electrogenic $Na^+/K^+$-ATPase pump maintains most of the monovalent cation gradient by transporting three $Na^+$ ions outward and two $K^+$ ions inward per ATP hydrolyzed. Other pumps transport $Ca^{2+}$ in exchange for $Na^+$ or $H+$.

In contrast to energy-requiring transport systems, ion channels allow ions to flow passively down their electrochemical gradients at rates roughly 1000-fold faster than transporters ($10^6$ per second vs. $10^3$ per second). Most ion channels are selectively permeable to one ion species, whereas some are nonselective and allow passage of a variety of cations and/or anions. The conductance of an ion channel quantifies the number of ions and the ease with which ions flow through the channel; it is expressed in units of charge per second per volt. A high-conductance channel allows more ions to flow for a particular driving voltage than does a low-conductance channel. Single-channel conductance γ as distinguished from the membrane conductance (G) of the entire population of channels, is defined as the ratio of single channel current amplitude (*i*) to driving voltage (V):

$$\gamma = \frac{i}{V}$$

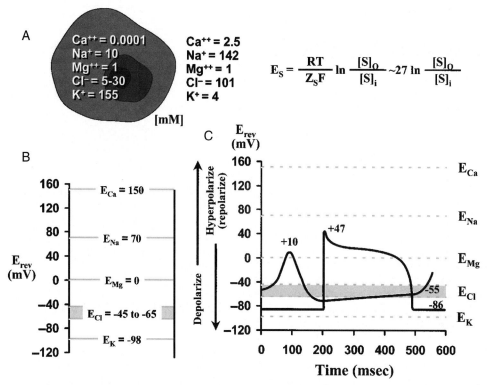

**FIGURE 18-1.** Basic concepts of the membrane potential. *A,* Physiologic ion concentrations for mammalian cells (concentrations in mmol) and the Nernst (equilibrium) equation. *B,* Nernst potentials for ion-selective channels. *C,* SA nodal and ventricular action potentials superimposed on ion channel reversal potentials.

The units of conductance are Siemens (ohms$^{-1}$). The biophysical properties of ion channels have been defined largely through the use of voltage clamp techniques and molecular biology (Fig. 18-2, Tables 18-1 and 18-2). Most ion channels present in cardiac cells have been cloned, and their primary structure is known.

The direction of ion movement through channels is governed by its Nernst equilibrium potential (Fig. 18-1*A*). Suppose a cell membrane contains only K$^+$-selective ion channels; the membrane potential at which no K$^+$ ions flow across the membrane is the equilibrium (Nernst) potential for K$^+$ ($E_K$). Equilibrium occurs when there is no energy difference, either chemical or electrical, for the ion across the membrane. Ions in solution diffuse from regions of high concentration to regions of low concentration, dissipating their chemical energy and achieving the highest entropy. Electrical energy arises from charge separation; transmembrane voltage differences drive charged ions down an electrical gradient. When only K$^+$-selective channels are open in the membrane under physiologic conditions, 155 mmol [K$^+$]$_i$ (inside) and 4 mmol [K$^+$]$_o$ (outside), K$^+$ ions flow down their concentration gradients until there is a slight excess of cations in the dilute solution. The excess K$^+$ ions are driven there by the high concentration gradient across the membrane and are forced to migrate alone by the ion-selectivity filter of the ion channel. The slight excess of positive charge on the outside of the cell creates a negative membrane potential. Equilibrium exists when the electrical forces exactly match and counteract the chemi-

cal forces. Thus, K$^+$ ions flow down their concentration gradient from inside the cell to outside the cell until a sufficient excess of charge develops to repel the excess cations. At this point, when electrical and chemical energy are exactly equal, no net current flows across the membrane, and the K$^+$ ions are at equilibrium ($E_K$). For a purely K$^+$-selective membrane, the Nernst potential is expressed as follows:

$$E_K = \frac{RT}{F}\ln[K]_0 / [K]_i$$

where $R$ is the gas constant, $T$ is the absolute temperature in degrees Kelvin, and $F$ is the Faraday constant. $RT/F$ is approximately 27 mV at body temperature, so that for this example:

$$E_K = 27 \text{ mV ln } (4/155) = -98 \text{ mV}$$

Thus, a cell with only K$^+$-selective channels would have an equilibrium, or resting membrane potential, equal to $-98$ mV.

Given the concentration of ions inside and outside the cells, the selectivity, voltage- and time-dependence, and the numbers of channels in the membrane, the cell's electrical behavior can be predicted. Figure 18-1*B* illustrates the equilibrium potentials for the principal ions. One should remember that, when only one type of ion channel opens, the selected ions flow and drive the cell's membrane potential toward its respective Nernst potential. Therefore, Na$^+$-selective channels permit the passive *influx* of Na$^+$ ions and drive the cell toward $E_{Na}$ (+70 mV). Calcium channels permit the passive *entry* of

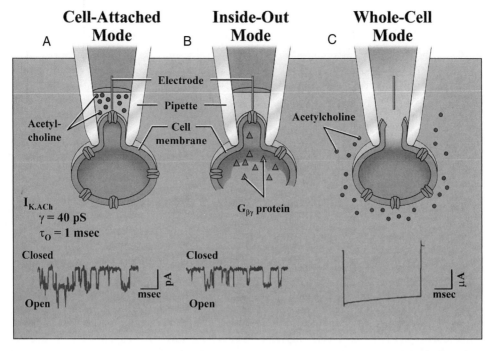

**FIGURE 18-2.** Electrophysiologic and biophysical profile of the cardiac potassium channel $I_{K.ACh}$. *A,* Cell-attached mode. A pipette is pressed tightly against the cell membrane, suction is applied, and a tight seal is formed between pipette and membrane. The seal ensures that the pipette captures current flowing through the channel. In the cell-attached membrane patch, the intracellular contents are undisturbed. Here, acetylcholine in the pipette activates $I_{K.ACh}$, which displays a characteristic open time ($\tau_o$) of 1 msec and a conductance ($\gamma$) of 40 picosiemens. *B,* Inside-out mode. After a cell-attached patch has been formed, the pipette is pulled away from the cell, ripping off a patch of membrane that forms an enclosed vesicle. Brief air exposure disrupts only the free hemisphere of the membrane, leaving the former intracellular surface of the membrane exposed to the bath. Now the milieu of the intracellular surface of the channels can be altered. In this arrangement, addition of purified $G_{\beta\gamma}$ protein to the exposed cytoplasmic surface activates $I_{K.ACh}$. *C,* Whole-cell mode. After formation of a cell-attached patch, a pulse of suction disrupts the membrane circumscribed by the pipette and the entire intracellular space is now accessible to the pipette. Instead of disrupting the patch by suction, a pore-forming molecule, amphotericin B or nystatin, can be incorporated into the intact patch, allowing ionic access to the interior of the cell but maintaining a barrier to larger molecules. In this particular whole-cell arrangement, the net current ($I_{K.ACh}$) after application of acetylcholine is shown. *(From Ackerman M, Clapham D: Mechanisms of disease: Ion channels–basic science and clinical disease. N Engl J Med 1997;336:1575–1586.)*

$Ca^{2+}$ ions into a cell, driving (depolarizing) the cell membrane potential toward $E_{Ca}$ (+150 mV). $K^+$ channels, on the other hand, allow the *efflux* of $K^+$ ions, driving the cell membrane potential toward $E_K$ (−98 mV). Finally, open chloride ion channels clamp the cell's membrane potential to $E_{Cl}$(−45 to −65 mV). Each type of ion channel "pulls" the cellular membrane potential toward its Nernst potential. The membrane potential at any moment is determined by the type of ion channel winning the tug-of-war. As in any tug-of-war, the

■ ■ ■

**TABLE 18-1**  ELECTROPHYSIOLOGY AND PHARMACOLOGY OF INWARD ION CURRENTS IN THE HUMAN CARDIAC ACTION POTENTIAL

| Ion Current | I-V Relationship | Activation Threshold (mV) | Peak Current (mV) | Relative Size $I_x/I_{Na}$ | Time to Peak (msec) | Blockers |
|---|---|---|---|---|---|---|
| $I_f$ | | −100, −35 | −60 | ~0.001 | | Cesium |
| $I_{Na}$ | | −55 | −20 | 1 | 1 | Tetrodotoxin (weak), cadmium, zinc<br>Class IA; quinidine, procainamide IB: lidocaine, tocainide, mexiletine IC: encainide, flecainide, propafenone |
| $I_{Ca.T}$ | | −50 | −20 | 0.004 | | Nickel, mibefradil (endothelin-1, activator) |
| $I_{Ca.L}$ | | −30 | +10 | 0.02 | ~3-5 | DHP (nifedipine)<br>Benzothiazepine (diltiazem)<br>Phenylalkylamines (verapamil) (BayK 8644, activator) |
| $I_{Na/Ca}$ | | 100 nM $[Ca]_i$<br>1 μM $[Ca]_i$ | | 0.003 | | |

■ ■ ■

**TABLE 18-2** ELECTROPHYSIOLOGY AND PHARMACOLOGY OF OUTWARD ION CURRENTS IN THE HUMAN CARDIAC ACTION POTENTIAL

| Ion Current | I-V Relationship | Activation Threshold (mV) | Peak Current (mV) | Relative Size $I_x/I_{Na}$ | Time to Peak (msec) | Blockers |
|---|---|---|---|---|---|---|
| $I_{to,fast}$ | | −75 | >0 | 0.03 | 5-10 | 4-AP, Quinidine, TEA, Terfenadine |
| $I_{Cl,Ca}$ | | | >0 | <0.001 | | SITS, DIDS, $Mn^{2+}$, Caffeine, Ryanodine |
| $I_{Kr}$ | | −40 | >0 $[K]_o$ dependent | 0.007 | >500 | E-4031, sotalol, propafenone, quinidine, UK-68, 798, dofetilide, clofilium, almokalant |
| $I_{Ks}$ | | −40 | >0 | 0.03 | >1000 | (−) E-4031, Clofilium, Amiodarone, NE 10064 |
| $I_{Kur}$ | | −30 | >0 | — | ~10 | 4-AP, Quinidine, Terfenadine, (−) TEA |
| $I_{K1}$ | | Always on | −75 $[K]_o$ dependent | 0.009 | Instantaneous | TEA, cesium, barium RP58866, RP62719, LY97241, LY97119, propafenone |

winners are on the side with the strongest (highest conductance) and/or the most numerous pullers. These four selective ion channel populations (plus one non-selective type) are responsible for the generation of the SA nodal and ventricular action potentials displayed in Figure 18-1C.

Armed with this basic understanding, several features of the cardiac action potential can be appreciated intuitively. First, because resting potentials are closest to $E_K$, the highest permeability of cardiac membranes at rest must be to $K^+$ ions. There must be a greater number of $K^+$ channels activated at rest in the ventricular myocyte than in the nodal cell to maintain the ventricular cell in a more hyperpolarized state (more negative, closer to $E_K$). Second, the ventricular myocyte depolarizes (moves toward positive potentials) much more quickly than nodal cells, suggesting that faster, more numerous depolarizing channels are present in the ventricle. Third, only $Na^+$ or $Ca^{2+}$ channels can drive a cell to membrane potentials above 0 mV. Fourth, there must be a balanced tug-of-war between depolarizing and repolarizing ion channels to account for the long plateau of the cardiac action potential. With this background, the specific biophysical fingerprints and the molecular blueprints of the ion channels responsible for the cardiac action potential are now examined (Tables 18-1 to 18-4).

## THE CARDIAC ACTION POTENTIAL IN THE NODAL SYSTEM AND THE MYOCARDIUM

### General Features

Cardiac action potentials have strikingly longer durations (200 to 400 msec) than either nerve or muscle (1 to 5 msec). The long plateau phase around 0 mV provides the sustained depolarization and contraction needed to empty the heart's chambers. Figure 18-3A shows the action potentials recorded from different parts of an adult heart.[1,2,4-6] Heart tissue is both electrically and mechanically specialized. The SA node, for example, consists of cells with very few contractile elements and a relatively simple action potential. As the pacemaker cells controlling the rate and rhythm of the beating heart, SA and AV nodal cells have ever-changing membrane potentials. In contrast, ventricular cells are packed with contractile elements and have more complex, triggered action potentials. The heart has its own independent rhythm. When removed from nervous system innervation and transplanted into another body, the heart continues to beat rhythmically. Nerves modulate the rate and rhythm of the heart but do not initiate or have fundamental control over heart rate.

The SA node membrane potential dips to −50 to −60 mV during diastole (Fig. 18-1C and 18-3A and B) but has no stable resting potential. After repolarization, the transmembrane potential depolarizes slowly and spontaneously. This pacemaker depolarization underlies the automaticity of sinus cells and is recorded from all specialized cardiac fibers capable of normal pacemaker activity. The rate of rise of the upstroke of the action potential is slow (1 to 10 V/sec) in SA nodal cells, resulting in slow propagation of the impulse (<0.05 m/sec). In the atria, the upstroke is rapid (100 to 200 V/sec) from the steady resting potential (~−90 mV). The peak of the action potential occurs around +40 mV, and the action potential propagates at 0.3 to 0.4 m/sec (~10 times faster than the nodal system). AV nodal action potentials are intermediate between the SA nodal and atrial action potentials. Slow conduction in the AV node is the result of a low rate of rise of the action potential and weak electrical coupling between AV nodal cells. When the SA node has been disabled either by congenital abnormalities or by the aging process, the AV node can take over as the primary pacemaker. From the AV node, the impulse spreads through the His-Purkinje system. In all remaining fibers of the heart, from the common bundle to ventricular muscle, the upstroke of the action potential is rapid (100 to 700 V/sec), and the action potential duration is long (200 to 500 msec).

**TABLE 18-3**    MOLECULAR ARCHITECTURE OF HUMAN CARDIAC ION CHANNELS (INWARD CURRENTS)

| Ion Current | Candidate Gene(s) | Gene Symbol | Chromosome Locus | Amino Acids (no.) | Channelopathy |
|---|---|---|---|---|---|
| $I_f/I_h$ | $I_{f,fast}$ | HCN2 | 19p13.3 | 889 | – |
| | $I_{f,slow}$ | HCN4 | 15q24-q25 | 1203 | – |
| $I_{Na}$ | $\alpha = Na_v\, 1.5$ | SCN5A | 3p21 | 2015 | + |
| | + $\beta1 = Na_v\, \beta1.1$ | SCN1B | 19q13.1 | 218 | – |
| $I_{Ca.T}$ | $\alpha1H = Ca_v\, T.2$ | CACNA1H | 16p13.3 | 2353 | – |
| $I_{Ca.L}$ (DHPR) | $\alpha1C = Ca_v\, 1.2$ | CACNA1C | 12p13.3 | 2157 | – |
| | + $\beta_{1-4}$ | CACNB1-4 | 17q/10p12/12q13/2q22 | – | |
| | + $\alpha2/\delta$ | CACNA2D1 | 7q21-q22 | 1091 | – |
| $I_{Na/Ca}$ | Na-Ca exchanger | NCX1 (SLC8A1) | 2p21-p23 | 973 | – |
| CRC | Ryanodine receptor | RyR2 | 1q42.1-q43 | 4967 | + |
| | + FK506 binding protein | FKBP12.6 (FKBP1B) | 2p25.1 | 108 | – |

**TABLE 18-4**    MOLECULAR ARCHITECTURE OF HUMAN CARDIAC ION CHANNELS (OUTWARD CURRENTS)

| Ion Current | Candidate Gene(s) | Gene Symbol | Chromosome Locus | Amino Acids (no.) | Channelopathy |
|---|---|---|---|---|---|
| $I_{to,slow}$ | ± Kv1.4 | KCNA4 | 11p14 | 653 | – |
| | hKvβ3 | KCNAB1 | 3q26.1 | 401 | – |
| $I_{to,fast}$ | Kv4.2 | KCND2 | 7q31 | 629 | – |
| | ± MiRP1 | KCNE2 | 21q22.12 | 123 | + |
| | ± KChIP2 | KCNIP2 | 10q24 | 252 | – |
| | or Kv4.3 | KCND3 | 1p13.2 | 656 | – |
| $I_{Kr}$ | + HERG | KCNH2 | 7q35-q36 | 1159 | + |
| | MiRP1 | KCNE2 | 21q22.12 | 123 | + |
| $I_{Ks}$ | + KvLQT1 | KCNQ1 | 11p15.5 | 676 | + |
| | MinK | KCNE1 | 21q22.12 | 129 | + |
| $I_{Kur}$ | Kv1.5 | KCNA5 | 12p13 | 611 | – |
| $I_{K1}$ | Kir2.1 | KCNJ2 | 17q23.1-q24.2 | 427 | + |

Under normal conditions, ventricular cells do not undergo pacemaker depolarization but have resting membrane potentials (−86 mV) close to $E_K$. Tissue-specific shapes of the action potential are shown in Figure 18-3$A$. The impulse must spread rapidly through-out the myocardium and at the same time allow enough delay between impulses so that all fibers in the tissue have time to contract. Atrial and ventricular action potentials provide the time needed to wring the blood from their respective chambers.

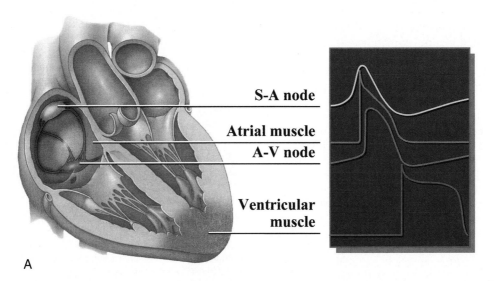

**S-A node**

**Atrial muscle**

**A-V node**

**Ventricular muscle**

A

**FIGURE 18-3.** The human cardiac action potential. $A$, Action potentials recorded from different parts of the heart.

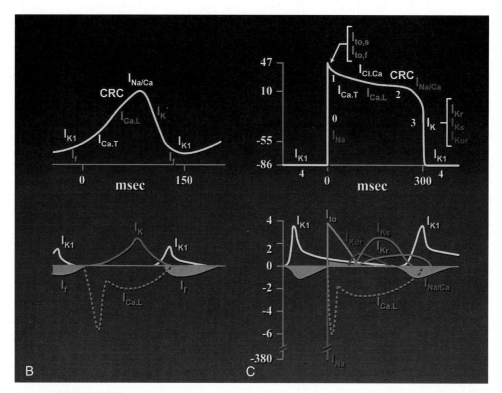

**FIGURE 18-3, cont'd** *B,* Principal currents responsible for the SA nodal *(left)* and ventricular *(right)* action potential. Note that $I_{Kur}$ is depicted here although it is predominantly present in atrial rather than ventricular myocytes. Time is depicted on the x-axis, and voltage (mV) on the y-axis. *C,* Model of the magnitude and duration of the principal currents in the generation of the SA nodal and ventricular action potentials. Here, magnitude of current in microamps/microfarad is depicted on the y-axis.

## Conduction

To efficiently pump blood, the heart tissue must maximize conduction of the action potential from pacing cells throughout the atrial and ventricular cells. The velocity with which the action potential spreads throughout the tissue is regulated by the speed of the upstroke of the action potential, the degree of insulation of individual heart cells (membrane resistance), and the conductivity between heart cells through gap junctions (Fig. 18-4). The upstroke of the action potential is much like that of nerve; large numbers of fast opening Na+-selective channels rapidly depolarize the membrane potential to approximately +50 mV. Calcium is needed for contraction and $Ca^{2+}$ entry is maximal around the peak of the L-type $Ca^{2+}$ selective ion channel's $(I_{Ca.L})$ current-voltage (I-V) relation. The rapid repolarization by the transient outward $(I_{to})$ K+ and Cl⁻ currents brings the action potential back to the start of the plateau around 0 mV, where the $Ca^{2+}$ current is largest. The second major parameter that limits conduction speed is the intercellular resistance, which in cardiac cells is largely determined by gap junctions between cells. The cardiac gap junction proteins (connexins) link across cells to form cell-to-cell channels of low resistance and selectivity.[7,8] Cardiac connexins (connexin40, connexin43, and connexin45) can close under adverse conditions, isolating cells from one another. Because cardiac muscle is not a true syncytium like skeletal muscle, individual cells are, in a sense, wired individually into the conduction system. This

may protect healthy myocardium from rogue or damaged cells. These mutinous cells can be set adrift by the closure of their gap junction channels (gap junction remodeling). Unfortunately, this mechanism may also underlie fibrillation in which islands of tissue become independent from pacemaking currents.

## Sinoatrial Nodal Action Potential

Figure 18-3*B* displays the 6 principal ion currents that underlie the nodal action potential and the 10

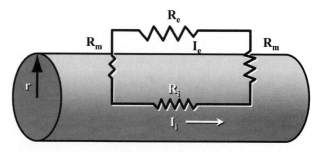

**Conduction velocity is proportional to** $R_m$, r, $\dfrac{dV}{dt}$, $\dfrac{I}{Ri}$, $\dfrac{I}{Re}$

**FIGURE 18-4.** Basic cable theory. Conduction velocity down an ideal cylindrical conductor will be faster for lower internal (large radii, r) and external resistances, higher membrane resistance (few open ion channels), and faster action potential upstroke velocities. These general principles also hold true for other tissue geometries.

predominant ion currents that orchestrate the myocardial action potential. Properties of these inward and outward conductances are summarized in Tables 18-1 and 18-2. The SA node is paced by the $I_f$ (f for *funny*) current (also known as the hyperpolarization-activated current [$I_h$] or human cyclic nucleotide-gated [HCN]) and by decreased opposition to depolarization by the inwardly rectifying $K^+$ conductance $I_{K1}$.[9] The designation *funny* current stemmed from its particularly unique property of slow activation on hyperpolarization. $I_f$ is a nonselective inward current that is *inactive* at depolarized potentials at which the action potentials are firing; however, $I_f$ is *activated* by hyperpolarization to the pacing range of potentials (–80 to –30 mV). Activation of $I_f$ drives the membrane potential toward $E_f$ (–20 mV; Fig. 18-3C). Thus, negative to its equilibrium voltage, $I_f$ permits both $K^+$ and sodium into the cell, slowly depolarizing the membrane potential, and deactivates on continued depolarization (Table 18-1). $I_f$ is opposed by $I_{K1}$, resulting in a slow but carefully timed pacemaker depolarization to –40 mV In addition, cAMP causes a positive shift in the current-voltage relationship and accelerates channel activation of $I_f$, in part accounting for the adrenaline-mediated increase in heart rate.[10]

At –40 mV, $Ca^{2+}$ channels begin to open, and the membrane is depolarized more rapidly. The slow upstroke of the action potential in nodal cells results from a relative lack of $Na^+$ channels and dependence of depolarization on the fewer, slower, inward $Ca^{2+}$ channels. Even if $Na^+$ channels were present, they would become inactivated by the depolarized resting membrane potentials of the SA node and, therefore, unable to participate significantly in depolarization. The first $Ca^{2+}$ current to activate is the transient $Ca^{2+}$ current $I_{Ca.T}$.[11] $I_{Ca.T}$ drives the cell's membrane potential toward $E_{Ca}$ and in the process triggers the activation of the L-type voltage-activated $Ca^{2+}$ current ($I_{Ca.L}$) at –30 mV. Properties of these two inward $Ca^{2+}$ currents are described in more detail in the section on the ventricular action potential. Almost simultaneous with the activation of these inward currents, competing outwardly conducting delayed rectifying $K^+$ currents ($I_K$) are triggered at membrane potentials depolarized to –40 mV (Fig. 18-3C). The result is again a tug-of-war between the inward conductances ($I_{Ca.T}$, $I_{Ca.L}$, and $I_{Na/Ca}$; collectively the forces of depolarization) and the outwardly conducting (hyperpolarizing) $K^+$ currents $I_K$. The balance is reached at a peak depolarization of +10 mV before the outward $K^+$ current $I_K$ slowly overcomes the inward currents, is joined by $I_{K1}$, and repolarizes the cell back toward $E_K$.

As the membrane potential is driven hyperpolarized to –35 mV, $I_f$ is activated again and $I_K$ turns off. Thus, the membrane potential never reaches $E_K$. Instead, the depolarizing $I_f$ pacemaker current gains the upper hand and slowly depolarizes the membrane potential away from the maximum diastolic potential. The inwardly rectifying behavior of $I_{K1}$ contributes significantly to this pacemaking activity. $I_{K1}$ has an unusual property: in the physiologic range of membrane potentials (above $E_K$), the net outward current has a negatively sloped I-V relation (negative conductance). Thus, $I_{K1}$ becomes smaller and smaller with depolarization (Table 18-2). $I_{K1}$ is not very time-dependent and does not inactivate significantly. If $I_{K1}$ were the only channel opening between –90 and –60 mV, any depolarization induced by an inward current of any kind would result in *less* outward current. In essence, the membrane potential is unstable and is driven in the depolarizing direction. The inward rectification of $I_{K1}$ ensures that a small inward current results in pacemaker depolarization. The reader is referred to an excellent review on cardiac pacemaking in the SA node by Irisawa et al.[9]

## Ventricular Action Potential

Figure 18-3 and Tables 18-1 and 18-2 summarize the key features of the 10 predominant currents involved in the generation of the ventricular myocardial action potential. Traditionally, this action potential has been divided into five phases: phase 0, action potential upstroke or rapid depolarization; phase 1, early phase of repolarization; phase 2, the plateau; phase 3, the late phase of rapid repolarization; and phase 4, resting membrane potential and diastolic depolarization.[2,4,6]

### Phase 0: Action Potential Upstroke, or Rapid Depolarization

In ventricular cardiocytes, the membrane potential at rest remains near $E_K$. Activation from pacemaker cells via the conduction system can stimulate another action potential. An excitatory stimulus or pacemaker potential that depolarizes the cell membrane beyond its threshold potential (~–70 mV) triggers an intricately woven cascade of channel openings and closings that generates the ventricular action potential shown in Figure 18-3B. The fast upstroke in atrial and ventricular cells is accomplished by $Na^+$ channels ($I_{Na}$). Once the threshold potential of –70 mV is reached, $Na^+$ channels are activated, resulting in an enormous (>–380 microamps/microfarad) albeit brief (<5 msec) inward $Na^+$ current. $I_{Na}$ is 50 to 1000 times larger in net conductance than any other population of ion channels. The depolarizing current carried by the influx of sodium drives the cell toward $E_{Na}$. More $Na_+$ channels are opened as the current peaks at –20 mV, producing the regenerative depolarization responsible for the propagation of the cardiac action potential.

As stated earlier, the increase in $Na^+$ conductance, although enormous, is short-lived (<5msec) because the $Na^+$ channels are inactivated as a function of time and voltage. Inactivation causes the current to shut down almost as quickly as it turns on. The rapidity whereby $Na^+$ channels recover from their voltage- and time-dependent inactivation is a key determinant of the refractory period of the ventricle (Fig. 18-5). Thus, the upstroke peaks at approximately +47 mV, short of the $Na^+$ equilibrium potential. The maximum upstroke velocity ($V_{max}$) reflects the density of $I_{Na}$. $I_{Na}$ is the major determinant of the velocity of impulse conduction throughout the ventricle. All the class I antiarrhythmics (e.g., quinidine [IA], lidocaine [IB], and encainide [IC]) block $I_{Na}$, thus slowing the conduction velocity and prolonging the action potential duration (IC agents can

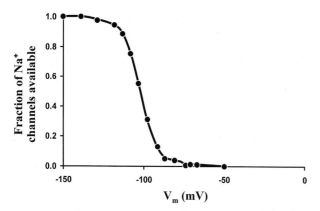

**FIGURE 18-5.** $I_{Na}$ channel activation and the membrane potential. The percentage of activatable sodium channels sharply decreases as the steady-state membrane potential ($E_m$) becomes more depolarized. For damaged or depolarized cardiac cells, lower membrane potentials will inactivate the sodium channels, thereby slowing action potential upstroke velocity and conduction of the cardiac impulse.

shorten the action potential duration (APD); see Table 18-1). Some agents, like quinidine, also block $K^+$ channels to prolong the action potential plateau. Reducing the amplitude and maximum upstroke velocity $V_{max}$ of the action potential upstroke may slow ventricular conduction too far, even to the point of arrhythmogenesis.

### Phase 1: Early Phase of Repolarization

Figure 18-3$C$ shows the predicted amplitude and time course of the ionic currents that underlie the cardiac action potential.[5] The threshold-dependent activation of $I_{Na}$ quickly depolarizes the membrane to the levels of activation of both inward $Ca^{2+}$ currents and outward $K^+$ currents. The $Ca^{2+}$ currents are substantially smaller than fully activated $I_{Na}$, but they also pull the membrane potential to very positive potentials. The final result (Fig. 18-3$B$) is that the upstroke terminates around +47 mV before reaching $E_{Na}$, followed by a phase of rapid repolarization to +10 mV. This phase 1 repolarization is a consequence of the rapid voltage-dependent inactivation of $I_{Na}$; the activation of the $Ca^{2+}$-independent transient outward $K^+$ current ($I_{to}$)[12]; and the activation of a second type of transient outward current ($I_{to2}$), the $Ca^{2+}$-activated chloride current $I_{Cl.Ca}$.[13]

Two kinetic variants of cardiac $I_{to}$ have been identified: fast $I_{to}$ ($I_{to'f}$) and slow $I_{to}$ ($I_{to's}$).[12] $I_{to}$ activates almost simultaneously at the threshold potential (−70 mV), reaching its peak current within 5 to 10 msec. However, $I_{to}$ carries approximately only 3% of the current carried by the depolarizing $Na^+$ current. $I_{to}$ is a $K^+$-selective channel blocked by 4-aminopyridine, tetraethylammonium (TEA), and terfenadine. $I_{to'f}$ is distinguished from $I_{to's}$ on the basis of relatively "fast" inactivation (25 to 80 msec vs. 80 to 200 msec) and recovery from inactivation (25 to 80 msec vs. 1 to 2 seconds), respectively. Notably, this current contributes outward current (efflux of $K^+$) well into the plateau (phase 2) of the action potential, markedly affecting the magnitude of the L-type $Ca^{2+}$ current and thereby modulating excitation-contraction and myocardial contractility (Fig. 18-3$C$). This modulatory

effect is dynamic throughout the myocardium because of the striking regional differences in the expression of $I_{to'f}$ and $I_{to's}$ current with fivefold greater $I_{to}$ currents in epicardial layers compared with endocardial layers.[14] In general, regions of the heart manifesting a longer APD (septum, LV endocardium, LV apex) display preferential expression of $I_{to,s}$, whereas $I_{to,f}$ expression predominates in the epicardial cells, right ventricle, and base of the heart.[15] Heterogeneous $I_{to}$ expression not only accounts for regional variations in the action potential but also tunes repolarization throughout the ventricle and may enable regional modulation of cardiac contractility.[16,17] Much less is known regarding the contribution of the 4-aminopyridine-insensitive, transient outward chloride current ($I_{Cl.Ca}$) to the human cardiac action potential. This current is small compared with $I_{to}$; is carried by chloride; activated by $Ca^{2+}$; and suppressed by manganese, caffeine, and ryanodine.[13]

### Phase 2: Action Potential Plateau

The plateau of the cardiac action potential is a unique feature of cardiac cells. Strikingly few channels are open during the plateau, and, thus, the total membrane conductance is low. The high resistance of the membrane during the plateau insulates the cardiac cells and allows rapid propagation of the action potential with little dissipation. The plateau phase is maintained by a finely tuned balance between two types of inward $Ca^{2+}$ currents and at least four types of outward $K^+$ currents (Fig. 18-3$B$ and $C$). Only a few hundred channels per cell are used to maintain this fine balance. Ultimately, $K^+$ channels dominate and the membrane potential is driven back toward $E_K$.

During the plateau, two distinct $Ca^{2+}$ currents, the low–voltage-activated, transient $Ca^{2+}$ current ($I_{Ca,T}$, T-type) and the high–voltage-activated, long-lasting $Ca^{2+}$ current ($I_{Ca,L}$, L-type), admit the $Ca^{2+}$ needed to initiate contraction.[18,19] Less is known about the contribution of the transient $Ca^{2+}$ current to the ventricular action potential[20] in comparison to its role as a slow depolarizing force in pacemaking cells.[11] In the normal heart, T-type $Ca^{2+}$ channels are found predominantly in atrial pacemaker cells, Purkinje fibers, and coronary artery smooth muscle. T-type $Ca^{2+}$ channels rapidly activate at approximately −50 mV, peak at −20 mV, inactivate with time, are blocked by nickel but are insensitive to dihydropyridines, and are selectively inhibited by a novel tetralol $Ca^{2+}$ channel blocker mibefradil (Table 18-1). $I_{Ca,T}$ is only one fifth of the size of $I_{Ca,L}$ (~0.3 microamps/microfarad density). Consequently, T-type $Ca^{2+}$ currents are expected to contribute relatively little to the $Ca^{2+}$ influx necessary for excitation-contraction coupling. For this reason, selective blockade of T-type $Ca^{2+}$ channels with mibefradil may be useful in the treatment of hypertension, angina pectoris, and heart failure without impeding cardiac inotropy.[21]

In contrast to $I_{Ca,T}$, the L-type $Ca^{2+}$ current ($I_{Ca,L}$) is the dominant $Ca^{2+}$ current found in virtually all cardiac cells in all species.[22] $I_{Ca,L}$ is activated at −30 mV; reaches its peak conductance at +10 mV within 3 to 5 msec; inactivates very slowly (hundred of milliseconds); and is sensitive to block by dihydropyridines (nifedipine), benzothiazepines (diltiazem), and phenylalkylamines (verapamil).[23] These channels carry inward current throughout the plateau phase and are crucial for coupling membrane excitability to myocardial contraction.

The terminal portion of the plateau is sustained by inward current through the electrogenic $Na^+/Ca^{2+}$ exchanger because $Ca^{2+}$ is transported out of the cell (Fig. 18-3C) at a ratio of one $Ca^{2+}$ ion per three $Na^+$ ions.[24] This electrogenic current (net charge transfer) is capable of providing inward current up to 50% of the size of $I_{Ca,L}$. During the action potential upstroke, the exchanger brings in $Ca^{2+}$ ions, increasing contractility. As the chief means of extruding $Ca^{2+}$ ions, the exchanger also modulates $[Ca^{2+}]_i$ and thus the $Ca^{2+}$ content of the sarcoplasmic reticulum.[25,26]

### Phase 3: Final Rapid Repolarization

Competing with the inward currents are at least four distinct populations of $K^+$ channels activated during the plateau phase (Fig. 18-3B and C). As the time-dependent inward currents inactivate, the outward $K^+$ currents (mostly $I_K$) rapidly drive the membrane potential toward $E_K$, thus repolarizing the cell.[2,27] However, these channels are unable to drive the cell completely to $E_K$ because they deactivate at membrane potentials less than −40 mV.

Delayed rectifying $K^+$ currents ($I_K$), consist of at least three distinct populations of $K^+$ channels: $I_{Kr}$ (rapid), $I_{Ks}$(slow), and $I_{Kur}$ (ultra-rapid), distinguished biophysically by their activation kinetics and pharmacologically by their sensitivity to class III antiarrhythmics (Table 18-2).[15,28,29] Rapidly activating $I_K$ ($I_{Kr}$) reaches its peak within 500 msec. Although an increase in $[K^+]_o$ decreases the electrochemical driving force, extracellular $K^+$ also directly increases $I_{Kr}$ by binding at the pore and relieving the partial block imposed by extracellular $Na^+$.[15] The much larger $I_{Ks}$ requires seconds to reach its peak and is insensitive to E-4031. $I_{Kur}$, the most recently described human cardiac $I_K$ subtype, is more abundant in atria than in ventricle and activates 50 times faster than $I_{Kr}$.[30] $I_{Kr}$ is insensitive to TEA but quite sensitive to 4-aminopyridine. $I_{Kur}$ is distinguished from the 4-aminopyridine-sensitive transient outward $K^+$ current ($I_{to}$) by limited slow inactivation, insensitivity to TEA, and 40-fold greater sensitivity to 4-aminopyridine. Selective inhibition of $I_{Kur}$ with 50-fM 4-aminopyridine prolongs the atrial action potential duration by nearly 70%, suggesting that $I_{Kur}$ plays a major role in phase 3 repolarization of the atrial action potential.[30]

### Phase 4: Resting Membrane Potential and Diastolic Depolarization

The delayed rectifying $K^+$ channels repolarize the membrane potential to approximately −40 mV, where the various $I_K$ currents deactivate. The inward rectifier $I_{K1}$, on the other hand, does not inactivate with time and ensures continued repolarization (see Fig. 18-3C). During most of repolarization, the heart cell cannot be triggered to fire another action potential (the absolute refractory period) because $Na^+$ channels remain inactivated. The voltage-dependent inactivation of $Na^+$ channels is a major mechanism for prevention of repetitive early firing and only hyperpolarization below approximately −70 mV can reprime $Na^+$ channels for activation.

Inward rectifier $K^+$ currents such as $I_{K1}$ are named for their ability to conduct $K^+$ more readily in the inward direction. This property is a consequence of the block of outward $K^+$ currents by intracellular magnesium and polyamines.[31] Physiologically, $I_{K1}$ current is always outward. Because $I_{K1}$ predominantly sets the membrane potential, raising $[K^+]_o$ shifts the resting membrane potential to more depolarized potentials. At both low and high $[K^+]_o$ concentrations, the membrane potential is depolarized compared with that in 4 mm $[K^+]_o$. Depolarization by high $[K^+]_o$ is explained by the shift of $E_K$ and its effect on $I_{K1}$. At low $[K^+]_o$, the Na/K-ATPase pump is slowly starved for $K^+$ substrate, $[K^+]_i$, falls, and again $E_K$ is shifted in the depolarized direction. Maintenance of serum $K^+$ levels in the 3.5- to 5-mmol range is crucial to prevention of cardiac arrhythmias. Outside this range, heart cells are depolarized. Depolarization enhances pacing currents, decreases the size of $Na^+$ and $Ca^{2+}$ currents through inactivation, and has broad effects on action potential duration.[15]

## Summary of the Cardiac Action Potential

By understanding the basic electrophysiology of the heart cell, the effects of antiarrhythmic agents on the heart can be appreciated more readily. Most class I antiarrhythmics block $I_{Na}$, decrease the speed and amplitude of upstroke, and thereby slow conduction velocity (decrease $V_{max}$) and prolong the action potential. Class IV antiarrhythmics ($Ca^{2+}$ channel blockers) delay conduction in $Ca^{2+}$ current-dependent cells by blocking currents contributing to the nodal upstroke. They also shorten the action potential duration in the atria and ventricle by decreasing the inward currents during the plateau. Class III antiarrhythmics targeting the delayed rectifier $K^+$ currents prolong the cardiac action potential by decreasing phase 3 repolarization and thereby terminate some reentry mechanisms. However, class III drugs are also potentially proarrhythmic because they prolong QT intervals and induce *torsades de pointes*.

The impact of disease processes on cardiac excitability by altering $K^+$ homeostasis can be anticipated intuitively. With hyperkalemia, the fast upstroke is slowed as a result of cell depolarization and the resulting partial inactivation of $Na^+$ channels at depolarized potentials (Fig. 18-5). In addition, the plateau is shortened because of increased $K^+$ currents (augmented $I_{Kr}$) and reduced $Ca^{2+}$ currents. Moderate hypokalemia slightly prolongs the action potential because of smaller plateau $K^+$ currents and decreased $I_{Kr}$.

## MOLECULAR ARCHITECTURE OF THE CARDIAC ACTION POTENTIAL

The preceding section described the ion currents that underlie the cardiac action potential. Over the past 10 years, the field of molecular cardiac electrophysiology has exploded as the proteins comprising ion channels have been discovered. Most of the principal ion channels have been cloned, and their structural design is being unraveled (Figs. 18-6 to 18-8). Molecular approaches to arrhythmogenesis using rational drug design and gene therapy are on the horizon. This section reviews some of the basic architectural features of cardiac ion channels (Figs. 18-6 and 18-7) and assigns the ionic conductances of the cardiac action potential to cloned proteins (Fig. 18-8 and Tables 18-3 and 18-4).

## Basic Ion Channel Design

The reader is referred to Chapter 1 to review general principles pertaining to molecular cloning strategies such as DNA hybridization screening and antibody immunoscreening. However, a brief review of expression cloning is warranted because most ion channel proteins were originally discovered or functionally assayed with this technique.[32] Oocytes from *Xenopus laevis* toads are large (1 mm) and can be injected easily with exogenous mRNA. In expression cloning, *in vitro* transcripts from a cDNA library derived from a source of tissue or cells known to be rich in a particular current are injected into individual oocytes. The proteins encoded by this library are allowed several days to be translated and processed before the oocyte currents are measured by voltage clamp techniques. The DNA library (with ~1 million unique clones) is serially subdivided until injected messenger RNA from a single cDNA clone that confers novel ion channel activity is isolated. Moreover, mutant clones with engineered alterations in the protein's primary structure can be expressed and the ion channel properties can be studied to implicate regions of the protein critical for channel activation, channel inactivation, ion permeation (the pore), and sites of drug interactions. Expression cloning and site-directed mutagenesis can also be accomplished by transfection of mammalian cell lines.

Figure 18-6*A* depicts the predicted transmembrane topology for a voltage-gated $K^+$ channel. Regions responsible for specific activities are highlighted.[1,2,33] The building blocks for most voltage-gated channel proteins are individual subunits or domains of subunits each containing six hydrophobic transmembrane regions labeled S1 through S6. The $Na^+$ and $Ca^{2+}$ channels are single $\alpha$ subunits comprised of four repeats of the six transmembrane-spanning domain motif. Voltage-gated $K^+$ channels ($K_v$; nomenclature refers to K channel, voltage-dependent) are encoded by a tetramer of *separate* six transmembrane-spanning motifs. Coassembly of the linked domains forms the central pore and confers the basic gating and permeation properties characteristic of the channel type. The peptide chain (H5 or P loop) juxtaposed between the membrane spanning segments S5

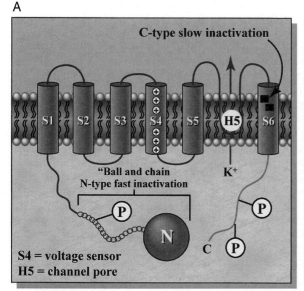
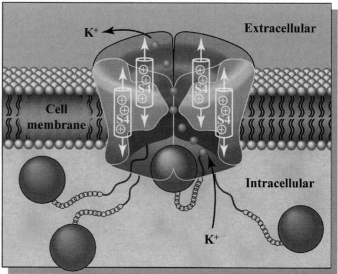

**FIGURE 18-6.** General ion channel architecture. *A,* Linear topology of voltage-gated potassium channel. Displayed is a six transmembrane-spanning motif, S1 through S6, that forms the core structure of sodium, calcium, and potassium channels. The ball and chain structure at the N-terminal portion of the protein is a region that participates in N-type "fast inactivation," occluding the ion selectivity filter. The circles containing *plus* signs in S4, the voltage sensor, are positively charged lysine and arginine residues. Critical residues responsible for the channel's ion selectivity filter/pore (H5) reside between S5 and S6. The genes for sodium and calcium channels encode a protein containing four repeats of this basic subunit, whereas the genes for voltage-activated potassium channels (Kv) encode a protein with only a single subunit. The genes for Kir channels encode a simplified subunit structure containing only the H5 (pore) loop juxtaposed between two transmembrane-spanning segments denoted M1 and M2 (similar to S5 and S6). *B,* Three-dimensional schematic of a cardiac potassium channel. Four such subunits (from panel A) assemble to form the tetrameric, voltage-gated potassium channel. Here, the pore region depicted here is based on data using high-affinity scorpion toxins and their structures (as determined by nuclear magnetic resonance imaging) as molecular calipers.[39] The pore region appears to have "wide" intracellular and extracellular vestibules (approximately 2.8 to 3.4 nm wide and 0.4 to 0.8 nm deep) that lead to a constricted pore 0.9 to 1.4 nm in diameter at its entrance, tapering to a diameter of 0.4 to 0.5 nm at a depth of 0.5 to 0.7 nm from the external vestibule. *(From Ackerman M, Clapham D: Mechanisms of disease: Ion channels–basic science and clinical disease. N Engl J Med 1997;336:1575–1586.)*

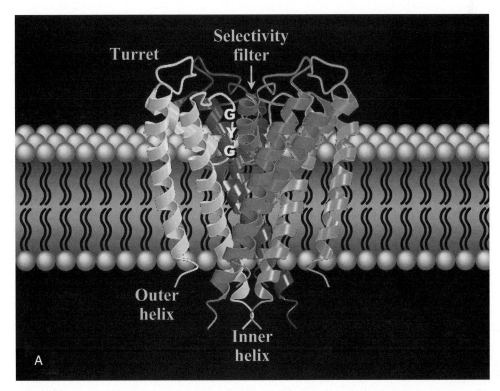

**FIGURE 18-7.** Molecular architecture and crystallographic structure of the KcsA bacterial potassium channel. *A,* Major functional features revealed by the 3.5-å resolution structure of the *Streptomyces lividans* K+-selective channel. The selectivity filter at the top with the signature GYG sequence excludes Na+ and divalent ions. Carbonyl oxygens from amino acids in the narrowest region of the pore substitute the H₂O molecules surrounding the K+ ion. The central cavity K+ ion's charge is stabilized in the polar environment by surrounding water molecules and by the four helical dipoles focused on the cavity. The bottom end of the α helices spanning the membrane are probably the major gate for channel activation.

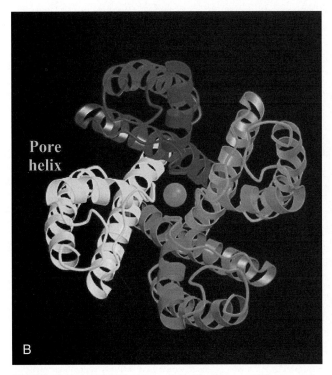

**FIGURE 18-7, cont'd** *B,* Top view of the KcsA pore; a K+ ion occupies the pore.

and S6 projects into the water-filled channel pore providing the channel's ion selectivity filter (pore). A highly conserved P loop in K+ channels, WWxxxxxxTVGYG, coordinates and selectively permeates K+ ions. S4, with its cluster of positively charged amino acids (arginines and lysines), is the major voltage sensor for the ion channel.[34] For some ion channels, voltage-dependent channel inactivation is mediated by a tethered amino terminal blocking particle (the ball and chain mechanism).[35-37] The cytoplasmic N-terminus "ball tethered to its chain" is somehow coupled to the voltage sensor (S4) and swings in to occlude the permeation pathway (N-type channel inactivation). Several amino acids in the S6 transmembrane segment participate in another inactivation pathway named carboxyl terminal (C)-type inactivation. Recently, structural details of this block have been discovered by a combination of mutagenesis and crystallography.[38]

The family of inward rectifier K+-selective channels (K channel, inward rectifier [Kir]) have a simplified architecture comprised of two transmembrane domains (M1 and M2) surrounding a P domain. Like the six transmembrane voltage-dependent channels, Kir channels are tetrameric. These channels slow heart rate and set the resting membrane potential. Their structural design is deceptively simple; heteromultimeric channel formation and interactions with other proteins considerably increase the versatility of this channel class.

Combined molecular biology and electrophysiology approaches have begun to reveal functional properties

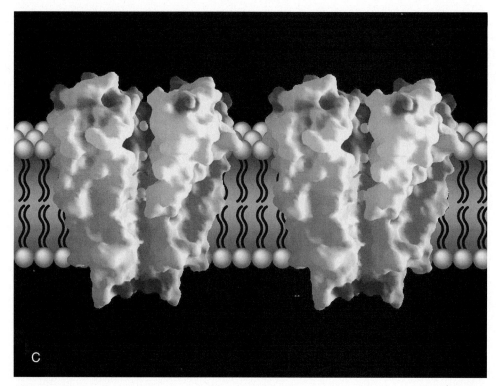

**FIGURE 18-7, cont'd** *C,* Molecular surface of KcsA and contour of the pore based on center of pore to the closest van der Waals protein contact. Three K$^+$ ions are queued in the selectivity filter. *(Modified from Doyle, Morais Cabral J, Pfuetzner RA, et al: The structure of the potassium channel: Molecular basis of K+ conduction and selectivity. Science 1998;280:69–77.)*

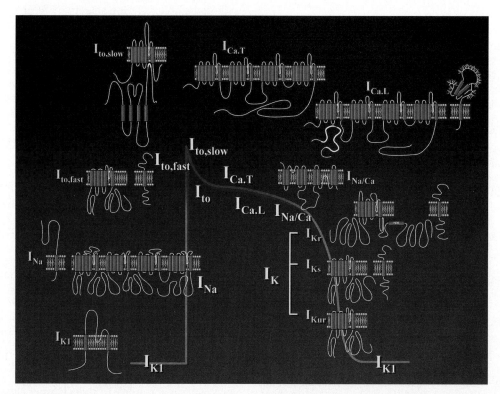

**FIGURE 18-8.** Linear models of the ion channels comprising the cardiac action potential. Again, I$_{Kur}$ is depicted here for this ventricular myocyte although it is primarily present in atrial myocytes. The linear topology of RyR2 is not shown. The number of amino acids in each subunit is shown in Tables 18-3 and 18-4.

and structural insights to these unseen electrical tunnels (Fig. 18-6B).[39] Before an ion enters the external entrance of the pore, it encounters a shallow ledge approximately 28 to 34 Å wide and 4 to 8 Å deep. The pore measures 9 to 14 Å in diameter at its entry point tapering to 4 to 5 Å at a depth of 5 to 7 Å from the vestibule. Although the primary amino acid blueprints for many ion channels are known, the actual three-dimensional physical architecture for ion channels remained a mystery until x-ray crystallographic images of a bacterial $K^+$ channel were obtained (Fig. 18-7).[40]

The crystal structure of the voltage-independent KcsA channel is a tetramer of two transmembrane-spanning α helices (M1 and M2) resembling an inverted teepee (Fig. 18-7A). The tent poles are the four M2 helices that lie in close apposition near the inner membrane and slant out to a broad base at the outer membrane. The M1 helices face the lipid membrane, and the shorter (30 amino acids) connecting pore helices (P loop) form the walls at the base of the teepee. At both inner and outer membrane faces, layers of aromatic amino acids (tryptophans and tyrosines) form a cuff around the pore, presumably pulling at the pore opening like a ring of springs (Fig. 18-7B). The selectivity filter is a narrow region near the outer face of the membrane lined by the carbonyl backbone of conserved P region amino acids (GYG). In theory, rings of carbonyl oxygen molecules act as surrogate water molecules to coordinate the two dehydrated $K^+$ ions sitting in line in the channel. The narrow channel in the selectivity filter rapidly broadens in hourglass fashion to form a large "lake" roughly halfway through the membrane, where 60 to 100 water molecules diffuse the charge of the $K^+$ ion residing in this cavity. The four short pore α helices run amino to carboxyl to focus their helix dipole negative electrostatic fields on the cavity. Finally, a long water-filled hydrophobic channel tunnels to the cytoplasm. $K^+$ ions migrate through the pore at 1Å/pS, and two to three ions are queued in the selectivity filter. After traversing the 18-Å long hydrophobic canal leading into the lake and moving into the wider 10-Å long cavity, the cation is surrounded by approximately 60 water molecules. The ion is also stabilized in the polar environment of the membrane by a negative field generated by the pore helical dipoles 8 Å above and focused in the middle of the lake (Fig. 18-7C).

The central theme for selectivity revealed by the KcsA structure is likely to be repeated for other types of cation-selective ion channels such as $Na^+$ and $Ca^{2+}$ channels. Probably the same theme of repulsion between two ions is used to push these ions through the pore. It seems likely that the inverted tip of the teepee, at the internal face of the channel, is the site of most channel gating.

## MOLECULAR BIOLOGY OF THE CARDIAC CHANNEL PROTEINS

Figure 18-8 correlates the cardiac action potential to the linear topologies of the channel proteins contributing to the cardiac action potential.[1,3,41] Tables 18-3 and 18-4 summarize the major properties of the cardiac ion channel genes.

## Inward Ion Channels

### $I_f$

There are two distinct kinetic components (fast and slow) to the hyperpolarization-activated cation current $I_f/I_h$. The human cardiac pacemaker channel ($I_{f,fast}$) is reproduced by expression of the protein encoded by the gene hyperpolarization-activated, cyclic nucleotide-gated channel (*HCN2*; chromosome 19p13.3), and $I_{f,slow}$ is encoded by *HCN4* (chromosome 15q24-q25).[42,43] The properties of cardiac $I_f$ partially overlap with the cyclic nucleotide-gated nonselective channels found in the cloned cyclic GMP-gated channel from rod photoreceptor.[44] *HCN2* encodes an 889 amino acid protein containing (1) a six transmembrane domain including an S4 voltage sensor like the voltage-gated $K^+$ channels (Fig. 18-6A), (2) a cyclic nucleotide-binding domain (cNBD) similar to *HERG*, and (3) a P loop sequence (CIGYGR) that is modified from the signature sequence of the $K^+$ selectivity filter (T[V/I]GYGD) and presumably permits entry and passage of sodium ions.[45]

*HCN4* encodes a 1203 amino acid protein, which is 90% identical to *HCN2* in the S1-S6, pore, and cNBD domains but divergent in its cytoplasmic N- and C-termini. The extra 250 amino acid segment at the C-terminus of *HCN2* may impart its distinctively slower activation kinetics. Sympathetic and parasympathetic nervous systems release transmitters onto pacing tissues. β-Adrenergic G-protein linked receptors activate adenylyl cyclases to generate cAMP that directly binds the *HCN2* and *HCN4* channels. Muscarinic receptors inhibit adenylyl cyclases to block this stimulatory effect.

### Sodium Channel

The cardiac $Na^+$ channel ($I_{Na}$) is comprised of a heavily glycosylated heterodimeric complex of α (260 kd) and β1 (36 kd) subunits.[46-48] Brain β2 $Na^+$ channel subunits are absent in cardiac $Na^+$ channels. The α subunit gene (*SCN5A*; chromosome 3p21) encodes a 2015 amino acid α subunit ($Na_v1.5$) containing four domains of six transmembrane spanning segments.[49] Unlike the brain or muscle $I_{Na}$ α subunit, the cardiac α subunit is much less sensitive to tetrodotoxin, presumably because of a single amino acid difference in the pore region of the first domain (C401Y).[50] $Na^+$ channel P loops each contribute one of the amino acids DEKA to line the pore.[51,52]

In general, $Na^+$ channels differ from $Ca^{2+}$ channels by misplacement or lack of negatively charged glutamic or aspartic acid residues in the pore. Rapid inactivation of the $Na^+$ channel involves the cytoplasmic loop between S6 of domain III and S1 of domain IV. The charged amino acids in this peptide loop shift as the membrane depolarizes, inactivating the channel by physically blocking the inner mouth of the channel pore (inactivation lid).[37,46,53] Interestingly, a three amino acid in-frame deletion (KPQ1505-1507del) within this peptide loop is responsible for one form of the hereditary long QT (LQT3) syndrome.[54] Expression of this mutant α subunit yields a $Na^+$ channel that fails to inactivate properly, resulting in a smaller but persistent $Na^+$ current during the plateau phase that prolongs the action potential duration.[55] C-type inactivation also contributes to $Na^+$ channel inactivation. The $\beta1$ subunit gene (*SCN1B*; chromosome 19q13.1) encodes a 218 amino acid intrinsic membrane protein ($Na_v\beta1.1$) that increases the peak current, accelerates activation and inactivation, and alters the voltage-dependence of inactivation of the $Na^+$ current.[56] Presently, no drugs or toxins are known to target $\beta1$ subunit activity, and the $\beta1$ subunit has not been identified as an arrhythmia susceptibility gene.

### Voltage-Gated Calcium Channels (Ca$_V$)

#### L-type Ca$^{2+}$ Channel I$_{Ca.L}$

The high–voltage-activated, long-lasting L-type $Ca^{2+}$ channel $I_{Ca.L}$ has been characterized extensively in skeletal muscle and more recently purified and photoaffinity-labeled in heart.[57-59] This voltage-dependent, dihydropyridine-sensitive $Ca^{2+}$ channel (also referred to as the dihydropyridine receptor [DHPR]) is a heterotetrameric complex comprised of $\alpha1$, $\beta$, and $\alpha2/\delta$ subunits (shown in Fig. 18-8). Cardiac $I_{Ca.L}$ lacks the 30-kd $\gamma$ subunit found in skeletal muscle. The 190-kd $\alpha1C$ subunit ($Ca_v1.2$) makes up the channel pore and has receptor sites that may be block by three classes of $Ca^{2+}$ channel drugs (dihydropyridines, benzothiazepines, and phenylalkylamines).

The human cardiac $\alpha1C$ (2157 amino acid) subunit is encoded by a single gene (*CACNA1C*; chromosome 12p13.3; Fig. 18-8).[60,61] Its H5 peptide (P loop, also referred to as SS1-SS2 segments between S5 and S6 of each of the four domains) lines the channel pore and contains four key glutamate residues that impart $Ca^{2+}$ selectivity to the channel.[62] Calcium channel blockers bind to separate, allosterically linked sites near this pore-lining region. The P loop of domain III and S6 of domains III and IV participate in dihydropyridine (e.g., nifedipine) binding. In contrast, the intracellular tail and a portion of S6 in domain IV participate in phenylalkylamine (verapamil) binding.[23,63,64] The cardiac $\alpha1c$ subunit and the vascular smooth muscle $\alpha1$ subunit are alternatively spliced products from the same gene, differing only in the S3 segment of domain IV. Marked differences in sensitivity to dihydropyridine may result from this alternative splicing. $I_{Ca.L}$ activation time is modified by mutations in S3 of domain I, whereas inactivation is influenced by the S6 segment of domain I. Excitation-contraction coupling uses the cytoplasmic loop between domains II and III.[58]

Although expression of the $\alpha1C$ subunit ($Ca_v1.2$) alone is sufficient to form a $Ca^{2+}$-selective, voltage-dependent channel, the $Ca_v1.2$ current kinetics are modulated significantly by the $\alpha2/\delta$ and $\beta$ subunits. Four distinct genes and their alternatively spliced products encode $\beta$ subunits, but the precise $\beta$ subunit composition of cardiac $I_{Ca.L}$ is unknown. The cytoplasmic $\beta$ subunit contains two highly conserved domains. The initial portion of the second domain interfaces with a highly conserved region in the $\alpha1c$ subunit's intracellular loop, just 24 amino acids distal to the I-S6 inactivation site. The $\beta$ subunit facilitates trafficking of the $I_{Ca.L}$ channel complex to the plasmalemma and modifies the gating properties of $I_{Ca.L}$, thus accelerating activation and shifting the activation threshold to more negative membrane potentials.[65] The $\alpha2/\delta$ subunit (chromosome 7q21-q22) is a 180-kd disulfide-linked protein complex that affects the current density and the number of drug receptor sites on $I_{Ca.L}$. The hydrophobic (30 kd, 146 amino acids) $\delta$ subunit spans the membrane and covalently anchors the extracellular glycosylated $\alpha2$ subunit (150 kd, 934 amino acids) via disulfide bridges. The L-type $Ca^{2+}$ channel is critical for multiple cellular functions and is regulated by multiple signaling pathways (PKA, PKC, and calmodulin [CaM]).[66] To date, no arrhythmia-causing mutations have been identified in any protein of the $Ca^{2+}$ channel complex.

#### T-type Ca$^{2+}$ Channel I$_{Ca.T}$

Although sharing the same basic architectural blueprint as the L-type $Ca^{2+}$ channel, the sequence of the low-voltage-activated, transient (T)-type $Ca^{2+}$ channel ($I_{Ca.T}$) has substantial differences. Virtually all the biophysical (voltage dependence, kinetics, and unitary conductance) and pharmacologic (mibefradil sensitivity) properties of $I_{Ca.T}$ are recapitulated by heterologous expression of the recombinant $\alpha1H$ subunit cloned from human heart.[67] *CACNA1H* (chromosome 16p13.3) encodes a 2353 amino acid protein ($\alpha1H$ or $Ca_vT.2$). The putative selectivity filter contains four negatively charged residues; two are glutamates as in the L-type channel, but the P loop of domains III and IV are aspartates. $\alpha1H$ does not possess the L-type $Ca^{2+}$ channel-binding motif for $\tilde\beta$ subunits.

### Excitation-Contraction Coupling (Local Control)

Once $I_{Na}$-mediated depolarization triggers $Ca^{2+}$ channel-mediated $Ca^{2+}$ influx, $Ca^{2+}$ increases dramatically beneath the sarcolemma (Fig. 18-9). This transient localized increase in subsarcolemmal $Ca^{2+}$ in turn activates the ryanodine receptor (RyR2) encoded calcium release channels (CRC) residing in the SR. This process, called $Ca^{2+}$-induced $Ca^{2+}$-release (CICR), amplifies and propagates $Ca^{2+}$ release throughout the myocardium. The efflux of $Ca^{2+}$ through CRCs from the SR into the cytoplasm is 10 to 65 times larger than that resulting from L-type $Ca^{2+}$ channels at the cell membrane.[68] As a result, $[Ca^{2+}]_i$ increases from approximately 100 nM in diastole to approximately 1000 nM in systole.[69] In addition, CICR indirectly mediates an increased inward current at the cell surface by fueling the electrogenic $Na^+/Ca^{2+}$ exchanger. $Ca^{2+}$ release from the SR is closely linked to the amplitude and duration of $I_{Ca.L}$. In animal model systems, $Ca^{2+}$ entering via reverse $Na^+/Ca^{2+}$ exchange or via the rapidly inactivating influx through $I_{Ca.T}$ is not sufficient to trigger normal phasic contractions. Contractions are controlled chiefly by $I_{Ca.L}$, RyR2, and CICR. Consequently, dihydropyridines, other $Ca^{2+}$ channel blockers, and interference with the ryanodine receptor can reduce contractile function to the point of producing congestive heart failure.

Because $Ca^{2+}$ mediates a myriad of cellular processes ranging from contraction to gene expression, it is no surprise that numerous elements are devoted to ensure

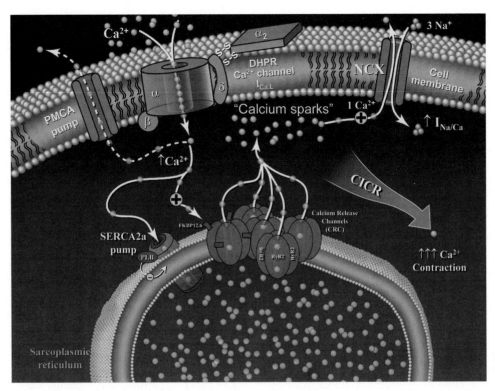

**FIGURE 18-9.** Cardiac excitation-contraction coupling relies on $Ca^{2+}$-induced $Ca^{2+}$ release. $Ca^{2+}$ entering through plasmalemma, dihydropyridine-sensitive (DHPR) voltage-activated $Ca^{2+}$ channels bind to cardiac ryanodine receptors (RyR2) on the SR, triggering RyR2 channel openings yielding $Ca^{2+}$ sparks. Release of stored $Ca^{2+}$ raises intracellular $[Ca^{2+}]$ to approximately 1 fM and initiates contraction. Plasma membrane $Ca^{2+}$ pumps (PMCA), SR $Ca^{2+}$ pumps (SERCA2a), and the $Na^+/Ca^{2+}$ exchanger (NCX1) remove $Ca^{2+}$ from the cytoplasm to lower intracellular $[Ca^{2+}]$ to 50 to 100 nM.

proper $Ca^{2+}$ homeostasis. $Ca^{2+}$ itself along with the ubiquitous $Ca^{2+}$-binding protein CaM modulate $I_{Ca,L}$ inactivation.[22] In addition, the SR $Ca^{2+}$ ATPase transporter (SERCA2a) pumps $Ca^{2+}$ back into the SR and thus controls relaxation of cardiocytes.[70] SERCA2a activity is controlled by phospholamban (PLB) and other proteins.[71] In patients with dilated cardiomyopathy and hypertrophic cardiomyopathy, decreased mRNA expression of SERCA2a, altered SERCA2a activity, or dysregulation of the phosphorylation status of PLB may underlie markedly abnormal force-frequency relationships.[72-74] $Ca^{2+}$ buffering proteins also modulate levels of free $[Ca^{2+}]_i$ in the heart, but these are understood poorly at present.

### Ryanodine Receptor

The cardiac ryanodine receptor *RyR2* (chromosome 1q42.1-q43) encodes a 4967 amino acid protein.[75] Four 565-kd RyR2 subunits assemble into a huge ion channel tetramer. As a macromolecular signaling complex, the cardiac ryanodine receptor is associated with the FK506 binding protein (FKBP12.6, a member of the immunophilin family of *cis-trans* peptidyl-prolyl isomerases that serve as cytosolic receptors for the immunosuppressants rapamycin and FK506), protein kinase A (PKA) catalytic and regulatory subunits, the anchoring protein mAKAP, protein phosphatase 1 (PP1), and protein phosphatase 2A (PP2A).[69] In fact, FKBP12.6 functionally couples neighboring RyR2 tetrameric com-

plexes to cooperatively gate these ion channels.[76] Single amino acid perturbations in *RyR2* may underlie catecholaminergic polymorphic ventricular tachycardia in a structurally normal heart or arrhythmogenic right ventricular cardiomyopathy type 2 (ARVD2).[77-79]

### $Na^+/Ca^{2+}$ Exchanger

After the voltage-dependent $Ca^{2+}$ channels have inactivated, the terminal portion of the plateau is sustained by inward current through the $Na^+/Ca^{2+}$ exchanger. *NCX1* (*SLC8A1*; chromosome 2p21-p23) encodes the 973 amino acid human cardiac $Na^+/Ca^{2+}$ exchanger.[80,81] NCX1 is a nine putative transmembrane segment protein containing a large hydrophilic cytoplasmic loop between S5 and S6 (Fig. 18-8). The ion transport pathway of the exchanger is poorly understood.[26]

In isolated SA nodal cells, the intracellular CRC and the plasmalemmal $Na^+/Ca^{2+}$ exchanger regulate diastolic depolarization (Fig. 18-9). $Ca^{2+}$ influx and CICR trigger NCX-mediated $Ca^{2+}$ efflux. The resulting exchanger current speeds diastolic depolarization and boosts $Ca^{2+}$ current activation. Interestingly, disruption of either CRC or $I_{Na/Ca}$ can eliminate SA node automaticity.[82] In one rabbit model of heart failure in which the ventricular $Na^+/Ca^{2+}$ exchanger is upregulated, sarcoplasmic reticular $[Ca^{2+}]$ falls, leading to contractile dysfunction. Delayed after-depolarizations are increased in this setting of poorly controlled cytoplasmic $[Ca^{2+}]$, resulting in triggered arrhythmias.[83]

## Outward Ion Channels

Unambiguous assignment of cloned K+ channel proteins to the outward K+ currents of the cardiac action potential has been a more difficult task than assignment for Na+ and Ca$^{2+}$ ion channels.[84-86] Except for identification of I$_{K1}$ current as IRK1 (Kir 2.1), there has been reluctance to assign genes to the other K+ currents because the expressed clones often fail to match precisely the biophysical and pharmacologic properties of the native currents. The possibility of heteromultimeric assembly and the existence of K+ channel-specific β subunits[56] dictates an enormous potential diversity of K+ channel composition. Figure 18-8 and Table 18-4 tentatively match cloned K+ channel proteins to the outward K+ currents of the human cardiac action potential.

### Transient Outward I$_{to}$

Although no known genes encode proteins that explain the 4-aminopyridine-insensitive component of the transient outward current $_{\alpha}$to2), several K+ channel gene products are candidates for I$_{to,s}$ and I$_{to,f}$. *HK1* (Kv1.4) encodes a 653 amino acid K+ channel in human ventricle.[87] Kv1.4 exhibits many I$_{to,s}$-like properties but fails to explain the time course of recovery from inactivation.[88] Coexpression of hKvβ3 with Kv1.4 produced an I$_{to,s}$-like current with recovery from inactivation that resembled the recovery of the endogenous I$_{to,s}$ current.[89,90] I$_{to,s}$ may also be a heteromultimer of different α subunits, such as Kv1.4 and Kv1.2.[84,88]

The properties of rat I$_{to,f}$ are reproduced largely by expression of the 629 amino acid *Shal* homolog Kv4.2 (*KCND2*, chromosome 7q31). In heterologous expression systems, coexpression of Kv4.2 with the minK-related peptide 1 (MiRP1) and the Kv channel-interacting protein (KChIP2) most closely approximated rat I$_{to,f}$.[91] KChIPs are Ca$^{2+}$-binding proteins that may be integral components of some Kv channels. A 656 amino acid human homolog Kv4.3 (*KCND3*, chromosome 1p13.2) appears to account for most human I$_{to,f}$.[92-95] *KCND3* mRNA is downregulated in human heart failure, which corresponds to a decrease in I$_{to,f}$ density.[94] To date, no arrhythmias are correlated with either *KCND2* or *KCND3*, although QT intervals are prolonged in *KCND2*-knockout mice.[96]

### Delayed Rectifier I$_K$

#### I$_{Kr}$

The rapidly activating delayed rectifying I$_{Kr}$ current results from coexpression of the human *ether-a-go-go-* related gene *(HERG)* α subunits[97,98] and *MiRP1* (minK-related protein1/*KCNE2*) β subunits.[99] *HERG* (*KCNH2*; chromosome 7q35-36) is expressed chiefly in the heart, but it is also found in neural crest derived neurons and microglia.[100]

*HERG/KCNH2* encodes an 1159 amino acid polypeptide with the characteristic K+ channel topology shown in Figure 18-6. Presumably, the I$_{Kr}$ channel is a homotetramer of HERG α subunits combined with four auxiliary MiRP1 β subunits. The HERG P loop amino acid sequence (**YFxxxxxxxxGFG**) differs from many K+ channels. These differences are postulated to produce a narrower but more flexible external vestibule and may explain why external Na+ blocks the HERG pore.[15] Interestingly, HERG's inner vestibule appears to be larger than other voltage-gated K+ channels, perhaps because of the absence of two proline residues highly conserved in virtually all other voltage-gated K+ channel α subunits. In theory, these proline residues reduce the size of the inner vestibule by causing a kink in S6.[101] In addition, the HERG S6 domain contains two aromatic residues (tyrosine at 652 and phenylalanine at 656) that are conspicuously absent in other K+ channels. These aromatic residues face the internal vestibule and may bind large aromatic drugs in a φ-stacking interaction.[102] Sanguinetti and colleagues postulate that the HERG inner vestibule may accommodate and trap larger drugs, perhaps accounting for the plethora of diverse medications causing drug-induced QT interval prolongation.[103,104]

HERG has large N- and C-termini, and the C-terminus contains a cyclic nucleotide binding domain. HERG's first 135 amino acids show structural similarity to the gene products of Per-Arnt-Sim (PAS) motifs that regulate a variety of biochemical processes by serving as light and chemical sensors in prokaryotic cells.[105] The N-terminal PAS motif is instrumental in HERG's uniquely slow deactivation, presumably stabilizing N-terminal domain binding to the activation gate.[105,106] Mutations occurring in the PAS motif accelerate HERG deactivation to the closed state. Mutations in *HERG* are responsible for the chromosome 7q35-36 linked form of inherited long QT syndrome (LQT2),[100] whereas *MiRP1* perturbations are present in a less common long QT syndrome (LQT6).[99]

Coexpression of *HERG* and *MiRP1* recapitulates the biophysical and pharmacologic properties of cardiac I$_{Kr}$.[99] HERG-I$_{Kr}$ displays a bell-shaped current-voltage relationship, the result of inward rectification caused by C-type inactivation (Table 18-2).[107] This fast inactivation process limits the amount of outward current through the channel when the membrane potential is greater than 0 mV. During phase 3 repolarization as the membrane potential drops below 0 mV, HERG channels rapidly recover from inactivation, and outward I$_{Kr}$ resurges.[15,108] This peculiarity of HERG current may safeguard the heart against early after-depolarizations and premature beats.[107] Patients lacking this protection because of genetically disrupted (LQT2) or pharmacologically blocked HERG channels are susceptible to sudden cardiac arrhythmias.

#### I$_{Ks}$

I$_{Ks}$, the largest phase 3 repolarization current, results from the coassembly of the 676 amino acid *KVLQT1* (*KCNQ1*; chromosome 21q22.1) and a single transmembrane-spanning 129 amino acid subunit *minK* (*KCNE1*; chromosome 11p15.5).[109-113] The stoichiometric relationship between *KVLQT1* and *minK* necessary to reconstitute the I$_{Ks}$ channel has not been determined but is presumably a complex of four *KVLQT1* α subunits and four *minK* β subunits. *KVLQT1* resides in a chromosomal region associated with Beckwith-Wiedemann syndrome and is subject to imprinting with paternal silencing in most tissues except the heart.[114]

Heterozygous mutations in *KVLQT1* result in the most common form of autosomal dominant long QT syndrome (LQT1).[115,116] No clinical phenotype in other organs has been described for heterozygous mutations. However, homozygous mutations in either *KVLQT1* or *KCNE1* (*minK*) result in autosomal recessive Jervell and Lange-Nielsen syndrome (QT interval prolongation and sensorineural deafness).[117,118] Arrhythmia predisposition is inherited as a semidominant trait, whereas congenital deafness is inherited as an autosomal recessive trait. Both *KVLQT1* and *minK* are expressed in the inner ear and produce the $K^+$-rich endolymph bathing the organ of Corti.

Even further complexity in the orchestration and tuning of the cardiac action potential is provided by the marked heterogeneity of ion channel expression throughout the ventricular myocardium. Action potential duration varies widely between the various layers of the myocardium, that is, endocardium, midmyocardial M cells, and epicardium. M cells possess a longer APD and a steep dependence of APD on rate chiefly resulting from a reduced density of *KVLQT1/minK*-$I_{Ks}$ channels.[14,28] The reader is referred to an excellent review by Antzelevitch[119] on the impact of channel expression heterogeneity on transmural dispersion of repolarization and arrhythmogenesis.

### $I_{Kur}$

The atria's shorter action potential duration may be the result of $I_{Kur}$'s localization to atrial tissue. Kv1.5/*KCNA5* (chromosome 12p13) encodes a 611 amino acid protein with typical Kv channel topography. Expression in heterologous systems yields $K^+$ currents that are virtually indistinguishable from $I_{Kur}$.[30,87]

### Inward Rectifier $I_{K1}$

$I_{K1}$ enables the formation of the plateau phase, provides significant phase 3 repolarization, and establishes the cell's resting membrane potential (phase 4). Cardiac $I_{K1}$ is recapitulated by expression of recombinant IRK1 (Kir 2.1) channels. IRK1/Kir2.1/*KCNJ2* (chromosome 17q23.1-q24.2) encodes a 427 amino acid two membrane-spanning domain protein lacking a voltage sensor (Fig. 18-8).[31,120] Multiple promoter elements have been shown to control the transcription of the *KCNJ2* gene,[121] and specific export signals in the endoplasmic reticulum may provide differential regulation of $I_{K1}$ channel density in the plasma membrane.[122] Other $K^+$ channel subunits (Kir5.1/*KCNJ16*) may act as negative regulators of the $I_{K1}$ channel.[123] Andersen's syndrome, a rare disorder characterized by periodic paralysis, cardiac arrhythmias including QT interval prolongation, and dysmorphic features, has been associated with *KCNJ2* mutations.[124]

## MODULATORY ION CHANNELS

Roughly 6 currents in pacemaking cells and 10 currents in atria/ventricle are sufficient to explain the normal car-

diac action potential. However, heart rate is modulated by neurotransmitters and other ligands via several additional channels. This section highlights features of four important modulatory ion channels: $I_{Cl.cAMP}$, $I_{Cl.swell}$, $K_{ATP}$, and $I_{K.ACh}$. Their influence on the action potential and the opportunity they provide for novel antiarrhythmic approaches are discussed.

## Modulatory Chloride Channels

Although there is a small contribution from a calcium-sensitive chloride channel ($I_{Cl.Ca}$ or $I_{to2}$) on a beat-to-beat basis, there are additional chloride channels that may be recruited during sympathetic stimulation ($I_{Cl.cAMP}$) or during cell swelling ($I_{Cl.swell}$).[125,126] Chloride currents may provide novel targets for antiarrhythmic agents, especially during states of myocardial swelling, pronounced sympathetic tone, and histaminergic (H2) activation of $I_{Cl.cAMP}$ (a possible mechanism for histamine-induced ventricular tachyarrhythmias).[127] Because $E_{Cl}$ ranges from $-45$ to $-65$ mV (Fig. 18-1), chloride currents are poised to fine tune the cardiac action potential. At membrane potentials negative to $E_{Cl}$, chloride channels pass inward current (chloride efflux) causing a diastolic depolarization of the resting membrane potential. During the plateau, when membrane potentials are positive to $E_{Cl}$, activated $Cl^-$ currents contribute outward current ($Cl^-$ influx) and assist $K^+$ channels in repolarizing the membrane (Fig. 18-10*A*). Properties of $I_{Cl.cAMP}$ and $I_{Cl.swell}$ are summarized in Table 18-5.

Sympathetic stimulation of the heart increases intracellular cAMP and initiates PKA-mediated phosphorylation of $I_{Cl.cAMP}$ (Fig. 18-10*B*).[128,129] Rapid activation of $I_{Cl.cAMP}$ current during depolarization may help maintain a relatively more hyperpolarized plateau potential, enhancing $Ca^{2+}$ entry and preventing an excessive increase in action potential duration.[130] $I_{Cl.cAMP}$ is most likely cystic fibrosis transmembrane regulator (CFTR). CFTR is a transporter family protein with 12 putative transmembrane spanning domains (Fig. 18-10*C*). In cystic fibrosis patients, mutant epithelial CFTR (commonly F508del) diminishes cAMP-stimulated $Cl^-$ conductance. The cardiac CFTR isoform is an alternatively spliced version of the epithelial CFTR gene (lacking exon 5) found on chromosome 7q.[131] Activation of CFTR $Cl^-$ current is complex, requiring both ATP hydrolysis and PKA-mediated phosphorylation of five key serine residues within the regulatory domain.[132] It is unknown whether cardiac CFTR protein yields a physiologically active $Cl^-$ conductance in normal human cardiac currents or whether cardiac CFTR channels function properly in individuals with cystic fibrosis.

$I_{Cl.swell}$ has been observed in both human atria and ventricle and may become unmasked during pathologic states that initiate cell swelling (e.g., ischemia). The protein(s) responsible for $I_{Cl.swell}$ has not been established, but possible candidates are summarized in Table 18-6.

## Modulatory Potassium Channels

In addition to the five principal $K^+$ currents ($I_{K1}$, $I_{to}$, $I_{Kr}$, $I_{Ks}$, and $I_{Kur}$), the heart contains at least five other modu-

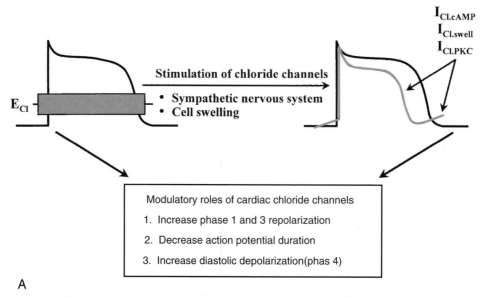

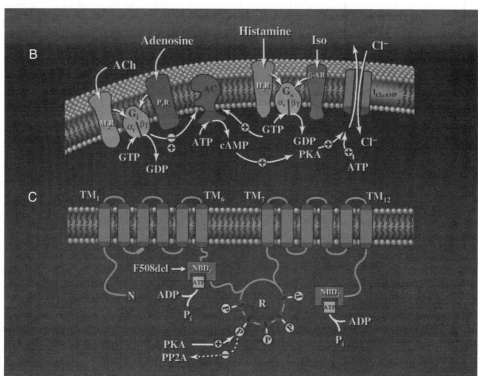

**FIGURE 18-10.** Modulation of the cardiac action potential by chloride channels. *A*, Effect of increasing Cl⁻ current on the action potential. *B*, Signal transduction cascade for activation of $I_{Cl.cAMP}$. AC, adenylyl cyclase; ACh, acetylcholine; β-AR, beta adrenergic receptor; $G_i$, inhibitory G-protein subunit; $G_s$, stimulatory G-protein subunit; $H_2R$, type 2 histaminergic receptor; Iso, isoproterenol; $M_2R$, type 2 muscarinic receptor; PKA, protein kinase A; $P_1R$, type 1 purinergic receptor. *C*, Model of cardiac CFTR. CFTR contains 1480 amino acids throughout 12 transmembrane (TM) spanning domains and two nucleotide binding domains (NBD). NBD1 is juxtaposed between the sixth and seventh transmembrane domain and contains the most common cystic fibrosis mutation, F508del. PP2A, protein phosphatase 2A; R, regulatory domain with multiple serine (S) phosphorylation sites (P).

latory K⁺ currents[41,133]: (1) $K_{ATP}$ normally inhibited by ATP but potentially activated during ischemia; (2) $I_{KACh}$ activated by G-protein βγ subunits in response to vagal stimulation (ACh) and/or adenosine; (3) $I_{K.Ca}$ activated by high cytosolic Ca²⁺ concentrations, perhaps accelerating repolarization in the Ca²⁺-overloaded heart; (4) $I_{K.Na}$ activated by high cytosolic Na⁺ concentrations and perhaps promoting repolarization and QT shortening in the Na⁺-overloaded heart (e.g., digitalis treatment); and (5) $I_{K.AA}$ activated by arachidonic acid and other fatty acids, particularly at acid pH. $I_{K.ATP}$ and $I_{K.ACh}$ are now understood in some biophysical and molecular detail.[1,134,135]

**TABLE 18-5   ELECTROPHYSIOLOGY OF REGULATORY ION CHANNELS IN THE HEART**

| Ion Current | I-V Relationship | Activation Threshold (mV) | Peak Current (mV) | Relative Size $I_x/I_{Na}$ | Time to Peak (msec) | Blockers | Activators |
|---|---|---|---|---|---|---|---|
| $I_{Cl.cAMP}$ | | −55 | >0 | Varies | | 9-AC<br>DPC<br>DNDS | |
| $I_{Cl.swell}$ | | −100, −35 | >0 | Varies | | 9-AC<br>NPPB | |
| $I_{K.ATP}$ | | | >0 | Varies | Instantaneous | ATP, phentolamine bretylium, glyburide, glipizide | Pinacidil cromakalim nicorandil minoxidil diazoxide |
| $I_{K.ACh}$ | | | −75 [K]$_o$ dependent | 0.02 | Instantaneous | $Ba^{2+}$ | Acetylcholine adenosine somatostatin |

## $K_{ATP}$

The cardiac adenosine triphosphate (ATP)-sensitive $K^+$ ($K_{ATP}$) channel is postulated to be an octameric complex comprised of four inwardly rectifying $K^+$ channel subunits (Kir 6.2/*KCNJ11*) and the cardiac sulfonylurea receptor isoform (*SUR2A*, Fig. 18-11A).[136-138] Kir 6.2/*KCNJ11* (chromosome 11p15.1) is a 390 amino acid protein comprising two transmembrane-spanning segments with 46% identity to IRK1 (Kir 2.1/*KCNJ2*) and 44% identity to GIRK4 (Kir 3.4/*KCNJ5*). SUR is a 12 transmembrane-spanning domain member of the ATP-binding cassette superfamily (including CFTR and P-glycoprotein). Containing two nucleotide-binding domains (NBD1 and NBD2; located between the eleventh and twelfth transmembrane regions and in the carboxyl terminus), SUR avidly binds sulfonylureas (e.g., glibenclamide). Coexpression of the human Kir 6.2 and SUR2A subunits recapitulates cardiac $K_{ATP}$ channel properties from human ventricular cells. These properties include an approximately 80-pS inwardly rectifying $K^+$ conductance, inhibition by ATP in the absence of magnesium, inhibition by glibenclamide, recovery by MgATP, stimulation by ADP when previously inhibited by ATP, and activation by pinacidil and cromakalim (but insensitive to diazoxide).[137]

$K_{ATP}$ channels are present in other tissues such as skeletal muscle, blood vessels (Kir6.2 + SUR2B), and the pancreas (Kir6.2 + SUR1). Pancreatic $K_{ATP}$ channels play a pivotal role in the regulation of insulin secretion.[135] Oral hypoglycemics, such as glibenclamide and glipizide used in the treatment of type II diabetes, bind the sulfonylurea receptor and inhibit $K_{ATP}$. Inhibition of $K_{ATP}$ reduces hyperpolarizing currents so that active inward currents depolarize the cell, promoting $Ca^{2+}$ influx and $Ca^{2+}$-dependent insulin secretion. $K_{ATP}$ channels are the targets of the pharmaceutical class of $K^+$ channel openers including nicorandil, pinacidil, aprikalim, levcromakalim, and diazoxide that hyperpolarize and relax blood vessels. Thus, these agents are potentially cardioprotective and may provide novel therapeutic strategies for angina, ischemia, cardiac bypass, transplantation, coronary angioplasty, and hypertension.[139-142]

In the heart, the precise physiologic role of $K_{ATP}$ is less clear (Fig. 18-11B). Cardiac $K_{ATP}$ channels are regulated by the heart's metabolic state.[139] Surprisingly, there are roughly 20-fold more $K_{ATP}$ channels in ventricle (~45,000 per cell) than $I_{K1}$ (~2500 per cell) or $I_K$ (~3000 per cell) channels. During ischemia, intracellular ATP levels may decrease to the point at which ATP-sensitive $K^+$ channels activate. Under these circumstances, $K_{ATP}$ channels theoretically shorten the plateau, attenuate action potential duration, and may mediate ST segment elevation (Fig. 18-11B).[143] Kir6.2-knockout mice manifest a marked reduction in ST segment elevation during ischemia suggesting that opening of sarcolemmal $K_{ATP}$ channels

**TABLE 18-6   MOLECULAR ARCHITECTURE OF REGULATORY ION CHANNELS IN THE HEART**

| Ion Current | Candidate Gene(s) | Candidate Symbol | Chromosome Location | Amino Acids (no.) | Channelopathy |
|---|---|---|---|---|---|
| $I_{Cl.cAMP}$ | Cystic fibrosis transmembrane regulator | CFTR | 7q31.2 | 1,480 | – |
| $I_{Cl.swell}$ | P-glycoprotein<br>or $I_{Cln}$<br>or ClC-3 | MDR1 (ABCB1)<br>CLNS1A/CLNS1B<br>CLCN3 | 7q21.1<br>11q/6p<br>4q33 | 1,279<br>237<br>820 | –<br><br>– |
| $I_{K.ATP}$ | Kir6.2 sulfonylurea receptor 2A | KCNJ11<br>SUR2A | 11p15.1<br>12p12.1 | 390<br>1,407 | –<br> |
| $I_{K.ACh}$ | Kir3.1 (GIRK1)<br>Kir3.4 (GIRK4) | KCNJ3<br>KCNJ5 | 2q24.1<br>11q24 | 501<br>419 | –<br> |

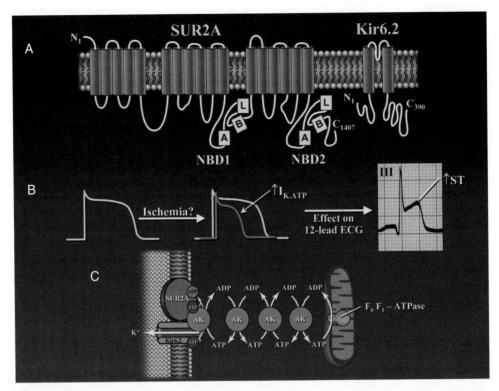

**FIGURE 18-11.** The ATP-sensitive $K^+$ channel, $K_{ATP}$. *A,* The $K_{ATP}$ ion channel. Cardiac $K_{ATP}$ is an octameric complex comprised of four Kir6.2 subunits and four SUR2A. Tissue specificity is determined by specific SUR coassembly. Pancreatic $K_{ATP}$ results from coassembly with SUR1. The SUR contains two nucleotide binding domains (NBD1 and NBD2) having highly conserved Walker motifs (A, B, L). *B,* Modulatory effect of $K_{ATP}$ on the action potential. During ischemia, activation of $K_{ATP}$ could shorten the action potential and may underlie ST segment elevation. *C,* Cellular and molecular regulation of $K_{ATP}$ adenylate kinase (AK) associates with the $K_{ATP}$ channel complex and provides a phosphorelay mechanism that efficiently couples cellular/mitochondrial energetics to the surface membrane $K_{ATP}$ channels. *(A, modified from Zingman, Alekseev AE, Bienengraeber M, et al: Signaling in channel/enzyme multimers: ATPase transitions in SUR module gate ATP-sensitive $K^+$ conductance. Neuron 2001;31:233–245; C, modified from Carrasco, et al: Adenylate kinase phosphotransfer communicates cellular energetic signals to ATP-sensitive potassium channels. PNAS 2001;98:7623–7628.)*

underlies ischemia-induced ST segment elevation.[144] *In vitro* studies demonstrate that recombinant cardiac $K_{ATP}$ channels confer resistance to hypoxia-reoxygenation injury and suggest a possible role in cardioprotection.[145,146] In humans, the use of sulfonylurea drugs has been associated with an increased (nonarrhythmogenic) risk for early mortality in diabetic patients undergoing coronary angioplasty for acute myocardial infarction.[147] Thus, inhibition of cardiac $K_{ATP}$ channels may adversely affect myocardial tolerance for ischemia and reperfusion.

Cellular and molecular regulation of $K_{ATP}$ channels is not understood fully. Recent studies suggest that the Kir6.2/SUR2A complex is not only a passive ion channel but a dynamic enzyme as well. SUR2A has intrinsic ATPase activity that serves a catalytic function for controlling $K_{ATP}$ channel opening.[148,149] Moreover, the $K_{ATP}$ channels may actively monitor the metabolic status of the cell through a series of phosphotransferase relays (Fig. 18-11*C*).[150] Finally, $K_{ATP}$ channels reside on the inner membrane of mitochondria and may participate in signaling networks that transduce intracellular metabolic events.[151]

*$I_{K.ACh}$*

A critical modulator of atrial, SA, and AV nodal excitability is the acetylcholine (ACh)-sensitive $K^+$ channel

$(I_{K.ACh})$.[134,152] $I_{K.ACh}$ activation slows heart rate by hyperpolarizing pacemaker cells in the SA and AV nodes and is a therapeutic target for the treatment of supraventricular tachycardia (SVT) (Fig. 18-12A and B). Secreted from the vagus nerve, acetylcholine binds to cardiac muscarinic type 2 receptors (m2) to activate pertussis toxin-sensitive G-proteins. The released $G\beta\gamma$ subunits directly bind and activate the channel.[153,154] $I_{K.ACh}$ is a heteromultimer of two inwardly rectifying K-channel subunits GIRK1 (Kir 3.1/*KCNJ3*) and GIRK4 (Kir 3.4/*KCNJ5*).[155] GIRK1, a 56-kd protein of 501 amino acids (chromosome 2q24.1), is expressed throughout the nervous system, whereas GIRK4 (chromosome 11q24; 419 amino acids) is fairly cardiac specific. Figure 18-12*C* depicts the $I_{K.ACh}$ channel as a tetramer of GIRK1/GIRK4, with presumably two subunits of each subtype per channel. GIRK4-knockout mice completely lack cardiac $I_{K.ACh}$ and display abnormal heart rate regulation. In particular, GIRK4 knockout mice manifest a dramatic reduction in heart rate variability, especially in response to vasopressor challenge.[156]

In addition to mediating the vagal-induced slowing of heart rate, $I_{K.ACh}$ is a major therapeutic target of intravenous adenosine. Adenosine, like acetylcholine, decreases spontaneous depolarization or pacemaker activity in the sinus node (Fig. 18-12*B*) and slows conduction velocity in the AV node.[157-159] The direct

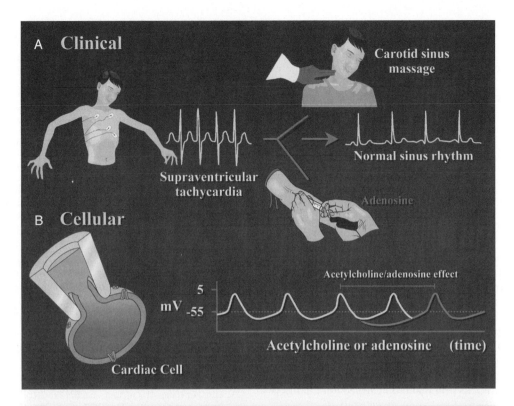

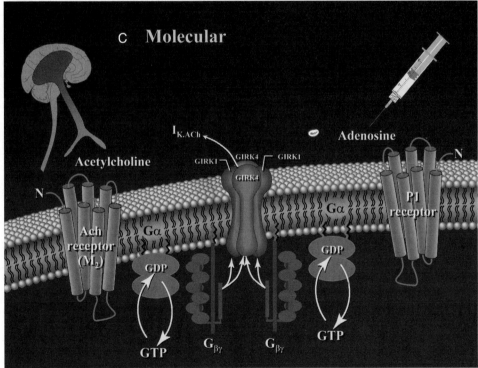

**FIGURE 18-12.** The acetylcholine/adenosine-activated K$^+$ channel, I$_{K.ACh}$. *A,* Clinical role in treatment of SVT by targeting I$_{K.ACh}$. Clinically, a patient's SVT can be terminated by vagotonic maneuvers such as carotid sinus massage or by intravenous administration of adenosine. *B,* Cellular effect of acetylcholine or adenosine on the SA nodal action potential results in prolongation and hyperpolarization. Carotid sinus massage causes the release of acetylcholine from the vagus nerve (tenth cranial nerve). Either acetylcholine or adenosine produces cellular hyperpolarization. *C,* Signal transduction pathway for I$_{K.ACh}$. At a molecular level, acetylcholine and adenosine bind to their respective receptors and activate the G-protein complex. Released G$_{\beta\gamma}$ directly binds to and activates I$_{K.ACh}$. I$_{K.ACh}$ is comprised of two GIRK1 and two GIRK4 subunits. Activation of this potassium channel results in hyperpolarization of the membrane potential shown in *B* as the open channel attempts to drive the membrane potential to E$_K$.

negative chronotropic and dromotropic properties form the basis for adenosine's broad diagnostic and therapeutic application in individuals with SVT. Adenosine binds to type 1 purinergic receptors in the heart and initiates the same set of steps demonstrated for $I_{K.ACh}$ activation. $G_{\beta\gamma}$ directly activates the GIRK1/GIRK4 channel (Fig. 18-12*C*). Human arrhythmia-causing mutations in cardiac $I_{K.ACh}$ (either *KCNJ3* or *KCNJ5*) have not been identified. However, $I_{K.ACh}$-deficient knockout mice are resistant to the profibrillatory effects of vagal stimulation on the atria and do not manifest carbachol-induced atrial fibrillation.[160]

# CONCLUSIONS

This chapter reviewed the cellular and molecular components of normal human cardiac electrophysiology. Ion channels are the proteins that shape the action potential by permitting restricted passage of selected ions across the cell membrane. Opening a specific ion channel drives the membrane potential to the Nernst potential for that channel. The effect on the action potential caused by block, deletion, or stimulation of a specific population of ion channels can be anticipated. Practically all the building blocks that make up cardiac ion channels are now known.

As a first approximation, 6 ion currents describe nodal pacing action potentials, and 10 discrete conductances are needed for atria and ventricle. Additional ion channels are activated by neurotransmitters or other stimuli to modulate heart rate. Current research in this area is focused on precise identification of the constituents of ion channels, the distribution of these channels in heart tissue, and the effects of genetic alterations on channel activity. Hopefully, understanding the basic architecture of these cardiac ion channels will lead to new molecular targets to improve the function of both normal and diseased hearts.

## REFERENCES

1. Ackerman MJ, Clapham DE: Ion channels: Basic science and clinical disease. N Engl J Med 1997;336:1575-1586.
2. Ackerman MJ: The long QT syndrome: Ion channel diseases of the heart. Mayo Clin Proc 1998;73:250-269.
3. Keating MT, Sanguinetti MC: Molecular and cellular mechanisms of cardiac arrhythmias. Cell 2001;104:569-580.
4. Shih HT: Anatomy of the action potential in the heart. Tex Heart Inst J 1994;21(1):30-41.
5. Luo CH, Rudy Y: A dynamic model of the cardiac ventricular action potential. I. Simulations of ionic currents and concentration changes. Circ Res 1994;74:1071-1096.
6. Coraboeuf E, Nargeot J: Electrophysiology of human cardiac cells. Cardiovasc Res 1993;27:1713-1725.
7. Kumar NM, Gilula NB: The gap junction communication channel. Cell 1996;84:381-388.
8. Jongsma HJ, Wilders R: Gap junctions in cardiovascular disease. Circ Res 2000;86:1193-1197.
9. Irisawa H, Brown HF, Giles W: Cardiac pacemaking in the sinoatrial node. Physiol Rev 1993;73(1):197-227.
10. Brown HF, DiFrancesco D, Noble SJ: How does adrenaline accelerate the heart? Nature 1979;280:235-236.
11. Vassort G, Alvarez J: Cardiac T-type calcium current: Pharmacology and roles in cardiac tissues. J Cardiovasc Electrophysiol 1994;5:376-393.
12. Oudit GY, Kassiri Z, Sah R, et al: The molecular physiology of the cardiac transient outward potassium current (I(to)) in normal and diseased myocardium. J Mol Cell Cardiol 2001;33:851-872.
13. Zygmunt AC, Gibbons WR: Properties of the calcium-activated chloride current in heart. J Gen Physiol 1992;99:391-414.
14. Liu DW, Gintant GA, Antzelevitch C: Ionic bases for electrophysiological distinctions among epicardial, midmyocardial, and endocardial myocytes from the free wall of the canine left ventricle. Circ Res 1993;72:671-687.
15. Tseng GN: I(Kr): The hERG channel. J Mol Cell Cardiol 2001; 33:835-849.
16. Volk T, et al: Relationship between transient outward K⁺ current and Ca²⁺ influx in rat cardiac myocytes of endo- and epicardial origin. J Physiol 1999;519(Pt 3):841-850.
17. Baker LC, et al: Enhanced dispersion of repolarization and refractoriness in transgenic mouse hearts promotes reentrant ventricular tachycardia. Circ Res 2000;86:396-407.
18. Balke CW, Gold MR: Calcium channels in the heart: An overview. Heart Dis Stroke 1992;1:398-403.
19. Poole-Wilson PA: Calcium channels in the heart. Postgrad Med J 1991;67(Suppl 3):S16-19.
20. Nilius B, et al: A novel type of cardiac calcium channel in ventricular cells. Nature 1985;316:443-446.
21. Hermsmeyer K: Role of T channels in cardiovascular function. Cardiology 1998;89(Suppl 1):2-9.
22. Anderson ME: Ca²⁺-dependent regulation of cardiac L-type Ca²⁺ channels: Is a unifying mechanism at hand? J Mol Cell Cardiol 2001;33:639-650.
23. Luft FC, Haller H: Calcium channel blockers in current medical practice: An update for 1993. Clin Exp Hypertens 1993;15:1263-1276.
24. Schouten VJ, ter Keurs HE, Quaegebeur JM: Influence of electrogenic Na/Ca exchange on the action potential in human heart muscle. Cardiovasc Res 1990;24:758-767.
25. Schulze D, et al: Sodium/calcium exchanger in heart muscle: Molecular biology, cellular function, and its special role in excitation-contraction coupling. Cardiovasc Res 1993;27:1726-1734.
26. Shigekawa M, Iwamoto T: Cardiac Na(+)-Ca(2+) exchange: Molecular and pharmacological aspects. Circ Res 2001;88:864-876.
27. Carmeliet E: K⁺ channels and control of ventricular repolarization in the heart. Fundam Clin Pharmacol 1993;7(1):19-28.
28. Viswanathan PC, Shaw RM, Rudy Y: Effects of IKr and IKs heterogeneity on action potential duration and its rate dependence: A simulation study. Circulation 1999;99:2466-2474.
29. Kurokawa J, Abriel H, Kass RS: Molecular basis of the delayed rectifier current I(ks) in heart. J Mol Cell Cardiol 2001;33:873-882.
30. Wang Z, Fermini B, Nattel S: Sustained depolarization-induced outward current in human atrial myocytes: Evidence for a novel delayed rectifier K⁺ current similar to Kv1.5 cloned channel currents. Circ Res 1993;73:1061-1076.
31. Lopatin AN, Nichols CG: Inward rectifiers in the heart: An update on I(K1). J Mol Cell Cardiol 2001;33:625-638.
32. Soreq H: The biosynthesis of biologically active proteins in mRNA-microinjected Xenopus oocytes. CRC Crit Rev Biochem 1985; 18(3):199-238.
33. Lawrence JH, Tomaselli GF, Marban E: Ion channels: Structure and function. Heart Dis Stroke 1993;2:75-80.
34. Sigworth FJ: Voltage gating of ion channels. Q Rev Biophys 1994;27(1):1-40.
35. Hoshi T, Zagotta WN, Aldrich RW: Biophysical and molecular mechanisms of Shaker potassium channel inactivation. Science 1990;250:533-538.
36. Lopez-Barneo J, et al: Effects of external cations and mutations in the pore region on C-type inactivation of Shaker potassium channels. Receptors Channels 1993;1(1):61-71.
37. Stuhmer W, et al: Structural parts involved in activation and inactivation of the sodium channel. Nature 1989;339:597-603.
38. Zhou M, et al: Potassium channel receptor site for the inactivation gate and quaternary amine inhibitors. Nature 2001;411:657-661.

39. Aiyar J, et al: Topology of the pore-region of a K⁺ channel revealed by the NMR-derived structures of scorpion toxins. Neuron 1995; 15:1169-1181.

40. Doyle DA, et al: The structure of the potassium channel: Molecular basis of K⁺ conduction and selectivity. Science 1998;280:69-77.

41. Katz AM: Cardiac ion channels. N Engl J Med 1993;328: 1244-1251.

42. Vaccari T, et al: The human gene coding for HCN2, a pacemaker channel of the heart. Biochim Biophys Acta 1999;1446:419-425.

43. Ludwig A, et al: Two pacemaker channels from human heart with profoundly different activation kinetics. EMBO J 1999;18: 2323-2329.

44. Kaupp UB, et al: Primary structure and functional expression from complementary DNA of the rod photoreceptor cyclic GMP-gated channel. Nature 1989;342:762-766.

45. Kaupp UB, Seifert R: Molecular diversity of pacemaker ion channels. Annu Rev Physiol 2001;63:235-257.

46. Catterall WA: From ionic currents to molecular mechanisms: The structure and function of voltage-gated sodium channels. Neuron 2000;26:13-25.

47. Goldin AL: Resurgence of sodium channel research. Annu Rev Physiol 2001;63:871-894.

48. Balser JR: The cardiac sodium channel: Gating function and molecular pharmacology. J Mol Cell Cardiol 2001;33:599-613.

49. Gellens ME, et al: Primary structure and functional expression of the human cardiac tetrodotoxin-insensitive voltage-dependent sodium channel. Proc Natl Acad Sci USA 1992;89:554-558.

50. Backx PH, et al: Molecular localization of an ion-binding site within the pore of mammalian sodium channels. Science 1992; 257:248-251.

51. Heinemann SH, et al: Calcium channel characteristics conferred on the sodium channel by single mutations. Nature 1992;356: 441-443.

52. Yamagishi T, et al: Topology of the P segments in the sodium channel pore revealed by cysteine mutagenesis. Biophys J 1997;73: 195-204.

53. Kellenberger S, Scheuer T, Catterall WA: Movement of the Na⁺ channel inactivation gate during inactivation. J Biol Chem 1996;271:30971-30979.

54. Wang Q, et al: SCN5A mutations associated with an inherited cardiac arrhythmia, long QT syndrome. Cell 1995;80:805-811.

55. Bennett PB, et al: Molecular mechanism for an inherited cardiac arrhythmia. Nature 1995;376:683-685.

56. Isom LL, De Jongh KS, Catterall WA: Auxiliary subunits of voltage-gated ion channels. Neuron 1994;12:1183-1194.

57. Kuniyasu A, et al: Structural characterization of the dihydropyridine receptor-linked calcium channel from porcine heart. J Biochem (Tokyo) 1992;112:235-242.

58. Hofmann F, Biel M, Flockerzi V: Molecular basis for Ca²⁺ channel diversity. Annu Rev Neurosci 1994;17:399-418.

59. Varadi G, et al: Molecular determinants of Ca²⁺ channel function and drug action. Trends Pharmacol Sci 1995;16(2):43-49.

60. Mikami A, et al: Primary structure and functional expression of the cardiac dihydropyridine-sensitive calcium channel. Nature 1989;340:230-233.

61. Wakamori M, et al: Single-channel analysis of a cloned human heart L-type Ca²⁺ channel alpha 1 subunit and the effects of a cardiac beta subunit. Biochem Biophys Res Commun 1993;196: 1170-1176.

62. Koch SE, et al: Architecture of Ca(2+) channel pore-lining segments revealed by covalent modification of substituted cysteines. J Biol Chem 2000;275:34493-34500.

63. Godfraind T: Cardioselectivity of calcium antagonists. Cardiovasc Drugs Ther 1994;8(Suppl 2):353-364.

64. Singh BN: Antiarrhythmic actions of calcium antagonists. Coron Artery Dis 1994;5(1):27-36.

65. Birnbaumer L, et al: Structures and functions of calcium channel beta subunits. J Bioenerg Biomembr 1998;30:357-375.

66. Kamp TJ, Hell JW: Regulation of cardiac L-type calcium channels by protein kinase A and protein kinase C. Circ Res 2000;87: 1095-1102.

67. Cribbs LL, et al: Cloning and characterization of alpha1H from human heart, a member of the T-type Ca²⁺ channel gene family. Circ Res 1998;83:103-109.

68. Wier WG, Balke CW: Ca(2+) release mechanisms, Ca(2+) sparks, and local control of excitation-contraction coupling in normal heart muscle. Circ Res 1999;85:770-776.

69. Marks AR: Ryanodine receptors/calcium release channels in heart failure and sudden cardiac death. J Mol Cell Cardiol 2001;33: 615-624.

70. Periasamy M, Huke S: Serca pump level is a critical determinant of ca(2+)homeostasis and cardiac contractility. J Mol Cell Cardiol 2001;33:1053-1063.

71. Simmerman HK, Jones LR: Phospholamban: Protein structure, mechanism of action, and role in cardiac function. Physiol Rev 1998;78:921-947.

72. Pieske B, et al: Ca²⁺ handling and sarcoplasmic reticulum Ca²⁺ content in isolated failing and nonfailing human myocardium. Circ Res 1999;85:38-46.

73. Munch G, et al: SERCA2a activity correlates with the force-frequency relationship in human myocardium. Am J Physiol Heart Circ Physiol 2000;278:H1924-1932.

74. Somura F, et al: Reduced myocardial sarcoplasmic reticulum Ca(2+)-ATPase mRNA expression and biphasic force-frequency relations in patients with hypertrophic cardiomyopathy. Circulation 2001;104:658-663.

75. Tunwell RE, et al: The human cardiac muscle ryanodine receptor-calcium release channel: Identification, primary structure and topological analysis. Biochem J 1996;318(Pt 2):477-487.

76. Marx SO, et al: Coupled gating between cardiac calcium release channels (ryanodine receptors). Circ Res 2001;88:1151—1158.

77. Priori SG, et al: Mutations in the cardiac ryanodine receptor gene (hRyR2) underlie catecholaminergic polymorphic ventricular tachycardia. Circulation 2001;103:196-200.

78. Laitinen PJ, et al: Mutations of the cardiac ryanodine receptor (RyR2) gene in familial polymorphic ventricular tachycardia. Circulation 2001;103:485-490.

79. Tiso N, et al: Identification of mutations in the cardiac ryanodine receptor gene in families affected with arrhythmogenic right ventricular cardiomyopathy type 2 (ARVD2). Hum Mol Genet 2001;10(3):189-194.

80. Komuro I, et al: Molecular cloning and characterization of the human cardiac Na⁺/Ca²⁺ exchanger cDNA. Proc Natl Acad Sci USA 1992;89:4769-4773.

81. Kraev A, Chumakov I, Carafoli E: The organization of the human gene NCX1 encoding the sodium-calcium exchanger. Genomics 1996;37(1):105-112.

82. Bogdanov KY, Vinogradova TM, Lakatta EG: Sinoatrial nodal cell ryanodine receptor and Na(+)-Ca(2+) exchanger: Molecular partners in pacemaker regulation. Circ Res 2001;88: 1254-1258.

83. Pogwizd SM, et al: Arrhythmogenesis and contractile dysfunction in heart failure: Roles of sodium-calcium exchange, inward rectifier potassium current, and residual beta-adrenergic responsiveness. Circ Res 2001;88:1159-1167.

84. Roberds SL, et al: Molecular biology of the voltage-gated potassium channels of the cardiovascular system. J Cardiovasc Electrophysiol 1993;4(1):68-80.

85. Honore E, Lesage F, Romey G: Molecular biology of voltage-gated K⁺ channels in heart. Fundam Clin Pharmacol 1994;8(2): 108-116.

86. Tristani-Firouzi M, et al: Molecular biology of K(+) channels and their role in cardiac arrhythmias. Am J Med 2001;110:50-59.

87. Tamkun MM, et al: Molecular cloning and characterization of two voltage-gated K⁺ channel cDNAs from human ventricle. FASEB J 1991;5:331-337.

88. Po S, et al: Functional expression of an inactivating potassium channel cloned from human heart. Circ Res 1992;71:732-736.

89. England SK, et al: Characterization of a voltage-gated K⁺ channel beta subunit expressed in human heart. Proc Natl Acad Sci USA 1995;92:6309-6313.

90. Majumder K, et al: Molecular cloning and functional expression of a novel potassium channel beta-subunit from human atrium. FEBS Lett 1995;361:13-16.

91. Zhang M, Jiang M, Tseng GN: minK-related peptide 1 associates with Kv4.2 and modulates its gating function: Potential role as beta subunit of cardiac transient outward channel? Circ Res 2001;88:1012-1019.

92. Dixon JE, et al: Role of the Kv4.3 K$^+$ channel in ventricular muscle. A molecular correlate for the transient outward current. Circ Res 1996;79:659-668.

93. Kong W, et al: Isolation and characterization of the human gene encoding Ito: Further diversity by alternative mRNA splicing. Am J Physiol 1998;275(6 Pt 2):H1963-1970.

94. Kaab S, et al: Molecular basis of transient outward potassium current downregulation in human heart failure: A decrease in Kv4.3 mRNA correlates with a reduction in current density. Circulation 1998;98:1383-1393.

95. Postma AV, et al: Genomic organisation and chromosomal localisation of two members of the KCND ion channel family, KCND2 and KCND3. Hum Genet 2000;106:614-619.

96. Barry DM, et al: Functional knockout of the transient outward current, long-QT syndrome, and cardiac remodeling in mice expressing a dominant-negative Kv4 alpha subunit. Circ Res 1998;83: 560-567.

97. Warmke JW, Ganetzky B: A family of potassium channel genes related to eag in Drosophila and mammals. Proc Natl Acad Sci U S A 1994;91:3438-3442.

98. Trudeau MC, et al: HERG, a human inward rectifier in the voltage-gated potassium channel family. Science 1995;269:92-95.

99. Abbott GW, et al: MiRP1 forms IKr potassium channels with HERG and is associated with cardiac arrhythmia. Cell 1999;97:175-187.

100. Curran ME, et al: A molecular basis for cardiac arrhythmia: HERG mutations cause long QT syndrome. Cell 1995;80:795-803.

101. del Camino D, et al: Blocker protection in the pore of a voltage-gated K$^+$ channel and its structural implications. Nature 2000;403:321-325.

102. Mitcheson JS, Chen J, Sanguinetti MC: Trapping of a methanesulfonanilide by closure of the HERG potassium channel activation gate. J Gen Physiol 2000;115:229-240.

103. Mitcheson JS, et al: A structural basis for drug-induced long QT syndrome. Proc Natl Acad Sci USA 2000;97:12329-12333.

104. Roden DM: Mechanisms and management of proarrhythmia. Am J Cardiol 1998;82(4A):49I-57I.

105. Morais Cabral JH, et al: Crystal structure and functional analysis of the HERG potassium channel N terminus: A eukaryotic PAS domain. Cell 1998;95:649-655.

106. Chen J, et al: Long QT syndrome-associated mutations in the Per-Arnt-Sim (PAS) domain of HERG potassium channels accelerate channel deactivation. J Biol Chem 1999;274:10113-10118.

107. Smith PL, Baukrowitz T, Yellen G: The inward rectification mechanism of the HERG cardiac potassium channel. Nature 1996; 379:833-836.

108. Spector PS, et al: Fast inactivation causes rectification of the IKr channel. J Gen Physiol 1996;107:611-619.

109. Yang WP, et al: KvLQT1, a voltage-gated potassium channel responsible for human cardiac arrhythmias. Proc Natl Acad Sci USA 1997;94:4017-4021.

110. Sanguinetti MC, et al: Coassembly of KVLQT1 and minK (IsK) proteins to form cardiac IKs potassium channel. Nature 1996;384: 80-83.

111. Barhanin J, et al: KVLQT1 and IsK (minK) proteins associate to form the IKs cardiac potassium current. Nature 1996;384:78-80.

112. Varnum MD, et al: The min K channel underlies the cardiac potassium current IKs and mediates species-specific responses to protein kinase C. Proc Natl Acad Sci USA 1993;90:11528-11532.

113. Lai LP, et al: Polymorphism of the gene encoding a human minimal potassium ion channel (minK). Gene 1994;151:339-340.

114. Lee MP, et al: Human KVLQT1 gene shows tissue-specific imprinting and encompasses Beckwith-Wiedemann syndrome chromosomal rearrangements. Nat Genet 1997;15:181-185.

115. Wang Q, et al: Positional cloning of a novel potassium channel gene: KVLQT1 mutations cause cardiac arrhythmias. Nat Genet 1996;12:17-23.

116. Splawski I, et al: Spectrum of mutations in long-QT syndrome genes. KVLQT1, HERG, SCN5A, KCNE1, and KCNE2. Circulation 2000;102:1178-1185.

117. Splawski I, et al: Molecular basis of the long-QT syndrome associated with deafness. N Engl J Med 1997;336:1562-1567.

118. Neyroud N, et al: A novel mutation in the potassium channel gene KVLQT1 causes the Jervell and Lange-Nielsen cardioauditory syndrome. Nat Genet 1997;15:186-189.

119. Antzelevitch C: Basic mechanisms of reentrant arrhythmias. Curr Opin Cardiol 2001;16:1-7.

120. Kubo Y, et al: Primary structure and functional expression of a mouse inward rectifier potassium channel. Nature 1993;362: 127-133.

121. Redell JB, Tempel BL: Multiple promoter elements interact to control the transcription of the potassium channel gene, KCNJ2. J Biol Chem 1998;273:22807-22818.

122. Ma D, et al: Role of ER export signals in controlling surface potassium channel numbers. Science 2001;291:316-319.

123. Derst C, et al: Genetic and functional linkage of Kir5.1 and Kir2.1 channel subunits. FEBS Lett 2001;491:305-311.

124. Plaster NM, et al: Mutations in Kir2.1 cause the developmental and episodic electrical phenotypes of Andersen's syndrome. Cell 2001;105:511-519.

125. Ackerman MJ, Clapham DC: Cardiac chloride channels. Trends Cardiovascular Med 1993;3:23-28.

126. Hume JR, Horowitz B: A plethora of cardiac chloride conductances: Molecular diversity or a related gene family. J Cardiovasc Electrophysiol 1995;6:325-331.

127. Wolff AA, Levi R: Histamine and cardiac arrhythmias. Circ Res 1986;58:1-16.

128. Harvey RD, Hume JR: Autonomic regulation of a chloride current in heart. Science 1989;244:983-985.

129. Ono K, Noma A: Autonomic regulation of cardiac chloride current. Jpn J Physiol 1994;44:S193-S198.

130. Gadsby DC, Nagel G, Hwang TC: The CFTR chloride channel of mammalian heart. Annu Rev Physiol 1995;57:387-416.

131. Hart P, et al: Cystic fibrosis gene encodes a cAMP-dependent chloride channel in heart. Proc Natl Acad Sci USA 1996;93: 6343-6346.

132. Gadsby DC, Nairn AC: Regulation of CFTR channel gating. Trends Biochem Sci 1994;19:513-518.

133. Wallert MA, et al: Two novel cardiac atrial K$^+$ channels, IK.AA and IK.PC. J Gen Physiol 1991;98:921-939.

134. Wickman K, Clapham DE: Ion channel regulation by G proteins. Physiol Rev 1995;75:865-885.

135. Abraham MR, et al: Channelopathies of inwardly rectifying potassium channels. FASEB J 1999;13:1901-1910.

136. Inagaki N, et al: Reconstitution of IKATP: An inward rectifier subunit plus the sulfonylurea receptor. Science 1995;270:1166-1170.

137. Babenko AP, et al: Reconstituted human cardiac KATP channels: Functional identity with the native channels from the sarcolemma of human ventricular cells. Circ Res 1998;83: 1132-1143.

138. Lorenz E, Terzic A: Physical association between recombinant cardiac ATP-sensitive K+ channel subunits Kir6.2 and SUR2A. J Mol Cell Cardiol 1999;31:425-434.

139. Cavero I, Guillon JM: Membrane ion channels and cardiovascular ATP-sensitive K$^+$ channels. Cardiologia 1993;38(12 Suppl 1): 445-452.

140. Quast U: Potassium channel openers: Pharmacological and clinical aspects. Fundam Clin Pharmacol 1992;6(7):279-293.

141. Haeusler G, Lues I: Therapeutic potential of potassium channel activators in coronary heart disease. Eur Heart J 1994;15(Suppl C):82-88.

142. Challinor-Rogers JL, McPherson GA: Potassium channel openers and other regulators of KATP channels. Clin Exp Pharmacol Physiol 1994;21:583-597.

143. Noma A: ATP-regulated K$^+$ channels in cardiac muscle. Nature 1983;305:147-148.

144. Li RA, et al: Molecular basis of electrocardiographic ST-segment elevation. Circ Res 2000;87:837-839.

145. Jovanovic A, et al: Recombinant cardiac ATP-sensitive K$^+$ channel subunits confer resistance to chemical hypoxia-reoxygenation injury. Circulation 1998;98:1548-1555.

146. Terzic A: New frontiers of cardioprotection. Clin Pharmacol Ther 1999;66(2):105-109.

147. Garratt KN, et al: Sulfonylurea drugs increase early mortality in patients with diabetes mellitus after direct angioplasty for acute myocardial infarction. J Am Coll Cardiol 1999;33:119-124.

148. Bienengraeber M, et al: ATPase activity of the sulfonylurea receptor: A catalytic function for the KATP channel complex. FASEB J 2000;14:1943-1952.

149. Zingman LV, et al: ATPase transitions in SUR module gate ATP-sensitive K+ conductance. Neuron 2001;31:233–245.

150. Carrasco AJ, et al: Adenylate kinase phosphotransfer communicates cellular energetic signals to ATP-sensitive potassium channels. Proc Natl Acad Sci USA 2001;98:7623–7628.

151. Terzic A, Vivaudou M: Molecular pharmacology of ATP-sensitive K+ channels: How and why? In Rusch AA (ed): Potassium Channels in Cardiovascular Biology. New York, Kluwer Academic/Plenum Publishers, 2001, pp 257–277.

152. Ackerman MJ, Clapham DC: G proteins and ion channels. In Jalife ZA (ed): Cardiac Electrophysiology: From Cell to Bedside. Philadelphia, WB Saunders, 2000, pp 112–118.

153. Logothetis DE, et al: The beta gamma subunits of GTP-binding proteins activate the muscarinic K+ channel in heart. Nature 1987;325:321–326.

154. Krapivinsky G, et al: G beta gamma binds directly to the G protein-gated K+ channel, IKACh. J Biol Chem 1995;270:29059–29062.

155. Krapivinsky G, et al: The G-protein-gated atrial K+ channel IKACh is a heteromultimer of two inwardly rectifying K(+)-channel proteins. Nature 1995;374:135–141.

156. Wickman K, et al: Abnormal heart rate regulation in GIRK4 knockout mice. Neuron 1998;20:103–114.

157. Malcolm AD, Garratt CJ, Camm AJ: The therapeutic and diagnostic cardiac electrophysiological uses of adenosine. Cardiovasc Drugs Ther 1993;7(1):139–147.

158. Pelleg A, Belardinelli L: Cardiac electrophysiology and pharmacology of adenosine: Basic and clinical aspects. Cardiovasc Res 1993;27(1):54–61.

159. Shen WK, Kurachi Y: Mechanisms of adenosine-mediated actions on cellular and clinical cardiac electrophysiology. Mayo Clin Proc 1995;70:274–291.

160. Kovoor P, et al: Evaluation of the role of I(KACh) in atrial fibrillation using a mouse knockout model. J Am Coll Cardiol 2001;37:2136–2143.

## EDITOR'S CHOICE

An WF, Bowlby MR, Betty M, et al: Modulation of A-type potassium channels by a family of calcium sensors. Nature 2000;403:553–556.

Choe S: Potassium channel structures. Nat Rev Neurosci 200;23:115–121.

Du GG, Sandhu B, Khanna VK, et al: Topology of the Ca2+ release channel of skeletal muscle sarcoplasmic reticulum (RyR1). Proc Natl Acad Sci U S A 2002;99:16725–16730.

Jiang Y, Lee A, Chen J, et al: X-ray structure of a voltage-dependent K+ channel. Nature 2003;423:33–41.

Jiang Y, Ruta V, Chen J, et al: The principle of gating charge movement in a voltage-dependent K+ channel. Nature 2003;423:42–48.

Kass RS, Kurokawa J, Marx SO, Marks AR: Leucine/isoleucine zipper coordination of ion channel macromolecular signaling complexes in the heart. Roles in inherited arrhythmias. Trends Cardiovasc Med 2003;13:52–56.

Keating MT, Sanguinetti MC: Molecular and cellular mechanisms of cardiac arrhythmias. Cell 2001;104:569–580.

Kuo HC, Cheng CF, Clark RB, et al: A defect in the Kv channel-interacting protein 2 (KChIP2) gene leads to a complete loss of I(to) and confers susceptibility to ventricular tachycardia. Cell 2001;107:801–813.

Nishida M, MacKinnon R: Structural basis of inward rectification: Cytoplasmic pore of the G protein-gated inward rectifier GIRK1 at 1.8 Å resolution. Cell 2002;111:957–965.

Robinson RB, Siegelbaum SA: Hyperpolarization-activated cation currents: From molecules to physiological function. Annu Rev Physiol 2003;65:453–480.

Rosati B, Pan Z, Lypen S, et al: Regulation of KChIP2 potassium channel beta subunit gene expression underlies the gradient of transient outward current in canine and human ventricle. J Physiol 2001;533:119–125.

# Cardiac Arrhythmias: Inherited Molecular Mechanisms

*Steve A. N. Goldstein*
*Mark T. Keating*
*Michael C. Sanguinetti*

The heart is a pump controlled by electrical impulses (Fig. 19-1). A coordinated wave of excitation passing through the two atria results in their contraction and pumping of blood into the ventricles; subsequent excitation and contraction of the ventricles pumps blood out of the heart. The right ventricle moves deoxygenated blood to the lungs for gas exchange. The left ventricle pumps oxygen-rich blood returning from the lungs to the rest of the organs and maintains systemic blood pressure. The brain is particularly sensitive to blood pressure and flow. When coordinated cardiac contractions stop for only a few seconds, blood pressure drops and consciousness is lost. If pump function is lost for more than a few minutes, permanent brain damage and death ensue.

Electrical impulses are intrinsic to the heart and are modulated by the autonomic nervous system. Specialized cells in the sinoatrial node (SAN) of the right atrium normally act as a pacemaker firing spontaneously approximately 70 times per minute at rest and up to 200 times per minute during rigorous exercise (Fig. 19-1). The impulse is conveyed to all atrial myocytes because the cells are coupled via intercellular gap junctions producing coordinated depolarization (a positive shift in the transmembrane potential) and contraction. On a surface electrocardiogram (ECG) atrial depolarization is reflected in the P wave (Fig. 19-1). The impulse is also conveyed to the atrioventricular node (AVN); these cells delay transmission of the electrical activity for about 20 msec to give the atria time to pump blood into the ventricles. Next, the impulse is conveyed to the bundle branch conduction (Purkinje) fibers that allow for orderly depolarization and contraction of the ventricles from the cardiac apex toward the outflow tracts. Ventricular depolarization is observed on an ECG as the QRS complex. Repolarization (a return to negative resting membrane potential) of the ventricles is reflected on an ECG by the T wave and leads to muscular relaxation and completion of one cardiac cycle. Rhythmic activity of the human heart is apparent by ultrasound at only 5 weeks' gestation and continues for a lifetime with virtually no tolerance for failure.

Although most hearts beat with fidelity and resilience, under certain circumstances the rhythm of the heart can fail. This is known as a cardiac arrhythmia. When the heartbeat is too slow (bradyarrhythmia or bradycardia) or too rapid (tachyarrhythmia or tachycardia) blood pressure cannot be maintained. Bradyarrhythmias often result from disease of pacemaker or other specialized conducting cells and can be effectively treated with artificial, electronic pacemakers. The most dangerous tachyarrhythmias are focused in the ventricles and are called ventricular tachycardia, *torsades de pointes,* and ventricular fibrillation (Fig. 19-1).

Cardiac arrhythmias are a leading cause of morbidity and mortality. More than 300,000 individuals in the United States die suddenly every year, and in most cases it is suspected that the underlying cause is ventricular tachyarrhythmia.[1,2] Despite their importance, the ability to predict, prevent, and treat these disorders remains a major scientific and medical challenge. This chapter discusses how recent studies of ventricular tachyarrhythmias have (1) revealed that rare inherited mutations in genes for cardiac ion channels leads to susceptibility to these life-threatening disorders; (2) advanced the understanding of the molecular basis for normal cardiac electrical function; and (3) demonstrated that common "acquired" arrhythmias can also have a genetic basis, that is, individuals can inherit susceptibility to secondary inciting challenges such as drug exposure.

## ION CHANNELS AND THE CARDIAC ACTION POTENTIAL

Like other excitable cells, such as neurons, skeletal muscle cells, and smooth muscle cells, the electrical activity of cardiac myocytes is manifest in action potentials. The cardiac myocyte action potential is distinctive in its long duration, lasting approximately 300 msec (those in neurons and skeletal muscle are just a few milliseconds). The cardiac action potential is described in five phases, numbered 0 to 4 (Fig. 19-2). Phase 0 represents depolarization of the myocyte. This phase is initiated by the rapid opening (activation) of voltage-gated sodium channels ($I_{Na}$). Depolarization of ventricular myocytes is reflected by the QRS complex on the surface ECG. Phase 1 of the cardiac action potential occurs immediately after the peak of depolarization and is recognized as a partial repolarization of

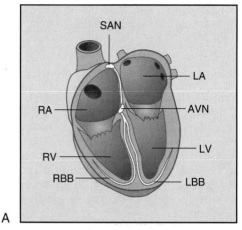

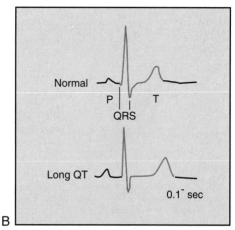

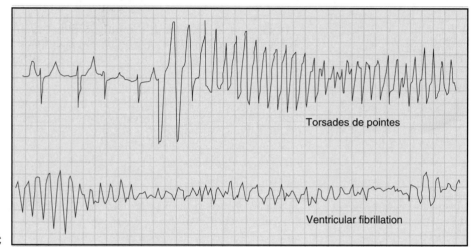

**FIGURE 19-1.** The heart is an electrically activated pump. *A,* Representation of a human heart including the SAN, the primary pacemaker; the AVN delays conduction to allow pumping of blood from the atria to ventricles; the right and left bundle branches (RBB, LBB) mediate coordinated excitation of the ventricles. LA, left atrium; LV, left ventricle; RA, right atrium; RV, right ventricle. *B,* Normal ECG and an ECG showing QT-interval prolongation. The y-axis indicates voltage, the x-axis is time. The P wave indicates atrial depolarization, the QRS complex indicates ventricular depolarization, and the T wave indicates ventricular repolarization. A normal QTc interval is approximately 0.40 seconds. *C,* ECG showing normal sinus rhythm converting to *torsades de pointes,* ventricular tachycardia, and ventricular fibrillation, a life-threatening cardiac arrhythmia because pumping is no longer sufficient to maintain systemic blood pressure. *(From Keating MT, Sanguinetti MC: Molecular and cellular mechanisms of cardiac arrhythmias. Cell 2001;104:569-580, with permission from Elsevier.)*

the membrane. This small repolarizing effect is due to the closure (inactivation) of cardiac sodium channels and activation of a transient outward potassium current ($I_{to}$). Phase 2 of the action potential is the plateau phase. This phase is especially long in ventricular myocytes and Purkinje fibers of the cardiac conduction pathway. The plateau is generated primarily by slowly decreasing inward calcium currents through L-type calcium channels and increasing outward currents through several types of potassium channels. The net current during the plateau phase of the cardiac action potential is small. As a consequence, relatively small changes in ion current during this phase can have a major impact on action potential duration, and the ECG during this phase is at baseline. Phase 3 represents myocellular repolarization and is mediated primarily by two outward potassium currents $I_{Kr}$ and $I_{Ks}$.[3] Other currents that contribute to repolarization are the plateau potassium currents ($I_{Kp}$) and the inward rectifier potassium current ($I_{K1}$), which also serves to determine diastolic membrane potential in atrial and ventricular myocytes.[4] Ventricular repolarization correlates with the T wave on the surface ECG. Phase 4 is the final phase of the action potential and signals a return of membrane potential to its resting level near −85 mV. This phase represents ventricular relaxation (or diastole) and again the ECG returns to baseline.

Thus, coordinated opening and closing of ion channels mediates the cardiac action potential, and duration of the QT interval on the ECG is a reflection of the length of the ventricular action potential. The genes associated with arrhythmia susceptibility encode ion channel subunits that contribute to these cardiac action potential currents or the process of excitation-contraction coupling: *SCN5A* ($I_{Na}$); *KvLQT1* and *KCNE1* ($I_{Ks}$); *HERG* and *KCNE1* ($I_{Kr}$); *KCNJ2* ($I_{K1}$); and *RYR2*, which mediates calcium-triggered release of calcium from the sarcoplasmic reticulum to produce cardiac contraction.

## LONG QT SYNDROME

Long QT syndrome (LQTS) is a group of disorders characterized by syncope and risk for sudden death because of episodic cardiac arrhythmias, particularly torsades de pointes and ventricular fibrillation.[5] Torsades de pointes means twisting around the point, an allusion to the alternating axis of the QRS complex around the isoelectric line of the ECG during this arrhythmia[6] (Fig. 19-1). Most individuals with LQTS have no other symptoms or signs of disease, and dangerous arrhythmias are relatively rare. Some cases are associated with congenital deafness and others with syndactyly, abnormal webbing of fingers or toes. Many

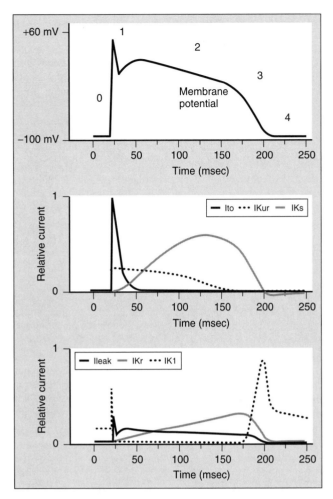

**FIGURE 19-2.** The cardiac action potential is mediated by ion currents. Schematic representation of a cardiac action potential with voltage on the y-axis and time on the x-axis. Inward sodium current mediates the rapid phase 0 depolarization (not shown). Transient outward potassium currents ($I_{to}$) mediate rapid phase 1 repolarization. The L-type inward calcium current contributes to the plateau duration (phase 2) as do $I_{Kr}$, $I_{Ks}$, $I_{K1}$, $I_{leak}$, and $I_{Kur}$ potassium currents (the last two appear to yield $I_{Kp}$); the potassium currents mediate repolarization (phase 2 and 3). The coordinated opening and closing of cardiac ion channels is responsible for cardiac excitability.

individuals have ECG abnormalities, particularly a prolonged QT interval, although changes can be subtle.[7]

The LQTSs have been divided on clinical grounds into two main types: familial and acquired. There are at least two familial forms of LQTS. One, the Jervell and Lange-Nielsen syndrome, was believed to be inherited as an autosomal recessive trait in association with congenital deafness.[8] A second, more common familial form is inherited as an autosomal dominant trait with no other phenotypic abnormalities. This form, sometimes referred to as the Romano Ward syndrome,[9,10] is usually associated with less arrhythmia risk than the autosomal recessive form.

The most common form of LQTS is acquired. Treatment with therapeutic medications (including certain antibiotics, antihistamines, and antiarrhythmics) is the most common cause of acquired LQTS.[11] There

are many additional causes of acquired LQTS including cardiomyopathy, cardiac ischemia, and electrolyte abnormalities.[12,13]

## A Case History: Inherited Long QT Syndrome

The presentation and course of inherited arrhythmia susceptibility in members of one family provides insight into these disorders.[14] A 25-year-old woman was seen for routine evaluation by her obstetrician. She was healthy and in her thirty-fifth week of gestation of a previously uncomplicated pregnancy when her physician noted a fetal heart rate of 70 to 80 beats per minute, approximately half the normal rate. Ultrasound examination revealed normal fetal development, and a male child was born spontaneously at 39 weeks.

During the first feeding the child became cyanotic and was rushed to the neonatal intensive care unit, where a series of tests were performed. All were normal except for the ECG, which showed a slow heart rate of 82 beats per minute and a prolonged rate corrected QT (QTc) interval of approximately 0.60 seconds. The QTc interval is a temporal measure of ventricular repolarization and is normally about 0.40 seconds. A pediatric cardiologist recommended audiographic evaluation. These tests showed severe bilateral hearing loss and a tentative diagnosis of Jervell and Lange-Nielsen syndrome was made. The child was placed on medications to reduce autonomic nervous activity of the heart (e.g., β-blockade), observed for several days without incident, and sent home after 10 days with a monitor. Because Jervell and Lange-Nielsen syndrome was thought to be purely recessive, no clinical evaluation of the child's parents or other family members was performed. However, several months later the patient's mother, who previously enjoyed excellent health, was awakened by her alarm clock and, on standing, had a cardiac arrest and died. Genetic evaluation of the family was undertaken.

## MUTATIONS IN CARDIAC ION CHANNEL GENES: ARRHYTHMIA SUSCEPTIBILITY

When molecular studies of LQTS began, there were two prominent theories for the pathogenesis of the disorder. One was the autonomic imbalance hypothesis based on studies showing that manipulation of the autonomic nervous system in dogs could produce QT prolongation and cardiac arrhythmia.[15] A second hypothesis, the cardiac ion channel hypothesis, suggested that inherited or acquired dysfunction of ion channels in the heart could be causative. Although it is clear that the autonomic nervous system plays a secondary role in many cardiac arrhythmias, the cardiac ion channel hypothesis has proved to be the primary mechanism of arrhythmia susceptibility in studies reported to date (Table 19-1, Fig. 19-2).

To define genes that contribute to arrhythmia susceptibility, familial forms of the disorder were examined,

■ ■ ■

**TABLE 19–1**    MOLECULAR AND CELLULAR MECHANISMS OF CARDIAC ARRHYTHMIA

| Arrhythmia | Inheritance | Protein (Gene) | Function | Abnormality |
|---|---|---|---|---|
| LQT1 | Autosomal dominant | KvLQT1 (KCNQ1) | $I_{Ks}$ K channel α subunit | Repolarization |
| LQT2 | Autosomal dominant | HERG (KCNH2) | $I_{Kr}$ K channel α subunit | Repolarization |
| LQT3 | Autosomal dominant | SCN5A (SCN5A) | $I_{Na}$ Na channel α subunit | Repolarization |
| LQT4 | Not identified | | | |
| LQT5 | Autosomal dominant | MinK (KCNE1) | $I_{Ks}$ K channel β subunit | Repolarization |
| LQT6 | Autosomal dominant | MiRP1 (KCNE2) | $I_{Kr}$ K channel β subunit | Repolarization |
| LQT7 | | Not identified | | |
| LQT8 (AS) | Autosomal dominant | Kir2.1 (KCNJ2) | $I_{K1}$ K channel α subunit | Repolarization |
| JLNS | Autosomal recessive | KvLQT1 (KCNQ1) | $I_{Ks}$ K channel α subunit | Repolarization |
| | With deafness | MinK (KCNE1) | $I_{Ks}$ K channel β subunit | Repolarization |
| IVF | Autosomal dominant | SCN5A (SCN5A) | $I_{Na}$ Na channel α subunit | Conduction |
| IVF2 | | Not identified | | |
| CVT | Autosomal dominant | RYR2 (RYR2) | Ryanodine receptor | Ca overload |
| ARVD | Autosomal dominant | RYR2 (RYR2) | Ca release channel | Ca overload |
| Drug-induced | None identified | HERG (KCNH2) | $I_{Kr}$ K channel α subunit | Repolarization |
| | Autosomal dominant | MiRP1 (KCNE1) | $I_{Kr}$ K channel β subunit | Repolarization |

ARVD, arrhythmogenic right ventricular dysplasia; AS, Andersen's syndrome; Ca, calcium CVT, catecholaminergic ventricular tachycardia; IVF, familial idiopathic ventricular fibrillation; JLNS, Jervell and Lange Nielson syndromes; K, potassium, LQT, long QT syndrome; Na, sodium.

particularly LQTS. Over the last 6 years, seven arrhythmia susceptibility genes, all encoding cardiac ion channel proteins, have been discovered: *KVLQT1* (or *KCNQ1*), *HERG* (or *KCNH2*), *SCN5A*, *KCNE1*, *KCNE2*, *RYR2*, and *KCNJ2* (Table 19-1).[16-23] *KVLQT1* was discovered by positional cloning, *HERG*, *SCN5A*, *RYR2*, and *KCNJ2* were discovered by using a positional cloning-candidate gene approach, and *KCNE1* and *KCNE2* were discovered by a pure candidate gene approach. Another LQTS locus mapped to chromosome 4 has yet to be identified,[24] and several additional arrhythmia genes appear to await discovery.

Jervell and Lange-Nielsen syndrome had been thought to be an autosomal recessive disorder; however, phenotypic evaluation of the family described previously revealed a more complicated picture.[14] Many members of the family, including the child's father, had subtle prolongation of the QT interval with normal hearing. Although the mother was the first family member to suffer a sudden cardiac death, some individuals gave a history of syncope. Furthermore, pedigree analyses revealed that the child was the product of a consanguineous union of second cousins. This led to the hypothesis, later confirmed by genetic analysis, that inheritance of two mutant alleles of an autosomal dominant LQTS produced Jervell and Lange-Nielsen syndrome. It is now clear that such homozygous mutations of either *KvLQT1* or *KCNE1* can cause the disorder.[20,25,26]

Congenital deafness, one aspect of Jervell and Lange-Nielsen syndrome, is inherited as an autosomal recessive trait; heterozygous carriers have no apparent hearing deficit (Table 19-1). However, arrhythmia susceptibility is inherited as a semidominant trait. Thus, both heterozygotes and homozygotes have susceptibility to arrhythmia, but the risk in homozygotes is much greater. Homozygous mutations of *HERG* have also been reported to increase the risk for arrhythmia but have not been associated with other abnormalities.[27]

## SODIUM CHANNEL DYSFUNCTION AND ARRHYTHMIA

Investigators had previously demonstrated that *SCN5A* encodes the pore-forming α subunits of the sodium channel responsible for initiating cardiac action potentials.[28] This gene is located on chromosome 3p21-p24, and the protein is predicted to have four major domains (Fig. 19-3). Each of these domains is believed to have a topology similar to a voltage-gated potassium channel with six membrane-spanning domains (S1 to S6) and a pore domain between S5 and S6. Although the α subunit can form functional channels, accessory β subunits have been identified that alter biophysical properties of the channel to produce behaviors like those recorded in native cells. To date, mutational analyses have revealed 14 distinct mutations of *SCN5A* associated with LQTS representing approximately 5% of known arrhythmia-associated mutations.[29]

Based on the location of these mutations and the physiology of the disease, it was hypothesized that gain-of-function mutations in *SCN5A* would cause LQTS for the following reasons. Normally, cardiac sodium channels open briefly in response to membrane depolarization. The channels then inactivate and remain closed for the remainder of the action potential. Sodium channel inactivation is mediated by an intracellular domain located between domains III and IV. This domain is referred to as the inactivation gate and is thought to physically block the inner mouth of the channel pore.[30] Several *SCN5A* mutations associated with LQTS were identified in this region. Physiologic characterization of one of these mutants (ΔKPQ) revealed that the mutations destabilized the inactivation gate.[31] Thus, activation of these mutant sodium channels is normal, and the rate of rapid inactivation is slightly faster than normal, but the channels reopen during the plateau phase of the action potential. The net effect is a small, maintained depolarizing current that lengthens action potential duration.[31,32]

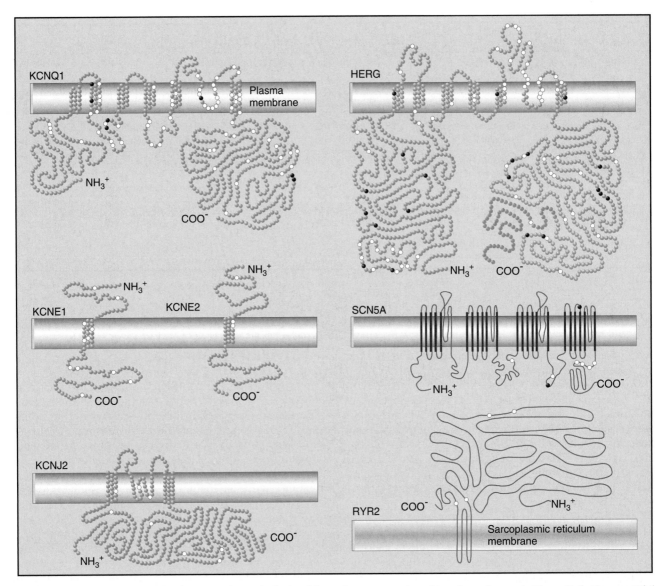

**FIGURE 19-3.** Ion channel mutations cause cardiac arrhythmias. Schematic representation of ion channels encoded by arrhythmia susceptibility genes including SCN5A sodium channel α subunits, KvLQT1 and HERG potassium channel α subunits, MinK and MiRP1 potassium channel β subunits, Kir2.1 potassium channel α subunits, and RYR2 ryanodine receptor/calcium release channels. Missense mutations are indicated by light dots, and the location of frameshifts or intragenic deletions are indicated by dark dots.

Although other LQTS-associated mutations of *SCN5A* had slightly different effects on channel function, all led to maintained depolarizing currents and action potential prolongation.

*SCN5A* mutations also cause familial ventricular fibrillation (Table 19-1).[17] As in LQTS, people with familial ventricular fibrillation often appear healthy without evidence of QT interval prolongation.[33] In other cases, subtle prolongation of the QRS complex or a distinct elevation of the ST segment can be demonstrated, for example, in Brugada's syndrome.[34] Inherited as an autosomal dominant trait with variable penetrance, these individuals are at increased risk for episodic ventricular fibrillation, a particularly lethal arrhythmia. In some cases, the mutations lead to loss-of-function,

whereas the effects of other changes are uncertain. Reduction of sodium current is predicted to shorten action potential duration and slow conduction velocity. Pharmacologic studies suggest that diminished sodium channel activity can be a substrate for development of re-entrant arrhythmias resulting from heterogeneity in the action potential as it traverses the right ventricular epicardium, leading to dispersion of myocardial repolarization and refractoriness.[35] Thus, gain- and loss-of-function mutations of *SCN5A* can both cause arrhythmia susceptibility. Gain of function causes prolongation of action potentials and is associated with LQTS; loss of function slightly shortens action potential duration, slows conduction velocity, and is linked to familial ventricular fibrillation.

## KVLQT1: A POTASSIUM CHANNEL SUBUNIT ASSOCIATED WITH LONG QT SYNDROME

*KVLQT1* (*KCNQ1*) is located on chromosome 11p5.5[36] in a region associated with Beckwith-Wiedemann syndrome.[37] Northern analyses indicate that *KVLQT1* is expressed in the heart, placenta, lung, kidney,[21] inner ear, and pancreas, with greatest expression in the pancreas.[38] *KVLQT1* and other genes in the region are imprinted, with paternal silencing in most tissues. However, *KVLQT1* is not imprinted in the heart.[37] Homologs of *KVLQT1* (*KCNQ2* and *KCNQ3*) have been identified in the brain and are associated with benign familial neonatal seizures, an inherited form of epilepsy.[39-41] Mutations in another homolog, *KCNQ4,* cause deafness.[42,43] KvLQT1 is a classical voltage-gated potassium channel pore-forming α subunit. It has six putative membrane spanning domains (S1 to S6) including a voltage sensor (S4) and a potassium channel pore "signature" sequence between S5 and S6 (Fig. 19-3). As of 2000, mutational analyses had revealed 85 mutations in the *KVLQT1* coding sequence, representing approximately 40% of known arrhythmia-associated mutations.[29] Most of these mutations are missense mutations located in membrane spanning and pore regions.

At least two molecular mechanisms account for reduced KvLQT1 function in LQTS.[44,45] In the first, disease-associated intragenic deletions of one KvLQT1 allele result in syntheses of abnormal subunits that do not assemble with normal subunits. As a result, only normal subunits form the functional tetrameric channels. This loss-of-function mechanism (haploinsufficiency) results in a 50% reduction in the number of functional channels. In the second mechanism, missense mutations result in synthesis of KvLQT1 subunits with subtle structural abnormalities. Many of these subunits can assemble with normal subunits, forming mixed heterotetrameric complexes with reduced function, or misfold and are degraded before trafficking to the plasma membrane. The net effect can be a greater than 50% reduction in channel activity, that is, a dominant negative effect. The severity of a dominant negative effect can vary considerably depending on the site and type of mutation. In some cases, the effect is relatively mild, whereas in others suppression of $I_{Ks}$ current is essentially complete. Missense mutations in pore sequences seem to be particularly potent. The severity of the dominant negative effect is suspected to impact the severity of arrhythmia susceptibility; however, many factors affect susceptibility, and phenotypic variability is seen among family members carrying the same *KVLQT1* mutation.

Expression studies of *KVLQT1* were also notable because the biophysical properties of the induced voltage-gated potassium channels were unlike any potassium current identified in cardiac myocytes.[46,47] This led to the hypothesis that KvLQT1 subunits might assemble with another subunit type to form native cardiac potassium channels.

## *KVLQT1* AND *KCNE1* PRODUCTS: SLOW DELAYED RECTIFIER POTASSIUM CHANNELS

The *KCNE1* gene located on chromosome 21q22.1 encodes MinK, so named because it appeared to encode a minimal potassium channel subunit.[48-50] Only 129 amino acids long, the protein has one membrane-spanning domain, no potassium channel pore signature sequence, and no voltage-sensing domain. Ten mutations of *KCNE1* have been associated with LQTS, representing approximately 5% of mutations identified to date.[29]

MinK was discovered by functional expression in *Xenopus* oocytes.[48] The biophysical properties of the current elicited by expression of *KCNE1* were similar to cardiac $I_{Ks}$, suggesting that MinK might form the cardiac channels on its own. However, the unusual structure of MinK, the failure of increasing amounts of the protein to produce increasing levels of current, and its failure to induce any currents in some cell types suggested it did not operate alone.[51-53] It is now clear that MinK is a required β subunit that assembles with KvLQT1 to form cardiac $I_{Ks}$ channels.[46,47] How is it that MinK alone can be functionally expressed in *Xenopus* oocytes? The explanation is that *XKVLQT1*, a homolog of *KVLQT1,* is constitutively expressed in *Xenopus* oocytes at a relatively low level and can interact with MinK to form $I_{Ks}$-like channels.[47] The stoichiometry of $I_{Ks}$ channels remains a matter of controversy; some argue that two MinK subunits assemble with four KvLQT1 α subunits[52,54] whereas others suggest that a variable number of MinK monomers (up to four) are present in each complex.[55]

The most apparent effect of MinK on KvLQT1 subunits is an approximately 10-fold slowing of activation kinetics, although MinK also alters inactivation and deactivation gating.[47,56] The unitary conductance of the MinK/KCNQ1 channels (in symmetric 140 mm potassium ions) is approximately fourfold greater than that of homomeric KCNQ1 channels.[56,57] MinK also alters selectivity for monovalent cations, sensitivity to both external and internal pore blockers, inhibition by class III antiarrhythmic agents (i.e., potassium channel blockers), and activation by small-molecule regulators.[58,59]

Inheritance of missense mutations in *KCNE1* leading to the replacement of serine at position 74 with leucine or aspartate at position 76 with asparagine have been associated with inherited LQTS. The changes in *KCNE1* reduce net potassium flux through $I_{Ks}$ channels because of a positive shift in the voltage dependence of activation (i.e., less current is generated at a given level of depolarization), a reduction in single channel conductance, and accelerated deactivation.[20,56]

KvLQT1 and MinK are both expressed in the inner ear where $I_{Ks}$ channels function to produce the potassium-rich fluid endolymph that bathes the organ of Corti, the cochlear organ responsible for hearing.[60] Individuals with Jervell and Lange-Nielsen syndrome have homozygous mutations of *KvLQT1* or *KCNE1* and, therefore, have no functional $I_{Ks}$ channels. As noted in the family described previously, these individuals have severe arrhythmia susceptibility and congenital sensorineural deafness. The mechanism of deafness is gleaned from *KCNE1* gene disruption in mice in which a lack of $I_{Ks}$ current leads to inadequate endolymph production and deterioration of the organ of Corti.[61]

## HERG: α-SUBUNIT OF CARDIAC $I_{Kr}$ POTASSIUM CHANNELS

*HERG (KCNH2),* located on chromosome 7q35-q36, is expressed primarily in the heart[18] but was originally identified in a human hippocampal cDNA library.[62] As of 2000, 94 distinct mutations of HERG had been identified.[29] These represent 45% of the total number of known LQTS mutations.[29]

*HERG* encodes a typical voltage-gated potassium channel α subunit with six membrane-spanning domains (S1 to S6), a voltage sensor (S4), and a potassium-selective pore-lining loop between S5 and S6. HERG subunits have a large intracellular C-terminal region containing a cyclic nucleotide binding domain and a large N-terminal domain, the first 135 amino acids of which are highly conserved in related channels. The structure of this N-terminal domain has been solved and has similarity to other Per-Arnt-Sim (PAS) domains known to be important for protein-protein interactions.[63] Proteins with PAS domains are often involved in signal transduction.

Expression of *HERG* in heterologous systems led to its identification as the α subunit of cardiac $I_{Kr}$ potassium channels, the channel that with $I_{Ks}$ is primarily responsible for termination of the plateau of the action potential.[64,65] One of the notable properties of $I_{Kr}$ channels reproduced by HERG is the bell-shaped current-voltage relationship caused by their rapid inactivation.[66] This behavior accounts for the importance of $I_{Kr}$ during phase 3 repolarization because recovery from inactivation followed by slow channel deactivation during the first half of phase 3 increases $I_{Kr}$ current despite a concurrent decrease in the electrochemical driving force for outward potassium flux.[67]

Many HERG mutations cluster around the membrane-spanning domains and the pore region. Some of these mutations, such as early nonsense mutations, have a pure loss-of-function effect. Oftentimes the encoded mutant proteins misfold and are rapidly degraded,[68] leading to a dominant negative effect, if they assemble with wild-type subunits, or haploinsufficiency, if they do not. Most LQTS-associated mutations in HERG are missense mutations. Expression studies support the idea that many of these mutations have a dominant negative effect. Analysis of LQTS-associated missense mutations[69] and engineered deletion mutants in HERG PAS domain[63] reveal that this region is important to the slow rate of $I_{Kr}$ channel deactivation, which is critical to its role in phase 3 repolarization.

Although many of the biophysical properties of HERG channels in heterologous systems are nearly identical to cardiac $I_{Kr}$, two properties are notably out of line.[16,64] First, deactivation of cardiac $I_{Kr}$ was slow but not so slow as HERG channels. Second, block of cardiac $I_{Kr}$ by methanesulfoanilide drugs was different from the block of HERG channels in both kinetics and voltage dependence. This led to the hypothesis that HERG, like KvLQT1, assembled with a β subunit to form native $I_{Kr}$ channels.

## *HERG* AND *KCNE2* PRODUCTS: FORMING CHANNELS THAT CONDUCT CARDIAC $I_{Kr}$

*KCNE2,* encoding MinK-related protein 1 (MiRP1), is located on chromosome 21q22.1, just 79 kb from MinK.[16] The two genes have significant homology at the DNA and amino acid level (27% identity) suggesting that they result from a recent duplication. Study of *KCNE2* resolved the disparity between native and cloned (i.e., homotetrameric) HERG channels: MiRP1 and HERG were found to form stable complexes that behave like native $I_{Kr}$ channels in their unitary conductance, sensitivity to external potassium ions, deactivation rate, and inhibition by the methanesulfoanilide E-4031. Thus, HERG channels were inhibited by E-4031 only in a use-dependent fashion during repetitive pulse cycles, whereas MiRP1/HERG and native $I_{Kr}$ channels showed tonic block (before the first activating pulse) and ready relaxation to equilibrium blockade. The distinctive gating attributes of HERG-containing channels that allow its significant contribution to phase 3 repolarization were maintained. MiRP1 has also been reported to coassemble with Kv4.2 transient outward potassium channel subunits[70] and HCN pacemaker channel subunits.[71] Thus, the possibility exists that arrhythmia-associated mutations in MiRP1 could be caused by dysfunction of multiple MiRP1-containing channels.

Consistent with a role in repolarization of the myocardium, four mutations in *KCNE2* have been found that correlate to a prolonged QT interval and arrhythmia susceptibility.[16,72] All four changes diminish baseline potassium flux through MiRP1/HERG channels because of shifts in voltage-dependent activation, acceleration of channel deactivation, compromised unitary current magnitude, or decreased cell surface half-life.

As discussed in greater detail later, patients with arrhythmia usually present with multiple inciting factors.[11,54,73] Of particular clinical relevance is the increased likelihood that individuals with a prolonged QT interval can develop acquired arrhythmia in response to drugs that block cardiac potassium channels,[74,75] because the drugs further impede already slowed cardiac repolarization. Recently, an inherited missense variant associated with LQTS and a common polymorphism of *KCNE2* that had no effect at baseline were shown to increase sensitivity of MiRP1/HERG channels to inhibition by drugs that block $I_{Kr}$ channels suggesting how a genetic predisposition can contribute to acquired arrhythmias.[16,72]

## KCNJ2: ENCODING AN INWARD RECTIFIER POTASSIUM CHANNEL LINKED TO ANDERSEN'S SYNDROME

Andersen's syndrome is characterized by periodic paralysis, LQTS, and other cardiac arrhythmias including bidirectional ventricular tachycardia. This disorder is also associated with short stature, scoliosis, and facial dysmorphic features such as wide-set eyes and small chin.[76] Positional cloning followed by a candidate gene approach has revealed seven missense and two deletion mutations in KCNJ2, the gene for the Kir2.1 potassium channel that maps to chromosome 17q23.[23] This channel mediates the cardiac $I_{K1}$ current that serves as the primary determinant of diastolic membrane potential in atrial and ventricular myocytes.[4] Each Kir2.1 subunit has just two transmembrane segments (M1 and M2) with an intervening pore-forming domain and forms channels through tetrameric association (like KvLQT1 and HERG subunits). Two mutations have been characterized by heterologous expression and found to cause loss-of-function in a dominant fashion, that is, they impede the operation of wild-type Kir2.1 subunits in mixed complexes to decrease potassium current. Mutations in Kir2.1 were not detected in several other Andersen's syndrome families indicating that at least one additional gene remains to be discovered as a cause of this disorder.[23]

## RYR2: THE SARCOPLASMIC RETICULUM CALCIUM RELEASE CHANNEL

Familial catecholaminergic ventricular tachycardia is a cardiac rhythm disorder characterized by syncope and sudden death in otherwise healthy young individuals. The genetic basis for arrhythmia susceptibility in these individuals appears to be mutations in RYR2, the ryanodine receptor gene mapped to chromosome 1q42.1q43.[19] RYR2 receptors are calcium-induced calcium release channels located in cardiac sarcoplasmic reticulum. These channels are activated by calcium that transiently enters the cell through plasma membrane L-type calcium channels during cardiac myocyte depolarization. When RYR2 channels open they allow release of calcium from the sarcoplasmic reticulum which, in turn, initiates activation of the contractile apparatus. Four RYR2 missense mutations have been reported in individuals with this disorder. More recently, two other RYR2 missense mutations were discovered in patients with familial arrhythmogenic right ventricular dysplasia, an autosomal dominant cardiomyopathy characterized by partial degeneration of the right ventricular myocardium, electrical instability, and sudden death.[77] The functional consequences of these six RYR2 mutations are not yet known; however, episodic, stress-induced calcium overload in cardiac myocytes may provide the substrate for arrhythmia.

## ARRHYTHMIAS RESULTING FROM BLOCKADE OF CARDIAC ION CHANNEL BY DRUGS

Abnormal cardiac repolarization, aberrant conduction, and frank arrhythmia are most often acquired rather than inherited. Common causes of acquired arrhythmia include medications; cardiac ischemia resulting from sudden disruption of blood flow to a region of the heart; cardiomyopathy leading to changes in cardiac structure; developmental abnormalities such as right ventricular dysplasia; and abnormal levels of serum potassium, calcium, or magnesium.

Acquired LQTS is a common side effect of numerous medications of diverse therapeutic and structural classes.[11,78] Drugs associated with LQTS include often used antiarrhythmics, anticonvulsants, antidepressants, antihistamines, antihypertensives, antimicrobials, antipsychotic, and antineoplastic agents. Most of these drugs block $I_{Kr}$ channels, leading to reduced potassium current and delayed repolarization. Two structural features of HERG channels appear to explain why cardiac $I_{Kr}$ currents are so susceptible to nonspecific blockade[79,80] (Fig. 19-4A). First, the inner cavity of the HERG channel may be larger than that found in other voltage-gated potassium channels because it lacks two proline residues in S6, which are thought to reduce the volume of other pores.[81] Second, the HERG S6 domain has two aromatic residues absent from other channels and these may enhance binding of aromatic drugs by π-stacking interactions. Of note, the affinity of drugs is enhanced by inactivation of HERG channels.[82] Comparative studies of HERG channel blockade and structure-activity relationships for medications should improve the ability to predict which drugs are likely to present a significant risk for cardiac arrhythmia by this mechanism.

## INHERITED DIFFERENCES IN CARDIAC ION CHANNELS: PREDISPOSITION TO DRUG-INDUCED ARRHYTHMIAS

Genetic predisposition had been suspected to play a role in drug-induced arrhythmias in individuals with ECG abnormalities at baseline (before drug exposure) and in individuals who appear free of any "inherent" risk of arrhythmia, that is, those with a normal ECG and without symptoms. Inherited differences were hypothesized to explain the small subset of people treated with arrhythmia-associated drugs who showed poor tolerance perhaps resulting from differences in drug metabolism or the structure or function of drug receptor molecules. Recent studies of KCNE2 have confirmed these ideas. Drug-induced arrhythmias have now been associated with rare inherited mutations (seen in less than 0.02% of the population) that cause abnormal repolarization at baseline[16] and with common, silent genetic polymorphisms (more frequent than 1% of individuals)[72] (Fig. 19-4B).

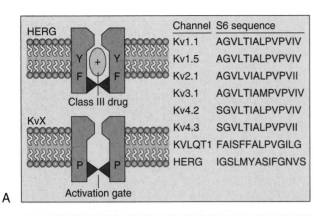

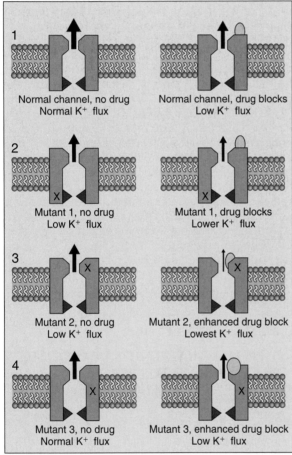

**FIGURE 19-4.** Arrhythmias resulting from unintended drug block: an inherited component. *A,* Two unusual structural features of HERG not shared by other voltage-gated potassium (Kv) channels appear to be explain its frequent, nonspecific drug interactions: a lack of conserved proline residues in the S6 transmembrane domain to increase the size of the HERG inner cavity and the presence of two aromatic residues (Y, F) in each subunit that contribute to the drug binding. *B,* Four drug effects: (1) unintended channel block of wild-type channels, (2) dysfunctional mutant channels and unintended block, (3) dysfunctional mutant channels with enhanced block, and (4) mutant channels with normal function but enhanced block. The precise mechanisms for altered drug block are not yet known.

First, it is known that individuals with a prolonged QT interval are at risk for dangerous arrhythmias in response to drug intake.[74,75] Thus, three individuals who carried M54T, I57T, and A116V missense variants of MiRP1 had long QT intervals before drug treatment and came to clinical attention after ingesting procainamide, oxatomide, or quinidine, respectively.[72] In these cases, myocardial repolarization was slow at baseline because of mutations that diminished $I_{Kr}$ currents, and drug therapy further inhibited $I_{Kr}$ potassium flux; these mutations did not alter sensitivity of the channels to the drugs. Conversely, a patient with the Q9E variant of MiRP1 presented with a long QT interval at baseline and clarithromycin-induced *torsade de pointes* and ventricular fibrillation; the mutation not only altered channel gating to reduce potassium flux at baseline but also increased sensitivity of $I_{Kr}$ channels to inhibition by the drug (Fig. 19-4*B*)[16]; this macrolide antibiotic had previously been associated with LQTS and $I_{Kr}$ blockade.[83] Of note, this patient was female and hypokalemic when she developed arrhythmia, two other factors associated with reduced $I_{Kr}$ current density emphasizing the need to consider LQTS in multifactorial terms (see next section).

Second, many individuals appear free of an inherent risk of arrhythmia (e.g., their ECG is normal) but are nevertheless prone to arrhythmia when exposed to certain drugs. Thus, the T8A polymorphism of MiRP1 is present in approximately 1.6% of the general population. Although the variant is associated with neither inherited LQTS nor changes in MiRP1/HERG channel function,[16] it increases sensitivity to blockade by sulfamethoxazole (a component of the common antibiotic Bactrim) leading to 50% current suppression at serum levels of the drug and is implicated in drug-induced arrhythmia (Fig. 19-4*B*).[72] This suggests that there is a common polymorphism that can carry important clinical implications for choice of drug therapy when alternatives exist and that should influence future drug development. Mutations in *KCNQ1* have also been implicated in predisposition to drug-induced LQTS.[84] Indeed, it seems likely that mutations or polymorphisms in all of the genes associated with the inherited forms of LQTS will eventually be shown to increase the risk of the acquired form of this disease.

## CARDIAC ARRHYTHMIAS: INDUCTION BY CUMULATIVE INSULTS

As is true of most common disorders, patients with LQTS and arrhythmia often present with multiple inciting factors that act cumulatively to impede cardiac repolarization.[11,13,54,85] This supports a multihit mechanism for this disease. Thus, individuals carrying only one mutant allele of an arrhythmia susceptibility gene have few, if any, arrhythmias. By contrast, individuals carrying two mutant alleles (e.g., Jervell and Lange-Nielson syndrome) have many arrhythmias and usually die during childhood unless effective treatment is implemented. Because these individuals do live into early childhood when untreated, there must be an additional event, such as introduction of a medication, required to produce arrhythmia. Conversely, it is also clear that a genetic predisposition is not a prerequisite for arrhythmia because rhythm disturbances can be induced in anyone exposed to high levels of certain medications, such as those that block cardiac potassium channels.

## RE-ENTRY: A FUNDAMENTAL MECHANISM OF ARRHYTHMIA

Together with previous physiologic studies, genetic advances offer a picture of cardiac arrhythmias at the molecular, cellular, and organ levels. Ion channels are expressed at varying levels in different regions of the heart in health and disease[86]; therefore, channel dysfunction produces excitation abnormalities with spatial variability. This is a substrate for arrhythmia. Thus, during a prolonged action potential, myocytes are relatively refractory to electrical excitation by neighboring myocytes. Such dispersion of refractoriness can lead to unidirectional block of a wave of electrical excitation (Fig. 19-5)[87] and pockets of cells that are temporarily unable to conduct the normal flow of electrical activity. Although unidirectional block can increase the risk of arrhythmia it is not sufficient—a triggering mechanism is required. The trigger for arrhythmia in LQTS is believed to be spontaneous secondary depolarizations that arise during or just following the plateau phase of action potentials. These depolarizations appear as premature, small action potentials and are mediated by depolarizing inward calcium currents. This mechanism predicts that the autonomic nervous system can have a significant impact on arrhythmia susceptibility because heightened sympathetic tone can increase spontaneous inward currents carried by L-type calcium channels to increase the likelihood that a spontaneous repolarization will trigger arrhythmia. This explains the utility of β-blockade therapy in patients with a long QT interval. Once triggered, arrhythmia is maintained by a regenerative circuit of electrical activity passing around relatively inexcitable tissue, a phenomenon known as re-entry (Fig. 19-5*A*). The development of multiple re-entrant circuits within the heart (Fig. 19-5*B*) causes ventricular fibrillation, the arrhythmia of sudden death.

## THE FUTURE: PREDICTION, PREVENTION, AND TREATMENT OF CARDIAC ARRHYTHMIAS

Despite recent advances, the fields of arrhythmia genetics, physiology, and therapy are still immature. Major problems include the identification of all genes that produce arrhythmia susceptibility, enumeration of common variants that contribute to arrhythmia risk in the general population, and the implementation of reliable, cost-effective genetic tests. Although early genetic studies involved cumbersome methods like positional cloning (because little of the human genome was mapped), the near future will bring detailed genetic maps of all human genes and rapid, inexpensive DNA

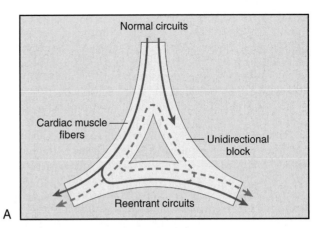

A

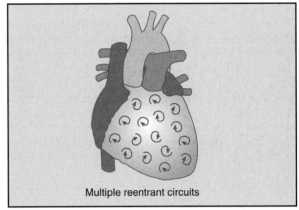

B

**FIGURE 19-5.** Unidirectional block and re-entry, a fundamental mechanism of arrhythmia. *A,* Abnormal cardiac repolarization, conduction, or intracellular calcium homeostasis can lead to episodic unidirectional block, a substrate for arrhythmia. Solid arrows represent the normal conduction in a bifurcated pathway. Conduction is blocked in an area of refractory tissue (unidirectional block). If conduction velocity is slowed, then re-entry through area of refractory tissue can occur *(dashed arrows). B,* Multiple re-entrant circuits *(multiple curved arrows)* is a mechanism of ventricular fibrillation, the cause of sudden death. *(From Keating MT, Sanguinetti MC: Molecular and cellular mechanisms of cardiac arrhythmias. Cell 2001;104:569–580, with permission from Elsevier.)*

sequence analysis to facilitate genetic testing for populations. Nonetheless, at least one significant hurdle remains—ascertainment and phenotypic characterization of individuals with arrhythmia susceptibility. The identification of novel arrhythmia genes and common arrhythmia susceptibility variants will involve genetic epidemiology, that is, genotypic characterization of large numbers of carefully phenotyped individuals. For the most part, phenotypic characterization has been slow, involving a great deal of one-on-one time in a process that is not easily scalable. Even here, however, technology holds the promise for improvement via Internet connection of individuals separated by large distances. Organizations and researchers are now using web sites to identify, organize, empower, and inform individuals with a variety of health care concerns, accelerating this step of human molecular genetic studies.

The new areas of functional genomics and proteomics will also have an impact on the field. Examining the expression of arrhythmia genes in tissues other than the heart can lead to testable hypotheses for other pathologies. Because ion channels are heteromultimers of many types of subunits and are modulated by signaling molecules, databases of protein-protein interactions will also be valuable.

Recent physiology studies also have important implications for the prevention and treatment of arrhythmias in addition to genetic testing. HERG channel current magnitude is paradoxically sensitive to extracellular potassium because of an interaction with extracellular sodium[88] highlights the importance of maintaining normal serum electrolyte levels and provides a new strategy for treatment.[89] Clearly, medications that prolong the QT interval should be avoided in patients with an abnormal ECG at baseline if a suitable alternative therapy exists. Caution is also in order based on the observation that both gain- and loss-of-function mutations of the cardiac sodium channels can cause arrhythmia susceptibility: drugs that modulate this channel may reduce the risk of one type of arrhythmia only to increase the risk of another. The future of arrhythmia therapy can, therefore, be expected to include use of devices that measure cardiac conduction and repolarization to deliver antiarrhythmic drugs only as needed and to provide a safety net in the form of automatic internal defibrillation.[90]

## SUMMARY

The known arrhythmia susceptibility genes encode cardiac ion channels. *SCN5A* encodes sodium channels that are responsible for initiating cardiac action potentials. The products of *HERG* and *KCNE2* combine, as do those encoded by *KvLQT1* and *KCNE1*, to form cardiac $I_{Kr}$ and $I_{Ks}$ channels, respectively. These potassium currents are responsible for termination of the plateau phase and contribute to final repolarization of the cardiac action potential. *KCNJ2* yields a potassium channel that contributes to both repolarization and diastolic electric activity. *RYR2* encodes the ryanodine receptor/calcium release channel crucial for excitation-contraction coupling. Mutations in these genes result in gain- or loss-of-function yielding abnormalities in action potential duration, repolarization time course, or conduction. Regional heterogeneity in these effects is a substrate for arrhythmia. In general, arrhythmia susceptibility is more severe in homozygotes than in heterozygotes. Although some familial forms of arrhythmia susceptibility are associated with phenotypic abnormalities (e.g., congenital neural deafness in Jervell and Lange-Nielsen syndrome), most patients go unrecognized until their first symptomatic arrhythmia. Genetic variation in ion channel genes has now been confirmed to contribute not only to familial arrhythmias but also to the occurrence of drug-induced (acquired) arrhythmia in patients with no ECG abnormalities before drug exposure. A multihit model for arrhythmogenesis has emerged that recognizes contributions of genetic susceptibility and secondary challenges. Studies of the genetics and physiology of

ion channels in episodic disorders of the heart are helping to define a new class of diseases, the "ion channelopathies."

Note: LQT4 has now been associated with mutation in *ANKB* on chromosome 4q25-27, a gene for an intracellular adapter protein involved in targeting proteins to membranes.[91]

## REFERENCES

1. Kannel W, Cupples A, D'Agostino R: Sudden death risk in overt coronary heart diseases: The Framingham study. Am Heart J 1987;113:799-804.
2. Willich S, Levy D, Rocco M, et al: Circadian variation in the incidence of sudden cardiac death in the Framingham heart study population. Am J Cardiol 1987;60:801-806.
3. Sanguinetti MC, Jurkiewicz NK: Two components of cardiac delayed rectifier K+ current. Differential sensitivity to block by class III antiarrhythmic agents. J Gen Physiol 1990;96:195-215.
4. Sanguinetti MC, Tristani-Firouzi M: Delayed and inward rectifier potassium channels. In Zipes DP, Jalife J (eds): Cardiac Electrophysiology: From Cell to Bedside. Philadelphia, WB Saunders, 2000, pp 79-86.
5. Schwartz P, Moss A, Vincent G, et al: Diagnostic criteria for the long QT syndrome. Circulation 1993;88:782-784.
6. Lazzara R: Twisting of the points. J Am Coll Cardiol 1997;29:843-845.
7. Moss AJ: ECG T-wave patterns in genetically distinct forms of the hereditary long QT syndrome. Circulation 1995;92:2929-2934.
8. Jervell A, Lange-Nielsen F: Congenital deaf-mutism, functional heart disease with prolongation of the QT interval, and sudden death. Am Heart J 1957;54:59-68.
9. Romano C, Gemme G, Pongiglione R: Artimie cardiach rare dell'eta pediatrica. II. Accessi sincopali per fibrillazione ventricolare parossitica. Clin Pediatr 1963;45:656-683.
10. Ward O: A new familial cardiac syndrome in children. J Ir Med Assoc 1964;54:103-106.
11. Roden DM: Mechanisms and management of proarrhythmia. Am J Cardiol 1998;82(4A):49I-57I.
12. Tomaselli GF, Beuckelmann DJ, Calkins HG, et al: Sudden cardiac death in heart failure: The role of abnormal repolarization. Circulation 1994;90:2534-2539.
13. Roden DM, Lazzara R, Rosen M, et al: Multiple mechanisms in the long-QT syndrome-current knowledge, gaps, and future directions. Circulation 1996;94:1996-2012.
14. Splawski I, Timothy KW, Vincent GM, et al: Molecular basis of the long-QT syndrome associated with deafness. N Engl J Med 1997;336:1562-1567.
15. Abildskov J: The sympathetic imbalance hypothesis of QT interval prolongation. J Cardiovasc Electrophysiol 1991;2:355-359.
16. Abbott GW, Sesti F, Splawski I, et al: MiRP1 forms IKr potassium channels with HERG and is associated with cardiac arrhythmia. Cell 1999;97:175-187.
17. Chen QY, Kirsch GE, Zhang DM, et al: Genetic basis and molecular mechanism for idiopathic-ventricular fibrillation. Nature 1998;392:293-296.
18. Curran ME, Splawski I, Timothy KW, et al: A molecular basis for cardiac arrhythmia: HERG mutations cause long QT syndrome. Cell 1995;80:795-803.
19. Priori SG, Napalitano C, Tiso N, et al: Mutations in the cardiac ryanodine receptor gene (hRyR2) underlie catecholamine polymorphic ventricular tachycardia. Circulation 2000;102:r49-53.
20. Splawski I, Tristani-Firouzi M, Lehmann MH, et al: Mutations in the hminK gene cause long QT syndrome and suppress IKs function. Nat Genet 1997;17:338-340.
21. Wang Q, Curran ME, Splawski I, et al: Positional cloning of a novel potassium channel gene: KVLQT1 mutations cause cardiac arrhythmias. Nat Genet 1996;12:17-23.
22. Wang Q, Shen J, Splawski I, et al: SCN5A mutations associated with an inherited cardiac arrhythmia, long QT syndrome. Cell 1995;80:805-811.

23. Plaster NM, Tawil R, Tristani-Firouzi M, et al: Mutations in Kir2.1 cause the developmental and episodic electrical phenotypes of Andersen's syndrome. Cell 2001;105:511-519.

24. Schott J, Charpentier F, Peltier S, et al: Mapping of a gene for long QT syndrome to chromosome 4q25-27. Am J Hum Genet 1995;57:1114-1122.

25. Duggal P, Vesely MR, Wattanasirichaigoon D, et al: Mutation of the gene for IsK associated with both Jervell and Lange-Nielsen and Romano-Ward forms of long-QT syndrome. Circulation 1998;97:142-146.

26. Neyroud N, Tesson F, Denjoy I, et al: A novel mutation in the potassium channel gene KVLQT1 causes the Jervell and Lange-Nielsen cardioauditory syndrome. Nat Genet 1997;15:186-189.

27. Hoorntje T, Alders M, van Tintelen P, et al: Homozygous premature truncation of the HERG protein: The human HERG knockout. Circulation 1999; 100:1264-1267.

28. Gellens M, George A, Chen L, et al: Primary structure and functional expression of the human cardiac tetrodotoxin-insensitive voltage-dependent sodium channel. Proc Natl Acad Sci USA 1992;89:554-558.

29. Splawski I, Shen J, Timothy KW, et al: Spectrum of mutations in long-QT syndrome genes: KVLQT1, HERG, SCN5A, KCNE1, and KCNE2. Circulation 2000;102:1178-1185.

30. Catterall WA: Molecular properties of voltage-sensitive sodium channels. Annu Rev Biochem 1986;55:953-985.

31. Bennett PB, Yazawa K, Makita N, et al: Molecular mechanism for an inherited cardiac arrhythmia. Nature 1995;376:683-685.

32. Dumaine R, Wang Q, Keating MT, et al: Multiple mechanisms of Na$^+$ channel-linked long-QT syndrome. Circ Res 1996;78:916-924.

33. Martini B: Wang Q, Keating Mt, Ventricular fibrillation without apparent heart disease: Description of six cases. Am Heart J 1989;118:1203-1209.

34. Brugada J, Brugada R, Brugada P: Right bundle branch block, ST segment elevation in leads V1-V3: A marker for sudden death in patients without demonstrable structural heart disease. Circulation 1997;96:1151.

35. Krishnan SC, Antzelevitch C: Sodium channel block produces opposite electrophysiological effects in canine ventricular epicardium and endocardium. Circ Res 1991;69:277-291.

36. Keating M, Atkinson D, Dunn C, et al: Linkage of a cardiac arrhythmia, the long QT syndrome, and the Harvey ras-1 gene. Science 1991:704-706.

37. Lee MP, Hu R-J, Johnson LA, et al: Human KVLQT1 gene shows tissue-specific imprinting and encompasses Beckwith-Wiedemann syndrome chromosomal rearrangements. Nat Genet 1997;15:181-185.

38. Yang WP, Levesque PC, Little WA, et al: KvLQT1, a voltage-gated potassium channel responsible for human cardiac arrhythmias. Proc Natl Acad Sci USA 1997;94:4017-4021.

39. Charlier C, Singh NA, Ryan SG, et al: A pore mutation in a novel KQT-like potassium channel gene in an idiopathic epilepsy family. Nat Genet 1998;18:53-55.

40. Singh NA, Charlier C, Stauffer D, et al: A novel potassium channel gene, KCNQ2, is mutated in an inherited epilepsy of newborns. Nat Genet 1998;18:25-29.

41. Yang WP, Levesque PC, Little WA, et al: Functional expression of two KvLQT1-related potassium channels responsible for an inherited idiopathic epilepsy. J Biol Chem 1998;273:19419-19423.

42. Coucke PJ, Van Hauwe P, Kelley PM, et al: Mutations in the KCNQ4 gene are responsible for autosomal dominant deafness in four DFNA2 familes. Hum Mol Genet 1999;8:1321-1328.

43. Kubisch C, Schroeder BC, Friedrich T, et al: KCNQ4, a novel potassium channel expressed in sensory outer hair cells, is mutated in dominant deafness. Cell 1999;96:437-446.

44. Wollnik B, Schroeder BC, Kubisch C, et al: Pathophysiological mechanisms of dominant and recessive KVLQT1 K$^+$ channel mutations found in inherited cardiac arrhythmias. Hum Mol Genet 1997;6:1943-1949.

45. Wang Z, Tristani-Firouzi M, Xu Q, et al: Functional effects of mutations in KvLQT1 that cause long QT syndrome. J Cardiovasc Electrophysiol 1999; 10:817-826.

46. Barhanin J, Lesage F, Guillemara E, et al: K(V)LQT1 and IsK (minK) proteins associate to form the I(Ks) cardiac potassium current. Nature 1996; 384:78-80.

47. Sanguinetti MC, Curran ME, Zou A, et al: Coassembly Of K(V)Lqt1 and Mink (Isk) proteins to form cardiac I-Ks potassium channel. Nature 1996; 384:80-83.

48. Takumi T, Ohkubo H, Nakanishi S: Cloning of a membrane protein that induces a slow voltage-gated potassium current. Science 1988;242:1042-1045.

49. Goldstein SA, Miller C: Site-specific mutations in a minimal voltage-dependent K$^+$ channel alter ion selectivity and open-channel block. Neuron 1991;7:403-408.

50. Freeman LC, Kass RS: Expression of a minimal K$^+$ channel protein in mammalian cells and immunolocalization in guinea pig heart. Circ Res 1993;73:968-973.

51. Blumenthal EM, Kaczmarek LK: The minK potassium channel exists in functional and nonfunctional forms when expressed in the plasma membrane of Xenopus oocytes. J Neurosci 1994; 14:3097-3105.

52. Wang KW, Goldstein SAN: Subunit composition of minK potassium channels. Neuron 1995;14:1303-1309.

53. Tai K-K, Wang K-W, Goldstein SAN: MinK potassium channels are heteromultimeric complexes. J Biol Chem 1997;272:1654-1658.

54. Abbott GW, Goldstein SAN: Potassium channel subunits encoded by the KCNE gene family: Physiology and pathophysiology of the MinK-related peptides (MiRPs). Mol Intervent 2001; 1:95-107.

55. Wang W, Xia J, Kass RS: MinK-KvLQT1 fusion proteins, evidence for multiple stoichiometries of the assembled IsK channel. J Biol Chem 1998;273:34069-34074.

56. Sesti F, Goldstein SAN: Single-channel characteristics of wild-type IKs channels and channels formed with two minK mutants that cause long QT syndrome. J Gen Physiol 1998; 112:651-664.

57. Yang Y, Sigworth F: Single-channel properties of IKs potassium channels. J Gen Physiol 1998;112:665-678.

58. Busch AE, Busch GL, Ford E, et al: The role of the IsK protein in the specific pharmacological properties of the IKs channel complex. Br J Pharmacol 1997;122:187-189.

59. Sesti F, Tai KK, Goldstein SAN: MinK endows the IKs potassium channel with sensitivity to internal TEA. Biophys J 2000; 79:1369-1378.

60. Marcus DC, Shen Z: Slowly activating voltage-dependent K$^+$ conductance is apical pathway for K$^+$ secretion in vestibular dark cells. Am J Physiol 1994;267(3 Pt 1):C857-864.

61. Vetter DE, Mann JR, Wangemann P, et al: Inner ear defects induced by null mutation of the isk gene. Neuron 1996;17:1251-1264.

62. Warmke J, Ganetzky B: A family of potassium channel genes related to eag in Drosophila and mammals. Proc Natl Acad Sci USA 1994;91:3438-3442.

63. Morais Cabral JH, Lee A, Cohen SL, et al: Crystal structure and functional analysis of the HERG potassium channel N terminus: A eukaryotic PAS domain. Cell 1998;95:649-655.

64. Sanguinetti MC, Jiang C, Curran ME, et al: A mechanistic link between an inherited and an acquired cardiac arrhythmia: HERG encodes the IKr potassium channel. Cell 1995;81:299-307.

65. Trudeau MC, Warmke JW, Ganetzky B, et al: HERG, a human inward rectifier in the voltage-gated potassium channel family. Science 1995;269:92-95.

66. Smith PL, Baukrowitz T, Yellen G: The inward rectification mechanism of the HERG cardiac potassium channel. Nature 1996; 379:833-836.

67. Spector PS, Curran ME, Zou A, et al: Fast inactivation causes rectification of the IKr channel. J Gen Physiol 1996;107:611-619.

68. Zhou Z, Gong Q, Ye B, et al: Properties of HERG channels stably expressed in HEK 293 cells studied at physiological temperature. Biophys J 1998;74:230-241.

69. Chen J, Zou A, Splawski I, et al: Long QT syndrome-associated mutations in the Per-Arnt-Sim (PAS) domain of HERG potassium channels accelerate channel deactivation. J Biol Chem 1999;274:10113-10118.

70. Zhang M, Jiang M, Tseng G: MiRP1 associates with Kv4.2 and modulates its gating function: A potential role as b subunit of cardiac transient outward channel? Circ Res 2001;88: 1012-1019.

71. Yu H, Wu J, Potapova I, et al: MinK-related peptide 1: A beta subunit for the HCN ion channel subunit family enhances expression and speeds activation. Circ Res 2001;88:E84-87.

72. Sesti F, Abbott GW, Wei J, et al: A common polymorphism associated with antibiotic-induced cardiac arrhythmia. Proc Natl Acad Sci 2000;97: 10613-10618.

73. Roden DM: Taking the "idio" out of "idiosyncratic": Predicting torsades de pointes. Pacing Clin Electrophysiol 1998;21: 1029-1034.

74. Minardo JD, Heger JJ, Miles WM, et al: Clinical characteristics of patients with ventricular fibrillation during antiarrhythmic drug therapy. N Engl J Med 1988;319:257-262.

75. Donger C, Denjoy I, Berthet M, et al: KVLQT1 C-terminal missense mutation causes a forme fruste long-QT syndrome. Circulation 1997;96:2778-2781.

76. Tawil R, Ptacek LJ, Pavlakis SG, et al: Andersen's syndrome: Potassium-sensitive periodic paralysis, ventricular ectopy, and dysmorphic features. [See comments]. Ann Neurol 1994;35: 326-330.

77. Tiso N, Stephan DA, Nava A, et al: Identification of mutations in the cardiac ryanodine receptor gene in families affected with arrhythmogenic right ventricular cardiomyopathy type 2 (ARVD2). Hum Mol Genet 2001;10(3):189-194.

78. Witchel HJ, Hancox JC: Familial and acquired long QT syndrome and the cardiac rapid delayed rectifier potassium current [Review]. Clin Exp Pharmacol Physiol 2000;27:753-766.

79. Mitcheson JS, Chen J, Lin M, et al: A structural basis for drug-induced long QT syndrome. Proc Natl Acad Sci USA 2000;97: 12329-12333.

80. Mitcheson JS, Chen J, Sanguinetti MC: Trapping of a methanesulfonanilide by closure of the HERG potassium channel activation gate. J Gen Physiol 2000;115:229-239.

81. del Camino D, Holmgren M, Liu Y, et al: Blocker protection in the pore of a voltage-gated K$^+$ channel and its structural implications. Nature 2000;403:321-325.

82. Ficker E: Molecular determinants of dofetilide block of HERG K+ channels. Circ Res 1998;82:386-395.

83. Lee KL, Jim MH, Tang SC, et al: QT prolongation and torsades de pointes associated with clarithromycin. Am J Med 1998;104: 395-396.

84. Napolitano C, Schwartz PJ, Brown AM, et al: Evidence for a cardiac ion channel mutation underlying drug-induced QT prolongation and life-threatening arrhythmias. J Cardiovasc Electrophysiol 2000l;11:691-696.

85. Drici MD, Knollmann BC, Wang WX, et al: Cardiac actions of erythromycin: Influence of female sex. JAMA 1998;280:1774-1776.

86. Nerbonne JM: Molecular basis of functional voltage-gated K$^+$ channel diversity in the mammalian myocardium. J Physiol 2000;525:285-298.

87. Keating MT, Sanguinetti MC: Molecular and cellular mechanisms of cardiac arrhythmias. Cell 2001;104:569-580.

88. Numaguchi H, Johnson Jr. JP, Peterson CI, et al: A sensitive mechanism for cation modulation of potassium current. Nat Neurosci 2000;3:429-430.

89. Compton SJ, Lux RL, Ramsey MR, et al: Genetically defined therapy of inherited long-QT syndrome: Correction of abnormal repolarization by potassium. Circulation 1996;94:1018-1022.

90. Moss AJ: Update on MADIT: The Multicenter Automatic Defibrillator Implantation Trial. The long QT interval syndrome. Am J Cardiol 1997;79:16-19.

91. Mohler PJ, Schott J-J, Gramolini AO, et al: Ankyrin-B mutation causes type 4 long-QT cardiac arrythmia and sudden cardiac death. Nature 2003; 421:634-639.

## EDITOR'S CHOICE

Arad M, Moskowitz IP, Patel VV, et al: Transgenic mice overexpressing mutant PRKAG2 define the cause of Wolff-Parkinson-White syndrome in glycogen storage cardiomyopathy. Circulation 2003;107: 2850-2856.

Chen YH, Xu SJ, Bendahhou S, et al: KCNQ1 gain-of-function mutation in familial atrial fibrillation. Science 2003;299:251-254.

Cheng CF, Kuo HC, Chien KR: Genetic modifiers of cardiac arrhythmias. Trends Mol Med 2003;9:59-66.

Gutstein DE, Morley GE, Tamaddon H, et al: Conduction slowing and sudden arrhythmic death in mice with cardiac-restricted inactivation of connexin43. Circ Res 2001;88:333-339.

Kuo HC, Cheng CF, Clark RB, et al: A defect in the Kv channel-interacting protein 2 (KChIP2) gene leads to a complete loss of I(to) and confers susceptibility to ventricular tachycardia. Cell 2001;107:801-813.

Mohler PJ, Schott JJ, Gramolini AO, et al: Ankyrin-B mutation causes type 4 long-QT cardiac arrhythmia and sudden cardiac death. Nature 2003;421:634-639.

Nguyen-Tran VT, Kubalak SW, Minamisawa S, et al: A novel genetic pathway for sudden cardiac death via defects in the transition between ventricular and conduction system cell lineages. Cell 2000;102: 671-682.

Priori SG, Schwartz PJ, Napolitano C, et al: Risk stratification in the long-QT syndrome. N Engl J Med 2003;348:1866-1874.

Rottbauer W, Baker K, Wo ZG, et al: Growth and function of the embryonic heart depend upon the cardiac-specific L-type calcium channel alpha1 subunit. Dev Cell 2001;1:265-275.

Splawski I, Timothy KW, Tateyama M, et al: Variant of SCN5A sodium channel implicated in risk of cardiac arrhythmia. Science 2002;297: 1333-1336.

Tanaka M, Berul CI, Ishii M, et al: A mouse model of congenital heart disease: Cardiac arrhythmias and atrial septal defect caused by haploin-sufficiency of the cardiac transcription factor Csx/Nkx2.5. Cold Spring Harb Symp Quant Biol 2002;67:317-325.

Wehrens XH, Lehnart SE, Huang F, et al: FKBP12.6 deficiency and defective calcium release channel (ryanodine receptor) function linked to exercise-induced sudden cardiac death. Cell 2003;113: 829-840.

■ ▦ ■ c h a p t e r **2 0**

# Inflammation and Immunity in Atherogenesis

*Peter Libby*
*Göran K. Hansson*
*Jordan S. Pober*

## CELL TYPES INVOLVED IN NORMAL VASCULAR HOMEOSTASIS AND IN ACUTE AND CHRONIC PATHOLOGIC REACTIONS OF ARTERIES

The pathologic changes in the arterial wall during atherogenesis result from a failure of normal homeostasis. Vascular homeostasis in turn depends largely on functions of the cell types resident within the normal vessel wall. Endothelial cells form a monolayer that lines the vessel's intima contacting the fluid phase of blood and serve as the semipermeable gateway that separates the blood compartment from the rest of the vessel wall in the macrocirculation, and the tissues in the microcirculation. Virtually unique among biologic or synthetic surfaces, a normal endothelial cell can maintain blood in a liquid state even during prolonged contact. The endothelium also interacts with the formed elements of blood—erythrocytes, platelets, and leukocytes. Endothelial cells normally produce a number of endogenous mediators that promote vascular homeostasis. Notable among these autacoids, nitric oxide (NO) and lipid mediators such as prostacyclin help to maintain normal vascular homeostasis by regulating the interactions of endothelial cells with blood cells and underlying smooth muscle cells alike.

The vascular smooth muscle cells, found in the intima of normal human arteries and representing the quasitotality of the cellular components of the tunica media, also contribute importantly to vascular homeostasis and hemodynamics. The contractile tone of smooth muscle cells regulates the caliber of vessels that they invest. The tone of arteriolar smooth muscle cells determines regional blood flow and systemic blood pressure. The contractile state of smooth muscle cells reflects local influences such as the vasodilator effect of endothelial-derived NO. Humoral vasoactive substances and vasoregulatory substances derived from vasomotor nerves also coordinate the contractile state of vascular smooth muscle cells.

Thus, normal vascular homeostasis depends on a tightly regulated and intricately interconnected network of functions of vascular endothelium and smooth muscle. In the diseased vessel, however, interactions with non-vascular cells frequently occur. For example, vascular thrombosis involves adherence and activation of blood platelets. Acute necrotizing vasculitides usually involve invasion of the vessel wall by polymorphonuclear leukocytes. Atherogenesis in particular represents a type of chronic inflammation and involves elements of the immune response. As in the case of chronic inflammatory lesions in other tissues, atherosclerotic lesions consistently contain accumulations of cells of the mononuclear phagocytic lineage as well as lymphocytes. Atheromas, like other inflammatory lesions and responses to tissue injury or wounding, involve not only infiltration by mononuclear leukocytes but also proliferation of stromal cells, accretion or remodeling of the extracellular matrix, and neovascularization. These aspects of atherogenesis recapitulate many features of granuloma formation or the histopathology of delayed-type hypersensitivity responses as well as formation of granulation tissue that occurs during wound healing (Fig. 20-1).

Recent research has identified a number of potential molecular mediators of these pathologic responses. We appreciate increasingly the importance of the exchange of signals among leukocytes and intrinsic vascular wall cells in the pathogenesis of this disease. We will therefore organize our discussion of the role of inflammation in atherogenesis by considering specific aspects of the interactions of various classes of leukocytes with vascular cells of the lineages (Table 20-1). In general, innate immune responses involve mononuclear phagocytes. Although T-lymphocytes orchestrate antigen-specific or adaptive immune responses, the mononuclear phagocyte acts as an effector in both innate and adaptive immunity (Fig. 20-2).

## MONONUCLEAR PHAGOCYTES

### Recruitment of Monocytes to Sites of Lesion Formation: A Special Case of Endothelial-Leukocyte Adhesion

As well substantiated by experimental studies and supported by observations in human tissues, the adhesion

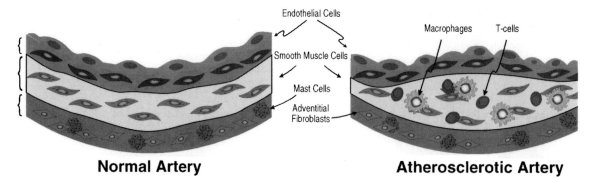

**Normal Artery**     **Atherosclerotic Artery**

**FIGURE 20-1.** Interactions of mononuclear leukocytes with intrinsic vascular wall cells characterize atherogenesis. The normal artery *(left)* has a relatively thin intimal layer and lacks a substantial leukocyte population. The intrinsic vascular wall cells, intimal endothelial cells, and medial smooth muscle cells generally do not display high levels of expression of adhesion molecules and cytokines involved in inflammatory responses. A few mast cells may reside in the normal adventitial layer. The atherosclerotic artery *(right)* contains numerous macrophage-derived foam cells and T lymphocytes. The macrophages congregate primarily in the central lipid-rich core of the lesion. T cells are most numerous in the shoulder region or leading edge of the atherosclerotic lesion, where it joins the more normal or uninvolved parts of the circumference of the arterial intima. The endothelial cells overlying atherosclerotic plaques may exhibit enhanced expression of cytokine-inducible adhesion molecules such as ICAM-1 or P-selectin. Smooth muscle cells and macrophages within the lesion may express class II major histocompatibility complex antigens, indicating their activation, and are consistent with exposure to gamma interferon. The macrophages and smooth muscle cells within atherosclerotic lesions both express pro-inflammatory cytokines such as tumor necrosis factor. They can also express chemoattractant chemokines such as macrophage chemoattractant protein I. The T cells within the lesion display evidence for a production of gamma interferon and bear markers of chronic activation as well, indicating an ongoing chronic immune response in the established atheroma. The intima of normal vessels contains no microvessels. The atherosclerotic intima characteristically develops a rich microvascular circulation connecting with the vasa vasorum (not shown).

## TABLE 20-1    LEUKOCYTE CLASSES POTENTIALLY INVOLVED IN ATHEROGENESIS

Mononuclear cells
  Mononuclear phagocytes
  Monocytes
  Macrophages
  Lymphocytes
    T cells
    CD4
    Th1
    Th2
    CD8
  B cells and plasma cells
Polymorphonuclear cells
  Granulocytes
  Eosinophils
Mast cells

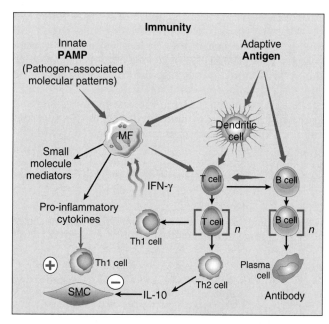

**FIGURE 20-2.** Interplay between adaptive and innate immunity during atherogenesis. The principal effector cell of innate immunity, the macrophage (MF), elaborates cytokines that critically regulate many functions of atheroma-associated cells involved with disease initiation, progression, and complication as well as thrombosis. IFN-γ, a product of the activated T cell, activates a number of these functions of the macrophage. In turn, the activated macrophage expresses high levels of MHC class II antigens, needed for antigen-dependent activation of T cells. (See color plate.) *(From Hansson GK, Libby P, Schonbeck U, et al: Innate and adaptive immunity in the pathogenesis of atherosclerosis Circ Res 2002;91:281–291.)*

of mononuclear phagocytes to the intact endothelium occurs very early in atherogenesis.[1-4] The molecular basis of the adhesive interaction between the mononuclear phagocyte and the endothelial cell likely involves the expression on the surface of the endothelium of a particular array of adhesion molecules that promote the local attachment of leukocytes (Table 20-2). The normal vascular endothelial cell displays little or no expression of these leukocyte adhesion molecules, except for low levels of constitutive expression of intercellular adhesion molecule-1 (ICAM-1). The endothelial cells overlying nascent atherosclerotic lesions show increased expression of vascular cell adhesion molecule-1 (VCAM-1), P-selectin, and increased levels of ICAM-1.[5-10] In established human atherosclerotic lesions, the plaque's microvasculature displays increased levels of leukocyte adhesion molecules that interact with mononuclear leukocytes.[7] Studies in genetically altered mice have shown that interruption of the func-

tion of P- and E-selectin and of VCAM-1 (but not ICAM-1) interfered with lesion formation in atherosclerosis-prone mice.[11,12]

Various types of inflammatory signals may account for the increased expression of leukocyte adhesion molecules

■ ■ ■

**TABLE 20-2**  EXAMPLES OF ADHESION MOLECULES POTENTIALLY INVOLVED IN ATHEROGENESIS

IgG superfamily members
  ICAM-1
  VCAM-1
Selectins
  P-selectin
Integrins
  AlphaV, beta 3

by endothelial cells overlying and within atherosclerotic lesions. Cytokines, protein mediators of inflammation and immunity, including those present in atherosclerotic lesions such as tumor necrosis factor (TNF) can induce leukocyte adhesion molecule expression by endothelial cells.[13-15] Moreover, constituents of modified lipoproteins such as lysophosphatidyl choline can transcriptionally regulate the expression of leukocyte adhesion molecules such as VCAM-1 and E-selectin.[16,17] These instigators of inflammatory responses may thus contribute to recruitment of mononuclear leukocytes to the atherosclerotic lesion.

Many of the systemic risk factors associated with the propensity to develop atherogenesis should exert their effects equally in all locales of the arterial tree. Such systemic risk factors include alterations in blood lipids such as hypercholesterolemia, hypertension, and elevated levels of such plasma factors as fibrinogen or lipoprotein (a). In stark contrast to this expected homogeneity of vascular lesion formation in space, atheromas typically occur focally and do not affect all portions of the arterial tree in an equal manner. What accounts for the focality of atheroma formation? Atheromas tend to form at predictable sites, particularly at those characterized by altered flow patterns. Branching points, for example, commonly show a predilection to atheroma development. Fluid dynamic analysis describes the flow characteristics in these regions as "disturbed," yielding low calculated shear stress on the endothelium at sites of lesion predilection.

Recent work has characterized some of the links between the local hydrodynamic environment and expression of particular genes that may mediate some of the inflammatory components of vascular lesion formation. Endothelial cells exposed to laminar shear stress exhibit increased transcription of certain genes of interest in the context of atherogenesis. A hexanucleotide motif GAGACC that binds members of the *rel* family of transcription factors occurs in the promoter regions of several of these genes, for example, platelet-derived growth factor B chain (PDGf B), ICAM-1, and the endothelial form of nitric oxide synthase.[18,19] In the case of PDGF B, this motif confers transcriptional regulability by shear stress. However, other molecules such as VCAM-1, known to be expressed by endothelial cells over nascent atheroma, lack this particular consensus motif, known as a shear stress response element. Undoubtedly, other such shear-regulated transcriptional elements exist in the promoters of other shear-regulated genes.

Interestingly, increased laminar shear stress does not appear to augment the transcription of VCAM-1.

Positive regulation may provide only one level of control of endothelial expression of adhesion molecules such as VCAM-1. As the laminar shear stress augments transcription of the constitutive nitric oxide synthase isoform found in endothelium and augments NO production by these cells, sites of disturbed flow where endothelial cells experience lower levels of shear stress should have reduced endogenous NO production NO can inhibit transcription of VCAM-1 and certain other genes regulated by the nuclear factor kappa B (NFκB) members of the *rel* family of transcription factors.[20,21] Therefore, a release from a tonic inhibition of VCAM-1 expression due to reduced local endothelial NO production might contribute to the augmented levels of this adhesion molecule at sites of low shear stress and hence lesion predilection in the arterial tree *in vivo*. Indeed, VCAM expression by aortic endothelium *in vivo* increases under conditions of experimentally disturbed shear stress.[22]

The traditional thinking about the focality of atheroma formation poses the question: What activates proatherogenic, inflammatory functions at loci of lesion formation? Another view turns this question around and asks: What normal protective mechanisms are inactivated at sites of atheroma formation? This concept of constitutive "atheroprotective" functions may prove a useful new framework for learning more about the key issue of focal expression of a disease influenced in large measure by systemic risk factors.[23]

## The Link between Hypercholesterolemia and Monocyte Recruitment

How might risk factors such as hypercholesterolemia influence local expression of leukocyte adhesion molecules and, hence, focal recruitment of mononuclear phagocytes to sites of lesion formation? We know that sites of lesion predilection in rabbits accumulate low-density lipoprotein (LDL) preferentially. Elegant studies of Schwenke and Carew documented that the local increased concentration of LDL in these regions depends on an increased residence time rather than simply an increase in permeability.[24,25] One explanation for the prolonged residence of LDL in these regions involves a local alteration in proteoglycan composition. LDL particles preferentially bind to certain proteoglycan classes including heparan sulfate proteoglycans elaborated by smooth muscle cells and endothelial cells.[26,27] An altered profile of proteoglycan synthesis at sites of altered hemodynamics or local release of inflammatory mediators could promote the retention of LDL in the subendothelial region of the intima. For example, cyclic strain augments elaboration of proteoglycans by cultured smooth muscle cells.[28] The protein moiety of LDL, apolipoprotein B100, contains a specific site that mediates binding to proteoglycans. A point mutation of this site results in production of LDL particles with little affinity for the extracellular matrix. Genetically engineered mice carrying this mutation on an atherogenic background have a substantially reduced tendency to develop atherosclerosis, implying that LDL binding to proteoglycans is an important step in early atherogenesis.[29]

LDL particles bound to proteoglycan in the intima may have heightened susceptibility to oxidative modification.[30] Several lines of evidence indicate that sites of lesion formation contain oxidatively modified LDL.[31] Constituents of such modified LDL particles may in turn regulate adhesion molecule gene expression. For example, as noted previously, lysophosphatidyl choline can transcriptionally activate VCAM-1 expression by human endothelial cells.[16] At certain concentrations, oxidatively modified LDL preparations can either augment or reduce cytokine expression by endothelial cells and mononuclear phagocytes *in vitro* and in mice *in vivo*.[31,32] In this manner, the retention of LDL and its subsequent oxidation might enhance local cytokine production at certain times during atherogenesis that would provide another potential stimulus for enhanced adhesion molecule gene expression. Some of the variability in the results obtained with various preparations of LDL oxidized *in vitro* may reflect heterogeneity in these poorly defined mixtures containing numerous biologically active components, including lipid peroxides, aldehydic short-chain hydrocarbons, oxysterols, and modified apoproteins and their fragments. A more rigorous understanding of the influences of altered gene expression in response to oxidatively modified lipoproteins will require isolation and characterization of the effects of specific chemical components that may trigger particular intracellular signaling pathways that regulate adhesion molecule and/or cytokine gene expression. It is unlikely that substantial further insight in this regard will emerge from *in vitro* studies of poorly characterized mixtures of oxidized lipoproteins. The chemical characterization of and attribution of specific biologic actions to certain isolated components of oxidized lipoproteins represents a step in this direction.[31,33]

In addition to diffusion of oxidatively modified lipids into cells as a pathway for gene regulation, the engagement of receptors on the surfaces of mononuclear phagocytes or intrinsic vascular cells by oxidatively modified lipoproteins may promote foam cell formation and, potentially, couple to signal transduction. The identification of a family of scavenger receptors that recognize modified LDL, among other ligands, provides an illustration of this concept. The first such scavenger receptors characterized structurally, the SRA series, bind acetylated LDL.[34,35] Recent work has identified a number of newly recognized molecules that may bind oxidatively modified lipoprotein particles, including CD36[36] and macrosialin/CD68.[37] Another member of the CD36 family, scavenger receptor B1 (SRB1), binds high-density lipoprotein (containing apolipoprotein AI) and apolipoprotein B containing particles.[38] A subset of macrophages expressed a scavenger receptor denoted MARCO.[39] Recent work has expanded knowledge of the *in vivo* function. Loss of function of SR-A or CD36 reduces experimental atherosclerosis in mice. Deletion or hypofunction of SRB1 can augment cholesterol levels and plasma HDL levels of mice when combined with the apolipoprotein E deficiency that augments atherosclerosis and promotes coronary artery thrombosis. More

recently described scavenger receptors include LOX-1 and SR-PSOX, which bind oxidized but not acetylated LDL.[40-42]

## The Site of Leukocyte Trafficking in Atheroma: Macrovascular or Microvascular?

Much of the model building regarding recruitment of leukocytes during atherogenesis has focused on the macrovascular luminal endothelium. Indeed, overexpression of leukocyte adhesion molecules on the endothelial surface of medium-sized or large arteries may prove crucial in the initial recruitment of monocytes to nascent atheroma. However, the endothelium overlying established human atheroma displays little or inconsistent augmentation of VCAM-1 expression. These cells often show augmented ICAM-1 expression and expression of P-selectin as well. However, the macrovascular lumen may contribute to leukocyte trafficking within the established atheroma to a lesser extent than the rich plexus of microvessels that develop in such lesions. The endothelial cells of such microvessels do display VCAM-1 expression.[7] Thus, indirect evidence suggests that the plaque's microvessels may provide an important locus for leukocyte trafficking during atherogenesis. These vessels do provide a considerably larger surface area for leukocyte trafficking than the macrovascular luminal endothelium.

## Chemoattraction of Adherent Monocytes into Lesions

Once the mononuclear phagocyte has adhered to the endothelium, it must penetrate into the intima. The engagement of the leukocyte adhesion molecules may activate certain functions of either leukocyte or endothelial cell that might facilitate transmigration of the leukocyte across the endothelial layer. The elaboration of chemotactic cytokines or other mediators may direct the migration of these leukocytes, promoting their accumulation at sites of local inflammation. One such cytokine, the chemokine monocyte chemoattractant protein-1 (MCP-1), provides a prototypical example of such a potential chemotactic stimulus for mononuclear phagocytes and T lymphocytes.[43] A variety of cell types in the atheroma can express MCP-1, including endothelium, macrophage, and smooth muscle cells when appropriately stimulated.[44-46] Human atherosclerotic lesions contain higher concentrations of MCP-1 messenger RNA and protein than do normal arteries.[47,48] Atherosclerosis-prone mice lacking MCP-1 or its receptor CCR2 have diminished lesion formation.[49,50] Chemokines, a superfamily of chemotactic cytokines, bind to a family of G protein-coupled heptahelical cell surface receptors. In addition to MCP-1, atheroma contain several other chemokines, including MCP-4, regulated on activation normal T cell expressed and secreted (RANTES), and interleukin-8 (IL-8). Lesions also exhibit CCR5, the receptor for MIP-1α and β.[51] *In vivo* studies in genetically modified mice have shown functional roles for the murine homologue of the IL-8 receptor CXCR2 in monocyte recruitment and retention in atherosclerotic lesions.

Thus, a variety of chemokines and their receptors may play critical roles in atherogenesis.

## Mechanisms of Macrophage Foam Cell Formation

Once the monocyte has taken up residence within the intima, it may take up the modified lipoproteins that have accumulated in the same locale. Scavenger receptors and the putative receptors for oxidized lipoproteins mentioned previously may mediate the entry of lipid into monocytes, leading to their conversion to foam cells. Inflammatory mediators may influence the expression by macrophages of these receptors for modified lipoproteins. For example, macrophage-colony stimulating factor (M-CSF), a cytokine found within plaques, can augment scavenger receptor expression by human macrophages.[52,53] Pro-inflammatory cytokines augment LOX-1 expression. However, gamma interferon, a product of the activated T-lymphocytes found within the atherosclerotic plaque (see below), can decrease expression of the scavenger receptor Type I on human macrophages *in vitro*.[54] The regulation of various receptors for modified lipoproteins on the macrophage surface may provide a link between inflammation, mediated by cytokines such as gamma interferon or M-CSF, and altered cholesterol economy within the plaque as manifested by monocyte transition to macrophage foam cells.

Such mediators of inflammation can also regulate other aspects of monocyte/macrophage function considered critical to atherogenesis. In addition to sequestering and potentially exporting lipid from the plaque, activated macrophages may produce reactive oxygen species that may participate in the oxidative modification of lipoproteins. Macrophages may also produce certain enzymes that metabolize lipoproteins, including acetyl cholesterol acyl transferase (ACAT) and lipoprotein lipase.[55-58]

## Products of Macrophages Resident in Lesions Modulate Latter Phases of Lesion Evolution

During the phase of transition of the foam cell-rich fatty streak to the more complex fibrous atheromatous lesion, mediators derived from lesional macrophages probably provide an important source of signals that regulate this aspect of lesion evolution. Macrophages can produce a number of growth factors that stimulate smooth muscle cell proliferation and/or migration and can alter extracellular matrix synthesis by smooth muscle cells. The smooth muscle cell probably migrates and proliferates within the intima during the transition from fatty streak to fibrous lesions. Moreover, the smooth muscle cell synthesizes most of the extracellular matrix components that accumulate within fibrous atherosclerotic plaques.

In addition to cytokines and growth factors, activated macrophages can elaborate small molecules such as nitric oxide, lipid mediators (including products of the arachidonate pathway), and oxygen species as previously noted. These biologically active, low-molecular-weight mediators may influence a number of aspects of smooth muscle behavior that contribute to lesion formation, evolution, and complication. For example, certain prostanoids and nitric oxide can inhibit smooth muscle cell proliferation and oppose inflammation providing a counterpoise for the pro-mitogenic and inflammatory stimuli found in atheroma. A balance between positive and negative regulators of smooth muscle cell growth may explain the low rates of smooth muscle cell proliferation (<< 1% of cells) noted in studies of advanced human atheroma.[59]

During the phase of lesion evolution, macrophages may participate in immune responses taking place within the atheroma. In particular, macrophages function very well as antigen-presenting cells. The macrophage can also provide costimulatory signals, both soluble and those requiring cell-cell contact, important in generating an immune response. The section on the lymphocyte elaborates on these ongoing cellular interactions in the immune response within atheroma.

## Roles of the Macrophage in Acute Complication of Atheroma

After a usually prolonged period of evolution, generally lasting decades, atherosclerotic plaques may often produce their first clinical manifestation. In the coronary arteries, a physical disruption of the atherosclerotic plaque with attendant thrombosis may provoke many of the acute clinical manifestations, including unstable angina pectoris episodes or acute myocardial infarction.[60] Products of the macrophage foam cell can destabilize atherosclerotic plaques.[61] These phagocytes elaborate enzymes that degrade macromolecules of the extracellular matrix including interstitial forms of collagen that provide the structural barrier between the blood and the thrombogenic contents of the plaque's center. Thus, enzymes such as collagenases, gelatinases, and stromelysin as well as non-metalloenzymes such as the cysteine proteinases cathepsins S and K can degrade matrix constituents and render a plaque vulnerable to disruption. Disrupted plaques provide a stimulus to blood coagulation and clot formation. A fracture of the plaque's fibrous cap allows contact of blood coagulation proteins with macrophages in the lipid core. Many of these macrophage foam cells express high levels of tissue factor, a potent pro-coagulant. Superficial erosions of atherosclerotic plaques uncover basement membrane forms of collagen that provide a stimulus for platelet aggregation and activation.[62] Matrix-degrading enzymes derived from macrophages may promote weakening of the fibrous cap and hence fracture of this structure. These same enzymes may promote desquamation of arterial endothelial cells by digesting the matrix links that tether the endothelial cell and the underlying extracellular matrix.[63] Matrix-degrading enzymes may thus promote both plaque rupture and superficial erosion of the atheroma, the two major anatomic substrates for the formation of inclusive coronary thrombosis. The macrophage not only furnishes a source of these hydrolytic enzymes but also provides the thrombogenic tissue factor that can incite local coagulation.[64] In this way, the macrophage plays a double role in promoting destabilization and thrombosis of the atherosclerotic plaque.

## Unanswered Questions Regarding Macrophage Involvement in Atherogenesis

Over the last dozen years, many studies such as those cited above have established critical functions for the macrophage in the biology of atherosclerosis. However, many questions remain unanswered in this regard. Knowledge regarding the kinetics of monocyte entry, monocyte/macrophage residence within the plaque, and the possibility of macrophage egress from plaques remains scanty. Elucidation of the leukokinetics in the atheroma will require much more work.

## The Macrophage: Beneficial or Deleterious during Atherogenesis?

The foregoing discussion of macrophage functions during atherogenesis highlighted primarily deleterious functions of the macrophage. However, the macrophage may also exert beneficial effects, potentially stemming or modulating atheroma progression. The ability of wild-type bone marrow transfer to "rescue" the atherosclerosis-prone phenotype of the apolipoprotein E-deficient mouse supports the ability of leukocyte-derived apolipoprotein E to modulate lesion formation.[65] This molecule has high affinity for peripheral LDL receptors. HDL particles may bind apolipoprotein E as they accumulate cholesterol within the atherosclerotic plaque. Association with apolipoprotein E may target HDL particles for peripheral catabolism. Macrophages in plaques also express the ABCA1 transporter, a molecule that appears critical in the exchange of cholesterol into HDL particles to effect reverse cholesterol transport. In this way, macrophages may promote net efflux of cholesterol ester from the atherosclerotic plaque.[66]

By sequestering modified lipoproteins and cholesterol ester within cells, macrophages may protect other denizens of the atheroma, such as the smooth muscle cell or the endothelial cell, from the ill-effects of these lipid constituents. Thus, one must conceive of macrophage functions as a balance, some potentially anti-atherogenic and others potentially deleterious in the course of atherogenesis. Further understanding of the regulation of these various macrophage functions might enable manipulation of the phenotype of macrophages within plaques emphasizing beneficial functions in a therapeutic manner.

## Heterogeneity of Macrophages in Atheroma

The literature generally treats lesional macrophages as a homogenous population and speaks globally of macrophage "activation." Actually, macrophages display considerable heterogeneity within the atherosclerotic plaque. Activation of macrophages does not occur in an "all or none" fashion but may display many subtle gradations depending on the activating stimuli and other aspects of the microenvironment of that particular macrophage. The oversimplifications implicit in most discussions of atheroma-associated macrophages obscure a great deal of ignorance about macrophage heterogeneity. Some mononuclear phagocytes within a plaque may

be recent arrivals, just beginning transformation into macrophages. Other lipid-rich foam cells expressing scavenger receptors, tissue factor, and class II histocompatibility antigens may exemplify longer-term residents of the atheromatous intima. Indeed, the more lipid-laden, scavenger-receptor-expressing macrophages may display lower levels of class II MHC molecule expression than the macrophages with lower lipid content. This tendency may reflect the ability of the T cell-derived cytokine gamma interferon to induce class II MHC gene expression on the one hand but to limit macrophage scavenger receptor expression on the other. Other macrophages appear to undergo cell death, some by an apoptotic pathway.[67,68] Thus, one may encounter many phases of the life span of a mononuclear phagocyte within the atheroma. Even among the "mature" foam cell population, there is considerable evidence for heterogeneity in the functions displayed by individual macrophages. This richer and more complex concept of plaque macrophages will require considerable more effort to unravel more completely.

## LYMPHOCYTES: AN ADDITIONAL LEUKOCYTIC CELL TYPE ABUNDANT IN ATHEROMA

Of the leukocytes found in atherosclerotic plaques, the monocyte/macrophage has received the most attention particularly until recently. However, lymphocytes comprise another important component of the leukocytic infiltrate in regions of the atherosclerotic plaque as well.[69-71] Both lymphocytes and macrophages bind to VCAM-1 on the endothelial surface. However, recruitment of T cells to lesions likely depends upon distinct chemoattractants, notably a trio of chemokines that bind to CXCR3 on their surface: interferon-inducible protein 10 (IP-10), monokine induced by interferon-gamma and interferon-inducible T cell alpha chemoattractant (I-TAC).[72]

## Subtyping of Lymphocytes in Atheromatous Lesions

Early studies demonstrated that T cells accounted for up to 20% of the cell population in the shoulder, or leading edge, region of established human carotid atherosclerotic plaques removed at therapeutic endarterectomy.[69] Atherosclerotic lesions in both humans and experimental animals, including rabbits and mice, also disclose the presence of lymphocytes early in the process of atherogenesis. Most of the lymphocytes in atheroma bear markers of T cells. B cells are rare in human atheroma, although advanced atheroma may contain immunoglobulin-secreting plasma cells.

Within the helper T cell population, further analysis has established that many of these cells have differentiated into more specialized Th1 lymphocytes That is, the profile of cytokines elaborated by lesion-derived cells includes higher levels of gamma interferon (ultimately promoting inflammation by activating macrophages as well as local vascular cells) than of the so-called Th2 cytokines such as IL-4 (which typically promote IgE synthesis by B lymphocytes, activation of mast cells, and recruitment and activation of eosinophils). These two extreme patterns of cytokine secretion from helper T cell populations represent two poles of a continuum. Complex chronic inflammatory lesions such as atheroma probably contain many gradations of helper T cell phenotypes that, as already suggested above, apply to lesional macrophages. In addition, the pattern of cytokine production by individual helper T cells may vary over time. For example, mice with prolonged and extreme hypercholesterolemia may undergo a shift to Th2 dominance.[73] The balance of Th1 versus Th2 cytokines may influence the degree of fibrogenic stimuli present during lesion evolution and may account for some of the heterogeneity in the histology of various individual atheromatous lesions characteristic of this disease in humans.

Most T cells in human atheroma express the alpha and beta chains of the T cell receptor for antigen.[71,74] Only a few cells use the gamma and delta chains of this receptor. This finding implies that the T cells recognize peptide antigens present in the groove of MHC class II molecules on the surface of antigen-resenting cells.

In principle, the T cells in atheroma could represent a population of bystander cells recruited nonspecifically by cytokines and chemokines generated during plaque formation, as described above. Alternatively, the T cells could participate actively in an immune and inflammatory response. To help distinguish between these possibilities, one can examine certain markers of T cell activation. The T cells within human atheroma exhibit markers of chronic activation. They display the RO isoform of CD45, indicating prior activation.[75] They also elaborate gamma interferon.[76] Expression of these markers indicates that the T cells indeed participate in the inflammatory reaction within the human atherosclerotic plaque. As noted above, the usual pathway for activation of T cells requires engagement of the T cell receptor for antigen by the cognate antigen, usually presented as a peptide in the groove of the self MHC II molecule on the surface of the antigen-presenting cell. Other pathways exist that bypass this traditional pathway. Notably, superantigens can activate T cells by binding to a site on the MHC II molecule distinct from the antigen cleft and nonetheless engage the T cell receptor. Other pathways for activating T cell behaviors independent of the T cell receptor may include exposure to constituents of modified LDL.

Additionally, accessory molecules expressed by the antigen-presenting cell can modulate the response of the T cells to antigen. Factors associated with atherogenesis, including cytokines and constituents of oxidatively modified lipoproteins, can modulate the expression of molecules with accessory functions including ICAM-1, VCAM-1, and CD 40, among others.

## Clonality of T cells in Atheroma

One way to garner more information about the potential stimuli for T cell activation involves examining the range of T cell receptors for antigen expressed by members of a population of lymphocytes. Restricted use of antigen receptors by T cells in the plaque would indicate that they participate in a local immune response directed against a correspondingly limited panel of specific antigens. Several strategies have shown that T cells from human carotid atheroma show no evidence of preferential use of certain T cell receptor variable region sequences.[77,78] Thus, at least in the advanced lesions sampled, the atheroma contain T cells capable of responding to a wide panel of antigens. This result, of course, cannot exclude an initial antigen-specific response directed against one or a small number of antigens at earlier stages in the history of the lesion. Indeed, CD 4 T cells in early atherosclerotic lesions of apolipoprotein E-deficient mice appear in clusters, consistent with activation and proliferation *in situ*.[79] Such a clone of T cells responding to a specific antigen could release mediators such as gamma interferon that could activate neighboring macrophages to secrete chemokines that could recruit T cells independent of their antigen specificity. This secondary recruitment might "dilute" the antigen-specific clone of T cells.

## Potential Antigens that Stimulate T cells in Atheromas

Although analysis of late-stage lesions shows no evidence that lesional T cells respond to a restricted set of antigens, antigen-specific stimuli remain a leading explanation for the presence of chronically activated T cells within the lesions. What antigens might then provoke this T cell activation? A number of candidates exist (Table 20-3). The strength of the evidence supporting involvement of these various candidates varies considerably.

### Oxidized Lipoproteins

Direct experimental evidence supports the concept that oxidatively modified LDL constitutes one such antigenic stimulus. T cell clones isolated from human carotid atheroma respond by proliferation and cytokine secretion when challenged with oxidatively modified LDL presented by autologous macrophages *in vitro*. T cell recognition oxidized LDL epitopes could induce local

■ ▪ ■

**TABLE 20-3** ANTIGENS POTENTIALLY INVOLVED IN STIMULATING T CELLS DURING ATHEROGENESIS

Modified lipoproteins
    Oxidatively modified LDL proteins/peptides
    Oxysterols or other lipids (involvement of CD1?)
Heat shock proteins
    HSP 65/60
Other autoantigens
    Cryptic or induced antigens
Infectious agents
    Herpesviridae
      Herpesvirus hominis
      Cytomegalovirus
    *Chlamydia pneumoniae* (TWAR)
    *Helicobacter* spp.

inflammation and provide help for antibody production. Thus, oxidized LDL is a potent autoantigen that elicits antibodies of both IgM and IgG classes. The appearance of such IgG antibodies, such as occurs in the atherosclerosis-prone, apolipoprotein E-deficient mouse, further supports a specific cellular immune response to these antigens, as production of the IgG antibodies implies the participation of T cell "help" as part of a T cell-dependent B cell response. Antibodies that bind to oxidized LDL recognize several epitopes, including adducts of amino acids on apolipoprotein B such as lysyl residues, whose epsilon-amino groups have undergone derivatization by reaction with malondialdehyde or 4-hydroxynonenol, both constituents of oxidized lipids.[80] Other antibodies recognize phospholipid structures that occur not only in oxidatively modified lipoproteins but also on apoptotic cells and in the cell wall of pneumococci.[80] The finding of a strong humoral antibody response to oxidized lipoproteins indicates a high degree of immunogenicity of the modified apolipoprotein B.[81,82] The titer of such antibodies appears to correlate with the degree of lesion progression. This finding points to the autoimmune response as a marker of disease activity. However, its pathogenic role remains obscure.

### Heat Shock Proteins

A portion of the T cell clones derived from atheromas does not respond to antigens associated with oxidized LDL, implying the existence of other types of antigenic stimuli. Heat shock proteins (HSP) may provide such alternative antigens to T cells within experimental and perhaps human atherosclerotic plaques. These proteins localize inside cells under normal circumstances. However, cellular injury of various sorts heightens the production and release of these proteins, whose accumulation accompanies many disease states. HSP can activate innate immunity via binding CD14 and toll-like receptor 4.[83,84] Immunization with HSP of the HSP65/60 family will potentiate lesion formation in rabbits in response to an atherogenic diet.[85] Circulating antibodies that react with HSP65/60 may damage endothelial cells and correlate with ultrasound evidence of carotid intimal thickening in humans.[86,87] The specific case of HSP exemplifies the general possibility of autoimmunity in atherosclerosis. Cell disruption during atherosclerosis could permit access to the immune surveillance system of antigens usually sequestered within cells. The cell debris in the so-called "necrotic" core of the atheroma provides a potential pool of such potential autoantigens. Immunization with HSP can limit experimental atherosclerosis, providing an example of immunomodulation affecting this process.[88]

### Other Potential "Autoantigens"

Alternatively, oxidative or other modification such as glycation of lipoproteins might provide neoepitopes for a localized immune response during atherogenesis. Another potential scenario involves an immune response directed against surface antigens on vascular cells usually not expressed but induced in response to inflammatory mediators present during atherogenesis. For example, we have already discussed a number of cytokine-inducible cell surface molecules expressed by vascular endothelial and/or smooth muscle cells during atherogenesis. An immune response to such induced antigens might provide another pathway of autoantigen production in atheroma. This mechanism has not yet been demonstrated to occur in atherosclerosis, but it does appear to contribute to another form of inflammatory vascular pathology, Kawasaki disease.[89,90]

### Infectious Agents as Antigenic Stimuli

Over many years, investigators have sought a connection between infectious agents and atherosclerosis. In certain well-defined experimental situations, notably Marek's disease in chickens (produced by an avian herpes virus) or exposure of atherosclerosis-prone mice with cytomegalovirus (CMV), viral infection can potentiate diet-induced atherogenesis.[91-95] Cell structure studies have revealed that CMV-encoded proteins can promote smooth muscle migration, which may be important in the formation of lesions.[96] Human atheromas can contain herpes virus DNA.[97] A number of studies have correlated evidence for herpes virus hominis or CMV in atherosclerosis or re-stenosis after arterial intervention.[98,99] Most particularly, several studies have attempted to correlate CMV infection with development of the accelerated form of arteriosclerosis that complicates organ transplantation.[100,101] In light of these findings, viral antigens constitute another potential source of stimulation to T cells during atherogenesis.

Nonviral microbial pathogens may also coexist with atherosclerotic lesions. Much recent interest has focused on *Chlamydia* and *Helicobacter* species in this regard.[102-104] As in the case of viruses, such microbial pathogens, whether or not causally related to instigation of atherosclerosis, may provide an antigenic stimulus for lesional T cells and thus contribute to the ongoing immune and inflammatory response characteristic of atherosclerosis.

## Transplantation Arteriosclerosis, An Example of Immune-Mediated Arterial Disease

The particular case of accelerated arteriosclerosis in transplanted coronary arteries provides an example of an alloimmune response potentiating the development of arterial intimal disease. We have postulated and presented evidence that a chronic allogeneic response to donor class II MHC antigens incites a cellular immune response that contributes to the pathogenesis of this accelerated arteriosclerosis.[105,106] Although the allogeneic response does not contribute to the common forms of atherosclerosis, this example illustrates how the immune response, and T cell-mediated immunity in particular, may contribute to arterial pathology.[107]

Recent experiments in genetically modified mice have explored the role of various components of the immune system in transplanted hearts, evaluating the responses of wild-type mice and in mutant mice with impaired function of various limbs of immunity. These studies have established a key role for gamma interferon in the development of arteriopathy but not parenchymal rejection, a process with distinct pathogenesis.[108] Deficiency in IL-4, TNF-α receptor 1, or CD40L does not prevent allograft arteriosclerosis.[109-111] Unexpectedly, IL-10 deficiency does not exacerbate allograft arteriopathy as it does in lipid-induced atherosclerosis in mice.[109] This seemingly paradoxical result highlights the differences between ordinary atherosclerosis and the accelerated transplantation-associated arteriosclerosis.

## IMMUNE FUNCTIONS OF CELLS IN "USUAL" ATHEROSCLEROSIS

In the transplantation situation, non-self (allogeneic) class II MHC antigen, probably presented by foreign endothelial cells, appears to incite the cellular immune response. What cells might perform these functions in the context of atherosclerosis affecting native, non-allogeneic arteries? Recognition of an antigen by T lymphocytes requires presentation of the nominal antigen in association with a class II MHC molecule. This antigen presentation usually requires cell-cell contact between the T cell and an "antigen-presenting cell" (APC). In classical cellular immunology, the macrophage or the B cell provides the antigen-presenting function by expressing class II MHC molecules. In addition, macrophages and B cells can express certain co-stimulatory molecules that potentiate and modulate the cellular immune response. Although atherosclerotic lesions contain few B cells, macrophages abound in these lesions. In addition to typical macrophages, plaques contain dendritic cells, cells of the monocyte lineage that appear specialized for antigen presentation.[112,113] Moreover, macrophages of various types within human atheroma often express MHC II antigens.[114] Plaque macrophages also express CD1 molecules on their surface. CD1 can present certain lipid antigens to T cells, and thus might play a special role in inciting immune responses in the atheromatous lesion.[115] Thus, macrophages provide a likely candidate for an APC in the context of T cell activation within atheroma in native arteries.

Endothelial cells can also serve as presenting cells for foreign antigens. They can express MHC II molecules and co-stimulatory molecules, and very effectively present antigen to T cells in vitro.[116] Although smooth muscle cells, like endothelial cells, can express class II MHC antigens in an inducible fashion, their role as APCs remains uncertain. Smooth muscle cells stimulate an allogeneic response much less efficiently than do endothelial cells from the same human donor.[106,117] This relative ineffectiveness of smooth muscle cells in engendering the allogeneic response appears to result from the elaboration by the smooth muscle cells of a poorly characterized, short-lived inhibitor.[118]

## Cytokines Activate Vascular and Immune Cells

Once T cells encounter antigen on a presenting cell and become activated, what functions might they subserve of pathophysiologic relevance to atherosclerosis? As discussed above, CD4 cells encountering the antigen elaborate cytokines, including the autocrine growth factor interleukin-2 (IL-2), gamma interferon, and TNF and the related molecule lymphotoxin. These cytokines can exert manifold actions on a variety of lesion-associated cell types. In particular, IL-2, by stimulating the proliferation of T cells, can expand the T cell population and also provide "help" to cytotoxic T cells. IL-2 release from activated CD4 cells can thus stimulate cytotoxic CD8 positive T cell functions. This pathway may be important to vascular diseases, in particular in the context of viral infections. For example, endothelial cells infected with herpes viruses such as CMV could undergo lytic injury mediated by CD8-positive T cells. Recent studies show that a CD8 attack on vascular smooth muscle cells dramatically aggravates atherosclerosis in hypercholesterolemic mice.[119]

Most agree that IL-2 has a narrow spectrum of activity, generally limited to lymphocytes. However, the other cytokines released by activated T lymphocytes act on a broader panel of cell types. TNF, lymphotoxin, and gamma interferon can all influence the expression of leukocyte adhesion molecules on endothelial and smooth muscle cells.[120] Gamma interferon can activate a number of macrophage functions that may be important in the pathogenesis of vascular diseases. For example, gamma interferon can augment the expression of class II histocompatibility antigens enhancing the antigen-presenting capacity of monocyte/macrophages. This lymphokine also inhibits scavenger receptor expression on macrophages, reducing their uptake of modified lipoproteins.[54] Gamma interferon acts on smooth muscle cells to reduce collagen and alpha actin synthesis and proliferation.[121,122] "Priming" of endothelial cells, smooth muscle cells, and macrophages by exposure to the lymphokine gamma interferon enables them to respond to the monokines TNF and IL-1 by enhancing NO production.[123] This route operates by transcriptionally activating the high capacity, inducible form of nitric oxide synthase (iNOS, or NOS II).

The local production of NO has diverse effects relevant to inflammation and atherosclerosis. The nitric oxide radical can inhibit smooth muscle cell contractility and proliferation and also reduce platelet aggregation. Increased iNOS expression at sites of arterial injury, as shown experimentally in rats, might compensate for the local loss of endothelium at these sites.[124] Nitric oxide radical can also inhibit cytokine-induced activation of both endothelial and smooth muscle cells (e.g., expression of adhesion molecule or cytokine gene expression) by augmenting the activity of IκB-α, an inhibitor of the NFκB transcriptional activation pathway.[20,21,125] However, the high concentration of NO produced by the high-capacity inducible form of this enzyme, particularly at sites of inflammation-induced increases in superoxide anion production, may promote cell injury or death by favoring production of the highly toxic species peroxynitrite (−ONOO).[126]

Exposure of endothelial cells, smooth muscle cells, and macrophages to TNF can enhance the production of cytokines of factors that promote smooth muscle cell growth, extracellular matrix biosynthesis, migration, and production of angiogenic peptides. Thus, T cell-derived cytokines may influence aspects of vascular cell and macrophage function that can contribute to lesion progression and complication.

T lymphocytes may also contribute to neovascularization of atherosclerotic plaques. We studied the development of intimal lesions in arteries of hearts transplanted heterotopically in rabbits that consumed an atherogenic diet. We found that the transplanted arteries developed accentuated intimal thickening compared with the native arteries of the recipient's own heart subjected to the same degree of hypercholesterolemia.[127] The transplanted arteries contained many more T cells than did the native arteries of the recipient. Moreover, there was a striking formation of microvessels within the lesions of the transplanted arteries compared with those of the recipients' own arteries. Activated T lymphocytes can elaborate angiogenic factors such as vascular endothelial cell growth factor (VEGF).[128,129] These results suggest that T cells may contribute importantly to plaque angiogenesis, at least in this special case of transplantation-associated arteriosclerosis.

## Multiple Roles for the T Cell-Derived Lymphokine Gamma Interferon in Atherogenesis

By activating macrophages, gamma interferon can indirectly promote smooth muscle cell proliferation and extracellular matrix synthesis. Gamma interferon may also have direct effects on smooth muscle cells. For example, this lymphokine modulates smooth muscle cell production of actin and limits interstitial collagen synthesis.[121,122] Initial studies suggested that gamma interferon acts primarily to inhibit the growth of cultured rat or human smooth muscle cells stimulated by serum or by PDGF.[130,131] A more recent study using porcine and human vascular smooth muscle cells instead found no effect on serum-induced proliferation and a pronounced potentiation of PDGF responses mediated in part through increased receptors for this growth factor.[132] The basis of this discrepancy is unclear but could relate to the heterogeneity of vascular smooth muscle cell types or to subtle differences in culture conditions. In vivo studies using human or pig coronary artery segments transplanted as aortic interposition grafts in immunodeficient mice have been informative. Gamma interferon is species specific so that the human cytokine does not act on mouse cells, and in this artificial system, administration of human gamma interferon does not affect mouse macrophages and other cell types. The unambiguous result is that human gamma interferon acts on human vascular smooth muscle cells to cause proliferation and net accumulation of cells in the intima. Increased levels of receptors for PDGF on the responding smooth muscle cells accompany this response.[132] The presence of other cytokines modulates the growth-promoting effects of gamma interferon on smooth muscle cells. A combination of gamma interferon plus TNF and interleukin-1 beta can induce apoptosis of rat and

human vascular smooth muscle cells.[133] Gamma interferon can also sensitize smooth muscle cells to killing by Fas ligand by inducing the translocation of CD95 (APO-1/Fas) from the Golgi to the cell surface.[134] Gamma interferon treatment also makes endothelial cells more susceptible to killing by Fas ligand, but in this case, the response involves de novo synthesis of CD95 and of caspase 8.[135]

In the early phases of atherogenesis, gamma interferon might reduce lesion progression by inhibiting smooth muscle cell growth, survival, and matrix production. However, the situation in advanced plaques may differ substantively. Late atherosclerotic lesions often contain hypocellular regions. Points of atherosclerotic plaques that tend to rupture have relatively few smooth muscle cells.[136,137] In contrast, the sites where plaques actually rupture contain relatively high numbers of T cells. Moreover, macrophages and smooth muscle cells in the vicinity of areas where human plaques have actually ruptured display high levels of class II MHC antigens.[137] Gamma interferon, but not a variety of other cytokines evaluated, can induce MHC class II antigen expression on these cells, particularly smooth muscle cells.[138] Thus, T cell-derived gamma interferon may contribute to loss of smooth muscle cells from regions of atheroma.

How might lack of smooth muscle cells, provoked by T cell-derived cytokines, promote plaque rupture? As noted previously, the integrity of the plaque's fibrous cap can regulate the exposure of blood coagulation factors to thrombogenic material in the plaque's central core. The smooth muscle cell manufactures the interstitial collagen that lends structural strength to the plaque's fibrous cap. At foci of T cell activation and consequent rarefaction of smooth muscle cells, matrix accretion and repair may suffer. In this manner, lesional T cells may promote plaque rupture by slowing growth or even causing death of smooth muscle cells and may enhance the formation and stability of thrombi that form in consequence.

Gamma interferon may also act directly on human smooth muscle cells to decrease the expression of interstitial collagen genes. Even smooth muscle cells exposed to the most potent stimulus for interstitial collagen gene expression yet identified, transforming growth factor beta, display marked inhibition of procollagen types I and III mRNA accumulation and protein synthesis when exposed to gamma interferon.[121] Thus, gamma interferon can both decrease the number of smooth muscle cells, as explained above, and interfere with their ability to synthesize this critical component of the plaque's extracellular matrix. In this way, T cell-derived gamma interferon may critically influence aspects of plaque biology related to the clinical manifestations associated with plaque disruption.[139] In addition, gamma interferon can directly provoke arteriosclerosis in vivo.[132]

## Unanswered Questions Regarding T Lymphocyte Involvement in Atherogenesis

Although we have learned much about T cell functions in relation to atherogenesis, many questions remain unanswered. We can generate a long list of antigens that potentially stimulate T cells within lesions, but there is no proof that any of these mechanisms actually acts *in vivo* in the plaque. In fact, the hunt for the culpable antigen may prove vain if the chronic activation of T cells, well-documented within human atheroma, proves independent of specific antigenic stimulation.

## The Cellular Immune Response: Pro- or Anti-Atherogenic?

As in the case of the macrophage, there is little consensus regarding the net effect of lymphocytes on lesion formation and complications. T cells exert certain functions that should augment lesion formation (e.g., activation of macrophages to produce growth factors, proteinases, and proinflammatory cytokines). On the other hand, by slowing smooth muscle cell proliferation, T cells might retard lesion formation even if the same effects can tend to favor local plaque disruption in more advanced atheroma. Using mice with genetically induced deficiencies in various immune functions, the tools to answer some of these questions have become available. Constructing compound mutants of atherosclerosis-prone animals and mice with targeted lack of certain immune functions should permit sorting out of the contribution of various immune functions to lesion formation and biology.

However, the information to date has engendered controversy. Apolipoprotein E-deficient mice lacking both humoral and cellular immunity develop atheroma when consuming an atherogenic diet.[140] On a chow diet, however, immunodeficient mice with less exaggerated hypercholesterolemia show attenuation of lesion formation. Adoptive transfer experiments have established a role for cellular immunity in experimental atherosclerosis.[141] For a more ample discussion of this complex debate, please see recent reviews.[71,142] Seemingly paradoxically, immunization of rabbits with modified LDL can inhibit lesion formation.[143] Immunization of mice with LDL induces T cell-dependent antibody formation and protects against atherosclerosis.[144] Some of the confusion in this area may result from a plethora of experimental protocols and differences in the preparations used or may reflect the complexity of the involvement of the immune response in atherogenesis. Fortunately, the tools provided by genetically altered mice may allow us to obviate the limitations of pharmacologic approaches and help to provide more definitive answers to questions regarding the role of the immune response and atherogenesis.[71,142]

The studies designed to probe this question thus far have generally measured lesion extent, an important but by itself insufficient variable to provide mechanistic insight into the biology of atherogenesis. Future studies should aim not only to measure the size of the lesions but also to probe aspects of the function of cells within the lesions themselves. We have illustrated how gamma interferon's inhibition of smooth muscle cell matrix elaboration might prove beneficial during the phase of lesion progression but disastrous when causing weakening of a vulnerable region of a complicated atherosclerotic plaque. The actual effect of aspects of the immune response in human atherogenesis may well differ depending on the stage of lesion evolution and the microanatomic location of a particular immune event. Such studies will doubtless require more subtle analysis than mere measurement of the lesion size to elucidate more completely the role of the immune system in atherogenesis.

## Mast Cells

Morphologists have long known that the adventitia of blood vessels contains mast cells. A number of recent studies have called attention to the presence of mast cells in the atherosclerotic intima.[145,146] These studies have employed a number of criteria for identification of mast cells, including reactivity with monospecific antibodies directed against characteristic mast cell granular enzymes such as chymase. The chemokines, discussed previously, and adhesion molecules that regulate the recruitment of other leukocyte subtypes may also participate in recruitment of mast cells. For example, cytokine-stimulated human smooth muscle cells produce eotaxin, and human atheroma contain both eotaxin and mast cells bearing CCR3, the receptor for eotaxin.[147] Mast cells classically participate in a specialized form of inflammatory response involving reaginic antibody. When appropriately stimulated by an IgE antibody, mast cells can release their granular contents. For example, recent work has suggested that hydrolytic enzymes released from mast cells might contribute to lipid deposition by modifying LDL and also to plaque disruption by activating matrix-degrading proteases. Mast cell chymase can inhibit smooth muscle cell growth and promote their apoptosis.[148,149] Despite these functions demonstrated by mast cells or their products *in vitro,* the pathogenic significance of these observations remains uncertain. The postulated functions of mast cells in atherogenesis overlap to a considerable extent with the functions of macrophages, a cell type considerably more numerous in typical atherosclerotic lesions than the mast cell. Much future work will be required to delineate the precise contribution of mast cells to atherogenesis. In particular, it is uncertain what mast cell-specific activating stimuli may prove pertinent to atherosclerosis.

## Polymorphonuclear Leukocytes

Most pathologic studies of chronic atherosclerotic lesions fail to show granulocytes as part of the leukocytic infiltrate within the atherosclerotic intima. In disrupted plaques complicated by thrombosis, polymorphonuclear leukocytes may associate with the clot. However, scant evidence supports the primary involvement of granulocytes in the chronic phases of atherosclerosis in relation to the acute complications of atheroma. Nonetheless, granulocytes clearly participate in acute necrotizing vasculitis, Arthus-like reactions, and other specific arterial pathologies. Although the role of granulocytes in usual atherosclerosis remains murky, previous involvement of arteries in some of these granulocyte-mediated acute inflammatory responses may potentiate atherogenesis.

Just because few granulocytes localize in late-stage atheroma, one cannot exclude a role for these cells in lesion initiation or potentiation in some cases. Kawsasaki disease illustrates an example of such a pathogenic pathway. A number of studies have documented that Kawsasaki arteritis in childhood may predispose to development of coronary atherosclerosis in adults.[150] The panarteritis of Kawsasaki disease typically involves granulocytic infiltration. In this particular case an early granulocyte-mediated damage to an artery may provide a nidus for initiating, augmenting, or hastening lesion formation in the presence of traditional risk factors for atherosclerosis.

Like the granulocyte, the basophil and eosinophil might accentuate atherogenesis under certain circumstances. For example, arteritides associated with eosinophil infiltration might interact with traditional risk factors to accelerate atherogenesis. However, most of these scenarios are uncommon. The roles of polymorphonuclear leukocytes, mast cells, and eosinophils remain much more speculative than the roles for macrophages and lymphocytes in atherogenesis. In populations with low levels of traditional atherogenic risk factors but more endemic parasitic or microbial diseases, atherosclerosis occurs less rather than more frequently. Thus, it seems unlikely that a large proportion of typical atherosclerosis results from initiation or amplification resulting from leukocytes of the granulocytic series.

## CLINICAL ASPECTS OF INFLAMMATION IN ATHEROSCLEROSIS

When this chapter was prepared for the previous edition of this book, there was little clinical information about, interest in, or utility of the concept of inflammation in atherosclerosis. Since then, the clinical application of inflammation biology in atherosclerosis has burgeoned.[151] The acute phase reactant C-reactive protein (CRP) has proven to be a robust readout and integrator of the inflammatory burden. One of the most exciting clinical advances in atherosclerosis in the last five years is the emergence of the utility of inflammatory markers as prognostic tools.[151,152] Elevated markers of inflammation predict outcomes of patients with acute coronary syndromes, independent of the amount of myocardial damage. Even in apparently well individuals, low-grade chronic inflammation, as indicated by levels of the inflammatory marker CRP in the upper ranges of normal, prospectively predict the risk of complications of atherosclerosis including acute myocardial infarction, stroke, and incident peripheral arterial disease. Moreover, the information provided by inflammatory markers such as CRP adds to the prognostic information provided by traditional risk factors such as the lipoprotein profile. Surprisingly, CRP levels predict future coronary events better than LDL levels.[153] Treatment with LDL-lowering drugs of the statin class that reduce coronary risk also limit inflammation as reflected in the CRP measurement.[154] These new insights into inflammation in atherosclerosis not only affirm the clinical importance of inflammation in atherosclerosis but also have practical clinical applications in risk stratification and targeting of therapy.[155]

The next iteration of the US guidelines for cardiovascular risk assessment and management may well incorporate biomarkers of inflammation. The clinical application of the concept of inflammation in atherosclerosis has also stimulated the design of a clinical trial that may change medical practice by selecting a group of patients for treatment with statins who do not merit drug therapy by current guidelines, criteria which are driven by classical risk factors.

## CONCLUSIONS

Until recently, most considered atherosclerosis a disease determined in the fluid phase of plasma. Prevailing opinion attributed atherogenesis to initiation by plasma-derived lipoproteins, relegating the arterial response to a secondary role if indeed acknowledging at all roles for the cells of the artery wall in this process. As appreciation of the cell biology has evolved, overwhelming evidence suggests that atherogenesis cannot be understood without taking to account the functions of the vascular wall cells; moreover, current thinking acknowledges many commonalties between atherogenesis and inflammation. Indeed, one may view atherogenesis as a special case of inflammation. This chapter has illustrated how inflammatory mediators can regulate a panoply of functions of vascular wall cells important for atherogenesis. In addition, this chapter has illustrated how infiltrating leukocytes, particularly the monocyte/macrophage and the T lymphocyte can interact with vascular wall cells by exchange of soluble mediators and by cell contact to affect many of these aspects of the inflammatory response during atherogenesis.

Although we lack much specific knowledge of the precise factors inciting inflammation during atherogenesis, we now possess a conceptual framework to focus our quest. Appreciation of the inflammatory aspects of atherosclerosis will doubtless increase our understanding of the molecular basis of atherogenesis. Moreover, such understanding may also yield insights useful for designing therapies to modulate this process. For example, we now know that lipid lowering can reduce coronary events. The recognition that certain lipid-lowering agents can limit inflammation provides a potential mechanism underlying these clinical benefits. Expanded knowledge of inflammatory pathways in atherosclerosis should identify novel targets for therapeutic intervention. The clinical application of these principles should permit more precise identification of individuals at risk for complications of this disease. Inflammatory markers may add to the panel of criteria that distinguish individuals who can benefit from particular preventive therapies and thus change clinical practice in the coming years.

## REFERENCES

1. Poole JCF, Florey HW: Changes in the endothelium of the aorta and the behavior of macrophages in experimental atheroma of rabbits. J Pathol Bacteriol 1958;75:245–253.

2. Gerrity RG, Naito HK, Richardson M, et al: Dietary induced atherogenesis in swine: Morphology of the intima in prelesion stages. Am J Pathol 1979;95:775–786.

3. Joris T, Nunnari JJ, Krolikowski FJ, et al: Studies on the pathogenesis of atherosclerosis. I. Adhesion and emigration of mononuclear cells in the aorta of hypercholesterolemic rats. Am J Pathol 1983;113:341–358.

4. Faggiotto A, Ross R, Harker: Studies of hypercholesterolemia in the nonhuman primate. I. Changes that lead to fatty streak formation. Arteriosclerosis 1984;4:323–340.

5. Cybulsky MI, Gimbrone MA Jr: Endothelial expression of a mononuclear leukocyte adhesion molecule during atherogenesis. Science 1991;251:788–791.

6. Li H, Cybulsky MI, Gimbrone MA Jr, et al: An atherogenic diet rapidly induces VCAM-1, a cytokine regulatable mononuclear leukocyte adhesion molecule, in rabbit endothelium. Arterioscler Thromb 1993;13:197–204.

7. O'Brien K, Allen M, McDonald T, et al: Vascular cell adhesion molecule-1 is expressed in human coronary atherosclerotic plaques: Implications for the mode of progression of advanced coronary atherosclerosis. J Clin Invest 1993;92:945–951.

8. Poston RN, Haskard DO, Coucher JR, et al: Expression of intercellular adhesion molecule-1 in atherosclerotic plaques. Am J Pathol 1992;140:665–673.

9. Printseva O, Peclo MM, Gown AM: Various cell types in human atherosclerotic lesions express ICAM-1: Further immunocytochemical and immunochemical studies employing monoclonal antibody 10F3. Am J Pathol 1992;140:889–896.

10. Wood KM, Cadogan MD, Ramshaw AL, et al: The distribution of adhesion molecules in human atherosclerosis. Histopathology 1993;22:437–444.

11. Dong ZM, Chapman SM, Brown AA, et al: The combined role of P- and E-selectins in atherosclerosis. J Clin Invest 1998;102:145–152.

12. Cybulsky MI, Iiyama K, Li H, et al: A major role for VCAM-1, but not ICAM-1, in early atherosclerosis. J Clin Invest 2001; 107:1255–1262.

13. Bevilacqua MP, Pober JS, Majeau GR, et al: Interleukin-1 acts on cultured human vascular endothelium to increase the adhesion of polymorphonuclear leukocytes, monocytes and related leukocyte cell lines. J Clin Invest 1985;76:2003–2011.

14. Bevilacqua MP, Pober JS, Mendrick DL, et al: Identification of an inducible endothelial-leukocyte adhesion molecule. Proc Natl Acad Sci USA 1987;84:9238–9242.

15. Dustin ML, Rothlein R, Bhan AK, et al: Induction by IL-1 and interferon-gamma: Tissue distribution, biochemistry, and function of a natural adherence molecule (ICAM-1). J Immunol 1986; 137:245–254.

16. Kume N, Gimbrone M Jr: Lysophosphatidylcholine transcriptionally induces growth factor gene expression in cultured human endothelial cells. J Clin Invest 1994;93:907–911.

17. Leitinger N, Tyner TR, Oslund L, et al: Structurally similar oxidized phospholipids differentially regulate endothelial binding of monocytes and neutrophils. Proc Natl Acad Sci USA 1999; 96:12010–12015.

18. Resnick N, Collins T, Atkinson W, et al: Platelet-derived growth factor B chain promoter contains a cis-acting fluid shear-stress-responsive element. Proc Natl Acad Sci USA 1993;90:4591–4595.

19. Khachigian LM, Resnick N, Gimbrone M Jr, et al: Nuclear factor-kappa B interacts functionally with the platelet-derived growth factor B-chain shear-stress response element in vascular endothelial cells exposed to fluid shear stress. J Clin Invest 1995; 96:1169–1175.

20. Peng HB, Libby P, Liao JK: Induction and stabilization of I kappa B alpha by nitric oxide mediates inhibition of NF-kappa B. J Biol Chem 1995;270:14214–14219.

21. Peng HB, Rajavashisth TB, Libby P, et al: Nitric oxide inhibits macrophage-colony stimulating factor gene transcription in vascular endothelial cells. J Biol Chem 1995;270:17050–17055.

22. Walpola PL, Gotlieb AI, Cybulsky MI, et al: Expression of ICAM-1 and VCAM-1 and monocyte adherence in arteries exposed to altered shear stress. Arterioscler Thromb Vasc Biol 1995;15:2–10.

23. Topper JN, Cai J, Falb D, et al: Identification of vascular endothelial genes differentially responsive to fluid mechanical stimuli: Cyclooxygenase-2, manganese superoxide dismutase, and endothelial cell nitric oxide synthase are selectively up-regulated by steady laminar shear stress. Proc Natl Acad Sci USA 1996;93: 10417–10422.

24. Schwenke DC, Carew TE: Initiation of atherosclerotic lesions in cholesterol-fed rabbits. I. Focal increases in arterial LDL concentration precede development of fatty streak lesions. Arteriosclerosis 1989;9:895–907.

25. Schwenke DC, Carew TE: Initiation of atherosclerotic lesions in cholesterol-fed rabbits. II. Selective retention of LDL vs. selective increases in LDL permeability in susceptible sites of arteries. Arteriosclerosis 1989;9:908–918.

26. Wight TN: The extracellular matrix and atherosclerosis. Curr Opin Lipidol 1995;6:326–334.

27. Hurt-Camejo E, Olsson U, Wiklund O, et al: Cellular consequences of the association of apoB lipoproteins with proteoglycans: Potential contribution to atherogenesis. Arterioscler Thromb Vasc Biol 1997;17:1011–1017.

28. Lee RT, Yamamoto C, Feng Y, et al: Mechanical strain induces specific changes in the synthesis and organization of proteoglycans by vascular smooth muscle cells. J Biol Chem 2001; 276:13847–13851.

29. Skalen K, Gustafsson M, Rydberg EK, et al: Subendothelial retention of atherogenic lipoproteins in early atherosclerosis. Nature 2002;417:750–754.

30. Lundstam U, Hurt-Camejo E, Olsson G, et al: Proteoglycans contribution to association of Lp(a) and LDL with smooth muscle cell extracellular matrix. Arterioscler Thromb Vasc Biol 1999; 19:1162–1167.

31. Witztum JL, Berliner JA: Oxidized phospholipids and isoprostanes in atherosclerosis. Curr Opin Lipidol 1998;9:441–448.

32. Glass CK, Witztum JL: Atherosclerosis: The road ahead. Cell 2001;104:503–516.

33. Subbanagounder G, Wong JW, Lee H, et al: Epoxyisoprostane and epoxycyclopentenone phospholipids regulate monocyte chemotactic protein-1 and interleukin-8 synthesis: Formation of these oxidized phospholipids in response to interleukin-1beta. J Biol Chem 2002;277:7271–7281.

34. Krieger M: The other side of scavenger receptors: Pattern recognition for host defense. Curr Opin Lipidol 1997;8:275–280.

35. Hajjar DP, Haberland ME: Lipoprotein trafficking in vascular cells: Molecular Trojan horses and cellular saboteurs. J Biol Chem 1997;272:22975–22978.

36. Endemann G, Stanton LW, Madden KS, et al: CD36 is a receptor for oxidized low density lipoprotein. J Biol Chem 1993; 268:11811–11816.

37. Ramprasad MP, Fischer W, Witztum JL, et al: The 94- to 97-kDa mouse macrophage membrane protein that recognizes oxidized low density lipoprotein and phosphatidylserine-rich liposomes is identical to macrosialin, the mouse homologue of human CD68. Proc Natl Acad Sci USA 1995;92:9580–9584.

38. Rigotti A, Trigatti BL, Penman M, et al: A targeted mutation in the murine gene encoding the high density lipoprotein (HDL) receptor scavenger receptor class B type I reveals its key role in HDL metabolism. Proc Natl Acad Sci USA 1997;94: 12610–12615.

39. Elomaa O, Kangas M, Sahlberg C, et al: Cloning of a novel bacteria-binding receptor structurally related to scavenger receptors and expressed in a subset of macrophages. Cell 1995;80:603–609.

40. Shimaoka T, Kume N, Minami M, et al: Molecular cloning of a novel scavenger receptor for oxidized low density lipoprotein, SR-PSOX, on macrophages. J Biol Chem 2000;275:40663–40666.

41. Kume N, Kita T: Roles of lectin-like oxidized LDL receptor-1 and its soluble forms in atherogenesis. Curr Opin Lipidol 2001;12:419–423.

42. Minami M, Kume N, Shimaoka T, et al: Expression of SR-PSOX, a novel cell-surface scavenger receptor for phosphatidylserine and oxidized LDL in human atherosclerotic lesions. Arterioscler Thromb Vasc Biol 2001;21:1796–1800.

43. Rollins BJ: JE/MCP-1: An early-response gene encodes a monocyte-specific cytokine. Cancer Cells 1991;3:517–524.

44. Rollins BJ, Stier P, Ernst T, et al: The human homolog of the JE gene encodes a monocyte secretory protein. Mol Cell Biol 1989; 9:468–695.

45. Rollins BJ, Yoshimura T, Leonard EJ, et al: Cytokine-activated human endothelial cells synthesize and secrete a monocyte chemoattractant, MCP-1/JE. Am J Pathol 1990;136:1229–1233.

46. Wang J, Sica A, Peri G, et al: Expression of monocyte chemotactic protein and interleukin-8 by cytokine-activated human vascular smooth muscle cells. Arterioscler Thromb 1991;11:1166-1174.

47. Nelken N, Coughlin S, Gordon D, et al: Monocyte chemoattractant protein-1 in human atheromatous plaques. J Clin Invest 1991;88:1121-1127.

48. Yla-Herttuala S, Lipton BA, Rosenfeld ME, et al: Expression of monocyte chemoattractant protein 1 in macrophage-rich areas of human and rabbit atherosclerotic lesions. Proc Natl Acad Sci USA 1991;88:5252-5256.

49. Gu L, Okada Y, Clinton S, et al: Absence of monocyte chemoattractant protein-1 reduces atherosclerosis in low-density lipoprotein-deficient mice. Mol Cell 1998;2:275-281.

50. Boring L, Gosling J, Cleary M, et al: Decreased lesion formation in CCR2-/-mice reveals a role for chemokines in the initiation of atherosclerosis. Nature 1998;394:894-897.

51. Schecter AD, Calderon TM, Berman AB, et al: Human vascular smooth muscle cells possess functional CCR5. J Biol Chem 2000;275:5466-5471.

52. Ishibashi S, Inaba T, Shimano H, et al: Monocyte colony-stimulating factor enhances uptake and degradation of acetylated low density lipoproteins and cholesterol esterification in human monocyte-derived macrophages. J Biol Chem 1990;265:14109-14117.

53. Clinton S, Underwood R, Sherman M, et al: Macrophage-colony stimulating factor gene expression in vascular cells and in experimental and human atherosclerosis. Am J Pathol 1992;140:301-316.

54. Geng YJ, Hansson GK: Interferon-gamma inhibits scavenger receptor expression and foam cell formation in human monocyte-derived macrophages. J Clin Invest 1992;89:1322-1330.

55. O'Brien KD, Gordon D, Deeb S, et al: Lipoprotein lipase is synthesized by macrophage-derived foam cells in human coronary atherosclerotic plaques. J Clin Invest 1992;89:1544-1550.

56. Yla-Herttuala S, Lipton BA, Rosenfeld ME, et al: Macrophages and smooth muscle cells express lipoprotein lipase in human and rabbit atherosclerotic lesions. Proc Natl Acad Sci USA 1991;88:10143-10147.

57. Fazio S, Major AS, Swift LL, et al: Increased atherosclerosis in LDL receptor-null mice lacking ACAT1 in macrophages. J Clin Invest 2001;107:163-171.

58. Accad M, Smith SJ, Newland DL, et al: Massive xanthomatosis and altered composition of atherosclerotic lesions in hyperlipidemic mice lacking acyl CoA:cholesterol acyltransferase 1. J Clin Invest 2000;105:711-719.

59. Gordon D, Reidy MA, Benditt EP, et al: Cell proliferation in human coronary arteries. Proc Natl Acad Sci USA 1990;87:4600-4604.

60. Davies MJ: Stability and instability: The two faces of coronary atherosclerosis: The Paul Dudley White Lecture, 1995. Circulation 1996;94:2013-2020.

61. Libby P: Current concepts of the pathogenesis of the acute coronary syndromes. Circulation 2001;104:365-372.

62. Virmani R, Burke AP, Farb A, et al: Pathology of the unstable plaque. Prog Cardiovasc Dis 2002;44:349-356.

63. Rajavashisth TB, Liao JK, Galis ZS, et al: Inflammatory cytokines and oxidized low density lipoproteins increase endothelial cell expression of membrane type 1-matrix metalloproteinase. J Biol Chem 1999;274:11924-11929.

64. Taubman MB, Fallon JT, Schecter AD, et al: Tissue factor in the pathogenesis of atherosclerosis. Thromb Haemost 1997;78:200-204.

65. Bellosta S, Mahley RW, Sanan DA, et al: Macrophage-specific expression of human apolipoprotein E reduces atherosclerosis in hypercholesterolemic apolipoprotein E-null mice. J Clin Invest 1995;96:2170-2179.

66. Chawla A, Boisvert WA, Lee CH, et al: A PPAR gamma-LXR-ABCA1 pathway in macrophages is involved in cholesterol efflux and atherogenesis. Mol Cell 2001;7:161-171.

67. Geng Y-J, Libby P: Evidence for apoptosis in advanced human atheroma: Co-localization with interleukin-1 β-converting enzyme. Am J Pathol 1995;147:251-266.

68. Geng YJ, Libby P: Progression of atheroma: A struggle between death and procreation. Arterioscler Thromb Vasc Biol 2002;22:1370-1380.

69. Jonasson L, Holm J, Skalli O, et al: Regional accumulations of T cells, macrophages, and smooth muscle cells in the human atherosclerotic plaque. Arteriosclerosis 1986;6:131-138.

70. Tsukada T, Rosenfeld M, Ross R, et al: Immunocytochemical analysis of cellular components in lesions of atherosclerosis in the Watanabe and fat-fed rabbit using monoclonal antibodies. Arteriosclerosis 1986;6:601-613.

71. Hansson GK: Immune mechanisms in atherosclerosis. Arterioscler Thromb Vasc Biol 2001;21:1876-1890.

72. Mach F, Sauty A, Iarossi AS, et al: Differential expression of three T lymphocyte-activating CXC chemokines by human atheroma-associated cells. J Clin Invest 1999;104:1041-1050.

73. Zhou X, Paulsson G, Stemme S, et al: Hypercholesterolemia is associated with a T helper (Th) 1/Th2 switch of the autoimmune response in atherosclerotic apo E-knockout mice. J Clin Invest 1998;101:1717-1725.

74. Hansson GK: Cell-mediated immunity in atherosclerosis. Curr Opin Lipidol 1997;8:301-311.

75. Stemme S, Holm J, Hansson GK: T lymphocytes in human atherosclerotic plaques are memory cells expressing CD45RO and the integrin VLA-1. Arterioscler Thromb 1992;12:206-211.

76. Hansson GK, Holm J, Jonasson L: Detection of activated T lymphocytes in the human atherosclerotic plaque. Am J Pathol 1989;135:169-175.

77. Stemme S, Rymo L, Hansson GK: Polyclonal origin of T lymphocytes in human atherosclerotic plaques. Lab Invest 1991;65:654-660.

78. Swanson S, Rosenzweig A, Seidman J, et al: Diversity of T-cell antigen receptor V beta gene utilization in advanced human atheroma. Arteriosclerosis 1994;14:1210-1214.

79. Zhou X, Stemme S, Hansson GK: Evidence for a local immune response in atherosclerosis: CD4+ T cells infiltrate lesions of apolipoprotein-E-deficient mice. Am J Pathol 1996;149:359-366.

80. Binder CJ, Chang MK, Shaw PX, et al: Innate and acquired immunity in atherogenesis. Nat Med 2002;8:1218-1226.

81. Palinski W, Tangirala RK, Miller E, et al: Increased autoantibody titers against epitopes of oxidized LDL in LDL receptor-deficient mice with increased atherosclerosis. Arterioscler Thromb Vasc Biol 1995;15:1569-1576.

82. Palinski W, Horkko S, Miller E, et al: Cloning of monoclonal autoantibodies to epitopes of oxidized lipoproteins from apolipoprotein E-deficient mice: Demonstration of epitopes of oxidized low density lipoprotein in human plasma. J Clin Invest 1996;98:800-814.

83. Kol A, Lichtman AH, Finberg RW, et al: Heat shock protein (HSP) 60 activates the innate immune response: CD14 is an essential receptor for HSP60 activation of mononuclear cells. J Immunol 2000;164:13-17.

84. Ohashi K, Burkart V, Flohe S, et al: Cutting Edge: Heat shock protein 60 is a putative endogenous ligand of the toll-like receptor-4 complex. J Immunol 2000;164:558-561.

85. Xu Q, Dietrich H, Steiner HJ, et al: Induction of arteriosclerosis in normocholesterolemic rabbits by immunization with heat shock protein 65. Arterioscler Thromb 1992;12:789-799.

86. Mayr M, Metzler B, Kiechl S, et al: Endothelial cytotoxicity mediated by serum antibodies to heat shock proteins of Escherichia coli and Chlamydia pneumoniae: Immune reactions to heat shock proteins as a possible link between infection and atherosclerosis. Circulation 1999;99:1560-1566.

87. Xu Q, Willeit J, Marosi M, et al: Association of serum antibodies to heat-shock protein 65 with carotid atherosclerosis. Lancet 1993;341:255-259.

88. Xu Q, Kleindienst R, Schett G, et al: Regression of arteriosclerotic lesions induced by immunization with heat shock protein 65-containing material in normocholesterolemic, but not hypercholesterolemic, rabbits. Atherosclerosis 1996;123:145-155.

89. Leung DYM, Geha RS, Newburger JW, et al: Two monokines, interleukin 1 and tumor necrosis factor, render cultured vascular endothelial cells susceptible to lysis by antibodies circulating during Kawasaki syndrome. J Exp Med 1986;164:1958-1972.

90. Leung DY, Collins T, Lapierre LA, et al: Immunoglobulin M antibodies present in the acute phase of Kawasaki syndrome lyse cultured vascular endothelial cells stimulated by gamma interferon. J Clin Invest 1986;77:1428-1435.

91. Hajjar DP: Warner-Lambert/Parke-Davis Award Lecture: Viral pathogenesis of atherosclerosis: Impact of molecular mimicry and viral genes. Am J Pathol 1991;139:1195-1211.

92. Epstein SE, Zhou YF, Zhu J: Potential role of cytomegalovirus in the pathogenesis of restenosis and atherosclerosis. Am Heart J 1999;138:S476-478.

93. O'Connor S, Taylor C, Campbell LA, et al: Potential infectious etiologies of atherosclerosis: A multifactorial perspective. Emerg Infect Dis 2001;7:780-788.

94. Zhu J, Nieto FJ, Horne BD, et al: Prospective study of pathogen burden and risk of myocardial infarction or death. Circulation 2001;103:45-51.

95. Hsich E, Zhou YF, Paigen B, et al: Cytomegalovirus infection increases development of atherosclerosis in apolipoprotein-E knockout mice. Atherosclerosis 2001;156:23-28.

96. Streblow DN, Soderberg-Naucler C, Vieira J, et al: The human cytomegalovirus chemokine receptor US28 mediates vascular smooth muscle cell migration. Cell 1999;99:511-520.

97. Benditt EP, Barrett T, McDougall JK: Viruses in the etiology of atherosclerosis. Proc Natl Acad Sci USA 1983;80:6386-6389.

98. Speir E, Modali R, Huang ES, et al: Potential role of human cytomegalovirus and p53 interaction in coronary restenosis. Science 1994;265:391-394.

99. Zhou YF, Leon MB, Waclawiw MA, et al: Association between prior cytomegalovirus infection and the risk of restenosis after coronary atherectomy. N Engl J Med 1996;335:624-630.

100. Grattan MT, Moreno-Cabral CE, Starnes VA, et al: Cytomegalovirus infection is associated with cardiac allograft rejection and atherosclerosis. JAMA 1989;261:3561-3566.

101. Koskinen PK, Nieminen MS, Krogerus LA, et al: Cytomegalovirus infection accelerates cardiac allograft vasculopathy: Correlation between angiographic and endomyocardial biopsy findings in heart transplant patients. Transpl Int 1993;6:341-347.

102. Danesh J: Coronary heart disease, Helicobacter pylori, dental disease, Chlamydia pneumoniae, and cytomegalovirus: Meta-analyses of prospective studies. Am Heart J 1999;138:S434-437.

103. Danesh J, Whincup P, Walker M, et al: Low grade inflammation and coronary heart disease: Prospective study and updated meta-analyses. BMJ 2000;321:199-204.

104. Danesh J, Whincup P, Lewington S, et al: Chlamydia pneumoniae IgA titres and coronary heart disease: prospective study and meta-analysis. Eur Heart J 2002;23:371-375.

105. Libby P, Salomon RN, Payne DD, et al: Functions of vascular wall cells related to the development of transplantation-associated coronary arteriosclerosis. Transplant Proc 1989; 21:3677-3684.

106. Salomon RN, Hughes CCW, Schoen FJ, et al: Human coronary transplantation-associated arteriosclerosis: Evidence for a chronic immune reaction to activated graft endothelial cells. Am J Pathol 1991;138:79-98.

107. Libby P, Pober JS: Chronic rejection. Immunity 2001;14:387-397.

108. Nagano H, Mitchell RN, Taylor MK, et al. Interferon-gamma deficiency prevents coronary arteriosclerosis but not myocardial rejection in transplanted mouse hearts. J Clin Invest 1997; 100:55-57.

109. Furukawa Y, Becker G, Stinn JL, et al: Interleukin-10 (IL-10) augments allograft arterial disease: Paradoxical effects of IL-10 in vivo. Am J Pathol 1999;155:1929-1939.

110. Nagano H, Tilney NL, Stinn JL, et al: Deficiencies of IL-4 or TNF-alpha receptor-1 do not diminish graft arteriosclerosis in cardiac allografts. Transplant Proc 1999;31:152.

111. Shimizu K, Schonbeck U, Mach F, et al: Host CD40 ligand deficiency induces long-term allograft survival and donor-specific tolerance in mouse cardiac transplantation but does not prevent graft arteriosclerosis. J Immunol 2000;165:3506-3518.

112. Bobryshev YV, Lord RS: Ultrastructural recognition of cells with dendritic cell morphology in human aortic intima: Contacting interactions of vascular dendritic cells in athero-resistant and athero-prone areas of the normal aorta. Arch Histol Cytol 1995;58:307-322.

113. Bobryshev YV, Lord RS: S-100 positive cells in human arterial intima and in atherosclerotic lesions. Cardiovasc Res 1995;29: 689-696.

114. Jonasson L, Holm J, Skalli O, et al: Expression of class II transplantation antigen on vascular smooth muscle cells in human atherosclerosis. J Clin Invest 1985;76:125-131.

115. Melian A, Geng YJ, Sukhova GK, et al: CD1 expression in human atherosclerosis: A potential mechanism for T cell activation by foam cells. Am J Pathol 1999;155:775-786.

116. Pober JS, Collins T, Gimbrone MAJ, et al: Lymphocytes recognize human vascular endothelial and dermal fibroblast Ia antigens induced by recombinant immune interferon. Nature 1983;305: 725-730.

117. Pober JS, Collins T, Gimbrone MA Jr, et al: Inducible expression of class II major histocompatibility complex antigens and the immunogenicity of vascular endothelium. Transplantation 1986; 41:141-146.

118. Murray AG, Libby P, Pober JS: Human vascular smooth muscle cells poorly co-stimulate and actively inhibit allogeneic CD4+ T cell proliferation in vitro. J Immunol 1995;154:151-161.

119. Ludewig B, Freigang S, Jaggi M, et al: Linking immune-mediated arterial inflammation and cholesterol-induced atherosclerosis in a transgenic mouse model. Proc Natl Acad Sci USA 2000; 97:12752-12757.

120. Pober JS, Gimbrone MAJ, Lapierre LA, et al: Overlapping patterns of activation of human endothelial cells by interleukin 1, tumor necrosis factor, and immune interferon. J Immunol 1986; 137:1893-1896.

121. Amento EP, Ehsani N, Palmer H, et al: Cytokines and growth factors positively and negatively regulate interstitial collagen gene expression in human vascular smooth muscle cells. Arterioscler Thromb Vasc Biol 1991;11:1223-1230.

122. Hansson GK, Hellstrand M, Rymo L, et al: Interferon-gamma inhibits both proliferation and expression of differentiation-specific alpha-smooth muscle actin in arterial smooth muscle cells. J Exp Med 1989;170:1595-1608.

123. Geng Y, Hansson GK, Holme E: Interferon-gamma and tumor necrosis factor synergize to induce nitric oxide production and inhibit mitochondrial respiration in vascular smooth muscle cells. Circ Res 1992;71:1268-1276.

124. Hansson GK, Geng YJ, Holm J, et al: Arterial smooth muscle cells express nitric oxide synthase in response to endothelial injury. J Exp Med 1994;180:733-738.

125. Shin W, Hong Y, Peng H, et al: Nitric oxide attenuates vascular smooth muscle cell activation by interferon-gamma: Role of constitutive NF-kappaB activity. J Biol Chem 1996;271:11317-11324.

126. Beckman JS, Chen J, Ischiropoulos H, et al: Oxidative chemistry of peroxynitrite. Methods Enzymol 1994;233:229-240.

127. Tanaka H, Sukhova G, Libby P: Interaction of the allogeneic state and hypercholesterolemia in arterial lesion formation in experimental cardiac allografts. Arterioscler Thromb 1994;14:734-745.

128. Klagsbrun M: Angiogenic factors: Regulators of blood supply-side biology. FGF, endothelial cell growth factors and angiogenesis: A keystone symposium, Keystone, Colorado, April 1-7, 1991. New Biol 1991;3:745-749.

129. Zhao XM, Hu Y, Miller GG, et al: Association of thrombospondin-1 and cardiac allograft vasculopathy in human cardiac allografts. Circulation 2001;103:525-531.

130. Hansson GK, Jonasson L, Holm J, et al: Gamma interferon regulates vascular smooth muscle proliferation and Ia expression in vivo and in vitro. Circ Res 1988;63:712-719.

131. Warner SJC, Friedman GB, Libby P: Immune interferon inhibits proliferation and induces 2'-5'-oligoadenylate synthetase gene expression in human vascular smooth muscle cells. J Clin Invest 1989;83:1174-1182.

132. Tellides G, Tereb DA, Kirkiles-Smith NC, et al: Interferon-gamma elicits arteriosclerosis in the absence of leukocytes. Nature 2000;403:207-211.

133. Geng Y-J, Wu Q, Muszynski M, et al: Apoptosis of vascular smooth muscle cells induced by in vitro stimulation with interferon-gamma, tumor necrosis factor-alpha, and interleukin-1-beta. Arterioscler Thromb Vasc Biol 1996;16:19-27.

134. Bennett M, Macdonald K, Chan SW, et al: Cell surface trafficking of Fas: A rapid mechanism of p53-mediated apoptosis. Science 1998;282:290-293.

135. Li JH, Kluger MS, Madge LA, et al: Interferon-gamma augments CD95(APO-1/Fas) and pro-caspase-8 expression and sensitizes human vascular endothelial cells to CD95-mediated apoptosis. Am J Pathol 2002;161:1485-1495.

136. Davies MJ, Richardson PD, Woolf N, et al: Risk of thrombosis in human atherosclerotic plaques: Role of extracellular lipid, macrophage, and smooth muscle cell content. Br Heart J 1993;69:377-381.

137. van der Wal AC, Becker AE, van der Loos CM, et al: Site of intimal rupture or erosion of thrombosed coronary atherosclerotic

plaques is characterized by an inflammatory process irrespective of the dominant plaque morphology. Circulation 1994;89: 36–44.

138. Warner SJC, Friedman GB, Libby P: Regulation of major histocompatibility gene expression in cultured human vascular smooth muscle cells. Arteriosclerosis 1989;9:279–288.

139. Libby P: The molecular bases of the acute coronary syndromes. Circulation 1995;91:2844–2850.

140. Dansky HM, Charlton SA, Harper MM, et al: T and B lymphocytes play a minor role in atherosclerotic plaque formation in the apolipoprotein E-deficient mouse. Proc Natl Acad Sci USA 1997;94:4642–4646.

141. Zhou X, Nicoletti A, Elhage R, et al: Transfer of CD4(+) T cells aggravates atherosclerosis in immunodeficient apolipoprotein E knockout mice. Circulation 2000;102:2919–2922.

142. Hansson GK, Libby P, Schonbeck U, et al: Innate and adaptive immunity in the pathogenesis of atherosclerosis. Circ Res 2002;91:281–291.

143. Palinski W, Miller E, Witztum JL: Immunization of low density lipoprotein (LDL) receptor-deficient rabbits with homologous malondialdehyde-modified LDL reduces atherogenesis. Proc Natl Acad Sci USA 1995;92:821–825.

144. Zhou X, Caligiuri G, Hamsten A, et al: LDL immunization induces T-cell-dependent antibody formation and protection against atherosclerosis. Arterioscler Thromb Vasc Biol 2001;21:108–114.

145. Kaartinen M, Penttila A, Kovanen PT: Mast cells of two types differing in neutral protease composition in the human aortic intima: Demonstration of tryptase- and tryptase/chymase-containing mast cells in normal intimas, fatty streaks, and the shoulder region of atheromas. Arterioscler Thromb 1994;14: 966–972.

146. Kovanen PT, Kaartinen M, Paavonen T: Infiltrates of activated mast cells at the site of coronary atheromatous erosion or rupture in myocardial infarction [see comments]. Circulation 1995; 92:1084–1088.

147. Haley KJ, Lilly CM, Yang JH, et al: Overexpression of eotaxin and the CCR3 receptor in human atherosclerosis: Using genomic technology to identify a potential novel pathway of vascular. Circulation 2000;102:2185–2189.

148. Wang Y, Shiota N, Leskinen MJ, et al: Mast cell chymase inhibits smooth muscle cell growth and collagen expression in vitro: Transforming growth factor-beta1-dependent and -independent effects. Arterioscler Thromb Vasc Biol 2001;21:1928–1933.

149. Leskinen M, Wang Y, Leszczynski D, et al: Mast cell chymase induces apoptosis of vascular smooth muscle cells. Arterioscler Thromb Vasc Biol 2001;21:516–522.

150. Kawasaki T: General review and problems in Kawasaki disease. Jpn Heart J 1995;36:1–12.

151. Libby P, Ridker PM, Maseri A: Inflammation and atherosclerosis. Circulation 2002;105:1135–1143.

152. Ridker PM: Role of inflammatory biomarkers in prediction of coronary heart disease. Lancet 2001;358:946–948.

153. Ridker PM, Rifai N, Rose L, et al: Comparison of C-reactive protein and low-density lipoprotein cholesterol levels in the prediction of first cardiovascular events. N Engl J Med 2002;347: 1557–1565.

154. Ridker PM, Rifai N, Pfeffer MA, et al: Long-term effects of pravastatin on plasma concentration of C-reactive protein: The Cholesterol and Recurrent Events (CARE) Investigators. Circulation 1999;100:230–235.

155. Ridker PM: Should statin therapy be considered for patients with elevated C-reactive protein? The need for a definitive clinical trial. Eur Heart J 2001;22:2135–2137.

## EDITOR'S CHOICE

Benagiano M, Azzurri A, Ciervo A, et al: T helper type 1 lymphocytes drive inflammation in human atherosclerotic lesions. Proc Natl Acad Sci USA 2003;100:6658–6663.
*T cells implicated in atherogenesis*

Boring L, Gosling J, Cleary M, Charo IF: Decreased lesion formation in CCR2-/-mice reveals a role for chemokines in the initiation of atherosclerosis. Nature 1998;394:894–897.
*First paper to document that the inhibition of chemokines could be a therapeutic target in atherosclerosis.*

Chawla A, Lee CH, Barak Y, et al: PPARdelta is a very low-density lipoprotein sensor in macrophages. Proc Natl Acad Sci USA 2003;100: 1268–1273.
*New pathway for the regulation of VLDL via the nuclear hormone receptor PPAR delta.*

Glass CK, Witztum JL: Atherosclerosis. the road ahead. Cell 2001;104:503–516.
*Thought leaders in the field provide a roadmap.*

Joseph SB, Castrillo A, Laffitte BA., et al: Reciprocal regulation of inflammation and lipid metabolism by liver X receptors. Nat Med 2003;9:213–219.
*LXR pathways are a therapeutic target but developing small molecules that can distinguish between liver and peripheral effects may be challenging.*

Lee CH, Chawla A, Urbiztondo N, et al: Transcriptional Repression of Atherogenic Inflammation: Modulation by PPAR{delta}. Science 2003.
*Lays out the molecular basis for PPAR delta pathways in atherogenesis.*

Li AC, Glass CK: The macrophage foam cell as a target for therapeutic intervention. Nat Med 2002;8:1235–1242.
*The macrophage is the focal point of new targets for atherogenesis.*

Libby P: Inflammation in atherosclerosis. Nature 2002;420:868–874.
*Pioneer in uncovering inflammatory pathways in atherogenesis makes the case.*

Ridker PM, Rifai N, Rose L, et al: Comparison of C-reactive protein and low-density lipoprotein cholesterol levels in the prediction of first cardiovascular events. N Engl J Med 2002;347:1557–1565.
*Seminal aper describes closse association between CRP and cardiac risk; question arises as to whether there are any new therapeutic implications, as well as whether the relationship is causal or casual.*

Spanbroek R, Grabner R, Lotzer K, et al: Expanding expression of the 5-lipoxygenase pathway within the arterial wall during human atherogenesis. Proc Natl Acad Sci USA 2003;100:1238–1243.
*Old pathway with new relevance in atherogenesis.*

# chapter 21

# Molecular Biology of Lipoproteins and Dyslipidemias

*Sotirios Tsimikas*
*Vincent Mooser*

Atherosclerotic cardiovascular disease is the major cause of morbidity and mortality in developed countries. The hallmark of early atherosclerotic lesions is the presence of macrophage-derived foam cells rich in oxidized lipids that are taken up by scavenger receptors in an unregulated manner.[1] A complex interplay between endothelial injury, continued lipid accumulation, oxidative modification of lipids and lipoproteins, inflammatory and immunologic mechanisms, smooth muscle cell migration, and foam cell necrosis and apoptosis results in formation of atheromas, the first recognized, clinically significant atherosclerotic lesion. Outward remodeling of the vessel wall accommodates the enlarging atherosclerotic lesion and preserves blood flow. Continued lipid accumulation, inward remodeling or shrinkage of the vessel, and disruption of the fibrous cap overlying a thrombogenic milieu results in obstruction of blood flow, tissue ischemia, and clinical manifestations of disease. The plasma lipoproteins provide the major source of lipid that accumulates in the vessel wall, and their role in transporting lipids between the small intestine, liver, and peripheral tissues is critically important in determining whether atherosclerotic lesions develop.

## NORMAL LIPOPROTEIN METABOLISM

There are three major pathways of lipoprotein metabolism in mammals: (1) exogenous fat metabolism including digestion, absorption, and packaging of dietary lipids for secretion into lymphatics and ultimately into the bloodstream; (2) endogenous fat metabolism including biosynthesis and secretion of lipids and apolipoproteins by the liver and small intestine; and (3) HDL metabolism mediating reverse cholesterol transport by transfer of cholesterol and lipids from peripheral cells back to the liver for disposal. Lipoproteins are composed of apolipoproteins containing a core of cholesterol, cholesterol esters, and triglycerides and an amphipathic phospholipid outer coat. They solubilize lipids via lipid-binding domains and provide lipids to various cells to enhance cell membrane permeability and fluidity, as precursors for steroid hormone synthesis and as a source of energy. Lipoproteins are taken up by receptors in the liver and other tissues and contain signal domains to control various aspects of cellular lipid metabolism. As lipoproteins circulate through the bloodstream, they are extensively remodeled by an interchange and removal of apolipoproteins and lipids.

## Exogenous Fat Metabolism

Dietary triglycerides are extensively hydrolyzed into free fatty acids by gastric and pancreatic lipases. Phospholipids are cleaved at the sn-2 position by phospholipase A2 releasing fatty acids. Cholesterol esters are cleaved by cholesterol esterase, which has broad specificity and also hydrolyzes triglycerides and phospholipids. Dietary cholesterol exists mostly as a free sterol with only 10% to 15% in the form of cholesterol esters. Emulsification of fats by bile acids results in fine lipid droplets that are taken up by intestinal enterocytes via brush border membranes. Recent data suggests that cholesterol absorption is an active process, possibly mediated by a yet-to-be-identified transporter.[2] The small intestine can discriminate among sterols with closely related structures and selectively absorbs cholesterol but not non-cholesterol sterols. In fact, patients with β-sitosterolemia, a disorder resulting from mutations in the adenosine triphosphate binding cassette (ABC) transporters ABCG5 and ABCG8, encoding proteins sterolin-1 and -2, absorb large quantities of plant sterols, particularly β-sitosterol, and develop xanthomatosis and accelerated atherosclerosis.[3-6] Sterolins are ABC half-transporters that may partner to generate a functional complex that extrudes non-cholesterol sterols from the enterocyte and promotes biliary excretion of sterols.[6] Additional studies suggest that the ABCA1 transporter also regulates absorption of dietary cholesterol via a retinoid X receptor (RXR) heterodimer mechanism.[7,8] This clearly suggests that specific molecular pathways regulate dietary cholesterol absorption and sterol excretion from the body, paving the way for novel preventive strategies and therapeutic targets.

After entering the enterocyte, lipids travel to the endoplasmic reticulum for resynthesis into triglycerides, cholesterol esters, and phospholipids. Cholesterol esters are formed by acyl coenzyme A:cholesterol acyltransferase (ACAT) enzymes that play a key regulatory role in intestinal cholesterol absorption and provide core lipid for packaging of chylomicrons and hepatic-derived lipoproteins. ACAT1 is ubiquitous but is notably expressed in macrophages, skin, brain, and adrenals. ACAT1 may be the predominant cholesterol ester enzyme in human liver, whereas ACAT2 is found primarily in the small intestine and liver.[9-12] ACAT enzymes appear to regulate cholesterol content of cell membranes by inducing storage of cholesterol esters as cytosolic droplets that protect cells from toxic free cholesterol. Selective ACAT1 knockouts in apolipoprotein E-deficient (apoE[-/-]) and LDL receptor–deficient (LDLR[-/-]) mice display lower plasma cholesterol levels and reduced cholesterol ester staining in macrophages. However, they demonstrate markedly increased brain and skin xanthomatosis with extensive cholesterol crystal deposition.[9,10,13] In addition, LDLR[-/-] mice reconstituted with ACAT1-deficient macrophages develop larger atherosclerotic lesions than control LDLR[-/-] mice suggesting that ACAT1 deficiency or inhibition may be proatherogenic by promoting cholesterol crystal deposition and its attendant cytotoxic properties in the arterial wall.[14] Lesion composition does seem to be affected with less staining for neutral lipid, but whether this will result in more "stable" lesions is unknown.

These intracellular lipids are then packaged into chylomicrons with the addition of apoB-48, apoA-I, and apoA-IV. During fasting, the small intestine secretes primarily VLDL, but in the fed state chylomicrons are preferentially secreted. An editing process introduces a stop-codon posttranscriptionally into the mRNA encoding apoB-100, producing an mRNA encoding apoB-48 that is about 48% of the full-length apoB-100.[15,16] As apoB is synthesized, it is cotranslationally given polar and neutral lipid by microsomal transfer protein (MTP), forming nascent (10 nm) apoB particles. MTP is primarily expressed in liver and intestine and plays a role in the folding and assembly of apoB and also functions as a chaperone by facilitating transfer of apoB across the endoplasmic reticulum.[17] Triglycerides are then added either as lipid droplets or by addition of lipid molecules to form chylomicrons (75 to 1200 nm). VLDL and chylomicrons containing the shortened apoB are assembled in the lumen of endoplasmic reticulum, transferred to the Golgi apparatus, and then secreted into lymph. The crucial role of MTP in lipoprotein assembly was recently delineated in the rare (approximately 100 cases have been documented, one third resulting from consanguineous marriages), autosomal recessive disorder abetalipoproteinemia in which there is almost a complete failure to make triglyceride-rich lipoproteins because of gene mutations of the large MTP subunit.[17] Patients with abetalipoproteinemia have normal apoB synthesis but a virtual absence of apoB in plasma and very low plasma cholesterol levels (total cholesterol ~20 to 50 mg/dL, triglycerides >10 mg/dL, and HDL-cholesterol decreased by 50%). As expected, these patients have normal digestion, absorption, and esterification of fatty acids back to triglycerides and phospholipids. MTP inhibitors significantly reduce plasma cholesterol and triglyceride levels in Watanabe heritable hyperlipidemic rabbits, implying a potential therapeutic role in patients with hyperlipidemia.[18]

After chylomicrons are secreted in lymph, they enter muscle and fat capillaries; lose apoA-I and apoA-IV; and acquire apolipoproteins CII, an activator of lipoprotein lipase, apoCIII, and apoE (Fig. 21-1). The triglycerides within chylomicrons are rapidly hydrolyzed by lipoprotein lipase, forming chylomicron remnants that are

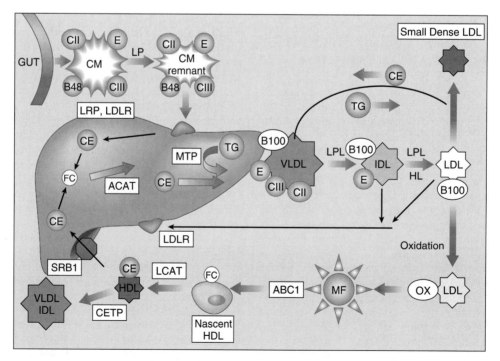

**FIGURE 21-1.** General overview of lipoprotein metabolism. CE, cholesteryl ester; FC, free cholesterol; HL, hepatic lipase; LPL, lipoprotein lipase; MΦ, macrophage; OxLDL, oxidized LDL; TG, triglycerides. (See color plate.)

removed by the LDL receptor, via apoE binding sites, and by the LDL receptor-related protein (LRP) receptor that acts in conjunction with proteoglycans. This is a necessary step for chylomicron remnant removal because apoB-48 does not contain an LDL receptor recognition domain. Because of this dual removal pathway, deficiency of either the LDL or LRP receptor does not result in accumulation of chylomicron remnants and explains why plasma chylomicrons are not elevated in familial hypercholesterolemia (FH). LRP is larger but structurally similar to the LDL receptor and has diverse biologic roles acting as a multifunctional scavenger receptor.[19,20] LRP is also expressed in neurons, which produce abundant apoE, raising the possibility that it mediates neuronal uptake of astrocyte-derived cholesterol and lipids and may have a role in Alzheimer's disease.[21] The importance of the physiologic role of LRP is suggested by the fact that LRP knockouts are lethal. In the rare apoE$_2$ deficiency or dysfunctional apoE$_2$ syndrome, increases in plasma chylomicrons are noted. Deficiency of apoCII or lipoprotein lipase results in increased plasma triglycerides in the form of chylomicrons, which confers an enhanced risk of pancreatitis.

## Endogenous Fat Metabolism

Lipoprotein transport systems are essential for survival and reproduction of all mammalian species. The major pathway for cellular cholesterol uptake is via the LDL receptor, which is regulated transcriptionally by cellular cholesterol levels through negative feedback inhibition. This complex process of controlling hepatic assembly and secretion of lipoproteins begins at the endoplasmic reticulum where the metabolic fate of de novo synthesized apoB is determined. ApoB-100 is a large (4536 amino acid, ~500,000 kd) highly lipophilic, secretory glycoprotein that transports two thirds of plasma cholesterol in humans. ApoB-100 contains lipid-binding domains through α-helices and β-sheets that interact directly with neutral lipid, which is added cotranslationally and is required for proper folding and stability. ApoB-100 is constitutively expressed in the liver and production is regulated posttranscriptionally and not at the gene transcription level. Newly synthesized apoB can undergo a concerted cotranslational translocation step coupled to lipoprotein particle assembly and secretion, or it can be arrested leading to ubiquitin conjugation and proteasomal degradation.[22,23] The rate-limiting step of apoB synthesis is movement out of the endoplasmic reticulum, and only a fraction of de novo synthesized apoB-100 is secreted while the rest is degraded within the hepatocyte. Therefore, plasma levels depend entirely on degradation.

The intrahepatic assembly and production of VLDL represents a complex interplay between protein and lipid biosynthesis, trafficking, and maturation and likely requires a specialized pattern of gene expression with multiple control points. The assembly of apoB-100 into triglyceride-rich VLDL (30 to 80 nm) is initiated by transfer of triglycerides by MTP during translation and then by fusion of nascent apoB with lipid droplets to form mature VLDL.[24] In the absence of apoB-100, there is translocation arrest. Phospholipases A and D2 mediate membrane transfer and addition of phospholipids to VLDL. ACAT enzymes provide the cholesterol esters for VLDL and chylomicrons. Assembly and secretion of apoB-100 and VLDL are coordinately regulated in response to nutritional state and is dependent on cholesterol levels and the bile synthetic pathway controlled by 7-α-hydroxylase (CYP7α), which regulates lipogenic enzymes through changes in cellular content of mature sterol regulatory-element binding proteins (SREBPs).

Triglyceride-rich VLDL is packaged with apoCII, apoCIII, and apoE and secreted into the bloodstream, where it is metabolized by lipoprotein lipase and hepatic lipase, causing release of fatty acids to be used for energy utilization or stored in adipose tissue. The resulting VLDL remnants are either taken up by liver LDL and LRP receptors or are progressively enriched in cholesterol esters from HDL lipid transfer to evolve into IDL and ultimately LDL, a cholesterol ester-rich particle containing only apoB-100 (Fig. 21-1). LDL has a long circulating half-life and is ultimately taken up by LDL receptors in the liver and peripheral tissues. In addition, LDL, VLDL, and chylomicron remnants may be oxidatively modified and removed by scavenger SRA or CD36 receptors on macrophages, leading to foam cell formation and development of atherosclerotic plaques. Targeted gene deletion of either the SRA or CD36 genes results in significant reduction in lesion development.[25,26]

Small, dense LDL particles are generated in patients with the metabolic syndrome that is characterized by insulin resistance, hypertension, obesity, low plasma HDL cholesterol, and elevated triglyceride levels. The triglycerides on VLDL are exchanged for cholesterol esters of LDL producing triglyceride-rich LDL, which then undergoes lipolysis by hepatic lipase to produce small, dense LDL particles (Fig. 21-1). Small, dense LDL is more amenable to oxidative modification and has been proposed as a more atherogenic particle than buoyant LDL.[27] Similar events occur on HDL, resulting in a small, dense HDL that is more easily catabolized by the kidney, resulting in lower HDL plasma levels.[28] In the FATS trial, treatment with colestipol/lovastatin and colestipol/niacin significantly decreased hepatic lipase activity with a concomitant conversion of small, dense LDL to buoyant LDL, which was the strongest predictor of angiographic regression.[29]

## HDL Metabolism

Excess cholesterol in peripheral tissues, either synthesized de novo (~9 mg/kg body weight per day)[30] or delivered by lipoproteins must be moved back to the liver through the process of reverse cholesterol transport. The balance between external and internal cellular cholesterol is maintained through the efflux of free cholesterol to pre-β-HDL at caveolae, small cholesterol-rich invaginations in the cell membrane.[31] HDL is secreted by the liver or small intestine as a lipid-poor, nascent particle containing apoAI and small amounts of phospholipids and triglycerides. Similar HDL particles may be formed by lipolysis of VLDL or chylomicron remnants by lipoprotein lipase or by the interconversion of $HDL_2$ to $HDL_3$ by cholesterol ester transfer protein (CETP), phospholipid transfer protein (PLTP), or hepatic lipase (Fig. 21-2). Unesterified cholesterol and phospholipids are transported out of cells via the ABCA1 transporter and loaded to nascent HDL. In cholesterol-loaded cells, the ABCA1 transporter is upregulated by oxysterols acting as ligands for nuclear receptors that activate the *ABCA1* gene. The ABCA1 transporter resides at the plasma membrane and may be the rate-limiting step for cellular cholesterol efflux.[32] However, studies have recently shown that plasma HDL levels and the HDL contribution to biliary cholesterol are minimally affected by macrophage ABCA1, suggesting that the cholesterol content of HDL, and thus reverse cholesterol transport, is also mediated by other cell types such as hepatocytes.[33-35] ABCA1 overexpression in both liver and macrophages leads to increased HDL and apoB levels and increased biliary cholesterol excretion.[36] However, the contribution of ABCA1 to prevention or reduction of atherosclerosis will not be known until animal atherosclerosis studies are reported. Mutations in the ABCA1 transporter result in Tangier disease, the hallmark of which is lack of lipid-rich α-HDL from plasma, the presence of cholesterol esters almost exclusively in macrophages, and an apparent increased risk of atherosclerosis.[32]

Lecithin-cholesterol acyl transferase (LCAT) esterifies free cholesterol present on nascent HDL with unsaturated fatty acids from the sn-2 position of lecithin (phospholipids) to create small, spherical $HDL_3$ particles.

LCAT also upregulates LDL receptors, lowers LDL, and raises HDL with ApoA1 acting as a major activator. PLTP-mediated acceptance of surface remnants (phospholipids, cholesterol) of triglyceride-rich lipoproteins to $HDL_3$ results in mature, lipid-rich, spherical $HDL_2$ particles. Absence of LCAT in humans leads to fish-eye disease, manifested by increased plasma triglycerides, low HDL (because of increased catabolism of nascent HDL), cloudy corneas, hemolytic anemia, and renal disease. LCAT knockout mice and LCAT deficient patients, however, do not have increased atherosclerosis, suggesting that reverse cholesterol transport may still proceed without spherical HDL.[37] PLTP deficiency results in a 60% to 70% reduction in HDL levels reflecting reduced transfer of phospholipids from triglyceride-rich lipoproteins.[38] PLTP overexpression results in increased pre-β-HDL activity and reduced cellular cholesterol accumulation.[39]

HDL transports cholesterol to the liver and steroidogenic tissues by three distinct pathways: (1) indirectly by transfer of cholesterol esters to VLDL and IDL, mediated by CETP, hepatic lipase, and endothelial lipase, which are then taken up by the LDL and LRP receptors; (2) by selective uptake via hepatic SR-B1 scavenger receptors; and (3) by apoE-rich HDL uptake via apoE and apoA-I binding sites.

In the indirect pathway, CETP transfers cholesterol esters from $HDL_2$ to triglyceride-rich VLDL, IDL, and LDL in exchange for triglycerides, resulting in smaller $HDL_3$ particles. In human CETP deficiency, reverse cholesterol transport is thought to be inhibited, and the HDL-cholesterol level is markedly elevated. However, clinical

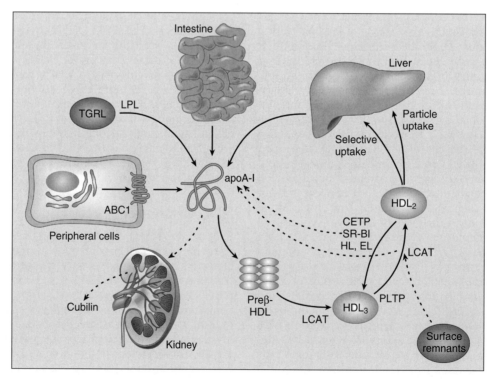

**FIGURE 21-2.** HDL lipoprotein metabolism. (See color plate.) *(Reproduced with permission from von Eckardstein A, Nofer JR, Assmann G: High density lipoproteins and artereosclerosis: Role of cholesterol efflux and reverse cholesterol transport. Arterioscler Thromb Vasc Biol 2001;21:13–27.)*

manifestation of CHD risk seems to depend on concomitant dyslipidemias, particularly hypertriglyceridemia.[40,41] Hepatic lipase hydrolyzes triglycerides and phospholipids in all lipoprotein classes and in concert with CETP regenerates phospholipid-rich, apoE-rich smaller HDL$_3$ particles. In addition, hepatic lipase acts as a cofactor for uptake of HDL lipids mediated by the SR-B1 receptor.[42,43] Hepatic lipase deficient mice have large, apoE-rich HDL, whereas hepatic lipase overexpressing mice have low HDL. In patients, hepatic lipase levels are inversely correlated with HDL$_2$ levels, but low levels of hepatic lipase are actually associated with the presence of atherosclerosis, implying inhibition of reverse cholesterol transport.[29,44]

The second pathway is mediated by SR-B1 receptors that are multiligand HDL receptors expressed in liver and steroidogenic tissues. SR-B1 receptors have broad specificity for a diverse group of ligands, including modified lipoproteins, and may also participate in innate immunity.[45] SR-B1 is member of the CD36 family, is found mainly in caveolae, and facilitates selective cellular uptake of cholesterol esters but not lipoproteins. After binding HDL, SR-B1 facilitates transfer of HDL lipid to the cell membrane, unlike the LDL receptor that mediates endocytosis of the intact LDL particle and hydrolysis by lysozymes. The lipid-poor HDL is then released back to the extracellular space and circulation. The expression of SR-B1 is coordinated with cholesterol homeostasis. SR-B1 knockout mice show elevated plasma cholesterol, which circulates as large, apoE-rich, HDL particles; a reduction in biliary cholesterol secretion but not bile acid or phospholipid content; and accelerated atherosclerosis. SR-B1 overexpression results in low HDL; increased biliary cholesterol; and paradoxically a reduction in atherosclerosis, implying enhanced reverse cholesterol transport.[46-49]

The third pathway involves catabolism of apolipoprotein A via endocytosis by the liver and kidney. ApoE-containing HDL particles can be internalized by LDL and LRP receptors. In the liver, cholesterol esters from these three pathways is hydrolyzed to free cholesterol and excreted as bile acids or free cholesterol in the gut.

## Regulatory Elements

SREBPs are three related membrane-bound transcription factors that mediate cellular cholesterol homeostasis.[50] SREBPs exist as precursors and have both a transcription factor DNA binding domain and a regulatory domain (Fig. 21-3). Cellular cholesterol is present mainly in cell membranes. When cholesterol or sterols are required by the cell, SREBPs undergo regulated transfer from the endoplasmic reticulum to the Golgi apparatus, escorted by the sterol sensor SREBP cleavage-activating protein SCAP.[51-53] The SREBP precursor is cleaved at two locations by site-1 and site-2 proteases to release the soluble transcription factor domain that translocates to the nucleus to stimulate the transcription of target genes for sterol synthesis, upregulation of LDL receptors, and fatty acid biosynthesis.[54,55] On the other hand, when cellular cholesterol accumulates, the SCAP/SREBP complex is retained in the endoplasmic reticulum because of the

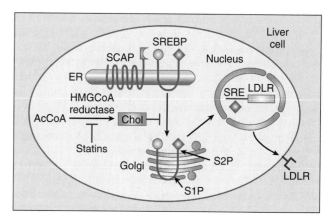

**FIGURE 21-3.** Regulation of cellular cholesterol metabolism by SREBPs. (See color plate.) *(Reproduced with permission from Rader DJ: A new feature on the cholesterol-lowering landscape. Nat Med 2001;7:1282-1284.)*

interaction between the sterol-sensing domain of SCAP and an unidentified protein present in the endoplasmic reticulum.[53,56] Ligands binding to the sterol-sensing domain of SCAP have been recently shown to upregulate the expression of LDL receptors, even in sterol-loaded cells, and to decrease plasma cholesterol and triglycerides in a hamster model.[57,58]

Nuclear receptors that regulate lipid metabolism are members of a large transcription factor superfamily characterized by both DNA- and ligand-binding domains that regulate genes that coordinate several metabolic pathways.[7] Nuclear receptors recognize and bind to DNA at specific response elements that activate or repress the expression of a target gene. Liver X receptors (LXR), bile acid receptors (FXR), and peroxisome proliferator activated receptors (PPARs) PPARγ and PPARα, when stimulated by their respective ligands, heterodimerize with the permissive retinoid X receptor (RXR), bind to DNA, and induce gene activation that influences cholesterol, bile acid, glucose, and triglyceride homeostasis, respectively. In contrast to classical endocrine steroid receptors, these nuclear receptors do respond to dietary lipids and glucose, and, therefore, their function is not controlled by simple feedback inhibition. Nuclear receptors function as lipid sensors by activating a feedforward cascade of lipid gene transcription such as cytochrome P450 that inactivates lipids,[59] intracellular lipid-binding proteins that buffer and transport hydrophobic ligands within cells,[60] and ABC1 transporters that mediate cellular cholesterol and lipid efflux to maintain lipid homeostasis.[8,61]

A unique class of oxysterols [22(R)-hydroxycholesterol, 24(S)-hydroxycholesterol, 24(S)-hydroxycholesterol, 27-hydroxycholesterol] regulate cellular cholesterol homeostasis by acting as ligands for nuclear receptors. Elevated oxysterol concentrations upregulate several genes involved in the catabolism and elimination of cholesterol, primarily through LXR receptor whose target genes include several ABC transporters mediating cellular cholesterol and phospholipid efflux.[62] Hepatic triglyceride and VLDL production is linked to the cholesterol and bile acid biosynthetic pathway via oxysterols. High consumption of cholesterol results in increased production of bile acids. When the enterohepatic concentration of bile acids is elevated, conversion of cholesterol to bile acids is reduced. The regulation of these processes is through FXR, which controls CYP7α1 the rate-limiting enzyme of neutral bile acid synthesis.[8] Activation of RXR receptors by synthetic ligands has been shown to inhibit cholesterol absorption and bile acid synthesis by regulating the expression of ABCA1 and CYP7α1[63] and to reduce development of atherosclerotic lesions in apoE[-/-] mice by upregulating ABCA1 expression and cholesterol efflux from macrophages.[64]

PPARα and PPARγ are expressed in all major cell types and are found in atherosclerotic tissue and regulate lipid metabolism, glucose homeostasis, and adipose cell differentiation.[65] PPARs display distinctive expression patterns, suggesting important functional differences. PPARα enhances fatty acid oxidation, and PPARγ promotes adipogenesis and fatty acid storage. PPARα ligands are fatty acids, eicosanoids, and fibrates. They stimulate lipoprotein lipase, repress apoCIII, regulate apoAI-II levels, and inhibit the expression of inflammatory genes. PPARγ ligands are arachidonic acid metabolites, oxidized LDL, and oxidized lipids and glitazones. PPARγ ligands exhibit both proatherogenic and antiatherogenic properties *in vitro*. PPARγ promotes cholesterol and phospholipid efflux from cells into HDL via the ABCA1 transporter and inhibits cell proliferation and migration, inflammatory processes, and cytokine release. However, it also upregulates CD36 and inhibits nitric oxide synthetase, which may be proatherogenic. In animal models, both PPARα and PPARγ agonists have been shown to reduce the progression of atherosclerosis.[66-68]

## DISORDERS OF LIPOPROTEIN METABOLISM

Disorders of lipoprotein metabolism result from abnormal synthesis, assembly, secretion, transport, processing, or catabolism of plasma lipoprotein particles. Twin studies indicate that plasma lipoprotein levels are under close genetic control.[69] Indeed, in most studies, more than 50% of the total variance in total-, LDL-, and HDL-cholesterol, triglycerides and Lp(a) could be explained by genetic factors[70] (Table 21-1). Moreover, more than half of patients with angiographically confirmed CAD

■ ■ ■

**TABLE 21-1**   HERITABILITY OF PLASMA LIIPID LEVELS IN TWIN STUDIES

|  | Heritability | Range |
|---|---|---|
| Total cholesterol | 0.64 | 0.28–0.80 |
| LDL-cholesterol | 0.85 | 0.22–1.00 |
| HDL-cholesterol | 0.71 | 0.24–0.82 |
| Triglycerides | 0.60 | 0–0.75 |
| Lp(a) | 0.94 | 0.67–0.98 |
| ApoA1 | 0.56 | 0.36–0.78 |
| ApoB | 0.73 | 0.48–0.91 |

These are the results from twin studies that have examined the heritability of total-, LDL-, and HDL-cholesterol and triglycerides (*n* = 13); apoA1 and apoB (*n* = 9); or Lp(a) (*n* = 6) as reviewed in (Snieder H, van Doornan LJP, Boomsma DI: Dissecting the genetic architechture of lipids, lipoproteins, and apolipoproteins: Lessons from twin studies. Arterioscler Thromb Vasc Biol 1999;19:2826–2834). The way heritability was estimated may have varied between studies, and median values are presented here.

before age 60 years have a familial lipoprotein disorder.[71] This association is most striking among younger patients and declines with increasing age at first MI. Finally, a high concordance for lipid abnormalities has been observed in sib-pairs affected with premature CAD.[72] Together, these observations suggest the presence of genetic factors that accelerate age-associated cardiovascular changes seen in the general population. Severe hyperlipidemia (total cholesterol >300 mg/dL or triglycerides >500 mg/dL) usually indicates a genetic disorder, and xanthomas always signal an underlying genetic defect. Such findings warrant examination of the patient's first-degree relatives.

Although genetic determinants make an important contribution to lipoprotein disorders, environmental factors such as diet, drugs, physical activity, and cigarette smoking or concomitant diseases may have a major impact on lipoprotein metabolism and in the determination of plasma lipoprotein levels, even in carriers of monogenic forms of dyslipidemia (Table 21-2). Accordingly, causes of secondary hyperlipidemia must be sought for in any hyperlipidemic patients. These persons may have a particular genetic susceptibility to the lipid-modifying effects of the environment. This is well-illustrated, for instance, by the close association between HIV-protease inhibitor-induced hypertriglyceridemia or

■ ■ ■

**TABLE 21-2**   COMMON CAUSES OF SECONDARY HYPERLIPIDEMIA

| Excess in LDL-Cholesterol | Excess in Triglycerides | Low HDL-Cholesterol |
|---|---|---|
| Hypothyroidism | Excessive alcohol consumption | Physical inactivity |
| Nephrotic syndrome | Obesity | Smoking |
| Chronic liver disease | Pregnancy | Diabetes mellitus |
| Cholestasis | Diabetes mellitus | Obesity |
| Dysglobulinemia | Hypothyroidism | Hypertriglyceridemia |
| Anorexia nervosa | Chronic renal failure | Anabolic steroids |
| | β-Blockers | |
| | Diuretics | |
| | Exogenous estrogens | |
| | Isotretinoin | |
| | Cushing's syndrome | |
| | Oral contraceptives | |

isotretinoin-associated hypertriglyceridemia and the apoE E2 and E4 alleles[73] or by the increased risk that carriers of such alleles have to develop hyperlipidemia when getting older.[74]

Six types of lipoprotein abnormalities are observed in association with atherosclerosis and CAD: elevated LDL-cholesterol levels, increased triglycerides and VLDL levels, reduced HDL-cholesterol levels, elevated levels of chylomicron remnants and IDL, elevated levels of Lp(a), and sitosterolemia. These disorders may result from single-gene defects (Table 21-3)[75,76] or may have a more complex origin. The severity and frequency of these disorders vary widely in the general population. As a rule of thumb, mild hyperlipidemia results from common (polygenic) hypercholesterolemia, familial combined hyperlipidemia, or hypertriglyceridemia associated with obesity and alcohol consumption, whereas severe hyperlipoproteinemia often results from FH or remnant hyperlipidemia. Genetic disorders of lipoprotein metabolism that are not associated with atherosclerosis (e.g., hypobetalipoproteinemia or excess HDL-cholesterol) are discussed briefly in this chapter.

## Elevated LDL-Cholesterol

Cholesterol levels higher than 240 mg/dL are associated with a threefold increased risk of death from ischemic heart disease in men relative to cholesterol levels less than 200 mg/dL, and there is a continuous risk gradient as cholesterol rises.[77-79] Elevated total cholesterol primarily reflects elevated LDL-cholesterol, which constitutes 70% of plasma cholesterol. Disorders characterized by elevation of cholesterol alone are classified as Fredrickson type IIa hyperlipoproteinemia. Moderate hypercholesterolemia is far more common than severe hypercholesterolemia and usually results from interactions between environment and multiple genes. In contrast,

severe hypercholesterolemia is often monogenic but may result from defects in separate genes, indicating genetic heterogeneity (Fig. 21-4). Given their low prevalence in the general population, these monogenic forms of severe hypercholesterolemia only account for approximately 5% of the general variance in plasma LDL-cholesterol levels[76]; nevertheless, they are discussed later in some detail, given the high risk for CAD in affected family members and the relevance of these disorders for understanding lipoprotein metabolism.

### Autosomal Dominant Familial Hypercholesterolemia

Autosomal dominant FH is the archetypal monogenic disorder of LDL excess and results from one of more than 600 reported mutations within the LDL receptor (LDLR) gene that reduce LDLR number and/or activities (Fig. 21-5).[80,81] In most populations, FH heterozygotes and homozygotes have frequencies of approximately 1:500 and approximately 1:1.000.000, respectively, with higher frequencies in some ethnic groups (such as French Canadians, Lebanese Christians, Jews of Lithuanian origin, Finns, and South African Afrikaners) because of founder effects. Heterozygous FH is present in approximately 5% of patients with MI.[82]

FH homozygotes typically have sixfold elevations in LDL-cholesterol, with total cholesterol levels of 650 to 1000 mg/dL; they can be identified at birth by markedly elevated cholesterol in umbilical cord blood. CAD is often clinically apparent before age 10 years, with MI occurring as early as 18 months of age; most homozygotes suffer fatal MI by age 30 years. A unique type of planar cutaneous xanthoma is present at birth or develops in childhood, often between the thumb and index finger, and many patients are first identified by dermatologists. However, diagnosis may be delayed until the appearance of angina pectoris or an episode of syncope

■ ■ ■

**TABLE 21-3**    SELECTED MONOGENIC DISORDERS AFFECTING PLASMA LIPOPROTEINS

| No | Lipoprotein Profile | Gene Product | Disease | Frequency | Risk of CAD |
|---|---|---|---|---|---|
| 1 | Excess in LDL-cholesterol | LDL-receptor | AD familial hypercholesterolemia | 1/500 (heterozygote) | Increased |
| 2 | | ApoB | Familial defective apoB | ~1/500 | Increased |
| 3 | | ARH | AR familial hypercholesterolemia | Rare | Increased |
| 4 | Low LDL-cholesterol | ApoB | Hypobetalipoproteinemia | ~1/1000 | Decreased? |
| 5 | | MTP | Abetalipoproteinemia | Rare | Decreased? |
| 6 | Elevated triglycerides | ApoC2 | ApoC2 deficiency, hyperchylomicronemia | Rare | Unchanged |
| 7 | | LPL | LPL deficiency, hyperchylomicronemia | Rare | Unchanged |
| 8 | Low HDL-cholesterol | ApoA1 | Analphalipoproteinemia | Rare | Increased? |
| 9 | | LCAT | Fish-eye disease, familial LCAT deficiency | Rare | Increased? |
| 10 | | ABCA1 | Tangier disease | Rare | Increased |
| 11 | Excess in HDL-cholesterol | CETP | CETP deficiency | 7% in Japan | Increased? |
| 12 | | HL | HL deficiency | Rare | Unchanged? |
| 13 | Excess remnants and IDL | ApoE | Dysbetalipoproteinemia | ~1/10.000 | Increased |
| 14 | | HL | HL deficiency | Rare | Increased? |
| 15 | Excess in Lp(a) | Apo(a) | Hyper-Lp(a)-proteinemia | ~20% | Increased |
| 16 | Sitosterolemia | ABCG5 | Sitosterolemia | Rare | Increased |
| 17 | | ABCG8 | Sitosterolemia | Rare | Increased |

ABCA1, ATP-binding cassette, subfamily A, member 1; ABCG5, ATP-binding cassette, subfamily G, member 5; AD, autosomal dominant; AR, autosomal recessive; FCHL, familial combined hyperlipidemia; HL, hepatic lipase; MPT, microsomal triglycerides transfer protein; LPL, lipoprotein lipase.

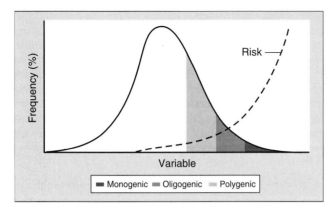

**FIGURE 21-4.** Hypothetical model to illustrate the contribution of genetics to a continuous variable associated with a certain risk. As an example, severely elevated levels of LDL-cholesterol are rare in the population, are associated with a markedly increased risk for CAD, and are most often due to monogenic defects like familial hypercholesterolemia (Table 21-1). In contrast, moderately elevated levels of LDL-cholesterol are much more prevalent and mostly result from interactions between a given environment and sequence variants in multiple genes.

resulting from xanthomatous aortic stenosis. A diagnosis of pediatric homozygous FH often serves as the impetus for further case finding in the family.

FH heterozygotes have LDL-cholesterol levels twice normal or approximately 140 mg/dL higher than family members with two normal genes. Before the statin era, approximately 5% of males had an MI by age 30 years; 25% died of MI by age 50 years; and 50% died by age 60 years. Onset of MI is typically delayed by 10 years in women. Heterozygous FH may be distinguishable from most other forms of hypercholesterolemia by the pres-

ence of nodular xanthomas of the Achilles' and other tendons, seen in up to 75% of heterozygotes. Diabetes and obesity are not associated with FH; a slender physique is typical. However, clinical presentation and outcome may be influenced by other genetic and lifestyle factors.[83]

At present, most FH patients are identified on the basis of lipoprotein profile and clinical findings. Cholesterol guidelines based on genetic testing have been developed for identifying possible FH heterozygotes.[84] Among first-degree relatives of known FH patients, a total cholesterol more than 220 mg/dL for patients younger than age 40 years or more than 290 mg/dL for age 40+ suggests FH. In the general population, total cholesterol higher than 270 mg/dL for patients younger than age 40 years or higher than 360 mg/dL for patients age 40+ suggests FH. Genetic testing is available from specialized clinics and may be useful to detect affected relatives of FH patients and to more successfully implement the prescription of lipid-lowering agents.[85] Patients with FH should receive genetic counseling.

Drug therapy is required to reduce cholesterol levels in FH heterozygotes. HMG CoA reductase inhibitors (statins) lower LDL cholesterol by 30% to 50% by reducing cholesterol synthesis and increasing LDL receptor synthesis from the normal gene. In this population, statins have led to a dramatic improvement in preventing the development of atherosclerosis[86] and expanding survival. Homozygous FH patients appear to be partly responsive to reduced cholesterol synthesis associated with HMG-CoA reductase inhibition[87]; however, LDL apheresis appears to be the treatment of choice. Liver transplantation may be an alternative, whereas gene therapy, which has been used so far on a few patients with limited reduction in plasma LDL levels, holds great promise.

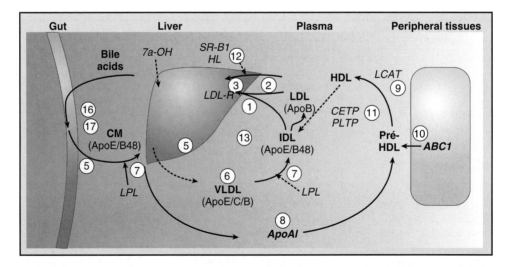

**FIGURE 21-5.** Schematic representation of the location of the defects responsible for monogenic forms of lipoprotein disorders. Numbers refer to Table 21-3. Lipoprotein particles are labeled in bold, apolipoproteins in plain text, and enzymes and receptors are italicized. ABCA1, ATP-binding cassette subfamily A, member 1; CETP, cholesterol-ester transfer protein; CM, chylomicrons; HL, hepatic lipase; LCAT, lecithin-cholesterol acyl transferase; LDL-R, LDL-receptor; LPL, lipoprotein lipase; PLTP, phospholipid transfer protein; 7α-OH, 7α-hydroxylase; SR-B1, scavenger receptor subfamily B, member 1. Lp(a) is not represented in this figure.

### Familial Defective ApoB

A second equally common single-gene disorder causing elevated LDL-cholesterol, familial defective apoB-100 (FDB), is due to a mutation at nucleotide 3500 in the *apoB* gene on chromosome 2. The resulting amino acid substitution disrupts apoB binding to the LDL receptor, impairing LDL uptake. Heterozygosity for this disorder increases LDL-cholesterol levels by at least 50% (60 to 80 mg/dL) relative to unaffected family members. In general, FDB may be clinically milder than FH, but many patients have tendon xanthomas and cholesterol levels may reach the FH range.[88] In some cases the two disorders are distinguishable only by genetic tests, and the approach to treatment is the same.

### Autosomal Recessive Familial Hypercholesterolemia

A third monogenic disorder causing elevated LDL-cholesterol has been characterized recently.[89] Children and adolescents carrying this disease have elevated LDL-cholesterol levels and early CAD, whereas their parents, unlike parents of children with autosomal dominant FH, have normal cholesterol levels. The disease is due to mutations within a gene encoding a putative adaptor protein ARH, which facilitates LDL receptor movement into coated pits.

### Other Genetic Factors Influencing LDL

As mentioned previously, excess in LDL-cholesterol levels results from a certain genetic heterogeneity. A series of loci on chromosomes 1, 3, 4, and 13 that are linked to LDL-cholesterol levels or LDL particle sizes have been identified using whole-genome scanning.[75] No LDL dyslipoproteinemic phenotype has been associated with mutations in candidate genes such as SREBPs, other members of the LDL-receptor superfamily, or apolipoproteins, with the exception of CYP7α and apoE that, in one study,[90] accounted for 15% and 11% of the variance in LDL-cholesterol levels. CYP7α is the limiting step in the generation of bile acid from cholesterol, whereas apoE mediates hepatic uptake of chylomicron remnants and IDL particles (Fig. 21-5). ApoE genotyping has revealed three common alleles in the population: *E3* (Caucasian frequency 77%), *E4* (15%), and *E2* (8%). Individuals with the *E4/3* genotype have mean LDL-cholesterol levels 5 to 10 mg/dL higher than subjects with the most common genotype *E3/3*; conversely, individuals with *E3/2* have LDL-cholesterol levels 10 to 20 mg/dL lower than those of *E3/3* subjects. Several mechanisms have been proposed to account for this. These include competition with LDL for clearance in the liver; *apoE4/3* or *apoE 3/3* might compete more effectively than *apoE 3/2*, leading to increased LDL-cholesterol levels.[91] Carriers of an *apoE E4* allele are at higher risk for the premature development of atherosclerosis, CAD,[92-94] and Alzheimer's disease[21] In contrast, carriers of an *apoE E2* allele [with the exception of the ~2% of homozygous *apoE 2/2* persons who develop Type III hyperlipoproteinemia (see later)] appear to be protected against these conditions. ApoE genotyping may assist in reassigning patients to higher risk strata than those predicted by traditional risk factors.

### Impact of Nongenetic Factors on Plasma LDL Levels

As mentioned previously, environmental conditions may modify the metabolism and the concentrations of lipoproteins and, hence, total- and LDL-cholesterol levels in plasma. These effects may be accounted for, at the molecular level, by overproduction of lipoprotein particles (as in nephrotic syndrome), reduced activity of the lipolytic pathway (as in physical inactivity), secondary to overproduction of apoCIII (an inhibitor of LPL) (as is the case during administration of isotretinoin), or reduction in the activity of the LDL-receptor (as in hypothyroidism).

## Elevated Triglycerides and Combined Hyperlipidemia

An elevation in plasma triglyceride levels is often encountered in the general population and in patients with CAD. This elevation usually reflects an accumulation of VLDL particles in plasma, in the context of familial combined hyperlipidemia, or in conjunction with environmental triggers (e.g., alcohol consumption) or concomitant diseases (e.g., chronic renal failure or diabetes). Type IV hyperlipoproteinemia is characterized by elevated VLDL, with triglycerides of 250 to 500 mg/dL, and LDL-cholesterol levels within the normal range, whereas in Type IIb hyperlipoproteinemia, the concentrations of both VLDL and LDL particles are increased. Hypertriglyceridemia may also result from accumulation of chylomicrons [Fredrickson type I; rare, resulting from complete lipoprotein lipase or apoCII deficiency) (Table 21-1 and Fig. 21-5) and type V (accumulation of VLDL and fasting chylomicrons, with fasting triglycerides >500 mg/dL)]. Elevated levels of VLDL in plasma are associated with a risk for CAD, which appears to add on the risk associated with low-HDL-cholesterol levels,[71] two conditions that are often encountered simultaneously,[78,79,95,96] whereas chylomicronemia is associated with an increased risk for pancreatitis but not CAD.

### Familial Combined Hyperlipidemia

Familial combined hyperlipidemia (FCHL)[82] is the most common form of genetic dyslipidemia (1% to 2% of the general population) and is characterized by elevated levels of VLDL and/or LDL (Table 21-3). FCHL is a potent cause of coronary heart disease and is present in about 5% of all subjects with premature CHD (age ≤60 years). This disorder was originally described as an inherited autosomal dominant trait[82]; however, this mode of inheritance has been challenged recently, and a more complex mode of transmission has been proposed.[96,97] The lipoprotein phenotype varies widely among affected individuals in a given family and even within one given subject over time, consistent with strong gene-environment interactions. This clinical heterogeneity has severely hampered the discovery of the molecular basis for FCHL. Hyperlipidemia usually does not appear until adulthood and is worsened by diabetes and obesity. Affected children display hypertriglyceridemia only, suggesting that the primary defect is in the metabolism of triglycerides-rich lipoproteins. In contrast to FH, xanthomas are not seen in FCHL.

Detailed characterization of the metabolic defects in FCHL shows that increased levels of apoB are always observed in association with the hyperlipidemia.[74] Metabolic turnover studies using radiolabeled VLDL have shown that the disease may be due to conjunction of increased production rates of VLDL apoB and reduced clearance of these triglycerides-rich lipoproteins.[98] Thus, defects in genes regulating the assembly of VLDL particles, their secretion, the interconversion of VLDL subclasses, their removal in the liver, and their conversion to IDL could be involved in FCHL.

As such, the molecular basis of FCHL remains incompletely understood. A series of evidences suggest that apoCIII, a strong inhibitor of lipoprotein lipase activity, is implicated in the pathogenesis of FCHL. First, apoCIII levels are augmented in this condition. Next, genetic studies have documented an association between the apoA-I/CIII/A-IV locus and FCHL.[96,99-101] Moreover, fibrates, which ameliorate the lipoprotein phenotype in FCHL, downregulate the expression of apoCIII.[102] Finally, mice genetically manipulated to overexpress apoCIII show a lipid phenotype similar to FCHL, when bred onto an LDL-R heterozygous knockout background.[103] Interestingly enough, comparative sequencing of the mouse and human apoA-1/CIII/A-IV locus has recently unraveled a new gene located approximately 30 kb from the apoA-I/CIII/A-IV gene cluster that shares strong homology with apoA-IV and was termed apoA-V. This new apolipoprotein has a role in triglyceride metabolism because mice overexpressing this protein have lower triglyceride levels than wild-type littermates, whereas conversely, homologous disruption of the gene encoding this protein is associated with a marked increase in plasma triglyceride levels. Moreover, single nucleotide polymorphisms within this gene are strongly associated with triglyceride levels in humans.[104] Evidence has also been provided that sequence variants within the genes encoding LCAT,[105] lipoprotein lipase,[106,107] hepatic lipase,[108] PPAR gamma,[109,110] and, more recently, tumor necrosis factor-receptor superfamily member 1B[111] are associated with triglyceride levels in plasma, consistent with multiple genetic variants that modify the phenotypic expression of the disease.

More promising are the results of recent linkage studies performed on independent FCHL families that provide evidence for a locus on chromosome 1q21-q23.[101,112] This region is synthenic to mouse chromosome 3, which harbors a murine combined-hyperlipidemia gene called Hyplip1.[113] Other loci have been identified, consistent with the suggestions that FCHL is genetically heterogeneous.

The apoB phenotype in FCHL is commonly associated with other metabolic abnormalities,[114] including the presence of small, dense LDL. The size of the LDL particles affects the atherogenic potential of these particles, because small, dense LDL particles are more susceptible to oxidation and thus accumulation within the vessel wall. Interestingly, the size of LDL particles is partly under complex genetic control.[115] Moreover, FCHL is often associated with insulin resistance.[116-118] As such, FCHL shares common features with metabolic syndrome, a multifaceted condition characterized by the presence of hyperlipidemia, hypertension, obesity, and diabetes whose primary defect appears to be a resistance to the effect of insulin.[118,119]

### Secondary Hypertriglyceridemia

Plasma triglyceride levels are highly susceptible to the effect of environmental factors like diet, obesity, lack of physical activity, alcohol consumption, and diabetes, and a cause for secondary hypertriglyceridemia should be sought for in every hypertriglyceridemic patient (Table 21-2). These conditions lead to an overproduction of VLDL particles by the liver, which translates into hypertriglyceridemia when delipidation of VLDL particles by lipoprotein lipase does not increase proportionally. This phenotype may respond well to correction of concomitant disorders and improvement in lifestyle and, if not sufficient, to administration of fibrates (see later).

## Low HDL-Cholesterol

Low HDL-cholesterol levels in plasma constitute the most frequent atherogenic dyslipidemia in the general population and in patients with CAD from Western countries[71] and are often associated with an elevation in plasma triglyceride levels.[71] An inverse relationship between plasma HDL-cholesterol level and risk for CAD has been amply demonstrated in large prospective studies in North America[77-79] and Europe,[31,120] with a continuous approximately 2.5% increased risk for each 1 mg/dL reduction in the plasma HDL-cholesterol level. Finally, fibrates, which increase HDL-cholesterol levels without modifying LDL-cholesterol levels, have been shown to be effective in preventing the development of CAD.[121] By convention, a low HDL-cholesterol level has been defined as less than 35 mg/dL (0.9 mmol/L) for men and 45 mg/dL (1.15 mmol/L) for women.

As mentioned previously (Table 21-1), the HDL-cholesterol level is under close genetic control, and several monogenic diseases responsible for markedly decreased HDL-cholesterol levels have been described (Table 21-2); Tangier disease is the most illustrative. Tangier disease is an exceedingly rare autosomal recessive disease characterized by almost complete absence of HDL particles in plasma and by accumulation in tissues (in particular tissues of the reticuloendothelial system) of cholesterol esters, which is responsible for peripheral neuropathy, enlarged tonsils, and hepatosplenomegaly. The molecular basis of Tangier disease has been elucidated simultaneously by three different groups using a candidate-gene approach[122-124] and by an additional group that used expression profiling.[125] Tangier disease is due to mutations in the ABCA1 gene, one member of an approximately 50-member family of genes that encode for proteins that use ATP to transport various substrates through plasma membrane. Defects in ABCA1 lead to impaired transmembrane cholesterol transport so that pre-HDL particles cannot form, and apoA1 is rapidly degraded. Plasma HDL-cholesterol levels are also decreased in heterozygote carriers of *ABCA1* mutations and are at increased risk for CAD.[126]

Other rare monogenic disorders responsible for low or absent HDL particles in plasma include homozygosity for *Apo A-1* null mutations,[76] LCAT deficiency (including the fish-eye syndrome),[127] Gaucher's disease type 1, and a subtype of Niemann-Pick disease, reinforcing the importance of the Niemann-Pick protein for intracellular cholesterol transport.[128] Modifier genes for HDL-cholesterol levels, that is, genes for which associations have been detected between allelic variants and plasma HDL-cholesterol levels include the ones encoding scavenger receptor B1,[129] hepatic lipase (this gene, in one study, accounted for 25% of the variance in HDL-cholesterol levels),[130] apoA-I/CIII/A-IV,[130] 7-α-hydroxylase (CYP7α),[90] PPAR gamma,[109] CETP (see later), and LCAT.[131,132] In addition, loci on various chromosomes have been identified that are linked to apoA1 and total- and HDL-cholesterol levels.[133] Finally, low HDL-cholesterol levels can be found in metabolic diseases of monogenic origin (e.g., diabetes) resulting in a defect in hepatocyte nuclear factor 1-a.[132]

The mechanism whereby low HDL-cholesterol levels are associated with an increased risk for CAD remains incompletely understood. A series of arguments indicates that this relationship is causal.[31] First, HDL particles have the ability to carry cholesterol from peripheral tissues back to the liver, a process called the reverse cholesterol transport. Moreover, HDL particles transport enzymes, such as paraoxonase[134] or phospholipase A-2, that may detoxify oxidatively modified lipoproteins and thus reduce their proatherogenic potential. Finally, HDL particles may have anticoagulant properties.[135,136] These mechanisms may explain why the protective effect of HDL particles is mostly apparent in industrialized countries, where LDL-cholesterol concentrations are high (and hence cholesterol deposition in the arterial walls is increased). The ability of HDL particles to perform reverse cholesterol transport may be related not only to their concentration in plasma but also to their structure and metabolism. In the mouse, for instance, overexpression of SR-B1 (which leads to accelerated excretion of cholesterol through the bile) is associated with a low HDL-cholesterol level, and, paradoxically, to reduced atherosclerotic lesions when these mice are bred onto a proatherogenic background.[48] Conversely, attenuated expression of SR-B1 in the mouse is associated with a higher HDL-cholesterol level and accelerated atherosclerosis.[137] A similar apparent paradox has been observed in humans: heterozygous carriers of CETP mutations (who represent ~7% of the Japanese population) have elevated plasma HDL-cholesterol levels, but their cardiovascular risk does not seem to be decreased,[138] possibly because of reduced ability of their HDL particles to extract cholesterol from peripheral tissues. Finally, persons who carry the apoA-1 Milano mutation have an approximately 70% reduction in plasma HDL-cholesterol levels; however, their risk for CAD is similar to that of the general population, and

their intima-media thickness at the carotid levels is less than that of age- and sex-matched individuals with similarly low LDL-cholesterol levels,[139] presumably because of an improved ability of these mutant particles to perform reverse cholesterol transport.[140]

## Elevated Chylomicrons and VLDL Remnant Cholesterol

Chylomicron and IDL remnant lipoproteins result from incomplete delipidation of these lipoproteins by lipoprotein lipase and form particles that migrate in the β-position on agarose gel electrophoresis. These particles are normally rapidly catabolized by apoE-mediated receptor mediated endocytosis to the LDL-R, the cell-surface heparan sulfate proteoglycans/LDL-R-related receptor complex, or the heparan sulfate proteoglycans alone. These remnants accumulate in Type III hyperlipoproteinemia resulting from an impairment in these processes.[141] Both cholesterol and triglycerides are elevated with mean levels of 450 mg/dL and 700 mg/dL, respectively. LDL-cholesterol level is generally low because of reduced conversion of VLDL to LDL and/or to upregulation of the LDL receptors. Patients are susceptible to severe premature CAD, strokes, and peripheral vascular disease.

The archetypal disorder of IDL excess is dysbetalipoproteinemia, which is due to the *apoE2* allele that encodes a protein with only 1% to 2% of normal receptor-binding activity. One percent of the population is homozygous for *ApoE E2* (*E2/2* genotype). These individuals do not generally exhibit fasting hyperlipidemia but have difficulty clearing chylomicron remnants from plasma postprandially. Approximately 1 in 50 *ApoE E2/2* individuals is unable to compensate for the defective apoE protein and develops the fasting lipid elevations characteristic of type III hyperlipoproteinemia. Xanthoma striatum palmare, orange or yellow discolorations of the palmar and digital creases, is pathognomonic of type III disease. The difference between ApoE *E2/2* individuals with or without fasting hyperlipidemia is presumably due to factors that affect IDL metabolism. These may include aging, exogenous estrogens, obesity, glucose intolerance, hypothyroidism, and heterozygosity for another genetic defect such as FH. Type III hyperlipoproteinemia has been reported in several patients with the *apoE E2/2* genotype who are also heterozygous for an *LPL* mutation, and there are almost certainly other mutant genes that can serve as a "second hit" resulting in type III disease. Recently, dominantly inherited forms of type III with almost full penetrance have been reported; they are caused by mutant apoE alleles aside from the common *ApoE E2* variant. Type III patients are highly diet- and weight-responsive, but drug therapy is often required.

Homozygous apoE mutations resulting in very low to undetectable levels of plasma apoE have been described. ApoE deficiency is associated with very high plasma levels of VLDL plus IDL cholesterol and with atherosclerosis. In mice, germline ablation of both copies of the apoE gene results in advanced atherosclerotic lesions similar to those observed in human CAD.[142]

## Elevated Lipoprotein(a)

Lp(a) is an enigmatic lipoprotein that is only present in humans, great apes, and hedgehogs.[143] In humans, approximately 10% of the population has no Lp(a) detectable in plasma, whereas others have levels higher than 100 mg/dL, with a distribution of plasma levels highly skewed toward lower values. Elevated plasma levels of Lp(a) have been associated with an increased risk for CAD, both in cross-sectional and in prospective studies. In a meta-analysis of 27 prospective studies published before 2000, there were 5436 deaths or nonfatal MIs. Comparison of individuals in the top third of baseline plasma Lp(a) levels with those in the bottom third in each study yielded a combined risk ratio of 1.6 (95% CI 1.4 to 1.8, 2P < 0.00001)[144] These observations have recently been confirmed in additional prospective studies.[78,145,146]

Plasma levels of Lp(a) are highly genetically determined[147,148] (Table 21-1) with approximately 90% of the interindividual variability in plasma Lp(a) levels being accounted for by sequences with the gene encoding apo(a), the distinctive, highly polymorphic glycoprotein that is attached to apoB-100 of LDL in a covalent fashion. Structurally, apo(a) is highly homologous to plasminogen, and both genes are located at the tip of the long arm of chromosome 6 (6q27-27).[149] Plasminogen comprises five pretzel-shaped motifs called kringles (K1-K5), followed by the protease domain. Tissue plasminogen activator cleaves plasminogen within the K4-K5 interkringle region to release the protease domain (plasmin) which is activated. In contrast to plasminogen, apo(a) does not contain any sequences homologous to K1-K3 but contains between 12 and 51 tandemly repeated copies of the K4 motif, followed by one K5 motif and the protease domain, which is functionally inactive. The size of the apo(a) glycoprotein is dictated by the number of K4-encoding units within the apo(a) gene. Larger apo(a) isoforms are usually associated with lower plasma Lp(a) levels, whereas smaller isoforms are usually associated with higher levels of Lp(a) in plasma. Overall, the size polymorphism of the apo(a) gene accounts for approximately 70% of the variability of plasma Lp(a) levels. Other sequences affect plasma Lp(a) levels,[150] in particular a G/A substitution within the intron separating the two exons encoding K4-type 8, which disrupts a splicing site and leads to a truncated apo(a) isoform that is unable to covalently attach apoB of LDL to form a Lp(a) particle and that leads to a "null" allele in whites.[151] Plasma Lp(a) levels are increased in chronic renal failure[152] and nephrotic syndrome[153] and after MI[154,163] and decrease dramatically, as other lipoproteins do, during sepsis.[155]

The mechanism whereby Lp(a) is atherogenic remains poorly understood. Given the homology between plasminogen and apo(a), Lp(a) may compete with plasminogen and partly inhibit fibrinolysis. This scenario is supported by in vitro[156] and in vivo[157] competition studies and by the demonstration that apo(a) co-deposits with fibrin in human arteries and inflammatory arthritides.[158] As such, Lp(a) may be thrombogenic, a possibility that is further supported by epidemiologic studies showing an association between elevated Lp(a) levels in plasma and an increased risk for venous thromboembolism.[159] This risk may be further increased in presence of a genetic predisposition to these conditions such as factor V Leiden.

The role of Lp(a) in promoting atherogenesis in animal models has been controversial,[160,161] and several studies even suggested that Lp(a) has protective effects in mediating wound healing by delivering lipids to the injured area and inhibiting tumor angiogenesis.[162] Recent observations have suggested the hypothesis that some of the atherogenic properties of Lp(a) may be due to its strong affinity for oxidized phospholipids, which may be preferentially transferred to and sequestered by Lp(a) after being released into the circulation.[163] Thus, the proatherogenic properties of Lp(a), particularly when plasma levels are elevated, may be due to its predilection for the vessel wall while accompanied by these oxidative byproducts resulting in enhanced inflammation and progression of atherosclerosis. Indeed, Lp(a) has been documented to exist in larger amounts in unstable coronary plaques compared with stable plaques and to co-localize with macrophages.[164]

This scenario may explain why Lp(a) appears to be particularly deleterious in presence of preexisting atherosclerosis,[165] additional risk factors[145] such as hyperhomocysteinemia,[166] or atherogenic conditions such as chronic renal failure.[167] In proatherogenic conditions, smaller apo(a) isoforms may be even more deleterious, irrespective of their association with higher plasma Lp(a) levels. Finally, the atherogenicity of Lp(a) may be enhanced in the presence of another genetically predisposing condition, such as the presence of an apoE E4 isoform.[94] Strikingly, a similar apoE-Lp(a) interaction was also recently observed for late-onset Alzheimer's disease.[168]

## Sitosterolemia

Sitosterolemia is a rare autosomal recessive disease,[169] but recent elucidation of the molecular basis of this disease[4,5] further illuminates the understanding of lipid metabolism and illustrates the power of molecular genetics in deciphering complex biologic systems. Phenotypically, sitosterolemia shares numerous features in common with FH, such as the development in childhood of tendon xanthomas and premature CAD. In contrast to FH, plasma cholesterol levels are subnormal or normal in sitosterolemia, but plant sterol levels are very elevated in this condition because of increased absorption of these sterols by the gut. In normal conditions, human gut is exquisitely able to distinguish between plant sterols (mostly represented by sitosterols) and cholesterol and to absorb approximately 5% and 50% of these compounds. Recently, a genetic mapping approach on locus 2p21 and expression mapping coupled to expression profiling[5] allowed scientists to identify two tandemly arranged new members of the ABC family ABCG5 (or sterolin-1) and ABCG8 (or sterolin-2)[170] that, when mutated, lead to increased sitosterol absorption by the gut and to sitosterolemia.

# DRUGS AFFECTING LIPID METABOLISM

## Drugs that Treat Lipid Disorders

### Statins

HMG-CoA reductase inhibitors, or statins, are used to treat patients with elevated plasma LDL-cholesterol. HMG-CoA reductase is the enzyme that controls the rate-limiting step for cholesterol biosynthesis in the liver and other tissues (Fig. 21-6). Gene expression of this enzyme is controlled by sterols and nonsterol products of the mevalonate metabolic pathway through negative feedback inhibition. Statins block cholesterol synthesis, reduce hepatocyte cholesterol content, and increase the expression of LDL receptors that take up circulating LDL into cells resulting in lower plasma LDL-cholesterol levels. A large number of angiographic progression and regression studies using statins in patients with hypercholesterolemia have shown very modest changes in angiographic dimensions but substantial clinical benefits, ascribed to plaque stabilization.[171,172] Subsequently, several prospective, placebo-controlled studies of primary[173,174] and secondary[175-177] prevention of CHD in subjects with hypercholesterolemia and even with "normal" cholesterol levels[178] have shown unequivocally that statins reduce the incidence of all-cause mortality, MI, stroke, and revascularization procedures.

The mechanisms behind these benefits are not completely understood but likely involve cholesterol and lipid removal from plaques (as has been shown in animal studies[179,180]) and possible pleiotropic properties of statins that are independent of cholesterol lowering.[181] Beneficial effects of statins such as improvement in endothelial function, plaque stabilization, reduction in oxidative stress, and vascular inflammation are mediated, in part, by inhibition of synthesis of isoprenoid intermediates, which play an important role in cell growth and signal transduction. Isoprenoids act as lipid anchors for many membrane-associated proteins and posttranslationally prenylate a variety of cellular proteins, such as Rho, Ras, and Rac, via mevalonate-dependent geranylgeranyl-, farnesyl-, and isopentyl pyrophosphates generated from this pathway.[182] For example, statins prevent the isoprenylation of the Rho G-protein that reduces nitric oxide production by inactivating eNOS mRNA. Statins also prevent isoprenylation of p21 Rac, which is involved in the assembly and function of superoxide-forming NADPH oxidase.[183,184] In aortic endothelial cells, statins decrease the basal expression of preproendothelin-1, a precursor to endothelin-1, which is a potent regulator of vascular tone and remodeling.[185] In addition, statins upregulate nitric oxide expression by decreasing caveolin-1 levels, which is present in caveolae and serves as a docking station for numerous signaling proteins including eNOS. Caveolin-1 is upregulated by LDL, but it inhibits eNOS function by preventing eNOS interaction with calcium and calmodulin.[186] In normal, but not eNOS-deficient mice, statins also reduce stroke size by upregulating eNOS expression, which is completely reversed by mevalonate and isoprenoids, supporting the concept that enhanced eNOS activity is the predominant mechanism of neuroprotection.[187]

Statins may also have an immunomodulatory and anti-inflammatory effects.[188,189] Statins inhibit interferon-γ-induced expression of class II major histocompatibility complexes on antigen-presenting cells, which are required for antigen presentation and T-cell receptor activation that may trigger T-cell proliferation, differentiation, and cytokine release.[190] Simvastatin has been shown to reduce acute inflammatory responses in a dose-dependent manner and similar in extent to indomethacin.[191] Statins also reduce monocyte chemotaxis and recruitment by inhibiting the expression of monocyte chemotactic protein-1 by peripheral blood monocytes and endothelial cells.[192] In vascular smooth muscle cells, statins induce apoptosis and inhibit migration and proliferation.[193-195] Statins also increase fibrinolytic activity through enhanced expression of tissue plasminogen activator and platelet activator inhibitor-1.[196] Although these cholesterol-independent effects have been well documented *in vitro* and in some animals models, their relevance to humans must be established.

### Bile Acid Sequestrants

Bile acid resins are generally used to treat elevated LDL-cholesterol levels as an adjunct to statins when additional LDL lowering is required. Bile acid resins are

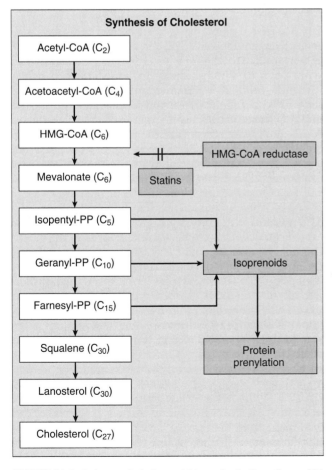

**FIGURE 21-6.** Pathway of cholesterol biosynthesis. Parentheses $(C_x)$ refers to the number of carbon atoms per molecule.

synthetic anion compounds that bind bile acids, but not cholesterol, in the intestinal lumen and prevent their absorption by interfering with the enterohepatic circulation. This, in turn, results in upregulation of hepatic CYP7α, which increases the synthesis of bile acids from cholesterol and results in upregulation of LDL receptors and a reduction in LDL-cholesterol levels.[23,80,197] However, bile acid resins induce increased cholesterol biosynthesis and increased synthesis and secretion of VLDL limiting their efficacy because of increased triglyceride concentrations.

### Fibric Acid Derivatives

Fibrates are drugs similar in chemical structure to short-chain fatty acids and are generally used to treat primary hypertriglyceridemia and type III dysbetalipoproteinemia, characterized by cholesterol-enriched VLDL that results from homozygosity of the rare apoE2 isoform. Fibrates increase lipoprotein lipase-mediated lipolysis, stimulate hepatic fatty acid uptake, and reduce hepatic triglyceride production. They convert fatty acids to acyl-CoA derivatives by stimulating β-oxidation of fatty acids, which results in decreased VLDL production and in reduced plasma triglyceride concentration. Fibrates are synthetic ligands for PPARα, which induces transcriptional synthesis of apoA-I and apoA-II resulting in increased $HDL_3$ concentration and augmented reverse cholesterol transport. Fibrates modestly increase HDL concentration and can lower LDL-cholesterol levels (particularly the number of atherogenic small, dense LDL particles that are more susceptible to oxidation) and reduce the extent of postprandial lipemia.[198] In addition, transcription of the *apoC-III* gene is suppressed resulting in decreased levels of apoC-III, which results in lipoprotein lipase activation.[199,200] Angiographic studies have shown that fibrates decrease the progression of coronary atherosclerosis and decrease coronary events.[201] The Helsinki Heart Study and the VA-HIT study have shown that fibrates reduce the number of clinical cardiovascular endpoints in primary and secondary prevention of CHD.[121,202]

### Niacin

Nicotinic acid is activated after oral ingestion by conversion to nicotinamide adenine dinucleotide. It reduces apoB-100, total cholesterol, VLDL and LDL-cholesterol, triglycerides, and Lp(a) and significantly raises HDL-cholesterol ($HDL_2/HDL_3$ ratio).[203] It also transforms small, dense LDL to more buoyant LDL.[29] Its mechanism of action is not well understood, but some of its beneficial actions may be through inhibition of release of free fatty acids from adipose and other peripheral tissues, increased lipoprotein lipase activity, decreased conversion of VLDL to LDL, and reduced apoA-I catabolism.[204,205] Niacin does not affect the fecal excretion of fats, sterols, or bile acids. The Coronary Drug Project showed that niacin reduces the incidence of nonfatal MI in middle-aged men.[206] The CLAS,[207] FATS,[208] and HATS[209] angiographic regression studies showed that niacin in combination with colestipol or simvastatin

reduced the rate of progression and/or induced regression of coronary atherosclerosis.

### Ezetimibe

Ezetimibe is a novel, selective cholesterol absorption inhibitor that prevents the uptake and absorption of dietary and biliary cholesterol at the intestinal brush border resulting in cholesterol excretion, without affecting the absorption of fatty acids or fat-soluble vitamins.[210] Ezetimibe undergoes enterohepatic recirculation and, therefore, repeatedly delivers its effect in reducing cholesterol reuptake. Results from preclinical studies in various animal models have demonstrated that ezetimibe lowers LDL levels, with a significant synergistic effect when combined with a statin.[211] It also reduces atherosclerosis in apoE-deficient mice.[212] This agent has recently been tested in randomized clinical trials and reduced LDL cholesterol as monotherapy by approximately 15% to 20% and as combination therapy with a statin by 50% to 60%.[213,214] Ezetimibe promises to be a viable option in the armamentarium for the pharmacologic treatment of hypercholesterolemia, particularly in patients not reaching target LDL cholesterol levels and in those with heterozygous FH.

## Drugs that Elevate Lipid Levels

### Protease Inhibitors

HIV-infected patients have been shown to sustain premature cardiovascular disease.[215,216] The use of protease inhibitors in HIV-infected patients has been shown to contribute to lipodystrophy, hyperinsulinemia, hyperglycemia, and dyslipidemic profiles manifested as increased LDL-cholesterol, triglycerides, and Lp(a) levels and decreased HDL-cholesterol levels.[217] The mechanisms underlying these disorders are not fully understood, but recent studies suggest a molecular basis for protease inhibitor-associated dyslipidemia. Protease inhibitors induce apoptosis in adipocytes resulting in release of massive quantities of fatty acids that reach the liver and result in hepatic synthesis of triglycerides and VLDL. Protease inhibitors also directly stimulate triglyceride synthesis and upregulate mRNA for key enzymes in the lipid biosynthetic pathway and increase apoB levels by inhibiting proteasomal degradation of nascent apolipoprotein B.[218] Patients with apoC-III polymorphisms of the −455C variant were recently shown to develop a 30% reduction in HDL-cholesterol levels compared with noncarriers and plasma triglycerides were shown to increase according to the number of variant alleles.[219]

### Immunosuppressive Agents

Treatment with cyclosporine or corticosteroids can lead to elevated lipid levels. Sirolimus, a new and potent immunosuppressive agent, has been shown to significantly increase plasma cholesterol and triglyceride levels and to exacerbate hyperlipidemia in patients taking other immunosuppressive agents. The mechanisms underlying these dyslipidemias are being evaluated, but sirolimus-induced hypertriglyceridemia is partly due to reduced catabolism of VLDL, and the effects are dose-dependent and rapidly reversible.[220]

## CONCLUSIONS

There has been rapid progress in the understanding of the molecular mechanisms underlying normal lipoprotein metabolism and lipoprotein disorders. This progress has been accelerated by molecular tools and techniques, (particularly transgenic mouse models), and has paved the way for defining novel pathways and regulatory processes in lipoprotein metabolism. Further research in this evolving area will undoubtedly illuminate novel physiologic and pathophysiologic pathways and will lead to new methods of prevention, diagnosis, and treatment of atherosclerosis.

## REFERENCES

1. Witztum JL, Steinberg D: The oxidative modification hypothesis of atherosclerosis: Does it hold for humans? Trends Cardiovasc Med 2001;11:93-102.
2. Nordskog BK, Phan CT, Nutting DF, et al: An examination of the factors affecting intestinal lymphatic transport of dietary lipids. Adv Drug Deliv Rev 2001;50:21-44.
3. Bhattacharyya AK, Connor WE: Beta-sitosterolemia and xanthomatosis: A newly described lipid storage disease in two sisters. J Clin Invest 1974;53:1033-1043.
4. Berge KE, Tian H, Graf GA, et al: Accumulation of dietary cholesterol in sitosterolemia caused by mutations in adjacent ABC transporters. Science 2000;290:1771-1775.
5. Lee MH, Lu K, Hazard S, et al: Identification of a gene, ABCG5, important in the regulation of dietary cholesterol absorption. Nat Genet 2001;27:79-83.
6. Hubacek JA, Berge KE, Cohen JC, et al: Mutations in ATP-cassette binding proteins G5 (ABCG5) and G8 (ABCG8) causing sitosterolemia. Hum Mutat 2001;18:359-360.
7. Chawla A, Repa JJ, Evans RM, et al: Nuclear receptors and lipid physiology: Opening the X-files. Science 2001;294:1866-1870.
8. Repa JJ, Turley SD, Lobaccaro J-MA, et al: Regulation of absorption and ABC1-mediated efflux of cholesterol by RXR heterodimers. Science 2000;289:1524-1529.
9. Meiner VL, Cases S, Myers HM, et al: Disruption of the acyl-CoA:cholesterol acyltransferase gene in mice: Evidence suggesting multiple cholesterol esterification enzymes in mammals. Proc Natl Acad Sci USA 1996;93:14041-14046.
10. Buhman KF, Accad M, Farese RV: Mammalian acyl-CoA:cholesterol acyltransferases. Biochim Biophys Acta 2000;1529:142-154.
11. Chang CCY, Sakashita N, Ornvold K, et al: Immunological quantitation and localization of ACAT-1 and ACAT-2 in human liver and small intestine. J Biol Chem 2000;275:28083-28092.
12. Lee RG, Willingham MC, Davis MA, et al: Differential expression of ACAT1 and ACAT2 among cells within liver, intestine, kidney, and adrenal of nonhuman primates. J Lipid Res 2000;41:1991-2001.
13. Accad M, Smith SJ, Newland DL, et al: Massive xanthomatosis and altered composition of atherosclerotic lesions in hyperlipidemic mice lacking acyl CoA:cholesterol acyltransferase 1. J Clin Invest 2000;105:711-719.
14. Fazio S, Major AS, Swift LL, et al: Increased atherosclerosis in LDL receptor-null mice lacking ACAT1 in macrophages. J Clin Invest 2001;107:163-171.
15. Chen SH, Habib G, Yang CY, et al: Apolipoprotein B-48 is the product of a messenger RNA with an organ-specific in-frame stop codon. Science 1987;238:363-366.
16. Innerarity TL, Borén J, Yamanaka S, et al: Biosynthesis of apolipoprotein B48-containing lipoproteins. J Biol Chem 1996;271:2353-2356.
17. Berriot-Varoqueaux N, Aggerbeck LP, Samson-Bouma ME, et al: The role of the microsomal triglyceride transfer protein in abetalipoproteinemia. Annu Rev Nutr 2000;20:663-697.
18. Shiomi M, Ito T: MTP inhibitor decreases plasma cholesterol levels in LDL receptor-deficient WHHL rabbits by lowering the VLDL secretion. Eur J Pharmacol 2001;431:127-131.
19. Herz J, Strickland DK: LRP: A multifunctional scavenger and signaling receptor. J Clin Invest 2001;108:779-784.
20. Shibata M, Yamada S, Kumar SR, et al: Clearance of Alzheimer's amyloid-{beta}1-40 peptide from brain by LDL receptor-related protein-1 at the blood-brain barrier. J Clin Invest 2000;106:1489-1499.
21. Strittmatter WJ, Weisgraber KH, Huang DY, et al: Binding of human apolipoprotein E to synthetic amyloid beta peptide: Isoform-specific effects and implications for late-onset Alzheimer disease. Proc Natl Acad Sci USA 1993;90:8098-8102.
22. Liao W, Yeung SC, Chan L: Proteasome-mediated degradation of apolipoprotein B targets both nascent peptides cotranslationally before translocation and full-length apolipoprotein B after translocation into the endoplasmic reticulum. J Biol Chem 1998;273:27225-27230.
23. Davis RA: Evolution of processes and regulators of lipoprotein synthesis: From birds to mammals. J Nutr 1997;127:795S-800S.
24. Shelness GS, Sellers JA: Very-low-density lipoprotein assembly and secretion. Curr Opin Lipidol 2001;12:151-157.
25. Suzuki H, Kurihara Y, Takeya M, et al: A role for macrophage scavenger receptors in atherosclerosis and susceptibility to infection. Nature 1997;386:292-296.
26. Febbraio M, Podrez EA, Smith JD, et al: Targeted disruption of the class B scavenger receptor CD36 protects against atherosclerotic lesion development in mice. J Clin Invest 2000;105:1049-1056.
27. Tribble DL, Rizzo M, Chait A, et al: Enhanced oxidative susceptibility and reduced antioxidant content of metabolic precursors of small, dense low-density lipoproteins. Am J Med 2001;110:103-110.
28. Kwiterovich PO: The metabolic pathways of high-density lipoprotein, low-density lipoprotein, and triglycerides: A current review. Am J Cardiol 2000;86:5-10.
29. Zambon A, Hokanson JE, Brown BG, et al: Evidence for a new pathophysiological mechanism for coronary artery disease regression: Hepatic lipase-mediated changes in LDL density. Circulation 1999;99:1959-1964.
30. Dietschy JM, Turley SD, Spady DK: Role of liver in the maintenance of cholesterol and low density lipoprotein homeostasis in different animal species, including humans. J Lipid Res 1993;34:1637-1659.
31. von Eckardstein A, Nofer JR, Assmann G: High density lipoproteins and arteriosclerosis: Role of cholesterol efflux and reverse cholesterol transport. Arterioscler Thromb Vasc Biol 2001;21:13-27.
32. Tall AR, Wang N: Tangier disease as a test of the reverse cholesterol transport hypothesis. J Clin Invest 2000;106:1205-1207.
33. Groen AK, Bloks VW, Bandsma RH, et al: Hepatobiliary cholesterol transport is not impaired in Abca1-null mice lacking HDL. J Clin Invest 2001;108:843-850.
34. Haghpassand M, Bourassa PA, Francone OL, et al: Monocyte/macrophage expression of ABCA1 has minimal contribution to plasma HDL levels. J Clin Invest 2001;108:1315-1320.
35. McNeish J, Aiello RJ, Guyot D, et al: High density lipoprotein deficiency and foam cell accumulation in mice with targeted disruption of ATP-binding cassette transporter-1. Proc Natl Acad Sci USA 2000;97:4245-4250.
36. Vaisman BL, Lambert G, Amar M, et al: ABCA1 overexpression leads to hyperalphalipoproteinemia and increased biliary cholesterol excretion in transgenic mice. J Clin Invest 2001;108:303-309.
37. Santamarina-Fojo S, Lambert G, Hoeg JM, et al: Lecithin-cholesterol acyltransferase: Role in lipoprotein metabolism, reverse cholesterol transport and atherosclerosis. Curr Opin Lipidol 2000;11:267-275.
38. Huuskonen J, Olkkonen VM, Jauhiainen M, et al: The impact of phospholipid transfer protein (PLTP) on HDL metabolism. Atherosclerosis 2001;155:269-281.

39. van Haperen R, van Tol A, Vermeulen P, et al: Human plasma phospholipid transfer protein increases the antiatherogenic potential of high density lipoproteins in transgenic mice. Arterioscler Thromb Vasc Biol 2000;20:1082-1088.

40. Hirano Ki, Yamashita S, Nakajima N, et al: Genetic cholesteryl ester transfer protein deficiency is extremely frequent in the Omagari area of Japan: Marked hyperalphalipoproteinemia caused by CETP gene mutation is not associated with longevity. Arterioscler Thromb Vasc Biol 1997;17:1053-1059.

41. Hirano Ki, Yamashita S, Kuga Y, et al: Atherosclerotic disease in marked hyperalphalipoproteinemia: Combined reduction of cholesteryl ester transfer protein and hepatic triglyceride lipase. Arterioscler Thromb Vasc Biol 1995;15:1849-1856.

42. Lambert G, Amar MJ, Martin P, et al: Hepatic lipase deficiency decreases the selective uptake of HDL-cholesteryl esters in vivo. J Lipid Res 2000;41:667-672.

43. Lambert G, Chase MB, Dugi K, et al: Hepatic lipase promotes the selective uptake of high density lipoprotein-cholesteryl esters via the scavenger receptor B1. J Lipid Res 1999;40:1294-1303.

44. Dugi KA, Brandauer K, Schmidt N, et al: Low hepatic lipase activity is a novel risk factor for coronary artery disease. Circulation 2001;104:3057-3062.

45. Krieger M: Scavenger receptor class B type I is a multiligand HDL receptor that influences diverse physiologic systems. J Clin Invest 2001;108:793-797.

46. Arai T, Wang N, Bezouevski M, et al: Decreased atherosclerosis in heterozygous low density lipoprotein receptor-deficient mice expressing the scavenger receptor BI transgene. J Biol Chem 1999;274:2366-2371.

47. Ueda Y, Gong E, Royer L, et al: Relationship between expression levels and atherogenesis in scavenger receptor class B, type I transgenics. J Biol Chem 2000;275:20368-20373.

48. Kozarsky KF, Donahee MH, Glick JM, et al: Gene transfer and hepatic overexpression of the HDL receptor SR-BI reduces atherosclerosis in the cholesterol-fed LDL receptor-deficient mouse. Arterioscler Thromb Vasc Biol 2000;20:721-727.

49. Trigatti B, Rayburn H, Vinals M, et al: Influence of the high density lipoprotein receptor SR-BI on reproductive and cardiovascular pathophysiology. Proc Natl Acad Sci USA 1999;96:9322-9327.

50. Brown MS, Goldstein JL: A proteolytic pathway that controls the cholesterol content of membranes, cells, and blood. Proc Natl Acad Sci U S A 1999;96:11041-11048.

51. Nohturfft A, Yabe D, Goldstein JL, et al: Regulated step in cholesterol feedback localized to budding of SCAP from ER membranes. Cell 2000;102:315-323.

52. DeBose-Boyd RA, Brown MS, Li WP, et al: Transport-dependent proteolysis of SREBP: Relocation of site-1 protease from Golgi to ER obviates the need for SREBP transport to Golgi. Cell 1999;99:703-712.

53. Yang T, Goldstein JL, Brown MS: Overexpression of membrane domain of SCAP prevents sterols from inhibiting SCAP.SREBP exit from endoplasmic reticulum. J Biol Chem 2000;275:29881-29886.

54. Sakai J, Rawson RB, Espenshade PJ, et al: Molecular identification of the sterol-regulated luminal protease that cleaves SREBPs and controls lipid composition of animal cells. Mol Cell 1998;2:505-514.

55. Rawson RB, Zelenski NG, Nijhawan D, et al: Complementation cloning of S2P, a gene encoding a putative metalloprotease required for intramembrane cleavage of SREBPs. Mol Cell 1997;1:47-57.

56. Nohturfft A, DeBose-Boyd RA, Scheek S, et al: Sterols regulate cycling of SREBP cleavage-activating protein (SCAP) between endoplasmic reticulum and Golgi. Proc Natl Acad Sci USA 1999;96:11235-11240.

57. Grand-Perret T, Bouillot A, Perrot A, et al: SCAP ligands are potent new lipid-lowering drugs. Nat Med 2001;7:1332-1338.

58. Rader DJ: A new feature on the cholesterol-lowering landscape. Nat Med 2001;7:1282-1284.

59. Waxman DJ: P450 gene induction by structurally diverse xenochemicals: Central role of nuclear receptors CAR, PXR, and PPAR. Arch Biochem Biophys 1999;369:11-23.

60. Storch J, Thumser AE: The fatty acid transport function of fatty acid-binding proteins. Biochim Biophys Acta 2000;1486:28-44.

61. Dean M, Hamon Y, Chimini G: The human ATP-binding cassette (ABC) transporter superfamily. J Lipid Res 2001;42:1007-1017.

62. Lu TT, Repa JJ, Mangelsdorf DJ: Orphan nuclear receptors as eLiXiRs and FiXeRs of sterol metabolism. J Biol Chem 2001;276:37735-37738.

63. Repa JJ, Mangelsdorf DJ: Nuclear receptor regulation of cholesterol and bile acid metabolism. Curr Opin Biotechnol 1999;10:557-563.

64. Claudel T, Leibowitz MD, Fievet C, et al: Reduction of atherosclerosis in apolipoprotein E knockout mice by activation of the retinoid X receptor. Proc Natl Acad Sci U S A 2001;98:2610-2615.

65. Willson TM, Brown PJ, Sternbach DD, et al: The PPARs: From orphan receptors to drug discovery. J Med Chem 2000;43:527-550.

66. Collins AR, Meehan WP, Kintscher U, et al: Troglitazone inhibits formation of early atherosclerotic lesions in diabetic and nondiabetic low density lipoprotein receptor-deficient mice. Arterioscler Thromb Vasc Biol 2001;21:365-371.

67. Chen Z, Ishibashi S, Perrey S, et al: Troglitazone inhibits atherosclerosis in apolipoprotein E-knockout mice: Pleiotropic effects on CD36 expression and HDL. Arterioscler Thromb Vasc Biol 2001;21:372-377.

68. Li AC, Brown KK, Silvestre MJ, et al: Peroxisome proliferator-activated receptor gamma ligands inhibit development of atherosclerosis in LDL receptor-deficient mice. J Clin Invest 2000;106:523-531.

69. Heller DA, de Faire U, Pedersen NL, et al: Genetic and environmental influences on serum lipid levels in twins. N Engl J Med 1993;328:1150-1156.

70. Snieder H, van Doornen LJP, Boomsma DI: Dissecting the genetic architecture of lipids, lipoproteins, and apolipoproteins. Lessons from twin studies. Arterioscler Thromb Vasc Biol 1999;19:2826-2834.

71. Genest JJ, Martin-Munley SS, McNamara JR, et al: Familial lipoprotein disorders in patients with premature coronary artery disease. Circulation 1992;85:2025-2033.

72. Jomini V, Oppliger-Pasquali S, Wietlisbach V, et al: Contribution of major cardiovascular risk factors to familial premature coronary artery disease-the GENECARD project. J Am Coll Cardiol. 2002;40:676-84.

73. Rodondi N, Darioli R, Ramelet AA, et al: High risk for hyperlipidemia and the metabolic syndrome after an episode of hypertriglyceridemia during 13-cis retinoic acid therapy for acne: A pharmacogenetic study. Ann Intern Med 2002;136:582-9.

74. McNeely MJ, Edwards KL, Marcovina SM, et al: Lipoprotein and apolipoprotein abnormalities in familial combined hyperlipidemia: A 20-year prospective study. Atherosclerosis 2001;159:471-481.

75. Hegele RA: Monogenic dyslipidemias: Window on determinants of plasma lipoprotein metabolism. Am J Hum Genet 2001;69:1161-1177.

76. Breslow JL: Genetics of lipoprotein abnormalities associated with coronary heart disease susceptibility. Annu Rev Genet 2000;34:233-254.

77. Wilson PW, D'Agostino RB, Levy D, et al: Prediction of coronary heart disease using risk factor categories. Circulation 1998;97:1837-1847.

78. Sharrett AR, Ballantyne CM, Coady SA, et al: Coronary heart disease prediction from lipoprotein cholesterol levels, triglycerides, lipoprotein(a), apolipoproteins A-1 and B, and HDL density subfractions: The Atherosclerosis Risk in Communities (ARIC) Study. Circulation 2001;104:1108-1113.

79. Stamler J, Daviglus ML, Garside DB, et al: Relationship of baseline serum cholesterol levels in 3 large cohorts of younger men to long-term coronary, cardiovascular, and all-cause mortality and to longevity. JAMA 2000;284:311-318.

80. Brown MS, Goldstein JL: A receptor-mediated pathway for cholesterol homeostasis. Science 1986;232:34-47.

81. Goldstein JL, Hobbs HH, Brown MS: The Metabolic and Molecular Bases of Inherited Disease. New York, McGraw Hill, 1995.

82. Goldstein JL, Schrott HG, Bierman EL, et al: Genetic analysis of lipid levels in 176 families and delineation of a new inherited disorder, combined hyperlipidemia. J Clin Invest 1973;52:1544-1568.

83. Sijsbrands ERG, Westendorp RGJ, Defesche JC, et al: Mortality over two centuries in large pedigrees with familial hypercholesterolaemia: Family tree mortality study. BMJ 2001;322:1019–1023.

84. Williams RR, Hunt SC, Schumacher MC, et al: Diagnosing heterozygous familial hypercholesterolemia using new practical criteria validated by molecular genetics. Am J Cardiol 1993;72: 171–176.

85. Umans-Eckenhausen MA, Defesche JC, Sijbrands EJ, et al: Review of first 5 years of screening for familial hypercholesterolaemia in the Netherlands. Lancet 2001;357:165–168.

86. Smilde TJ, van Wissen S, Wollersheim H, et al: Effect of aggressive versus conventional lipid lowering on atherosclerosis progression in familial hypercholesterolaemia (ASAP): A prospective, randomized, double-blind trial. Lancet 2001;357:577–581.

87. Raal FJ, Pappu AS, Illingworth DR, et al: Inhibition of cholesterol synthesis by atorvastatin in homozygous familial hypercholesterolaemia. Atherosclerosis 2000;150:421–428.

88. Miserez AR, Laager R, Chiodetti N, et al: High prevalence of familial defective apolipoprotein B-100 in Switzerland. J Lipid Res 1994;35:574–583.

89. Garcia CK, Wilund K, Arca M, et al: Autosomal recessive hypercholesterolemia caused by mutations in a putative LDL receptor adaptor protein. Science 2001;292:1394–1398.

90. Wang J, Freeman DJ, Grundy SM, et al: Linkage between cholesterol 7a-hydroxylase and high plasma low-density lipoprotein cholesterol concentrations. J Clin Invest 1998;101:1283–1291.

91. Kowal RC, Herz J, Weisgraber KH, et al: Opposing effects of apolipoprotein E and C on lipoprotein binding to low density lipoprotein receptor-related protein. J Biol Chem 1990;265: 10771–10779.

92. Wilson PW, Schaefer EJ, Larson MG, et al: Apolipoprotein E alleles and risk of coronary disease: A meta-analysis. Arterioscler Thromb Vasc Biol 1996;16:1250–1255.

93. Smith JD: Apolipoprotein E4: An allele associated with many diseases. Ann Med 2000;32:118–127.

94. Gerdes LU, Gerdes C, Kervinen K, et al: The apolipoprotein E4 allele determines prognosis and the effect on prognosis of simvastatin in survivors of myocardial infarction: A substudy of the Scandinavian Simvastatin Survival Study. Circulation 2000; 101:1366–1371.

95. Yarnell JW, Patterson CC, Sweetnam PM, et al: Do total and high density lipoprotein cholesterol and triglycerides act independently in the prediction of ischemic heart disease? Ten-year follow-up of Caerphilly and Speedwell cohorts. Arterioscler Thromb Vasc Biol 2001;21:1340–1345.

96. Austin MA, McKnight B, Edwards KL, et al: Cardiovascular disease mortality in familial forms of hypertriglyceridemia: A 20-year prospective study. Circulation 2000;101:2777–2782.

97. Cullen P, Farren B, Scott J, et al: Complex segregation analysis provides evidence for a major gene acting on serum triglyceride levels in 55 British families with familial combined hyperlipidemia. Arterioscler Thromb Vasc Biol 1994;14:1233–1249.

98. Reynisdottir S, Eriksson M, Angelin B, et al: Impaired activation of adipocyte lipolysis in familial combined hyperlipidemia. J Clin Invest 1995;95:2161–2169.

99. Dallinga-Thie GM, van Linde-Sibenius Trip M, Rotter JI, et al: Complex genetic contribution of the apo AI-CIII-AIV gene cluster to familial combined hyperlipidemia: Identification of different susceptibility haplotypes. J Clin Invest 1997;99:953–961.

100. Li W, Dammerman MM, Smith JD, et al: A mutation in the promoter of the human apoCIII gene abolishes regulation by insulin and may contribute to hypertriglyceridemia. J Clin Invest 1995;96:2601–2605.

101. Coon H, Myers RH, Borecki IB, et al: Replication of linkage of familial combined hyperlipidemia to chromosome 1q with additional heterogeneous effect of apolipoprotein A-1/C-III/A-IV locus: The NHLBI Family Heart Study. Arterioscler Thromb Vasc Biol 2000;20:2275–2280.

102. Staels B, Vu-Dac N, Kosykh VA, et al: Fibrates downregulate apolipoprotein C-III expression independent of induction of peroxisomal acyl coenzyme A oxidase: A potential mechanism for the hypolipidemic action of fibrates. J Clin Invest 1995;95: 705–712.

103. Masucci-Magoulas L, Goldberg IJ, Bisgaier CL, et al: A mouse model with features of familial combined hyperlipidemia. Science 1997;275:391–394.

104. Pennacchio LA, Olivier M, Hubacek JA, et al: An apolipoprotein influencing triglycerides in humans and mice revealed by comparative sequencing. Science 2001;294:169–173.

105. Aouizerat BE, Allayee H, Cantor RM, et al: Linkage of candidate gene locus to familial combined hyperlipidemia–lecithin-cholesterol acyltransferase on 16q. Arterioscler Thromb Vasc Biol 1999;19:2730–2736.

106. Nevin DN, Brunzell JD, Deeb SS: The LPL gene in individuals with familial combined hyperlipidemia and decreased LPL activity. Arterioscler Throm Vasc Biol 1994;14:869–873.

107. Reymer PWA, Groenemeyer BE, Gagné E, et al: A frequently occurring mutation in the lipoprotein lipase gene (Asn291Ser) contributes to the expression of familial combined hyperlipidemia. Hum Mol Gen 1995;4:1543–1549.

108. Allayee H, Dominguez KM, Aouizerat BE, et al: Contribution of the hepatic lipase gene to the atherogenic lipoprotein phenotype in familial combined hyperlipidemia. J Lipid Res 2000;41: 245–252.

109. Deeb SS, Fajas L, Nemoto M, et al: A Pro12Ala substitution in PPARg2 associated with decreased receptor activity, lower body mass index and improved insulin sensitivity. Nat Genet 1998;20:284–287.

110. Pihlajamäki J, Miettinen R, Valve R, et al: The Pro12Ala substitution in the peroxisome proliferator activated receptor gamma 2 is associated with an insulin-sensitive phenotype in families with familial combined hyperlipidemia and in nondiabetic elderly subjects with dyslipidemia. Atherosclerosis 2000;151: 567–574.

111. Geurts JM, Janssen RG, van Greevenbroek MM, et al: Identification of TNFRSF1B as a novel modifier gene in familial combined hyperlipidemia. Hum Mol Genet 2000;9:2067–2074.

112. Pajukanta P, Nuotio I, Terwilliger JD, et al: Linkage of familial combined hyperlipidaemia to chromosome 1q21-1q23. Nat Genet 1998;18:369–373.

113. Pajukanta P, Bodnar JS, Sallinen R, et al: Fine mapping of Hyplip1 and the human homolog, a potential locus for FCHL. Mamm Genome 2001;12:238–245.

114. Austin MA, Edwards KL: Small, dense low density lipoproteins, the insulin resistance syndrome and noninsulin-dependent diabetes. Curr Opin Lipidol 1996;7:167–171.

115. Austin MA, Stephens K, Walden CE, et al: Linkage analysis of candidate genes and the small, dense low-density lipoprotein phenotype. Atherosclerosis 1999;142:79–87.

116. Wahli W, Braissant O, Desvergne B: Peroxisome proliferator activated receptors: Transcriptional regulators of adipogenesis, lipid metabolism and more. Chem Biol 1995;2:261–266.

117. Ascaso JF, Lorente R, Merchante A, et al: Insulin resistance in patients with familial combined hyperlipidemia and coronary artery disease. Am J Cardiol 1997;80:1484–1487.

118. Purnell JQ, Kahn SE, Schwartz RS, et al: Relationship of insulin sensitivity and apoB levels to intra-abdominal fat in subjects with familial combined hyperlipidemia. Arterioscler Thromb Vasc Biol 2001;21:567–572.

119. Grundy SM: Hypertriglyceridemia, insulin resistance, and the metabolic syndrome. Am J Cardiol 1999;13:25F–29F.

120. Bolibar I, von Eckardstein A, Assmann G, et al: Short-term prognostic value of lipid measurements for coronary events in patients with angina pectoris. Thromb Haemost 2000;84: 955–961.

121. Rubins HB, Robins SJ, Collins D, et al: Gemfibrozil for the secondary prevention of coronary heart disease in men with low levels of high-density lipoprotein cholesterol: Veterans Affairs High-Density Lipoprotein Cholesterol Intervention Trial Study Group. N Engl J Med 1999;341:410–418.

122. Rust S, Rosier M, Funke H: Tangier disease is caused by mutations in the gene encoding ATP-binding cassette transporter 1. Nat Genet 1999;22:352–355.

123. Bodzioch M, Orso E, Klucken J, et al: The gene encoding ATP-binding cassette transporter 1 is mutated in Tangier disease. Nat Genet 1999;22:347–351.

124. Brooks-Wilson A, Marcil M, Clee SM, et al: Mutations in ABC1 in Tangier disease and familial high-density lipoprotein deficiency. Nat Genet 1999;22:336–345.

125. Lawn RM, Wade DP, Garvin MR, et al: The Tangier disease gene product ABC1 controls the cellular apolipoprotein-mediated lipid removal pathway. J Clin Invest 1999;104:R25–R31.

126. Clee SM, Kastelein JJ, van Dam M, et al: Age and residual cholesterol efflux affect HDL cholesterol levels and coronary artery disease in ABCA1 heterozygotes. J Clin Invest 2000;106:1263–1270.

127. Kuivenhoven JA, Pritchard H, Hill J, et al: The molecular pathology of lecithin:cholesterol acyltransferase (LCAT) deficiency syndromes. J Lipid Res 1997;38:191–205.

128. Dietschy JM, Turley SD: Cholesterol metabolism in the brain. Curr Opin Lipidol 2001;12:105–112.

129. Osgood-McWeeney D, Galluzzi JR, Ordovas JM: Allelic discrimination for single nucleotide polymorphisms in the human scavenger receptor class B type 1 gene locus using fluorescent probes. Clin Chem 2000;46:118–119.

130. Cohen JC, Wang Z, Grundy SM, et al: Variation at the hepatic lipase and apolipoprotein A1/CIII/AIV loci is a major cause of genetically determined variation in plasma HDL cholesterol levels. J Clin Invest 1994;94:2377–2384.

131. Rosset J, Wang J, Wolfe BM, et al: Lecithin:cholesterol acyl transferase G30S: Association with atherosclerosis, hypoalphalipoproteinemia and reduced in vivo enzyme activity. Clin Biochem 2001;34:381–386.

132. Hegele RA, Cao H, Harris SB, et al: The hepatocyte nuclear factor-1 alpha G319S variant is associated with early-onset type 2 diabetes in Canadian Oji-Cree. J Clin Endocrinol Metab 1999;84:1077–1082.

133. Klos KL, Kardia SL, Ferrell RE, et al: Genome-wide linkage analysis reveals evidence of multiple regions that influence variation in plasma lipid and apolipoprotein levels associated with risk of coronary heart disease. Arterioscler Thromb Vasc Biol 2001;21:971–978.

134. James RW, Glatter Garin MC, Calabresi L, et al: Modulated serum activities and concentrations of paraoxonase in high density lipoprotein deficiency states. Atherosclerosis 1998;139:77–82.

135. Lusis AJ: Atherosclerosis. Nature 2000;407:233–241.

136. Tall AR, Jiang XC, Luo Y, et al: 1999 George Lyman Duff memorial lecture: Lipid transfer proteins, HDL metabolism, and atherogenesis. Arterioscler Thromb Vasc Biol 2000;20:1185–1188.

137. Huszar D, Varban ML, Rinninger F, et al: Increased LDL cholesterol and atherosclerosis in LDL receptor-deficient mice with attenuated expression of scavenger receptor B1. Arterioscler Thromb Vasc Biol 2000;20:1068–1073.

138. Zhong S, Sharp DS, Grove JS, et al: Increased coronary heart disease in Japanese-American men with mutations in the cholesteryl ester transfer protein gene despite increased HDL levels. J Clin Invest 1996;97:2917–2923.

139. Sirtori CR, Calabresi L, Franceschini G, et al: Cardiovascular status of carriers of the apolipoprotein A-1Milano mutant: The Limone sul Garda Study. Circulation 2001;103:1949–1954.

140. Francheschini G, Calabresi L, Chiesa G, et al: Increased cholesterol efflux potential of sera from apoA-1 Milano carriers and transgenic mice. Arterioscler Thromb Vasc Biol 1999;19:1257–1262.

141. Mahley RW, Huang Y, Rall SC Jr: Pathogenesis of type III hyperlipoproteinemia (dysbetalipoproteinemia): Questions, quandaries, and paradoxes. J Lipid Res 1999;40:1933–1949.

142. Plump AS, Smith JD, Hayek T, et al: Severe hypercholesterolemia and atherosclerosis in apolipoprotein E-deficient mice created by homologous recombination in ES cells. Cell 1992;71:343–353.

143. Utermann G: The mysteries of lipoprotein(a). Science 1989;246:904–910.

144. Danesh J, Collins R, Peto R: Lipoprotein(a) and coronary artery disease: Metanalysis of prospective studies. Circulation 2000;102:1082–1085.

145. von Eckardstein A, Schulte H, Cullen P, et al: Lipoprotein(a) further increases the risk of coronary events in men with high global cardiovascular risk. J Am Coll Cardiol 2001;37:434–439.

146. Seed M, Ayres KL, Humphries SE, et al: Lipoprotein(a) as a predictor of myocardial infarction in middle-aged men. Am J Med 2001;110:22–27.

147. Boerwinkle E, Leffert CC, Lin J, et al: Apolipoprotein(a) gene accounts for greater than 90% of the variation in plasma lipoprotein(a) concentrations. J Clin Invest 1992;90:52–60.

148. Mooser V, Sheer D, Marcovina SM, et al: The apo(a) gene is the major determinant of variation in plasma Lp(a) levels in African-Americans. Am J Hum Gen 1997;61:402–417.

149. McLean JW, Tomlinson JE, Kuang WJ, et al: cDNA sequence of human apolipoprotein(a) is homologous to plasminogen. Nature 1987;330:132–137.

150. Mooser V, Mancini FP, Bopp S, et al: Sequence polymorphism in the apo(a) gene associated with specific levels of Lp(a) in plasma. Hum Mol Gen 1995;4:173–181.

151. Ogorelkova M, Gruber A, Utermann G: Molecular basis of congenital Lp(a) deficiency: A frequent apo(a) "null" mutation in Caucasians. Hum Mol Genet 1999;8:2087–2096.

152. Kronenberg F, Konig P, Neyer U, et al: Multicenter study of lipoprotein(a) and apolipoprotein(a) phenotypes in patients with end-stage renal disease treated by hemodialysis or continuous ambulatory peritoneal dialysis. J Am Soc Nephrol 1995;6:110–120.

153. Doucet C, Mooser V, Gonbert S, et al: Lipoprotein(a) in the nephrotic syndrome: Molecular analysis of lipoprotein(a) and apolipoprotein(a) fragments in plasma and urine. J Am Soc Nephrol 2000;11:507–513.

154. Slunga L, Johnson O, Dahlen GH, et al: Lipoprotein(a) and acute-phase proteins in acute myocardial infarction. Scand J Clin Invest 1992;52:95–101.

155. Mooser V, Berger MM, Tappy L, et al: Major reduction in plasma Lp(a) levels during sepsis and burns. Arterioscler Thromb Vasc Biol 2000;20:1137–1142.

156. Sangrar W, Koschinsky ML: Characterization of the interaction of recombinant apolipoprotein(a) with modified fibrinogen surfaces and fibrin clots. Biochem Cell Biol 2000;78:519–525.

157. Soulat T, Loyau S, Baudouin V, et al: Effect of individual plasma lipoprotein(a) variations in vivo on its competition with plasminogen for fibrin and cell binding: An in vitro study using plasma from children with idiopathic nephrotic syndrome. Arterioscler Thromb Vasc Biol 2000;20:575–584.

158. Busso N, Dudler J, Salvi R, et al: Plasma apolipoprotein(a) co-deposits with fibrin in inflammatory arthritic joints. Am J Pathol 2001;159:1445–1453.

159. Nowak-Göttl U, Junker R, Hartmeier M, et al: Increased lipoprotein(a) is an important risk factor for venous thromboembolism in childhood. Circulation 1999;100:743–748.

160. Fan J, Shimoyamada H, Sun H, et al: Transgenic rabbits expressing human apolipoprotein(a) develop more extensive atherosclerotic lesions in response to a cholesterol-rich diet. Arterioscler Thromb Vasc Biol 2001;21:88–94.

161. Sanan DA, Newland DL, Tao R, et al: Low density lipoprotein receptor-negative mice expressing human apolipoprotein B-100 develop complex atherosclerotic lesions on a chow diet: No accentuation by apolipoprotein(a). Proc Natl Acad Sci USA 1998;95:4544–4549.

162. Hobbs HH, White AL: Lipoprotein(a): Intrigues and insights. Curr Opin Lipidol 1999;10:225–236.

163. Tsimikas S, Bergmark C, Beyer RW, et al. Temporal increases in plasma markers of oxidized low-density lipoprotein strongly reflect the presence of acute coronary syndromes. J Am Coll Cardiol. 2003;41:360–370.

164. Dangas G, Mehran R, Harpel PC, et al: Lipoprotein(a) and inflammation in human coronary atheroma: Association with the severity of clinical presentation. J Am Coll Cardiol 1998;32:2035–2042.

165. Kronenberg F, Kronenberg MF, Kiechl S, et al: Role of lipoprotein(a) and apolipoprotein(a) phenotype in atherogenesis: Prospective results from the Bruneck study. Circulation 1999;100:1154–1160.

166. Foody JM, Milberg JA, Robinson K, et al: Homocysteine and lipoprotein(a) interact to increase CAD risk in young men and women. Arterioscler Thromb Vasc Biol 2000;20:493–499.

167. Kronenberg F, Neyer U, Lhotta K, et al: The low molecular weight apo(a) phenotype is an independent predictor for coronary artery disease in hemodialysis patients: A prospective follow-up. J Am Soc Nephrol 1999;10:1027–1036.

168. Mooser V, Helbecque N, Miklossy J, et al: Interactions between apolipoprotein E and apolipoprotein(a) in patients with late-onset Alzheimer disease. Ann Intern Med 2000;132:533–537.

169. Bkorkhem I, Boberg KM: Inborn errors in bile acid biosynthesis and storage of sterols other than cholesterol. In Scriver CR,

Beaudet AL, Sly WS, Valle D (eds): The Metabolic Basis of Inherited Disease. New York: McGraw Hill, 1995, pp 2073-2102.

170. Lu K, Lee MH, Hazard S, et al: Two genes that map to the STSL locus cause sitosterolemia: Genomic structure and spectrum of mutations involving sterolin-1 and sterolin-2, encoded by ABCG5 and ABCG8, respectively. Am J Hum Genet 2001;69: 278-290.

171. Superko HR, Krauss RM: Coronary artery disease regression: Convincing evidence for the benefit of aggressive lipoprotein management. Circulation 1994;90:1056-1069.

172. Libby P: Molecular bases of the acute coronary syndromes: Circulation 1995;91:2844-2850.

173. Shepherd J, Cobbe SM, Ford I, et al: Prevention of coronary heart disease with pravastatin in men with hypercholesterolemia. West of Scotland Coronary Prevention Study Group. N Engl J Med 1995;333:1301-1307.

174. Downs JR, Clearfield M, Weis S, et al: Primary prevention of acute coronary events with lovastatin in men and women with average cholesterol levels: Results of AFCAPS/TexCAPS. Air Force/Texas Coronary Atherosclerosis Prevention Study. JAMA 1998;279: 1615-1622.

175. Randomised trial of cholesterol lowering in 4444 patients with coronary heart disease: The Scandinavian Simvastatin Survival Study (4S). Lancet 1994;344:1383-1389.

176. Sacks FM, Pfeffer MA, Moye LA, et al: The effect of pravastatin on coronary events after myocardial infarction in patients with average cholesterol levels: Cholesterol and Recurrent Events Trial investigators. N Engl J Med 1996;335:1001-1009.

177. Prevention of cardiovascular events and death with pravastatin in patients with coronary heart disease and a broad range of initial cholesterol levels: The Long-Term Intervention with Pravastatin in Ischaemic Disease (LIPID) Study Group. N Engl J Med 1998;339:1349-1357.

178. MRC/BHF Heart Protection Study of cholesterol lowering with simvastatin in 20536 high-risk individuals: A randomised placebo-controlled trial. Lancet. 2002;360:7-22.

179. Small DM: George Lyman Duff Memorial Lecture: Progression and regression of atherosclerotic lesions. Arteriosclerosis 1988; 103-129.

180. Aikawa M, Rabkin E, Sugiyama S, et al: An HMG-CoA reductase inhibitor, cerivastatin, suppresses growth of macrophages expressing matrix metalloproteinases and tissue factor in vivo and in vitro. Circulation 2001;103:276-283.

181. Takemoto M, Liao JK: Pleiotropic effects of 3-hydroxy-3-methylglutaryl coenzyme A reductase inhibitors. Arterioscler Thromb Vasc Biol 2001;21:1712-1719.

182. Zhang FL, Casey PJ: Protein prenylation: Molecular mechanisms and functional consequences. Annu Rev Biochem 1996;65: 241-269.

183. Wagner AH, Kohler T, Ruckschloss U, et al: Improvement of nitric oxide-dependent vasodilation by HMG-CoA reductase inhibitors through attenuation of endothelial superoxide anion formation. Arterioscler Thromb Vasc Biol 2000;20:61-69.

184. Davis ME, Harrison DG: Cracking down on caveolin: Role of 3-hydroxy-3-methylglutaryl coenzyme A reductase inhibitors in modulating endothelial cell nitric oxide production. Circulation 2001;103:2-4.

185. Hernandez-Perera O, Perez-Sala D, Soria E, et al: Involvement of Rho GTPases in the transcriptional inhibition of preproendothelin-1 gene expression by simvastatin in vascular endothelial cells. Circ Res 2000;87:616-622.

186. Feron O, Dessy C, Desager JP, et al: Hydroxy-methylglutaryl-coenzyme A reductase inhibition promotes endothelial nitric oxide synthase activation through A decrease in caveolin abundance. Circulation 2001;103:113-118.

187. Endres M, Namura S, Shimizu-Sasamata M, et al: Attenuation of delayed neuronal death after mild focal ischemia in mice by inhibition of the caspase family. J Cereb Blood Flow Metab 1998;18:238-247.

188. Palinski W: Immunomodulation: A new role for statins? Nat Med 2000;6:1311-1312.

189. Palinski W: New evidence for beneficial effects of statins unrelated to lipid lowering. Arterioscler Thromb Vasc Biol 2001;21:3-5.

190. Kwak B, Mulhaupt F, Myit S, et al: Statins as a newly recognized type of immunomodulator. Nat Med 2000;6:1399-1402.

191. Sparrow CP, Burton CA, Hernandez M, et al: Simvastatin has anti-inflammatory and antiatherosclerotic activities independent of plasma cholesterol lowering. Arterioscler Thromb Vasc Biol 2001;21:115-121.

192. Romano M, Diomede L, Sironi M, et al: Inhibition of monocyte chemotactic protein-1 synthesis by statins. Lab Invest 2000;80: 1095-1100.

193. Guijarro C, Blanco-Colio LM, Ortego M, et al: 3-Hydroxy-3-methyl-glutaryl coenzyme a reductase and isoprenylation inhibitors induce apoptosis of vascular smooth muscle cells in culture. Circ Res 1998;83:490-500.

194. Laufs U, Marra D, Node K, et al: 3-Hydroxy-3-methylglutaryl-CoA reductase inhibitors attenuate vascular smooth muscle proliferation by preventing rho GTPase-induced down-regulation of p27(Kip1). J Biol Chem 1999;274:21926-21931.

195. Indolfi C, Cioppa A, Stabile E, et al: Effects of hydroxymethylglutaryl coenzyme A reductase inhibitor simvastatin on smooth muscle cell proliferation in vitro and neointimal formation in vivo after vascular injury. J Am Coll Cardiol 2000;35:214-221.

196. Essig M, Nguyen G, Prie D, et al: 3-Hydroxy-3-methylglutaryl coenzyme A reductase inhibitors increase fibrinolytic activity in rat aortic endothelial cells: Role of geranylgeranylation and Rho proteins. Circ Res 1998;83:683-690.

197. Angelin B, Einarsson K, Hellstrom K, et al: Bile acid kinetics in relation to endogenous tryglyceride metabolism in various types of hyperlipoproteinemia. J Lipid Res 1978;19:1004-1016.

198. Yoshida H, Ishikawa T, Ayaori M, et al: Beneficial effect of gemfibrozil on the chemical composition and oxidative susceptibility of low density lipoprotein: A randomized, double-blind, placebo-controlled study. Atherosclerosis 1998;139:179-187.

199. Staels B, Dallongeville J, Auwerx J, et al: Mechanism of action of fibrates on lipid and lipoprotein metabolism. Circulation 1998;98:2088-2093.

200. Auwerx J, Schoonjans K, Fruchart JC, et al: Transcriptional control of triglyceride metabolism: Fibrates and fatty acids change the expression of the LPL and apo C-III genes by activating the nuclear receptor PPAR. Atherosclerosis 1996;124 (Suppl):S29-S37.

201. Frick MH, Syvanne M, Nieminen MS, et al: Prevention of the angiographic progression of coronary and vein-graft atherosclerosis by gemfibrozil after coronary bypass surgery in men with Low levels of HDL cholesterol. Circulation 1997;96:2137-2143.

202. Manninen V, Elo MO, Frick MH, et al: Lipid alterations and decline in the incidence of coronary heart disease in the Helsinki Heart Study. JAMA 1988;260:641-651.

203. Knopp RH, Alagona P, Davidson M, et al: Equivalent efficacy of a time-release form of niacin (Niaspan) given once-a-night versus plain niacin in the management of hyperlipidemia. Metabolism 1998;47:1097-1104.

204. Knopp RH, Ginsberg J, Albers JJ, et al: Contrasting effects of unmodified and time-release forms of niacin on lipoproteins in hyperlipidemic subjects: Clues to mechanism of action of niacin. Metabolism 1985;34:642-650.

205. Grundy SM, Mok HY, Zech L, et al: Influence of nicotinic acid on metabolism of cholesterol and triglycerides in man. J Lipid Res 1981;22:24-36.

206. Canner PL, Berge KG, Wenger NK, et al: Fifteen year mortality in Coronary Drug Project patients: Long-term benefit with niacin. J Am Coll Cardiol 1986;8:1245-1255.

207. Blankenhorn DH, Nessim SA, Johnson RL, et al: Beneficial effects of combined colestipol-niacin therapy on coronary atherosclerosis and coronary venous bypass grafts. JAMA 1987; 257:3233-3240.

208. Brown BG, Zhao XQ, Chait A, et al: Simvastatin and niacin, antioxidant vitamins, or the combination for the prevention of coronary disease. N Engl J Med 2001;345:1583-1592.

209. Brown BG, Albers JJ, Fisher LD, et al: Regression of coronary artery disease as a result of intensive lipid-lowering therapy in men with high levels of apolipoprotein B. N Engl J Med 1990; 323:1289-1298.

210. Bays HE, Moore PB, Drehobl MA, et al: Effectiveness and tolerability of ezetimibe in patients with primary hypercholesterolemia:

Pooled analysis of two phase II studies. Clin Ther 2001;23:1209-1230.

211. Davis HR Jr, Pula KK, Alton KB, et al: The synergistic hypocholesterolemic activity of the potent cholesterol absorption inhibitor, ezetimibe, in combination with 3-hydroxy-3-methylglutaryl coenzyme a reductase inhibitors in dogs. Metabolism 2001;50:1234-1241.

212. Davis HR Jr, Compton DS, Hoos L, et al: Ezetimibe, a potent cholesterol absorption inhibitor, inhibits the development of atherosclerosis in apoE knockout mice. Arterioscler Thromb Vasc Biol 2001;21:2032-2038.

213. Ballantyne CM, Houri J, Notarbartolo A, et al: Effect of ezetimibe coadministered with atorvastatin in 628 patients with primary hypercholesterolemia: A prospective, randomized, double-blind trial. Circulation 2003;107:2409-2415.

214. Davidson MH, McGarry T, Bettis R et al. Ezetimibe coadministered with simvastatin in patients with primary hypercholesterolemia. J Am Coll Cardiol. 2002;40:2125-2134.

215. Depairon M, Chessex S, Sudre P, et al: Premature atherosclerosis in HIV-infected individuals–focus on protease inhibitor therapy. AIDS 2001;15:329-334.

216. Stein JH, Klein MA, Bellehumeur JL, et al: Use of human immunodeficiency virus-1 protease inhibitors is associated with atherogenic lipoprotein changes and endothelial dysfunction. Circulation 2001;104:257-262.

217. Periard D, Telenti A, Sudre P, et al: Atherogenic dyslipidemia in HIV-infected individuals treated with protease inhibitors: The Swiss HIV Cohort Study. Circulation 1999;100:700-705.

218. Mooser V, Carr A: Antiretroviral therapy-associated hyperlipidaemia in HIV disease. Curr Opin Lipidol 2001;12:313-319.

219. Fauvel J, Bonnet E, Ruidavets JB, et al: An interaction between apo C-III variants and protease inhibitors contributes to high triglyceride/low HDL levels in treated HIV patients. AIDS 2001;15:2397-2406.

220. Hoogeveen RC, Ballantyne CM, Pownall HJ, et al: Effect of sirolimus on the metabolism of apob100-containing lipoproteins in renal transplant patients. Transplantation 2001;72:1244-1250.

## EDITOR'S CHOICE

Berge KE, Tian H, Graf GA, et al: Accumulation of dietary cholesterol in sitosterolemia caused by mutations in adjacent ABC transporters. Science 2000;290:1771-1775.
*New pathway for cholesterol regulation uncovered by rare monogenic huma disorder.*
Bodnar JS, Chatterjee A, Castellani LW, et al: Positional cloning of the combined hyperlipidemia gene Hyplip1. Nat Genet 2002;30:110-116.
*New genetic link to hyperlipidemia.*
Bodzioch M, Orso E, Klucken J, et al: The gene encoding ATP-binding cassette transporter 1 is mutated in Tangier disease. Nat Genet 1999;22:347-351.
*First description of role of ABC transporters in atherogenesis.*
Brooks-Wilson A, Marcil M, Clee SM, et al: Mutations in ABC1 in Tangier disease and familial high-density lipoprotein deficiency. Nat Genet 1999;22:336-345.
*Companion paper by independent scientists to Bodzioch et al.*

Downes M, Verdecia MA, Roecker AJ, et al: A chemical, genetic, and structural analysis of the nuclear bile acid receptor FXR. Mol Cell 2003;11:1079-1092.
*A beautiful study of a nuclear hormone receptor that controls bile acid metabolism; likely to become a new therapeutic target for atherogenesis.*
Garcia CK, Wilund K, Arca M, et al: Autosomal recessive hypercholesterolemia caused by mutations in a putative LDL receptor adaptor protein. Science 2001;292:1394-1398.
*Uncovering the protein complexes that interact with lipoprotein receptors is leading to new clinical and scientific insight into atherogenesis.*
Goodwin B, Jones SA, Price RR, et al: A regulatory cascade of the nuclear receptors FXR, SHP-1, and LRH-1 represses bile acid biosynthesis. Mol Cell 2000;6:517-526.
*The FXR pathway and bile acid synthesis; new therapeutic approaches to regulating bile acid secretion could be in the offing.*
Hobbs HH, Graf GA, Yu L, et al: Genetic defenses against hypercholesterolemia. Cold Spring Harb Symp Quant Biol 2002;67:499-505.
Janowski BA, Willy PJ, Devi TR, et al: An oxysterol signalling pathway mediated by the nuclear receptor LXR alpha. Nature 1996;383:728-731.
*The de-orphanizing of LXR.*
Lu TT, Makishima M, Repa JJ, et al: Molecular basis for feedback regulation of bile acid synthesis by nuclear receptors. Mol Cell 2000;6:507-515.
*Nuclear hormone receptors have evolved a pivotal role in bile acid metabolism.*
Mi LZ, Devarakonda S, Harp JM, et al: Structural basis for bile acid binding and activation of the nuclear receptor FXR. Mol Cell 2003;11:1093-1100.
*Structural advances pave the way for rationale drug design in the FXR story.*
Rader DJ, Cohen J, Hobbs HH: Monogenic hypercholesterolemia: New insights in pathogenesis and treatment. J Clin Invest 2003;111:1795-1803.
*Excellent recent review highlights new insights.*
Rust S, Rosier M, Funke H, et al: Tangier disease is caused by mutations in the gene encoding ATP-binding cassette transporter 1. Nat Genet 1999;22:352-355.
*Companion paper from independent lab to the Bodzioch et paper.*
Shih DQ, Bussen M, Sehayek E, et al: Hepatocyte nuclear factor-1 alpha is an essential regulator of bile acid and plasma cholesterol metabolism. Nat Genet 2001;27:375-382.
*HNF pathways intersect with cholesterol metabolism.*
Sinal CJ, Tohkin M, Miyata M, et al: Targeted disruption of the nuclear receptor FXR/BAR impairs bile acid and lipid homeostasis. Cell 2000;102:731-744.
*Closes the loop on fingering FXR in bile acid metabolism in vivo.*
Tunaru S, Kero J, Schaub A, et al: PUMA-G and HM74 are receptors for nicotinic acid and mediate its anti-lipolytic effect. Nat Med 2003;9:352-355.
*The discovery of the nicotinic acid receptor provides direct molecular target for second generation agents with fewer problematic clinical side effects.*
Wang H, Chen J, Hollister K, et al: Endogenous bile acids are ligands for the nuclear receptor FXR/BAR. Mol Cell 1999;3:543-553.
*Independent work supporting pivotal role of FXR in bile acid metabolism.*

# chapter 22

# Lipoprotein Oxidation, Macrophages, Immunity, and Atherogenesis

*Sotirios Tsimikas*
*Christopher K. Glass*
*Daniel Steinberg*
*Joseph L. Witztum*

## NATURAL HISTORY OF THE ATHEROSCLEROTIC LESION

The earliest visible atherosclerotic lesion is the fatty streak, a lesion that occurs under an intact monolayer of endothelial cells. It consists primarily of an accumulation of cholesteryl ester-laden cells, mostly derived from circulating monocytes that have penetrated through the endothelial layer, but also derived from modified smooth muscle cells. This lesion, itself clinically silent, is now accepted to be the precursor of the more advanced lesions, which go on to become the sites of thrombosis. Consequently there is great interest in identifying the initiating factors that give rise to the fatty streak. Presumably, prevention of fatty streak formation would prevent the appearance of later lesions and of the clinical sequelae. The schema shown in Figure 22-1 summarizes the current consensus on the key processes contributing to the generation of the fatty streak. A more detailed discussion of inflammatory pathways and their relationship to atherosclerosis can be found in Chapter 20. This chapter deals primarily with the oxidative modification hypothesis of atherogenesis, that is, the hypothesis that LDL oxidation plays a quantitatively important role in the disease.[1] We also discuss the interrelated roles of the macrophage and the immune system.

As a disease that is almost always clinically silent until the fifth or sixth decade, atherosclerosis cannot exert any significant genetic pressure. Hypercholesterolemia and atherosclerosis have little or no effect on the ability to procreate. Thus, it makes no sense to expect that genes that might protect against atherosclerosis would be "selected." Teleologic thinking is out of place when discussing atherogenesis. To be sure, there are "good" genes and there are "bad" genes regulating lipoprotein metabolism and controlling the vascular responses to hypercholesterolemia, hypertension, and other factors that relate to atherogenesis. However, those genes are "good" or "bad" by chance, not by selection. This point is particularly important when thinking about the function of receptors for oxidatively modified LDL. It is also important when thinking about the many adhesion molecules, chemokines, inflammatory cytokines, and growth factors that contribute to the evolution of the atherosclerotic plaque.

## LDL PARADOX

The most compelling evidence that hypercholesterolemia can be in itself a sufficient cause for atherosclerosis is the remarkably premature disease in patients with the homozygous form of familial hypercholesterolemia (HFH).[2] These patients, with LDL cholesterol levels of 600 to 800 mg/dL, can have myocardial infarctions before age 10 and most have their first infarction before age 20. This is a monogenic disorder and, therefore, all of the phenotypic expression must ultimately be traceable to the direct or indirect effects of a single malfunctioning gene. The landmark studies of Drs. Joseph L. Goldstein and Michael S. Brown established that the affected gene encoded the LDL receptor, a membrane protein to which LDL binds with high affinity and which leads to its internalization and degradation within the cell.[3] Because patients with HFH have no LDL receptors at all or very few of them, the accumulation of cholesterol in their subcutaneous and tendon xanthomas and in their arterial lesions must be occurring by some pathway other than the LDL receptor pathway. However, their circulating LDL, although it does show some relatively minor differences in structure from that of normal LDL, behaves metabolically very much like LDL from normal subjects. Indeed, transfused into a normal subject it disappears from the plasma compartment at exactly the same rate as the endogenous normal LDL of the recipient.[4] Therefore, one is forced to conclude that the buildup of cholesterol in foam cells in these patients is not due to uptake of LDL by way of the native LDL receptor.

The second paradox is that incubation of monocytes and macrophages with native LDL *in vitro* does not lead to accumulation of cholesterol.[5] Even in the presence of very high concentrations of LDL in the medium, the monocyte or macrophage will only increase its cell cholesterol content by 20% or so. The same is true for smooth muscle cells.[6] Thus, one cannot

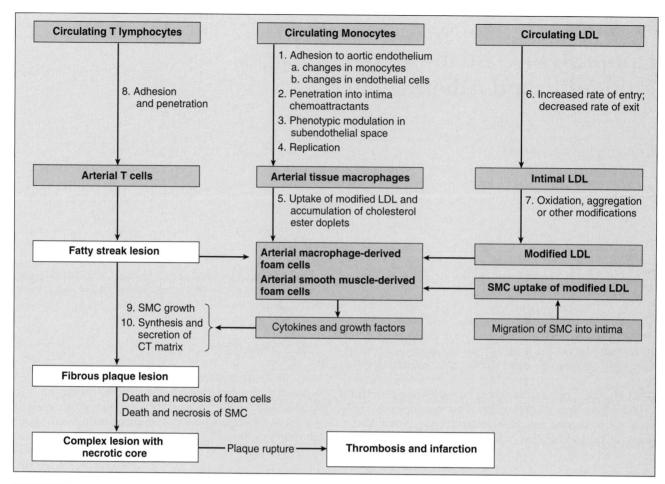

**FIGURE 22-1.** Proposed scheme of how hypercholesterolemia induces atherosclerosis. *(From Steinberg D: Oxidative modification of LDL and atherogenesis. Circulation 1997;9S:1062–1071.)*

explain the origin of either monocyte-derived or smooth muscle cell-derived foam cells on the basis of the uptake of native LDL.

One way to resolve the paradox would be to postulate that the structure of LDL must somehow be modified *in vivo* and that the modified form of LDL is what gave rise to foam cells (Fig. 22-2). Goldstein et al.[5] showed that treatment of LDL *in vitro* with acetic anhydride, such that a significant fraction of the lysine residues of apoB were modified, generated a modified form of LDL that was indeed taken up several times more rapidly than native LDL by cultured macrophages and taken up by way of a specific, saturable receptor, which they called the "acetyl LDL receptor." Moreover, unlike the LDL receptor, which downregulates as the cell cholesterol content increases, the acetyl LDL receptor was not downregulated, but continued to be fully active even as the cell cholesterol content increased markedly. Monocytes and macrophages from patients lacking the LDL receptor expressed normal levels of this new receptor. Studies by Kodama et al.[7] resulted in the cloning and sequencing of the acetyl LDL receptor, which was redesignated the scavenger receptor type A (SR-A). Acetoacetylation or conjugation with malondialdehyde (MDA) also generated modified LDLs

recognized by the acetyl LDL receptor or SR-A.[8,9] However, it seems unlikely that any of these chemically modified forms can be generated in any quantity under *in vivo* conditions. *In vitro*, MDA-LDL can be generated by platelets undergoing aggregation,[8,9] but the concentrations of MDA needed to generate MDA-LDL are likely to be much higher than those that would be achieved *in vivo* during platelet aggregation. So the question became: "What modifications can occur that are biologically plausible that would convert native LDL to a form recognized by the macrophage and taken up at a sufficiently high rate to account for foam cell formation?" In 1981 Henriksen et al.[10] reported that overnight incubation of LDL with a cultured monolayer of endothelial cells induced a number of striking alterations in the properties of the LDL. These included an increase in the electrophoretic mobility, an increase in hydrated density, a decrease in phospholipid and cholesterol content, and most importantly a marked increase in the rate of uptake and degradation by mouse peritoneal macrophages. The binding and uptake of the modified LDL was competitively inhibited by unlabeled acetyl LDL (to the extent of about 60%) indicating that a large part of the uptake was by way of the acetyl LDL receptor and implying that

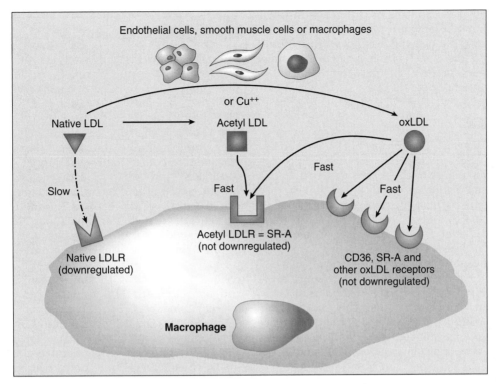

**FIGURE 22-2.** Mechanisms of OxLDL uptake by monocytes. Native LDL cannot induce foam cell formation because uptake is slow and because the LDL receptor downregulates. Either acetyl LDL or OxLDL can induce cholesterol accumulation in macrophages resulting in foam cell formation because uptake is rapid and the scavenger receptors do not downregulate in response to an increase in cellular cholesterol. (See color plate.) *(Reproduced with permission from Steinberg D: Atherogenesis in perspective: Hypercholesterolemia and inflammation as partners in crime. Nat Med 2002;8:1211–1217.)*

additional receptors must be involved. Similar changes could be induced by incubating the LDL with vascular smooth muscle cells[11] or peritoneal macrophages.[12,13] Later studies by Steinbrecher et al.[14] showed that all of these cell-induced changes are blocked by including an antioxidant such as vitamin E in the medium and that all of these changes could be reproduced by simply incubating the LDL with copper to catalyze nonenzymatic oxidation. Morel et al.[15] had previously observed that oxidatively modified LDL was cytotoxic for cultured endothelial cells and that antioxidants prevented generation of that cytotoxicity. Thus, oxidative modification of LDL seemed to be a biologically plausible way of changing its properties so that it could induce foam cell formation.

Any one of a large number of antioxidants can prevent copper-mediated or cell-induced oxidative modification of LDL *in vitro*. Even the addition of 5% or 10% serum into the medium is sufficient to protect LDL. Consequently there was understandable skepticism at first about the occurrence of oxidative modification under *in vivo* conditions. If only 5% or 10% serum (v/v) can inhibit, one would not expect oxidation *in vivo* when there are many antioxidants available at all times in plasma and, at a lesser but substantial concentration, in extracellular fluid. However, subsequent studies have provided ample evidence that oxidative modification *does* indeed occur *in vivo* (see the section on evidence that oxidation of LDL takes place *in vivo*).

## ALTERNATIVE WAYS TO ACCOUNT FOR FOAM CELL FORMATION

This chapter deals primarily with oxidative modification of LDL. However, it is important to recognize that there are a number of alternative mechanisms by which foam cells might be generated. None of these has been as extensively studied nor as well documented as oxidative modification, but it remains a possibility that one or more of these mechanisms could contribute as much as, or even more than, oxidative modification of LDL does.

### βVLDL and Other Lipoproteins Rich in Apoprotein E

βVLDL is a minor component of normal plasma but accumulates as a result of cholesterol feeding.[16] It has a density like that of VLDL but electrophoretic mobility like that of LDL, that is, beta mobility. Because of its high content of apoprotein E it shows a very high affinity for the LDL receptor, probably because each βVLDL contains several molecules of apoprotein E on its surface, and thus, one βVLDL can bind simultaneously to several LDL receptors.[17] βVLDL binds avidly to macrophages and is taken up at a sufficiently rapid rate to increase the cell cholesterol content.[18] Why the macrophage LDL receptor does not downregulate effectively to prevent this buildup of cholesterol is not clear. In any case, animals or patients with high levels of βVLDL might generate foam cells by way of the LDL receptor (although this has not been demonstrated *in vivo*). Uptake of βVLDL may occur via other receptors as well, such as LRP, perhaps assisted by binding of lipoprotein lipase (LPL).[19]

## Aggregated LDL

As shown by Khoo et al.[20] aggregates of LDL created by denaturation (vigorous mixing) are taken up by macrophages much more avidly than is native LDL and can lead to accumulation of intracellular cholesterol. This uptake occurs by phagocytosis, rather than endocytosis, and occurs by way of the native LDL receptor rather than the acetyl LDL receptor. Studies by Nievelstein et al.[21] using electron microscopy have demonstrated the presence of large aggregates of LDL in the matrix of the rabbit arterial intima soon after an intravenous injection of a large single bolus of LDL. Thus, it is quite conceivable that this mechanism plays a role in foam cell formation, but there is so far little direct evidence for its participation in the atherogenic process either in experimental animals or in humans.

## LDL-Autoantibody Immune Complexes

Complexes of LDL or of aggregated LDL with IgG antibodies are taken up by macrophages at a markedly increased rate.[22,23] This is partly because the complex can now be taken up both by way of the LDL receptor and by way of the Fc receptor and perhaps partly because the LDL is further aggregated in the presence of a sufficient concentration of antibody. Again, *in vivo* evidence is scanty.

## Complex Formation between LDL and Proteoglycans

LDL binds tightly to certain forms of proteoglycans.[24,25] Indeed this may in part account for the trapping of LDL in the matrix and the generation of aggregates discussed previously. In addition, LDL that has formed a complex with soluble forms of proteoglycan, and is then separated from it, is more susceptible to subsequent oxidative modification.[26] Complexes of LDL with dextran sulfate are taken up more avidly by the macrophage, and there may be a similar phenomenon involving sulfated matrix components.

## Enzymatically Modified LDL

A variety of modifications to LDL have been described that alter the LDL so that the enzyme-modified LDL has enhanced uptake by macrophages. Examples include sphingomyelinase and trypsin/cholesterol esterase induced modifications.[27,28] Whether these occur *in vivo* to an extent that promotes atherogenesis is unknown.

# MECHANISMS OF LDL OXIDATION

## Nonenzymatic Mechanisms

The LDL particle is exquisitely sensitive to oxidative damage. LDL stored in plasma is reasonably stable, but once it has been purified it begins to deteriorate rapidly. It was recognized very early that copper and other divalent cations were particularly dangerous and for that reason a chelating agent must be present whenever possible during the preparation of LDL.[29] Even very minute concentrations of copper or iron are able to catalyze rather rapid oxidative degradation. Both the protein and the lipid moieties undergo oxidative damage, and the overall process is enormously complex.

Each LDL particle contains about 700 molecules of phospholipids, 600 of free cholesterol, 1600 of cholesterol esters, 185 of triglycerides, and 1 of apoprotein B-100, which in turn is made of 4536 amino acid residues! Oxidation sufficient to make LDL a good ligand for the acetyl LDL receptor can be effected by overnight incubation in the presence of $5\mu M$ $Cu^{2+}$.[14] Oxidized LDL (OxLDL) produced in this way has undergone a number of fairly drastic changes. As much as 40% of the phosphatidylcholine has been degraded by oxidative attack on the polyunsaturated fatty acids (PUFAs) in the *sn*-2 position and has been converted to lysophosphatidylcholine. The hydrated density of the LDL particle increases markedly, in some cases even to a density as high as that of HDL. Fifty percent or even 75% of the PUFAs has been destroyed by attacks at the double bonds.[30,31] Finally, the apoprotein also undergoes drastic alteration, partly resulting from direct oxidative attack and partly because of conjugation of lipid fragments with the protein. The recognition of OxLDL by scavenger receptors probably depends in part on the generation of neoepitopes created by the masking of epsilon amino groups of lysine residues by aldehyde fragments generated from the PUFAs. This may explain why chemically acetylated LDL and biologically OxLDL are both recognized by the scavenger receptors, that is, in both cases the chemical changes include the masking of lysine amino groups and generation of neoepitopes.

Nonenzymatic oxidation catalyzed by $Cu^{2+}$ is believed to depend on the presence of lipid hydroperoxides in the starting material.[32] These hydroperoxides are degraded to peroxy radicals and alkoxy radicals by $Cu^{2+}$, and in turn those radicals can initiate a cyclic chain reaction that can generate many more hydroperoxides. The fatty acid side chains of cholesterol esters are susceptible to oxidative damage, and cholesterol's polycyclic sterol ring structure is also subject to oxidative attack. Further discussion of the chemical mechanisms involved are to be found in the excellent review by Esterbauer et al.[32] Incubation of LDL with $Cu^{2+}$ for even a few hours is sufficient to oxidize it to the point that it develops important new biologic properties.[33] This form of LDL, designated mm-LDL or "minimally OxLDL," is still recognized by the LDL receptor, and at this stage of oxidation it is not a ligand for the scavenger receptors.[33,34] *In vitro* experiments have indicated a large number of biologic properties that could in principle make it proatherogenic, as discussed later.

From the previous discussion it is clear that there exists a broad spectrum of forms of "OxLDL" with widely differing structures.[35] Thus, the term "*OxLDL*" by no means designates a specific or homogenous molecular form. The complexity of the LDL particle is so great that there has been no attempt yet to classify "OxLDLs" more narrowly. For the present, perhaps the best that can be done is to specify as carefully as possible the conditions under which a given preparation was made and to describe its biologic properties.

## Enzymatic and Cell-mediated Mechanisms

Incubation of LDL with any of several cell types *in vitro* accelerates its oxidative modification. Included among these are endothelial cells, smooth muscle cells, and monocytes and macrophages, that is, all of the cell types that are found in an atherosclerotic lesion. However, a number of other cell types can also oxidize LDL *in vitro*, including neutrophils and fibroblasts. Thus, there is good reason to believe that LDL is oxidized not only within the artery wall but also at other sites, particularly at sites of inflammation.[36]

There are also many postulated mechanisms by which LDL could become oxidized within the artery wall. One mechanism that has gained strong support is that the enzyme 12/15-lipoxygenase (LO) initiates the "seeding" of LDL in the tissue fluids with hydroperoxides, leading to the subsequent initiation of lipid peroxidation and the changes that render OxLDL proinflammatory and lead to its subsequent enhanced uptake by macrophages. Evidence to support this hypothesis includes the observations that incubation of LDL with isolated soybean LO leads to oxidation of LDL[37]; that inhibitors of macrophage 12/15-LO decrease the ability of macrophages to initiate oxidation of LDL[38]; and that LDL incubated with fibroblasts transfected with LO become "seeded" with fatty acid hydroperoxides, which can then propagate lipid peroxidation under the proper conditions.[39,40] Both mRNA and protein of 15-LO (the homologous enzyme in rabbits and humans) are found in atherosclerotic lesions of rabbits and humans but not in normal arteries.[41] Moreover, stereospecific products of the LO reaction can be found in lesions, consistent with enzymatic oxidation.[42,43] Treatment of hypercholesterolemic rabbits with specific inhibitors of 15-LO reduces the progression of atherosclerosis,[44,45] and, as described later, genetic studies in which 12/15-LO was deleted reduced lesion formation.

A number of different enzyme systems such as LOs,[37-39,46,47] myeloperoxidase (MPO),[48] NADPH oxidase,[49] and other peroxidases[50] have been shown to have the potential of contributing to the oxidation of LDL. Macrophages and/or other phagocytes express these enzymes and, in particular, use MPO-inducible NO synthase and NADPH oxidase as mechanisms for generating antimicrobial reactive oxygen species essential for native immunity.[51] Although macrophages may not be required to initiate LDL oxidation, they are likely to amplify oxidative reactions in macrophage-rich areas of atherosclerotic lesions.

The leukocyte 5-LO has recently been identified as a significant modifier of susceptibility to atherosclerosis in inbred strains of mice.[52] This observation may be linked to LDL modification, but a direct association has not yet been established. There is strong evidence for a role of the 12/15-LO in contributing to OxLDL formation and atherosclerosis in animal models based on experiments assessing the effects of both gain and loss of 12/15-LO activity in atherosclerosis-prone mice[53,54] and protective effects of 15-LO inhibitors in rabbits.[44,45] However, overexpression of 15-LO in the rabbit paradoxically reduced atherosclerosis.[55] Similarly, conflicting results have been observed for the contributions of endothelial and inducible NO synthases to the development of atherosclerosis in mouse models.[56-59] It is possible that mechanisms responsible for LDL oxidation differ between humans and animal models. For example, MPO is a heme enzyme secreted by neutrophils and monocytes that generates a number of oxidants, including hypochlorous acid (HOCl), which can initiate lipid oxidation and peroxidation. MPO has been identified in human atherosclerotic lesions and is of particular interest because lipid modifications found in human atherosclerosis bear similarities to HOCl-mediated derivation of lipoprotein constituents *in vitro*.[60] However, in bone marrow transplantation experiments in which LDLR-/- mice received MPO-deficient bone marrow progenitor cells, larger lesions were observed than in LDLR-/- mice transplanted with wild type progenitor cells. Similar results were seen when MPO-deficient mice were crossed into LDLR-/- mice. However, there was no evidence for the presence of MPO in murine lesions, and the types of MPO-dependent oxidation products found in human lesions were not present in murine lesions,[61] suggesting that MPO could not be directly related to lesion formation in mice.

# MACROPHAGE FOAM CELL FORMATION

## Macrophage Scavenger Receptors

Macrophages express several scavenger receptors that mediate binding and uptake of OxLDL, including SR-A, CD36, SR-BI, CD68, and scavenger receptor for phosphatidylserine and oxidized lipoprotein (SR-PSOX)[62-64] (Fig. 22-3). It is unlikely that scavenger receptors evolved as a mechanism for clearing OxLDL because atherosclerosis is a disease essentially limited to humans, whereas these receptors are found in lower mammals and, at least functionally, as far back as *Drosophila*.[65] As a class, these proteins tend to recognize polyanionic macromolecules and have been proposed to play physiologic roles in the recognition and clearance of pathogens and apoptotic cells. For example, the SR-A receptor has been shown to bind certain gram-positive and gram-negative bacteria,[66] and mice generated with SR-A deletion were found to be more susceptible to infections.[67] Sambrano et al.[68] postulated

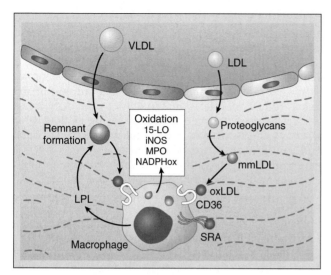

**FIGURE 22-3.** Mechanisms contributing to foam-cell formation. LDL penetrates into the artery wall where it is trapped after adhering to proteoglycans. It is then highly susceptible to oxidation by enzymes such as LOs, MPO, and iNOS. VLDL particles are subject to modification by LPL. The resulting remnant particles are also subject to trapping by proteoglycans, oxidative modification, and uptake by macrophages. mmLDL, minimally modified LDL; SR-A, scavenger receptor class A. (See color plate.) *(Reproduced with permission from Li AC, Glass CK: The macrophage foam cell as a target for therapeutic intervention. Nat Med 2002;8:1235–1242.)*

that the properties of an oxidatively damaged plasma membrane might be analogous to those of an oxidatively modified LDL. Both present a phospholipid-protein domain, which on oxidation can lead to lipid-protein and lipid-lipid interactions, possibly generating closely related structures. They tested the hypothesis by comparing the binding of an oxidatively damaged red blood cell (OxRBC) with that of OxLDL. OxRBC bound tightly to freshly plated macrophages (whereas native RBC did not), and that binding was almost completely blocked in the presence of OxLDL. The ability of CD36 to participate in uptake of apoptotic cells has been known for some time.[69-71] Additional functions have been ascribed for some scavenger receptors. For example, CD36 has also been demonstrated to function as a fatty acid transport protein in adipose tissue and muscle,[63] and SR-BI mediates selective uptake of HDL cholesterol esters in liver and steroidogenic tissues.[72-74]

In contrast to the native LDL receptor, scavenger receptors are not downregulated as the cholesterol content of the cell increases and can, therefore, mediate massive cholesterol accumulation in the macrophage. Gene deletion and bone marrow transplantation experiments suggest that SR-A and CD36 play quantitatively important roles in mediating uptake of OxLDL and promoting the development of atherosclerosis.[67,75,76] A comparison of OxLDL binding and internalization by macrophages from SR-A knockout mice and macrophages from wild-type mice suggests that only 20% to 30% of OxLDL uptake is attributable to SR-A.[67] A comparison of monocytes and macrophages from patients with a total

deficiency of CD36 with normal monocytes and macrophages suggests that about 50% of the uptake of OxLDL is attributable to this receptor under the conditions studied.[77] Studies of the *SR-BI* gene indicate that it plays an antiatherogenic role,[78,79] presumably because of its function in mediating reverse cholesterol transport by HDL. Although SR-BI may inhibit net ABCA1-mediated cholesterol efflux in macrophages by facilitating cholesterol ester reuptake,[80] the overall actions of SR-BI in the arterial wall appear to be protective. Macrophages from mice with combined SR-A and CD36 deficiency show a 75% decrease in uptake of OxLDL *in vitro.*[81] SR-BI/apo E double knockout mice exhibit severe atherosclerosis with evidence of plaque rupture and acute myocardial infarction, complications that are rare in other murine models of atherosclerosis.[78]

The relative contributions of additional scavenger receptors to foam cell formation have not yet been addressed through genetic loss of function experiments, although several of these proteins are expressed in human atherosclerotic lesions. Although inhibition of macrophage scavenger receptor activity could potentially provide the basis of an antiatherogenic therapy, it may be the case that several classes of proteins will have to be targeted simultaneously. Because these receptors are also involved in clearing microorganisms, enhanced susceptibility to specific infectious pathogens may also occur. Finally, it is also possible that inhibition of scavenger receptor function could have deleterious effects if they play an important role in the clearance of apoptotic cells. Lesions that have a large necrotic lipid core are the favored sites for terminal thrombosis.[82] Necrosis of lipid-laden foam cells might tend to favor the formation of a large lipid core, whereas apoptosis of foam cells followed by phagocytosis might prevent such an outcome (i.e., favor the formation of a predominantly fibrous lesion).

## Cholesterol Homeostasis and Foam Cell Formation

The role of macrophages in the uptake of apoptotic cells places special demands on phospholipid and cholesterol homeostasis. Maintenance of cholesterol homeostasis following phagocytosis of an apoptotic cell cannot be achieved simply by negative feedback regulation of the LDL receptor and of the enzymes involved in cholesterol biosynthesis. Macrophages possess robust feedforward mechanisms for preserving cholesterol homeostasis that involve its export to extracellular acceptors and conversion to cholesterol esters. These pathways appear to be overwhelmed in the setting of atherosclerosis through scavenger receptor-mediated uptake of modified lipoproteins. When cholesterol uptake exceeds the capacity of cholesterol efflux pathways, cholesterol esterification results in the formation of lipid droplets that are characteristic of macrophage foam cells.

Cholesterol esterification is carried out by acyl coenzyme A:acylcholesterol transferase (ACAT). Two *ACAT* genes have been identified; ACAT-1 is expressed in a variety of cells, including macrophages, whereas ACAT-2 is primarily expressed in the liver and intestine.[83] The actions of ACAT are opposed by neutral cholesterol esterases, exemplified by hormone-sensitive lipase (HSL), which hydrolyzes cholesterol esters and also functions as the rate-limiting enzyme for hydrolysis of triglycerides in adipocytes. Altering the expression or activities of these enzymes to favor the formation of free cholesterol was hypothesized to be of therapeutic benefit by inhibiting foam cell formation. However, in the setting of severe hypercholesterolemia, both ACAT-1/apoE and ACAT-1/LDLR double knockout mice developed similar or only slightly reduced extents of atherosclerosis as compared with control apo E-/-or LDLR-/- mice[84] but did exhibit severe skin xanthomas and cholesterol deposits in the brain. Reconstitution of LDL-/- mice with ACAT-1-/- macrophages resulted in no difference in serum cholesterol levels but larger lesions than LDL receptor-deficient mice receiving wild type macrophages.[85] However, enhanced hydrolysis of cholesterol esters by overexpression of rat HSL in murine macrophages paradoxically resulted in thicker aortic lesions in transgenic mice.[86] Collectively, these studies suggest that cholesterol esterification is a protective response to excess free cholesterol under conditions in which cholesterol efflux pathways become saturated. Although these findings argue against the use of ACAT inhibitors in the prevention or treatment of atherosclerosis, studies of an inhibitor of ACAT-1 and ACAT-2 in apoE-/-mice demonstrated a significant decrease in serum lipoprotein levels and extent of atherosclerosis without evidence of toxicity,[87] suggesting that partial inhibition of these pathways may be beneficial.

Disposal of excess cholesterol can be achieved by delivery to extracellular acceptors, such as lipid-poor apo AI, or by conversion to more soluble forms. Cultured macrophages and endothelial cells have been reported to secrete 27-oxygenated metabolites of cholesterol. This is not observed in macrophages derived from monocytes of patients with sterol 27-hydroxylase deficiency, demonstrating that sterol 27-hydroxylase is the critical enzyme for the conversion of cholesterol into the 27-oxygenated steroids.[88] Mutations in the 27-hydroxylase gene are the cause of the autosomal recessive disease cerebrotendinous xanthomatosis (CTX),[89] characterized by progressive dementia, xanthomatosis, and accelerated atherosclerosis. Recent studies indicate that members of the ABC family of transport proteins, including ABCA1, also play an important role in the mechanism by which cells transfer excess cholesterol to HDL acceptors. Loss of ABCA1 results in Tangier disease, a condition in which patients have extremely low levels of circulating HDL and massive accumulation of cholesterol in macrophage-rich organs.[90-93] ABCA1 is required for effective transport of cholesterol from cells to apo AI, suggesting a critical role in reverse cholesterol transport.[83,94] Homozygous subjects have extremely low LDL levels that appear to partially protect them from accelerated atherogenesis, but subjects heterozygous for ABCA1 deficiency who have normal LDL levels appear to be at increased risk.[95]

## Roles of Peroxisome Proliferators-Activated Receptors (PPARs) and Liver X Receptors (LXRs) in Regulating Scavenger Receptor Activity and Cholesterol Homeostasis

PPARs are members of the nuclear receptor superfamily of ligand-activated transcription factors. The PPAR subfamily consists of PPARα, PPARγ, and PPARδ (also known as PPARβ).[96] The endogenous ligands that regulate PPAR activity remain poorly characterized but are presumed to include fatty acids and their metabolites. Recent studies indicate that PPARα and PPARδ are regulated by fatty acids liberated from triglyceride-rich lipoproteins by LPL.[97,98] The prostaglandin 15-deoxy $\Delta^{12,14}$ prostaglandin $J_2$ and LO products including 12 HETE and 13 HODE present in OxLDL have been suggested to be endogenous ligands for PPARγ in macrophages.[99-102]

PPARα plays an important physiologic role in the liver regulating fatty acid metabolism and lipoprotein biosynthesis. Fibrates such as gemfibrozil reduce circulating triglyceride levels and raise HDL levels and have been demonstrated to reduce incidence of coronary heart disease in clinical trials.[103] PPARγ is highly expressed in adipose tissue and is required for adipocyte differentiation.[104,105] PPARγ is also the molecular target of thiazolidinediones (TZDs) that are widely used in the management of patients with type 2 diabetes mellitus.[106] PPARγ is also highly expressed in macrophages and foam cells of atherosclerotic lesions. Several lines of evidence suggest that PPARγ agonists can exert both atherogenic and antiatherogenic effects on patterns of gene expression.[102,107-109] PPARγ stimulates expression of the scavenger receptor CD36.[109] PPARγ agonists also inhibit the program of macrophage activation in response to inflammatory mediators such as IFN-γ and lipopolysaccharide (LPS).[108,110,111] In addition, PPARα and PPARγ have been reported to induce the expression of LXRα, suggesting that PPARs may exert antiatherogenic effects through secondary activation of LXR target genes,[112,113] as described later. The net effects of TZDs in mouse models of atherosclerosis are protective.[114-117] In addition, LDLR-/- mice transplanted with PPARγ-/- bone marrow progenitor cells develop more extensive atherosclerosis than animals transplanted with wild-type bone marrow, demonstrating a protective role of PPARγ in monocyte-derived macrophages.[112] Although clinical data assessing the impact of TZD therapy on risk of acute coronary events is not yet available, a recent study of diabetic patients demonstrated that treatment with the TZD rosiglitazone significantly reduced circulating CRP and matrix metalloproteinase levels.[118]

LXRs α and β comprise a second subfamily of nuclear receptors that have more recently emerged as transcription factors that function in concert with SREBPs to regulate cholesterol homeostasis.[119] At least three important classes of LXR target genes have been identified that influence cholesterol homeostasis and foam cell formation in macrophages. First, LXRs induce the expression of ABC transporters that have been linked to cholesterol efflux.[120] Second, LXRs induce the expression of apo E, which can potentially serve as an acceptor of cholesterol transported by ABCA1-dependent processes.[121] Third, LXRα appears to induce synthesis of fatty acids that are preferential substrates of ACAT in cholesterol esterification reactions.[119] Thus, these genes act in concert to reduce free cholesterol levels and protect macrophages from its cytotoxic effects. The ability of LXR/RXR heterodimers to regulate *ABCA1* and other genes involved in cholesterol homeostasis raises the possibility that they may be important new targets for the development of antiatherogenic drugs. Consistent with this, the use of LXR agonists indicates that LXRs exert antiatherogenic effects in mouse models of atherosclerosis.[115,122] An important caveat to the use of currently available LXR agonists is that they cause a marked increase in circulating triglyceride levels, apparently as a consequence of inducing the expression and activity of SREBP-1c.[119,123] These observations suggest that it will be necessary to develop selective modulators of RXRs and LXRs if they are to become useful targets for the development of antiatherogenic drugs.

## PROPERTIES OF OXIDIZED LDL THAT MAKE IT POTENTIALLY MORE ATHEROGENIC THAN NATIVE LDL

A partial list of biologic properties of OxLDL that may make it more atherogenic than native LDL is shown in Table 22-1. The full list would include as many as 15 different proatherogenic properties, but we discuss only four well-documented examples.

## The Ability to Induce Foam Cell Formation from Monocyte/Macrophages and from Smooth Muscle Cells

As discussed previously, the ability to cause cholesterol accumulation in macrophages *in vitro* was the first observation that called attention to the possible impor-

tance of OxLDL in atherogenesis.[10,50] That uptake was due partly to interaction with SR-A, which was cloned by Kodama et al.[7,124] Recent studies have shown that under certain conditions smooth muscle cells can be induced to express SR-A,[125] and this may then account for foam cell formation from smooth muscle cells. As discussed earlier, there are probably several other macrophage receptors that may also play a role in foam cell formation.

## Recruitment of Monocytes from the Circulation into the Artery Wall

OxLDL is itself a chemoattractant for monocytes[126] and T lymphocytes[127] but not for B lymphocytes. This specificity is consonant with the finding that circulating cells recruited to atherosclerotic lesions are predominantly monocytes and T lymphocytes.[128] OxLDL is actually an inhibitor of the motility of tissue macrophages[129] and might, therefore, suppress any tendency for macrophages to exit from an atherosclerotic lesion. Furthermore, minimally OxLDL can indirectly participate in the recruitment of monocytes by stimulating the release from endothelial cells of monocyte chemoattractant protein-1 (MCP-1)[130] and macrophage-colony stimulating factor (M-CSF).[131] Recent studies suggest that some of the biologic effects of OxLDL are in large part attributable to oxidized phospholipids in which the fatty acids in the *sn*-2 position have been partially degraded.[132] Lysophosphatidylcholine, a major component of more extensively OxLDL,[14] can induce the expression of adhesion molecules and, thus, contribute to monocyte recruitment.[133]

## Cytotoxicity

Hessler et al.[134] and Henriksen et al.[135] independently noted that endothelial cells or smooth muscle cells incubated in the presence of LDL showed signs of toxicity going on to cell death in 24 to 48 hours. This toxicity was only evident if other serum proteins were

■ ▪ ■

**TABLE 22-1** POTENTIAL MECHANISMS BY WHICH OXIDIZED FORMS OF LDL MAY INFLUENCE ATHEROGENESIS

OxLDL has enhanced uptake by macrophages leading to foam cell formation.
Products of OxLDL are chemotactic for monocytes and T cells and inhibit the motility of tissue macrophages.
Products of OxLDL are cytotoxic, in part because of oxidized sterols, and can induce apoptosis.
OxLDL, or products, are mitogenic for smooth muscle cells and macrophages.
OxLDL, or products, can alter gene expression of vascular cells (e.g., induction of MCP-1, colony-stimulating factors, IL-1, and expression of adhesion molecules).
OxLDL, or products, can increase expression of macrophage scavenger receptors, thereby enhancing its own uptake.
OxLDL, or products, can induce proinflammatory genes (e.g., hemoxygenase, SAA, and ceruloplasmin).
OxLDL can induce expression and activate PPARγ, thereby influencing many gene functions.
OxLDL is immunogenic and elicits autoantibody formation and activated T cells.
Oxidation renders LDL more susceptible to aggregation, which independently leads to enhanced uptake. Similarly, OxLDL is a better substrate for sphingomyelinase, which also aggregates LDL.
OxLDL may enhance procoagulant pathways (e.g., by induction of tissue factor and platelet aggregation).
Products of OxLDL can adversely affect arterial vasomotor properties.
OxLDL is involved in acute coronary syndromes and may potentially lead to plaque disruption.

Modified from Witztum JL, Steinberg D: The oxidative modification hypothesis of atherosclerosis: Does it hold for humans? Trends Cardiovasc Med 2001;11:93–102.

absent or present at low concentrations. Subsequent work established that the cytotoxicity depended on the fact that the cells were converting the LDL in the medium to OxLDL during the course of the incubation.[136] The addition of antioxidants completely prevented the cytotoxicity as did the addition of whole serum. Recent work has documented that certain oxidized sterols are chiefly responsible for this cytotoxicity. Whether or not the concentrations of OxLDL generated *in vivo* ever reach the level needed to damage cells is not known. Obviously, damage to the endothelium could have profound implications for atherogenesis.[137]

## Inhibition of Vasodilation in Response to Nitric Oxide

The classical studies of Furchgott and Zawadzki[138] showed that the relaxation of aortic rings *in vitro* in response to acetylcholine and a number of other vasoactive compounds depended on their interaction with the endothelial lining and the release of a potent vasodilator from that lining. Endothelial-derived relaxing factor (EDRF) is now generally recognized to be NO or a compound closely related to it. This phenomenon is strongly inhibited in the presence of OxLDL.[139] Indeed, in some instances the vasorelaxation is converted into a paradoxical vasoconstriction! Clinical studies show that human coronary arteries and brachial arteries of patients with hypercholesterolemia, with or without obvious atherosclerotic lesions, can show this paradoxical response to vasodilators.[140] Moreover, pretreatment with antioxidant compounds can partially restore the normal response. Lowering of LDL levels acutely by apheresis restores normal vasodilatory responses, and this correction is best correlated to acute reduction of OxLDL levels.[141] This is one of the better documented toxic effects of OxLDL at the clinical level.[142]

## Other Properties

There are many additional biologic effects of OxLDL not shared by native LDL. Most, but not all, are proatherogenic. As discussed previously, some, such as the stimulation of the release of M-CSF and MCP-1 from endothelial cells, can be elicited by even very minimally OxLDL. Others, including recognition by scavenger receptors, only become apparent after more extensive oxidation. So far *in vivo* evaluation of these potentially proatherogenic properties is relatively limited.

## EVIDENCE THAT OXIDATION OF LDL TAKES PLACE *IN VIVO*

When isolated LDL is incubated *in vitro* with a transition metal such as copper or with cultured cells, it undergoes rapid oxidation after its endogenous content of antioxidants is depleted. However, if one simply supplements the medium with 5% serum or even albumin, oxidation can be completely inhibited. Because of the ubiquitous presence of proteins and/or aqueous antioxidants in plasma and because the concentrations of these components in the extracellular fluid appears to be sufficient to confer antioxidant protection under ordinary circumstances,[143] there was much skepticism that oxidation of LDL could actually occur *in vivo*. However, there are now many lines of evidence that oxidation of lipoproteins does occur *in vivo* and that this process is quantitatively important. This evidence has been extensively reviewed elsewhere[144,145] and can be summarized as follows:

1. When LDL undergoes oxidative modification a variety of profound structural changes occur in the particle. It was shown many years ago that even as subtle a modification of LDL as the nonenzymatic glycation of apoB resulted in adduct formation that rendered autologous LDL immunogenic.[146] Similarly, the many changes induced in the LDL by oxidation generate a variety of neoepitopes that render even autologous LDL immunogenic. For example, one of the common breakdown products of the oxidation of PUFAs is MDA, which is a highly reactive dialdehyde. MDA can form adducts with adjacent ε-amino groups of lysine residues leading to the generation of MDA-lysine adducts. Similarly, 4-hydroxynonenal (4-HNE) is a highly reactive α, β-unsaturated aldehyde that can form both Schiff base adducts and Michael-type adducts with lysine residues and thiols and histidine, yielding yet another class of epitopes resulting from the oxidation process. Many other similar modifications can be generated, yielding both lipid-protein and lipid-lipid adducts. We have termed these "oxidation-specific" epitopes. To develop antibodies that would recognize these epitopes we prepared models such as MDA-LDL and 4-HNE-LDL, prepared from homologous LDL and used these to immunize animals (e.g., murine LDL was modified with MDA and then used to generate murine monoclonal antibodies). A variety of different "oxidation-specific" antibodies were generated.[147,148] All of these demonstrated the presence of such epitopes in atherosclerotic lesions in rabbits, nonhuman primates, and humans but not in normal arterial tissue. Other investigators have developed similar antibodies that immunostain atherosclerotic lesions in a similar manner.[149,150]

2. Many of the "oxidation-specific" antibodies were specific for the adduct itself (e.g. MDA-lysine or 4-HNE-lysine) and would recognize this epitope to some degree even when present on other similarly modified proteins other than apolipoprotein B. Thus, to prove that the immunostaining was due to OxLDL itself, LDL was gently extracted from atherosclerotic tissue of rabbits and humans and shown to have all of the physical, biologic, and immunologic properties observed with LDL oxidized *in vitro*.[151] Of particular importance was the demonstration that LDL particles isolated from fatty streak lesions had enhanced uptake by macrophage scavenger receptors and that this uptake could be competed for by *in vitro* OxLDL.

3. Oxidized lipids, including oxidized sterols are routinely demonstrable in atherosclerotic tissue but not in normal aortic tissue.[152] In addition, stereospecific products of the 15-LO pathway are found in atherosclerotic tissue but not normal tissue.[43] Studies *in vitro* have demonstrated that cells overexpressing 15-LO mRNA and protein could "seed" LDL in the medium with hydroperoxides and thus render the LDL more susceptible to oxidation.[39,40] Because 15-LO mRNA and protein have been previously demonstrated to be present in atherosclerotic tissue by *in situ* hybridization and immunocytochemistry,[41] the presence of 15-LO products documents 15-LO activity and suggests at least one mechanism (among many others) by which macrophages might mediate the oxidation of LDL *in vivo*.

4. As noted previously, there are abundant antioxidant defenses in plasma and extracellular fluid that would make it highly unlikely that LDL could be oxidized in the circulation. However, as first described by Schwenke and Carew,[153,154] LDL undoubtedly circulates through a variety of tissues, including the artery wall itself, and may well undergo minimal or early degrees of modification during such passage. Indeed, numerous reports now document that circulating LDL displays chemical indices of early stages of oxidation,[155,156] and oxidation-specific epitopes can be demonstrated in LDL particles by immunochemical techniques.[157-159]

5. Even minimal modifications of autologous LDL render it immunogenic. Because OxLDL occurs *in vivo* in atherosclerotic tissues, one would expect that autoantibodies to oxidation-specific epitopes should exist. Indeed, it has been demonstrated that autoantibodies to a variety of epitopes of OxLDL can be found in sera of experimental animal models with atherosclerosis.[147,158,160] For example, titers of autoantibodies to epitopes of OxLDL correlated significantly with the extent of atherosclerosis in apoE-/- and LDLR-/- mice.[158,160,161] Furthermore, as noted in greater detail later, preliminary data suggests that the titers of such autoantibodies are related to the presence and/or the rate of progression of disease in animal models[162-164] and possibly humans as well.

6. Autoantibodies to OxLDL epitopes are not only found in the circulation but also are found in atherosclerotic lesions of mice,[165] rabbits, and humans, where they are in immune complexes with OxLDL.[166]

7. Recent human and animal studies on the fetal origins of atherosclerosis support a role for oxidation of LDL in the pathogenesis of lesion formation even in fetal life. OxLDL was present even in the earliest human fetal lesions, most often before the presence of monocytes and macrophages. Strong correlations were noted between fetal and maternal plasma cholesterol levels up to the second trimester, which in turn were proportional to the extent of lesion formation in the fetus. In animal models, these lesions can be significantly diminished by treating hypercholesterolemic pregnant mothers with cholestyramine or antioxidants. Follow-up studies of aortic atherosclerosis in children of mothers who were hypercholesterolemic during pregnancy showed significantly enhanced progression of atherosclerosis compared with children of mothers who had been normocholesterolemic, despite the fact that plasma cholesterol levels of the children were similar.[167]

8. Physical evidence for the presence of OxLDL in the vessel wall has been obtained by imaging techniques using radiolabeled oxidation-specific antibodies *in vivo*.[168,169] Radiolabeled oxidation-specific antibodies (Ox-AB) specifically accumulated *in vivo* within lipid-rich atherosclerotic lesions but not in normal arteries. Attempts are being made to exploit this to provide a quantitative measure of the lesion content of OxLDL and, hopefully, to allow detection of atherosclerosis progression and regression (Figs. 22-4 and 22-5). In addition, human OxLDL antibodies have been developed, which may have significant advantages over murine antibodies in clinical applications.[170]

## OXIDIZED LDL AND THE IMMUNE SYSTEM IN ATHEROGENESIS

The appreciation that inflammation is a fundamentally important component of atherosclerotic lesion initiation and progression has fundamentally altered the view of the pathogenesis of atherogenesis. Inflammation is a process whereby blood leukocytes migrate from the vascular space into a tissue site in response to a perceived pathogen. With the exception of the absence of neutrophils, the chronic atherosclerotic lesion has all the pathologic components of a typical inflammatory response, including the presence of monocytes and macrophages, dendritic cells, T cells, antigen-specific immunoglobulins, activated complement, and even mast cells. Immune activation that occurs in the atherosclerotic lesion must be viewed in the context of a coordinated response to perceived pathogens. In the case of the atherosclerotic lesion, the nature of the inciting pathogen(s) is not so clear. There are a variety of candidate pathogens, including microbial and viral agents; aberrant expression of endogenous proteins, such as heat shock proteins; and other modifications of proteins, such as the generation of nonenzymatic glycation and advanced glycation endproducts that occur secondary to hyperglycemia. Chief among the potential pathogens are the presence of various forms of minimally and heavily OxLDL. The generation of a wide spectrum of oxidized moieties that occur when LDL is oxidized creates bioactive molecules that have many and diverse proinflammatory effects, and, as described previously, such oxidation-specific epitopes are immunogenic and result in a profound cellular and humoral immune response. In turn, there is a coordinated inflammatory response, as indicated by elevated CRP, IL-6, serum amyloid A, and soluble adhesion molecules, which have been shown to be independent predictors of coronary disease.[171]

A wide variety of both adaptive and innate immune responses have been shown to be capable of modulating

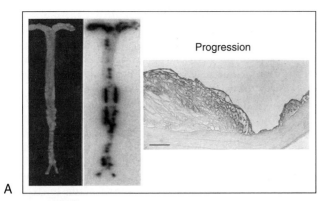

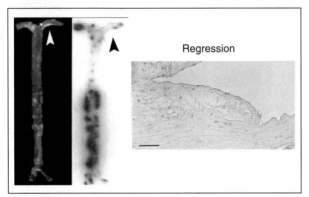

FIGURE 22-4. *In vivo* uptake of [125]I-MDA2, a prototype oxidation-specific antibody that was intravenously injected in LDLR-/- mice with pre-existing atherosclerotic lesions. These mice were subsequently placed on either a dietary atherosclerosis progression diet *(A)* or a regression diet *(B)*. The aorta (left panels of each figure) represents the presence of plaque accentuated by Sudan IV staining and the aorta in the middle panels represents the corresponding autoradiograph. In the progression aorta, there is nearly 100% concordance of Sudan staining and *in vivo* distribution and plaque uptake of [125]I-MDA2. Immunostaining for OxLDL (far right panel) shows strong staining pattern. In contrast in a regression mouse *(B)*, the arrowheads depict an area in the aortic arch where a Sudan-stained lesion does not take up [125]I-MDA2. Immunostaining of this segment, which is similar in size to the area in the progression mouse, shows essentially absent OxLDL staining following a regression antioxidant diet.[169] (See color plate.) *(Reproduced with permission from Tsimikas S, Shortal BP, Witztum JL, Palinski W: In vivo uptake of radiolabeled MDA2, an oxidation-specific monoclonal antibody, provides an accurate measure of atherosclerotic lesions rich in oxidized LDL and is highly sensitive to their regression. Arterioscler Thromb Vasc Biol 2000;20:689-697.)*

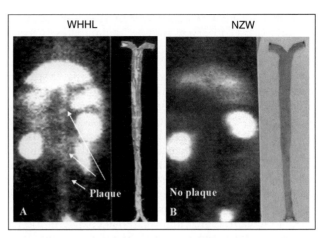

FIGURE 22-5. Noninvasive imaging of atherosclerosis with [99m]Tc-MDA2. Panel A represents an atherosclerotic WHHL rabbit in which antibody uptake and signal is visible in the abdominal aorta. Next to the image is the *ex vivo* aorta stained with Sudan IV. In contrast, no signal is generated in a nonatherosclerotic New Zealand White (NZW) rabbit. The rabbits are viewed in the supine position. *(Reproduced with permission from Tsimikas S, Palinski W, Halpern SE, et al: Radiolabeled MDA2, an oxidation-specific, monoclonal antibody, identifies native atherosclerotic lesions in vivo. J Nucl Cardiol 1999;6:41-53.)*

lesion formation in animal models of atherosclerosis. It is now apparent that many of the immune responses found in atherosclerosis are, in fact, aspects of specific components of inflammatory responses in general. The role of the immune system in atherogenesis has been recently reviewed in depth.[172-174] For example, both apoE-/- and LDLR-/- models have been crossed into RAG-deficient mice, which lack both T and B cells. When such mice are fed an atherogenic diet, achieving very high cholesterol levels, the extent of lesion formation is not altered. However, when these same mice are examined at very early time points or even over more extended periods of time, but in the presence of more

modest elevations of plasma cholesterol, immune deficiency resulted in a 40% to 80% decrease in lesion formation. This data indicates that immune cells are not obligatory for lesion formation in the presence of the extreme atherogenic pressure generated by marked hypercholesterolemia. However, in the presence of a lesser atherogenic pressure, these immune responses are capable of importantly modulating the progress of the atherogenic process. Although these studies indicate a net proatherogenic effect of adaptive immunity, there are many examples in which specific components of adaptive immunity can be protective as well. For example, immunization of mice with OxLDL has been shown to reduce the extent of lesion formation despite very high plasma cholesterol levels.[171] The net impact of a given perturbation of the immune system on atherogenesis is very complex and is likely to be both context and antigen dependent.

Adaptive immunity represents a somewhat delayed but precise response of the immune system to newly exposed antigens. Adaptive immunity is mediated by somatic mutations of antigen receptors, such as T cell receptors and B cell receptors, which give rise to specific and high-affinity cellular and humoral immunity. In contrast, innate immunity is mediated by highly conserved and phylogenetically ancient pattern recognition receptors (PRRs) that provide a rapid if less precise response to a given pathogen. Macrophages and dendritic cells are central mediators of innate immunity and also provide links to adaptive responses as well. Scavenger receptors on macrophages specific for OxLDL, such as CD36, are in fact typical PRRs, and not only bind OxLDL but many other conserved motifs, which are termed pathogen-associated molecular patterns (PAMPs). Natural antibodies, which are usually IgM or IgA, are so-called germ-line encoded antibodies that arise without known antigenic stimulation and contain evolutionarily conserved antigen binding sites that are thought to provide rapid recognition of PAMPs on pathogens.

We have recently uncovered an example of a common PAMP that is found on OxLDL, apoptotic cells and on the cell wall of many common pathogens. The IgM autoantibody EO6 was cloned from apoE-deficient mice for its ability to bind to OxLDL.[158] Subsequently it was shown to bind to oxidized phospholipids and specifically to the phosphorylcholine (PC) moiety of the oxidized phospholipid. Interestingly, EO6 did not bind to PC-containing phospholipids that were not oxidized, even though it had the same PC motif.[175] Thus, oxidation caused a specific conformational change in the PC headgroup that "exposed" the PC for EO6 binding.[176] Subsequently, it was shown that cells undergoing apoptosis, which are also subjected to enhanced oxidative stress, also "expose" the PC moiety of their oxidized phospholipids and enable binding of EO6. EO6 does not bind to viable cells.[177] It was also shown that EO6 could inhibit the binding and uptake of OxLDL and apoptotic cells by macrophages and CD36 transfected cells.[62] Thus, the oxidized phospholipid containing the PC moiety is a ligand on OxLDL and apoptotic cells that mediates binding and uptake by macrophage scavenger receptors (e.g., PC is a PAMP on OxLDL and apoptotic cells recognized by the PRR CD36). Cloning and sequencing studies of the antigen-binding domains of EO6 revealed that this antibody was identical to an antibody named T15 that was studied more than 30 years ago.[165] T15 is an anti-PC antibody that binds to the PC moiety that is covalently linked to the cell wall polysaccharide of common pathogens, such as *Streptococcus pneumoniae,* and in mice this single antibody class provides the optimal protection to mice against lethal infection with this pathogen. Thus, there is molecular mimicry between the exposed PC of OxLDL and apoptotic cells and the PC of many pathogens.

CRP, which is a highly primitive innate immune PRR has been long known to bind to the PC of *S. pneumoniae*. In recent studies we have shown that CRP also binds specifically to the exposed PC of OxLDL and apoptotic cells in a similar manner[178] (Fig. 22-6). Thus, EO6/T15, certain scavenger receptors of macrophages, and CRP are all highly conserved innate immune responses to the PC moiety of these structures. Because oxidation is undoubtedly a common accompaniment of inflammatory responses, it is likely that these innate PRRs to PC have been conserved to respond to this common PAMP. With respect to atherogenesis, the enhanced uptake of OxLDL by CD36 for example, although providing for removal of damaged and potentially

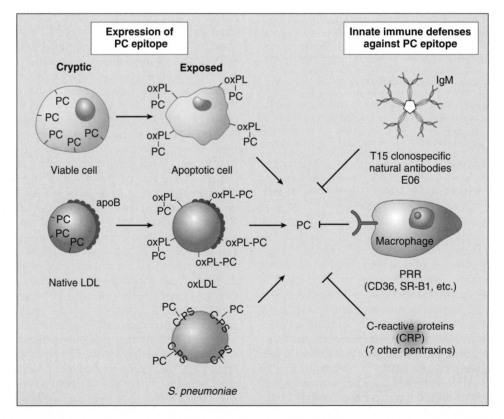

**FIGURE 22-6.** Molecular mimicry between epitopes of OxLDL, apoptotic cells, and the PC of the cell wall polysaccharide (C-PS) of pathogens. For native LDL and viable cells, the PC-containing phospholipids need to be oxidized (OxPL) to have the PC moiety exposed for recognition by innate immune defenses, represented by natural antibodies of the T15/EO6 type; macrophage scavenger receptors, such as CD36 and SR-B1; and CRP. *(Reproduced with permission from Binder CJ, Chang MK, Shaw PX, et al: Innate and acquired immunity in atherogenesis. Nat Med 2002;8:1218–1226.)*

proinflammatory lipids, if sustained nevertheless leads to foam cell formation. In contrast, EO6 can block uptake of OxLDL and should decrease atherogenesis. Indeed, immunization of LDLR-negative mice with a heat-killed pneumococcus was recently shown to reduce the progression of atherogenesis. It is not yet clear whether CRP will have a similar effect, but these observations suggest that CRP may not simply be a marker of inflammation but may be an active participant in a concerted immune response. In a similar manner, it is likely that there is a logic behind many of the immune responses that occur in the atherogenic process.

## EVIDENCE THAT OXIDATION OF LDL IS RELEVANT IN ANIMAL MODELS OF ATHEROSCLEROSIS

### Evidence *Other* than Antioxidant Intervention Studies

There are by now many published studies in animal models demonstrating that a variety of antioxidants retard the progression of atherosclerosis[179-215] (Table 22-2). This is discussed in detail below. There are additional experimental models that support an important role for OxLDL. For example, Colin Funk's laboratory has provided strong evidence for an important role of 12/15-LO in murine atherogenesis. They showed that crossing 12/15-LO deficient mice into apoE-deficient mice caused a significant reduction (~50%) in the extent of early lesions up to 15 months of age, despite similar blood lipid profiles in both groups.[53,163,216] Urinary and plasma levels of $F_2$-isoprostanes, nonenzymatic breakdown products resulting from lipid peroxidation of arachidonic acid, and OxLDL autoantibodies were also reduced, and both highly correlated with plaque burden and with each other. In 12/15-LO deficient mice crossed into LDLR-/- mice, there was also less atherosclerosis.[217] Although it is possible that LO affected atherogenesis by other mechanisms, these studies lend strong support to the concept that a major mechanism by which LO deficiency decreased atherosclerosis was by decreasing the extent of lipid peroxidation and, specifically, the generation of OxLDL. Conversely, overexpression of 15-LO in endothelial cells led to an enhancement of atherosclerosis in LDLR-negative mice.[54] However, in contrast is a report that macrophage-specific overexpression of 15-LO led to protection against atherosclerosis in cholesterol-fed rabbits. The 12/15-LO deletion was global, although the studies with 15-LO overexpression were tissue specific. Whether this explains the difference in the latter two studies is unclear. Of course, it is likely that *in vivo* there are many mechanisms, beside LO, by which LDL is oxidized within the artery wall.[218] Additional studies have shown that combined paraoxonase/apoE-deficient knockout mice have enhanced LDL oxidation detected by enhanced clearance of intravenously injected LDL and faster generation of plasma levels of circulating OxLDL and immune complexes and attendant enhanced atherosclerosis.[219]

■ ▪ ■

**TABLE 22-2  EFFECTS OF ANTIOXIDANTS IN ANIMAL MODELS OF ATHEROSCLEROSIS**

| Type of Study | Result | Reference |
|---|---|---|
| Probucol in LDLR-/- rabbits | + | 179 |
| | + | 180 |
| | + | 181 |
| | +/− | 182 |
| | + | 183 |
| | + | 184 |
| | + | 185 |
| | + | 186 |
| | + | 187 |
| Probucol analogs in LDLR-/- rabbits | + | 188 |
| | − | 183 |
| | − | 185 |
| Probucol in cholesterol-fed rabbits | − | 189 |
| | + | 190 |
| | + | 191 |
| | + | 192 |
| | + | 193 |
| | + | 187 |
| *Other antioxidants in rabbits* | | |
| DPPD | + | 194 |
| BHT | + | 195 |
| Vitamin E | + | 196 |
| | − | 197 |
| | − | 198 |
| | − | 192 |
| | − | 199 |
| | − | 186 |
| *Vitamin E analogs* | | |
| TMG | + | 187 |
| Carvedilol | + | 184 |
| Vitamin E/C | + | 193 |
| Ubiquinone-10 | −* | 186 |
| *Antioxidants in rodents* | | |
| *Hamsters* | | |
| Probucol | + | 200 |
| Probucol | − | 201 |
| Vitamin E | + | 200 |
| Vitamin E | − | 201 |
| *ApoE-/- mice* | | |
| DPPD | + | 202 |
| Probucol | −* | 203 |
| Probucol | +/−* | 204 |
| Probucol | −* | 205 |
| Probucol | +/−* | 206 |
| Vitamin E | + | 207 |
| AGI-1067 | + | 208 |
| *LDLR-/- mice* | | |
| Probucol | −* | 209 |
| Probucol | −* | 210 |
| Probucol | − | 211 |
| Probucol | − | 206 |
| Probucol analog | + | 210 |
| Dietary antioxidants | + | 212 |
| AGI-1067 | + | 208 |
| *LDLR-/- /ApoE-/- mice* | | |
| Probucol metabolite | + | 213 |
| *Antioxidants in nonhuman primates* | | |
| Probucol | + | 214 |
| Vitamin E | +/− | 215 |

+, positive study (atherosclerosis decreased); −, negative study (atherosclerosis unchanged);
+/−, atherosclerosis equivocal; −*, atherosclerosis enhanced.
Modified from Witztum JL, Steinberg D: The oxidative modification hypothesis of atherosclerosis: Does it hold for humans? Trends Cardiovasc Med 2001;11:93–102

Conversely, in experimental studies of atherosclerosis regression, evidence has accumulated that, in conjunction with dietary lipid lowering, reduced OxLDL content in the vessel wall has been strongly associated with plaque regression and possibly plaque stabilization. For example, Tsimikas et al.[169] have shown that the OxLDL content of the vessel wall, measured by the uptake of an intravenously injected [125]I-labeled antibody against OxLDL (MDA2, an oxidation-specific antibody binding to MDA-lysine epitopes of OxLDL), is significantly reduced following dietary and/or antioxidant intervention and enhanced significantly following a high-fat and high-cholesterol diet. Remarkably, the vessel wall OxLDL content was strongly correlated with OxLDL autoantibody titers, which also correlated with extent of atherosclerosis progression and regression.[53,162,164] This observation was subsequently confirmed and extended by Aikawa et al.[162] in cholesterol-fed rabbits by showing that OxLDL immunostaining with MDA2 was reduced to a greater extent than was apoB-100 staining, indicative of a preferential depletion of plaque OxLDL. In support of this, OxLDL autoantibody titers were also reduced. Reduction in OxLDL markers was also associated with features of plaque stabilization, such as reduction in expression of VCAM-1 and MCP-1 and improvement in eNOS expression.

## Evidence that Antioxidants Slow the Progression of Lesions in Animal Models of Atherosclerosis

The data presented previously leaves little doubt that oxidation of LDL occurs in atherosclerotic tissue. However, this data does not directly address the issue of whether the oxidation of LDL is a quantitatively important accompaniment of the atherogenic process nor whether it is causally related. If oxidation of LDL promotes atherogenesis, the most convincing evidence would be the direct demonstration that inhibition of oxidation leads to inhibition of the progression of atherosclerosis and that this occurs independently of any effects on plasma lipoprotein levels. As originally shown by Carew et al.[179] and by Kita et al.[180] the use of the potent antioxidant compound probucol, which is a highly lipophilic antioxidant strategically located within the LDL particle, effectively inhibited atherogenesis, independent of any effects on plasma lipoprotein levels. In several different rabbit studies, probucol inhibited atherosclerosis by 40% to 80%, despite the fact that it lowered HDL levels. A recent study with AGI-1067, a probucol analog that does not reduce HDL levels to the same extent and does not significantly prolong QTc compared with probucol, has shown significant reductions in atherosclerosis in both LDLR-/- and apoE-/- mice. These reductions in atherosclerosis were also associated with reduced expression of inflammatory genes such as VCAM-1 and MCP-1.[208]

By now, there have been a whole series of different studies using a variety of antioxidants that also show that inhibition of atherosclerosis can be achieved independent of lowering of plasma cholesterol lev-

els. These antioxidant compounds have been used successfully in both spontaneously hypercholesterolemic WHHL rabbits and in cholesterol-fed rabbits, cholesterol-fed hamsters, and cholesterol-fed nonhuman primates. In most of the studies shown in Table 22-2 the inhibition of atherosclerosis ranged from 40% to 80%. It should be appreciated, however, that those studies in which potent inhibition of atherosclerosis was achieved were almost always associated with the use of a very potent antioxidant such as probucol, which conferred maximal protection on LDL, much greater than that achieved with a natural antioxidant such as vitamin E (as discussed in greater detail later).

However, a number of major questions remain unanswered about the exact mechanisms by which these compounds inhibit atherosclerosis. Do these antioxidants achieve this protective effect by their direct protection of the LDL, by altering the redox potential within the cells of the artery (such as endothelial cells), or both? In addition it is also possible that these compound effect protection against atherogenesis by some nonantioxidant properties. For example, probucol can inhibit release of IL-1 from macrophages under certain conditions[220] and can elevate levels of cholesterol-ester-transfer protein.[221] However, there is considerable evidence that antioxidant mechanisms are responsible for the protective effect. First, antioxidants of widely differing structure, such as probucol and diphenylphenylenediamine, have proved effective and are unlikely to share biologic properties other than their antioxidant effect. Second, those compounds that have conferred the most potent antioxidant protection to LDL, such as probucol or probucol analogs, almost universally inhibit the progression of atherosclerosis, whereas those compounds that are weaker, such as vitamin E, have often failed to inhibit atherosclerosis in some experimental animal models although they were very effective in others.[207] In a study of the effects of probucol in nonhuman primates by Sasahara et al.[214] there was a significant correlation between the extent of antioxidant protection of plasma LDL and the extent of inhibition of atherosclerosis.

Not all studies in animals have shown a positive benefit of antioxidant therapy. For example Fruebis et al.[183] tested probucol and a probucol analog in LDL receptor-negative rabbits, which have marked hypercholesterolemia even on a chow diet. Probucol provided very potent protection to the LDL from oxidation, prolonging the lag time for conjugated diene formation of the LDL (an index of the extent of antioxidant protection) by as much as eightfold, whereas the probucol analog only prolonged the lag time by fourfold. Although probucol strongly inhibited atherosclerosis, the probucol analog did not. On the one hand, this suggests that for a given degree of prooxidant stress (e.g., marked hypercholesterolemia) a certain threshold of antioxidant protection may need to be achieved. However, other experiments strongly suggest that under some circumstances that the degree of *ex vivo* protection observed in the circulating LDL may not necessarily be a reflection of an antioxidant compound's antiatherogenic potential. For example, it may well be that it is the antioxidant protection at the tissue level or at the intracellular level that counts most. In addition, these experiments raise the very important possibility that for any given level of prooxidant stress there is a given level of antioxidant protection required. Further support for this latter hypothesis can be found in the studies of Parker et al.[200] who looked at the ability of probucol and vitamin E to protect against atherosclerosis in a cholesterol-fed hamster model. When the hamsters were fed sufficient cholesterol to result in marked hypercholesterolemia, neither probucol nor vitamin E was able to prevent progression of early lesions. However, at lower levels of hypercholesterolemia vitamin E and probucol were both effective. Praticó et al.[207] showed that large doses of vitamin E retarded the progression of lesion formation in apoE-/- mice. This protection was directly correlated with plasma vitamin E levels, and the degree of lesion formation was inversely related to aortic levels. Further studies are needed in animal models to test this "threshold hypothesis" because it has obvious and important clinical relevance to studies in humans. For example, it might suggest that the antioxidant protection required for a nonsmoking, normocholesterolemic individual may be quite different than the degree of antioxidant protection required for a hypercholesterolemic individual who is a smoker. Thus, supplemental vitamin E might be sufficient in the case of the former but therapeutic doses of a potent lipophilic antioxidant, such as a probucol analog, may be required for the latter.

As noted previous there are now many proposed mechanisms by which products of OxLDL may promote inflammation and atherogenesis. Thus, antioxidants may protect against atherosclerosis and adverse clinical events, by means other than simple direct protection of LDL from oxidation.[222] For example, in the presence of hypercholesterolemia or even as a result of some other factor leading to an altered redox state (e.g., infection), endothelial cells may be activated, leading to increased expression of adhesion molecules such as VCAM-1, which in turn would bind monocytes and T cells leading to their ingress into the intima. A prooxidant state within the cell favors induction of VCAM-1, and antioxidants may abrogate this induction.[223,224] Similarly, it is known that hypercholesterolemia may impair the normal EDRF activity of endothelial cells, which has been demonstrated to occur as a result of products of OxLDL. Antioxidants may restore normal EDRF activity of endothelial cells by inhibiting the oxidation of LDL and by directly affecting the intracellular redox state of the endothelial cell.

# EVIDENCE THAT OXIDATION OF LDL IS RELEVANT TO HUMAN ATHEROSCLEROSIS

## Evidence that Oxidative Modification Occurs in Humans

With the exception of intervention trials, all of the previously summarized evidence that describes the presence of OxLDL in animal models of atherosclerosis applies equally well to humans. In brief

1. Immunocytochemical studies using antibodies directed against oxidation-specific epitopes demonstrate the presence of such epitopes in atherosclerotic lesions of human tissues.[151]
2. LDL extracted from atherosclerotic tissue of humans has all of the physical, immunologic, and biologic properties of LDL oxidized in vitro.[151]
3. Although heavily OxLDL per se is not found in the plasma, investigators at several laboratories have now shown that a small fraction of circulating LDL particles display a number of chemical indices consistent with early stages of OxLDL.[155,156] Oxidation-specific epitopes can also be demonstrated on some LDL particles by highly sensitive immunocytochemical techniques.[225] Furthermore, as recently shown by Tamai et al.[141] improvement of endothelial function achieved by LDL apheresis was best correlated with a decrease in the presence of oxidation-specific epitopes on LDL particles.

Recent studies from several laboratories have shown that increased levels of circulating OxLDL are found in the plasma of patients with cardiovascular disease (CVD), previous myocardial infarction, and acute coronary syndromes (ACS).[159,226-229] Nishi et al.[230] documented that vulnerable carotid plaques from humans are greatly enriched in OxLDL. Plasma levels of OxLDL correlated with plaque content of OxLDL, but the concentrations in the wall were 70 times that of the plasma levels. In addition, plasma levels of OxLDL have been shown to correlate with endothelial dysfunction[141,231] and increased carotid intima-media thickness.[232] Recent studies have also shown an association between plasma OxLDL levels and acute cerebral infarction,[233] and strong immunostaining for OxLDL (MDA-LDL) has been reported in the brains of patients with Alzheimer's disease.[234]

In humans pretreated with pravastatin to lower plasma cholesterol levels, significantly reduced OxLDL immunostaining has been noted in carotid plaques removed during carotid endarterectomy (stained with our monoclonal antibody NA59, which recognizes 4-hydroxynonenal epitopes of OxLDL).[235] In addition, simvastatin has been shown to reduce plasma levels of OxLDL and urinary levels of 8-Iso-prostagalndin $F_{2a}$ (an in vivo index of oxidative stress) in hypercholesterolemic subjects.[236] Interestingly, addition of 800 IU of vitamin E did not affect either OxLDL or 8-Iso-$F_{2a}$ levels. Other studies have shown that circulating OxLDL has been associated with functional changes such as endothelial dysfunction and progression of carotid disease.[141,231,232,237] An interesting study by Iuliano et al.[238] has shown that radiolabeled LDL, which was injected into patients with carotid plaques who are undergoing endarterectomy, accumulates within the plaques, and its uptake is markedly decreased by treatment with vitamin E (900 mg/day) for 4 weeks.

These human studies (and animal studies cited previously) assessing plaque morphology and stability strongly suggest that OxLDL is closely associated with atherosclerosis progression and possibly plaque instability. Removal or absence of OxLDL from the vessel wall seems to accompany stabilization of plaques. Thus, OxLDL in the vessel wall seems to be a marker of active disease. Additional human studies will be needed to confirm this.

4. Oxidized lipids that were found in animals, including oxidized sterols and products of the LO pathway, are also found in human atherosclerotic tissue.[42]

5. OxLDL is immunogenic, and autoantibodies to a variety of epitopes of OxLDL are found in human subjects. As originally reported, the autoantibody titer to MDA-LDL, an epitope of OxLDL, was a highly significant predictor of the progression of carotid intimal-medial thickness in a group of middle-aged Finnish males[237] and in a recent Swedish cohort.[239] There have now been a large number of studies in humans suggesting that the titer of antibodies to epitopes of OxLDL are associated with manifestations of atherosclerosis or with traditional risk factors for atherosclerosis such as hypertension, diabetes, and smoking.[240]

6. As in animals, autoantibodies to OxLDL epitopes are found in atherosclerotic lesions of humans and are present as part of immune complexes with OxLDL.[240]

In summary, all of the different lines of evidence supporting the existence of OxLDL in animal models of atherosclerosis apply also in humans, with the exception of the intervention studies.

## Epidemiologic Correlations between Antioxidant Vitamin Intake and CHD Risk

The subject of antioxidant intake and its association with CVD is a popular one, and there are many epidemiologic studies exploring this relationship. This has been reviewed recently in great detail.[241] There are many epidemiologic studies demonstrating an inverse relationship between dietary intake and/or serum levels of antioxidants and CAD. For example, in a summary of a large multicenter cross-sectional study of European countries, Gey et al.[242] demonstrated a strong inverse relationship between intake of vitamin C and vitamin E and rates of CAD. In another study, a 14-year follow-up of Finnish men and women initially free from heart disease demonstrated that the relative risk of heart disease was 32% lower for men and 65% lower for women who were in the highest tertile of vitamin E intake compared with the lowest tertile. In women in the highest tertile for both dietary vitamin E and carotenoids the relative risk of CAD was 84% lower than that for women in the lowest tertile; similarly it was 83% lower in women with both vitamin C and vitamin E intakes in the highest tertile.[243]

There have many such association studies in men and women in the United States, with some mixed results.[241] However, two large prospective cohort studies in the United States, which studied female nurses[244] and male health professionals,[245] found that those who had the highest self-reported intake of vitamin E had the lowest incidence of CAD risk. For example, in the group of 39,910 male health professionals, men who took vitamin E supplements of greater than 100 IU per day for at least 2 years had a 37% lower risk of CHD, compared with men who did not take supplements. In this study, however, a high intake of vitamin C was not associated with a lower risk of CAD. In an even larger study of 87,245 female nurses, women who had been taking vitamin E supplements for more than 2 years had a 41% lower relative risk of major CAD. In contrast, women who had taken vitamin E supplements for less than 2 years showed no significant reduction in risk. In this study the protection was only seen in those nurses who took supplemental vitamin E, and no protection was seen in nurses who had the highest intake of vitamin E supplied only by diet, as judged by dietary records. In another study, the 10-year follow-up of the First National Health and Nutrition Survey, vitamin C intake was inversely related to CAD and overall mortality, but this study was not controlled for vitamin E intake.[246]

Epidemiologic studies are important and suggestive of relationships, but unfortunately they do not demonstrate cause and effect and they do not substitute for prospective intervention trials. It seems likely that health professionals who would take vitamin E supplements would have other lifestyle behaviors that could influence CAD development, and, therefore, only prospective intervention trials can truly test the hypothesis that antioxidant intervention will inhibit CAD and its sequelae.

## Factors Affecting the Oxidation of LDL *in Vivo* That Would Be Amenable to Intervention

Factors potentially affecting the oxidation of LDL *in vivo* are listed in Table 22-3.[247] One may group these factors into those intrinsic to LDL and those extrinsic to LDL (e.g., conditions in the tissue spaces where LDL oxidation occurs). With factors intrinsic to LDL, a major determinant is fatty acid composition. Because PUFAs are more susceptible to oxidation, one would expect that LDL enriched in such PUFAs would be more susceptible than LDL with a high saturated fatty acid content or even LDL enriched in monounsaturated fatty acids (MUFAs). Of course diets rich in saturated fatty acids would raise plasma cholesterol levels, which would be undesirable, but substitution of MUFAs, as opposed to PUFAs, in place of saturated fat would lead not only to lowered plasma cholesterol levels but also theoretically to LDL with a reduced susceptibility to oxidation. Indeed this is what was found.[248,249] A second major determinant of the susceptibility to oxidation would be the endogenous content of antioxidants, including natural antioxidants such as beta carotene, vitamin E, or ubiquinol-10. Studies from many laboratories have now shown that increased dietary content of vitamin E can increase LDL content of vitamin E and confer a 40% to 50% increase in the resistance of LDL to oxidation (as measured by *in vitro* assays). However, it should be emphasized that this leads to an extension

■ ■ ■

**TABLE 22-3**   FACTORS POTENTIALLY AFFECTING OXIDATION OF LDL IN VIVO*

**Factors intrinsic to LDL**

Fatty acid composition (polyunsaturated fatty acid content in particular)
Content of antioxidants: natural (e.g., beta-carotene, vitamin E, ubiquinol-10), pharmacologic (e.g., probucol)
Phospholipase $A_2$ activity (PAF-acetylhydrolase activity)
Others: including size of particle, inherent properties of apoB-100, distribution of fatty acids (e.g., in surface phospholipids or in core
    triglycerides or cholesteryl esters), carbohydrate content, degree of nonenzymatic glycation

**Factors extrinsic to LDL**

Potential variation in cellular prooxidant activity (e.g., genetically or environmentally induced variation in macrophage expression
    of 15-lipoxygenase, myeloperoxidase, or NADPH oxidase activity)
Concentrations of plasma and extracellular fluid pro-oxidant components (e.g., trace metal concentrations)
Concentrations of plasma and extracellular fluid antioxidant components (e.g., ascorbate, urate)
Concentrations of extracellular HDL and HDL content of paraoxonase and PAF-acetylhydrolase
Concentrations of other factors influencing LDL oxidation (e.g., ceruloplasmin)
Factors influencing residence time of LDL in intima (e.g., factors that increase binding such as Lp(a), nonenzymatic glycosylation of LDL or
    matrix, differences in localized matrix proteins that bind LDL)

*apoB, apolipoprotein B; Lp(a), lipoprotein a; PAF, platelet-activating factor.
Modified from Steinberg D, Witztum JL: Lipoproteins, lipoprotein oxidation, and atherogenesis. In Chien KR (ed): Molecular Basis of Cardiovascular Disease. Philadelphia, WB Saunders Company, 1999, pp 458–475.

of the lag time for oxidation by only 20 minutes or so, whereas a potent antioxidant such as probucol prolongs lag time by 10 to 20 hours! However, enrichment of LDL as a consequence of dietary supplementation with beta carotene, even though LDL beta carotene levels can be increased 20-fold, does not increase the resistance of LDL to oxidation at least as measured by *in vitro* assays.[250] Synthetic lipophilic antioxidants such as probucol, which is one of the most powerful antioxidants known, can also be introduced into LDL. Probucol, in sufficient quantities, can nearly completely protect LDL from *in vitro* oxidation.[251] Finally, as noted in Table 22-3 there are a number of other properties of the LDL that may influence its susceptibility to oxidation including its endogenous content of phospholipase $A_2$ activity, which appears to be attributable to its PAF acetylhydrolase activity.[132] Other properties that influence oxidation susceptibility include the size of the particle, because small, dense LDL often found in patients with mild hypertriglyceridemia and "syndrome X" show enhanced susceptibility to oxidation.[252,253] In this category are likely to be LDL from diabetic patients, which may also show a similar enhanced susceptibility to oxidation.[254]

Table 22-3 also lists a variety of factors extrinsic to LDL that may influence tissue modification of LDL. Little is known about which if any of these processes are important *in vivo*. However, eventually, one may want to intervene and modify these factors. Because the ability of cells to express cellular prooxidant activity and reactive oxygen species may be of crucial importance in fighting infections, for example, one would want to be cautious in intervening to alter these factors. One attractive target for modification would be the concentration of extracellular HDL. In a variety of *in vitro* assays, HDL has been shown to protect LDL from oxidation and to inhibit the release of a variety of bioactive molecules from minimally OxLDL. This latter property appears to be due to the presence of paraoxonase in HDL, an enzyme capable of hydrolyzing oxidized short-chain fatty acids in the *sn*-2 position

of phospholipids.[255-257] These phospholipids may play an important role in a number of the proinflammatory properties of minimally modified LDL.[132] PAF-acetylhydrolase on HDL may also play a similar role, although as noted previously the major content of this enzyme is found on plasma LDL.

## Randomized, Placebo-Controlled Clinical Trials Assessing Plaque Morphology

Over the last few years, measurements of plaque dimensions have been reported as the endpoint in antioxidant trials. Similar to clinical intervention trials, the data is mixed, and differences in dose, baseline risk, and agents are suggested to explain the disparities. Table 22-4 lists the major randomized placebo trials with antioxidants.[258-265]

The Probucol Quantitative Regression Swedish Trial (PQRST) evaluated the effects of probucol superimposed on cholestyramine and diet therapy and used angiographic assessment of femoral atherosclerosis as an endpoint.[258] Despite the fact that probucol markedly increased the resistance of circulating LDL to oxidation *ex vivo*, there was no effect on the rate of progression of femoral stenosis. It should be noted that disease in the femoral arteries is generally more advanced, and the lesions tend to be more fibrotic. The studies in experimental animals, in which probucol has had marked beneficial effects, have largely dealt with fatty streak lesions. Also, the observed 24% reduction in HDL levels may have masked any beneficial effect of the antioxidant.

The Study to Evaluate Carotid Ultrasound changes (SECURE) trial was a substudy of the Heart Outcomes Prevention Evaluation (HOPE) trial evaluating 400 IU natural vitamin E on changes in carotid intima-media thickness (IMT) in 732 patients with established CAD or diabetes after 4 to 6 years of treatment.[259,266] Vitamin E did not have any impact on the progression of mean carotid IMT, whereas ramipril reduced progression despite only modest changes in blood pressure. Statins

■ ▪ ■

**TABLE 22-4**  EFFECTS OF ANTIOXIDANT SUPPLEMENTATION ON PLAQUE PROGRESSION AND REGRESSION

| Study/Year | N | Imaging Modality | Antioxidant | Duration | Effect on CVD |
|---|---|---|---|---|---|
| PQRST 1994[258] | 303 | Femoral QCA | Probucol 500 mg bid | 3 years | No benefit |
| SECURE 2001[259] | 732 | B-mode US carotid IMT | Vit E (N) 400 IU | 4–6 years | No benefit |
| HATS 2001[260] | 160 | Coronary QCA | Vit E (N) 800 IU Vit C 1000 mg BetaC 25 mg Selenium 100 μg | 3 years | No benefit |
| FAST 2002[261] | 246 | B-mode US carotid IMT | Probucol 500 mg/day or pravastatin 10 mg/day | 2 years | −14% reduction in IMT with both probucol and pravastatin. Probucol reduced cardiac events |
| Transplant-Associated Atherosclerosis 2002[262] | 40 | Coronary IVUS | Vit E (N) 400 IU Vit C 500 mg | 1 year | Reduced intimal index 0.8% vs. 8%, P = 0.008 |
| VEAPS 2002[263] | 332 | B-mode US carotid IMT | Vit E (S) 400 IU | 3 years | No benefit |
| CART-1 2003[264] | 305 | Coronary IVUS | AGI-1067 280 mg qd | 6 months | AGI induced regression of reference segments |
| ASAP 2003[265] | 440 | B-mode US carotid IMT | Vit E (N) 136 IU Vit C 250 mg both bid | 6 years | −26%, P = 0.014 |

BetaC, beta carotene; IVUS, intravascular ultrasound. Intimal index defined as plaque area divided by vessel area; QCA, quantitative coronary angiography; Vit C, vitamin C; Vit E (N), natural vitamin E; Vit E (S), synthetic vitamin E.

were used in 32% of patients. No changes in clinical outcomes were noted in this subgroup. This study suggests that vitamin E is not effective for secondary prevention in unselected patients with vascular disease.

The HDL-Atherosclerosis Treatment Trial (HATS) recruited patients with low HDL and documented CAD.[267] The HATS study evaluated simvastatin-niacin, antioxidants (vitamin E, vitamin C, beta carotene, and selenium), or both combined and showed, using quantitative coronary angiography, that simvastatin-niacin resulted in a net regression of coronary stenosis (−0.4% vs. +3.9%, P < 0.001, compared with placebo). The progression in the antioxidant arm was +1.8% (P = 0.16 compared with placebo), that is, the progression in the antioxidant group was only about one half of that in the placebo group, but the difference did not reach statistical significance possibly because of the small sample size (approximately 40 patients in each group). In the combination arm, there was some degree of progression, +0.7% (P = 0.004 compared with placebo), and the authors concluded that the antioxidants had a deleterious effect. They suggested that the antioxidant regimen reduced the expected rise in $HDL_{2c}$ and $apoA_1$ levels by niacin (Slo-Niacin). The effect of antioxidant vitamins on $HDL_{2c}$ and $apoA_1$ levels will need to be confirmed in larger studies.

The Vitamin E Atherosclerosis Prevention Study (VEAPS) evaluated subclinical atherosclerosis progression using carotid IMT in patients without known CVD after 3 years treatment with 400 IU vitamin E.[267] They showed no benefit in men or women, despite the fact that the levels of circulating OxLDL were reduced.

However, four other recent randomized, double-blind studies have shown significant reduction in plaque dimensions with antioxidants. In the FAST trial, Sawayama et al.[261] showed that probucol and pravastatin

independently reduced carotid IMT by 14%. The effect of probucol was independent of cholesterol levels. In addition, there was a lower incidence of cardiac events in the probucol group compared with placebo (2.4% vs. 13.6%, P = 0.016). Fang et al.[262,268] showed that a combination of vitamin E (400 IU) and vitamin C (500 mg) given twice daily slowed the progression of intravascular ultrasound (IVUS)-measured transplant-associated atherosclerosis, a condition accepted to be associated with increased oxidative stress. All of these patients were being treated with statins. Recently, the Antioxidant Supplementation in Atherosclerosis Prevention Study (ASAP)[269] reported the 6-year follow-up data and showed a persistent decrease in the rate of carotid IMT progression using natural vitamin E and slow-release vitamin C given twice daily. Significant decreases in plasma $F_2$-isoprostane levels were noted, similar to animal studies that were correlated with atherosclerosis regression. No effects on HDL-C were noted. The recently reported CART-1 trial[264] tested the effects of probucol versus AGI-1067, a novel probucol-analog antioxidant that does not reduce HDL levels or prolong the QTc interval, on the ability to inhibit restenosis following coronary stenting. Using intracoronary ultrasound, the authors noted improved lumen dimensions in the reference segment outside the stented area suggesting an antiatherosclerotic effect.

## Randomized, Placebo-Controlled Clinical Trials Assessing Restenosis

A potential role of antioxidants in preventing restenosis following percutaneous coronary intervention was first suggested by animal and small clinical studies and subsequently confirmed by the Multivitamins and Probucol Study (MVP)[270-272] (Table 22-5). Probucol (500 mg twice

■ ▩ ■

**TABLE 22-5**  EFFECTS OF ANTIOXIDANT SUPPLEMENTATION ON ANGIOGRAPHIC CORONARY RESTENOSIS

| Study/Year | N | Modality | Antioxidant | Duration | Effect on CVD |
|---|---|---|---|---|---|
| MVP 1997[270] Balloon | 317 | Coronary QCA | Vit E (N) 700 IU Vit C 500 mg BetaC 30,000 IU Probucol 500 mg All bid | 6 months | Restenosis reduced with probucol 20.7% vs. 38.9%, P = 0.003 |
| PART 1997[271] Balloon | 101 | Coronary QCA | Probucol 1000 mg qd | 6 months | Restenosis reduced with probucol 23% vs. 58%, P = 0.001 |
| EUROCARE 2000[272] Atherectomy | 292 | Coronary QCA | Carvedilol 25 mg bid | 6 months | No reduction in restenosis |
| CART-1 2003[264] Stent | 305 | Coronary QCA IVUS | AGI-1067 280 mg qd or probucol 500 mg bid | 6 months | AGI and probucol reduced restenosis |

IVUS, intravascular ultrasound; QCA, quantitative coronary angiography; Vit E (N), natural vitamin E.

daily), given 1 month before balloon angioplasty (stents were not used), resulted in significant reduction in late lumen loss (0.22 mm vs. 0.38 mm, P = 0.006) and angiographic restenosis (21% vs. 39%, P = 0.009) that resulted in reduced need for target lesion revascularization (11% vs. 27%). The multivitamin group results were similar to placebo. The benefit of probucol was noted despite a 40% decrease in HDL levels. Although LDL was also decreased, other studies with statins have shown no benefit in reducing the rate of restenosis in balloon-treated vessels.[273] However, statins have been shown to reduce major cardiac adverse events in patients treated with balloon angioplasty in the first 6 months independent of the lack of effect on restenosis. An IVUS substudy of MVP showed that the mechanism of benefit was not reduction in neointimal proliferation, but rather reduction in constrictive vessel remodeling following balloon angioplasty.[274] The results of the MVP study were confirmed by the Probucol Angioplasty Restenosis Trial (PART)[271] that also showed a reduction in restenosis (23% vs. 58%, P = 0.001).

Carvedilol, an agent with nonselective β-adrenergic, α-1 blocking properties and antioxidant effects (the antioxidant moiety mimics vitamin E), was not successful in reducing restenosis in a cohort undergoing coronary atherectomy when given 24 hours before the procedure.[272]

In the CART-1 trial,[264] the beneficial effects of probucol and three doses of AGI-1067 on in-stent restenosis (85% of patients received stents) were documented with IVUS. AGI-1067 showed a dose-dependent benefit on in-stent lumen area at 6 months (2.66 ± 1.58 mm² for placebo, 3.69 ± 2.69 mm² for probucol, 2.75 ± 1.76 mm² for AGI-1067 70 mg, 3.17 ± 2.26 mm² for AGI-1067 140 mg, and 3.36 ± 2.12 mm² for AGI-1067 280 mg, P = 0.046 for AGI-1067 280 mg vs. placebo; P = 0.01 for probucol vs. placebo). An increase in QTc was noted in 4.8% of placebo patients, 17.4% of probucol patients, and 2.5% in the AGI-1067 patients (P = 0.02). HDL did not change in placebo patients, decreased by 35% in probucol patients, and by 17.4% in AGI-1067 patients (P

< 0.01). As mentioned previously, significant improvements were noted in the reference segment lumen area, suggesting reduction in atherosclerosis. This will be studied further in a larger phase III study.

## Clinical Endpoint Intervention Trials

In 1991, a workshop of leading experts convened by the National Heart, Lung and Blood Institute[275] reviewed the available data on antioxidants and suggested that clinical trials were justified, primarily based on a large body of epidemiologic data and animal data, mostly with probucol. They recommended that the first trials be done with naturally occurring antioxidants on the premise that they would be safe. Unfortunately, the mechanisms underlying any potential reduction in atherosclerosis or clinical events were inferred, and not proven, as would be required for any other drug undergoing evaluation. In addition, dietary antioxidants were assumed to share similar biologic properties and could be used interchangeably. This has proven to be a false assumption. For example, beta carotene is a potent trap for singlet oxygen but much less effective in terminating free-radical chain reactions. Vitamin E, on the other hand, is an excellent terminator of chain reactions. Beta carotene does not significantly protect LDL against *ex vivo* oxidation,[250] but vitamin E is moderately effective.[253] However, this reduction in plasma LDL oxidation is not anywhere near the rate of reaction of superoxide radicals in initiating oxidation.[222] Presumably inhibiting oxidation in the vessel wall is much more important than inhibiting oxidation in plasma, which is enriched in antioxidants. In addition, because of the uncertainty about where and how LDL gets oxidized *in vivo* it is not possible to make meaningful comparisons of these various antioxidants. There are also large differences in the pharmacokinetics of the several nutrient antioxidants. For example, vitamin C is distributed exclusively in the aqueous phase, whereas vitamin E is lipophilic and is transported in lipoproteins.

## Beta Carotene Trials

Three large-scale trials of beta carotene have been reported.[276-278] None of them showed a beneficial effect with respect to CVD or cancer. The doses ranged from 20 to 30 mg of beta carotene daily, enough to markedly increase plasma levels of the antioxidant but without any protection conferred on circulating LDL. In one study,[278] 25,000 units of vitamin A daily was combined with 30 mg of beta carotene daily. In this latter study the relative risk of death from CVD was actually 26% *higher* than in the placebo group, for reasons not yet clear. In another study administration of beta carotene, 50 mg every other day did not result in a decrease in CAD, but no adverse consequences were reported.[277]

## Vitamin E and Combination Antioxidant Studies

Seven double-blind, placebo-controlled interventional trials with vitamin E, alone or combined with other antioxidants, have been performed to date. Most of these studies, and all of the very large trials, have shown no benefit of vitamin E in secondary prevention settings (Table 22-6).[279-285] Following is a discussion of the possible reasons.

The alpha-tocopherol beta carotene (ATBC) study in Finland[276] included 29,133 male smokers (36 pack-years) who were treated with 20 mg per day of beta carotene, 50 mg per day of vitamin E, both, or neither and followed for 5 to 8 years. There was no significant effect on either cancer endpoints or CVD endpoints. However, this dose of vitamin E was likely too low. Prolongation of diene conjugation lag time, a measure of protection against LDL oxidation *ex vivo,* becomes significant only at about 150 mg/day and becomes maximal at about 800 to 1200 mg/day.[253,286]

A retrospective analysis of the cholesterol-lowering atherosclerosis study (CLAS), which was a randomized placebo-controlled angiographic trial evaluating cholesterol-niacin treatment, suggests a beneficial effect of vitamin E.[267] In this analysis it was shown that patients who had initiated dietary intake of vitamin E (>100 IU/day) showed significant reduction in angiographic progression over the 2-year follow-up period.

The CHAOS trial (Cambridge Heart Antioxidant Study) tested the effect of vitamin E on cardiovascular events in 2002 patients with angiographically proved CAD randomized to either placebo or to 800 IU/day of vitamin E (first 546 patients) or 400 IU/day (next 489 patients) for a mean follow-up of only 1.4 years. The primary composite endpoint (cardiovascular death or nonfatal myocardial infarction) was reduced by 47% (P = 0.005), and there was an overall 74% decrease in the risk of nonfatal myocardial infarction. A confounding observation, however, was that total mortality from CVD was slightly, although not significantly, greater in the vitamin E supplemented group.[280]

The GISSI trial[281] enrolled patients who had had a myocardial infarction within the past 3 months. Patients, followed over 3.5 years, received either vitamin E (300 mg/day) or omega-3-PUFAs (1 g/day), both, or neither. There was no vitamin E effect on the composite primary endpoint.

In the HOPE[282] trial, patients who had advanced symptomatic CVD were given either 400 IU vitamin E daily or an angiotensin-converting enzyme inhibitor (ramipril), neither, or both. The primary endpoint was a composite of nonfatal infarction, stroke, or death from CVD. Ramipril conferred significant protection, but vitamin E was without effect.

In the SPACE[283] (Secondary Prevention with Antioxidants of CVD in End stage renal disease) study, patients were randomized to receive 800 IU/day of vitamin E or placebo and followed for an average of only 1.4 years. Although only 196 patients were randomized, the number of cardiovascular endpoints was high; almost 50% of these patients had a primary endpoint (myocardial infarction, ischemic stroke, peripheral vascular disease, or unstable angina). Events were reduced by 54% in the vitamin E group (P = 0.014), and myocardial infarction was reduced by 70% (P = 0.016). This study strongly suggests that such a high-risk population may benefit from antioxidant intervention, and further trials in such populations are clearly warranted. It is generally accepted that these patients have a high risk of CVD and are exposed to increased oxidative stress for a variety of reasons, including the fact that free-radical oxygen species are generated at the surface of the membranes used in hemodialysis.[287]

The Primary Prevention Project[284] (PPP) randomized 4495 subjects with classical risk factors for CVD or diabetes mellitus in a 2 × 2 factorial design to open-label aspirin (100 mg/day) and vitamin E (300 mg/day), both,

■ ▪ ■

**TABLE 22-6    EFFECTS OF ANTIOXIDANT SUPPLEMENTATION ON CVD ENDPOINTS**

| Study/Year | N | Prevention | Dose/antioxidant t | Duration | Effect on CVD |
|---|---|---|---|---|---|
| ATBC 1994[279] | 29,133 | Primary | 50 mg Vit E (S) 20 mg BetaC | 5–8 years | No benefit |
| CHAOS 1996[280] | 2,002 | Secondary | 400/800 IU Vit E (N) | 510 days | −47% (P = 0.005) |
| GISSI 1999[281] | 11,324 | Secondary | 300 mg Vit E (S) | 3.5 years | No benefit |
| HOPE 2000[282] | 9,541 | Secondary | 400 IU Vit E (N) | 4–6 years | No benefit |
| SPACE 2000[283] | 196 | Secondary | 400 IU Vit E (N) | 519 days | −46% (P = 0.014) |
| PPP 2001[284] | 4,495 | Primary | 300 mg Vit E (S) | 3.6 years | No benefit |
| HPS 2002[285] | 20,536 | Secondary | 400 IU Vit E (N) 250 mg Vit C 20 mg BetaC | 5 years | No benefit |

BetaC, beta carotene; Vit E (N), natural vitamin E; Vit E (S), synthetic vitamin E.

or neither. After a mean follow-up of 3.6 years, aspirin, but not vitamin E, lowered major CVD events.

The Heart Protection Study[285] (HPS) enrolled 20,536 adults with documented CVD or diabetes and randomized to simvastatin, antioxidant vitamins (600 mg/day vitamin E, 250 mg/day vitamin C, and 20 mg/day beta carotene), both, or neither. No reduction in cardiovascular events was noted with the antioxidant vitamin cocktail.

In a randomized nutritional intervention trial in Linxian, China, intervention with low doses of beta carotene, vitamin E, and selenium produced a 10% lowering of cerebrovascular disease.[288] This has been corroborated with epidemiologic studies showing reduced risk of Alzheimer's disease in patients with increased dietary intake of antioxidant vitamins.[289]

Taking these trials as a whole, one would conclude that in unselected patients with established, well-advanced CVD, vitamin E at doses up to 800 IU/day does not have any measurable benefit in preventing cardiovascular events over 5 years of treatment. The patients in CHAOS, HOPE, and GISSI were more or less comparable in severity of CVD, and the dosages were similar. Additional studies with vitamin E in unselected patients of this description (elderly patients with advanced, well-established CVD; particularly those without evidence of enhanced oxidative stress) would seem unlikely to lead to any different conclusion.[290]

The patients studied in SPACE represent a special subset: patients at high risk for CVD and patients exposed to high oxidative stress during their periodic hemodialysis. The numbers are small, but the magnitude of the effect is significant. Is the benefit due to the increased oxidative stress, which makes it easier to see the effects of an antioxidant in a short period of time in patients at high risk? It is intriguing that such a dramatic effect on *clinical endpoints* was seen in such a short period of time. This raises the possibility that the antioxidant effects of vitamin E might be working through effects on stabilization of vulnerable plaques, improvement in oxidatively induced abnormalities in vasomotor function, or disturbances in coagulation and platelet function. Clearly, further studies are needed in patients with high oxidative stress.

## Why Have the Vitamin E Clinical Endpoint Trials Been Largely Negative?

It is unlikely that the pathogenesis in the human disease is fundamentally different from that in animals. From mouse to rabbit to primate the appearance and the evolution of the lesions appears to be similar. Moreover, oxidation of LDL occurs in humans, OxLDL is present in human lesions, and titers of autoantibodies against OxLDL and plasma levels of OxLDL predict risk. Why then are the results negative so far?

As discussed elsewhere in great detail,[145,290] there are many reasons, which are briefly summarized in the following:

1. Treatment may need to be started earlier and continued longer. Most of the animal model studies deal

with early lesions. Oxidation may have less of an effect on the late, clinically dangerous lesions.

2. The wrong antioxidants and/or the wrong dose are being used. There is little information about the pharmacokinetics of the antioxidants used so far. Moreover, there is no independent measure of the effectiveness of these compounds *in vivo*. In almost none of the clinical endpoint studies is there any marker that would determine whether a desired antioxidant effect was being obtained.

3. In humans, the rate of generation of reactive oxygen species (free radicals) is much lower per unit body weight than in small mammals. The role of oxidation in atherogenesis may be less robust, and, thus, it may take longer to demonstrate the effectiveness of antioxidant intervention.

4. We still do not know where in the body and exactly how LDL is oxidized. Thus they are shooting in the dark when choosing this or that antioxidant. Moreover, it is not known exactly what to measure *in vivo* to get an independent measure of effectiveness. Would we do a statin trial without measuring the magnitude of the effect on blood cholesterol?

5. Of course it is possible, but unlikely, that the human disease really is different enough to explain the discordance.

## THE ROLE OF OXIDIZED LDL IN ACUTE CORONARY SYNDROMES

Most data on OxLDL has been derived from animal studies and from human epidemiologic and vitamin antioxidant intervention studies. However, only recently has progress been made in understanding the pathophysiologic role of OxLDL in acute CVD. Human pathologic studies of patients dying of acute myocardial infarction or sudden death have shown that most ACS result from ruptured or disrupted coronary plaques.[291-293] Unstable coronary plaques generally involve vessel remodeling, inflammation, and disruption of thin weakened fibrous caps overlying a large pool of extracellular lipid. Because of the difficulties in obtaining access to freshly disrupted plaques in patients and the lack of techniques to easily image these lesions, a deficiency of knowledge exists regarding the contents of these lipid pools. However, several postmortem studies have shown that oxidized cholesterol, cholesterol esters, and phospholipids and their breakdown products are present within this lipid gruel in substantial quantities.[166,294,295] It is generally accepted that fully OxLDL does not exist in the circulation because it is rapidly cleared by the reticuloendothelial system, particularly in the liver.[296] By contrast, circulating minimally modified LDL (mmLDL), in which oxidative modification has not been sufficient to cause changes recognized by scavenger receptors, has been clearly documented.[155,297]

Recent studies from several laboratories have shown that circulating OxLDL was associated with an increased risk of CAD. In addition, elevated plasma levels of OxLDL (measured by several different antibodies) have shown a strong association with ACS. For example, Ehara et al.[226] showed that circulating OxLDL-DLH3 (OxLDL detected by monoclonal antibody DLH3) levels, measured on isolated LDL rather than plasma, reflected the presence of immunochemically detected OxLDL in coronary atherectomy specimens and, to some extent, appeared to differentiate the severity of the underlying clinical presentation.[227] Studies by Holvoet et al.[227] using other antibodies to MDA-LDL and Cu-OxLDL showed that OxLDL measured in the emergency room setting was a strong predictor of the presence of ACS in conjunction with troponin measurements. We recently documented a consistent association of a comprehensive panel of 11 OxLDL markers with ACS in a prospective study with a 7-month follow-up period. In addition, we recently documented the association of Lp(a) with OxLDL-E06, a minimally-modified phospholipid epitopes of OxLDL. Remarkably, the correlation of plasma levels of OxLDL-E06 and Lp(a) was 0.91 (P < 0.0001). In addition, both of these lipid moieties were noted to acutely elevate in concert following acute myocardial infarction. This data provides a pathophysiologic link between OxLDL, ACS, and the atherogenicity of Lp(a). Future studies in this area will determine if OxLDL plasma measurements provide independent diagnostic or prognostic information above and beyond any easily measured lipoprotein parameter.

## SUMMARY

The concepts of initiation and clinical expression of atherosclerosis are evolving rapidly.[287,298–300] Current research has focused on inflammation[301] and oxidation.[302] These are not necessarily mutually exclusive. Current data best supports the hypothesis that atherosclerosis is a chronic inflammatory disease that finds expression almost exclusively in the context of hypercholesterolemia. Hypercholesterolemia, on the other hand, is strongly correlated with vessel wall oxidation, which is one of the strongest inflammatory influences in the vessel wall. In that regard, although these processes can be conceptualized separately, it is unlikely that these mechanisms function independently. Targeting only one aspect of this complex disease, for example, specifically treating inflammation or oxidation, is not likely to be as fruitful as targeting all aspects, particularly upstream targets such as the substrate for inflammation and oxidation. This in fact, may be the basis for the astonishing success with statins. By removing the LDL substrate, inflammation and oxidation become less relevant to clinical expression. It is clear from the statin trials that more than 60% to 70% of the treated patients nevertheless experience major clinical events during a 5- to 7-year trial.[303] Starting treatment earlier and continuing it for a longer time may reduce event rates still further, but investigators must keep looking for additional targets. As investigators search for new insights into the pathogenesis of atherogenesis and try to develop new therapies, it will be important to better understand the interactions between hypercholesterolemia, inflammation, and oxidation.

## REFERENCES

1. Steinberg D, Parthasarathy S, Carew TE, et al: Beyond cholesterol: Modifications of low-density lipoprotein that increase its atherogenicity. N Engl J Med 1989;320:915–924.
2. Goldstein JL, Kita T, Brown MS: Defective lipoprotein receptors and atherosclerosis: Lessons from an animal counterpart of familial hypercholesterolemia. N Engl J Med 1983;309:288–296.
3. Brown MS, Goldstein JL: A receptor-mediated pathway for cholesterol homeostasis. Science 1986;232:34–47.
4. Simons LA, Reichl D, Myant NB, Mancini M: The metabolism of the apoprotein of plasma low density lipoprotein in familial hyper-betalipoproteinaemia in the homozygous form. Atherosclerosis 1975;21:283–298.
5. Goldstein JL, Ho YK, Basu SK, Brown MS: Binding site on macrophages that mediates uptake and degradation of acetylated low density lipoprotein, producing massive cholesterol deposition. Proc Natl Acad Sci USA 1976;76:333–337.
6. Weinstein DB, Carew TE, Steinberg D: Uptake and degradation of low density lipoprotein by swine arterial smooth muscle cells with inhibition of cholesterol biosynthesis. Biochim Biophys Acta 1976;424:404–421.
7. Kodama T, Freeman M, Rohrer L, et al: Type I macrophage scavenger receptor contains alpha-helical and collagen-like coiled coils. Nature 1990;343:531–535.
8. Fogelman AM, Shechter I, Seager J, et al: Malondialdehyde alteration of low density lipoproteins leads to cholesteryl ester accumulation in human monocyte-macrophages. Proc Natl Acad Sci USA 1980;77:2214–2218.
9. Mahley RW, Innerarity TL, Weisgraber KB, Oh SY: Altered metabolism (in vivo and in vitro) of plasma lipoproteins after selective chemical modification of lysine residues of the apoproteins. J Clin Invest 1979;64:743–750.
10. Henriksen T, Mahoney EM, Steinberg D: Enhanced macrophage degradation of low density lipoprotein previously incubated with cultured endothelial cells: Recognition by receptors for acetylated low density lipoproteins. Proc Natl Acad Sci USA 1981;78:6499–6503.
11. Henriksen T, Mahoney EM, Steinberg D: Interactions of plasma lipoproteins with endothelial cells. Ann NY Acad Sci 1982;401:102–116.
12. Cathcart MK, Morel DW, Chisolm GM III: Monocytes and neutrophils oxidize low density lipoprotein making it cytotoxic. J Leukoc Biol 1985;38:341–350.
13. Parthasarathy S, Printz DJ, Boyd D, et al: Macrophage oxidation of low density lipoprotein generates a modified form recognized by the scavenger receptor. Arteriosclerosis 1986;6:505–510.
14. Steinbrecher UP, Parthasarathy S, Leake DS, et al: Modification of low density lipoprotein by endothelial cells involves lipid peroxidation and degradation of low density lipoprotein phospholipids. Proc Natl Acad Sci USA 1984;81:3883–3887.
15. Morel DW, Hessler JR, Chisolm GM: Low density lipoprotein cytotoxicity induced by free radical peroxidation of lipid. J Lipid Res 1983;24:1070–1076.
16. Mahley RW: Atherogenic lipoproteins and coronary artery disease: Concepts derived from recent advances in cellular and molecular biology. Circulation 1985;72:943–948.
17. Pitas RE, Innerarity TL, Mahley RW: Cell surface receptor binding of phospholipid. protein complexes containing different ratios of receptor-active and -inactive E apoprotein. J Biol Chem 1980;255:5454–5460.
18. Goldstein JL, Ho YK, Brown MS, et al: Cholesteryl ester accumulation in macrophages resulting from receptor-mediated uptake and degradation of hypercholesterolemic canine beta-very low density lipoproteins. J Biol Chem 1980;255:1839–1848.
19. Chappell DA, Inoue I, Fry GL, et al: The carboxy-terminal domain of lipoprotein lipase induces cellular catabolism of normal very low density lipoproteins via the low density lipoprotein receptor-related protein/alpha 2-macroglobulin receptor. Ann NY Acad Sci 1994;737:434–438.

20. Khoo JC, Miller E, McLoughlin P, Steinberg D: Enhanced macrophage uptake of low density lipoprotein after self-aggregation. Arteriosclerosis 1988;8:348-358.

21. Nievelstein PF, Fogelman AM, Mottino G, Frank JS: Lipid accumulation in rabbit aortic intima 2 hours after bolus infusion of low density lipoprotein: A deep-etch and immunolocalization study of ultrarapidly frozen tissue. Arterioscler Thromb 1991;11:1795-1805.

22. Khoo JC, Miller E, Pio F, et al: Monoclonal antibodies against LDL further enhance macrophage uptake of LDL aggregates. Arterioscler Thromb 1992;12:1258-1266.

23. Lopes-Virella MF, Griffith RL, Shunk KA, Virella GT: Enhanced uptake and impaired intracellular metabolism of low density lipoprotein complexed with anti-low density lipoprotein antibodies. Arterioscler Thromb 1991;11:1356-1367.

24. Camejo G: The interaction of lipids and lipoproteins with the intercellular matrix of arterial tissue: Its possible role in atherogenesis. Adv Lipid Res 1982;19:1-53.

25. Kaplan M, Aviram M: Retention of oxidized LDL by extracellular matrix proteoglycans leads to its uptake by macrophages: An alternative approach to study lipoproteins cellular uptake. Arterioscler Thromb Vasc Biol 2001;21:386-393.

26. Hurt E, Camejo G: Effect of arterial proteoglycans on the interaction of LDL with human monocyte-derived macrophages. Atherosclerosis 1987;67:115-126.

27. Marathe S, Choi Y, Leventhal AR, Tabas I: Sphingomyelinase converts lipoproteins from apolipoprotein E knockout mice into potent inducers of macrophage foam cell formation. Arterioscler Thromb Vasc Biol 2000;20:2607-2613.

28. Torzewski M, Klouche M, Hock J, et al: Immunohistochemical demonstration of enzymatically modified human LDL and its colocalization with the terminal complement complex in the early atherosclerotic lesion. Arterioscler Thromb Vasc Biol 1998;18:369-378.

29. Schuh J, Fairclough GF Jr, Haschemeyer RH: Oxygen-mediated heterogeneity of apo-low-density lipoprotein. Proc Natl Acad Sci USA 1978;75:3173-3177.

30. Esterbauer H, Jurgens G, Quehenberger O, Koller E: Autoxidation of human low density lipoprotein: Loss of polyunsaturated fatty acids and vitamin E and generation of aldehydes. J Lipid Res 1987;28:495-509.

31. Reaven P, Parthasarathy S, Grasse BJ, et al: Effects of oleate-rich and linoleate-rich diets on the susceptibility of low density lipoprotein to oxidative modification in mildly hypercholesterolemic subjects. J Clin Invest 1993;91:668-676.

32. Esterbauer H, Gebicki J, Puhl H, Jurgens G: The role of lipid peroxidation and antioxidants in oxidative modification of LDL. Free Radic Biol Med 1992;13:341-390.

33. Berliner JA, Territo MC, Sevanian A, et al: Minimally modified low density lipoprotein stimulates monocyte endothelial interactions. J Clin Invest 1990;85:1260-1266.

34. Navab M, Berliner JA, Watson AD, et al: The Yin and Yang of oxidation in the development of the fatty streak. Arterioscler Thromb Vasc Biol 1996;16:831-842.

35. Steinberg D: Oxidized low density lipoprotein: An extreme example of lipoprotein heterogeneity. Isr J Med Sci 1996;32:469-472.

36. Liao F, Andalibi A, Qiao JH, et al: Genetic evidence for a common pathway mediating oxidative stress, inflammatory gene induction, and aortic fatty streak formation in mice. J Clin Invest 1994;94:877-884.

37. Sparrow CP, Parthasarathy S, Steinberg D: Enzymatic modification of low density lipoprotein by purified lipoxygenase plus phospholipase A2 mimics cell-mediated oxidative modification. J Lipid Res 1988;29:745-753.

38. Rankin SM, Parthasarathy S, Steinberg D: Evidence for a dominant role of lipoxygenase(s) in the oxidation of LDL by mouse peritoneal macrophages. J Lipid Res 1991;32:449-456.

39. Benz DJ, Mol M, Ezaki M, et al: Enhanced levels of lipoperoxides in low density lipoprotein incubated with murine fibroblast expressing high levels of human 15-lipoxygenase. J Biol Chem 1995;270:5191-5197.

40. Ezaki M, Witztum JL, Steinberg D: Lipoperoxides in LDL incubated with fibroblasts that overexpress 15-lipoxygenase. J Lipid Res 1995;36:1996-2004.

41. Ylä-Herttuala S, Rosenfeld M, Sigal E, et al: Gene expression in macrophage-rich human atherosclerotic lesions. 15-lipoxygenase and acetyl low density lipoprotein receptor messenger RNA colocalize with oxidation specific lipid-protein adducts. J Clin Invest 1991;87:1146-1152.

42. Folcik VA, Nivar-Aristy RA, Krajewski LP, Cathcart MK: Lipoxygenase contributes to the oxidation of lipids in human atherosclerotic plaques. J Clin Invest 1995;96:504-510.

43. Kuhn H, Belkner J, Zaiss S, et al: Involvement of 15-lipoxygenase in early stages of atherogenesis. J Exp Med 1994;179:1903-1911.

44. Sendobry SM, Cornicelli JA, Welch K, et al: Attenuation of diet-induced atherosclerosis in rabbits with a highly selective 15-lipoxygenase inhibitor lacking significant antioxidant properties. Br J Pharmacol 1997;120:1199-1206.

45. Bocan TM, Rosebury WS, Mueller SB, et al: A specific 15-lipoxygenase inhibitor limits the progression and monocyte-macrophage enrichment of hypercholesterolemia-induced atherosclerosis in the rabbit. Atherosclerosis 1998;136:203-216.

46. Parthasarathy S, Wieland E, Steinberg D: A role for endothelial cell lipoxygenase in the oxidative modification of low density lipoprotein. Proc Natl Acad Sci USA 1989;86:1046-1050.

47. Cathcart MK, McNally AK, Chisolm GM: Lipoxygenase-mediated transformation of human low density lipoprotein to an oxidized and cytotoxic complex. J Lipid Res 1991;32:63-70.

48. Savenkova ML, Mueller DM, Heinecke JW: Tyrosyl radical generated by myeloperoxidase is a physiological catalyst for the initiation of lipid peroxidation in low density lipoprotein. J Biol Chem 1994;269:20394-20400.

49. McNally AK, Chisolm GM III, Morel DW, Cathcart MK: Activated human monocytes oxidize low-density lipoprotein by a lipoxygenase-dependent pathway. J Immunol 1990;145:254-259.

50. Wieland E, Parthasarathy S, Steinberg D: Peroxidase-dependent metal-independent oxidation of low density lipoprotein in vitro: A model for in vivo oxidation? Proc Natl Acad Sci USA 1993;90:5929-5933.

51. Babior BM: Phagocytes and oxidative stress. Am J Med 2000;109:33-44.

52. Mehrabian M, Allayee H, Wong J, et al: Identification of 5-lipoxygenase as a major gene contributing to atherosclerosis susceptibility in mice. Circ Res 2002;91:120-126.

53. Cyrus T, Witztum JL, Rader DJ, et al: Disruption of the 12/15-lipoxygenase gene diminishes atherosclerosis in apo E-deficient mice. J Clin Invest 1999;103:1597-1604.

54. Harats D, Shaish A, George J, et al: Overexpression of 15-lipoxygenase in vascular endothelium accelerates early atherosclerosis in LDL receptor-deficient mice. Arterioscler Thromb Vasc Biol 2000;20:2100-2105.

55. Shen J, Herderick E, Cornhill JF, et al: Macrophage-mediated 15-lipoxygenase expression protects against atherosclerosis development. J Clin Invest 1996;98:2201-2208.

56. Detmers PA, Hernandez M, Mudgett J, et al: Deficiency in inducible nitric oxide synthase results in reduced atherosclerosis in apolipoprotein E-deficient mice. J Immunol 2000;165:3430-3435.

57. Ihrig M, Dangler CA, Fox JG: Mice lacking inducible nitric oxide synthase develop spontaneous hypercholesterolaemia and aortic atheromas. Atherosclerosis 2001;156:103-107.

58. Niu XL, Yang X, Hoshiai K, et al: Inducible nitric oxide synthase deficiency does not affect the susceptibility of mice to atherosclerosis but increases collagen content in lesions. Circulation 2001;103:1115-1120.

59. Shi W, Wang X, Shih DM, et al: Paradoxical reduction of fatty streak formation in mice lacking endothelial nitric oxide synthase. Circulation 2002;105:2078-2082.

60. Daugherty A, Dunn JL, Rateri DL, Heinecke JW: Myeloperoxidase, a catalyst for lipoprotein oxidation, is expressed in human atherosclerotic lesions. J Clin Invest 1994;94:437-444.

61. Brennan ML, Anderson MM, Shih DM, et al: Increased atherosclerosis in myeloperoxidase-deficient mice. J Clin Invest 2001;107:419-430.

62. Boullier A, Gillotte KL, Horkko S, et al: The binding of oxidized low density lipoprotein to mouse CD36 is mediated in part by oxidized phospholipids that are associated with both the lipid and protein moieties of the lipoprotein. J Biol Chem 2000;275:9163-9169.

63. Febbraio M, Hajjar DP, Silverstein RL: CD36: A class B scavenger receptor involved in angiogenesis, atherosclerosis, inflammation, and lipid metabolism. J Clin Invest 2001;108:785–791.

64. Linton MF, Fazio S: Class A scavenger receptors, macrophages, and atherosclerosis. Curr Opin Lipidol 2001;12:489–495.

65. Krieger M, Herz J: Structures and functions of multiligand lipoprotein receptors: Macrophage scavenger receptors and LDL receptor-related protein (LRP). Annu Rev Biochem 1994;63:601–637.

66. Krieger M, Acton S, Ashkenas J, et al: Molecular flypaper, host defense, and atherosclerosis: Structure, binding properties, and functions of macrophage scavenger receptors. J Biol Chem 1993;268:4569–4572.

67. Suzuki H, Kurihara Y, Takeya M, et al: A role for macrophage scavenger receptors in atherosclerosis and susceptibility to infection. Nature 1997;386:292–296.

68. Sambrano GR, Parthasarathy S, Steinberg D. Recognition of oxidatively damaged erythrocytes by a macrophage receptor with specificity for oxidized low density lipoprotein. Proc Natl Acad Sci USA. 1994;91:3265–3269.

69. Fadok VA, Savill JS, Haslett C, et al: Different populations of macrophages use either the vitronectin receptor or the phosphatidylserine receptor to recognize and remove apoptotic cells. J Immunol 1992;149:4029–4035.

70. Fadok VA, Voelker DR, Campbell PA, et al: Exposure of phosphatidylserine on the surface of apoptotic lymphocytes triggers specific recognition and removal by macrophages. J Immunol 1992;148:2207–2216.

71. Savill J, Fadok V, Henson P, Haslett C: Phagocyte recognition of cells undergoing apoptosis. Immunol Today 1993;14:131–136.

72. Acton S, Rigotti A, Landschulz KT, et al: Identification of scavenger receptor SR-BI as a high density lipoprotein receptor. Science 1996;271:518–520.

73. Ji Y, Wang N, Ramakrishnan R, et al: Hepatic scavenger receptor BI promotes rapid clearance of high density lipoprotein free cholesterol and its transport into bile. J Biol Chem 1999;274:33398–33402.

74. Kozarsky KF, Donahee MH, Rigotti A, et al: Overexpression of the HDL receptor SR-BI alters plasma HDL and bile cholesterol levels. Nature 1997;387:414–417.

75. Febbraio M, Podrez EA, Smith JD, et al: Targeted disruption of the class B scavenger receptor CD36 protects against atherosclerotic lesion development in mice. J Clin Invest 2000;105:1049–1056.

76. Sakaguchi H, Takeya M, Suzuki H, et al: Role of macrophage scavenger receptors in diet-induced atherosclerosis in mice. Lab Invest 1998;78:423–434.

77. Nozaki S, Kashiwagi H, Yamashita S, et al: Reduced uptake of oxidized low density lipoproteins in monocyte-derived macrophages from CD36-deficient subjects. J Clin Invest 1995;96:1859–1865.

78. Braun A, Trigatti BL, Post MJ, et al: Loss of SR-BI expression leads to the early onset of occlusive atherosclerotic coronary artery disease, spontaneous myocardial infarctions, severe cardiac dysfunction, and premature death in apolipoprotein E-deficient mice. Circ Res 2002;90:270–276.

79. Huszar D, Varban ML, Rinninger F, et al: Increased LDL cholesterol and atherosclerosis in LDL receptor-deficient mice with attenuated expression of scavenger receptor B1. Arterioscler Thromb Vasc Biol 2000;20:1068–1073.

80. Chen W, Silver DL, Smith JD, Tall AR: Scavenger receptor-BI inhibits ATP-binding cassette transporter 1-mediated cholesterol efflux in macrophages. J Biol Chem 2000;275:30794–30800.

81. Kunjathoor VV, Febbraio M, Podrez EA, et al: Scavenger receptors class A-I/II and CD36 are the principal receptors responsible for the uptake of modified low density lipoprotein leading to lipid loading in macrophages. J Biol Chem 2002;277:49982–49988.

82. Davies MJ: Anatomic features in victims of sudden coronary death: Coronary artery pathology. Circulation 1992;85:I19–I24.

83. Brewer HB Jr: The lipid-laden foam cell: An elusive target for therapeutic intervention. J Clin Invest 2000;105:703–705.

84. Accad M, Smith SJ, Newland DL, et al: Massive xanthomatosis and altered composition of atherosclerotic lesions in hyperlipidemic mice lacking acyl CoA:cholesterol acyltransferase 1. J Clin Invest 2000;105:711–719.

85. Fazio S, Major AS, Swift LL, et al: Increased atherosclerosis in LDL receptor-null mice lacking ACAT1 in macrophages. J Clin Invest 2001;107:163–171.

86. Escary JL, Choy HA, Reue K, et al: Paradoxical effect on atherosclerosis of hormone-sensitive lipase overexpression in macrophages. J Lipid Res 1999;40:397–404.

87. Kusunoki J, Hansoty DK, Aragane K, et al: Acyl-CoA:cholesterol acyltransferase inhibition reduces atherosclerosis in apolipoprotein E-deficient mice. Circulation 2001;103:2604–2609.

88. Babiker A, Andersson O, Lund E, et al: Elimination of cholesterol in macrophages and endothelial cells by the sterol 27-hydroxylase mechanism: Comparison with high density lipoprotein-mediated reverse cholesterol transport. J Biol Chem 1997;272:26253–26261.

89. Cali JJ, Hsieh CL, Francke U, Russell DW: Mutations in the bile acid biosynthetic enzyme sterol 27-hydroxylase underlie cerebrotendinous xanthomatosis. J Biol Chem 1991;266:7779–7783.

90. Bodzioch M, Orso E, Klucken J, et al: The gene encoding ATP-binding cassette transporter 1 is mutated in Tangier disease. Nat Genet 1999;22:347–351.

91. Brooks-Wilson A, Marcil M, Clee SM, et al: Mutations in ABC1 in Tangier disease and familial high-density lipoprotein deficiency. Nat Genet 1999;22:336–345.

92. Lawn RM, Wade DP, Garvin MR, et al: The Tangier disease gene product ABC1 controls the cellular apolipoprotein-mediated lipid removal pathway. J Clin Invest 1999;104:R25–R31.

93. Rust S, Rosier M, Funke H: Tangier disease is caused by mutations in the gene encoding ATP-binding cassette transporter 1. Nat Genet 1999;22:352–355.

94. Tall AR, Wang N: Tangier disease as a test of the reverse cholesterol transport hypothesis. J Clin Invest 2000;106:1205–1207.

95. Clee SM, Zwinderman AH, Engert JC, et al: Common genetic variation in ABCA1 is associated with altered lipoprotein levels and a modified risk for coronary artery disease. Circulation 2001;103:1198–1205.

96. Willson TM, Brown PJ, Sternbach DD, Henke BR: The PPARs: From orphan receptors to drug discovery. J Med Chem 2000;43:527–550.

97. Chawla A, Lee CH, Barak Y, et al: PPAR delta is a very low-density lipoprotein sensor in macrophages. Proc Natl Acad Sci USA 2003;100:1268–1273.

98. Ziouzenkova O, Perrey S, Asatryan L, et al: Lipolysis of triglyceride-rich lipoproteins generates PPAR ligands: Evidence for an antiinflammatory role for lipoprotein lipase. Proc Natl Acad Sci USA 2003;100:2730–2735.

99. Forman BM, Tontonoz P, Chen J, et al: 15-Deoxy-delta 12, 14-prostaglandin J2 is a ligand for the adipocyte determination factor PPAR gamma. Cell 1995;83:803–812.

100. Kliewer SA, Lenhard JM, Willson TM, et al: A prostaglandin J2 metabolite binds peroxisome proliferator-activated receptor gamma and promotes adipocyte differentiation. Cell 1995;83:813–819.

101. Huang JT, Welch JS, Ricote M, et al: Interleukin-4-dependent production of PPAR-gamma ligands in macrophages by 12/15-lipoxygenase. Nature 1999;400:378–382.

102. Nagy L, Tontonoz P, Alvarez JG, et al: Oxidized LDL regulates macrophage gene expression through ligand activation of PPARgamma. Cell 1998;93:229–240.

103. Barbier O, Torra IP, Duguay Y, et al: Pleiotropic actions of peroxisome proliferator-activated receptors in lipid metabolism and atherosclerosis. Arterioscler Thromb Vasc Biol 2002;22:717–726.

104. Barak Y, Nelson MC, Ong ES, et al: PPAR gamma is required for placental, cardiac, and adipose tissue development. Mol Cell 1999;4:585–595.

105. Rosen ED, Sarraf P, Troy AE, et al: PPAR gamma is required for the differentiation of adipose tissue in vivo and in vitro. Mol Cell 1999;4:611–617.

106. Lehmann JM, Moore LB, Smith-Oliver TA, et al: An antidiabetic thiazolidinedione is a high affinity ligand for peroxisome proliferator-activated receptor gamma (PPAR gamma). J Biol Chem 1995;270:12953–12956.

107. Ricote M, Huang J, Fajas L, et al: Expression of the peroxisome proliferator-activated receptor gamma (PPARgamma) in human atherosclerosis and regulation in macrophages by colony stimulating factors and oxidized low density lipoprotein. Proc Natl Acad Sci USA 1998;95:7614–7619.

108. Ricote M, Li AC, Willson TM, et al: The peroxisome proliferator-activated receptor-gamma is a negative regulator of macrophage activation. Nature 1998;391:79–82.

109. Tontonoz P, Nagy L, Alvarez JG, et al: PPARgamma promotes monocyte/macrophage differentiation and uptake of oxidized LDL. Cell 1998;93:241-252.

110. Jiang C, Ting AT, Seed B: PPAR-gamma agonists inhibit production of monocyte inflammatory cytokines. Nature 1998;391:82-86.

111. Marx N, Schonbeck U, Lazar MA, et al: Peroxisome proliferator-activated receptor gamma activators inhibit gene expression and migration in human vascular smooth muscle cells. Circ Res 1998;83:1097-1103.

112. Chawla A, Boisvert WA, Lee CH, et al: A PPAR gamma-LXR-ABCA1 pathway in macrophages is involved in cholesterol efflux and atherogenesis. Mol Cell 2001;7:161-171.

113. Chinetti G, Lestavel S, Bocher V, et al: PPAR-alpha and PPAR-gamma activators induce cholesterol removal from human macrophage foam cells through stimulation of the ABCA1 pathway. Nat Med 2001;7:53-58.

114. Chen Z, Ishibashi S, Perrey S, et al: Troglitazone inhibits atherosclerosis in apolipoprotein E-knockout mice: Pleiotropic effects on CD36 expression and HDL. Arterioscler Thromb Vasc Biol 2001;21:372-377.

115. Claudel T, Leibowitz MD, Fievet C, et al: Reduction of atherosclerosis in apolipoprotein E knockout mice by activation of the retinoid X receptor. Proc Natl Acad Sci USA 2001;98:2610-2615.

116. Collins AR, Meehan WP, Kintscher U, et al: Troglitazone inhibits formation of early atherosclerotic lesions in diabetic and nondiabetic low density lipoprotein receptor-deficient mice. Arterioscler Thromb Vasc Biol 2001;21:365-371.

117. Li AC, Brown KK, Silvestre MJ, et al: Peroxisome proliferator-activated receptor gamma ligands inhibit development of atherosclerosis in LDL receptor-deficient mice. J Clin Invest 2000;106:523-531.

118. Haffner SM, Greenberg AS, Weston WM, et al: Effect of rosiglitazone treatment on nontraditional markers of cardiovascular disease in patients with type 2 diabetes mellitus. Circulation 2002; 106:679-684.

119. Repa JJ, Liang G, Ou J, et al: Regulation of mouse sterol regulatory element-binding protein-1c gene (SREBP-1c) by oxysterol receptors, LXRalpha and LXRbeta. Genes Dev 2000;14:2819-2830.

120. Chawla A, Repa JJ, Evans RM, Mangelsdorf DJ: Nuclear receptors and lipid physiology: Opening the X-files. Science 2001;294:1866-1870.

121. Laffitte BA, Repa JJ, Joseph SB, et al: LXRs control lipid-inducible expression of the apolipoprotein E gene in macrophages and adipocytes. Proc Natl Acad Sci USA 2001;98:507-512.

122. Joseph SB, McKilligin E, Pei L, et al: Synthetic LXR ligand inhibits the development of atherosclerosis in mice. Proc Natl Acad Sci USA 2002;99:7604-7609.

123. Schultz JR, Tu H, Luk A, et al: Role of LXRs in control of lipogenesis. Genes Dev 2000;14:2831-2838.

124. Resnick D, Pearson A, Krieger M: The SRCR superfamily: A family reminiscent of the Ig superfamily. Trends Biochem Sci 1994;19:5-8.

125. Pitas RE: Expression of the acetyl low density lipoprotein receptor by rabbit fibroblasts and smooth muscle cells: Up-regulation by phorbol esters. J Biol Chem 1990;265:12722-12727.

126. Quinn MT, Parthasarathy S, Fong LG, Steinberg D: Oxidatively modified low density lipoproteins: A potential role in recruitment and retention of monocyte/macrophages during atherogenesis. Proc Natl Acad Sci USA 1987;84:2995-2998.

127. McMurray HF, Parthasarathy S, Steinberg D: Oxidatively modified low density lipoprotein is a chemoattractant for human T lymphocytes. J Clin Invest 1993;92:1004-1008.

128. Jonasson L, Holm J, Skalli O, et al: Regional accumulations of T cells, macrophages, and smooth muscle cells in the human atherosclerotic plaque. Arteriosclerosis 1986;6:131-138.

129. Quinn MT, Parthasarathy S, Steinberg D: Endothelial cell-derived chemotactic activity for mouse peritoneal macrophages and the effects of modified forms of low density lipoprotein. Proc Natl Acad Sci USA 1985;82:5949-5953.

130. Cushing SD, Berliner JA, Valente AJ, et al: Minimally modified low density lipoprotein induces monocyte chemotactic protein 1 in human endothelial cells and smooth muscle cells. Proc Natl Acad Sci USA 1990;87:5134-5138.

131. Rajavashisth TB, Andalibi A, Territo MC, et al: Induction of endothelial cell expression of granulocyte and macrophage colony-stimulating factors by modified low-density lipoproteins. Nature 1990;344:254-257.

132. Watson AD, Navab M, Hama SY, et al: Effect of platelet activating factor-acetylhydrolase on the formation and action of minimally oxidized low density lipoprotein. J Clin Invest 1995;95:774-782.

133. Kume N, Cybulsky MI, Gimbrone MA Jr: Lysophosphatidylcholine, a component of atherogenic lipoproteins, induces mononuclear leukocyte adhesion molecules in cultured human and rabbit arterial endothelial cells. J Clin Invest 1992;90:1138-1144.

134. Hessler JR, Morel DW, Lewis LJ, Chisolm GM: Lipoprotein oxidation and lipoprotein-induced cytotoxicity. Arteriosclerosis 1983;3:215-222.

135. Henriksen T, Evensen SA, Carlander B: Injury to human endothelial cells in culture induced by low density lipoproteins. Scand J Clin Lab Invest 1979;39:361-368.

136. Morel DW, DiCorleto PE, Chisolm GM: Endothelial and smooth muscle cells alter low density lipoprotein in vitro by free radical oxidation. Arteriosclerosis 1984;4:357-364.

137. Colles SM, Maxson JM, Carlson SG, Chisolm GM: Oxidized LDL-induced injury and apoptosis in atherosclerosis: Potential roles for oxysterols. Trends Cardiovasc Med 2001;11:131-138.

138. Furchgott RF, Zawadzki JV: The obligatory role of endothelial cells in the relaxation of arterial smooth muscle by acetylcholine. Nature 1980;288:373-376.

139. Kugiyama K, Kerns SA, Morrisett JD, et al: Impairment of endothelium-dependent arterial relaxation by lysolecithin in modified low-density lipoproteins. Nature 1990;344:160-162.

140. Kinlay S, Selwyn AP, Delagrange D, et al: Biological mechanisms for the clinical success of lipid-lowering in coronary artery disease and the use of surrogate end-points. Curr Opin Lipidol 1996;7:389-397.

141. Tamai O, Matsuoka H, Itabe H, et al: Single LDL apheresis improves endothelium-dependent vasodilation in hypercholesterolemic humans. Circulation 1997;95:76-82.

142. Anderson TJ, Meredith IT, Yeung AC, et al: The effect of cholesterol-lowering and antioxidant therapy on endothelium-dependent coronary vasomotion. N Engl J Med 1995;332:488-493.

143. Dabbagh AJ, Frei B: Human suction blister interstitial fluid prevents metal ion-dependent oxidation of low density lipoprotein by macrophages and in cell-free systems. J Clin Invest 1995;96:1958-1966.

144. Tsimikas S, Witztum JL: The oxidative modification hypothesis of atherosclerosis. In Keaney JF (ed): Oxidative Stress and Vascular Disease. Boston, Kluwer Academic Publishers, 2000, pp 49-74.

145. Witztum JL, Steinberg D: The oxidative modification hypothesis of atherosclerosis: Does it hold for humans? Trends Cardiovasc Med 2001;11:93-102.

146. Witztum JL, Steinbrecher UP, Kesaniemi YA, Fisher M: Autoantibodies to glucosylated proteins in the plasma of patients with diabetes mellitus. Proc Natl Acad Sci USA 1984;81:3204-3208.

147. Palinski W, Rosenfeld ME, Yla-Herttuala S, et al: Low density lipoprotein undergoes oxidative modification in vivo. Proc Natl Acad Sci USA 1989;86:1372-1376.

148. Palinski W, Ylä-Herttuala S, Rosenfeld ME, et al: Antisera and monoclonal antibodies specific for epitopes generated during oxidative modification of low density lipoprotein. Arteriosclerosis 1990;10:325-335.

149. Haberland ME, Fong D, Cheng L: Malondialdehyde-altered protein occurs in atheroma of Watanabe heritable hyperlipidemic rabbits. Science 1988;241:215-218.

150. Boyd HC, Gown AM, Wolfbauer G, Chait A: Direct evidence for a protein recognized by a monoclonal antibody against oxidatively modified LDL in atherosclerotic lesions from a Watanabe heritable hyperlipidemic rabbit. Am J Pathol 1989;135:815-825.

151. Ylä-Herttuala S, Palinski W, Rosenfeld ME, et al: Evidence for the presence of oxidatively modified low density lipoprotein in atherosclerotic lesions of rabbit and man. J Clin Invest 1989;84:1086-1095.

152. Hulten LM, Lindmark H, Diczfalusy U, et al: Oxysterols present in atherosclerotic tissue decrease the expression of lipoprotein

lipase messenger RNA in human monocyte-derived macrophages. J Clin Invest 1996;97:461–468.

153. Schwenke DC, Carew TE: Initiation of atherosclerotic lesions in cholesterol-fed rabbits. I. Focal increases in arterial LDL concentration precede development of fatty streak lesions. Arteriosclerosis 1989;9:895–907.

154. Schwenke DC, Carew TE: Initiation of atherosclerotic lesions in cholesterol-fed rabbits. II. Selective retention of LDL vs. selective increases in LDL permeability in susceptible sites of arteries. Arteriosclerosis 1989;9:908–918.

155. Hodis HN, Kramsch DM, Avogaro P, et al: Biochemical and cytotoxic characteristics of an in vivo circulating oxidized low density lipoprotein (LDL-). J Lipid Res 1994;35:669–677.

156. Sevanian A, Hwang J, Hodis H, et al: Contribution of an in vivo oxidized LDL to LDL oxidation and its association with dense LDL subpopulations. Arterioscler Thromb Vasc Biol 1996;16:784–793.

157. Itabe H, Yamamoto H, Suzuki M, et al: Oxidized phosphatidylcholines that modify proteins: Analysis by monoclonal antibody against oxidized low density lipoprotein. J Biol Chem 1996; 271:33208–33217.

158. Palinski W, Hörkkö S, Miller E, et al: Cloning of monoclonal autoantibodies to epitopes of oxidized lipoproteins from apolipoprotein E-deficient mice: Demonstration of epitopes of oxidized low density lipoprotein in human plasma. J Clin Invest 1996;98:800–814.

159. Tsimikas S, Witztum JL: Measuring circulating oxidized low-density lipoprotein to evaluate coronary risk. Circulation 2001;103:1930–1932.

160. Palinski W, Tangirala RK, Miller E, et al: Increased autoantibody titers against epitopes of oxidized LDL in LDL receptor-deficient mice with increased atherosclerosis. Arterioscler Thromb Vasc Biol 1995;15:1569–1576.

161. Freigang S, Hörkkö S, Miller E, et al: Immunization of LDL receptor-deficient mice with homologous malondialdehyde-modified and native LDL reduces progression of atherosclerosis by mechanisms other than induction of high titers of antibodies to oxidative neoepitopes. Arterioscler Thromb Vasc Biol 1998; 18:1972–1982.

162. Aikawa M, Sugiyama S, Hill CC, et al: Lipid lowering reduces oxidative stress and endothelial cell activation in rabbit atheroma. Circulation 2002;106:1390–1396.

163. Cyrus T, Praticó D, Zhao L, et al: Absence of 12/15-lipoxygenase expression decreases lipid peroxidation and atherogenesis in apolipoprotein E-deficient mice. Circulation 2001;103:2277–2282.

164. Tsimikas S, Palinski W, Witztum JL: Circulating autoantibodies to oxidized LDL correlate with arterial accumulation and depletion of oxidized LDL in LDL receptor-deficient mice. Arterioscler Thromb Vasc Biol 2001;21:95–100.

165. Shaw PX, Hörkkö S, Chang MK, et al: Natural antibodies with the T15 idiotype may act in atherosclerosis, apoptotic clearance, and protective immunity. J Clin Invest 2000;105:1731–1740.

166. Ylä-Herttuala S, Palinski W, Butler SW, et al: Rabbit and human atherosclerotic lesions contain IgG that recognizes epitopes of oxidized LDL. Arterioscler Thromb 1994;14:32–40.

167. Palinski W, Napoli C: The fetal origins of atherosclerosis: Maternal hypercholesterolemia, and cholesterol-lowering or antioxidant treatment during pregnancy influence in utero programming and postnatal susceptibility to atherogenesis. FASEB J 2002; 16:1348–1360.

168. Tsimikas S, Palinski W, Halpern SE, et al: Radiolabeled MDA2, an oxidation-specific, monoclonal antibody, identifies native atherosclerotic lesions in vivo. J Nucl Cardiol 1999;6:41–53.

169. Tsimikas S, Shortal BP, Witztum JL, Palinski W: In vivo uptake of radiolabeled MDA2, an oxidation-specific monoclonal antibody, provides an accurate measure of atherosclerotic lesions rich in oxidized LDL and is highly sensitive to their regression. Arterioscler Thromb Vasc Biol 2000;20:689–697.

170. Shaw PX, Hörkkö S, Tsimikas S, et al: Human-derived anti-oxidized LDL autoantibody blocks uptake of oxidized LDL by macrophages and localizes to atherosclerotic lesions in vivo. Arterioscler Thromb Vasc Biol 2001;21:1333–1339.

171. Binder CJ, Chang MK, Shaw PX, et al: Innate and acquired immunity in atherogenesis. Nat Med 2002;8:1218–1226.

172. Glass CK, Witztum JL: Atherosclerosis. the road ahead. Cell 2001;104:503–516.

173. Hansson GK: Immune mechanisms in atherosclerosis. Arterioscler Thromb Vasc Biol 2001;21:1876–1890.

174. Hansson GK, Libby P, Schonbeck U, Yan ZQ: Innate and adaptive immunity in the pathogenesis of atherosclerosis. Circ Res 2002;91:281–291.

175. Hörkkö S, Bird DA, Miller E, et al: Monoclonal autoantibodies specific for oxidized phospholipids or oxidized phospholipid-protein adducts inhibit macrophage uptake of oxidized low-density lipoproteins. J Clin Invest 1999;103:117–128.

176. Friedman P, Hörkkö S, Steinberg D, et al: Correlation of antiphospholipid antibody recognition with the structure of synthetic oxidized phospholipids: Importance of Schiff base formation and Aldol condensation. J Biol Chem 2001;277:7010–7020.

177. Chang MK, Bergmark C, Laurila A, et al: Monoclonal antibodies against oxidized low-density lipoprotein bind to apoptotic cells and inhibit their phagocytosis by elicited macrophages: Evidence that oxidation-specific epitopes mediate macrophage recognition. Proc Natl Acad Sci USA 1999;96:6353–6358.

178. Chang MK, Binder CJ, Torzewski M, Witztum JL: C-reactive protein binds to both oxidized LDL and apoptotic cells through recognition of a common ligand: Phosphorylcholine of oxidized phospholipids. Proc Natl Acad Sci USA 2002;99:13043–13048.

179. Carew TE, Schwenke DC, Steinberg D: Antiatherogenic effect of probucol unrelated to its hypocholesterolemic effect: Evidence that antioxidants in vivo can selectively inhibit low density lipoprotein degradation in macrophage-rich fatty streaks and slow the progression of atherosclerosis in the Watanabe heritable hyperlipidemic rabbit. Proc Natl Acad Sci USA 1987;84: 7725–7729.

180. Kita T, Nagano Y, Yokode M, et al: Probucol prevents the progression of atherosclerosis in Watanabe heritable hyperlipidemic rabbit, an animal model for familial hypercholesterolemia. Proc Natl Acad Sci USA 1987;84:5928–5931.

181. Mao SJ, Yates MT, Rechtin AE, et al: Antioxidant activity of probucol and its analogues in hypercholesterolemic Watanabe rabbits. J Med Chem 1991;34:298–302.

182. Daugherty A, Zweifel BS, Schonfeld G: The effects of probucol on the progression of atherosclerosis in mature Watanabe heritable hyperlipidaemic rabbits. Br J Pharmacol 1991;103:1013–1018.

183. Fruebis J, Steinberg D, Dresel HA, Carew TE: A comparison of the antiatherogenic effects of probucol and of a structural analogue of probucol in low density lipoprotein receptor-deficient rabbits. J Clin Invest 1994;94:392–398.

184. Donetti E, Soma MR, Barberi L, et al: Dual effects of the antioxidant agents probucol and carvedilol on proliferative and fatty lesions in hypercholesterolemic rabbits. Atherosclerosis 1998; 141:45–51.

185. Witting P, Pettersson K, Ostlund-Lindqvist AM, et al: Dissociation of atherogenesis from aortic accumulation of lipid hydro(pero)xides in Watanabe heritable hyperlipidemic rabbits. J Clin Invest 1999;104:213–220.

186. Brasen JH, Koenig K, Bach H, et al: Comparison of the effects of alpha-tocopherol, ubiquinone-10 and probucol at therapeutic doses on atherosclerosis in WHHL rabbits. Atherosclerosis 2002;163:249–259.

187. Yoshida N, Murase H, Kunieda T, et al: Inhibitory effect of a novel water-soluble vitamin E derivative on atherosclerosis in rabbits. Atherosclerosis 2002;162:111–117.

188. Mao SJ, Yates MT, Parker RA, et al: Attenuation of atherosclerosis in a modified strain of hypercholesterolemic Watanabe rabbits with use of a probucol analogue (MDL 29,311) that does not lower serum cholesterol. Arterioscler Thromb 1991;11:1266–1275.

189. Stein Y, Stein O, Delplanque B, et al: Lack of effect of probucol on atheroma formation in cholesterol-fed rabbits kept at comparable plasma cholesterol levels. Atherosclerosis 1989;75:145–155.

190. Daugherty A, Zweifel BS, Schonfeld G: Probucol attenuates the development of aortic atherosclerosis in cholesterol-fed rabbits. Br J Pharmacol 1989;98:612–618.

191. Prasad K, Kalra J, Lee P: Oxygen free radicals as a mechanism of hypercholesterolemic atherosclerosis: Effects of probucol. Int J Angio 1994;3:100–112.

192. Shaish A, Daugherty A, O'Sullivan F, et al: Beta-carotene inhibits atherosclerosis in hypercholesterolemic rabbits. J Clin Invest 1995;96:2075–2082.

193. Schwenke DC, Behr SR: Vitamin E combined with selenium inhibits atherosclerosis in hypercholesterolemic rabbits independently of effects on plasma cholesterol concentrations. Circ Res 1998;83:366–377.

194. Sparrow CP, Doebber TW, Olszewski J, et al: Low density lipoprotein is protected from oxidation and the progression of atherosclerosis is slowed in cholesterol-fed rabbits by the antioxidant N,N'-diphenyl-phenylenediamine. J Clin Invest 1992;89:1885–1891.

195. Bjorkhem I, Henriksson-Freyschuss A, Breuer O, et al: The antioxidant butylated hydroxytoluene protects against atherosclerosis. Arterioscler Thromb 1991;11:15–22.

196. Mantha SV, Prasad M, Kalra J, Prasad K. Antioxidant enzymes in hypercholesterolemia and effects of vitamin E in rabbits. Atherosclerosis 1993;101:135–144.

197. Morel DW, Llera-Moya M, Friday KE. Treatment of cholesterol-fed rabbits with dietary vitamins E and C inhibits lipoprotein oxidation but not development of atherosclerosis. J Nutr 1994;124:2123–2130.

198. Kleinveld HA, Hak-Lemmers HL, Hectors MP, et al: Vitamin E and fatty acid intervention does not attenuate the progression of atherosclerosis in Watanabe heritable hyperlipidemic rabbits. Arterioscler Thromb Vasc Biol 1995;15:290–297.

199. Fruebis J, Carew TE, Palinski W: Effect of vitamin E on atherogenesis in LDL receptor-deficient rabbits. Atherosclerosis 1995;117:217–224.

200. Parker RA, Sabrah T, Cap M, Gill BT: Relation of vascular oxidative stress, alpha-tocopherol, and hypercholesterolemia to early atherosclerosis in hamsters. Arterioscler Thromb Vasc Biol 1995;15:349–358.

201. El Swefy S, Schaefer EJ, Seman LJ, et al: The effect of vitamin E, probucol, and lovastatin on oxidative status and aortic fatty lesions in hyperlipidemic-diabetic hamsters. Atherosclerosis 2000;149:277–286.

202. Tangirala RK, Casanada F, Miller E, et al: Effect of the antioxidant N,N'-diphenyl 1,4-phenylenediamine (DPPD) on atherosclerosis in apoE-deficient mice. Arterioscler Thromb Vasc Biol 1995;15:1625–1630.

203. Zhang SH, Reddick RL, Avdievich E, et al: Paradoxical enhancement of atherosclerosis by probucol treatment in apolipoprotein E-deficient mice. J Clin Invest 1997;99:2858–2866.

204. Witting PK, Pettersson K, Letters J, Stocker R: Anti-atherogenic effect of coenzyme Q10 in apolipoprotein E gene knockout mice. Free Radical Biol Med 2000;29:295–305.

205. Moghadasian MH, McManus BM, Godin DV, et al: Proatherogenic and antiatherogenic effects of probucol and phytosterols in apolipoprotein E-deficient mice: Possible mechanisms of action. Circulation 1999;99:1733–1739.

206. Yoshikawa T, Shimano H, Chen Z, et al: Effects of probucol on atherosclerosis of apoE-deficient or LDL receptor-deficient mice. Horm Metab Res 2001;33:472–479.

207. Praticó D, Tangirala RK, Rader DJ, et al: Vitamin E suppresses isoprostane generation in vivo and reduces atherosclerosis in ApoE-deficient mice. Nat Med 1998;4:1189–1192.

208. Sundell CL, Somers PK, Meng CQ, et al: AGI-1067: A multifunctional phenolic antioxidant, lipid modulator, anti-inflammatory and anti-atherosclerotic agent. J Pharmacol Exp Ther 2003. 305:1116–1123.

209. Bird DA, Tangirala RK, Fruebis J, et al: Effect of probucol on LDL oxidation and atherosclerosis in LDL receptor-deficient mice. J Lipid Res 1998;39:1079–1090.

210. Cynshi O, Kawabe Y, Suzuki T, et al: Antiatherogenic effects of the antioxidant BO-653 in three different animal models. Proc Natl Acad Sci USA 1998;95:10123–10128.

211. Benson GM, Schiffelers R, Nicols C, et al: Effect of probucol on serum lipids, atherosclerosis and toxicology in fat-fed LDL receptor deficient mice. Atherosclerosis 1998;141:237–247.

212. Crawford RS, Kirk EA, Rosenfeld ME, et al: Dietary antioxidants inhibit development of fatty streak lesions in the LDL receptor-deficient mouse. Arterioscler Thromb Vasc Biol 1998;18:1506–1513.

213. Witting P, Pettersson K, Ostlund-Lindqvist AM, et al: Dissociation of atherogenesis from aortic accumulation of lipid hydro(pero)xides in Watanabe heritable hyperlipidemic rabbits. J Clin Invest 1999;104:213–220.

214. Sasahara M, Raines EW, Chait A, et al: Inhibition of hypercholesterolemia-induced atherosclerosis in the nonhuman primate by probucol. I. Is the extent of atherosclerosis related to resistance of LDL to oxidation? J Clin Invest 1994;94:155–164.

215. Verlangieri AJ, Bush MJ: Effects of d-alpha-tocopherol supplementation on experimentally induced primate atherosclerosis. J Am Coll Nutr 1992;11:131–138.

216. Steinberg D: At last, direct evidence that lipoxygenases play a role in atherogenesis. J Clin Invest 1999;103:1487–1488.

217. George J, Afek A, Shaish A, et al: 12/15-Lipoxygenase gene disruption attenuates atherogenesis in LDL receptor-deficient mice. Circulation 2001;104:1646–1650.

218. Heinecke JW: Is lipid peroxidation relevant to atherogenesis? J Clin Invest 1999;104:135–136.

219. Shih DM, Xia YR, Wang XP, et al: Combined serum paraoxonase knockout/apolipoprotein E knockout mice exhibit increased lipoprotein oxidation and atherosclerosis. J Biol Chem 2000;275:17527–17535.

220. Jackson RL, Barnhart RL, Mao SJ: Probucol and its mechanisms for reducing atherosclerosis. Adv Exp Med Biol 1991;285:367–372.

221. Quinet EM, Huerta P, Nancoo D, et al: Adipose tissue cholesteryl ester transfer protein mRNA in response to probucol treatment: Cholesterol and species dependence. J Lipid Res 1993;34:845–852.

222. Landmesser U, Harrison DG: Oxidant stress as a marker for cardiovascular events: Ox marks the spot. Circulation 2001;104:2638–2640.

223. Khan BV, Parthasarathy SS, Alexander RW, Medford RM: Modified low density lipoprotein and its constituents augment cytokine-activated vascular cell adhesion molecule-1 gene expression in human vascular endothelial cells. J Clin Invest 1995;95:1262–1270.

224. Khan BV, Harrison DG, Olbrych MT, et al: Nitric oxide regulates vascular cell adhesion molecule 1 gene expression and redox-sensitive transcriptional events in human vascular endothelial cells. Proc Natl Acad Sci USA 1996;93:9114–9119.

225. Itabe H, Yamamoto H, Imanaka T, et al: Sensitive detection of oxidatively modified low density lipoprotein using a monoclonal antibody. J Lipid Res 1996;37:45–53.

226. Ehara S, Ueda M, Naruko T, et al: Elevated levels of oxidized low density lipoprotein show a positive relationship with the severity of acute coronary syndromes. Circulation 2001;103:1955–1960.

227. Holvoet P, Collen D, van de Werf F: Malondialdehyde-modified LDL as a marker of acute coronary syndromes. JAMA 1999;281:1718–1721.

228. Valgimigli M, Agnoletti L, Curello S, et al: Serum from patients with acute coronary syndromes displays a proapoptotic effect on human endothelial cells: A possible link to pan-coronary syndromes. Circulation 2003;107:264–270.

229. Tsimikas S, Bergmark C, Beyer RW, et al: Temporal increases in plasma markers of oxidized low-density lipoprotein strongly reflect the presence of acute coronary syndromes. J Am Coll Cardiol 2003;41:360–370.

230. Nishi K, Itabe H, Uno M, et al: Oxidized LDL in carotid plaques and plasma associates with plaque instability. Arterioscler Thromb Vasc Biol 2002;22:1649–1654.

231. Penny WF, Ben Yehuda O, Kuroe K, et al: Improvement of coronary artery endothelial dysfunction with lipid-lowering therapy: Heterogeneity of segmental response and correlation with plasma-oxidized low density lipoprotein. J Am Coll Cardiol 2001;37:766–774.

232. Hulthe J, Fagerberg B: Circulating oxidized LDL is associated with subclinical atherosclerosis development and inflammatory cytokines (AIR Study). Arterioscler Thromb Vasc Biol 2002;22:1162–1167.

233. Uno M, Kitazato KT, Nishi K, et al: Raised plasma oxidised LDL in acute cerebral infarction. J Neurol Neurosurg Psychiatry 2003;74:312–316.

234. Dei R, Takeda A, Niwa H, et al: Lipid peroxidation and advanced glycation end products in the brain in normal aging and in Alzheimer's disease. Acta Neuropathol (Berl) 2002;104:113–122.

235. Crisby M, Nordin-Fredriksson G, Shah PK, et al: Pravastatin treatment increases collagen content and decreases lipid content,

inflammation, metalloproteinases, and cell death in human carotid plaques: Implications for plaque stabilization. Circulation 2001;103:926-933.

236. De Caterina R, Cipollone F, Filardo FP, et al: Low-density lipoprotein level reduction by the 3-hydroxy-3-methylglutaryl coenzyme-A inhibitor simvastatin is accompanied by a related reduction of F2-isoprostane formation in hypercholesterolemic subjects: No further effect of vitamin E. Circulation 2002;106:2543-2549.

237. Salonen JT, Ylä-Herttuala S, Yamamoto R, et al: Autoantibody against oxidised LDL and progression of carotid atherosclerosis. Lancet 1992;339:883-887.

238. Iuliano L, Mauriello A, Sbarigia E, et al: Radiolabeled native low-density lipoprotein injected into patients with carotid stenosis accumulates in macrophages of atherosclerotic plaque: Effect of vitamin E supplementation. Circulation 2000;101:1249-1254.

239. Hulthe J, Bokemark L, Fagerberg B: Antibodies to oxidized LDL in relation to intima-media thickness in carotid and femoral arteries in 58-year-old subjectively clinically healthy men. Arterioscler Thromb Vasc Biol 2001;21:101-107.

240. Palinski W, Witztum JL: Immune responses to oxidative neoepitopes on LDL and phospholipids modulate the development of atherosclerosis. J Intern Med 2000;247:371-380.

241. Jha P, Flather M, Lonn E, et al: The antioxidant vitamins and cardiovascular disease: A critical review of epidemiologic and clinical trial data. Ann Intern Med 1995;123:860-872.

242. Gey KF, Moser UK, Jordan P, et al: Increased risk of cardiovascular disease at suboptimal plasma concentrations of essential antioxidants: An epidemiological update with special attention to carotene and vitamin C. Am J Clin Nutr 1993;57:787S-797S.

243. Knekt P, Reunanen A, Jarvinen R, et al: Antioxidant vitamin intake and coronary mortality in a longitudinal population study. Am J Epidemiol 1994;139:1180-1189.

244. Stampfer MJ, Hennekens CH, Manson JE, et al: Vitamin E consumption and the risk of coronary disease in women. N Engl J Med 1993;328:1444-1449.

245. Rimm EB, Stampfer MJ, Ascherio A, et al: Vitamin E consumption and the risk of coronary heart disease in men. N Engl J Med 1993;328:1450-1456.

246. Enstrom JE, Kanim LE, Klein MA: Vitamin C intake and mortality among a sample of the United States population. Epidemiology 1992;3:194-202.

247. Steinberg D, Witztum JL: Lipoproteins, lipoprotein oxidation, and atherogenesis. In Chien KR (ed): Molecular Basis of Cardiovascular Disease. Philadelphia, WB Saunders, 1999, pp 458-475.

248. Tsimikas S, Philis-Tsimikas A, Alexopoulos S, et al: LDL isolated from Greek subjects on a typical diet or from American subjects on an oleate-supplemented diet induces less monocyte chemotaxis and adhesion when exposed to oxidative stress. Arterioscler Thromb Vasc Biol 1999;19:122-130.

249. Tsimikas S, Reaven PD: The role of dietary fatty acids in lipoprotein oxidation and atherosclerosis. Curr Opin Lipidol 1998;9:301-307.

250. Reaven PD, Khouw A, Beltz WF, et al: Effect of dietary antioxidant combinations in humans: Protection of LDL by vitamin E but not by beta-carotene. Arterioscler Thromb 1993;13:590-600.

251. Reaven PD, Parthasarathy S, Beltz WF, Witztum JL: Effect of probucol dosage on plasma lipid and lipoprotein levels and on protection of low density lipoprotein against in vitro oxidation in humans. Arterioscler Thromb 1992;318-324.

252. Tribble DL, Thiel PM, van den Berg JJ, Krauss RM: Differing alpha-tocopherol oxidative lability and ascorbic acid sparing effects in buoyant and dense LDL. Arterioscler Thromb Vasc Biol 1995;15:2025-2031.

253. Reaven PD, Witztum JL: Comparison of supplementation of RRR-alpha-tocopherol and racemic alpha-tocopherol in humans: Effects on lipid levels and lipoprotein susceptibility to oxidation. Arterioscler Thromb 1993;13:601-608.

254. Kawamura M, Heinecke JW, Chait A: Pathophysiological concentrations of glucose promote oxidative modification of low density lipoprotein by a superoxide-dependent pathway. J Clin Invest 1994;94:771-778.

255. Watson AD, Berliner JA, Hama SY, et al: Protective effect of high density lipoprotein associated paraoxonase: Inhibition of the bio-

logical activity of minimally oxidized low density lipoprotein. J Clin Invest 1995;96:2882-2891.

256. Van Lenten BJ, Hama SY, de Beer FC, et al: Anti-inflammatory HDL becomes pro-inflammatory during the acute phase response: Loss of protective effect of HDL against LDL oxidation in aortic wall cell cocultures. J Clin Invest 1995;96:2758-2767.

257. Mackness MI, Durrington PN: HDL, its enzymes and its potential to influence lipid peroxidation. Atherosclerosis 1995;115:243-253.

258. Walldius G, Erikson U, Olsson AG, et al: The effect of probucol on femoral atherosclerosis: The Probucol Quantitative Regression Swedish Trial (PQRST). Am J Cardiol 1994;74:875-883.

259. Lonn E, Yusuf S, Dzavik V, et al: Effects of ramipril and vitamin E on atherosclerosis: The study to evaluate carotid ultrasound changes in patients treated with ramipril and vitamin E (SECURE). Circulation 2001;103:919-925.

260. Brown BG, Zhao XQ, Chait A, et al: Simvastatin and niacin, antioxidant vitamins, or the combination for the prevention of coronary disease. N Engl J Med 2001;345:1583-1592.

261. Sawayama Y, Shimizu C, Maeda N, et al: Effects of probucol and pravastatin on common carotid atherosclerosis in patients with asymptomatic hypercholesterolemia: Fukuoka atherosclerosis trial (FAST). J Am Coll Cardiol 2002;39:610-616.

262. Fang JC, Kinlay S, Beltrame J, et al: Effect of vitamins C and E on progression of transplant-associated arteriosclerosis: A randomized trial. Lancet 2002;359:1108-1113.

263. Hodis HN, Mack WJ, LaBree L, et al. for the VEAPS Research Group: Alpha-tocopherol supplementation in healthy individuals reduces low-density lipoprotein oxidation but not atherosclerosis: The Vitamin E Atherosclerosis Prevention Study (VEAPS). Circulation 2002;106:1453-1459.

264. Tardif JC, Gregoire J, Schwartz L, et al: Effects of AGI-1067 and probucol after percutaneous coronary interventions. Circulation 2003;107:552-558.

265. Salonen RM, Nyyssonen K, Kaikkonen J, et al: Six-year effect of combined vitamin C and E supplementation on atherosclerotic progression: The Antioxidant Supplementation in Atherosclerosis Prevention (ASAP) Study. Circulation 2003;107:947-953.

266. Brown BG, Albers JJ, Fisher LD, et al: Regression of coronary artery disease as a result of intensive lipid-lowering therapy in men with high levels of apolipoprotein B. N Engl J Med 1990;323:1289-1298.

267. Hodis HN, Mack WJ, LaBree L, et al: Alpha-tocopherol supplementation in healthy individuals reduces low-density lipoprotein oxidation but not atherosclerosis: The Vitamin E Atherosclerosis Prevention Study (VEAPS). Circulation 2002;106:1453-1459.

268. Fang JC, Kinlay S, Behrendt D, et al: Circulating autoantibodies to oxidized LDL correlate with impaired coronary endothelial function after cardiac transplantation. Arterioscler Thromb Vasc Biol 2002;22:2044-2048.

269. Salonen RM, Nyyssonen K, Kaikkonen J, et al: Six-year effect of combined vitamin C and E supplementation on atherosclerotic progression: The Antioxidant Supplementation in Atherosclerosis Prevention (ASAP) Study. Circulation 2003;107:947-953.

270. Tardif JC, Cote G, Lesperance J, et al: Probucol and multivitamins in the prevention of restenosis after coronary angioplasty. Multivitamins and Probucol Study Group. N Engl J Med 1997;337:365-372.

271. Yokoi H, Daida H, Kuwabara Y, et al: Effectiveness of an antioxidant in preventing restenosis after percutaneous transluminal coronary angioplasty: The Probucol Angioplasty Restenosis Trial. J Am Coll Cardiol 1997;30:855-862.

272. Serruys PW, Foley DP, Hofling B, et al: Carvedilol for prevention of restenosis after directional coronary atherectomy: Final results of the European carvedilol atherectomy restenosis (EUROCARE) trial. Circulation 2000;101:1512-1518.

273. Serruys PW, Foley DP, Jackson G, et al: A randomized placebo-controlled trial of fluvastatin for prevention of restenosis after successful coronary balloon angioplasty; final results of the fluvastatin angiographic restenosis (FLARE) trial. Eur Heart J 1999;20:58-69.

274. Cote G, Tardif JC, Lesperance J, et al: Effects of probucol on vascular remodeling after coronary angioplasty: Multivitamins and Protocol Study Group. Circulation 1999;99:30-35.

275. Steinberg D: Antioxidants in the prevention of human atherosclerosis: Summary of the proceedings of a National Heart, Lung, and

Blood Institute Workshop, September 5-6, 1991, Bethesda, Maryland. Circulation 1992;85:2337-2344.

276. The effect of vitamin E and beta carotene on the incidence of lung cancer and other cancers in male smokers: The Alpha-Tocopherol, Beta Carotene Cancer Prevention Study Group. N Engl J Med 1994;330:1029-1035.

277. Hennekens CH, Buring JE, Manson JE, et al: Lack of effect of long-term supplementation with beta carotene on the incidence of malignant neoplasms and cardiovascular disease. N Engl J Med 1996;334:1145-1149.

278. Omenn GS, Goodman GE, Thornquist MD, et al: Effects of a combination of beta carotene and vitamin A on lung cancer and cardiovascular disease. N Engl J Med 1996;334:1150-1155.

279. Beta Carotene Cancer Prevention Study Group The Alpha-Tocopherol: The effect of vitamin E and beta carotene on the incidence of lung cancer and other cancers in male smokers. N Engl J Med 1994;330:1029-1035.

280. Stephens NG, Parsons A, Schofield PM, et al: Randomised controlled trial of vitamin E in patients with coronary disease: Cambridge Heart Antioxidant Study (CHAOS). Lancet 1996;347:781-786.

281. Dietary supplementation with n-3 polyunsaturated fatty acids and vitamin E after myocardial infarction: Results of the GISSI-Prevenzione trial. Lancet 1999;354:447-455.

282. The Heart Outcomes Prevention Evaluation Study Investigators. Vitamin E Supplementation and Cardiovascular Events in High-Risk Patients. N Engl J Med 2000;342:154-160.

283. Boaz M, Smetana S, Weinstein T, et al: Secondary prevention with antioxidants of cardiovascular disease in endstage renal disease (SPACE): Randomised placebo-controlled trial. Lancet 2000;356:1213-1218.

284. Roncaglioni MC: Low-dose aspirin and vitamin E in people at cardiovascular risk: A randomised trial in general practice. Lancet 2001;357:89-95.

285. MRC/BHF Heart Protection Study of cholesterol lowering with simvastatin in 20536 high-risk individuals: A randomised placebo-controlled trial. Lancet 2002;360:7-22.

286. Esterbauer H, Dieber-Rotheneder M, et al: Role of vitamin E in preventing the oxidation of low-density lipoprotein. Am J Clin Nutr 1991;53:314S-321S.

287. Boaz M, Green M, Fainauru M, Smetana S: Oxidative stress and cardiovascular disease in hemodialysis. Clin Nephrol 2001;55:93-100.

288. Blot WJ, Li JY, Taylor PR, et al: Nutrition intervention trials in Linxian, China: Supplementation with specific vitamin/mineral combinations, cancer incidence, and disease-specific mortality in the general population. J Natl Cancer Inst 1993;85:1483-1492.

289. Engelhart MJ, Geerlings MI, Ruitenberg A, et al: Dietary intake of antioxidants and risk of Alzheimer disease. JAMA 2002;287:3223-3229.

290. Steinberg D, Witztum JL: Is the oxidative modification hypothesis relevant to human atherosclerosis? Do the antioxidant trials conducted to date refute the hypothesis? Circulation 2002;105:2107-2111.

291. Falk E, Shah PK, Fuster V: Coronary plaque disruption. Circulation 1995;92:657-671.

292. Davies MJ: Glagovian remodelling, plaque composition, and stenosis generation. Heart 2000;84:461-462.

293. Virmani R, Kolodgie FD, Burke AP, et al: Lessons from sudden coronary death: A comprehensive morphological classification scheme for atherosclerotic lesions. Arterioscler Thromb Vasc Biol 2000;20:1262-1275.

294. Carpenter KL, Taylor SE, van der Veen C, et al: Lipids and oxidised lipids in human atherosclerotic lesions at different stages of development. Biochim Biophys Acta 1995;1256:141-150.

295. Piotrowski JJ, Shah S, Alexander JJ: Mature human atherosclerotic plaque contains peroxidized phosphatidylcholine as a major lipid peroxide. Life Sci 1996;58:735-740.

296. Steinbrecher UP, Witztum JL, Parthasarathy S, Steinberg D: Decrease in reactive amino groups during oxidation or endothelial cell modification of LDL: Correlation with changes in receptor-mediated catabolism. Arteriosclerosis 1987;7:135-143.

297. Avogaro P, Bon GB, Cazzolato G: Presence of a modified low density lipoprotein in humans. Arteriosclerosis 1988;8:79-87.

298. Steinberg D: The cholesterol controversy is over. Why did it take so long? Circulation 1989;80:1070-1078.

299. Gould AL, Rossouw JE, Santanello NC, et al: Cholesterol reduction yields clinical benefit: Impact of statin trials. Circulation 1998;97:946-952.

300. Randomised trial of cholesterol lowering in 4444 patients with coronary heart disease: The Scandinavian Simvastatin Survival Study (4S). Lancet 1994;344:1383-1389.

301. Libby P, Ridker PM, Maseri A: Inflammation and atherosclerosis. Circulation 2002;105:1135-1143.

302. Steinberg D: Atherogenesis in perspective: Hypercholesterolemia and inflammation as partners in crime. Nat Med 2002;8:1211-1217.

303. Tsimikas S, Witztum JL: Shifting the diagnosis and treatment of atherosclerosis to children and young adults: A new paradigm for the 21st century. J Am Coll Cardiol 2002;40:2122-2124.

## EDITOR'S CHOICE

Chawla A, Boisvert WA, Lee CH, et al: A PPAR gamma-LXR-ABCA1 pathway in macrophages is involved in cholesterol efflux and atherogenesis. Mol Cell 2001;7:161-171.
*The PPAR gamma-LXR connection intersects within macrophages, developing agents that can selectively target this pathway in macrophages versus other tissues is the next challenge.*

Chawla A, Lee CH, Barak Y, et al: PPAR delta is a very low-density lipoprotein sensor in macrophages. Proc Natl Acad Sci USA 2003;100:1268-1273.
*Nuclear hormone receptors now linked to regulation of VLDL metabolism.*

Glass CK, Witztum JL: Atherosclerosis. the road ahead. Cell 2001;104:503-516.
*Excellent review from thought leaders in the field.*

Joseph SB, Castrillo A, Laffitte BA, et al: Reciprocal regulation of inflammation and lipid metabolism by liver X receptors. Nat Med 2003;9:213-219.
*LXR has effects in the peripheral vascular system and more centrally in the liver, can these effects be segregated by a refined class of small molecules?*

Lee CH, Chawla A, Urbiztondo N, et al: Transcriptional Repression of Atherogenic Inflammation: Modulation by PPAR{delta}. Science 2003.
*Molecular basis for PPAR delta effects on atherogenesis.*

Li AC, Glass CK: The macrophage foam cell as a target for therapeutic intervention. Nat Med 2002;8:1235-1242.
*Unraveling the biology of macrophages is crucial for the development of new therapeutic approaches to influence inflammatory pathways in atherogenesis.*

Welch JS, Ricote M, Akiyama TE., et al: PPARgamma and PPARdelta negatively regulate specific subsets of lipopolysaccharide and IFN-gamma target genes in macrophages. Proc Natl Acad Sci USA 2003;100:6712-6717.
*Distinct roles for PPAR isoforms in cytokine activation of macrophages; implies specificity of downstream pathways and effectors.*

# Cellular Cholesterol Metabolism in Health and Disease

*Ira Tabas*

All cells of higher organisms require cholesterol for several critical functions, including structural roles in cellular membranes and as precursors to steroid hormones, bile acids, and activators of nuclear hormone receptors. Cells acquire cholesterol by two routes: internalization of exogenous cholesterol via uptake of plasma-derived lipoproteins, which is a major source of cholesterol for the liver and steroidogenic cells, and biosynthesis of endogenous cholesterol, which is the primary source in most other tissues.[1] The former route—cellular lipoprotein uptake—can occur by various mechanisms, but the best understood mechanism involves cell-surface receptors, such as the LDL receptor, and occurs via receptor-mediated endocytosis or phagocytosis.[2] The second route That cells use to acquire cholesterol—endogenous cholesterol biosynthesis—involves a complex, multienzyme pathway that is subject to many levels of physiologic regulation.[3,4] Regulation of both the LDL receptor and the cholesterol biosynthetic pathway is critical in keeping cellular cholesterol levels from getting too high or too low, which is important because excessively high or low cholesterol levels can be harmful to cells. Cells possess additional mechanisms to control cellular cholesterol levels, including cholesterol esterification and cholesteryl ester hydrolysis, cholesterol efflux, and, in the liver, bile acid synthesis and secretion of cholesterol into the bile.

Intracellular cholesterol metabolic events in specific cell types play important roles in atherogenesis, the disease process responsible for the most common causes of death in industrialized societies. In particular, cellular cholesterol metabolism in the intestine and liver influences plasma levels of atherogenic lipoproteins, and cholesterol metabolic pathways in arterial-wall cells, particularly macrophages, determine how these lipoproteins influence atherosclerotic lesion development once they enter the arterial wall. For example, cholesterol metabolism in hepatocytes determines liver LDL receptor expression, which is the most important determinant of plasma LDL levels. The level of plasma LDL determines the degree to which these lipoproteins accumulate in the subendothelial matrix of critical arteries, which, in turn, leads to a series of biologic responses that result in atherosclerotic lesion formation.[5,6] An example of the importance of cellular cholesterol metabolism in arterial-wall cells that participate in atherogenesis is the loading of lesional macrophages with massive amounts of cholesterol ("foam cell" formation). These foam cells are prominent features of both early and late lesions and contribute to the formation and progression of atheromas.[7,8]

Thus, a thorough understanding of both lipoprotein metabolism and atherogenesis requires knowledge of cellular pathways involved in cholesterol trafficking and metabolism. In this light, the goals of this chapter are to summarize the current knowledge of cellular cholesterol distribution, trafficking, and metabolism; to describe cellular cholesterol metabolism in arterial wall cells; and to discuss antiatherogenic therapeutic strategies related to cellular cholesterol trafficking and metabolism.

## DISTRIBUTION OF CELLULAR CHOLESTEROL

The cholesterol derived from lipoprotein uptake and endogenous synthesis is distributed in cells and organelles in a nonuniform fashion.[9,10] The bulk of unesterified (free) cellular cholesterol is in the plasma membrane; the exact percentage varies according to cell type and method of measurement but is in the range of 65% to 90%.[9,10] Although cholesterol is present in both bilayers of the plasma membrane and readily flip-flops between these bilayers, lateral distribution of cholesterol is not uniform.[11,12] The presence of cholesterol-rich and cholesterol-poor lateral domains within the plasma membrane may have important implications in several cellular processes, including cholesterol efflux,[13] localization of glycosylphospatidylinositol (GPI)-anchored proteins and caveolae,[14] and distribution of cellular proteins with different-sized membrane-spanning regions.[15] The subcellular distribution of most of the non-plasma-membrane cholesterol is a subject of controversy and probably varies according to cell type. Endosomes, which are derived from the plasma membrane, have a relatively high cholesterol content, and, thus, cells with a high steady-state level of endosomal vesicles have a substantial amount of cholesterol in these intracellular structure.[16] In other cells, the Golgi apparatus probably contains most of the non-plasma-membrane cholesterol, and there is some evidence that Golgi cholesterol is enriched in a cis-to-trans gradient.[17] The endoplasmic reticulum (ER), particularly the ribosome-studded rough ER, is relatively cholesterol poor, and this property may be important for certain ER functions and proteins distribution.[10]

Neither the mechanism of cellular cholesterol distribution nor the means of intracellular cholesterol transport have been definitively characterized at the molecular level. Cholesterol-rich membranes and membrane domains (i.e., rafts) in the cell are often enriched with the phospholipid sphingomyelin, which is known to have a high affinity for cholesterol in biologic and artificial membranes.[18] Furthermore, depletion of plasma membrane sphingomyelin by treatment of cells with exogenous sphingomyelinase causes some redistribution of cholesterol to the cell interior.[19] Thus, the sphingomyelin content of cellular membranes and membrane domains may be one determinant of cellular cholesterol localization. Other determinants must affect cholesterol distribution, however, because the correlation between membrane sphingomyelin content and cholesterol content in cells is far from exact. The means by which cholesterol is transported to the plasma membrane and to sites of metabolism is also not known. The three general mechanisms that could potentially mediate this process include vesicular transport, protein-carrier-mediated transport, and diffusion. As discussed in more detail later, it is likely that different mechanisms are involved in the various cholesterol transport pathways that exist in cells.

## CHOLESTEROL DELIVERY TO CELLS

The most widely studied process for cellular cholesterol delivery is via cellular uptake of lipoproteins followed by delivery to lysosomes.[2] The particles may enter the cells by receptor-mediated endocytosis involving specific lipoprotein receptors (Fig. 23-1, Pathway 1). However, other uptake processes, such as phagocytosis, pinocytosis, and nonspecific absorptive endocytosis may also lead to lysosomal delivery of lipoproteins and other cholesterol-rich particles. (Fig. 23-1, Pathway 2). In cells other that hepatocytes and steroidogenic cells (see later), LDL receptor-independent uptake can be substantial, and this process can become important even in the liver when plasma LDL levels are high.[1] Once in lysosomes, the cholesteryl ester (CE) in the core of lipoproteins is hydrolyzed by a 41-kd acidic lysosomal CE hydrolase to liberate unesterified (free) cholesterol (FC) and free fatty acid.[20] The CE-derived FC and the FC originally in the lipopro-tein particle are then exported from the lysosome, as described in detail later.

Although the lysosomal pathway is quantitatively the most important route for delivery of lipoprotein-cholesterol to cells, recent work with cultured cells has revealed the presence of cell-surface pathways that may play an important role in intracellular cholesterol metabolism. Lipoprotein-CE can be selectively internalized (i.e., not accompanied by whole particle uptake and degradation) when they interact with certain cell-surface receptors (Fig. 23-1, Pathway 3). The best studied pathway is that involving the selective uptake of HDL-CE by steroidogenic cells and liver via SR-BI.[21] The CE delivered by this pathway appears to be hydrolyzed by a non-lysosomal CE hydrolase.[22] Morphologic studies by Reavan et al.[23] have revealed that HDL is localized at the base of

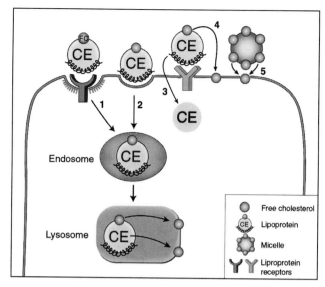

**FIGURE 23-1.** Cholesterol delivery to cells. Pathways 1 to 4 depict processes involving lipoproteins, which contain most of their cholesterol in the core as CE but also have a significant portion on the surface as FC. In Pathway 1, lipoproteins are internalized by receptor-mediated endocytosis and delivered via endosomes to lysosomes, where the CE moiety is hydrolyzed by acid CE hydrolase. The CE-derived FC and the original lipoprotein-FC are then distributed to the cell. In Pathway 2, lipoproteins enter this lysosomal pathway by receptor-independent processes, such as absorptive endocytosis or pinocytosis. Pathway 3 demonstrates selective CE uptake, and Pathway 4 demonstrates direct transfer of lipoprotein-FC to the cell surface. Pathway 5 schematizes the uptake of FC from nonlipoprotein particles, such as occurs with the absorption of micellar cholesterol by intestinal mucosal cells.

microvilli on the surface of these cells, and this may represent specialized sites where SR-BI-mediated selective lipid uptake occurs. A related pathway, also involving cell-surface invaginations, may occur when macrophages encounter aggregated LDL bound to extracellular matrix.[24] Another cell-surface pathway, described by Fielding and Fielding,[25] is a high-capacity, low-affinity process that results in the uptake of FC from LDL to the plasma membrane (Fig. 23-1, Pathway 4). This pathway, which is present in LDL receptor-negative cells, is sensitive to inhibitors of vesicular transport. The cholesterol derived from this pathway is readily esterified inside the cell.

Non-lipoprotein cholesterol may also deliver cholesterol to cells (Fig. 23-1, Pathway 5); the most important example of this process is the absorption of dietary and biliary cholesterol by intestinal mucosal cells. Dietary cholesterol is initially in the form of both FC and CE, and the CE is subsequently converted to FC by pancreatic CE hydrolase; biliary cholesterol is entirely in the form of FC. In both cases, the cholesterol is dissolved in bile salt micelles, which are thought to facilitate the diffusion of cholesterol through an unstirred water layer into plasma membrane of the intestinal mucosal cell.[26] On entering the mucosal cell, the cholesterol becomes rapidly esterified by acyl-coenzyme A:cholesterol acyltransferase-2 (ACAT-2; see later) and packaged into chylomicrons, which are transported through lymphatics into the circulation (see later). Whether a transport protein facilitates intestinal cholesterol uptake is not yet known. However, an azetidinone-based cholesterol absorption inhibitor, which has recently been shown to be an effective cholesterol-lowering agent in humans, appears to function by interacting with an as-yet-unidentified intestinal brush border membrane protein.[27]

Sterol uptake by mucosal cells is relatively selective for cholesterol. Recently, ABCG5 and ABCG8, members of the ATP-binding cassette (ABC) transporter family, have been identified as the defective molecules in the disease β-sitosterolemia, in which large amounts of plant sterols, especially sitosterol, are absorbed.[28,29] Thus, these two molecules somehow function to limit the absorption of plant sterols by intestinal epithelial cells and appear also to function in biliary sterol excretion. Importantly, patients with β-sitosterolemia develop xanthomas and are at increased risk for coronary artery disease even though total plasma sterol levels that are not markedly elevated.

## INTRACELLULAR CHOLESTEROL TRAFFICKING

### Lysosome-to-Plasma Membrane Trafficking

As mentioned previously, the bulk cholesterol delivered to many cells from exogenous sources is routed through lysosomes. Under usual conditions, this cholesterol is rapidly (half-life = 40 minutes) exported from the lysosomes to the plasma membrane by an energy-independent process.[9] Recent data from two separate laboratories supports the following model for this transport pathway[30,31] (Fig. 23-2): first, there is very rapid lysosome-to-plasma membrane cholesterol transport; next, this pool of plasma membrane cholesterol is rapidly internalized into a "cholesterol sorting organelle"; finally, cholesterol is transported from this putative sorting organelle to peripheral cellular sites, including the plasma membrane and ER (see later).

The most important advance in the understanding of cholesterol trafficking through the lysosomal pathway has been the cloning of npc1, the protein that is defective in humans with Niemann-Pick C (NPC) disease and in an NPC mouse model.[32,33] In NPC disease, there is intracellular accumulation of cholesterol and other lipids in lamellar bodies, resulting in multiorgan dysfunction, especially in the central nervous system and lungs.[34] Although the precise mechanism of the clinical abnormalities is not yet known, cells from these affected individuals have a defect in the trafficking of cholesterol derived from the lysosomal pathway.[32,33]

The npc1 protein is a multispanning integral membrane protein with a so-called cholesterol-sensing domain, homologous to that which occurs in HMG-CoA reductase and SREBP cleavage-activating protein (SCAP) (see later). Mutations in the cholesterol sensing domain of npc1 result in cholesterol trafficking defects.[35] Under normal conditions, npc1 is in late endosomal structures, but the protein accumulates in lysosomes and Golgi

when cells are loaded with cholesterol.[36] Chang and Lange propose that npc1 functions in cholesterol transport from the previously mentioned cholesterol sorting compartment[30,31] (Fig. 23-2), but the precise mechanism of how npc1 facilitates cholesterol transport is not known. Approximately 5% of patients with NPC disease (so-called NPC type 2 disease) have a defect not in npc1 but in a protein called HE1.[37] HE1 is a lysosomal protein that is known to bind cholesterol, but, as is the case with npc1, its mechanism of action is not known.

Two other molecules that have been implicated in the trafficking of cholesterol derived from the lysosomal pathway are lysobisphosphatidic acid (LBPA) and sphingomyelin (SM). Cells injected with neutralizing antibodies against LBPA have defects in cholesterol trafficking similar to that observed with defective npc1.[38] It has been proposed that this acidic phospholipid, which is located in the inner membrane of late endosomes, may be involved in internal vesiculation or tubulation, which in turn may be a necessary step in cholesterol transport.[38,39] SM is a cholesterol-binding lipid that normally is degraded in lysosomes by acidic sphingomyelinase. However, when this enzyme is genetically absent (i.e., types A and B Niemann-Pick disease) or inactivated (e.g., by oxysterols or free cholesterol accumulation), cholesterol trafficking is defective, probably resulting from sequestration of cholesterol by the accumulated SM.[40,41]

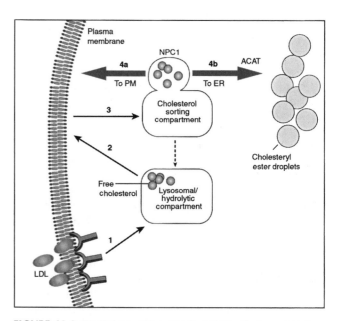

**FIGURE 23-2.** Trafficking of lysosomal cholesterol. According to a model proposed by Chang et al., lipoprotein delivery to lysosomes (Pathway 1) and lipoprotein-CE hydrolysis is followed by a very rapid lysosome-to-plasma membrane cholesterol transport (Pathway 2). Next, there is rapid internalization of this pool of plasma membrane cholesterol into a cholesterol sorting compartment (Pathway 3). Cholesterol is transported from this putative sorting organelle to peripheral cellular sites, including the plasma membrane and ACAT in the endoplasmic reticulum, by an npc1-dependent process (Pathways 4a and 4b, respectively). *(Adapted from Cruz JC, Sugii S, Yu C, Chang TY: Role of Niemann-Pick type C1 protein in intracellular trafficking of low density lipoprotein-derived cholesterol. J Biol Chem 2000;275: 4013–4021.)*

## Plasma Membrane-to-Endoplasmic Reticulum Trafficking

The trafficking of plasma membrane cholesterol to the ER is important for two critically important processes in intracellular cholesterol metabolism: ACAT (see later), leading to cholesterol esterification; and transcriptional and posttranscriptional regulation of the LDL receptor and cholesterol biosynthetic enzymes. Plasma membrane-to-ER transport of cholesterol, unlike the transport of cholesterol from lysosomes, is energy dependent and is blocked by several different types of inhibitors of membrane vesicle trafficking.[10,42] Importantly, transport is stimulated when cellular cholesterol levels are increased above a certain threshold level.[43,44] According to one model, this threshold corresponds with saturation of raft cholesterol in the plasma membrane, and the subsequent increase of cholesterol in non-raft, or liquid-disordered, domains enables or activates cholesterol transport to the ER.[12,44,45] Although the detailed cellular and molecular mechanisms of plasma membrane-to-ER cholesterol transport remain to be elucidated, this overall scheme allows the cell to sense and then regulate its cellular FC content, most of which is in the plasma membrane. Failure of this mechanism can lead to FC-induced cytotoxicity.[46]

## ENDOPLASMIC RETICULUM-TO-PLASMA MEMBRANE TRAFFICKING

Cholesterol is synthesized in the ER (see later) and then transported to the plasma membrane. This process is energy- and microtubule-dependent but is distinct from that used by secretory proteins.[47,48] For example, collapse of the Golgi complex with brefeldin A totally blocks protein transport but only partially blocks the transport of newly synthesized cholesterol.[48] Interestingly, appearance of newly synthesized cholesterol in membrane rafts occurs before its appearance on the cell surface, but whether or not these rafts actually participate in the transport process is not known.[48] Also unknown is whether vesicular transport or protein-mediated transport is involved. Studies suggesting involvement of specific proteins, such as sterol carrier protein-2 or a caveolin-chaperone complex, have been suggested from some experimental studies but questioned by others.[12] Whatever the mechanism, the trafficking is very rapid (half-life ~15 minutes), which may account for the finding that only a very small percentage of newly synthesized cholesterol is esterified by ACAT despite the localization of ACAT in the same vicinity as the cholesterol biosynthetic enzymes.[49]

## Cholesterol Efflux

An important mechanism to prevent cellular cholesterol levels from getting too high is cellular cholesterol efflux. Cholesterol efflux, by mediating the removal of cholesterol from cells in atherosclerotic lesions, may be an important antiatherogenic process.[50] Recently, the role of specific cell-surface proteins has come to the forefront in this field of research. Although covered in detail in another chapter, a brief mention here is necessary to integrate these new findings with intracellular cholesterol transport.

One cell-surface protein that likely plays an important role in cholesterol efflux is the ABC transporter ABCA1. Dysfunctional ABCA1 is the cause of Tangier disease, which is characterized by the accumulation of cholesterol in peripheral tissues, low plasma HDL, and increased risk for coronary artery disease.[51] According to the most recent data, the interaction of lipid-free or lipid-poor apolipoprotein A-1 (apoA-1) with cell-surface ABCA1 results in cellular phospholipid efflux, which in turn results in the formation of apoA-1-phosholipid complexes (Fig. 23-3, Pathway 1). These complexes, which are ideal cholesterol acceptors because of their very low cholesterol-to-phospholipid ratio, then interact with the cells by an unknown mechanism to cause cholesterol efflux.[52,53] Apolipoprotein E may act by a similar mechanism as apoA-1, and there is evidence that both proteins play an antiatherogenic role *in vivo* by promoting cholesterol efflux from lesional foam cell macrophages.[54,55] The scavenger receptor SR-B1, known to play an important role in selective cholesterol uptake can also mediate HDL-mediated cholesterol efflux from certain cell types, including macrophages[56] (Fig. 23-3, Pathway 2).

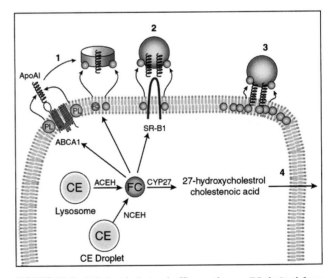

**FIGURE 23-3.** Cellular cholesterol efflux pathways. FC derived from the hydrolysis of lysosomal CE by acidic CE hydrolase (ACEH) or from CE in cytoplasmic lipid droplets by neutral CE hydrolase (NCEH) is transported to the plasma membrane, where efflux can occur if extracellular acceptors are present. In Pathway 1, free apoA-1 interacts with ABCA1, leading to phospholipid (PL) efflux and the formation of PL-rich disks. These disks, in turn, promote the efflux of cellular FC. In Pathway 2, HDL can interact with SR-B1 in certain cell types and result in cholesterol efflux. Pathway 3 depicts the release of plasma membrane cholesterol to HDL by receptor-independent mechanisms, such as desorption through the unstirred water layer. In Pathway 4, which may play a role in macrophage sterol efflux, cholesterol is converted by cholesterol 27-hydroxylase (CYP27) to 17-hydroxychoesterol (27OH-C) and 3β-hydroxy-5-cholestenoic acid, which are readily exported by cells. *(Depiction of Pathway 3 adapted from Rothblat GH, Mahlberg FH, Johnson WJ, Phillips MC: Apolipoproteins, membrane cholesterol domains, and the regulation of cholesterol efflux. J Lipid Res 1992;33:1091-1097.)*

Cholesterol efflux to HDL, particularly the subfraction $HDL_2$, is not mediated by ABCA1 and, in many cells, does not involve SR-B1.[50] Whether this efflux pathway involves a specific cell-surface protein is not known. In one model (Fig. 23-3, Pathway 3), cholesterol is desorbed from the plasma membrane, perhaps from liquid-disordered domains. Then the cholesterol diffuses through the unstirred water layer surrounding the cell until it collides with and is absorbed by the HDL or other acceptor particles.[57] Both desorption and diffusion determine the rate of cholesterol efflux at relatively low acceptor concentrations, but, at high acceptor levels, cholesterol desorption becomes the rate-limiting step. In a related pathway, the α-helical portions of HDL-associated apolipoproteins directly interact with specific lipid domains of the plasma membrane, resulting in increased cholesterol desorption.

Finally, Björkhem et al.[58] have proposed that cholesterol efflux in macrophages can be achieved by conversion of cholesterol to 27-hydroxycholesterol and 3β-hydroxy-5-cholesteroic acid, which are readily transported out of cells by sterol 27-hydroxylase (Fig. 23-3, Pathway 4). This pathway may be particularly important when extracellular HDL levels are low or absent. Indeed, 27-hydroxycholesterol is a prominent oxysterol found in lesions, and some studies have shown an inverse correlation between 27-hydroxylase levels and atherosclerosis.[59] Future studies with mice genetically engineered to have macrophage-specific deficiency of 27-hydroxylase should shed further light on the physiologic importance of this pathway.

## INTRACELLULAR CHOLESTEROL METABOLISM

### Sterol-Mediated Gene Regulation

Cholesterol and oxysterol metabolites of cholesterol can regulate many genes in a variety of cells. It is beyond the scope of this chapter to review this vast topic in detail, and the reader is referred to several excellent reviews on these topics.[60-62] In brief, cholesterol-induced activation of the transcription factor sterol response element binding protein (SREBP) regulates genes encoding cholesterol biosynthetic enzymes, the LDL receptor, enzymes involved in fatty acid metabolism, cholesteryl ester transfer protein, and CTP:phosphocholine cytidylyltransferase. For the purpose of this chapter, the key concept is that cholesterol/SREBP-mediated regulation of cholesterol biosynthetic enzymes and the LDL receptor represents a homeostatic response to keep cellular cholesterol levels high enough during sterol starvation and low enough during sterol excess.

SREBPs are encoded by two genes (SREBP-1 and SREBP-2), and SREBP-1 has two isoforms (a and c). The three forms of SREBP (1a, 1c, and 2) have different cell specificities and different functions with regard to cholesterol versus fatty acid metabolism. In sterol-replete cells, SREBP is retained in the ER via its interaction with SREBP-cleavage activating protein (SCAP) (Fig. 23-4). SCAP has a sterol-sensing domain, and, when cells are

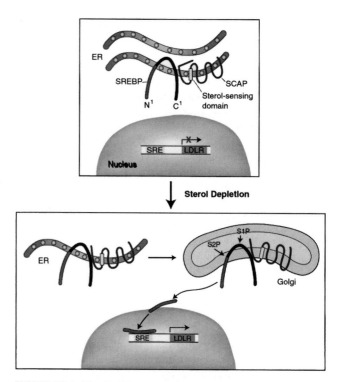

**FIGURE 23-4.** The SREBP/SCAP pathway of cholesterol regulation. In sterol-replete cells *(top panel)*, SREBP is retained in the ER via its interaction with SREBP-cleavage activating protein (SCAP). SCAP has a sterol-sensing domain, and, when cells are depleted of sterols, a conformational change in SCAP results in the transport of SREBP to the Golgi *(bottom panel)*. In the Golgi, SREBP is hydrolyzed by two proteases *(S1P and S2P)* that result in the release of an N-terminal domain from SREBP. This protein fragment enters the nucleus and regulates transcription by interacting with SRE elements in the promoters of a variety of genes, such as the LDL receptor *(LDLR)* depicted here and HMG-CoA reductase.

depleted of sterols, a conformational change in SCAP results in the transport of SREBP to the Golgi. In the Golgi, SREBP is hydrolyzed by two proteases that result in the release of an N-terminal domain from SREBP. This protein fragment enters the nucleus and regulates transcription by interacting with SRE elements in the promoters of the aforementioned genes.

Oxysterol metabolites of cholesterol, such as 25-hydroxycholesterol and 7-ketocholesterol, are also able to regulate the SCAP/SREBP pathway,[61] but it remains to be determined whether these oxysterols are abundant enough in cells to have a significant effect on this pathway. Moreover, exciting recent work has revealed that certain oxysterols are activators of nuclear transcription factors.[62] In particular, three oxysterols found *in vivo*, 24,25 epoxycholesterol, 24-hydroxycholesterol, and 22-hydroxycholesterol (but not cholesterol) activate the nuclear hormone receptors LXRα, LXRβ, and FXR. Once activated, these molecules heterodimerize with activated RXR, forming active transcription factors that translocate to the nucleus and induce several genes important in atherosclerosis and hepatic lipid metabolism (see later). In particular, a set of genes important in the reverse cholesterol transport pathway are activated by this pathway.[63] The proteins encoded by these genes include macrophage ABCA1 and apolipoprotein E, which promote cholesterol efflux from foam cells; plasma cholesteryl ester transfer protein, which transfers HDL-cholesterol to lipoproteins that can be internalized by hepatocytes; and liver 7α-hydroxylase, which is the key enzyme that converts hepatocyte cholesterol into bile acids for excretion (see later). Recent studies with genetically manipulated mice have demonstrated the importance of the LXR pathway *in vivo*. For example, activation of RXR reduces atherosclerosis in apolipoprotein E knockout mice,[64] and the livers of cholesterol-fed LXRα knockout mice accumulate very large amounts of cholesterol.[65] Finally, a direct connection between the LXR pathway and the SREBP pathway was revealed by Mangelsdorf and colleagues, who showed that LXR/RXR induces the transcription of SREBP-1c, which regulates genes involved in fatty acid metabolism.[66]

## Cholesterol Biosynthesis

The cholesterol requirements for cells are substantial, particularly for membrane synthesis during cell division, and most cells meet this requirement primarily through endogenous cholesterol biosynthesis.[1] Cholesterol is synthesized in all cells of the body through a complex series of reactions in which the key intermediate, mevalonate, is first synthesized from three acetate molecules (Fig. 23-5, Pathway 1); mevalonate is then converted to an isoprenoid unit, six of which condense to form squalene. Cyclization of squalene forms lanosterol, which is finally converted to cholesterol. Importantly, this pathway leads to the synthesis of a number of nonsterol compound that have roles in electron transport, glycoprotein biosynthesis, and cell growth. Cell growth effects are mediated through the isoprenylation of several key cellular proteins, including small GTP-binding proteins and heterotrimeric G proteins.[3,4] A rate-limiting enzyme in this pathway involves the conversion of HMG-CoA into mevalonate by the enzyme HMG-CoA reductase.[3,4] It is this enzyme that is inhibited by the potent statin-class of LDL-lowering drugs. Inhibition of the reductase enzyme and cholesterol biosynthesis leads to a compensatory rise in hepatic LDL receptors, which mediate an increase in clearance of plasma LDL.

HMG-CoA reductase is a 97-kd ER protein that consists of a membrane-spanning domain and a soluble catalytic domain.[3,4] The enzyme activity is maximally suppressed by incubating cells with both cholesterol and mevalonate, which mediates its regulatory effect through farnesol.[3,4,67] Cholesterol alone cannot completely downregulate the enzyme, thus ensuring continued synthesis of nonsterol products. The mechanisms of cholesterol-mediated downregulation include decreased transcription of the reductase gene via the SREB pathway (see previous discussion) and accelerated degradation of the protein itself by cholesterol and farnesol. By interacting with the sterol-sensing domain in the membrane-spanning region of HMG-CoA reductase, cholesterol and farnesol cause a conformational change that renders the enzyme more susceptible to degradation by a cathepsin L-type cysteine protease that resides in the ER membrane.[68] HMG-CoA reductase activity is also subject to diurnal and hormonal regulation and changes in the

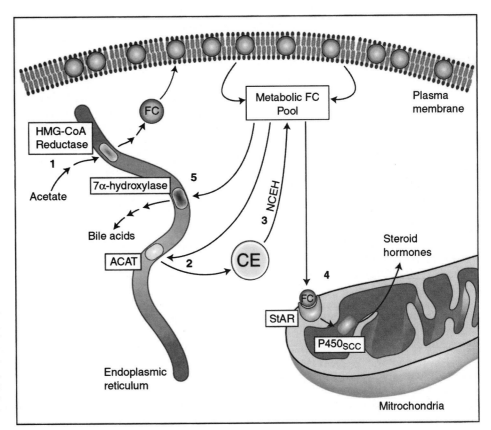

**FIGURE 23-5.** Major metabolic pathways involving cellular cholesterol. Pathway 1 shows the synthesis of cholesterol from acetate via the rate-limiting enzyme HMG-CoA reductase. Cholesterol from this pathway and exogenously derived cholesterol are rapidly transported to the plasma membrane (see Fig. 23-2). Subsequent reactions involve various metabolic pools of cholesterol, some of which are derived from the plasma membrane as shown in this model. These reactions include esterification by ACAT in the ER (Pathway 2) coupled with hydrolysis of ACAT-derived CE by NCEH (Pathway 3); transfer to the inner mitochondrial membrane by StAR, leading to conversion to steroid hormones via cytochrome P450scc (Pathway 4); and conversion to bile acids via the rate-limiting enzyme 7α-hydroxylase (Pathway 5).

phosphorylation state of the enzyme affect its activity as well.[3,4] These multiple mediators and levels of regulation are necessary to ensure that the various sterol and nonsterol products derived from mevalonate are finely controlled, both acutely and chronically, in response to changing levels and needs of these products in cells.

## Cholesterol Esterification and Hydrolysis

Intracellular cholesterol esterification, catalyzed by the enzyme ACAT (see previous discussion), is an important mechanism to prevent excessive cellular levels of FC, which can be toxic to cells.[46,69,70] The cholesterol esterification pathway begins when exogenous supplies of cholesterol are transported to the plasma membrane or to a plasma membrane-associated compartment, as described previously. After a threshold increment in cellular cholesterol mass has been reached, mixed pools of cellular and lipoprotein-cholesterol come into contact with ACAT in the ER (see previous discussion) (Fig. 23-5, Pathway 2). The mechanism and regulation of ACAT stimulation are incompletely understood.[69] Monocyte-to-macrophage differentiation is associated with a marked increase in ACAT mRNA,[71] and long-term cholesterol-feeding of animals can modestly increase ACAT mRNA levels in the liver.[72] The major form of regulation, however, appears to be posttranslational: control over intracellular "delivery" of cholesterol to ACAT, which can affect the enzyme's activity by both substrate provision and allosteric activation.[69] As the ACAT molecule is studied in more detail, other forms or regulation, such as changes in phosphorylation state, multimerization, or protein-protein interactions, may shed more light on the properties and control of this important intracellular reaction.

There are two ACAT genes.[70,73,74] In mice, ACAT-1 is enriched in macrophages and steroidogenic tissues, whereas ACAT-2 is found in the liver and intestine. In humans, ACAT-1 is the major hepatic ACAT.[74] Thus, ACAT-1 is likely involved in atherosclerotic foam cell formation and, in humans, hepatic lipoprotein assembly. ACAT-2 plays roles in hepatic lipoprotein assembly in mice and in intestinal cholesterol absorption in all species examined.[70,73,74] ACAT-1 knockout mice show markedly decreased ACAT activity in the adrenal and macrophages and massive xanthomatosis when crossed onto a hyperlipidemic background.[75,76] Bone marrow transplantation studies with these mice have shown that a deficiency of ACAT in macrophages leads to increased atherosclerosis and increased apoptosis of lesional macrophages.[77] This latter finding is likely due to FC-induced macrophage death.[46,77] In ACAT-2 knockout mice, there is decreased intestinal cholesterol absorption and increased cholesterol gallstone formation, consistent with the localization of ACAT-2 in mice.[78]

The CE formed by the ACAT pathway is present in the form of membrane-bound cytoplasmic lipid droplets, which can be hydrolyzed by a neutral, cytoplasmic CE hydrolase[79] (Fig. 23-5, Pathway 3). There is evidence, at least in macrophages, that this enzyme is activated by cAMP-dependent protein kinase and is identical to hor-mone-sensitive lipase.[80] Cells that have CE stores undergo a continuous cycle of esterification and hydrolysis that appears to be important for both cholesterol efflux and retrieval of cellular cholesterol for metabolic pathways.[81] This latter point is particularly relevant to adrenal cells, where there may be an acute need for cholesterol to make stress-induced steroid hormones (see later). Interestingly, mice overexpressing hormone-sensitive lipase in macrophages have increased atherosclerosis,[82] which may be due to increased levels on intracellular FC (see previous discussion).

Cellular cholesterol esterification has physiologic and pathophysiologic relevance to three other tissues. In the intestine, dietary cholesterol absorbed by enterocytes is esterified and packaged in chylomicrons, which are then secreted in the lymph for delivery to the plasma compartment. As stated previously, the role of ACAT-2-mediated esterification in intestinal cholesterol absorption has been demonstrated in ACAT-2 knockout mice.[78] In the liver, cholesteryl esters are incorporated into newly synthesized lipoproteins, and some studies, but not all, have shown that inhibition of cholesterol esterification blocks lipoprotein secretion.[83] Cholesterol esterification in the liver may also be important in preventing the saturation of bile with cholesterol, which is the cause of cholesterol gallstones.[78] Moreover, CE metabolism in the liver may explain why a diet rich in saturated fats leads to an increase in plasma LDL levels[84]: saturated fatty acids inhibit the cholesterol esterification pathway, which raises intracellular FC levels. The increase in FC, in turn, downregulates hepatic LDL receptor levels and diminishes clearance of plasma LDL. Finally, as discussed in more detail later, cholesterol esterification is the key process leading to macrophage and smooth muscle cell (SMC) foam cell formation in the arterial wall during atherogenesis.

## Steroidogenesis

The rate-limiting step in steroid hormone synthesis in adrenocortical, gonadal, and placental cells is transfer of cholesterol to the inner mitochondrial membrane, where the cholesterol is converted to pregnenolone by the side-chain cleavage cytochrome P450 (P450scc)[85] (Fig. 23-5, Pathway 4). Most of the cholesterol used for this pathway in rodents originates from selective uptake of CE from plasma lipoproteins, including SR-BI-mediated uptake of HDL-cholesterol. In humans, the LDL receptor pathway may play some role in steroidogenesis because patients with homozygous LDL receptor-negative familial hypercholesterolemia demonstrate a diminished, but not absent, cortisol response to prolonged ACTH stimulation.[86] In unstimulated cells, the CE is stored as cytoplasmic lipid droplets. On activation of the cells with the appropriate anterior pituitary peptide hormone, however, the CE is hydrolyzed to liberate FC. The mechanism involves hormone-induced stimulation of adenylate cyclase, which leads to elevated cAMP levels; cAMP, in turn, results in the phosphorylation and activation of neutral CE hydrolase.[85]

Although the mechanism or transport of newly hydrolyzed cholesterol to the mitochondria is not known, a 30-kd phosphorylated cAMP-regulated protein, termed steroidogenic acute regulatory protein (StAR), plays an essential role in the transfer of cholesterol from the outer to the inner mitochondrial membrane.[85] Humans with functionally defective StAR mutations have a disorder called congenital lipoid adrenal hyperplasia, which is characterized by defective steroid hormone synthesis. Recent data suggests that StAR facilitates this process by inducing a change in the mitochondrial membranes that alters sterol domain structure.[87] Other proteins that may play a role in the process of cholesterol delivery to cytochrome P450scc in the inner mitochondrial membrane include $SCP_2$ (although $SCP_2$-knockout mice do not appear to have major defects in steroidogenesis), a small polypeptide termed steroidogenesis activator polypeptide (SAP), and diazepam-binding inhibitor.[88,89] In addition, apolipoprotein E is abundantly expressed in steroidogenic tissues, and Williams and colleagues have shown that this protein has several effects in cultured adrenal cells, including inhibition of cholesterol efflux, enhancement of LDL-CE selective uptake, and inhibition of steroidogenesis by suppression of cAMP-mediated signal transduction.[90-92]

## Bile Acid Synthesis

A major route for eliminating cholesterol from the body is secretion of cholesterol and cholesterol-derived bile acids from the liver (Fig. 23-5, Pathway 5). Direct secretion of unesterified cholesterol appears to be tightly coupled to phospholipid secretion into bile, because disruption of the latter process in *mdr2* P-glycoprotein-knockout mice results in a 15-fold decrease in biliary FC.[93] Regarding the trafficking of cholesterol, the ABC transporters ABCG8 and ABCG5 (see previous discussion) appear to be involved, because defects in these proteins are the cause of sitosterolemia, which is characterized by decreased biliary excretion of dietary sterols.[28] These transporters are expressed in the liver and in the intestine, and their expression is induced by cholesterol feeding, consistent with a role in the biliary excretion of cholesterol.[28] In addition, as part of the reverse cholesterol transport pathway (see previous discussion), Tall and colleagues have implicated a role for SR-B1 in biliary cholesterol secretion by showing that SR-B1 transgenic mice have increased delivery of HDL-derived FC into bile[94]. Moreover, SR-B1 appears to be involved in the movement of HDL-derived cholesterol from the basolateral surface to apical bile canaliculi in cultured primary hepatocytes.[95] Interestingly, increasing biliary cholesterol in mice by a high-cholesterol diet or by overexpression of SR-B1 revealed a strong and inverse relationship between biliary cholesterol excretion and dietary cholesterol absorption.[96]

The most abundant sterol component in normal bile, however, is cholesterol-derived bile acids. Bile acid synthesis represents the major cholesterol metabolic pathway in the liver and accounts for almost all of whole-body cholesterol catabolism.[97] In humans, the liver converts approximately 0.5 g of cholesterol into bile acids per day, principally cholate and chenodeoxycholate. Bile acids are conjugated with glycine and tau-

rine and then excreted by the bile salt export pump (BSEP) into the small intestine, where they emulsify dietary lipids. Excess bile acids are eventually reabsorbed in the distal ileum by the ileal bile acid transporter. In a complex with the ileal bile acid binding protein (IBABP), the bile acids are transported to the liver in the portal circulation and are taken up by hepatocytes by an apical transporter. This recirculation pathway leads to the overall loss of about 0.5 g of bile acids per day (~5% of total bile acids), which accounts for the daily conversion rate of cholesterol stated previously. In the course of their synthesis, excretion, and recirculation, bile acids serve several important functions in reverse cholesterol transport; absorption of fats and fat-soluble vitamins in the intestines; solubilization of hepatic metabolites such as bilirubin; and regulation of genes involved in cholesterol, fat, and bile acid metabolism.[97]

Cholesterol is converted to bile acids, primarily cholic acid and chenodeoxycholic acid in humans through the action of at least 14 hepatic enzymes.[98] The first and rate-limiting enzyme in the pathway is liver-specific cholesterol 7α-hydroxylase (CYP7A), a 504 amino acid cytochrome P450 enzyme located in the ER.[97] Homozygous disruption of the *Cyp7a* gene in mice leads to neonatal fat malabsorption, wasting, skin abnormalities, visual defects, decreased plasma vitamin $D_3$ and E, and a high incidence of postnatal death that is correctable by supplementation with vitamins of bile acids.[99,100] Serum lipoprotein levels, however, were found to be normal, presumably because of other homeostatic regulatory mechanisms and other means of cholesterol excretion and metabolism. Interestingly, there was marked decrease in both fecal fat excretion and symptoms after 3 weeks of age, which was associated with the induction of a hepatic oxysterol 7α-hydroxylase (CYP7B). This enzyme, which oxidizes 25- and 27-hydroxycholesterol, was also found in wild-type mice. The 27-hydroxycholesterol pathway is the major precursor in liver, and CYP27, the enzyme that converts cholesterol to this oxysterol, is coordinately regulated with CYP7B.[101] Thus, this alternative cholesterol metabolic pathway can serve to back up the major CYP7A pathway and, under normal circumstances, may contribute to bile acid diversity and oxysterol catabolism. This latter function may be critical, because oxysterols are important regulators of lipid-related genes, as mentioned previously. The importance of the CYP7B pathway in humans is indicated by the finding that its deficiency leads to severe neonatal liver disease.[101]

As might be expected of the rate-limiting enzyme of the major cholesterol catabolic pathway in the liver, CYP7A is subject to multiple levels of regulation. Most of the regulation occurs at the transcriptional level, including diurnal and hormonal regulation, downregulation by bile acids and upregulation by bile acid-binding resins, and regulation by cholesterol that depends on the species studied. Most studies have studied rodent CYP7A, which is induced by cholesterol.[97] In this case, the liver is responding to excess cholesterol by routing it to an elimination pathway. In monkeys and rabbits, however, increased dietary cholesterol has been associated with downregulation of the enzyme. The resulting decreased secretion of bile acids is thought to be part of a negative-feedback system that results in decreased absorption of dietary cholesterol, a process that is facilitated by intestinal bile acids.[102]

In mice, the induction of the *Cyp7a* gene by cholesterol is mediated by a heterodimer of nuclear hormone receptors RXR and LXRα (see previous discussion). LXRα is activated by the cholesterol metabolites 24-hydroxycholesterol and 24,25-epoxycholesterol.[97] As expected LXRα-knockout mice have very low levels of Cyp7A activity and accumulate large amounts of cholesterol in the liver.[65] Another orphan nuclear receptor called liver response homolog-1 (LRH-1; also known as CBF for *Cyp7a* promoter binding factor) is responsible for both basal liver-specific expression of the *Cyp7a* gene and for participating in LXRα-induced transcription of *Cyp7a*.[103]

Bile acids regulate homeostatic transcription of *Cyp7a* and *IBABP* (see previous discussion). This regulation is mediated by another nuclear hormone receptor called FXR, which, when activated by bile acids and coupled with RXR, blocks transcription of *Cyp7a* and induces transcription of *IBABP*. Inhibition of Cyp7a transcription involves a pathway in which activated FXR induces another nuclear hormone receptor called small heterodimer partner (SHP), which in turn antagonizes LRH-1 (see previous discussion).[104] FXR knockout mice are healthy under normal conditions but, when fed a cholate-containing diet, accumulate bile in the liver and plasma and develop hepatotoxicity.[105] Other changes on this diet include markedly decreased expression of *BSEP, IBABP,* and *SHP* but lack of suppression of *Cyp7a*. These findings establish the importance of FXR in the regulation of bile acid metabolic genes *in vivo*.

Knowledge of hepatic bile acid metabolism, particularly of how the bile acid pathway is integrated with other cholesterol metabolic pathways, leads to important insight into disease mechanisms and therapeutic strategies. For example, the relationship between hepatic LDL receptor regulation and bile acid metabolism explains how bile acids resins lower plasma LDL and why these drugs complement the effect of reductase inhibitors in lowering plasma LDL. Bile acid resins can also have the undesired effect of raising plasma triglycerides, which is related to the normal suppressive activity of bile acids on secretion of VLDL triglyceride by the liver.[106]

The lack of stimulation of CYP7A by dietary cholesterol in certain species, such as monkeys and humans (see previous discussion), may have important implications in disease mechanisms. For example, this phenomenon may explain some cases of cholesterol gallstone formation, because it would tend to promote the formation of bile with a relatively high cholesterol-to-bile-salt ratio.[102] Lack of stimulation of CYP7A by dietary cholesterol would also promote relatively high FC levels in the hepatocyte, which, in turn, would lead to downregulation of hepatocyte LDL receptors and decreased clearance of LDL from the plasma compartment. Support for this concept was obtained by showing that adenovirus-

mediated transfer of the *Cyp7a* in hamsters, a species that does not increase *Cyp7a* expression or bile acid synthesis in response to dietary cholesterol, resulted in lower plasma LDL levels.[107] Finally, a defect in CYP27 causes the disease cerebrotendinous xanthomatosis (CTX).[108] Patients with CTX accumulate the sterol cholestanol and develop tendon xanthomas, neurologic defects, cataracts, and, occasionally, premature atherosclerosis.[109]

# CELLULAR CHOLESTEROL METABOLISM IN ATHEROSCLEROSIS

## Macrophages

Macrophages enter nascent atherosclerotic lesions and become a major cellular component of the intima.[110] Lesional Mφs progressively accumulate both FC and ACAT-derived CE, and these so-called foam cells influence both early atherogenesis and late lesional complications, including plaque rupture and acute thrombosis.[8,110,111] In this context, the important areas related to macrophage cholesterol metabolism are mechanisms of cholesterol loading, consequences of cholesterol loading, and cholesterol efflux, which was covered in a previous section of this chapter. Much of what is known about the mechanisms and consequences of cellular cholesterol loading comes from studies using cultured macrophages from various species, particularly mouse and human. Thus, one must exercise caution in applying the conclusions from these studies to human lesional cells. Nonetheless, many of the basic observations are likely to have physiologic relevance, as demonstrated by recent *in vivo* studies in which macrophage-specific gene expression has been altered via bone marrow transplantation or via the cre-lox system in mice.[112,113]

### Mechanisms of Cholesterol Loading in Macrophages

The two major types of atherogenic lipoproteins that probably contribute most to macrophage foam cell formation are forms of LDL that are modified in the subendothelium and chylomicron remnant-like particles (Fig. 23-6). Native LDL is a poor inducer of foam cells in culture.[114] Although this finding is generally ascribed to poor uptake of LDL by these cells, the mechanism of this effect is also related to the manner in which LDL-cholesterol is trafficked and metabolized by macrophages.[111] The LDL modification that has received the most attention is oxidation. Oxidized LDL is present in lesions and likely plays important roles in atherogenesis. Moreover, oxidized LDL is avidly internalized by macrophages via a number of receptors that are not subject to cholesterol-mediated repression. However, studies using several types of *in vitro* oxidized LDL have shown that the oxidized LDL-derived cholesterol is poorly esterified by ACAT in macrophages.[115] As mentioned previously, this phenomenon may result form inhibition of lysosomal sphingomyelinase by oxidized LDL lipids, leading to sequestration of oxidized LDL cholesterol away from

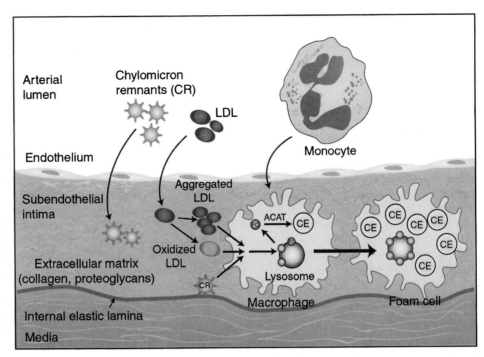

**FIGURE 23-6.** Macrophage foam cell formation during atherogenesis. Circulating LDL and chylomicron remnants (CR) enter the subendothelial intima of arteries and are retained on extracellular matrix in areas destined to become atherosclerotic. LDL is modified into several atherogenic forms, including oxidized LDL and aggregated LDL. These particles are taken up by macrophages, and the FC derived from these lipoproteins is esterified by ACAT to form CE. Eventually, ACAT-derived CE is sequestered in numerous membrane-bound cytoplasmic lipid droplets, forming the foam cells. Note also that in advanced lesions, the cells become loaded with FC, which appears to accumulate mainly in lysosomes. Lysosomal FC accumulation, as opposed to massive CE accumulation, may be particularly important during the interaction of macrophages with oxidized forms of LDL (see text).

ACAT.[41] Thus, it remains to be established whether or not oxidized LDL is a major inducer of macrophage foam cells in atherosclerotic lesions.

Aggregated LDL represents another type of modified LDL that is known to occur in atherosclerotic lesions (Fig. 23-6) and, unlike oxidized LDL, is a potent stimulator of CE accumulation in cultured macrophages.[115] The mechanism of LDL aggregation *in vivo* is not known. Extensive oxidation can lead to LDL aggregation, but it probably cannot explain LDL aggregation that occurs in very early lesions.[116] Lipases and proteases known to be in the arterial wall can also cause LDL aggregation *in vitro*.[115,117] Recently, data obtained from cell culture studies, human atherosclerotic lesions, and genetically altered mouse models has supported a role for a form of sphingomyelinase, called S-SMase, that is secreted by macrophages and endothelial cells.[118]

Chylomicron remnant-like particles, including postprandial lipoproteins and β-VLDL found in patients with familial dysbetalipoproteinemia are highly atherogenic and lead to massive foam cell formation[119,120] (Fig. 23-6). These lipoproteins, through their apolipoprotein E moieties, are internalized by LDL receptors and possibly other LDL-related receptors such as LRP. The observation that LDL receptors are downregulated in lesional macrophages[121] does not preclude a role for ligands for these receptors, such as chylomicron remnants and aggregated nonoxidized LDL, in foam cell formation. First, the methods used in these studies may not be sensitive enough to detect low but substantial LDL receptor activity. LDL receptors in cultured macrophages have been shown to be resistant to complete downregulation, which may be due to diversion of regulatory cholesterol into an active cholesterol esterification pathway.[111] Second, LDL receptors in macrophages that have recently entered the arterial wall are likely to be at a relatively

high level of expression, and, thus, these atherogenic particles may play a particularly important role in the initiation of foam cell formation. Indeed, a bone marrow transplantations study in mice has shown a direct role for the macrophage LDL receptor in atherosclerosis.[122]

An important consideration in the interpretation of cell culture experiments vis-à-vis foam cell formation *in vivo* is that most of these experiments use monomeric soluble lipoproteins, which is a model that favors receptor-mediated endocytosis. *In vivo*, however, a substantial portion of lesional lipoproteins are aggregated (see previous discussion) and avidly bound to extracellular matrix[123] (Fig. 23-4). The interaction of macrophages with matrix-retained and aggregated LDL may have several important implications that would be missed by the typical cell culture model. For example, another cell culture model in which macrophages are plated on top of matrix-retained and aggregated LDL has demonstrated prolonged cell-surface contact between the macrophages and the lipoproteins before complete internalization and lysosomal delivery is achieved.[24] Prolonged cell-surface contact, which has been observed to occur in cell-surface invaginations on macrophages, creates a situation that favors both cell-surface transfer of the lipoprotein-FC and selective lipoprotein-CE uptake.[24,111,124] The FC content of certain lipoproteins can be substantial in lipoprotein-FC transfer, and there appears to be a relationship between lipoprotein-FC content and atherogenesis.[125,126] In addition, the interaction of cultured macrophages with matrix-bound lipoproteins is more like phagocytosis than receptor-mediated endocytosis, and it involves cytoskeletal processes and receptors that appear to differ from those involved in receptor-mediated endocytosis.[127] Thus, the understanding of fundamental aspects of macrophage-lipoprotein interactions that occur *in vivo* is far from complete.

## Accumulation of Free Cholesterol in Macrophages

After extensive delivery of lipoprotein cholesterol, macrophages accumulate progressively large amounts of ACAT-derived CE using the trafficking pathways described previously (Fig. 23-4). As mentioned previously, this metabolic reaction probably represents a defense mechanism to protect the cells from excessive accumulation of FC. However, foam cells in advanced atherosclerotic lesions accumulate large amounts of FC, suggesting defects in one or more components of the cholesterol esterification pathway (e.g., cholesterol trafficking to ACAT or ACAT itself).[46] Interestingly, lesional foam cells also accumulate large amount of phospholipid (PL), as evidenced by intracellular membrane whorl-like structures, and have increased PL synthesis.[111] Cell culture studies have suggested a link between FC and PL accumulation, because FC loading of macrophages leads to increased synthesis of both phosphatidylcholine (PC) and sphingomyelin.[111] FC-induced PC synthesis is increased by post-translational activation of the rate-limiting enzyme in PC biosynthesis, CTP:phosphocholine cytidylyltransferase.[111] The increase in PL biosynthesis probably represents a final "line of defense" to protect macrophages from the toxic effects of FC loading. Macrophages from mice that have been genetically altered to have decreased PC biosynthesis are extremely susceptible to FC-induced death.[113]

With progressive FC loading of cultured macrophages, the PL adaptive mechanism eventually fails, resulting in macrophage death.[46] These events may mimic events in atherosclerotic lesions, because macrophage death becomes increasingly apparent in advanced lesions.[128,129]

Macrophage death likely contributes to lesional necrosis, which is a predisposing factor for plaque rupture, acute thrombosis, and acute clinical events[8]. The mechanisms of FC-induced death have, therefore, been an important area of investigation. On one hand, high levels of FC can block the action of critical membrane-bound proteins, such as enzymes and ion transport proteins, and intracellular cholesterol crystals that may form in the setting high cellular FC can physically damage cells.[46] On the other hand, FC loading of macrophages can activate specific apoptosis pathways, including activation of Fas ligand and induction of Bax, which triggers the mitochondrial apoptosis pathway.[130,131] Many questions remain unanswered, however, about the inducers, pathways, and consequences of macrophage death in atherosclerosis. For example, the relative importance of FC-induced macrophage death versus death caused by other means, such as toxic oxysterols, is not known. Moreover, macrophage death in lesions probably involves both apoptotic and necrotic pathways,[128] and the consequences of these different modes of death on atherogenesis and plaque rupture remain to be determined.

## Consequences of Cholesterol Loading in Macrophages

In addition to the stimulation of ACAT activity and PC biosynthesis, cholesterol loading of macrophages is likely to have other important consequences on cellular physiology (Table 23-1). Examples include induction of apolipoprotein E synthesis and ABCA1, which play a role in cholesterol efflux (see previous discussion)[132,133];

■ ▪ ■

## TABLE 23-1    CONSEQUENCES OF CHOLESTEROL LOADING OF ARTERIAL WALL CELLS

| Event | Possible Significance |
| --- | --- |
| *Macrophages* | |
| ↑ Expression of ABCA1 | Cholesterol efflux |
| ↑ Expression of ABCG1 (ABC8) | ? Cholesterol efflux |
| Altered expression of other ABC transporters | Altered efflux of lipids and other hydrophobic molecules |
| ↑ Synthesis and secretion of apolipoprotein E | Cholesterol efflux |
| ↑ Phospholipid biosynthesis | Prevention of FC-mediated toxicity |
| ↑ Secretion of lipoxygenase products | SMC migration |
| ↑ Expression of a receptor for lipoprotein(a) | ? |
| ↑ Expression of plasminogen activator | Plasmin-mediated proteolysis |
| ↑ Expression of interleukin-8 | Chemoattraction; mitogenesis |
| ↑ Expression of CCR2 in monocytes | Monocyte chemoattraction to MCP-1 |
| ↑ Expression of CD36 | ? Increased uptake of oxidized LDL |
| ↑ Expression of vigilin (HDL-binding protein) | ? |
| ↓ Expression of types IV and VII fucosyltransferase | ↓ CD15 and CD15s → decreased adhesion |
| *Smooth muscle cells* | |
| ↓ Prostacyclin synthesis | Thrombosis; vasoconstriction |
| ↓ CE hydrolysis | CE accumulation |
| ↑ Synthesis and secretion of b-FGF | SMC proliferation |
| ↑ Calcium uptake | ? SMC proliferation |
| ↑ NO synthesis and sensitivity to NO | Vasodilation |
| *Endothelial cells* | |
| ↑ LDL transport | Promote atherogenesis |

ABC, ATP-binding cassette; b-FGF, basic fibroblast growth factor; CE, cholesteryl ester; HDL, high-density lipoprotein; LDL, low-density lipoprotein; MCP-1, monocyte chemoattractant-1; NO, nitric oxide; SMC, smooth muscle cell.

increased secretion of specific lipoxygenase products that may induce SMC migration[134]; induction of a receptor for the atherogenic lipoprotein, lipoprotein(a)[135]; increased expression of membrane-bound urokinase-type plasminogen activator, leading to increased plasmin-mediated proteolysis[136]; and induction of interleukin-8 secretion, which may contribute to the chemoattraction of T cells and to the mitogenesis of SMCs.[137] Some of these consequences of cholesterol loading, such as increased apolipoprotein E secretion and ABCA1 expression, are likely to be adaptive and possibly antiatherogenic, whereas others, such as induction of CD36, may be promote lesion complications. The physiologic relevance of these findings and the net effect on atherogenesis *in vivo* remain to be determined and represents an important avenue of research. Related to this issue is a more fundamental issue surrounding foam cell formation, namely, whether the massive uptake of atherogenic lipoproteins by subendothelial macrophages is atherogenic or protective.[138] One might imagine that, at least initially, macrophage scavenging of potentially harmful subendothelial lipoproteins is adaptive. In macrophage-deficient mice, however, atherosclerosis was found to be substantially diminished.[7] Furthermore, macrophage secretory products and macrophage necrosis (see previous discussion) may promote late lesion complications, such as plaque rupture.[8] Thus, although early and subtle protective effects might have been missed by these studies, this most recent data supports the idea that macrophage foam cell formation promotes lesion formation.

## Smooth Muscle Cells

The other cell type in atherosclerotic lesions that accumulates large amounts of cholesterol is the SMC.[139,140] Compared with macrophages, much less is known about the mechanisms of SMC foam cell formation. SMCs have LDL receptors, but, as with macrophages, native LDL does not lead to substantial cholesterol accumulation. Inducers of foam cell formation in cultured SMCs include cationized LDL,[141] β-VLDL,[142] CE emulsions,[143] cholesterol-rich activated platelets,[144] aggregated LDL and aggregated lipoprotein-proteoglycan complexes,[145,146] and complexes of LDL and mast cell granule remnants.[147]

Several receptors have been implicated in the interaction of SMCs with modified forms of LDL. Scavenger receptors, which can mediate foam cell formation in cultured macrophages (see previous discussion), have been demonstrated on cytokine-treated cultured human SMCs and on SMCs in rabbit lesions.[148,149] The receptor is regulated by oxidant stress via activation of AP-1/c-Jun and CCAAT enhancer-binding protein-β (C/EBPβ).[150] Possible ligands for these receptors include oxidized LDL and a naturally occurring multiple modified form of LDL.[151] However, these receptors have not been found on SMCs in human lesions,[152] and the ability of scavenger receptor lipoprotein ligands (e.g., acetyl-LDL or oxidized LDL) to effect substantial cholesterol loading of cells has not yet been demonstrated. Other receptors implicated in SMC-lipoprotein interactions have been LDL receptor-

related protein (LRP), the VLDL receptor, CD36, and the lectin-like oxidized LDL receptor (LOX-1).[153-155]

CE accumulation in SMCs depends not only on lipoprotein uptake but also on cellular cholesterol metabolism (see previous discussion). For example, oxidative stress might be able to promote CE loading of SMCs by inhibiting CE hydrolysis and cholesterol efflux, and insulin and insulin growth factor-1 can also inhibit neutral CE hydrolase activity in SMCs.[156,157] Protective effects may be mediated by prostacyclin, which stimulates CE hydrolysis and cholesterol efflux in cultured SMCs, and calcium channel blockers, which also stimulate CE hydrolase activity in SMCs.[158,159]

As with macrophages, SMC physiology is likely to be substantially altered by cellular cholesterol loading (Table 23-1). Hajjar and Pomerantz[158] have shown that cholesterol accumulation in these cells inhibits HDL-induced stimulation of prostacyclin synthesis and CE hydrolysis. Another potentially atherogenic effect may be related to the observation that cholesterol and oxysterol loading of cultured SMCs stimulates the synthesis and secretion of basic fibroblast growth factor, a SMC mitogen.[141] FC loading of SMC also stimulates basal, serum-induced, and serotonin-stimulated calcium uptake.[160] This increased calcium uptake may mediate several atherogenic responses, such as SMC proliferation and CE accumulation (see previous discussion). A possible antiatherogenic effect of SMC cholesterol loading is the observed increase in cytokine- and endotoxin-mediated induction of NO synthesis in these cells and increased sensitivity to the vasodilatory effect of NO.[161,162] It is important to note that all of the observations described previously were made with cultured SMCs or tissue, and, as with macrophages, the physiologic relevance of net effect of these findings on the atherogenic process *in vivo* remains to be determined.

## Endothelial Cells

Most endothelial cells, like macrophages and SMCs, can internalize LDL and β-VLDL via LDL receptors and acetylated and oxidized LDL via scavenger receptors. Several receptors on endothelial cells are candidates for the uptake of oxidized LDL. Daugherty et al.[163] showed that the type A scavenger receptor is present on rabbit aortic endothelium *in vivo*. On the other hand, Adachi et al.[164] cloned a novel scavenger receptor from human endothelial cells. Human coronary endothelial cells also express LOX-1 (see previous discussion), which may play a role in oxidized LDL-induced apoptosis of endothelial cells.[157] Endothelial cells undergo they same basic cholesterol metabolic pathways described for other cell types, and inflammatory cytokines may regulate these pathways, but they do not become massively loaded with CE. Nonetheless, enrichment of these cells with FC may have important functional consequences, particularly in the setting of high plasma cholesterol levels (Table 23-1). For example, cholesterol loading of cultured endothelial cells has been demonstrated to increase transport of LDL,[165] which is a key process in atherogenesis. On the other hand, treatment of endothelial cells and endothelial cell membranes with HDL activates endothelial NOS, which may explain the ability of this lipoprotein to enhance endothelium- and NO-dependent relaxation in aortae.[156] Whether this effect, which requires binding to SR-B1, involves selective HDL-CE uptake, cellular cholesterol efflux, or an SR-B1-mediated signal transduction pathway remains to be determined.

## THERAPEUTIC STRATEGIES RELATED TO CELLULAR CHOLESTEROL TRAFFICKING AND METABOLISM

The impact of basic studies of cellular cholesterol metabolism on therapeutic strategies has already been substantial (Table 23-2). The mechanism of action of two major classes of LDL-lowering drugs, the HMG-CoA reductase inhibitors (statins) and the bile acid-binding resins, and the use of liver transplantation therapy for homozygous familial hypercholesterolemia is based on specific interacting pathways of hepatocyte cholesterol metabolism. A new type of drug that inhibits cholesterol absorption (ezetimibe) has shown substantial progress in clinical trials and was released in 2002.[166] The future holds promise for other interventions in this area, and many of these are currently being tested in animal models.[167] For example, investigators are developing gene therapy strategies for directly enhancing hepatic LDL receptor activity.[168] ACAT inhibitors may be beneficial in decreasing intestinal absorption, lipoprotein production by the liver, and atheroma foam cell formation.[169] Some caution is needed in considering the latter effect, however, because the FC that would be expected to accumulate in ACAT-inhibited macrophages and SMCs may promote atherogenic changes and necrosis in these cells (see previous discussion).

The cellular cholesterol efflux pathway presents another potential opportunity for intervention. Studies in animals showed that intravenous injections of compounds that induce cholesterol efflux, such as liposomes, HDL, or apoA-I, have marked antiatherogenic effects.[170,171] In mouse models of atherosclerosis, overexpression of apolipoprotein AI by transgenesis or gene therapy significantly retards atherogenesis, most likely by induction of cholesterol efflux from arterial wall cells.[54,172] Strategies to induce ABCA1, the receptor for apoA-I-mediated efflux, may hold future promise in this area. Activation of LXR may be an even more promising target, because activated LXR induces a set of genes involved in reverse cholesterol transport, including ABCA1, apoE, cholesteryl ester transfer protein, and CYP7A.[63] Similarly, apolipoprotein E expression in the arterial wall of apolipoprotein E knockout mice diminishes lesions,[173] and this effect may also be related to induction of cellular cholesterol efflux (see previous discussion). Thus, methods to induce apolipoprotein E production may have beneficial effects not only in whole-body lipoprotein metabolism but also on cholesterol metabolism in the arterial wall. Finally, as mentioned previously, hepatic bile acid synthesis is a major route for cholesterol excretion by the body. Thus, pharmacologic or gene-mediated stimulation of cholesterol 7α-hydroxylase may promote this process, as demonstrated by the LDL-lowering effect of adenovirus-mediated transfer to the *Cyp7a* gene in hamsters.[107]

## CONCLUSIONS

This chapter reviewed the major pathways of cellular cholesterol delivery, trafficking, and metabolism, including cholesterol biosynthesis, cholesterol esterification and CE hydrolysis, steroidogenesis, and bile acid synthesis. These pathways play important roles in a wide variety of physiologic and pathophysiologic processes. In particular, intracellular cholesterol metabolic pathways function in virtually all aspects of atherogenesis, from lipoprotein metabolism to arterial-wall events. Likewise,

■ ■ ■

**TABLE 23-2** ANTIATHEROGENIC THERAPEUTIC STRATEGIES RELATED TO INTRACELLULAR CHOLESTEROL METABOLISM

| Strategy | Postulated Mechanisms |
|---|---|
| *Currently Available* | |
| Inhibit HMG-CoA reductase (statins) | ↓ Cholesterol synthesis → ↑ hepatic LDL receptors → ↓ plasma LDL |
| Inhibit reabsorption of bile acids (bile acid resins) | ↑ Bile acid synthesis → ↑ hepatic LDL receptors → ↓ plasma LDL |
| Liver transplantation for homozygous FH | ↑ Hepatic LDL receptors → ↓ plasma LDL |
| Inhibit intestinal cholesterol absorption (ezetimibe) | ↓ Plasma cholesterol directly; ↓ hepatic cholesterol → ↑ hepatic LDL receptors → ↓ plasma LDL |
| *In Progress or Proposed* | |
| Inhibit ileal Na+/bile acid cotransporter | ↑ Bile acid synthesis → ↑ hepatic LDL receptors → ↓ plasma LDL |
| Inject HDL, liposomes, or apoA-I; enhance apoA-I or apoE synthesis or secretion; stimulate ABCA1 or SR-B1 | ↑ Cholesterol efflux from foam cells → ↑ reverse cholesterol transport |
| LDL receptor gene therapy | ↑ Hepatic LDL receptors → ↓ plasma LDL |
| Inhibit ACAT | ↓ Intestinal cholesterol absorption; ↓ hepatic lipoprotein secretion; ↓ foam cell formation (although may promote FC-induced cytotoxicity) |
| Stimulate CYP7A | ↑ bile acid synthesis → ↑ hepatic LDL receptors → ↓ plasma LDL |

ABC, ATP-binding cassette; ACAT, acyl-coenzyme A, cholesterol acyltransferase; apo, apolipoprotein; CYP7A, cholesterol 7α-hydroxylase; FC, free (i.e., unesterified) cholesterol; FH, familial hypercholesterolemia; HDL, high-density lipoprotein; HMG-CoA, hydroxymethylglutaryl coenzyme A; LDL, low-density lipoprotein; SR-B1, scavenger receptor B1.

knowledge of these pathways has lead to the discovery and implementation of valuable new drugs, the most important of which are the HMG-CoA reductase inhibitors. Knowledge of atherogenesis and other processes affected by the molecules and reactions described in this chapter will undoubtedly grow as additional information is gained about the molecular and regulatory details of intracellular cholesterol metabolism. With this new knowledge comes the exciting prospect of novel therapeutic strategies to combat atherosclerosis and possibly other disease processes.

## REFERENCES

1. Dietschy JM, Turley SD, Spady DK: Role of the liver in the maintenance of cholesterol and low density lipoprotein homeostasis in different animal species, including humans. J Lipid Res 1993;34:1637–1659.
2. Goldstein JL, Brown MS, Anderson RGW, et al: Receptor-mediated endocytosis: Concepts emerging from the LDL receptor system. Annu Rev Cell Biol 1985;1:1–39.
3. Goldstein JL, Brown MS: Regulation of the mevalonate pathway. Nature 1990;343:425–430.
4. Russell DW: Cholesterol biosynthesis and metabolism. Cardiovasc Drugs Ther 1992;6:103–110.
5. Williams KJ, Tabas I: The response-to-retention hypothesis of early atherogenesis. Arterioscler Thromb Vasc Biol 1995;15:551–561.
6. Williams KJ, Tabas I: The response-to-retention hypothesis of atherogenesis, reinforced. Curr Opin Lipidol 1998;9:471–474.
7. Smith JD, Trogan E, Ginsberg M, et al: Decreased atherosclerosis in mice deficient in both macrophage colony-stimulating factor (op) and apolipoprotein E. Proc Natl Acad Sci USA 1995; 92:8264–8268.
8. Libby P, Clinton SK: The role of macrophages in atherogenesis. Curr Opin Lipidol 1993;4:355–363.
9. Liscum L, Munn NJ: Intracellular cholesterol transport. Biochim Biophys Acta 1999;1438:19–37.
10. Lange Y: Intracellular cholesterol movement and homeostasis. In Chang TY, Freeman DA (eds): Intracellular Cholesterol Trafficking. Boston, Kluwer; 1998, 15–27.
11. Schroeder F, Frolov AA, Murphy EJ, et al: Recent advances in membrane cholesterol domain dynamics and intracellular cholesterol trafficking. Proc Soc Exp Biol Med 1996;213:150–177.
12. Simons K, Ikonen E: How cells handle cholesterol. Science 2000;290:1721–1726.
13. Fielding PE, Fielding CJ: Plasma membrane caveolae mediate the efflux of cellular free cholesterol. Biochemistry 1995; 34:14288–14292.
14. Brown DA, London E: Functions of lipid rafts in biological membranes. Annu Rev Cell Dev Biol 1998;14:111–136.
15. Munro S: Localization of proteins to the Golgi apparatus. Trends Cell Biol 1998;8:11–15.
16. Allan D, Kallen KJ: Is plasma membrane lipid composition defined in the exocytic or the endocytic pathway? Trends Cell Biol 1994;4:350–353.
17. Orci L, Montesano R, Meda P, et al: Heterogeneous distribution of filipin–cholesterol complexes across the cisternae of the Golgi apparatus. Proc Natl Acad Sci USA 1981;78:293–297.
18. Ridgway ND: Interactions between metabolism and intracellular distribution of cholesterol and sphingomyelin. Biochim Biophys Acta 2000;1484:129–141.
19. Porn MI, Slotte JP: Localization of cholesterol in sphingomyelinase-treated fibroblasts. Biochem J 1995;308:269–274.
20. Du H, Duanmu M, Witte D, Grabowski GA: Targeted disruption of the mouse lysosomal acid lipase gene: Long-term survival with massive cholesteryl ester and triglyceride storage. Hum Mol Genet 1998;7:1347–1354.
21. Rigotti A, Trigatti B, Babitt J, et al: Scavenger receptor BI–a cell surface receptor for high density lipoprotein. Curr Opin Lipidol 1997;8:181–188.

22. Sparrow CP, Pittman RC: Cholesterol esters selectively taken up from high-density lipoproteins are hydrolyzed extralysosomally. Biochim Biophys Acta 1990;1043:203–210.
23. Reaven E, Spicher M, Azhar S: Microvillar channels: A unique plasma membrane compartment for concentrating lipoproteins on the surface of rat adrenal cortical cells. J Lipid Res 1989;30:1551–1560.
24. Buton X, Mamdouh Z, Ghosh R, et al: Unique cellular events occurring during the initial interaction of macrophages with matrix-retained or methylated aggregated low density lipoprotein (LDL): Prolonged cell-surface contact during which LDL-cholesteryl ester hydrolysis exceeds LDL-protein degradation. J Biol Chem 1999;274:32112–32121.
25. Fielding CJ, Fielding PE: Role of N-ethylmaleimide-sensitive factor in the selective cellular uptake of low-density lipoprotein free cholesterol. Biochemistry 1995;34:14237–14244.
26. Dawson PA, Rudel LL: Intestinal cholesterol absorption. Curr Opin Lipidol 1999;10:315–320.
27. Van Heek M, France CF, Compton DS, et al: In vivo metabolism-based discovery of a potent cholesterol absorption inhibitor, SCH58235, in the rat and rhesus monkey through the identification of the active metabolites of SCH48461. J Pharmacol Exp Ther 1997;283:157–163.
28. Berge KE, Tian H, Graf GA, et al: Accumulation of dietary cholesterol in sitosterolemia caused by mutations in adjacent ABC transporters. Science 2000;290:1771–1775.
29. Lee MH, Lu K, Hazard S, et al: Identification of a gene, ABCG5, important in the regulation of dietary cholesterol absorption. Nat Genet 2001;27:79–83.
30. Cruz JC, Sugii S, Yu C, Chang TY: Role of Niemann-Pick type C1 protein in intracellular trafficking of low density lipoprotein-derived cholesterol. J Biol Chem 2000;275:4013–4021.
31. Lange Y, Ye J, Rigney M, Steck TL: Cholesterol movement in Niemann-Pick type C cells and in cells treated with amphiphiles. J Biol Chem 2000;275:17468–17475.
32. Liscum L, Klansek JJ: Niemann-Pick disease type C. Curr Opin Lipidol 1998;9:131–135.
33. Pentchev PG, Blanchette-Mackie EJ, Liscum L: Biological implications of the Niemann-Pick C mutation. SubCell Biochem 1997;28:437–451.
34. Pentchev PG, Vanier MT, Suzuki K, Patterson MC: Niemann-Pick disease type C: A cellular cholesterol lipidosis. In Scriver CR, Beaudet AL, Sly WS, Valle D (eds): Metabolic Basis of Inherited Disease. New York, McGraw-Hill, 1995, 2625–2639.
35. Watari H, Blanchette-Mackie EJ, Dwyer NK, et al: Mutations in the leucine zipper motif and sterol-sensing domain inactivate the Niemann-Pick C1 glycoprotein. J Biol Chem 1999;274: 21861–21866.
36. Neufeld EB, Wastney M, Patel S, et al: The Niemann-Pick C1 protein resides in a vesicular compartment linked to retrograde transport of multiple lysosomal cargo. J Biol Chem 1999;274: 9627–9635.
37. Naureckiene S, Sleat DE, Lackland H, et al: Identification of HE1 as the second gene of Niemann-Pick C disease. Science 2000; 290:2298–2301.
38. Kobayashi T, Beuchat MH, Lindsay M, et al: Late endosomal membranes rich in lysobisphosphatidic acid regulate cholesterol transport. Nat Cell Biol 1999;1:113–118.
39. Ory DS: Niemann-Pick type C: A disorder of cellular cholesterol trafficking. Biochim Biophys Acta 2000;1529:331–339.
40. Leventhal AR, Chen W, Tall AR, Tabas I: Acid sphingomyelinase-deficient macrophages have defective cholesterol trafficking and efflux. J Biol Chem 2001;276:44976-83.
41. Maor I, Mandel H, Aviram M: Macrophage uptake of oxidized LDL inhibits lysosomal sphingomyelinase, thus causing the accumulation of unesterified cholesterol-sphingomyelin-rich particles in the lysosomes: A possible role for 7-ketocholesterol. Arterioscler Thromb Vasc Biol 1995;15:1378–1387.
42. Skiba PJ, Zha X, Schissel SL, et al: The distal pathway of lipoprotein-induced cholesterol esterification, but not sphingomyelinase-induced cholesterol esterification, is energy-dependent. J Biol Chem 1996;271:13392–13400.
43. Xu X, Tabas I: Lipoproteins activate acyl coenzyme A: Cholesterol acyl transferase in macrophages only after cellular cholesterol

pools are expanded to a critical threshold level. J Biol Chem 1991;266:17040–17048.

44. Lange Y, Ye J, Rigney M, Steck TL: Regulation of endoplasmic reticulum cholesterol by plasma membrane cholesterol. J Lipid Res 1999;40:2264–2270.

45. Radhakrishnan A, Anderson TG, McConnell HM: Condensed complexes, rafts, and the chemical activity of cholesterol in membranes. Proc Natl Acad Sci USA 2000;97:12422–12427.

46. Tabas I: Free cholesterol-induced cytotoxicity: A possible contributing factor to macrophage foam cell necrosis in advanced atherosclerotic lesions. Trends Cardiovasc Med 1997;7:256–263.

47. Kaplan MR, Simoni RD: Transport of cholesterol from the endoplasmic reticulum to the plasma membrane. J Cell Biol 1985;101:446–453.

48. Heino S, Lusa S, Somerharju P, et al: Dissecting the role of the Golgi complex and lipid rafts in biosynthetic transport of cholesterol to the cell surface. Proc Natl Acad Sci USA 2000;97:8375–8380.

49. Lange Y, Strebel F, Steck TL: Role of the plasma membrane in cholesterol esterification in rat hepatoma cells. J Biol Chem 1993;268:13838–13843.

50. Tall AR. An overview of reverse cholesterol transport. Eur Heart J 1998;19:A31–A35.

51. Hayden MR, Clee SM, Brooks-Wilson A, et al: Cholesterol efflux regulatory protein, Tangier disease and familial high-density lipoprotein deficiency. Curr Opin Lipidol 2000;11:117–122.

52. Wang N, Silver DL, Thiele C, Tall AR: ATP-binding cassette transporter A1 (ABCA1) functions as a cholesterol efflux regulatory protein. J Biol Chem 2001;276:23742–23747.

53. Fielding PE, Nagao K, Hakamata H, et al: A two-step mechanism for free cholesterol and phospholipid efflux from human vascular cells to apolipoprotein A-1. Biochemistry 2000;39:14113–14120.

54. Dansky HM, Charlton SA, Barlow CB, et al: Apo A-I inhibits foam cell formation in apo E-deficient mice after monocyte adherence to endothelium. J Clin Invest 1999;104:31–39.

55. Hasty AH, Linton MF, Brandt SJ, et al: Retroviral gene therapy in ApoE-deficient mice: ApoE expression in the artery wall reduces early foam cell lesion formation. Circulation 1999;99:2571–2576.

56. Ji Y, Jian B, Wang N, et al: Scavenger receptor BI promotes high density lipoprotein-mediated cellular cholesterol efflux. J Biol Chem 1997;272:20982–20985.

57. Rothblat GH, Llera-Moya M, Atger V, et al: Cell cholesterol efflux: Integration of old and new observations provides new insights. J Lipid Res 1999;40:781–796.

58. Björkhem I, Andersson O, Diczfalusy U, et al: Atherosclerosis and sterol 27-hydroxylase: Evidence for a role of this enzyme in elimination of cholesterol from human macrophages. Proc Natl Acad Sci USA 1994;91:8592–8596.

59. Shanahan CM, Carpenter KL, Cary NR: A potential role for sterol 27-hydroxylase in atherogenesis. Atherosclerosis 2001; 154:269–276.

60. Brown MS, Goldstein JL: A proteolytic pathway that controls the cholesterol content of membranes, cells, and blood. Proc Natl Acad Sci USA 1999;96:11041–11048.

61. Edwards PA, Tabor D, Kast HR, Venkateswaran A: Regulation of gene expression by SREBP and SCAP. Biochim Biophys Acta 2000;1529:103–113.

62. Peet DJ, Janowski BA, Mangelsdorf DJ: The LXRs: A new class of oxysterol receptors. Curr Opin Genet Dev 1998;8:571–575.

63. Tall AR, Costet P, Luo Y: 'Orphans' meet cholesterol. Nat Med 2000;6:1104–1105.

64. Claudel T, Leibowitz MD, Fievet C, et al: Reduction of atherosclerosis in apolipoprotein E knockout mice by activation of the retinoid X receptor. Proc Natl Acad Sci USA 2001;98:2610–2615.

65. Peet DJ, Turley SD, Ma W, et al: Cholesterol and bile acid metabolism are impaired in mice lacking the nuclear oxysterol receptor LXRa. Cell 1998;93:693–704.

66. Repa JJ, Liang G, Ou J, et al: Regulation of mouse sterol regulatory element-binding protein-1c gene (SREBP-1c) by oxysterol receptors, LXRalpha and LXRbeta. Genes Dev 2000;14:2819–2830.

67. Meigs TE, Simoni RD: Farnesol as a regulator of HMG-CoA reductase degradation: Characterization and role of farnesyl pyrophosphatase. Arch Biochem Biophys 1997;345:1–9.

68. Moriyama T, Wada M, et al: 3-Hydroxy-3-methylglutaryl coenzyme A reductase is sterol-dependently cleaved by cathepsin L-type cysteine protease in the isolated endoplasmic reticulum. Arch Biochem Biophys 2001;386:205–212.

69. Chang TY, Chang CCY, Cheng D: Acyl-coenzyme A:cholesterol acyltransferase. Annu Rev Biochem 1997;66:613–638.

70. Buhman KF, Accad M, Farese RV: Mammalian acyl-CoA:cholesterol acyltransferases. Biochim Biophys Acta 2000;1529:142–154.

71. Wang H, Germain SJ, Benfield PP, Gillies PJ: Gene expression of acyl-coenzyme A:cholesterol acyltransferase is upregulated in human monocytes during differentiation and foam cell formation. Arterioscler Thromb Vasc Biol 1996;16:809–814.

72. Pape ME, Schultz PA, Rea TJ, et al: Tissue specific changes in acyl-CoA:cholesterol acyltransferase (ACAT) mRNA levels in rabbits. J Lipid Res 1995;36:823–838.

73. Rudel LL, Lee RG, Cockman TL: Acyl coenzyme A: cholesterol acyltransferase types 1 and 2: Structure and function in atherosclerosis. Curr Opin Lipidol 2001;12:121–127.

74. Chang TY, Chang CC, Lin S, et al: Roles of acyl-coenzyme A:cholesterol acyltransferase-1 and -2. Curr Opin Lipidol 2001; 12:289–296.

75. Meiner VL, Cases S, Myers HM, et al: Disruption of the acyl CoA:cholesterol acyltransferase (ACAT) gene in mice: Evidence suggesting multiple cholesterol esterification enzymes in mammals. Proc Natl Acad Sci USA 1996;93:14041–14046.

76. Accad M, Smith SJ, Newland DL, et al: Massive xanthomatosis and altered composition of atherosclerotic lesions in hyperlipidemic mice lacking acyl CoA:cholesterol acyltransferase 1. J Clin Invest 2000;105:711–719.

77. Fazio S, Major AS, Swift LL, et al: Increased atherosclerosis in LDL receptor-null mice lacking ACAT1 in macrophages. J Clin Invest 2001;107:163–171.

78. Buhman KK, Accad M, Novak S, et al: Resistance to diet-induced hypercholesterolemia and gallstone formation in ACAT2-deficient mice. Nat Med 2000;6:1341–1347.

79. Hajjar DP: Regulation of cholesteryl ester hydrolases. Adv Enzymol Rel Areas Mol Biol 1994;69:45–82.

80. Escary JL, Choy HA, Reue K, Schotz MC: Hormone-sensitive lipase overexpression increases cholesteryl ester hydrolysis in macrophage foam cells. Arterioscler Thromb Vasc Biol 1998;18:991–998.

81. Brown MS, Ho YK, Goldstein JL: The cholesteryl ester cycle in macrophage foam cells: Continual hydrolysis and re-esterification of cytoplasmic cholesteryl esters. J Biol Chem 1980; 255:9344–9352.

82. Escary JL, Choy HA, Reue K, et al: Paradoxical effect on atherosclerosis of hormone-sensitive lipase overexpression in macrophages. J Lipid Res 1999;40:397–404.

83. Burnett JR, Wilcox LJ, Huff MW: Acyl coenzyme A: cholesterol acyltransferase inhibition and hepatic apolipoprotein B secretion. Clin Chim Acta 1999;286:231–242.

84. Dietschy JM: Dietary fatty acids and the regulation of plasma low density lipoprotein cholesterol concentrations. J Nutr 1998;128:444S–448S.

85. Christenson LK, Strauss JF III: Steroidogenic acute regulatory protein (StAR) and the intramitochondrial translocation of cholesterol. Biochim Biophys Acta 2000;1529:175–187.

86. Illingworth DR, Lees AM, Lees RS: Adrenal cortical function in homozygous familial hypercholesterolemia. Metabol Clin Exper 1983;32:1045–1052.

87. Petrescu AD, Gallegos AM, Okamura Y, et al: Steroidogenic acute regulatory protein binds cholesterol and modulates mitochondrial membrane sterol domain dynamics. J Biol Chem 2001; 276:36970-82

88. Xu TS, Bowman EP, Glass DB, Lambeth JD: Stimulation of adrenal mitochondrial cholesterol side-chain cleavage by GTP, steroidogenesis activator polypeptide (SAP), and sterol carrier protein2. GTP and SAP act synergistically. J Biol Chem 1991;266:6801–6807.

89. Papadopoulos V, Amri H, Boujrad N, et al: Peripheral benzodiazepine receptor in cholesterol transport and steroidogenesis. Steroids 1997;62:21–28.

90. Prack MM, Rothblat GH, Erickson SK, et al: Apolipoprotein E expression in Y1 adrenal cells is associated with increased intracellular cholesterol content and reduced free cholesterol efflux. Biochemistry 1994;33:5049–5055.

91. Swarnakar S, Beers J, Strickland DK, et al: The apolipoprotein E-dependent low density lipoprotein cholesteryl ester selective uptake pathway in murine adrenocortical cells involves chondroitin sulfate proteoglycans and an alpha 2-macroglobulin receptor. J Biol Chem 2001;276:21121-21128.

92. Reyland ME, Gwynne JT, Forgez P, et al: Expression of the human apolipoprotein E gene suppresses steroidogenesis in mouse Y1 adrenal cells. Proc Natl Acad Sci USA 1991;88:2375-2379.

93. Smit JJ, Schinkel AH, Oude Elferink RP, et al: Homozygous disruption of the murine mdr2 P-glycoprotein gene leads to a complete absence of phospholipid from bile and to liver disease. Cell 1993;75:451-462.

94. Ji Y, Wang N, Ramakrishnan R, et al: Hepatic scavenger receptor BI promotes rapid clearance of high density lipoprotein free cholesterol and its transport into bile. J Biol Chem 1999; 274:33398-33402.

95. Silver DL, Wang N, Xiao X, Tall AR: High density lipoprotein (HDL) particle uptake mediated by scavenger receptor class B type 1 results in selective sorting of HDL cholesterol from protein and polarized cholesterol secretion. J Biol Chem 2001; 276:25287-25293.

96. Sehayek E, Ono JG, Shefer S, et al: Biliary cholesterol excretion: A novel mechanism that regulates dietary cholesterol absorption. Proc Natl Acad Sci USA 1998;95:10194-10199.

97. Russell DW: Nuclear orphan receptors control cholesterol catabolism. Cell 1999;97:539-542.

98. Russell DW, Setchell KD: Bile acid biosynthesis. Biochemistry 1992;31:4737-4749.

99. Ishibashi S, Schwarz M, Frykman PK, et al: Disruption of cholesterol 7a-hydroxylase gene in mice. I. Postnatal lethality reversed by bile acid and vitamin supplementation. J Biol Chem 1996;271:18017-18023.

100. Schwarz M, Lund EG, Setchell KDR, et al: Disruption of cholesterol 7a-hydroxylase gene in mice. II. Bile acid deficiency is overcome by induction of oxysterol 7a-hydroxylase. J Biol Chem 1996; 271:18024-18031.

101. Schwarz M, Lund EG, Russell DW: Two 7 alpha-hydroxylase enzymes in bile acid biosynthesis. Curr Opin Lipidol 1998; 9:113-118.

102. Rudel L, Deckelman C, Wilson M, et al: Dietary cholesterol and downregulation of cholesterol 7 alpha-hydroxylase and cholesterol absorption in African green monkeys. J Clin Invest 1994;93:2463-2472.

103. Nitta M, Ku S, Brown C, et al: CPF: An orphan nuclear receptor that regulates liver-specific expression of the human cholesterol 7alpha-hydroxylase gene. Proc Natl Acad Sci USA 1999; 96:6660-6665.

104. Chawla A, Saez E, Evans RM: Don't know much bile-ology. Cell 2000;103:1-4.

105. Sinal CJ, Tohkin M, Miyata M, et al: Targeted disruption of the nuclear receptor FXR/BAR impairs bile acid and lipid homeostasis. Cell 2000;102:731-744.

106. Beil U, Crouse JR, Einarsson K, Grundy SM: Effects of interruption of the enterohepatic circulation of bile acids on the transport of very low density-lipoprotein triglycerides. Metabolism 1982; 31:438-444.

107. Spady DK, Cuthbert JA, Willard MN, Meidell RS: Adenovirus-mediated transfer of a gene encoding cholesterol 7 alpha-hydroxylase into hamsters increases hepatic enzyme activity and reduces plasma total and low density lipoprotein cholesterol. J Clin Invest 1995;96:700-709.

108. Cali JJ, Hsieh C-L, Francke U, Russell DW: Mutations in the bile acid biosynthetic enzyme sterol 27-hydroxylase underlie cerebrotendinous xanthomatosis. J Biol Chem 1991;266:1179-1183.

109. Björkhem I, Boberg KM: Inborn errors in bile acid biosynthesis and storage of sterols other than cholesterol. In Scriver CR, Beaudet AL, Sly WS, Valle D (eds): The Metabolic and Molecular Bases of Inherited Disease. New York, McGraw-Hill, 1995, 2073-2099.

110. Ross R: Cell biology of atherosclerosis. Annu Rev Physiol 1995;57:791-804.

111. Tabas I: Cholesterol and phospholipid metabolism in macrophages. Biochim Biophys Acta 2000;1529:164-174.

112. Linton MF, Fazio S: Macrophages, lipoprotein metabolism, and atherosclerosis: Insights from murine bone marrow transplantation studies. Curr Opin Lipidol 1999;10:97-105.

113. Zhang D, Tang W, Yao PM, et al: Macrophages deficient in CTP: Phosphocholine cytidylyltransferase-alpha are viable under normal culture conditions but are highly susceptible to free cholesterol-induced death: Molecular genetic evidence that the induction of phosphatidylcholine biosynthesis in free cholesterol-loaded macrophages is an adaptive response. J Biol Chem 2000;275:35368-35376.

114. Brown MS, Goldstein JL: Lipoprotein metabolism in the macrophage: Implications for cholesterol deposition in atherosclerosis. Annu Rev Biochem 1983;52:223-261.

115. Tabas I: Nonoxidative modifications of lipoproteins in atherogenesis. Annu Rev Nutr 1999;19:123-139.

116. Nievelstein PFEM, Fogelman AM, Mottino G, Frank JS: Lipid accumulation in rabbit aortic intima 2 hours after bolus infusion of low density lipoprotein. Arterioscl Thromb 1991;11:1795-1805.

117. Oorni K, Pentikainen MO, Ala-Korpela M, Kovanen PT: Aggregation, fusion, and vesicle formation of modified low density lipoprotein particles: Molecular mechanisms and effects on matrix interactions. J Lipid Res 2000;41:1703-1714.

118. Tabas I: Secretory sphingomyelinase. Chem Phys Lipids 1999;102:131-139.

119. Goldstein JL, Ho YK, Brown MS, et al: Cholesteryl ester accumulation in macrophages resulting from receptor-mediated uptake and degradation of hypercholesterolemic canine b -very low density lipoproteins. J Biol Chem 1980;255:1839-1848.

120. Zilversmit DB: Atherogenesis: A postprandial phenomenon. Circulation 1979;60:473-485.

121. Ylä-Herttuala S, Rosenfeld ME, Parthasarathy S, et al: Gene expression in macrophage-rich human atherosclerotic lesions. J Clin Invest 1991;87:1146-1152.

122. Linton MF, Babaev VR, Gleaves LA, Fazio S: A direct role for the macrophage low density lipoprotein receptor in atherosclerotic lesion formation. J Biol Chem 1999;274:19204-19210.

123. Smith EB, Massie IB, Alexander KM: The release of an immobilized lipoprotein fraction from atherosclerotic lesions by incubation with plasmin. Atherosclerosis 1976;25:71-84.

124. Kruth HS, Chang J, Ifrim I, Zhang WY: Characterization of patocytosis: Endocytosis into macrophage surface-connected compartments. Eur J Cell Biol 1999;78:91-99.

125. Miller KW, Small DM: Structure of triglyceride-rich lipoproteins: An analysis of core and surface phases. In Neuberger A, van Deenen LLM (eds): New Comprehensive Biochemistry. Amsterdam, Elsevier, 1987, 1-75.

126. Fielding CJ: The origin and properties of free cholesterol potential gradients in plasma, and their relation to atherogenesis. J Lipid Res 1984;25:1624-1628.

127. Sakr S, Eddy RJ, Barth H, et al: The uptake and degradation of matrix-retained and aggregated LDL by macrophages is uniquely dependent on the cytoskeleton: New insight into foam cell formation as it likely occur in vivo. J Biol Chem. 2001;276:37649-58.

128. Mitchinson MJ, Hardwick SJ, Bennett MR: Cell death in atherosclerotic plaques. Curr Opin Lipidol 1996;7:324-329.

129. Kockx MM: Apoptosis in the atherosclerotic plaque: Quantitative and qualitative aspects. Arterioscler Thromb Vasc Biol 1998;18:1519-1522.

130. Yao PM, Tabas I: Free cholesterol loading of macrophages induces apoptosis involving the Fas pathway. J Biol Chem 2000; 275:23807-23813.

131. Yao PM, Tabas I: Free cholesterol loading of macrophages is associated with widespread mitochondrial dysfunction and activation of the mitochondrial apoptosis pathway. J Biol Chem 2001; 276:42468-76.

132. Basu SK, Ho YK, Brown MS, et al: Biochemical and genetic studies of the apolipoprotein E secreted by mouse macrophages and human monocytes. J Biol Chem 1982;257:9788-9795.

133. Langmann T, Klucken J, Reil M, et al: Molecular cloning of the human ATP-binding cassette transporter 1 (hABC1): Evidence for sterol-dependent regulation in macrophages. Biochem Biophys Res Commun 1999;257:29-33.

134. Mathur SN, Field FJ: Effect of cholesterol enrichment on 12-hydroxyeicosatetraenoic acid metabolism by mouse peritoneal macrophages. J Lipid Res 1987;28:1166–1176.

135. Bottalico LA, Keesler GA, Fless GM, Tabas I: Cholesterol loading of macrophages leads to marked enhancement of native lipoprotein(a) and apoprotein(a) internalization and degradation. J Biol Chem 1993;268:8569–8573.

136. Falcone DJ, McCaffrey TA, Haimovitz-Friedman A, et al: Macrophage and foam cell release of matrix-bound growth factors: Role of plasminogen activation. J Biol Chem 1993;268:11951–11958.

137. Wang N, Tabas I, Winchester R, et al: Interleukin-8 is induced by cholesterol loading of macrophages and expressed by macrophage foam cells in human atheroma. J Biol Chem 1996;271:8837–8842.

138. Steinberg D: Lipoproteins and atherosclerosis: A look back and a look ahead. Arteriosclerosis 1983;3:283–301.

139. Haley JN, Shio H, Fowler S: Characterization of lipid-laden aortic cells from cholesterol-fed rabbits. I. Resolution of aortic cell populations by metrizamide density gradient centrifugation. Lab Invest 1977;37:287–296.

140. Stein O, Stein Y: Smooth muscle cells and atherosclerosis. Curr Opin Lipidol 1995;6:269–274.

141. Kraemer R, Pomerantz KB, Joseph-Silverman J, Hajjar DP: Induction of basic fibroblast growth factor mRNA and protein synthesis in smooth muscle cells by cholesteryl ester enrichment and 25-hydroxycholesterol. J Biol Chem 1993;268:8040–8045.

142. Campbell JH, Reardon MF, Campbell GR, Nestel PJ: Metabolism of atherogenic lipoproteins by smooth muscle cells of different phenotype in culture. Arteriosclerosis 1985;5:318–328.

143. Wolfbauer G, Glick JM, Minor LK, Rothblat GH: Development of the smooth muscle foam cell: Uptake of macrophage lipid inclusions. Proc Natl Acad Sci USA 1986;83:7760–7764.

144. Kruth HS: Platelet-mediated cholesterol accumulation in cultured aortic smooth muscle cells. Science 1985;227:1243–1245.

145. Llorente-Cortes V, Martinez-Gonzalez J, Badimon L: Esterified cholesterol accumulation induced by aggregated LDL uptake in human vascular smooth muscle cells is reduced by HMG-CoA reductase inhibitors. Arterioscler Thromb Vasc Biol 1998;18:738–746.

146. Vijayagopal P, Glancy DL: Macrophages stimulate cholesteryl ester accumulation in cocultured smooth muscle cells incubated with lipoprotein-proteoglycan complex. Arterioscler Thromb Vasc Biol 1996;16:1112–1121.

147. Wang Y, Lindstedt KA, Kovanen PT: Phagocytosis of mast cell granule remnant-bound LDL by smooth muscle cells of synthetic phenotype: A scavenger receptor-mediated process that effectively stimulates cytoplasmic cholesteryl ester synthesis. J Lipid Res 1996;37:2155–2166.

148. Pitas RE: Expression of the acetyl low density lipoprotein receptor by rabbit fibroblasts and smooth muscle cells. J Biol Chem 1990;265:12722–12727.

149. Li H, Freeman MW, Libby P: Regulation of smooth muscle cell scavenger receptor expression in vivo by atherogenic diets and in vitro by cytokines. J Clin Invest 1995;95:122–133.

150. Mietus-Snyder M, Glass CK, Pitas RE: Transcriptional activation of scavenger receptor expression in human smooth muscle cells requires AP-1/c-Jun and C/EBPbeta: Both AP-1 binding and JNK activation are induced by phorbol esters and oxidative stress. Arterioscler Thromb Vasc Biol 1998;18:1440–1449.

151. Tertov VV, Orekhov AN: Metabolism of native and naturally occurring multiple modified low density lipoprotein in smooth muscle cells of human aortic intima. Exp Mol Pathol 1997;64:127–145.

152. Luoma J, Hiltunen T, Sarkioja T, et al: Expression of alpha 2-macroglobulin receptor/low density lipoprotein receptor-related protein and scavenger receptor in human atherosclerotic lesions. J Clin Invest 1994;93:2014–2021.

153. Hiltunen TP, Luoma JS, Nikkari T, Yla-Herttuala S: Expression of LDL receptor, VLDL receptor, LDL receptor-related protein, and scavenger receptor in rabbit atherosclerotic lesions: Marked induction of scavenger receptor and VLDL receptor expression during lesion development. Circulation 1998;97:1079–1086.

154. Matsumoto K, Hirano K, Nozaki S, et al: Expression of macrophage scavenger receptor, CD36, in cultured human aortic smooth muscle cells in association with expression of peroxisome proliferator activated receptor-g, which regulates gain of macrophage-like phenotype in vitro, and its implication in atherogenesis. Arterioscler Thromb Vasc Biol 2000;20:1027–1032.

155. Draude G, Hrboticky N, Lorenz RL: The expression of the lectin-like oxidized low-density lipoprotein receptor (LOX-1) on human vascular smooth muscle cells and monocytes and its down-regulation by lovastatin. Biochem Pharmacol 1999;57:383–386.

156. Yuhanna IS, Zhu Y, Cox BE, et al: High-density lipoprotein binding to scavenger receptor-BI activates endothelial nitric oxide synthase. Nat Med 2001;7:853–857.

157. Li D, Mehta JL: Upregulation of endothelial receptor for oxidized LDL (LOX-1) by oxidized LDL and implications in apoptosis of human coronary artery endothelial cells: Evidence from use of antisense LOX-1 mRNA and chemical inhibitors. Arterioscler Thromb Vasc Biol 2000;20:1116–1122.

158. Hajjar DP, Pomerantz KB: Signal transduction in atherosclerosis: Integration of cytokines and the eicosanoid network. FASEB J 1992;6:2933–2941.

159. Etingin OR, Hajjar DP: Calcium channel blockers enhance cholesteryl ester hydrolysis and decrease total cholesterol accumulation in human aortic tissue. Circ Res 1990;66:185–190.

160. Bialecki RA, Tulenko TN, Colucci WS: Cholesterol enrichment increases basal and agonist-stimulated calcium influx in rat vascular smooth muscle cells. J Clin Invest 1991;88:1894–1900.

161. Pomerantz KB, Hajjar DP, Levi R, Gross SS: Cholesterol enrichment of arterial smooth muscle cells upregulates cytokine-induced nitric oxide synthesis. Biochem Biophys Res Comm 1993;191:103–109.

162. Bialecki RA, Tulenko TN: Acute exposure to cholesterol increases arterial nitroprusside- and endothelium-mediated relaxation. Am J Physiol 1993;264(Pt 1):C32–39.

163. Daugherty A, Cornicelli JA, Welch K, et al: Scavenger receptors are present on rabbit aortic endothelial cells in vivo. Arterioscler Thromb Vasc Biol 1997;17:2369–2375.

164. Adachi H, Tsujimoto M, Arai H, Inoue K: Expression cloning of a novel scavenger receptor from human endothelial cells. J Biol Chem 1997;272:31217–31220.

165. Navab M, Hough GP, Berliner JA, et al: Rabbit beta-migrating very low density lipoprotein increases endothelial macromolecular transport without altering electrical resistance. J Clin Invest 1986;78:389–397.

166. Stein E: Results of phase I/II clinical trials with ezetimibe, a novel selective cholesterol absorption inhibitor. Eur Heart J 2001;3:E11–E16.

167. Brown WV: Therapies on the horizon for cholesterol reduction. Clin Cardiol 2001;24:III24–III27.

168. Pakkanen TM, Laitinen M, Hippelainen M, et al: Enhanced plasma cholesterol lowering effect of retrovirus-mediated LDL receptor gene transfer to WHHL rabbit liver after improved surgical technique and stimulation of hepatocyte proliferation by combined partial liver resection and thymidine kinase–ganciclovir treatment. Gene Ther 1999;6:34–41.

169. Nicolosi RJ, Wilson TA, Krause BR: The ACAT inhibitor, CI1011 is effective in the prevention and regression of aortic fatty streak area in hamsters. Atherosclerosis 1998;137:77–85.

170. Williams KJ, Werth VP, Wolff JA: Intravenously administered lecithin liposomes: A synthetic antiatherogenic lipid particle. Perspect Biol Med 1984;27:417–431.

171. Badimon JJ, Badimon L, Fuster V: Regression of atherosclerotic lesions by high density lipoprotein plasma fraction in the cholesterol-fed rabbit. J Clin Invest 1990;85:1234–1241.

172. Tangirala RK, Tsukamoto K, Chun SH, et al: Regression of atherosclerosis induced by liver-directed gene transfer of apolipoprotein A-I in mice. Circulation 1999;100:1816–1822.

173. Bellosta S, Mahley RW, Sanan DA, et al: Macrophage-specific expression of human apolipoprotein E reduces atherosclerosis in hypercholesterolemic apolipoprotein E-null mice. J Clin Invest 1995;96:2170–2179.

## EDITOR'S CHOICE

Binder CJ, Chang MK, Shaw PX, et al: Innate and acquired immunity in atherogenesis. Nat Med 2002;8:218-1226.
*Eloquently makes the case for atherogenesis as an immune-mediated disease.*
Boucher P, Gotthardt M, Li WP, et al: LRP: Role in vascular wall integrity and protection from atherosclerosis. Science 2003;300:329-332.
*New role for lipoprotein related receptors uncovered by a leader in the field.*
Braun A, Zhang S, Miettinen HE, et al: Probucol prevents early coronary heart disease and death in the high-density lipoprotein receptor SR-BI/apolipoprotein E double knockout mouse. Proc Natl Acad Sci U S A 2003;100:7283-7288.
*One of the few mouse models that actually displays coronary disease and events documents the utility of probucol, an inhibitor of LDL oxidation. Ongoing clinical trials of a probucol related drug should provide a definitive answer in the next few years.*
Breslow JL: Genetics of lipoprotein abnormalities associated with coronary artery disease susceptibility. Annu Rev Genet 2000;34:233-254.
*Genetics of atherogenesis moving from disease causing genes to genetic modifiers of disease.*
Feng B, Yao PM, Li Y, et al: The endoplasmic reticulum is the site of cholesterol-induced cytotoxicity in macrophages. Nat Cell Biol 5, 781-792.
Herz, J. (2001). The LDL receptor gene family: (Un)expected signal transducers in the brain. Neuron 2003;29:571-581.
*A new twist on cholesterol and macrophages.*
Horton JD, Goldstein JL, Brown MS: SREBPs: Transcriptional mediators of lipid homeostasis. Cold Spring Harb Symp Quant Biol 2002;67:491-498.
*The undisputed pioneers in cholesterol regulation highlight the role of SREBP pathways in the control of lipid metabolism that now extends from atherogenesis to diabetes and obesity*
Russell DW: The Enzymes, Regulation, and Genetics of Bile Acid Synthesis. Annu Rev Biochem 2003;72:137-174.
*Excellent review and update on new pathways that have been uncovered in the regulation of bile acid metabolism that highlights new therapeutic targets.*
Williams KJ, Tabas I: Atherosclerosis and inflammation. Science 2002;297:521-522.
*Atherogenesis as an inflammatory disease.*

■ ▨ ■ c h a p t e r **2 4**

# Angiogenesis in Cardiovascular Disease

*Karen S. Moulton*
*Judah Folkman*

Angiogenesis is one biologic response enacted by endothelial cells. Several cardiovascular conditions including atherosclerosis, myocardial infarction, and cardiac growth and hypertrophy are accompanied by angiogenesis that can repair injury or facilitate pathologic progression when it is sustained. Information concerning general mechanisms of angiogenesis, therefore, provides new insights into these cardiovascular diseases. At a more fundamental level, the analysis of endothelial cell behavior during the orchestrated events of angiogenesis reveals how these and other vascular wall cells respond to mechanical forces, soluble growth factors and inhibitors, inflammation, and coagulation factors. Thus, angiogenesis can be viewed as a specialized response that uses basic cellular mechanisms related to general endothelial cell and vascular biology.

The cellular events of angiogenesis are also related to the more broadly defined concept of vascular remodeling. Vascular remodeling involves changes in proliferation, apoptosis, and migration of vascular wall cells and changes in the turnover of extracellular matrix (ECM).[1] These adaptive vascular remodeling events are observed during angiogenesis and arteriogenesis but are also widely observed in cardiovascular conditions of systemic and pulmonary hypertension, restenosis after angioplasty or stenting, closure of the ductus arteriosus, arterial remodeling of saphenous vein bypass grafts, and compensatory enlargement of an atherosclerotic vessel by flow disturbances associated with an atheroma. The mechanisms of angiogenesis regulation by ECM and soluble factors can, therefore, also operate in nonangiogenic cardiovascular conditions.

## ANGIOGENESIS, VASCULOGENESIS, AND ARTERIOGENESIS

The formation of new blood vessels is a fundamental process involved in development, reproduction, inflammation, and wound repair.[2] Physiologic growth, tumor growth, and remodeling and regeneration of adult tissues can only occur when accompanied by angiogenesis.[3] During early development, endothelial cells arise by *in situ* differentiation of precursor angioblasts to form the primary vascular plexus in the embryo and blood islands in the yolk sac—a process termed *vasculogenesis*.[4] The term *angiogenesis* refers to the formation of new vessels from preexisting blood vessels. Its broadened definition encompasses the mechanisms of sprouting, intussusception, bridging, and intercalation of endothelial cells to increase the length and diameter enlargement of blood vessels.[5] The vascular plexus formed by these basic mechanisms must be further remodeled to create mature three-dimensional vascular networks with appropriate arterial and venous patterns and optimal circulation. During the maturation phase, some newly formed vessels regress and become filled-in with matrix, and other vessels are fortified. The molecular factors involved in vascular pruning during development are just being discovered. Vascular pattern formation requires ephrin B2-Eph B4 signaling, Tie2 receptors and their angiopoietic ligands, activin receptor-like kinase 1, and neuropilins.[6-10] However, the abundance of soluble factors and receptor signaling pathways alone cannot fully account for the pruned vascular network, because regression and fortification of adjacent vessels occur simultaneously in a saturated growth factor-rich tissue environment. Normal vascular patterning requires that vascular cells integrate and exhibit differential responses to multiple factors. ECM molecules in the vascular basement membrane can exert mechanical control over endothelial cell behavior.[11] Hemodynamic forces and the flow of blood through a newly perfused capillary can further remodel the vascular plexus. Signals for vascular pattern formation also arise outside the vasculature—from nerves and mesenchymal cells adjacent to developing blood vessels.[12] Ultimately, these diverse signals converge on vascular cells to determine whether any individual cell proliferates, migrates, differentiates, or dies.

Arteriogenesis is the formation of larger more complex blood vessels, which consist of an endothelium but also incorporate smooth muscle cells and ECM to form the media, elastin fibers, and adventitia. Although the term angiogenesis is often applied to the formation of collateral vessels, it is useful to distinguish arteriogenesis from angiogenesis because the mechanisms to create large blood vessels *de novo* or to remodel existing vessels into larger conductance vessels are different than the mechanisms to create more simple capillary structures comprised of an endothelium, basement membrane, and fewer mural cells. The processes of angiogenesis and arteriogenesis may share common endothelial cell regulators, but the molecular mechanisms and spatial cues to generate or remodel large caliber conduit vessels capable must be different. Many current therapeutic collateral trials have used factors that primarily target endothelial cell proliferation and migration. However, it is not yet clear how these single agents alone achieve collateral growth. Do these factors expand the capillary bed, which then indirectly signals for the expansion of conduit arterioles and veins in this circuit? What are the cascades of signals and cellular events activated by a single endothelial growth factor that recruits inflammatory and mural cells and remodels the vascular basement membrane to create collaterals? Signals derived from the local ischemic tissue are necessary to complete arteriogenesis. Placental growth factor (PlGF) and monocyte chemotactic protein-1 promote arteriogenesis more than angiogenesis because of their added effects on inflammatory cells that cooperate with endothelial cells in collateral growth. Future advances will expand the molecular understanding of angiogenesis and arteriogenesis mechanisms so that refined strategies to modulate each process selectively may be developed.

## Embryonic Vascular Development

Vascular development in the embryo, reviewed more extensively elsewhere, involves both vasculogenesis and angiogenesis.[5] The prevalence of both developmental processes varies temporally and spatially in different regions of the embryo. For instance, the dorsal aorta forms by vasculogenesis, and the cerebral vasculature develops predominantly by mechanisms of angiogenesis.[13] At early phases of fetal development, endothelial cell precursors (angioblasts) and hematopoietic precursor cells arise from a common progenitor termed the *hemangioblast* found in the yolk sac. During vasculogenesis, angioblasts migrate to various sites of vessel origin in the embryo, differentiate, and adhere to one another to form cords of endothelial cells that comprise a primitive vascular network. Gene deletion studies have shown that VEGF and VEGFR-2 are important for angioblast differentiation.[14-16] Endothelial cell differentiation is also regulated by GATA transcription factors with their cofactors and inhibits differentiation (Id) members of the basic helix-loop-helix (bHLH) class of transcription factors.[17,18] The primitive endothelial cell plexus then recruits mural cells and synthesizes ECM. Important molecular mediators of endothelial cell interactions with pericytes and matrix components include the Tie2 receptor and its angiopoietic ligands, integrins, platelet-derived growth factor (PDGF-BB), PDGF receptor β, and TGF-β and its activin receptor-like kinase receptors. The fate of vascular cells to become arteries or veins is regulated by the bHLH factor gridlock and ephrin family members.[7,19] It is noteworthy that the arterial and venous pattern in the embryo develops before the start of circulation, which indicates that arterial and venous identity and function can be determined by molecular events independent of blood flow. This finding does not diminish the impact of hemodynamic factors on the postnatal regulation of vascular patterns. The biologic signals integrated by arterial and venous markers will be useful in understanding the modifications that occur in venous bypass grafts exposed to arterial blood flow, arteriovenous fistulas, vascular malformations, and vascular remodeling events after arterial occlusion or thrombosis.

During late stages of fetal development until adulthood, new blood vessels originate predominantly by mechanisms of angiogenesis.[20] Smaller vessels may be derived as sprouts that branch from a parent vessel or form as subdivisions from larger parent vessel by intussusception. During bridging, connections between endothelial cells develop across the lumen to create smaller subdivision. Angiogenesis in the embryo requires subsequent remodeling to create the mature pruned vascular network. Arteriogenesis in the embryo proceeds by increasing layers of smooth muscle cells and matrix in the media that are proportional to the diameter and flow conditions of the expanding vessel. Large arteries and veins elongate and continue to remodel during fetal growth.

In the embryo, the process of vascular development must also be coordinated with organogenesis because the vascular architecture in many organs such as the lung, liver, kidney, and endocrine glands is closely integrated with the physiology of that organ. Organ-specific factors can regulate angiogenesis in conjunction with organogenesis in specific tissues of the embryo. For example, the transcription factor FOG (friend of GATA)-2 is expressed in the myocardium but is required for the migration and differentiation of cells to form the coronary arteries.[17] An endocrine gland-specific endothelial cell growth factor and its receptor postnatally regulate the proliferation and migration of endothelial cells derived from the capillaries of endocrine glands but not from other tissues.[21] Blood vessels induce the development of the pancreas.[22] Other organ-specific factors may still be identified to link the formation of vascular anatomy with different types of organogenesis.

## Postnatal Vasculogenesis: Endothelial Precursor Cells

Early investigations showed that endothelial cell colonies that seeded impermeable endovascular grafts implanted in dogs after bone marrow transplantation were derived from the donor bone marrow cells.[23] These and other studies proposed that a small number of endothelial precursor stem cells persist in the adult.[24] Several studies now demonstrate that endothelial precursor cells can be mobilized from the bone marrow by VEGF, bFGF, granulocyte-monocyte colony-stimulating factor, insulin-like growth factor (IGF-1), and PlGF via its activation of VEGF receptor 1(VEGFR-1).[25] Likewise, some inhibitors of angiogenesis impair release of endothelial precursors from the bone marrow. Endothelial precursor cells home to sites of angiogenesis, intercalate into vascular structures, and differentiate into mature endothelial cells (Fig. 24-1). When local angiogenesis in suppressed as in Id-deficient mice, implanted tumors do not grow because of suppressed tumor angiogenesis, but tumor growth and angiogenesis (comprised of wild-type donor endothelial cells) is supported after these Id-deficient mice receive wild-type bone marrow stem cells or endothelial precursor cells.[18,26] The number of precursor-cell-derived

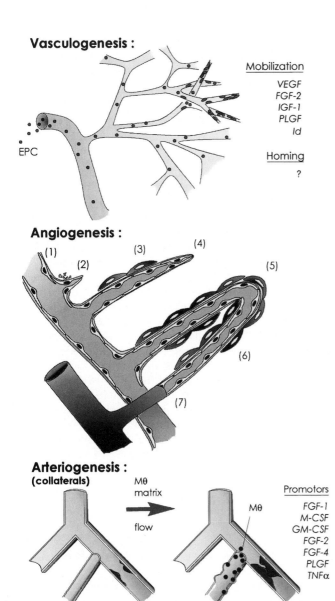

**Vasculogenesis :**

Mobilization

VEGF
FGF-2
IGF-1
PLGF
Id

EPC

Homing

?

**Angiogenesis :**

(1) (2) (3) (4) (5) (6) (7)

**Arteriogenesis :**
(collaterals)

Mθ
matrix

flow

Mθ

Promotors

FGF-1
M-CSF
GM-CSF
FGF-2
FGF-4
PLGF
TNFα

**FIGURE 24-1.** Mechanisms of postnatal angiogenesis and/or arteriogenesis. Vasculogenesis can occur in the adult via mobilization of endothelial precursor cells from the bone marrow. The fate of these cells in circulation are not fully understood, but these cells can home to sites of angiogenesis, where they differentiate, migrate, and incorporate into newly formed vessels or repair areas of injured endothelium. Several growth factors promote the release of these cells, but the mechanisms of homing are not known. Angiogenesis sprouting is diagramed showing seven stages as outlined in the text: (1) vasodilation of the parent vessel. (2) degradation of basement membrane, (3) endothelial cell migration and proliferation, (4) lumen formation, (5) capillary loop formation, (6) synthesis of new basement membrane, and (7) stabilization and incorporation of pericytes. Arteriogenesis involves the expansion or formation of new larger caliber vessels that can act as conduit vessels to supply blood flow into capillary beds. Macrophages (Mθ) and flow can significantly enhance collateral growth. Several angiogenic factors promote both angiogenesis (capillary formation) and collateral development. The listed factors provide additional signals that are necessary to complete the arteriogenesis program. *(Illustration by Silvia Sonn.)*

arrived cells have critical functions for activating angiogenesis in quiescent endothelium.[27] Endothelial cells derived from the circulation may be especially important for recanalization of thrombosed arteries and veins or for the regrowth of the endothelium after balloon and stent injury.

The findings for endothelial progenitors are consistent with the effects of other circulating stem cells that self-renew and differentiate into other cell types including liver, skin, and muscle. In atherosclerosis and cardiac transplantation, several studies showed that vascular smooth muscle cells in the neointima can arise from circulating precursor cells not just from medial wall cells.[28,29]

## Postnatal Angiogenesis: Mechanisms

Mechanisms of postnatal vessel formation and remodeling in the adult involve postnatal vasculogenesis (in which endothelial precursor cells mobilize and home to sites of vascular remodeling), angiogenesis (most commonly sprouting), and arteriogenesis (Fig. 24-1). Despite potential differences in the nature of various angiogenic stimuli involved in physiologic and pathologic examples of neovascularization, the process of angiogenesis and sprouting generally adheres to the following series of morphologic and biochemical events:

1. Vasodilation of the parent vessel. Vasodilation is mediated through the production of nitric oxide. The permeability of angiogenic vessels is enhanced by VEGF and its downstream signaling targets and VE-cadherin. These early vascular responses promote the extravasation of plasma proteins that can act as a provisional matrix to support cell migration.
2. Remodeling of basement membrane. Endothelial cells in the parent vessel must alter their attachment to basement membrane and pericytes. Changes in flow and mechanical factors transmitted through the endothelium activates proteases such as plasminogen activator and metalloproteases that remodel the vascular basement membrane causing it to thin and change its composisition.[30,31] Matrix remodeling mediated by proteases and their inhibitor complexes have several consequences for regulating angiogenesis: (1) mechanical forces may converge in the regions of thinned basement membrane to facilitate sprouting; (2) the remodeled ECM may alter endothelial cell responsiveness to soluble growth factors; and (3) growth factors or inhibitors sequestered in the matrix may be released to potentiate or limit a burst of angiogenesis.[32,33]
3. Endothelial cell migration and proliferation. Endothelial cell proliferation and migration contribute to the increasing length of the developing vessel, but the migrating endothelial cells tend to form the tip of the capillary sprout.[34] In the absence of DNA proliferation blocked by high-dose radiation, significant vessels can form by migrating endothelial cells. Most angiogenesis factors including members of the VEGF and fibroblast growth factor (FGF) families and PlGF modulate both proliferation and migration of endothelial cells. Complexes of activated metalloproteases and

endothelial cells at sites of postnatal angiogenesis is variable depending on the tissue and tumor type, the presence of ongoing injury, and the disease model studied. Sometimes there is less than 3% of these cells in angiogenic sites; however, it is possible that these newly

$\alpha_v\beta_3$ integrins on endothelial cells coordinate migration with the exposure of matrix molecules to their cell surface adhesion receptors.[35]

4. Lumen formation. As the endothelial cells align themselves in the developing capillary, they form attachments to each other and the ECM in a manner that creates a lumen. The lumen typically develops proximally in the developing sprout as a continuation of the lumen from the parent vessel. However, lumen formation can also occur by vacuolization within the endothelial cell. Lumen formation requires the production of fibronectin and laminin[36,37] and depends on critical adhesion events using adhesion molecules and cell surface glycoproteins.[38,39] Lumen caliber is increased as endothelial cells spread or new cells are added. Angiopoietin-1 has little mitogenic activity but increases the diameters of newly formed vessels.[40]

5. Loop formation. Parallel capillaries fuse and coalesce along their length or at their tips to form a loop capable of handling blood flow. Blood flow can cause further vascular remodeling. Blood cells such as platelets carry several endothelial factors that could mature the developing newly perfused vessel.[41]

6. Maturation of the basement membrane. The newly developed capillary continues to remodel the basement membrane by enhancing the composition comprised of collagen type IV, collagen XV, and collagen XVIII.[42]

7. Stabilization and incorporation of pericytes. In the final stages of capillary development, maturation of the new vessel requires the recruitment of pericytes.[43] Pericytes have long protruding cytoplasmic processes that run lengthwise and around the capillary wall. Pericyte functions include the synthesis of basement membrane; regulation of blood flow and permeability; and the production of paracrine signals VEGF, PDGF, TGF-$\beta$ and angiopoietin-1 that promote endothelial cell and pericyte interactions and may recruit other cells to form the medial and adventitial layers of larger blood vessels.[44,45] Several studies have shown that pericytes stabilize the newly formed blood vessel and inhibit regression if angiogenic growth factors are withdrawn.[46]

## Endothelial Cell Survival

In quiescent blood vessels, the endothelial cells can survive with little cell turnover. In an angiogenic environment, several soluble factors and remodeled ECM may affect endothelial cell survival and apoptosis. The regulation of endothelial cell apoptosis is a natural mechanism for controlling the growth and regression of blood vessels that is required for vascular pattern formation. Endothelial cells die when cell attachments to matrix or other endothelial cells (VE-cadherin) are disrupted, growth factors VEGF and angiopoietin-1 are withdrawn, or nitric oxide and hemodynamic shear forces are changed.[47,48] Angiogenic growth factors VEGF and FGF promote endothelial survival and resist apoptosis by distinct pathways.[49] Several angiogenesis inhibitors such as thrombospondin-1 (TSP-1), angiostatin, antagonists of $\alpha_v\beta_3$, endostatin, and VEGF antagonists induce endothe-

lial cell apoptosis.[50-52] The regulation of the apoptotic pathway in endothelial cells or circulating endothelial precursor cells is, therefore, an important control point for the regulation of angiogenesis and vascular injury.

## Postnatal Angiogenesis: Physiologic and Pathologic

In the adult, endothelial cell turnover is relatively quiescent, with only 0.01% of cells in the cell division cycle at any given time.[53] During physiologic processes such as ovulation, postnatal growth, menstrual cycle changes of the endometrium, wound healing, and tissue regeneration, angiogenesis is stimulated for a short period.[54] In contrast, pathologic angiogenesis persists for a longer duration and is abnormally sustained in a variety of disease states such as tumor growth, diabetic retinopathy, synovial pannus formation in rheumatoid arthritis, psoriasis, cardiac hypertrophy, ischemia, and in the neointima of atherosclerotic plaques.[2,55] Although many cellular events and regulatory molecules are common to both types of angiogenesis, there are emerging differences that distinguish angiogenesis regulation in these different physiologic and pathologic tissue environments. Another main difference is that inflammation accompanies most forms of postnatal pathologic angiogenesis. Immune cells including macrophages, mast cells, and T cells release matrix-associated proteases to initiate angiogenesis, activate endothelial cells to remodel the basement membrane and vessel wall, facilitate endothelial cell invasion, and provide systemic signals to recruit precursor cells from the bone marrow.[56-59] The angiogenesis-related molecules PlGF, e-NOS, chemokines, and cyclooxygenase-2 have few effects on embryonic angiogenesis or ovulation but have significant effects on postnatal angiogenesis particularly in inflammation-related models.[60-62]

Differences between physiologic and pathologic angiogenesis can be exploited for selective treatments. For example, tumor vasculature differs by the formation of dilated saccular capillaries with arteriovenous connections and abnormal flow and shunting. Tumor vessels often have gaps of incomplete endothelium between endothelial cells and transcellular holes, which account for their unregulated permeability. Tumor cells can transit through these spaces or reside within the mosaic tumor vasculature where they are exposed to blood cells and plasma proteins.[63,64] Tumor endothelium expresses unique markers that may be exploited for drug delivery and targeting to specific vascular addresses.[65,66] Additional molecular distinctions of other types of pathologic angiogenesis could provide more specific therapeutic targets that will regulate pathologic angiogenesis but not physiologic angiogenesis. Angiogenesis associated with chronic inflammation in atherosclerosis and rheumatoid arthritis may be more responsive to agents that target chemokines, TNF-$\alpha$, Cox-2, or other factors regulated by immune cells.

Diseases characterized by pathologic angiogenesis can be further divided into those that involve angiogenesis (angiogenic) and those that require angiogenesis for pathologic progression (angiogenesis-dependent).[67] This separation is determined empirically with interventions that block the neovascular component of the disease model to distinguish pathologic conditions amenable to treatments that target angiogenesis. For example, wound healing is an angiogenic process that is only modestly inhibited by a number of direct angiogenesis inhibitors,[68] whereas the dependence of tumor growth on angiogenesis has been demonstrated in animal models of tumor progression and has been validated by genetic, molecular, and clinical studies.[18,48]

## ASSAYS OF ANGIOGENESIS

Advances in the understanding of angiogenesis were facilitated by the establishment of culture techniques for the isolation and growth of endothelial cells.[69,70] *In vitro* angiogenesis assays have been developed to measure the effects of regulators on proliferation, migration, tube formation, and endothelial cell survival or apoptosis, which are important endothelial cell responses evoked during the angiogenesis program. The methods, advantages, and limitations of a wide variety of assays have been extensively reviewed.[71] The aortic ring assay, originally developed for the rat aorta but adapted to mice with targeted mutations, allows for the analysis of specific genes on mechanisms of endothelial cell sprout formation.[72,73]

Although *in vitro* assays examine the effects of soluble or matrix factors on specific endothelial cell responses that relate to angiogenesis, assessments of molecular regulators of angiogenesis require validation *in vivo*. First, culture conditions sometimes have increased oxygen, saturated growth factors, and serum that do not represent the *in vivo* angiogenesis environment. Second, agents that regulate endothelial cell function *in vivo* may be metabolized differently *in vivo* or may require additional cofactors for activity. Third, agents with endothelial cell activity may have secondary effects on other cell types that cooperate with endothelial cells during angiogenesis. Fourth, the endothelial cells used in some *in vitro* arrays are often derived from mature large vessel endothelium, which may differ significantly from microvascular or less differentiated endothelial cells. Lastly, the effects of matrix turnover and mechanical factors may not be represented in tissue culture conditions. Common *in vivo* methods include the corneal micropocket and matrigel or sponge implant assays, in which a growth factor is implanted in the avascular cornea or implant material and the extent of vascular ingrowth is quantified.[74] These methods are particularly useful experimental tools to study postnatal angiogenesis mechanisms in mice with genetic mutations. Specialized videomicroscopy chambers have been developed to study the temporal patterns of cellular and molecular events during angiogenesis *in vivo*.[75]

## ANGIOGENIC GROWTH FACTORS

The importance of angiogenesis in normal development and under certain pathologic conditions has prompted investigators to look for factors influencing angiogenesis. Table 24-1 lists a number of identified naturally occurring factors that promote angiogenesis.[3] Selected angiogenesis stimulators and inhibitors with expression relevant to the cardiovascular system are discussed in this section.

### Fibroblast Growth Factors

FGFs constitute a large family of related polypeptide growth factors that are potent endothelial cell mitogens and that also have effects on other cell types. Basic FGF (FGF-2) was the first isolated angiogenesis factor followed quickly by acidic FGF (FGF-1).[76,77] Acidic and basic FGF sequences do not contain a secretion signal sequence, suggesting that cell injury is one mechanism for their release.[78] FGF association with heparan sulfate glycosaminoglycans on the cell surface facilitates the binding of FGF ligand to its native receptors. This heparin-binding property mediates binding to ECM and creates a growth factor reservoir that may be released under wounding or inflammatory conditions.[79] Mast cells associated with wounds and sites of angiogenesis release heparin and mobilize basic FGF.[80] In full-thickness wounds, basic FGF levels increase fourfold by day 8, temporally preceding the time of highest vascular density. Applications of basic FGF increase angiogenesis and the healing rate of wounds.[81] Similarly, locally administered neutralizing antibodies to basic FGF delay

■ ▪ ■

## TABLE 24-1 ENDOGENOUS ANGIOGENIC FACTORS

| Factor | Molecular Weight | Endothelial I Mitogen | Year Reported |
| --- | --- | --- | --- |
| Basic fibroblast growth factor | 18,000 | Yes | 1984 |
| Acidic fibroblast growth factor | 16,400 | Yes | 1984 |
| Angiogenin | 14,100 | No | 1985 |
| Transforming growth factor α | 5,500 | Yes | 1986 |
| Transforming growth factor β | 25,000 | No | 1986 |
| Tumor necrosis factor α | 17,000 | No | 1987 |
| Vascular endothelial growth factor | 45,000 | Yes | 1983 |
| Platelet-derived endothelial cell growth factor | 45,000 | Yes | 1989 |
| Granulocyte colony-stimulating factor | 17,000 | Yes | 1991 |
| Placental growth factor | 25,000 | Weak | 1991 |
| Interleukin-8 | 40,000 | Yes | 1992 |
| Hepatocyte growth factor | 92,000 | Yes | 1993 |
| Proliferin | 35,000 | Yes | 1993 |

wound closure, wound collagen content, cell proliferation, and microvessel density.

The effects of acidic and basic FGF have been evaluated in vascular diseases. Adventitial delivery of basic FGF augments neointimal smooth muscle cell proliferation and neovascularization after balloon injury of the carotid artery.[82] Direct gene transfer of acidic FGF in endothelial cells of porcine arteries promoted intimal hyperplasia and stimulated intimal neovascularization.[83] Human atherosclerotic tissues showed enhanced expression of acidic FGF compared with normal vessels, whereas basic FGF transcripts were abundant in both normal and atherosclerotic vessels.[84] Increased levels of acidic FGF in atherosclerotic plaques may contribute to the development of neovascularization that is seen in advanced atherosclerotic lesions. The role of acidic and basic FGF in intimal hyperplasia has suggested strategies to control restenosis. However, clinical trials have not confirmed these findings, possibly because of the presence of preexisting lesions in patients compared with the normal vessels treated in animal studies.

In models of myocardial or limb ischemia discussed later, acidic FGF and basic FGF administration has enhanced the development of collateral vessels.[85-87] The additional effects of FGF on smooth muscle cells in collateral vessels may have theoretical advantages in arteriogenesis programs.

## Vascular Endothelial Growth Factor and Placental Growth Factor

VEGF, also known as vascular permeability factor, is a potent cytokine that exerts multiple effects on the vascular endothelium.[88] The VEGF family of growth factors includes the prototype member VEGF-A and other members VEGF-B, VEGF-C, VEGF-D, and VEGF-E, which differ by their tissue distribution and affinities for different VEGF receptors. Similar to FGF, VEGF stimulates endothelial cell proliferation and migration and has a high heparin-binding affinity. As its alternative name implies, VEGF increases the permeability of developing capillaries and is important for the development of fenestrated endothelium in the kidney.[89] Increased permeability of capillaries may facilitate angiogenesis via the extravasation of plasma proteins that form a provisional matrix favoring cell migration.[90]

VEGF and its receptors are required for blood vessel growth during development. Interestingly, interruption of only one allele of the *VEGF* gene was embryonic lethal, showing that VEGF expression in development is tightly regulated.[15,16] VEGF binds to tyrosine kinase receptors VEGFR-1, also known as *fms*-like tyrosine kinase-1 (Flt-1), and VEGFR-2, also known as kinase insert domain containing receptor (Kdr) or fetal liver kinase (Flk-1).[91] These receptors bind VEGF with high affinity and are expressed in vascular endothelial cells but are also present on some hematopoietic and precursor cell types. During development, VEGFR-2 is localized to the yolk sac and intraembryonic mesoderm, from which the endothelium derives. VEGFR-2 is later expressed on angioblasts and all endothelial cells, especially proliferating cells of vascular sprouts.[92] A targeted homozygous null mutation of VEGFR-2 blocked the formation of blood

islands, hematopoiesis, and vasculogenesis.[14,93] VEGFR-2 is required for later stages of endothelial cell differentiation. In comparison, VEGFR-1 is similarly expressed during early vascular development and in postnatal angiogenesis, but VEGFR-1 expression persists in some adult organs and inflammatory cells.[94] Deletion of the *VEGFR-1* gene allowed the formation of differentiated endothelial cells but resulted in the assembly of endothelial cells into abnormal vascular channels.[95] Later studies then showed that VEGFR-1 deficiency resulted in increased hemangioblast commitment and that VEGFR-1 signaling was not directly required for endothelial cell differentiation and embryonic angiogenesis.[96,97]

Because of the embryonic lethality of the absence of VEGF and its receptors, the functions of these molecules during postnatal angiogenesis have been evaluated with conditional knockout mice and the use of pharmacologic inhibitors. Soluble VEGF receptors, VEGF receptor neutralizing antibodies, and other VEGF antagonists have demonstrated that VEGF is an important regulator of ovarian angiogenesis coupled with ovulation, bone vascularization, postnatal growth, and retinal neovascularization.[46,98,99] VEGF is more abundant as atherosclerotic lesions progress and functions to recruit both monocytes and neovascularization.[62,100] VEGF agents have been tested in several clinical trials for therapeutic angiogenesis.[101]

VEGF-A has several common isoforms $VEGF_{121}$, $VEGF_{165}$, and $VEGF_{189}$ and less abundant isoforms $VEGF_{145}$ and $VEGF_{206}$, which form as a result of alternative splicing from the same gene. These distinct splice variants all stimulate endothelial cell proliferation but have different affinities for cell-surface heparan sulfate proteoglycans.[102] The isoform $VEGF_{121}$ exists mostly in soluble form and shows little binding to ECM components, whereas the isoforms $VEGF_{189}$ and $VEGF_{206}$ are primarily associated with matrix. The most ubiquitously expressed isoform $VEGF_{165}$ is detected as both soluble and matrix-associated protein. $VEGF_{165}$ also binds neuropilin receptors that may function in development to coordinate neural axon and vascular patterning.[103] Interestingly, $VEGF_{121}$ does not bind neuropilin; therefore, various VEGF isoforms may have differential functions. Mice that only express the soluble murine $VEGF_{120}$ isoform (comparable to the human splice variant $VEGF_{121}$) die early in the postnatal period because of impaired myocardial angiogenesis and ischemic cardiomyopathy.[104] Retinal vessel development is severely impaired in $VEGF_{120}$ mice. $VEGF_{188}$ mice have normal retinal veins but abnormal retinal arterioles, which typically express neuropilin receptors.

The complexity of VEGF activity has been further increased by the finding that VEGF can circulate as a heterodimer in combination with a homologous protein PlGF. Compared with VEGF homodimers, VEGF-PlGF heterodimers are equally chemotactic for endothelial cells but are relatively less mitogenic and, therefore, may inhibit the activity of VEGF homodimers.[105] The relative distribution of VEGF as homodimers or heterodimers in tissues may differentially regulate angiogenesis.[106]

## Tie2 Receptors and Angiopoietins

The endothelial cell receptors Tie1 and Tie2 are important for vascular development.[107] Vascular integrity is abnormal in Tie1-deficient embryos that develop edema and hemorrhage. The physiologic ligands for Tie1 receptors are not yet identified. Tie2-deficient embryos have abnormal angiogenesis with a failure to produce mature vascular networks. Angiopoietins comprise a family of ligands that bind Tie2 receptors and have effects on blood vessel development, particularly in the interactions between endothelial cells themselves or with periendothelial cells and basement membrane.[108,109] The most abundant angiopoietic members are angiopoietin-1 (Ang1) and angiopoietin-2 (Ang2), which function as an agonist and relative antagonists, respectively. In the adult Ang1 inhibits vascular permeability.[110] Although Ang1 has little mitogenic activity on endothelial cells itself, in combination with VEGF it can enhance angiogenesis and collateral formation while blocking permeability and inflammatory cell recruitment associated with increased expression of VEGF alone.[111,112]

## EphrinB2 and EphB4 Receptors

The pathologic differences between arteries and veins have been assumed to be due to differences in the physiologic environment such as oxygen levels and blood pressure and flow. Genetic deletion of ephrinB2, a transmembrane ligand for EphB4 receptor, identifies arterial but not venous endothelial cells.[7] Conversely, the EphB4 receptor is expressed on veins. This pattern exists before the onset of angiogenesis and before blood circulates in the embryo, indicating that arterial and venous identities are determined by molecular mediators independent of hemodynamic signals, however, flow-related signals may later provide essential physiologic cues. EphrinB2-deficient mice develop abnormal capillary networks in the brain and yolk sac and abnormal myocardial trabeculation. The phenotype of embryos that lack the EphB4 receptor is similar to the effects associated with deletion of its ligand, showing that normal capillary patterns require reciprocal signaling by the receptor and transmembrane ligand pair.[113] Smooth muscle cells acquire the ephrinB2 transmembrane ligand as they incorporate into arterial structures, which suggests that it may regulate the media of growing or remodeling arteries.[114] EphrinB2 is also important for neural cell guidance and provides a mechanism for the parallel development of nerves and blood vessels.[12,115] The extracellular domains of ephrinB2 provide sufficient guidance cues for nerves, but internal signals generated by this receptor on endothelial cells are required for normal vascular patterning.[116] The biologic effects of these arterial and venous markers during postnatal angiogenesis and responses of vein grafts implanted into arterial circuits are subjects of future investigations. Strategies to promote functional new blood vessels may need to consider the signals that provide guidance cues and the signals that quantitatively regulate angiogenesis.

## Matrix Metalloproteases

Proteases of the matrix metalloprotease (MMP), heparanase, and plasminogen activator families regulate angiogenesis by a variety of mechanisms. These proteases may be used by endothelial cells and other cells to migrate and invade tissues during stages of angiogenesis and sprouting. In some cases, MMPs associate with integrins in complexes on the endothelial cell surface to coordinate adhesion and matrix remodeling during directed cell migration.[35] Protease activation correlates with the angiogenic switch in some tissue, partly because of changes in the ECM and partly because of mobilization of growth factors VEGF, bFGF, and IGF-1, which then become accessible to endothelial cell receptors.[56,117] At the same time, these same proteases may release fragments of parent molecules that have negative effects on angiogenesis. MMP activity correlates with the inflammatory content of atherosclerotic lesions and may play an important role in the destabilization of atheromas that trigger a myocardial infarction or stroke.[118]

## Chemokines and Other Angiogenic Molecules

Several other factors including leptin, chemokines, hepatocyte growth factor, Thy-1, and interleukins can induce angiogenesis when provided exogenously in various models of angiogenesis, but their endogenous role in blood vessel regulation remains unknown. Different chemokine members can act as inhibitors or stimulators of angiogenesis.[119] Stromal cell-derived factor-1 binds to the chemokine receptor CXCR-4 and can participate in the mobilization of endothelial cell precursors.[25,120]

## INHIBITORS OF ANGIOGENESIS

Control of angiogenesis also involves negative regulators, some of which are listed in Table 24-2.[3] Endothelial cells in capillaries may be maintained in a quiescent state by the effects of endogenous endothelial inhibitors. In some conceptual models, the net effect on angiogenesis may be determined by the balance of both angiogenic growth factors and inhibitors observed in some tissues.[121]

## Interferon α

Previously, interferon-α was shown to inhibit angiogenesis in the cornea assay, and it inhibited both endothelial cell proliferation and migration in culture.[122] Currently, this inhibitor is administered at low doses to inhibit growth of life-threatening hemangiomas and certain tumors.[123] Interferon-α can act as an indirect inhibitor of angiogenesis, in part because of its inhibition of basic FGF release.

## Thrombospondin-1

TSP-1 is a component of ECM that acts as a negative regulator of angiogenesis. The antiangiogenesis function of TSP-1 was noted in a tumor progression model, in which inactivation of the tumor suppressor gene *p53* resulted in loss of TSP-1 and increased tumorigenicity of the parent tumor cell line.[124] TSP-1 was purified and shown to inhibit endothelial cell migration and neovascularization in the cornea assay. Differential TSP-1 expression regu-

■ ■ ■

**TABLE 24-2**   ENDOGENOUS NEGATIVE REGULATORS OF ENDOTHELIAL-CELL PROLIFERATION

| Factor | Inhibits Proliferation | Inhibits Chemotaxis | In Circulation | In Matrix |
|---|---|---|---|---|
| Platelet factor 4 | Yes | Yes | Yes | No |
| Thrombospondin-1 | Yes | Yes | Yes | Yes |
| TIMP-1 | No | Yes | Yes | — |
| TIMP-2 | Yes | Yes | Yes | — |
| TIMP-3 | — | — | — | Yes |
| Prolactin (16-kd fragment) | Yes | Yes | — | — |
| Angiostatin (38-kd fragment of plasminogen) | Yes | Yes | Yes | — |
| Basic FGF soluble receptor | Yes | — | Yes | — |
| Transforming growth factor β | Yes | Yes | Yes | — |
| Placental proliferin-related protein | Yes | Yes | Yes | — |
| Endostatin | Yes | — | Yes | Yes |

lated by progesterone modulates the development and regression of endometrial vessels during the menstrual cycle.[125] The effects of TSP-1 on endothelial cell apoptosis are mediated by the CD36 receptor, which also functions as a scavenger receptor important for the clearance of apoptotic bodies and lipids.[52,126] Atherosclerotic tissues and intimal lesions associated with vascular injury express TSP-1.[127] Functional studies in a rat carotid balloon injury model showed that neutralizing antibodies to TSP-1 enhanced reendothelialization and inhibited smooth muscle cell proliferation.[128]

## Tissue Inhibitors of Metalloproteases (TIMPs)

The activities of metalloproteases are tightly regulated during angiogenesis at many levels, including activation by proteolytic processing of a proenzyme precursor protein and complex association with a specific inhibitor, which itself is a protease that requires activation.[129] The stoichiometric ratio of the metalloprotease members and their respective family of inhibitors known as TIMPs are closely regulated in tissues. The tissue complexes of TIMPs and MMPs may be altered under conditions of tissue remodeling such as in neoplasia, inflammation, tissue growth, and injury. Based on their interactions with specific metalloproteases and the presence of inernal peptide domains within specific TMP family members that directly regulate angiogenesis, the TIMPs can function as angiogenesis inhibitors.[130]

## Cryptic Regulators of Angiogenesis

A growing number of cryptic angiogenesis regulators are released by proteolysis of parent molecules, which suggests another level of control. TSP-1 and platelet factor 4 parent molecules are angiogenesis inhibitors themselves, but they can be modified to truncated forms with more potent inhibitory activity.[32,131] Plasminogen, fibronectin, and prolactin have no initial effect on angiogenesis but can release peptides that are potent angiogenesis inhibitors.[132-134] The angiogenesis inhibitor angiostatin is derived from its precursor plasminogen by elastases and metalloprotease-2, which themselves are activated during tissue remodeling.[135] Endostatin and tumastatin are fragments of basement membrane proteins collagen XVIII and collagen IV, respectively.

Endostatin and tumastatin promote endothelial cell apoptosis and inhibit endothelial cell proliferation.[33,136] In some cases, these truncated molecules could act as a dominant negative agent that inhibits endothelial cell interactions with the basement membrane. Normal endothelium is maintained in a quiescent state, and stored angiogenic growth factors and inhibitors are reserved for conditions such as wounding. Sequestered growth factors such as FGF and VEGF with short half-lives can potentiate angiogenesis, whereas ECM molecules with longer half-lives may help terminate angiogenesis.

## Switch to the Angiogenic Phenotype

Analysis of tumor progression models in transgenic mice and premalignant stages of human breast, skin, and cervical cancers have shown that angiogenesis is a regulated and rate-limiting step important in the development of a solid tumor. VEGF levels are already elevated in the preangiogenic phase, but the angiogenic switch corresponds to the entry of MMP-9 expressing inflammatory cells.[56,117] The MMP-9 activity may induce several effects critical for the angiogenic switch in this experimental model including activation of growth factors, matrix remodeling, and processing of kit-ligand to recruit other cells important for angiogenesis.[58] In a second model, comparisons of angiogenic and avascular chondrosarcoma nodules show that VEGF levels are higher and that hypoxia inducing factor 1-α (HIF-1α) has a nuclear location pattern in avascular nodules. These examples demonstrate the limitations of a reductionist approach and the simplified assumption that angiogenic growth factors are more abundant in tissues with ongoing angiogenesis. Switch mechanisms must consider complex integration of several regulators and conditions that exist in the tissue microenvironment. Understanding the molecular basis of the angiogenic switch in different tissues may also be relevant to cardiovascular diseases. For example, several angiogenesis stimulators are expressed in inflammatory and smooth muscle cells present in early atherosclerotic lesions, but angiogenesis is not prevalent until later stages. VEGF abundance and distribution do not correlate with the localized regions of neovascularization present only in some atheromas.[137]

# LYMPHANGIOGENESIS

The mechanisms of lymphangiogenesis are becoming defined as markers of lymphatic endothelium and specific growth factors for these cells are identified. VEGFR-3 is expressed on lymphatic endothelium in the embryo and adult. VEGFR-3 deficient mice have defects in the lumens of large vessels that cause pericardial fluid accumulation and cardiovascular failure before the onset of lymphatic development.[138] VEGFR-3 mutations result in lymphedema and abnormal lymphatic development. In addition, mutations found in patients with hereditary congenital lymphedema syndromes map to the *VEGFR-3* gene.[139,140] VEGFR-3 is activated by VEGF-C and VEGF-D. Overexpression of VEGF-C can induce lymphangiogenesis via activation of VEGFR-3 but also has effects on angiogenesis mediated by binding to other VEGF receptors.[141-143] This data illustrates the importance of VEGFR-3 and its ligands VEGF-C and VEGF-D in lymphatic development. Other receptors important for normal lymphangiogenesis include the neuropilin-2 receptor. Neuropilin-2 expression is restricted to veins and lymphatic vessels in mice, and null mutants show abnormal formation of small lymphatic vessels without obvious changes in the larger collecting lymphatics channels.[10]

Although some factors may exert dual regulation of angiogenesis and lymphangiogenesis during development or in postnatal conditions of inflammation and disease, specificity can be obtained.[144] The *Prox1* homeobox gene is necessary for lymphatic development and sprouting but does not interfere with angiogenesis.[145]

Understanding the regulation of lymphangiogenesis may be important in tumor metastasis, lymphatic malformations, and cardiovascular diseases characterized by lymphedema. Animal models that stimulate lymphangiogenesis have been developed to understand the cellular events and signals involved in this process compared with angiogenesis. Some circulating endothelial cell precursors express VEGFR-3, which raises questions regarding how and from what point of entry these cells might leave the blood circulation to incorporate into lymphatic channels.[146] Delivery of VEGF-C induces angiogenesis and lymphangiogenesis that may ameliorate lymphedema syndromes.[140,142] Mutations in VEGF-C have also been designed that are specific for VEGFR-3 and produce selective effects on lymphatic development without inducing angiogenesis.[147]

# ANGIOGENESIS IN CARDIAC GROWTH AND HYPERTROPHY

During late fetal and early postnatal periods of development, rapid growth of cardiac myocytes is accompanied by a proportional growth of capillaries and some degree of growth in larger coronary vessels.[148] The cardiac growth rate decreases rapidly with maturity, but under specific hormonal, hemodynamic, and pathologic circumstances, cardiomyocyte hypertrophy and hyperplasia can be stimulated in the adult. These changes in myocardial mass occur along with changes in the coronary vasculature, suggesting that there may be paracrine signals that coordinate changes in the endothelial and myocardial compartments. An ischemic myocardium and cardiomyopathy resulted from inadequate development of coronary arteries as seen in genetically modified mice that only express VEGF$_{120}$.[104] A cardiomyocyte-specific knockout of VEGF resulted in an abnormal heart with reduced capillary density, myocardial thinning, ventricular dysfunction, and induction of hypoxia-responsive genes involved in energy metabolism. These two examples of impaired myocardial angiogenesis or coronary artery development during stages of postnatal heart growth show that normal myocardial function and dimensions require coordinated changes in the vasculature.[149]

Angiogenesis in the adult heart and coronary circulation during cardiac hypertrophy is mostly observed at the capillary level. Larger coronary vessels do not significantly increase in number or density after birth, but they can adapt to changes in hemodynamics and produce significant enlargement of coronary arterioles and coronary artery branches. The growth of coronary vessels and capillaries in the heart can be assessed by a variety of methods: (1) measurements of capillary density in heart tissue fixed at the same systolic or diastolic period, the capillary : myofibril ratio, or the endothelial cell incorporation of bromodeoxyuridine[150] can be made; (2) the functional capacity of the vascular bed can also be determined by measuring maximal blood flow after maximal vasodilation relative to resting blood flow; and (3) nuclear medicine perfusion technologies or endothelial cell targeted microbubbles can be used to quantify changes in collateral circulation or regional tissue perfusion.[151]

## Postnatal Changes in Coronary Vessels

In early postnatal development, the ventricle is exposed to increased stretch and pressure load, resulting in hypertrophy and hyperplasia of cardiac myocytes. At the same time, the coronary capillary density increases by sprouting and intussusception mechanisms of angiogenesis. During this rapid phase of cardiac growth, capillary diameters decrease, which maximize oxygen transport because the endothelial surface area relative to vessel volume increases.[152]

After birth, the number of main coronary arteries remains fixed and the number of arterioles does not increase. Actually, arteriole density slowly declines during aging, resulting in a modest increase in minimal coronary vascular resistance.[148] Large vessels remodel in response to mechanical and humoral factors. During growth to maturity, the length and diameter of coronary vessels increase.[150] Large vessels incorporate endothelial cells to increase the intimal surface area, remodel the basement membrane, recruit pericytes and smooth muscle cells to expand the media, and develop adventitial vessels known as vaso vasorum to provide the necessary blood supply to the thicker vessel wall.

At older ages, hearts may be exposed to hypertension, age-related changes in vascular resistance, or valvular abnormalities that can alter pressure or volume loads to the heart and induce myocyte hypertrophy. The molecular mechanisms regulating cardiac hypertrophy will not be fully reviewed, but it is important to evaluate changes in coronary vessels and capillaries in the context of concomitant changes in the cardiac myocyte compartment. Limited capillary growth can occur in younger hypertrophied hearts, but typically less capillary growth is seen in older individuals. The increased capillary density may be inadequate to meet the demands of hypertrophied myocytes, thereby contributing to later myocardial dysfunction.[153] An inadequate response of the coronary microcirculation could induce hypoxia-related changes or may diminish paracrine factors that sustain myocyte and endothelial cell interactions.

## FACTORS INFLUENCING MYOCARDIAL ANGIOGENESIS

### Hormonal and Pharmacologic Factors

Cardiac growth and changes in the cardiac vasculature can be influenced by hormonal and certain physiologic conditions. Elevated thyroxin increases myocardial size and increases capillary density, but endothelial cell proliferation is not significantly altered by thyroxin excess or deficiency, suggesting that the increased capillary density may be due to elongation of existing cells.[154]

### Mechanical Factors Affecting Cardiac Angiogenesis

Mechanical influences exerted under dynamic flow conditions are important in vessel development and remodeling. The endothelium can modulate flow-mediated vasorelaxation by inducing the synthesis of prostacyclins, epoxyeicosatrienoic acids, and nitric oxide or by inhibiting the production of the vasoconstrictor endothelin-l.[1,155] The molecular mechanisms that transmit these mechanical stimuli are complex and may involve integrin molecules and their signaling pathways, activation of flow-sensitive ion channels, and regulation of other cell-cell and cell-matrix interactions.[156,157] Endothelial cells respond to shear stress and stretch with altered patterns of gene expression and cell shape.[158] Changes in endothelial cell shape can alter cellular responsiveness to growth factors, and distortions of the cytoskeleton initiated from the luminal surface can be transmitted to the abluminal side of vessels.[159] Endothelial cell production of nitric oxide by eNOS contributes to angiogenesis and collateral formation in the ischemic hindlimb model.[60] The mechanism of the eNOS effect may depend partly on flow and mechanical signals generated *in vivo* and partly on downstream signaling mediated by nitric oxide that is initiated by VEGF.

Mechanical factors triggered by changes in coronary blood flow, heart rate, and inotropy can modify capillary growth in the adult heart.[150] Long-term administration of vasodilators increases coronary blood flow and the capillary density in myocardium but has little effect on the diameter or length of large vessels. A decreased heart rate increases capillary growth caused by the increased capillary diameters and wall tension forces

generated during longer diastolic periods. Lastly, pharmacologic interventions that increase cardiac inotropy without altering heart rate or coronary blood flow have been shown to increase capillary density.

### Hypoxia

Hypoxia in tissues is a potent inducer of angiogenesis. VEGF transcript levels are increased in hypoxia, mostly because of posttranscriptional stabilization of VEGF mRNA by factors induced by hypoxia.[160] Hypoxia or hypoglycemia activate the HIF-1α transcription factor to regulate a number of genes including VEGF that are involved in angiogenesis or erythropoiesis to restore homeostasis in tissues deprived of oxygen or nutrients.[161] Because these factors activate transcriptional programs for several genes involved in angiogenesis, they have been tested in experimental models of arteriogenesis and angiogenesis. The HIF-1α induced blood vessels show more advanced stages of remodeling with a greater number of larger caliber vessels that incorporate smooth muscle cells compared with the patterns of capillaries induced by VEGF alone.[162] HIF-1α also regulates genes involved in cell cycle and apoptosis, which affect cell responses in hypoxic microenvironments. Clinical trials will examine the effectiveness of these agents to induce collaterals in the desired tissue without causing incidental effects that could activate angiogenesis in clinically undetected dormant tumors. This theoretical undesirable effect has not been seen in single growth factor trials on smaller numbers of patients, but this risk may be different for factors that regulate more general programs of gene expression.[163-165]

The effects of hypoxia on coronary vessels and the heart *in vivo* are more complex, because chronic hypoxia in patients induces other physiologic adaptations. For example, chronic hypoxia induces pulmonary hypertension and right ventricular hypertrophy, which may increase capillary density in the right ventricle because of the altered pressure load rather than reduced oxygen delivery in the right ventricle. Hypoxia results in microscopic foci of myocardial necrosis and inflammation that secondarily stimulate angiogenesis or the development of collaterals. Patients with chronic megaloblastic and iron deficiency anemia have a compensatory increased heart rate and cardiac output and acquire more numerous coronary anastomoses and collaterals.[166] Hypoxic tissues can, therefore, trigger mechanical factors, release cytokines and growth factors, and mobilize precursor cells to enhance local sites of angiogenesis.[167]

## ANGIOGENESIS AFTER MYOCARDIAL INFARCTION

In myocardial infarction, abrupt closure of the coronary vessels results in myocardial necrosis and elevated levels of angiogenic growth factors such as basic FGF and VEGF. Serial angiography examinations of patients with acute myocardial infarction followed the temporal changes of coronary collateral vessels after an infarction. Either collateral growth or regression can occur after an infarction. A significant fraction of patients with acute infarcts have preexisting established collateral vessels, which developed in the setting of chronic ischemia caused by flow-limiting obstructions of the coronary arteries present before the acute infarction.[168] Angiographic studies showed the prevalence of coronary collaterals in patients with a persistently occluded coronary artery increased from 33% at baseline to 90% by 10 to 14 days after the acute event. In comparison, the incidence of collaterals decreased from 38% to 7% in those patients with sustained reperfusion.[169,170] These observations suggest that collateral vessels can develop within 10 days in the setting of persistent ischemia. Even though some collateral vessels appear to regress on an angiogram, some of these collateral channels may still be patent but show selective contrast filling caused by alternative blood flow patterns in conduit vessels.

Following a myocardial infarction, significant myocardial remodeling must occur in conjunction with remodeling of the coronary circulation. Strategies to deliver bone marrow derived stem cells after a myocardial infarction to repair injured myocardium, stimulate coronary collaterals and myocardial angiogenesis, and rescue hibernating myocardium in the periphery of the infarct zone show benefits in animal studies.[171]

# FORMATION OF COLLATERAL VESSELS

The functional importance of coronary collateral circulation has been demonstrated in multiple studies that assess preserved left-ventricular function after myocardial infarction. In clinical thrombolysis trials, collaterals had a protective effect that limited infarct size and maintained myocardial viability in those patients with documented unsuccessful reperfusion.[168,172] The presence of collateral vessels is associated with an earlier peak release of cardiac enzymes and a reduced total level of creatine kinase.[173] Collateral vessels reduce the extent of transmural infarction and the incidence of left-ventricular aneurysm following myocardial infarction. It is also possible that the healing response of infarcted tissues is improved when collateral vessels are available to provide perfusion, metabolic substrates, leukocytes, and precursor cells.

## Animal Models and Preclinical Studies

Given this demonstrated protective effect of coronary collateral vessels, there is natural interest in understanding the mechanisms of collateral development.[174] The canine and porcine animal models of collateral development have important differences related to the anatomic variations of these two species. The dog has large previously formed epicardial collateral vessels that can dilate 20-fold when the left circumflex artery is gradually constricted. In comparison, the porcine coronary vessels are predominantly end vessels with little overlapping collateral circulation. Progressive occlusion of native coronary vessels in the pig results in the development of intramyocardial collateral vessels. These intramyocardial collateral vessels have diameters ranging from 20 to 200 μ, structurally resemble capillaries, usually lack smooth muscle cell layers, and are associated with microscopic foci of myocardial necrosis induced by impaired perfusion. Both models are relevant to the human coronary circulation in which large epicardial collaterals and intramyocardial capillary networks can be induced.[175]

The expansion of epicardial collateral vessels occurs at a site separated from the myocardial tissue that is rendered ischemic by chronic occlusion of the left circumflex artery. Humoral factors released by the subendocardial ischemic tissue cannot account for the alterations in epicardial vessels. Pressure gradients across the collateral network and altered shear stresses on endothelial cells may initiate cellular and ECM remodeling events.[174] The expanding anastomoses sites of stimulated collaterals show the following microscopic changes: (1) the vessel diameter increases, as do the proliferation rates of endothelial cells and smooth muscle cells; (2) the surface of the endothelium looks ruffled and adhesion by monocytes increases; (3) monocytes release proteases and express several mitogenic factors that can influence smooth muscle and endothelial cell proliferation; (4) the wall of the remodeling arteriole becomes thinned as the internal elastic lamina and medial layers are reorganized; and (5) eventually the medial wall thickness increases as smooth muscle cells proliferate and are incorporated, but often the expanded internal elastic lamina has a helical orientation around the enlarged collateral accounting for its tortuosity.[175] The tortuous expansion of collateral vessels is also seen in human coronary arteries exposed to high cardiac flow states associated with chronic anemia and arteriovenous fistulas.

The collaterals induced in the porcine model are associated with focal areas of myocardial ischemic and necrosis. The stimulated new vessels resemble capillaries and develop through mechanisms typical of angiogenesis in other tissues. Endothelial growth factors acidic FGF, IGF-1, and VEGF are expressed in ischemic muscle or myocardium and by infiltrating macrophages.[176] Recent studies have demonstrated the importance of monocytes, macrophages, and possibly other inflammatory cell types in the formation of collaterals. Mice that lack macrophage colony-stimulating factor (op/op mice) and that have few macrophages show impaired arteriogenesis. Agents that directly activate these cells, including granulocyte-monocyte colony-stimulating factor (GM-CSF), PlGF, monocyte chemotactic protein-1, IGF-1, and TNF-α, show enhanced arteriogenesis.[59,62,176] A randomized double-blind placebo-controlled clinical trial using short-term administration of GM-CSF showed improved coronary collateral blood flow index.[177]

Agents that target smooth muscle cell differentiation and recruitment to form the muscular and matrix components of the blood vessel wall can also augment collaterals. Because the arteriogenesis program requires more complex remodeling and smooth muscle cell incorporation into enlarged or new collaterals, factors such as basic FGF, PDGF-B, and TGF-β may have added effects compared with factors with primary or more exclusive effects on endothelial cells alone.

## Clinical Trials for Myocardial and Limb Ischemia and Future Directions

The therapeutic uses of acidic FGF, basic FGF, and VEGF have been most widely studied. Enhancement of collaterals by these factors has been demonstrated in several animal models of hindlimb and myocardial ischemia. Basic FGF was shown to increase collateral flow and improve myocardial function in pigs with chronic myocardial ischemia. Endovascular transfection of an expression plasmid encoding $VEGF_{165}$ into the iliac artery of rabbits with an ischemic hindlimb resulted in a significant increase in collateral vessels.[178] Clinical trials based on these preclinical studies have been performed with some promising results. Several studies show improved exercise capacity and relief of angina scores, but similar improvements were sometimes seen in placebo-control patients.[101,179] Endpoint assessments of collateral blood flow and perfusion, however, have been less dramatic.

Therapeutic arteriogenesis trials for peripheral vascular disease are also being tested. Treatment endpoints in these studies included improved exercise tolerance without claudication symptoms, ankle-brachial blood pressure index, and in some instances improved healing of ischemic ulcers or improved neural sensation.[180] Although initial phase 1 clinical studies evaluated dose and delivery schedules and did not always have placebo-control patients, one placebo-control trial (TRAFFIC) showed improved peak walking time 90 days after a single intraarterial injection of basic FGF.[181]

The strategies used in these early therapeutic arteriogenesis trials have tested the delivery of a single agent by either protein or gene expression methods. The delivery method and level of expression of a single factor are important variables in these strategies. Unregulated and enhanced local expression of VEGF, for example, stimulated the local proliferation of endothelial cells without guidance cues and resulted in the formation of hemangioma-like vascular structures.[182] In an attempt to augment collateral responses, some clinical trials use tools to map the ischemic regions and deliver angiogenesis factors to those targeted regions.[183] Although the agents may be delivered locally, factors may quickly redistribute or extend into the systemic circulation. Systemic effects are seen in patients who received local agents including changes in blood pressure and increased mobilization of endothelial precursors in peripheral blood samples.[184] The delivery of growth factor agents as protein versus gene expression vector affects the duration and dose level achieved, but ultimately the delivery methods may be less important than the design of strategies that activate other target molecules and other cell types involved in the arteriogenesis cascade. The shortcomings of single-agent clinical trials may be best addressed by the use of combined agents.

The underlying limitation of current arteriogenesis strategies is probably related to the limited understanding about the complex cascade of events required for collateral growth. The strategies have mostly focused on the role of angiogenesis stimulators. Ischemic tissue itself is a source of these factors, so it is unclear why incremental increases in these factors provide a sufficient stimulus for collateral growth. Is there a threshold effect? Do the ischemic tissues provide other unidentified cofactors that complement these added stimulants? What is the prerequisite role for signals derived from the distal ischemic microenvironment that induce responses in the physically separated proximal conduit vessels? Local expansion of the capillary bed in the ischemic tissues may provide proximal and distal acting signals to the circulation to increase the conduit arteriole and venous vessels that supply this region. Future answers to these basic questions and mechanisms may provide clues to design optimal arteriogenesis treatments or determine why collateral responses in some patients are blunted.

The enhancement of collaterals by single growth factors in experimental ischemia models was observed in young adult animals, but these same interventions are less effective when clinical factors such as hypercholesterolemia, hypertension, nitric oxide endothelial cell dysfunction, diabetes, increased age, and concurrent vascular disease are present.[185-188] Another approach to augment the collateral response in patients is to correct these clinical conditions or compensate for suboptimal steps in the process.

The transcription regulator gene HIF-1α activates broader gene programs. HIF-1α expression stimulated larger vascular structures with more mural cells and stabilized permeability.[162] Increased formation of larger caliber vessels was also observed in the ischemic hindlimb model treated with exogenous PlGF.[62] These and other agents cited previously stimulate inflammatory cells and smooth muscle cells that cooperate with vascular endothelial cells in arteriogenesis programs. In the future, organ-specific growth factors may be identified that regulate the coronary vasculature while having limited effects on other vascular beds.[21] Further improvements may be seen by the reversal of clinical conditions that impair collateral growth and the use of angiogenic factors in combination to enhance multiple target molecules involved in arteriogenesis or angiogenesis.

Despite the potential advantages of augmenting coronary collateral circulation to protect tissue viability after acute vascular occlusion and to enhance perfusion to ischemic myocardium or limbs, there are a number of limitations of such therapeutic strategies. First, although the magnitude of collateral expansion can be significant, it is often an inadequate adaptation that does not compensate for the primary loss of coronary flow capacity. Fortunately, sometimes only an incremental improvement of perfusion by collaterals can be sufficient to maintain tissue viability or heal ischemic ulcers that threaten amputation. These palliative goals for advanced disease can have significant clinical impact, but collateral interventions should not be relied on to the exclusion of preventive treatments for the progression of the systemic disease that causes the need for collaterals in the first place. Second, it remains to be shown whether collateral treatments will improve cardiovascular mortality and morbidity. Collateral treatments obviate the effects of flow-limiting stenosis similar to the goals of coronary and peripheral artery bypass grafting, stents, and angioplasty. These established revascularization procedures produce marked enhancement of coronary and peripheral limb perfusion, but improved cardiovascular mortality can only be demonstrated in subsets of patients with severe coronary artery disease.[189] Third, at this time the long-term duration of new collaterals is not fully known. Many collateral vessels remain stable because of enhanced pericyte or smooth muscle cell coverage.[46] Collaterals at the site of vascular stenosis may not fill after angioplasty is performed in the native coronary, but they are often present when restenosis develops several months later. Despite these observations made over months, long-term evaluations of collateral vessels formed in experimental animals suggest that even these established collaterals may remodel and regress over a few years. Prophylactic attempts to induce collaterals to ameliorate the consequences of an acute vascular occlusion will need to address this question. Fourth, collaterals may have limited benefits for the treatment of proximal left main coronary artery lesions, where a large ischemic myocardial territory is at risk and where bridging collaterals from the thick-walled proximal aorta beyond the left main obstruction are less often seen. Lastly, the benefits of angiogenic growth factors may be offset by the theoretical but potential side effects of enhancing angiogenesis in other tissues—such as an occult neoplasm, a retina affected by diabetic proliferative retinopathy, or intimal capillaries associated with primary atherosclerotic plaques. Selection of patients eligible for these therapeutic strategies will need to consider these potential issues.

## ANGIOGENESIS IN ATHEROSCLEROTIC PLAQUES AND CHRONIC VASCULAR INFLAMMATION

Normal vessels have a microvasculature, known as the vaso vasorum, which is confined to the adventitial and outer medial layers (Fig. 24-2). Earlier observations by Virchow, Koester, Winternitz, and others demonstrated the association of intimal neovascularization and the presence of atherosclerotic plaques.[190] More recently, the neovascularization within the intimal layer of atherosclerotic plaques was demonstrated by cinematography after injection of silicone polymer in the coronary arter-

ies.[55] Plaque capillaries arise as branches from the native adventitial vasa vasorum more often than from the large vessel lumen and are often observed in the shoulder regions and base of plaques near areas with abundant macrophages and T cells.[191] Mast cell infiltrates in atherosclerotic plaques are similarly located in regions of intimal neovascularization.[192] The proliferation of vasa vasorum is not unique to atherosclerosis and not unique to arteries. Intimal neovascularization is also observed in giant cell arteritis, in vascular lesions associated with chronic rejection, and in association with thromboembolic involvement of veins and arteries.[193,194]

The clinical importance of plaque microvessels is suggested by studies showing their higher prevalence in cellular and inflammatory lesions that produce a greater degree of luminal stenosis and have a higher incidence of plaque rupture.[195] The pathologic consequences of neovascularization in primary atherosclerotic lesions may, therefore, be important in the genesis of late ischemic complications of atherosclerosis. Because these microvessels are fragile, similar to the vessels in proliferative diabetic retinopathy, they may be a source for intraplaque hemorrhage observed in some acute ischemic events. The endothelium of the intimal microvasculature binds endothelin-1 and responds by vasoconstriction, which may play a role in generating hypoxia of the vessel wall, regulating plaque blood flow, or altering plaque stability.[196] Finally, intimal neovascularization may indirectly affect plaque stability because of its association with inflammatory cells that promote rupture by degrading the fibrous cap over necrotic lipid collections in some vulnerable plaques.[197]

## Functions of Plaque Angiogenesis

Plaque neovascularization may promote the growth of atherosclerotic lesions by a variety of mechanisms. It may sustain growth of plaque tissue beyond a critical mass by providing nutrients, plasma components, and inflammatory cells. Atherectomy specimens from primary atherosclerotic lesions show a correlation between proliferating endothelial cells in plaque capillaries and the proliferation of other cells, which suggests that plaque angiogenesis may be a marker of growing lesions.[198] Several studies suggest that vasa vasorum function to provide

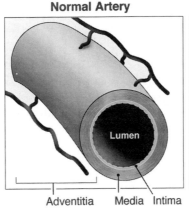
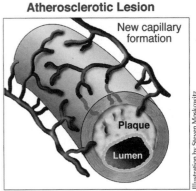

**Normal Artery**    **Atherosclerotic Lesion**

New capillary formation

Plaque

Lumen

Lumen

Illustration by Steven Moskowitz

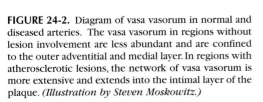

**FIGURE 24-2.** Diagram of vasa vasorum in normal and diseased arteries. The vasa vasorum in regions without lesion involvement are less abundant and are confined to the outer adventitial and medial layer. In regions with atherosclerotic lesions, the network of vasa vasorum is more extensive and extends into the intimal layer of the plaque. *(Illustration by Steven Moskowitz.)*

Adventitia    Media    Intima

perfusion to the thickened vessel wall; vaso vasorum are observed in the arteries of humans and other species when the wall thickness exceeds approximately 300 μ.[199,200] Interruption of vasa vasorum results in medial necrosis.[201] Diffusible tracers in the circulation localize near these capillaries and intimal tissue is hypoxic, even in the presence of neovascularization and arterial blood flow in the main vessel.[202] The functional association between plaque growth and plaque neovascularization has also been tested in intervention studies that showed that some inhibitors of angiogenesis impaired plaque growth in atherosclerosis-prone mice.[203] Conversely, two separate angiogenesis stimulators promoted plaque growth.[204,205] These positive and negative endothelial cell regulators may alter plaque growth via diverse mechanisms, but together these results support the hypothesis that plaque neovascularization promotes the progression of atherosclerosis.

Although larger plaques are more likely to have intimal neovascularization, this does not mean the plaque size is the sole determinant for their distribution and abundance. Extents of neovascularization show a poor linear correlation with plaque size and some advanced lesions contain no intimal neovascularization. Instead plaque neovascularization shows a strong linear and spatial correlation with regions of inflammatory cell infiltrates.[73] The correlation of plaque neovascularization with the inflammatory content in atherosclerotic lesions supports the hypothesis that these small vessel networks may act as conduits for leukocyte exchange or deposition of plasma constituents into advanced plaques, similar to their roles in other diseases of chronic inflammation such as rheumatoid arthritis.[62] Alternatively, or in addition to this potential mechanism, plaque capillaries may develop around these inflammatory cells because they elaborate angiogenic factors necessary for their formation. Macrophages are present in early lesions before the ingrowth of vasa vasorum; however, once initiated a positive feedback loop may operate in atherosclerosis whereby intimal neovascularization may propagate inflammatory cell recruitment. The endothelial cells of the intimal microvasculature have been shown to express increased levels of the leukocyte adhesion molecules E-selectin, VCAM-1, and ICAM-1 that are known to affect monocyte recruitment in atherosclerosis-prone mice.[206,207] If plaque capillaries function to regulate leukocyte exchange, then atheromas that acquire neovascularization may progress at different rates compared with atheromas that lack it. The plaque microvascular network may have additional significance because of recent data that other cell types in atheromas such as smooth muscle cell and endothelial precursors may be derived from the circulation.[29]

The role of plaque angiogenesis in mechanisms of plaque rupture is a subject of speculation. Plaque capillaries may directly promote plaque rupture as a source of intraplaque hemorrhage. During angiogenesis, endothelial cells may elaborate proteases that could alter the mechanical properties of lesions.[208] Plaque neovascularization can indirectly promote plaque disruption through its correlation with inflammatory cells, which are more abundant in lesions with vulnerable plaque morphologies.[209] Regulation of the neovascular component in atherosclerotic lesions may be a potential strategy to modify plaque stability, but these strategies require experimental verification in basic investigations. The effects of different angiogenesis inhibitor on atherosclerosis may not be similar, because of their diverse mechanisms of action. Known plaque-stabilizing agents such as HMG-CoA reductase are now recognized to have antiangiogenic effects; however, these properties alone may not account for the mechanisms of plaque stabilization observed in their widespread clinical use.[210,211]

## Regulation of Plaque Angiogenesis

Despite the intriguing significance of intimal neovascularization in atherosclerotic plaques, the mechanisms controlling intimal angiogenesis are not fully known.[212] Several angiogenic factors including VEGF, FGF family members, chemokines, PlGF, and platelet-derived endothelial cell growth factor are abundantly expressed in human atherosclerotic lesions.[84,100,137] Macrophages in atherosclerotic lesions also express interleukin-8, TGF-β, and other cytokines that can further augment the production of some angiogenic factors by smooth muscle cells in the vascular wall. In addition, increased expression and activity of MMP-2 and MMP-9 are present in atherosclerotic plaques, which may be important in plaque stability and may also influence plaque angiogenesis.[208] VEGF is abundant in atheromas, but VEGFR-2 antagonists did not inhibit plaque neovascularization when provided for a short period.[62] VEGF may regulate plaque angiogenesis via different VEGF receptors, or other angiogenic factors in the plaque can overcome the inhibitory effects on this receptor alone.

Many angiogenic factors are abundant even in early atheromas before the onset of plaque angiogenesis. In addition, the expression patterns and tissue abundance do not spatially coincide with regions of plaque angiogenesis. Thus, the presence of angiogenic stimulators may be necessary but not sufficient to initiate angiogenesis. A more complex understanding of the regulation of plaque angiogenesis must also consider the role of matrix or endogenous factors that antagonize the proliferation of vasa vasorum. Factors such as TSP-1 and endostatin, a component of collagen XVIII, are abundant factors in the vessel wall, but their functions in the regulation of plaque angiogenesis are not yet known.[213] These and other molecules in the vessel wall may impede the inward growth of vasa vasorum or may be modified in the presence of atherosclerosis.

## Making Arteries Grow and Blocking Plaque Angiogenesis

The potential use of both endothelial cell growth factors and inhibitors for patients with cardiovascular disease raises a number of important and clinically relevant questions. Will exogenous growth factor treatments have an untoward effect to enhance intimal angiogenesis or destabilize lesions? Atheromas already have a significant reservoir of local angiogenic growth factors, so systemic growth factors may have a limited local effect. On the other hand, it can be argued that ischemic limbs and myocardium also have increased expression of VEGF and basic FGF, yet systemic delivery of these growth factors results in arteriogenesis. In addition, bolus delivery of VEGF to mice with hypercholesterolemia-enhanced disease progression over a short time interval, although it is not known if these effects were sustained or related to the acute permeability effects of VEGF.[205] Given the relatively short period of time required for collaterals to grow, alterations in plaque size, inflammation, and angiogenesis could be controlled or be self-limited during this short phase of collateral stimulation. Use of selective arteriogenesis factors may also minimize this theoretical negative effect at other sites of neovascularization.

The converse question also arises. Will angiogenesis inhibitors block collateral development? Angiogenesis inhibitors such as TSP and platelet factor 4 can inhibit collateral development when provided at the time of a vascular occlusion, but they are not effective if the treatments are delayed.[214] Long-term evaluations of collaterals have shown that once formed, collateral vessels can remain patent even after growth factor levels reduce, which occurs after revascularization is achieved. Currently, applications of angiogenesis inhibitors for cardiovascular conditions are restricted to basic investigations to validate the functions and significance of plaque angiogenesis. Clinical applications of angiogenesis inhibitors for cancer, macular degeneration, and arthritis are being tested, and the use of these agents requires chronic treatments. Given the prevalence of cardiovascular disease in the population, these agents are likely to have concurrent effects on vascular diseases. Thus, understanding the functions and regulation of plaque angiogenesis will be important as the clinical use of these agents expands. In addition, the diverse mechanisms of action of various angiogenesis inhibitors directed at different stages in angiogenesis need to be evaluated for their likely diverse effects on cardiovascular diseases.

## RESTENOSIS

The subject of coronary artery restenosis and its therapeutic management is discussed in the chapter on restenosis. Only a few comments on the use of angiogenesis regulators to modify restenosis are provided. After balloon injury or stent placement, the endothelium on the surface of the large vessel is damaged or removed.[215] In addition, vasa vasorum in the adventitia proliferate.[216,217] Thus, animal studies have tested endothelial cell regulators in attempts to either enhance the regrowth of functional endothelium or inhibit the proliferation of vasa vasorum, sometimes with conflicting results. Administration of VEGF promoted the re-endothelialization of injured rabbit arteries.[218] However, when VEGF was provided in a canine coronary ischemia model at doses sufficient to induce collaterals, it significantly exacerbated neointimal formation after angioplasty.[219] Experimental differences in the model and method of VEGF delivery could account for these differ-

ent findings. Furthermore, the extensions of these findings to interventions on diseased vessels will add another layer of complexity to the mechanistic basis of these applications. Selective strategies might be used to deliver inhibitors to the adventitia while promoting the healing of functional endothelium on the surface of the main vessel.[128]

## HEMANGIOMAS AND VASCULAR MALFORMATIONS

Hemangioma of infancy is a benign tumor of endothelial cells characterized by the proliferation of capillary endothelium; the development of large vascular channels with multilaminated basement membranes; and the accumulation of mast cells, platelets, fibroblasts, and macrophages. Hemangiomas occur in about 10% of white infants and about 22% of preterm babies. The tumors most often involve the skin but can be generalized and involve other organs to cause bleeding and clinical complications that require intervention. Hemangiomas can cause severe hypothyroidism because of expression of type 3 iodothyronine deiodinase; hypothyroidism must be corrected to avoid neurologic problems in the infant.[220] Most hemangiomas resolve spontaneously and require no treatment. The natural history of hemangioma growth is characterized by a proliferative phase of growth lasting for 8 to 18 months after birth, followed by slow regression over 5 to 8 years during an involution phase. The primary defects that cause hemangioma have not been elucidated, but genetic studies have shown that hemangiomas are composed of clonal endothelial cells that exhibit abnormal properties *in vitro* and may arise when a somatic mutation occurs in a progenitor cell. These changes in the endothelial cells can lead to altered proliferation and response to angiogenesis regulators and may also induce changes in the adjacent tissue.[221] In contrast, vascular malformations, which include arteriovenous malformations and capillary telangiectasias, do not proliferate and do not involute spontaneously. Cellular markers can distinguish the various stages of hemangiomas and can differentiate hemangiomas from vascular malformations.[222]

The primary defects associated with other vascular malformations are being evaluated in genetic studies. Activating mutations in the Tie2 receptor are associated with familial cases of venous malformations that are made up of dilated venous channels with reduced and abnormal layers smooth muscle cells.[223] Defects in activin-like kinase receptors, which are receptors for TGF-β growth factors, are associated with hereditary hemorrhagic telangiectasia, or Osler-Rendu-Weber syndrome. Defects of activin receptors in mice result in abnormal fistulous connections and fusions between arteries and veins.[8,224]

## PULMONARY VASCULAR REMODELING

Pulmonary hypertension is a complex condition associated with vascular remodeling in the pulmonary circulation, either as a primary intrinsic defect or as a secondary response to hemodynamic changes associated with cardiac defects, pulmonary embolus, or hypoxic conditions. The pathologic changes in the pulmonary vessels include endothelial cell and smooth muscle cell proliferation associated with enhanced growth factors. These changes can occur in response to endothelial cell injury or activation of proteases.[225,226] Plexiform lesions associated with some forms of pulmonary hypertension can consist of clonal endothelial cell populations; however, clonal expansion may result from local proliferation and not be caused by acquired mutations in these cells. Areas of intimal hyperplasia in pulmonary arteries can also develop neovascularization. Many of these properties are also evident in atherosclerotic lesions of systemic arteries. Characterization of the responses of endothelial cells and smooth muscle cells during pathologic angiogenesis may provide further understanding of potential mediators of pulmonary vascular diseases.

## Pulmonary Arteriovenous Malformations after Glenn Shunt

Glenn shunt procedures involve the anastomosis of the superior vena cava to the right pulmonary artery to increase pulmonary blood flow in patients with cyanotic heart disease. Initial theoretical advantages of the Glenn procedure compared with systemic artery to pulmonary artery shunts were increased pulmonary blood flow, an absolute reduction in intracardiac right-to-left shunt, and less excessive pulmonary blood flow. This procedure subsequently reported increased mortality resulting from superior vena cava syndrome, progressive cyanosis from the development of systemic venous collaterals to the inferior vena cava, and the development of abnormal pulmonary arteriovenous malformations (PAVMs) in the right lung.[227] The histology of PAVMs show dilated tortuous networks of vessels: some have thin elastic lamina and thin smooth muscle cell collars, and some have thickened medial layers containing hyalinized connective tissue.[228] The incidence of PAVMs after Glenn procedures ranges from 25% to 31% and increases with the time interval following surgery.[229] Selected PAVMs may be treated with coil embolization, but often the PAVMs are distributed diffusely in the affected lung.

The conditions favoring the development of PAVMs have been postulated to be low pulsatile pulmonary flow, abnormal distribution of pulmonary flow, and the presence or absence of circulating factors. The occurrence and similarity of PAVMs in patients with liver disease and the regression of some PAVMs after liver transplantation have suggested the possibility that the loss of a hepatic factor or decreased hepatic clearance of a systemic vascular malformation promoting factor may be important in the development of PAVMs.[228] Patients treated with Fontan procedures have low pulsatile lung blood flow but rarely develop PAVMs. The rare observation of PAVMs in a few reported cases of patients receiving modified Fontan operations with shunts that excluded hepatic flow adds support to the hypothesis that the loss of a hepatic factor is important in the pathogenesis of PAVMs.[230] Further data is required to confirm

the predisposing conditions for PAVMs. Clinicians should look for early evidence of PAVMs in their patients with Glenn anastomoses and in patients who have had diversion of hepatic venous blood flow away from the lungs. The role of adjunctive procedures that provide some source of normal hepatic blood to the lungs as an attempt to palliate the progression of PAVMs has not been determined.

## FUTURE APPLICATIONS

The study of angiogenesis in the field of tumor biology has improved the understanding of mechanisms of angiogenesis and has identified a number of important growth factors, inhibitors, and ECM molecules that are important in regulating this process. This information is now providing new insights into cardiovascular diseases that involve mechanisms of vascular remodeling; the development of collateral vessels; and the stimulation of angiogenesis in atherosclerotic plaques, chronic rejection in transplant organs, and inflammatory conditions of arteries such as in Kawasaki's disease or temporal arteritis. Understanding the contributions of angiogenesis to many of these pathologic processes may provide new options for therapeutic interventions.

## REFERENCES

1. Gibbons GH, Dzau VJ: The emerging concept of vascular remodeling. N Engl J Med 1994;330:1431–1438.
2. Folkman J: Angiogenesis in cancer, vascular, rheumatoid and other disease. Nat Med 1995;1:27–31.
3. Folkman J: Seminars in Medicine of the Beth Israel Hospital, Boston: Clinical applications of research on angiogenesis. N Engl J Med 1995;333:1757–1763.
4. Risau W, Sariola H, Zerwes HG, et al: Vasculogenesis and angiogenesis in embryonic-stem-cell-derived embryoid bodies. Development 1988;102:471–478.
5. Carmeliet P: Mechanisms of angiogenesis and arteriogenesis. Nat Med 2000;6:389–395.
6. Suri C, Jones PF, Patan S, et al: Requisite role of angiopoietin-1, a ligand for the TIE2 receptor, during embryonic angiogenesis [see comments]. Cell 1996;87:1171–1180.
7. Wang HU, Chen ZF, Anderson DJ: Molecular distinction and angiogenic interaction between embryonic arteries and veins revealed by ephrin-B2 and its receptor Eph-B4 [see comments]. Cell 1998;93:741–753.
8. Urness LD, Sorensen LK, Li DY: Arteriovenous malformations in mice lacking activin receptor-like kinase-1. Nat Genet 2000;26:328–331.
9. Oh SP, Seki T, Goss KA, et al: Activin receptor-like kinase 1 modulates transforming growth factor-beta 1 signaling in the regulation of angiogenesis. Proc Natl Acad Sci USA 2000;97:2626–2631.
10. Yuan L, Moyon D, Pardanaud L, et al: Abnormal lymphatic vessel development in neuropilin 2 mutant mice. Development 2002;129:4797–4806.
11. Ingber DE: Mechanical signaling and the cellular response to extracellular matrix in angiogenesis and cardiovascular physiology. Circ Res 2002;91:877–887.
12. Mukouyama YS, Shin D, Britsch S, et al: Sensory nerves determine the pattern of arterial differentiation and blood vessel branching in the skin. Cell 2002;109:693–705.
13. Drexler H, Schnurch H, Breier G, Risau W: Regulation of embryonic blood vessel formation. In Maragoudakis M, Gullino P, Lelkes P (eds): Angiogenesis in Health and Disease. New York, Plenum Press, 1992, pp 17–26.

14. Shalaby F, Rossant J, Yamaguchi TP, et al: Failure of blood-island formation and vasculogenesis in Flk-1-deficient mice. Nature 1995;376:62-66.

15. Carmeliet P, Ferreira V, Breier G, et al: Abnormal blood vessel development and lethality in embryos lacking a single VEGF allele. Nature 1996;380:435-439.

16. Ferrara N, Carver-Moore K, Chen H, et al: Heterozygous embryonic lethality induced by targeted inactivation of the VEGF gene. Nature 1996;380:439-442.

17. Tevosian SG, Deconinck AE, Tanaka M, et al: FOG-2, a cofactor for GATA transcription factors, is essential for heart morphogenesis and development of coronary vessels from epicardium. Cell 2000;101:729-739.

18. Lyden D, Young AZ, Zagzag D, et al: Id1 and Id3 are required for neurogenesis, angiogenesis and vascularization of tumour xenografts. Nature 1999;401:670-677.

19. Zhong TP, Rosenberg M, Mohideen MA, et al: Gridlock, an HLH gene required for assembly of the aorta in zebrafish. Science 2000;287:1820-1824.

20. Wilting J, Christ B: Embryonic angiogenesis: A review. Naturwissenschaften 1996;83:153-164.

21. LeCouter J, Kowalski J, Foster J, et al: Identification of an angiogenic mitogen selective for endocrine gland endothelium. Nature 2001;412:877-884.

22. Lammert E, Cleaver O, Melton D: Induction of pancreatic differentiation by signals from blood vessels. Science 2001;294:564-567.

23. Shi Q, Rafii S, Wu MH, et al: Evidence for circulating bone marrow-derived endothelial cells. Blood 1998;92:362-367.

24. Asahara T, Murohara T, Sullivan A, et al: Isolation of putative progenitor endothelial cells for angiogenesis. Science 1997;275:964-967.

25. Peichev M, Naiyer AJ, Pereira D, et al: Expression of VEGFR-2 and AC133 by circulating human CD34(+) cells identifies a population of functional endothelial precursors. Blood 2000;95:952-958.

26. Lyden D, Hattori K, Dias S, et al: Impaired recruitment of bone-marrow-derived endothelial and hematopoietic precursor cells blocks tumor angiogenesis and growth. Nat Med 2001;7:1194-1201.

27. Asahara T, Masuda H, Takahashi T, et al: Bone marrow origin of endothelial progenitor cells responsible for postnatal vasculogenesis in physiological and pathological neovascularization. Circ Res 1999;85:221-228.

28. Quaini F, Urbanek K, Beltrami AP, et al: Chimerism of the transplanted heart. N Engl J Med 2002;346:5-15.

29. Sata M, Saiura A, Kunisato A, et al: Hematopoietic stem cells differentiate into vascular cells that participate in the pathogenesis of atherosclerosis. Nat Med 2002;8:403-409.

30. Liotta LA, Steeg PS, Stetler-Stevenson WG: Cancer metastasis and angiogenesis: An imbalance of positive and negative regulation. Cell 1991;64:327-336.

31. Gross JL, Moscatelli D, Rifkin DB: Increased capillary endothelial cell protease activity in response to angiogenic stimuli in vitro. Proc Natl Acad Sci USA 1983;80:2623-2627.

32. Tolsma SS, Volpert OV, Good DJ, et al: Peptides derived from two separate domains of the matrix protein thrombospondin-1 have anti-angiogenic activity. J Cell Biol 1993;122:497-511.

33. O'Reilly MS, Boehm T, Shing Y, et al: Endostatin: An endogenous inhibitor of angiogenesis and tumor growth. Cell 1997;88:277-285.

34. Ausprunk DH, Folkman J: Migration and proliferation of endothelial cells in preformed and newly formed blood vessels during tumor angiogenesis. Microvasc Res 1977;14:53-65.

35. Brooks PC, Stromblad S, Sanders LC, et al: Localization of matrix metalloproteinase MMP-2 to the surface of invasive cells by interaction with integrin alpha v beta 3. Cell 1996;85:683-693.

36. Ingber DE, Folkman J: Mechanochemical switching between growth and differentiation during fibroblast growth factor-stimulated angiogenesis in vitro: Role of extracellular matrix. J Cell Biol 1989;109:317-330.

37. Grant DS, Tashiro K, Segui-Real B, et al: Two different laminin domains mediate the differentiation of human endothelial cells into capillary-like structures in vitro. Cell 1989;58:933-943.

38. Leavesley DI, Schwartz MA, Rosenfeld M, Cheresh DA: Integrin beta 1- and beta 3-mediated endothelial cell migration is triggered through distinct signaling mechanisms. J Cell Biol 1993;121:163-170.

39. Nguyen M, Strubel NA, Bischoff J: A role for sialyl Lewis-X/A glycoconjugates in capillary morphogenesis. Nature 1993;365:267-269.

40. Suri C, McClain J, Thurston G, et al: Increased vascularization in mice overexpressing angiopoietin-1. Science 1998;282:468-471.

41. Mohle R, Green D, Moore MA, et al: Constitutive production and thrombin-induced release of vascular endothelial growth factor by human megakaryocytes and platelets. Proc Natl Acad Sci USA 1997;94:663-668.

42. Ausprunk DH, Dethlefsen S, Higgins E: Distribution of fibronectin, laminin and type IV collagen during development of blood vessels in the chick chorioallantoic membrane. In Feinberg R, Sherer G, Auerbach R (eds): The Development of the Vascular System. Basel, Karger, 1991, pp 93-108.

43. Hirschi KK, D'Amore PA: Pericytes in the microvasculature. Cardiovasc Res 1996;32:687-698.

44. Nakamura H: Electron microscopic study of the prenatal development of the thoracic aorta in the rat. Am J Anat 1988;181:406-418.

45. Leveen P, Pekny M, Gebre-Medhin S, et al: Mice deficient for PDGF B show renal, cardiovascular, and hematological abnormalities. Genes Dev 1994;8:1875-1887.

46. Benjamin LE, Hemo I, Keshet E: A plasticity window for blood vessel remodelling is defined by pericyte coverage of the preformed endothelial network and is regulated by PDGF-B and VEGF. Development 1998;125:1591-1598.

47. Carmeliet P, Lampugnani MG, Moons L, et al: Targeted deficiency or cytosolic truncation of the VE-cadherin gene in mice impairs VEGF-mediated endothelial survival and angiogenesis. Cell 1999;98:147-157.

48. Hood JD, Bednarski M, Frausto R, et al: Tumor regression by targeted gene delivery to the neovasculature. Science 2002;296:2404-2407.

49. Friedlander M, Brooks PC, Shaffer RW, et al: Definition of two angiogenic pathways by distinct alpha v integrins. Science 1995;270:1500-1502.

50. Brooks PC, Montgomery AM, Rosenfeld M, et al: Integrin alpha v beta 3 antagonists promote tumor regression by inducing apoptosis of angiogenic blood vessels. Cell 1994;79:1157-1164.

51. Holmgren L, O'Reilly MS, Folkman J: Dormancy of micrometastases: Balanced proliferation and apoptosis in the presence of angiogenesis suppression [see comments]. Nat Med 1995;1:149-153.

52. Jimenez B, Volpert OV, Crawford SE, et al: Signals leading to apoptosis-dependent inhibition of neovascularization by thrombospondin-1. Nat Med 2000;6:41-48.

53. Engerman RL, Pfaffenbach D, Davis MD: Cell turnover of capillaries. Lab Invest 1967;17:738-743.

54. Reynolds LP, Killilea SD, Redmer DA: Angiogenesis in the female reproductive system. FASEB J 1992;6:886-892.

55. Barger AC, Beeuwkes R 3rd, Lainey LL, Silverman KJ: Hypothesis: Vasa vasorum and neovascularization of human coronary arteries: A possible role in the pathophysiology of atherosclerosis. N Engl J Med 1984;310:175-177.

56. Bergers G, Brekken R, McMahon G, et al: Matrix metalloproteinase-9 triggers the angiogenic switch during carcinogenesis. Nat Cell Biol 2000;2:737-744.

57. Polverini PJ, Cotran RS, Gimbrone MA Jr, Unanue ER: Activated macrophages induce vascular proliferation. Nature 1977;269:804-806.

58. Heissig B, Hattori K, Dias S, et al: Recruitment of stem and progenitor cells from the bone marrow niche requires MMP-9 mediated release of kit-ligand. Cell 2002;109:625-637.

59. Arras M, Ito WD, Scholz D, et al: Monocyte activation in angiogenesis and collateral growth in the rabbit hindlimb. J Clin Invest 1998;101:40-50.

60. Murohara T, Asahara T, Silver M, et al: Nitric oxide synthase modulates angiogenesis in response to tissue ischemia. J Clin Invest 1998;101:2567-2578.

61. Jones MK, Wang H, Peskar BM, et al: Inhibition of angiogenesis by nonsteroidal anti-inflammatory drugs: Insight into mechanisms and implications for cancer growth and ulcer healing [see comments]. Nat Med 1999;5:1418-1423.

62. Luttun A, Tjwa M, Moons L, et al: Revascularization of ischemic tissues by PlGF treatment, and inhibition of tumor angiogenesis, arthritis and atherosclerosis by anti-Flt1. Nat Med 2002; 8:831-840.

63. Maniotis A J, Folberg R, Hess A, et al: Vascular channel formation by human melanoma cells in vivo and in vitro: Vasculogenic mimicry. Am J Pathol 1999;155:739-752.

64. McDonald DM, Munn L, Jain RK: Vasculogenic mimicry: How convincing, how novel, and how significant? Am J Pathol 2000; 156:383-388.

65. St Croix B, Rago C, Velculescu V, et al: Genes expressed in human tumor endothelium. Science 2000;289:1197-1202.

66. Arap W, Kolonin MG, Trepel M, et al: Steps toward mapping the human vasculature by phage display. Nat Med 2002;8:121-127.

67. Folkman J: Angiogenesis. In Braunwald E, Fauci AS, Kasper DL, et al. (eds): Harrison's Textbook of Internal Medicine. New York, McGraw-Hill, 2001, pp 517-530.

68. Clark RA, Tonnesen MG, Gailit J, Cheresh DA: Transient functional expression of alphaVbeta 3 on vascular cells during wound repair. Am J Pathol 1996;148:1407-1421.

69. Jaffe EA, Nachman RL, Becker CG, Minick CR: Culture of human endothelial cells derived from umbilical veins: Identification by morphologic and immunologic criteria. J Clin Invest 1972; 52:2745-2756.

70. Folkman J, Haudenschild C, Zetter BR: Long-term culture of capillary endothelial cells. Proc Natl Acad Sci USA 1979;76: 5217-5221.

71. Angiogenesis Protocols. Totowa, New Jersey, Humana Press, 2001.

72. Nicosia RF, Ottinetti A: Growth of microvessels in serum-free matrix culture of rat aorta: A quantitative assay of angiogenesis in vitro. Lab Invest 1990;63:115-122.

73. Moulton KS, Vakili K, Zurakowski D, et al: Inhibition of plaque neovascularization reduces macrophage accumulation and progression of advanced atherosclerosis. PNAS 2003;100:4736-4741.

74. Kenyon BM, Browne F, D'Amato RJ: Effects of thalidomide and related metabolites in a mouse corneal model of neovascularization. Exp Eye Res 199764:971-978.

75. Leunig M, Yuan F, Menger M, et al: Angiogenesis, microvascular architecture, microhemodynamics, and interstitial fluid pressure during early growth of human adenocarcinoma LS174T in SCID mice. Cancer Res 1992;52:6553-6560.

76. Shing Y, Folkman J, Sullivan R, et al: Heparin affinity: Purification of a tumor-derived capillary endothelial cell growth factor. Science 1984;223:1296-1299.

77. Thomas KA, Rios-Candelore M, Fitzpatrick S: Purification and characterization of acidic fibroblast growth factor from bovine brain. Proc Natl Acad Sci USA 1984;81:357-361.

78. Vlodavsky I, Folkman J, Sullivan R, et al: Endothelial cell-derived basic fibroblast growth factor: Synthesis and deposition into subendothelial extracellular matrix. Proc Natl Acad Sci USA 1987;84:2292-2296.

79. Maciag T, Mehlman T, Friesel R, Schreiber AB: Heparin binds endothelial cell growth factor, the principal endothelial cell mitogen in bovine brain. Science 1984;225:932-935.

80. Meininger C J, Zetter BR: Mast cells and angiogenesis. Semin Cancer Biol 1992;3:73-79.

81. Ono I: The effects of basic fibroblast growth factor (bFGF) on the breaking strength of acute incisional wounds. J Dermatol Sci 2002;29:104-113.

82. Edelman ER, Nugent MA, Smith LT, Karnovsky MJ: Basic fibroblast growth factor enhances the coupling of intimal hyperplasia and proliferation of vasa vasorum in injured rat arteries. J Clin Invest 1992;89:465-473.

83. Nabel EG, Yang ZY, Plautz G, et al: Recombinant fibroblast growth factor-1 promotes intimal hyperplasia and angiogenesis in arteries in vivo. Nature 1993;362:844-846.

84. Brogi E, Winkles JA, Underwood R, et al: Distinct patterns of expression of fibroblast growth factors and their receptors in human atheroma and nonatherosclerotic arteries: Association of acidic FGF with plaque microvessels and macrophages. J Clin Invest 1993;92:2408-2418.

85. Baffour R, Berman J, Garb JL, et al: Enhanced angiogenesis and growth of collaterals by in vivo administration of recombinant basic fibroblast growth factor in a rabbit model of acute lower limb ischemia: Dose-response effect of basic fibroblast growth factor. J Vasc Surg 1992;16:181-191.

86. Pu LQ, Sniderman AD, Brassard R, et al: Enhanced revascularization of the ischemic limb by angiogenic therapy. Circulation 1993;88:208-215.

87. Yanagisawa-Miwa A, Uchida Y, Nakamura F, et al: Salvage of infarcted myocardium by angiogenic action of basic fibroblast growth factor. Science 1992;257:1401-1403.

88. Ferrara N, Houck KA, Jakeman LB, et al: The vascular endothelial growth factor family of polypeptides. J Cell Biochem 1991; 47:211-218.

89. Roberts WG, Palade GE: Increased microvascular permeability and endothelial fenestration induced by vascular endothelial growth factor. J Cell Sci 1995;108(Pt 6):2369-2379.

90. Dvorak HF, Brown LF, Detmar M, Dvorak AM: Vascular permeability factor/vascular endothelial growth factor, microvascular hyperpermeability, and angiogenesis. Am J Pathol 1995; 146:1029-1039.

91. Mustonen T, Alitalo K: Endothelial receptor tyrosine kinases involved in angiogenesis. J Cell Biol 1995;129:895-898.

92. Millauer B, Wizigmann-Voos S, Schnurch H, et al: High affinity VEGF binding and developmental expression suggest Flk-1 as a major regulator of vasculogenesis and angiogenesis. Cell 1993;72:835-846.

93. Shalaby F, Ho J, Stanford WL, et al: A requirement for Flk1 in primitive and definitive hematopoiesis and vasculogenesis. Cell 1997;89:981-990.

94. Peters KG, De Vries C, Williams LT: Vascular endothelial growth factor receptor expression during embryogenesis and tissue repair suggests a role in endothelial differentiation and blood vessel growth. Proc Natl Acad Sci USA 1993;90:8915-8919.

95. Fong GH, Rossant J, Gertsenstein M, Breitman ML: Role of the Flt-1 receptor tyrosine kinase in regulating the assembly of vascular endothelium. Nature 1995;376:66-70.

96. Fong GH, Zhang L, Bryce DM, Peng J: Increased hemangioblast commitment, not vascular disorganization, is the primary defect in flt-1 knock-out mice. Development 1999;126:3015-3025.

97. Hiratsuka S, Minowa O, Kuno J, et al: Flt-1 lacking the tyrosine kinase domain is sufficient for normal development and angiogenesis in mice. Proc Natl Acad Sci USA 1998;95:9349-9354.

98. Ferrara N, Chen H, Davis-Smyth T, et al: Vascular endothelial growth factor is essential for corpus luteum angiogenesis. Nat Med 1998;4:336-340.

99. Gerber HP, Vu TH, Ryan AM, et al: VEGF couples hypertrophic cartilage remodeling, ossification and angiogenesis during endochondral bone formation [see comments]. Nat Med 1999; 5:623-628.

100. Inoue M, Itoh H, Ueda M, et al: Vascular endothelial growth factor (VEGF) expression in human coronary atherosclerotic lesions: Possible pathophysiological significance of VEGF in progression of atherosclerosis. Circulation 1998;98:2108-2116.

101. Henry TD, Annex BH, McKendall GR, et al: The VIVA trial: Vascular endothelial growth factor in ischemia for vascular angiogenesis. Circulation 2003;107:1359-1365.

102. Ng YS, Rohan R, Sunday ME, et al: Differential expression of VEGF isoforms in mouse during development and in the adult. Dev Dyn 2001;220:112-121.

103. Soker S, Takashima S, Miao HQ, et al: Neuropilin-1 is expressed by endothelial and tumor cells as an isoform-specific receptor for vascular endothelial growth factor. Cell 1998;92:735-745.

104. Carmeliet P, Ng YS, Nuyens D, et al: Impaired myocardial angiogenesis and ischemic cardiomyopathy in mice lacking the vascular endothelial growth factor isoforms VEGF164 and VEGF188 [see comments]. Nat Med 1999;5:495-502.

105. Cao Y, Chen H, Zhou L, et al: Heterodimers of placenta growth factor/vascular endothelial growth factor. Endothelial activity, tumor cell expression, and high affinity binding to Flk-1/KDR. J Biol Chem 1996;271:3154-3162.

106. Eriksson A, Cao R, Pawliuk R, et al: Placenta growth factor-1 antagonizes VEGF-induced angiogenesis and tumor growth by the formation of functionally inactive PlGF-1/VEGF heterodimers. Cancer Cell 2002;1:99-108.

107. Sato TN, Tozawa Y, Deutsch U, et al: Distinct roles of the receptor tyrosine kinases Tie-1 and Tie-2 in blood vessel formation. Nature 1995;376:70-74.

108. Davis S, Aldrich TH, Jones PF, et al: Isolation of angiopoietin-1, a ligand for the TIE2 receptor, by secretion-trap expression cloning [see comments]. Cell 1996;87:1161-1169.

109. Maisonpierre PC, Suri C, Jones PF, et al: Angiopoietin-2, a natural antagonist for Tie2 that disrupts in vivo angiogenesis [see comments]. Science 1997;277:55-60.

110. Thurston G, Rudge JS, Ioffe E, et al: Angiopoietin-1 protects the adult vasculature against plasma leakage. Nat Med 2000; 6:460-463.

111. Shyu KG, Manor O, Magner M, et al: Direct intramuscular injection of plasmid DNA encoding angiopoietin-1 but not angiopoietin-2 augments revascularization in the rabbit ischemic hindlimb. Circulation 1998;98:2081-2087.

112. Thurston G, Suri C, Smith K, et al: Leakage-resistant blood vessels in mice transgenically overexpressing angiopoietin-1. Science 1999;286:2511-2514.

113. Gerety SS, Wang HU, Chen ZF, Anderson DJ: Symmetrical mutant phenotypes of the receptor EphB4 and its specific transmembrane ligand ephrin-B2 in cardiovascular development. Mol Cell 1999;4:403-414.

114. Shin D, Garcia-Cardena G, Hayashi S, et al: Expression of ephrinB2 identifies a stable genetic difference between arterial and venous vascular smooth muscle as well as endothelial cells, and marks subsets of microvessels at sites of adult neovascularization. Dev Biol 2001;230:139-150.

115. Wang HU, Anderson DJ: Eph family transmembrane ligands can mediate repulsive guidance of trunk neural crest migration and motor axon outgrowth. Neuron 1997;18:383-396.

116. Adams RH, Diella F, Hennig S, et al: The cytoplasmic domain of the ligand ephrinB2 is required for vascular morphogenesis but not cranial neural crest migration. Cell 2001;104:57-69.

117. Coussens LM, Raymond WW, Bergers G, et al: Inflammatory mast cells up-regulate angiogenesis during squamous epithelial carcinogenesis. Genes Dev 1999;13:1382-1397.

118. Aikawa M, Rabkin E, Okada Y, et al: Lipid lowering by diet reduces matrix metalloproteinase activity and increases collagen content of rabbit atheroma: A potential mechanism of lesion stabilization. Circulation 1998;97:2433-2444.

119. Strieter RM, Polverini PJ, Kunkel SL, et al: The functional role of the ELR motif in CXC chemokine-mediated angiogenesis. J Biol Chem 1995;270:27348-27357.

120. Naiyer AJ, Jo DY, Ahn J, et al: Stromal derived factor-1-induced chemokinesis of cord blood CD34(+) cells (long-term culture-initiating cells) through endothelial cells is mediated by E-selectin. Blood 1999;94:4011-4019.

121. Hanahan D, Folkman J: Patterns and emerging mechanisms of the angiogenic switch during tumorigenesis. Cell 1996; 86:353-364.

122. Brouty-Boye D, Zetter BR: Inhibition of cell motility by interferon. Science 1980;208:516-518.

123. Ezekowitz RA, Mulliken JB, Folkman J: Interferon alfa-2a therapy for life-threatening hemangiomas of infancy. N Engl J Med 1992;326:1456-1463.

124. Rastinejad F, Polverini PJ, Bouck NP: Regulation of the activity of a new inhibitor of angiogenesis by a cancer suppressor gene. Cell 1989;56:345-355.

125. Iruela-Arispe ML, Porter P, Bornstein P, Sage EH: Thrombospondin-1, an inhibitor of angiogenesis, is regulated by progesterone in the human endometrium. J Clin Invest 1996;97:403-412.

126. Febbraio M, Hajjar DP, Silverstein RL: CD36: A class B scavenger receptor involved in angiogenesis, atherosclerosis, inflammation, and lipid metabolism. J Clin Invest 2001;108:785-791.

127. Roth JJ, Gahtan V, Brown JL, et al: Thrombospondin-1 is elevated with both intimal hyperplasia and hypercholesterolemia. J Surg Res 1998;74:11-16.

128. Chen D, Asahara T, Krasinski K, et al: Antibody blockade of thrombospondin accelerates reendothelialization and reduces neointima formation in balloon-injured rat carotid artery [see comments]. Circulation 1999;100:849-854.

129. Kleiner DE Jr, Tuuttila A, Tryggvason K, Stetler-Stevenson WG: Stability analysis of latent and active 72-kDa type IV collagenase: The role of tissue inhibitor of metalloproteinases-2 (TIMP-2). Biochemistry 1993;32:1583-1592.

130. Moses MA, Sudhalter J, Langer R: Identification of an inhibitor of neovascularization from cartilage. Science 1990;248:1408-1410.

131. Gupta SK, Hassel T, Singh JP: A potent inhibitor of endothelial cell proliferation is generated by proteolytic cleavage of the chemokine platelet factor 4. Proc Natl Acad Sci USA 1995; 92:7799-7803.

132. O'Reilly MS, Holmgren L, Shing Y, et al: Angiostatin: A novel angiogenesis inhibitor that mediates the suppression of metastases by a Lewis lung carcinoma. Cell 1994;79:315-328.

133. Homandberg GA, Williams JE, Grant D, et al: Heparin-binding fragments of fibronectin are potent inhibitors of endothelial cell growth. Am J Pathol 1985;120:327-332.

134. Clapp C, Martial JA, Guzman RC, et al: The 16-kilodalton N-terminal fragment of human prolactin is a potent inhibitor of angiogenesis. Endocrinology 1993;133:1292-1299.

135. O'Reilly MS, Wiederschain D, Stetler-Stevenson WG, et al: Regulation of angiostatin production by matrix metalloproteinase-2 in a model of concomitant resistance. J Biol Chem 1999;274:29568-29571.

136. Maeshima Y, Sudhakar A, Lively JC, et al: Tumstatin, an endothelial cell-specific inhibitor of protein synthesis. Science 2002;295: 140-143.

137. Couffinhal T, Kearney M, Witzenbichler B, et al: Vascular endothelial growth factor/vascular permeability factor (VEGF/VPF) in normal and atherosclerotic human arteries. Am J Pathol 1997;150:1673-1685.

138. Dumont DJ, Jussila L, Taipale J, et al: Cardiovascular failure in mouse embryos deficient in VEGF receptor-3. Science 1998;282:946-949.

139. Irrthum A, Karkkainen MJ, Devriendt K, et al: Congenital hereditary lymphedema caused by a mutation that inactivates VEGFR3 tyrosine kinase. Am J Hum Genet 2000; 67:295-301.

140. Karkkainen MJ, Saaristo A, Jussila L, et al: A model for gene therapy of human hereditary lymphedema. Proc Natl Acad Sci USA 2001;98:12677-12682.

141. Jeltsch M, Kaipainen A, Joukov V, et al: Hyperplasia of lymphatic vessels in VEGF-C transgenic mice. [erratum appears in Science 1997;277:463]. Science 1997;276:1423-1425.

142. Cao Y, Linden P, Farnebo J, et al: Vascular endothelial growth factor C induces angiogenesis in vivo. Proc Natl Acad Sci USA 1998; 95:14389-14394.

143. Saaristo A, Veikkola T, Enholm B, et al: Adenoviral VEGF-C overexpression induces blood vessel enlargement, tortuosity, and leakiness but no sprouting angiogenesis in the skin or mucous membranes. FASEB J 2002;16:1041-1049.

144. Chang LK, Farnebo F, Fannon M, et al: Lymphangiogenesis in the absence of angiogenesis. 2003 (submitted).

145. Wigle JT, Oliver G: Prox1 function is required for the development of the murine lymphatic system. Cell 1999;98:769-778.

146. Salven P, Mustjoki S, Alitalo R, et al: VEGFR-3 and CD133 identify a population of CD34+ lymphatic/vascular endothelial precursor cells. Blood 2003;101:168-172.

147. Saaristo A, Veikkola T, Tammela T, et al: Lymphangiogenic gene therapy with minimal blood vascular side effects. J Exp Med 2002; 196:719-730.

148. Rakusan K, Cicutti N, Flanagan MF: Changes in the microvascular network during cardiac growth, development, and aging. Cell Mol Biol Res 1994;40:117-122.

149. Giordano FJ, Gerber HP, Williams SP, et al: A cardiac myocyte vascular endothelial growth factor paracrine pathway is required to maintain cardiac function. Proc Natl Acad Sci USA 2001; 98:5780-5785.

150. Hudlicka O, Brown MD: Postnatal growth of the heart and its blood vessels. J Vasc Res 1996;33:266-287.

151. Leong-Poi H, Christiansen J, Klibanov AL, et al: Noninvasive assessment of angiogenesis by ultrasound and microbubbles targeted to alpha(v)-integrins. Circulation 2003;107:455-460.

152. van Groningen JP, Wenink AC, Testers LH: Myocardial capillaries: Increase in number by splitting of existing vessels. Anat Embryol (Berl) 1991;184:65-70.

153. Tomanek RJ, Torry RJ: Growth of the coronary vasculature in hypertrophy: Mechanisms and model dependence. Cell Mol Biol Res 1994;40:129-136.

154. Heron MI, Rakusan K: Geometry of coronary capillaries in hyperthyroid and hypothyroid rat heart. Am J Physiol 1994; 267: H1024-1031.

155. Node K, Huo Y, Ruan X, et al: Anti-inflammatory properties of cytochrome P450 epoxygenase-derived eicosanoids. Science 1999;285:1276-1279.

156. Shen J, Luscinskas FW, Connolly A, et al: Fluid shear stress modulates cytosolic free calcium in vascular endothelial cells. Am J Physiol 1992;262:C384-390.

157. Cooke JP, Rossitch E Jr, Andon NA, et al: Flow activates an endothelial potassium channel to release an endogenous nitrovasodilator. J Clin Invest 1991;88:1663-1671.

158. Topper JN, Cai J, Falb D, Gimbrone MA Jr: Identification of vascular endothelial genes differentially responsive to fluid mechanical stimuli: Cyclooxygenase-2, manganese superoxide dismutase, and endothelial cell nitric oxide synthase are selectively up-regulated by steady laminar shear stress. Proc Natl Acad Sci USA 1996;93:10417-10422.

159. Wang N, Butler JP, Ingber DE: Mechanotransduction across the cell surface and through the cytoskeleton. Science 1993; 260:1124-1127.

160. Shweiki D, Itin A, Soffer D, Keshet E: Vascular endothelial growth factor induced by hypoxia may mediate hypoxia-initiated angiogenesis. Nature 1992;359:843-845.

161. Carmeliet P, Dor Y, Herbert JM, et al: Role of HIF-1alpha in hypoxia-mediated apoptosis, cell proliferation and tumour angiogenesis. Nature 1998;394:485-490.

162. Elson DA, Thurston G, Huang LE, et al: Induction of hypervascularity without leakage or inflammation in transgenic mice overexpressing hypoxia-inducible factor-1alpha. Genes Dev 2001;15:2520-2532.

163. Harada K, Grossman W, Friedman M, et al: Basic fibroblast growth factor improves myocardial function in chronically ischemic porcine hearts. J Clin Invest 1994;94:623-630.

164. Takeshita S, Zheng LP, Brog, E, et al: Therapeutic angiogenesis. A single intraarterial bolus of vascular endothelial growth factor augments revascularization in a rabbit ischemic hind limb model. J Clin Invest 1994;93:662-670.

165. Fang J, Yan L, Shing Y, Moses MA: HIF-1alpha-mediated up-regulation of vascular endothelial growth factor, independent of basic fibroblast growth factor, is important in the switch to the angiogenic phenotype during early tumorigenesis. Cancer Res 2001;61:5731-5735.

166. Pepler W, Meyer B: Interarterial coronary anastomoses and coronary artery pattern: A comparative study of South African Bantu and European hearts. Circulation 1960;22:14-24.

167. Takahashi T, Kalka C, Masuda H, et al: Ischemia- and cytokine-induced mobilization of bone marrow-derived endothelial progenitor cells for neovascularization. Nat Med 1999;5:434-438.

168. Rentrop KP, Thornton JC, Feit F, Van Buskirk M: Determinants and protective potential of coronary arterial collaterals as assessed by an angioplasty model. Am J Cardiol 1988;61:677-684.

169. Rentrop K P, Feit F, Sherman W, Thornton JC: Serial angiographic assessment of coronary artery obstruction and collateral flow in acute myocardial infarction: Report from the second Mount Sinai-New York University Reperfusion Trial. Circulation 1989;80:1166-1175.

170. Schwartz H, Leiboff RH, Bren GB, et al: Temporal evolution of the human coronary collateral circulation after myocardial infarction. J Am Coll Cardiol 1984;4:1088-1093.

171. Kocher AA, Schuster MD, Szabolcs MJ, et al: Neovascularization of ischemic myocardium by human bone-marrow-derived angioblasts prevents cardiomyocyte apoptosis, reduces remodeling and improves cardiac function. Nat Med 2001;7:430-436.

172. Frye RL, Gura GM, Chesebro JH, Ritman EL: Complete occlusion of the left main coronary artery and the importance of coronary collateral circulation. Mayo Clin Proc 1977;52:742-745.

173. Habib GB, Heibig J, Forman SA, et al: Influence of coronary collateral vessels on myocardial infarct size in humans: Results of phase I thrombolysis in myocardial infarction (TIMI) trial. The TIMI Investigators. Circulation 1991;83:739-746.

174. Kass RW, Kotler MN, Yazdanfar S: Stimulation of coronary collateral growth: Current developments in angiogenesis and future clinical applications. Am Heart J 1992;123:486-496.

175. Schaper W: Control of coronary angiogenesis. Eur Heart J 1995;16:66-68.

176. Kluge A, Zimmermann R, Munkel B, et al: Insulin-like growth factor I is involved in inflammation linked angiogenic processes after microembolisation in porcine heart. Cardiovasc Res 1995;29:407-415.

177. Seiler C, Pohl T, Wustmann K, et al: Promotion of collateral growth by granulocyte-macrophage colony-stimulating factor in patients with coronary artery disease: A randomized, double-blind, placebo-controlled study. Circulation 2001;104:2012-2017.

178. Takeshita S, Rossow ST, Kearney M, et al: Time course of increased cellular proliferation in collateral arteries after administration of vascular endothelial growth factor in a rabbit model of lower limb vascular insufficiency. Am J Pathol 1995;147:1649-1660.

179. Simons M, Annex BH, Laham RJ, et al: Pharmacological treatment of coronary artery disease with recombinant fibroblast growth factor-2: Double-blind, randomized, controlled clinical trial. Circulation 2002;105:788-793.

180. Baumgartner I, Pieczek A, Manor O, et al: Constitutive expression of phVEGF165 after intramuscular gene transfer promotes collateral vessel development in patients with critical limb ischemia [see comments]. Circulation 1998;97:1114-1123.

181. Lederman R J, Mendelsohn FO, Anderson RD, et al: Therapeutic angiogenesis with recombinant fibroblast growth factor-2 for intermittent claudication (the TRAFFIC study): A randomised trial. Lancet 2002;359:2053-2058.

182. Springer ML, Chen AS, Kraft PE, et al: VEGF gene delivery to muscle: Potential role for vasculogenesis in adults. Mol Cell 1998; 2:549-558.

183. Garcia L, Baim DS, Post M, et al: Therapeutic angiogenesis using endocardial approach to administration: Techniques and results. Curr Intervent Cardiol Rep 1999;1:222-227.

184. Kalka C, Masuda H, Takahashi T, et al: Vascular endothelial growth factor(165) gene transfer augments circulating endothelial progenitor cells in human subjects. Circ Res 2000;86:1198-1202.

185. Couffinhal T, Silver M, Kearney M, et al: Impaired collateral vessel development associated with reduced expression of vascular endothelial growth factor in ApoE-/-mice. Circulation 1999; 99:3188-3198.

186. Rivard A, Fabre JE, Silver M, et al: Age-dependent impairment of angiogenesis. Circulation 1999;99:111-120.

187. Rivard A, Silver M, Chen D, et al: Rescue of diabetes-related impairment of angiogenesis by intramuscular gene therapy with adeno-VEGF. Am J Pathol 1999;154:355-363.

188. Van Belle E, Rivard A, Chen D, et al: Hypercholesterolemia attenuates angiogenesis but does not preclude augmentation by angiogenic cytokines. Circulation 1997;96:2667-2674.

189. Investigators B: Comparison of coronary bypass surgery with angioplasty in patients with multivessel disease: The Bypass Angioplasty Revascularization Investigation (BARI) Investigators [see comments] [published erratum appears in N Engl J Med 1997;336:147]. N Engl J Med 1996;335:217-225.

190. Koester W: Endarteritis and arteritis. Berl Klin Wochenschr 1876;13:454-455.

191. Kumamoto M, Nakashima Y, Sueishi K: Intimal neovascularization in human coronary atherosclerosis: Its origin and pathophysiological significance. Hum Pathol 1995;26:450-456.

192. Kaartinen M, Penttila A, Kovanen PT: Mast cells accompany microvessels in human coronary atheromas: Implications for intimal neovascularization and hemorrhage. Atherosclerosis 1996;123:123-131.

193. Kaiser M, Younge B, Bjornsson J, et al: Formation of new vasa vasorum in vasculitis: Production of angiogenic cytokines by multinucleated giant cells. Am J Pathol 1999;155:765-774.

194. Tanaka H, Sukhova GK, Libby P: Interaction of the allogeneic state and hypercholesterolemia in arterial lesion formation in experimental cardiac allografts. Arterioscler Thromb 1994;14:734-745.

195. Paterson JC: Capillary rupture with intimal hemorrhage as a causative factor in coronary thrombosis. Arch Pathol 1938;25:474-487.

196. Dashwood MR, Barker SG, Muddle JR, et al: [125I]-Endothelin-1 binding to vasa vasorum and regions of neovascularization in human and porcine blood vessels: A possible role for endothelin in intimal hyperplasia and atherosclerosis. J Cardiovasc Pharmacol 1993;22:S343-347.

197. Libby P: Molecular bases of the acute coronary syndromes. Circulation 1995;91:2844-2850.

198. O'Brien ER, Garvin MR, Dev R, et al: Angiogenesis in human coronary atherosclerotic plaques. Am J Pathol 1994;145:883-894.

199. Wolinsky H, Glagov S: A lamellar unit of aortic medial structure and function in mammals. Circ Res 1967;20:99–111.

200. Geiringer E: Intimal vascularization and atherosclerosis. J Pathol Bacteriol 1951;63:210–211.

201. Werber AH, Armstrong ML, Heistad DD: Diffusional support of the thoracic aorta in atherosclerotic monkeys. Atherosclerosis 1987;68:123–130.

202. Williams JK, Armstrong ML, Heistad DD: Vasa vasorum in atherosclerotic coronary arteries: Responses to vasoactive stimuli and regression of atherosclerosis. Circ Res 1988;62:515–523.

203. Moulton KS, Heller E, Konerding MA, et al: Angiogenesis inhibitors endostatin or TNP-470 reduce intimal neovascularization and plaque growth in apolipoprotein E-deficient mice [see comments]. Circulation 1999;99:1726–1732.

204. Heeschen C, Jang JJ, Weis M, et al: Nicotine stimulates angiogenesis and promotes tumor growth and atherosclerosis. Nat Med 2001;7:833–839.

205. Celletti FL, Waugh JM, Amabile PG, et al: Vascular endothelial growth factor enhances atherosclerotic plaque progression. Nat Med 2001;7:425–429.

206. O'Brien KD, McDonald TO, Chait A, et al: Neovascular expression of E-selectin, intercellular adhesion molecule-1, and vascular cell adhesion molecule-1 in human atherosclerosis and their relation to intimal leukocyte content. Circulation 1996;93:672–682.

207. Cybulsky MI, Iiyama K, Li H, et al: A major role for VCAM-1, but not ICAM-1, in early atherosclerosis. J Clin Invest 2001; 107:1255–1262.

208. Galis ZS, Sukhova GK, et al: Increased expression of matrix metalloproteinases and matrix degrading activity in vulnerable regions of human atherosclerotic plaques. J Clin Invest 1994; 94:2493–2503.

209. Burke AP, Farb A, Malcom GT, et al: Coronary risk factors and plaque morphology in men with coronary disease who died suddenly [see comments]. N Engl J Med 1997;336:1276–1282.

210. Park HJ, Kong D, Iruela-Arispe L, et al: 3-Hydroxy-3-methylglutaryl coenzyme A reductase inhibitors interfere with angiogenesis by inhibiting the geranylgeranylation of RhoA. Circ Res 2002; 91:143–150.

211. Wilson SH, Herrmann J, Lerman LO, et al: Simvastatin preserves the structure of coronary adventitial vasa vasorum in experimental hypercholesterolemia independent of lipid lowering. Circulation 2002;105:415–418.

212. Moulton KS: Plaque angiogenesis: Its functions and regulation. Cold Spring Harbor Symp Quant Biol 2003;LXVIII:471–482.

213. Miosge N, Sasaki T, Timpl R: Angiogenesis inhibitor endostatin is a distinct component of elastic fibers in vessel walls. FASEB J 1999;13:1743–1750.

214. Couffinhal T, Silver M, Zheng LP, et al: Mouse model of angiogenesis. Am J Pathol 1998;152:1667–1679.

215. Clowes AW, Collazzo RE, Karnovsky MJ: A morphologic and permeability study of luminal smooth muscle cells after arterial injury in the rat. Lab Invest 1978;39:141–150.

216. Kwon HM, Sangiorgi G, Ritman EL, et al: Adventitial vasa vasorum in balloon-injured coronary arteries: Visualization and quantitation by a microscopic three-dimensional computed tomography technique [see comments]. J Am Coll Cardiol 1998; 32:2072–2079.

217. Pels K, Labinaz M, Hoffert C, O'Brien ER: Adventitial angiogenesis early after coronary angioplasty: Correlation with arterial remodeling. Arterioscl Thromb Vasc Biol 1999;19:229–238.

218. Asahara T, Bauters C, Pastore C, et al: Local delivery of vascular endothelial growth factor accelerates reendothelialization and attenuates intimal hyperplasia in balloon-injured rat carotid artery [see comments]. Circulation 1995;91:2793–2801.

219. Lazarous DF, Shou M, Scheinowitz M, et al: Comparative effects of basic fibroblast growth factor and vascular endothelial growth factor on coronary collateral development and the arterial response to injury. Circulation 1996;94:1074–1082.

220. Huang SA, Tu HM, Harney JW, et al: Severe hypothyroidism caused by type 3 iodothyronine deiodinase in infantile hemangiomas. N Engl J Med 2000;343:185–189.

221. Boye E, Yu Y, Paranya G, et al: Clonality and altered behavior of endothelial cells from hemangiomas. J Clin Invest 2001; 107:745–752.

222. Takahashi K, Mulliken JB, Kozakewich HP, et al: Cellular markers that distinguish the phases of hemangioma during infancy and childhood. J Clin Invest 1994;93:2357–2364.

223. Vikkula M, Boon LM, Carraway KL 3rd, et al: Vascular dysmorphogenesis caused by an activating mutation in the receptor tyrosine kinase TIE2 [see comments]. Cell 1996;87:1181–1190.

224. Johnson DW, Berg JN, Baldwin MA, et al: Mutations in the activin receptor-like kinase 1 gene in hereditary haemorrhagic telangiectasia type 2. Nat Genet 1996;13:189–195.

225. Cowan KN, Jones PL, Rabinovitch M: Elastase and matrix metalloproteinase inhibitors induce regression, and tenascin-C antisense prevents progression, of vascular disease. J Clin Invest 2000; 105:21–34.

226. Rosenberg HC, Rabinovitch M: Endothelial injury and vascular reactivity in monocrotaline pulmonary hypertension. Am J Physio 1988;255:H1484–1491.

227. McFaul RC, Tajik AJ, Mair DD, et al: Development of pulmonary arteriovenous shunt after superior vena cava-right pulmonary artery (Glenn) anastomosis: Report of four cases. Circulation 1977;55:212–216.

228. Srivastava D, Preminger T, Lock JE, et al: Hepatic venous blood and the development of pulmonary arteriovenous malformations in congenital heart disease. Circulation 1995;92:1217–1222.

229. Kopf GS, Laks H, Stansel HC, et al: Thirty-year follow-up of superior vena cava-pulmonary artery (Glenn) shunts. J Thorac Cardiovasc Surg 1990;100:662–670; discussion 670–661.

230. Moore JW, Kirby WC, et al: Development of pulmonary arteriovenous malformations after modified Fontan operations. J Thorac Cardiovasc Surg 1989;98:1045–1050.

## EDITOR'S CHOICE

Carmeliet P: Angiogenesis in health and disease. Nat Med 2003;9:653–660.

*Excellent review by thought leader in the field.*

Carmeliet P: Blood vessels and nerves: common signals, pathways and diseases. Nat Rev Genet 2003;4:710–720.

*Growing links between nerve and vessels.*

Ema M, Rossant J: Cell fate decisions in early blood vessel formation. Trends Cardiovasc Med 2003;13:254–259.

*The hemangioblast and beyond.*

Fernando NH, Hurwitz HI: Inhibition of vascular endothelial growth factor in the treatment of colorectal cancer. Semin Oncol 2003;30:39–50.

*Avastin clinical trial provides first evidence that anti-angiogenesis strategy, in this case anti-VEGF, can be effective chemotherapy in human cancer.*

Ferrara N, Gerber HP, LeCouter J: The biology of VEGF and its receptors. Nat Med 2003;9:669–676.

*Pioneer in VEGF biology provides excellent review of area.*

Giordano FJ, Gerber HP, Williams SP, et al: A cardiac myocyte vascular endothelial growth factor paracrine pathway is required to maintain cardiac function. Proc Natl Acad Sci USA 2001;98:5780–5785.

*VEGF from cardiac myocytes is critical to maintain cardiac function; likely to be mediated via effect on promoting coronary vessel maturation.*

Jain RK: Molecular regulation of vessel maturation. Nat Med 2003;9:685–693.

*From angiogenesis to vasculogenesis.*

Kocher AA, Schuster MD, Szabolcs MJ, et al: Neovascularization of ischemic myocardium by human bone-marrow-derived angioblasts prevents cardiomyocyte apoptosis, reduces remodeling and improves cardiac function. Nat Med 2001;7:430–436.

*Cellular transplantation can affect cardiac angiogenesis; primary versus secondary role remains unclear; as does long term benefits.*

Mukouyama YS, Shin D, Britsch S, et al: Sensory nerves determine the pattern of arterial differentiation and blood vessel branching in the skin. Cell 2002;109:693–705.

*Seminal study providing direct link between the peripheral nervous system and angiogenesis.*

Nagy JA, Dvorak AM, Dvorak HF: VEGF-A(164/165) and P1GF: roles in angiogenesis and arteriogenesis. Trends Cardiovasc Med 2003;13:169–175.

*PIGF is a new player in angiogenesis; its role reviewed herein.*

Rebar EJ, Huang Y, Hickey R, et al: Induction of angiogenesis in a mouse model using engineered transcription factors. Nat Med 2002;8:1427–1432.

*New strategy to promote angiogenesis with designer transcription factors that impinge on HIF pathways.*

Schaper W, Scholz D: Factors regulating arteriogenesis. Arterioscler Thromb Vasc Biol 2003;23:1143–1151.

*Pioneer in the field of coronary collateralization provides update.*

Stalmans I, Lambrechts D, De Smet F, et al: VEGF: a modifier of the del22q11 (DiGeorge) syndrome? Nat Med 2003;9:173–182.

*Angiogenic pathways may modify congenital heart malformations particularly in the outflow tract.*

Yang JC, Haworth L, Sherry RM, et al: A randomized trial of bevacizumab, an anti-vascular endothelial growth factor antibody, for metastatic renal cancer. N Engl J Med 2003;349:427–434.

*Additional encouraging data supporting the concept that anti-VEGF therapy can be efficacious as an adjunct in a subset of human cancers.*

# chapter 25

# Coronary Restenosis

*Hiroshi Ashikaga*
*Ori Ben-Yehuda*
*Kenneth R. Chien*

Over the last decade, percutaneous coronary interventions (PCIs) have become the standard therapeutic approach to symptomatic coronary artery disease. Currently, more than 1 million PCI procedures, including coronary balloon angioplasty, stenting, and rotational atherectomy, are performed every year worldwide, with one half conducted in the United States.[1] Compared with bypass surgery for multivessel disease, PCIs offer similar protection against major ischemic events and are less expensive.[2] Despite great advances in device technology and adjunctive pharmacotherapy, restenosis (i.e., late renarrowing of the target lesion) remains as the limitation of PCI.

The incidence of *angiographic restenosis* (greater than 50% reduction in luminal diameter) is 40% to 50%.[3] Approximately one half of patients with angiographic restenosis experience *clinical restenosis* with recurrent symptoms that lead to major adverse cardiac events (MACEs) or target vessel revascularization (TVR).[4] Thus, stent implantation, which decreases the rate of angiographic restenosis to 20% to 30%, has become the mainstream intervention, currently used in more than 70% of PCIs.[5] Nevertheless, the rate of repeat revascularization is still unacceptably high (9% to 15%) with intracoronary stents.[6-9]

There are four primary pathologic processes responsible for restenosis after overdistension of the diseased vessel by angioplasty: *elastic recoil, thrombogenesis, neointimal formation,* and *remodeling.* The results of intravascular ultrasound studies suggest that coronary stenting reduces restenosis rate, compared with coronary balloon angioplasty, by preventing both elastic recoil and negative remodeling as luminal scaffolds.[10-12] In addition, aggressive antiplatelet therapy and various stent coating materials have reduced subacute thrombosis that had once been the major issue with early stent devices. Neointimal formation, however, has remained a major obstacle. Neointimal formation is responsible for both in-stent restenosis (ISR) and postballoon angioplasty restenosis (Fig. 25-1). This chapter reviews molecular and cellular events involved in neointimal formation.

## NEOINTIMAL FORMATION

The neointima is rich in smooth muscle cells (SMCs) that are surrounded by extensive extracellular matrix.[13-16]

Neointimal formation is believed to be an exaggerated wound healing process in response to various forms of vascular injuries associated with PCI, including vascular wall distension, endothelial denudation, atherosclerotic plaque rupture, medial dissection, and fracture of the internal elastic lamina.[17-20] Balloon injury induces apoptosis of medial SMCs in an early phase, which may exacerbate subsequent neointimal formation by provoking a greater wound healing response to overcome the cellular deficit.[21] Neointimal formation is seen in coronary artery bypass grafts, transplanted hearts, arteriovenous fistulas, and angioplastied vessels.[22-25] Although this complex process is not completely understood, longstanding research efforts have provided critical clues about the therapeutics of restenosis that have led to a number of ongoing clinical trials.

## Inflammation

Leukocytes and other mediators of inflammation appear to play a major role in the development of the neointima. In balloon-injured coronary arteries, leukopenia decreases neointimal formation and adventitial fibrosis.[26] Balloon angioplasty upregulates selectins, integrins, VCAM-1, and ICAM-1 on the remaining endothelium of the injured artery, resulting in leukocyte adhesion to the injured vessel wall within 24 to 48 hours.[27,28] Leukocytes, recruited by selectin-mediated attachment and rolling, activate and express surface integrins that facilitate the adherence to ICAMs on the endothelial cells, thereby promoting leukocyte transendothelial migration to the sites of inflammation.[29,30] Perturbation of the selectin-mediated process reduces the adhesion of platelets and leukocytes to injured arteries and prevents subsequent neointimal formation, adventitial inflammation, and negative vascular remodeling.[31-35] ICAM-1 and VCAM-1 are receptors that mediate adhesion of leukocytes to endothelial cells. The serum levels of ICAM-1 and also a neutrophil integrin Mac-1 (CD11b/CD18) after PCI correlate with the late restenotic lumen loss.[36] Coronary stenting is associated with a persistent increase in plasma ICAM-1 levels, which may explain the mechanism of increased neointimal formation with stent devices compared with balloon angioplasty.[37] Inhibition of ICAM-1 or Mac-1 diminishes medial leukocyte accumulation, SMC proliferation, and neointimal formation after PCI.[38-41] In addition, a single nucleotide polymorphism of the Mac-1 gene is associated with a lower

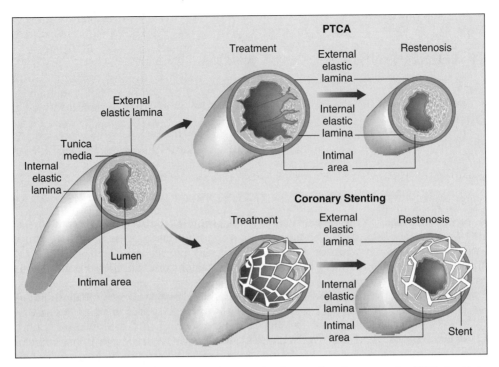

**FIGURE 25-1.** Restenosis after PTCA and coronary stenting. Serial intravascular ultrasound studies suggest that PTCA almost always disrupts plaque without reducing the total intimal area; often causes dissections that penetrate into the tunica media through the internal elastic lamina; and transiently enlarges the vessel, measured as the cross-sectional area subtended by the external elastic lamina. Restenosis is caused by pathologic arterial remodeling, characterized by shrinkage of the area circumscribed by the external elastic lamina, and to a lesser extent by neointimal thickening. Coronary stenting also enlarges the cross-sectional area of the vessel. The radial force of the stent prevents vessel shrinkage, but neointimal proliferation can be excessive. *(From Bittl JA: Advances in coronary angioplasty. N Engl J Med 1996;335:1290–1302 Copyright ©1996 Massachusetts Medical Society. All rights reserved.)*

incidence of angiographic restenosis after coronary stenting.[42] These observations suggest that neutrophil activation plays a critical role in the pathogenesis of neointimal formation. Neutrophils may also promote platelet-derived growth factor (PDGF) and cell proliferation through oxygen free radical production.[43,44]

Mononuclear leukocytes, which account for more than 20% of coronary plaque cells in human atherectomy tissues, also appear to play a major role in neointimal formation.[45] Monocytes turn into activated macrophages when recruited at the injured vessel after PCI, and the magnitude of macrophage infiltration in injured arteries parallels the magnitude of the subsequent SMC proliferation and neointimal formation. Disruption of the monocyte adhesion process by inhibiting monocyte chemoattractant protein (MCP)-1, a monocyte integrin, decreases neointimal formation in injured rat carotid arteries.[46] Macrophage infiltration and subsequent neointimal growth are reduced by a potent monocyte deactivator IL-10 or monoclonal antibodies against a mononuclear leukocyte integrin, very late antigen (VLA)-4.[47,48] The level of soluble IL-2 receptor, a marker of activated T lymphocytes, immediately after balloon angioplasty correlates linearly with the rate of subsequent restenosis.[49]

The development of the neointima is also mediated by various inflammatory cytokines. Balloon angioplasty upregulates IL-1 and TNF-α, which increase adhesiveness of cultured endothelial monolayers for circulating immature bone marrow cells and mature leukocytes and promote transendothelial migration of leukocytes.[50-52] Both IL-1α and TNF-α stimulate SMC proliferation by inducing PDGF.[53-55] In experimental models, external application of IL-1 and TNF-α increases the endothelial expression of both ICAM-1 and VCAM-1, thereby promoting leukocyte adhesion to the vessel wall and neointimal thickening and luminal narrowing.[56,57] There is also a positive correlation between the restenosis rate and the preprocedural plasma level of IL-6 or C-reactive protein. In addition, inhibition of IL-6 significantly reduces TNF-α-induced SMC proliferation *in vitro*.[55,58,59]

## Thrombogenesis

The role of thrombogenesis in neointimal formation has been recognized since an early study reported that thrombocytopenic rats develop little neointimal formation in balloon-injured carotid artery.[60] Platelet adherence and aggregation occur at the vascular surface components that are exposed by angioplasty, such as collagen, von Willebrand factor, fibronectin, and laminin. Thrombus formation is observed on stent struts within 10 days after stent deployment.[15,61,62] Thrombus formation is stimulated by tissue factor (TF), an endogenous procoagulant upregulated in balloon-injured vessels.[63,64] TF initiates the extrinsic coagulation pathway by activating factor VII, which subsequently activates factors IX and X, resulting in thrombin formation. Thrombin stimulates release of PDGF, proliferation of SMCs, and alteration of extracellular matrix composition.[65,6] Thrombin, monocytes, and SMCs upregulate the gene expression of TF, further perpetuating the thrombogenic cycle.[67] Termination of the thrombogenic cycle with the recombinant TF pathway inhibitor (rTFPI) or with hirudin, a direct thrombin inhibitor, has been demonstrated in experimental models. rTFPI markedly inhibits fibrin formation and subsequent neointimal development on the balloon-injured arteries, whereas hirudin curtails persistent expression of TF following balloon injury and diminishes restenosis.[67-69] However, hirudin did not affect the late luminal loss or event-free survival in patients treated with coronary angioplasty.[70] In addition to hirudin, a number of agents that interrupt thrombogenesis, including glycoprotein IIb/IIIa inhibitors, were examined in clinical trials and failed to show benefit in preventing postangioplasty restenosis.[71,72] Failure of the antithrombotic approach to affect the outcome of restenosis may reflect the complexity of the pathogenesis of the human neointima.

## Growth Factors

Growth factors released after arterial injury play critical roles in neointimal formation. Thrombus formation and endothelial denudation promote platelet degranulation within the thrombi, releasing growth factors such as PDGF, FGF, and TGF-β. These factors act in a complementary and interdependent fashion. PDGF is a potent mitogen that is immediately released in response to injury or inflammation, and thus regarded as one of the most important initiators of neointimal formation. In carotid artery injured rats, PDGF increases the migration of SMC from the media to the intima and the proliferation of medial SMC.[60,73] PDGF also induces expression of MCP-1, which may contribute to monocyte activation. Overexpression of PDGF-B by direct gene transfer into porcine arteries induces neointimal formation *in vivo* with prominent SMC proliferation.[74] In animal balloon injury models, disruption of the interaction between PDGF and its receptors decreases neointimal formation.[75-77] A clinical trial has shown that PDGF antagonists prevented angiographic and clinical restenosis after balloon angioplasty, but the benefit was modest.[78] FGF is another potent mitogen that initiates SMC proliferation. Augmentation of acidic FGF (aFGF) or basic FGF (bFGF) results in neointimal formation with accentuated intimal angiogenesis *in vivo*.[79,80] Antibodies against bFGF before balloon injury significantly decrease SMC proliferation but do not affect subsequent neointimal formation.[81,82] TGF-β, another putative culprit of neointimal formation, is believed to be a cell-type-specific regulator of proteoglycan synthesis in human blood vessels. TGF-β stimulates synthesis of proteoglycans specifically in human adult arterial SMCs *in vitro* but does not significantly stimulate proliferation of quiescent SMCs or inhibit proliferating cells.[83] Overexpression of TGF-β1 *in vivo* promotes procollagen synthesis and neointimal formation, both of which are inhibited by ribozyme oligonucleotides against TGF-β.[84,85] Human neointimal SMCs from atherectomy tissues contain a high level of another growth factor IGF-1 and type 1 IGF receptor and IGF binding proteins.[86] IGF-1 promotes cell-cycle progression and mitogenesis, resulting in SMC proliferation and migration.[87-91] IGF-1 stimulates SMC proliferation synergistically with PDGF, and overexpression of IGF-1 in SMCs leads to SMC hyperplasia *in vivo*.[92,93] Contribution of IGF-1 in neointimal formation is also suggested by elevated levels of insulin and IGF-1 in diabetic patients, who have a significantly high incidence of restenosis after PCI.[94,95] Although IGF-1 inhibitors, such as somatostatin analogs octreotide and angiopeptin, inhibit SMC proliferation and neointimal formation in animal studies, clinical trials with IGF-1 inhibitors failed to show consistent benefits.[96-102]

## Smooth Muscle Cells

### Origins of Neointimal Smooth Muscle Cells

Neointimal SMCs appear to represent a distinct cell population of heterogenous origins. Neointimal SMCs are different from medial SMCs in phenotype and gene-expression patterns[103-105]; neointimal SMCs *(synthetic phenotype)* appear less mature than medial SMCs *(contractile phenotype)*. The synthetic phenotype is epithelioid shaped as opposed to the spindle-shaped contractile phenotype and contains prominent endoplasmic reticulum and Golgi complex, which suggests active protein synthesis and cell proliferation.[106,107] The synthetic phenotype also exhibits a reduced expression of α-smooth muscle actin (α-SMA) and laminin, and an increase in fibronectin, tropoelastin, and α1 procollagen (type I). In addition, the synthetic phenotype expresses a large number of growth factor receptors and produces PDGF-B, TGF-β1, IGF-1, and osteopontin.[108,109]

These observations have led to the concept of *phenotypic modulation* or *dedifferentiation*, that is, neointimal SMCs originate from normal SMCs in the tunica media at the injury site through regression to a less mature phenotype, followed by proliferation, migration, and synthesis of extracellular matrix in the tunica intima.[103,104,110,111] Neointimal SMCs may also derive from remnant precursor cells in the tunica media that become activated in response to injury.[112]

Fibroblasts in the tunica adventitia have also been suggested as another possible origin of neointimal SMCs. Fibroblasts are relatively undifferentiated and can assume a particular phenotype in response to physiologic needs and/or microenvironmental stimuli.[113] Adventitial fibroblasts acquire α-SMA after angioplasty and are transformed into myofibroblasts, which are phenotypically similar to synthetic SMCs and proliferate earlier than medial SMCs.[114-117] Fibroblasts, myofibroblasts, and synthetic SMCs may be part of the same spectrum of cells, deriving from a common progenitor cell as well.[113,118-121] In fact, both SMCs and fibroblasts originate from epicardially derived mesenchymal cells in the developing coronary arteries.[122] A number of cytokines and growth factors influence proliferation and phenotypic transitions of fibroblasts and myofibroblasts, including TGF-β1, IFN-γ, and heparin.[120,121,123-125] In rats, TGF-β receptor antagonists almost completely inhibit the induction of α-SMA expression in adventitial cells and decrease neointimal formation after balloon injury, primarily through prevention of negative remodeling, in parallel with reduced adventitial fibrosis and collagen deposition.[126] The migratory capacity of myofibroblasts in injured vessels, however, has not been definitively established. Although early studies have suggested that at least some of the neointimal SMCs may originate from the adventitia, two recent studies have reached opposite conclusions.[114,115] When lacZ-transfected myofibroblasts are introduced into the adventitia after balloon injury in rat carotid arteries, β-galactosidase expression is observed in the adventitia, media, and neointima, suggesting that myofibroblasts have a viable migratory capacity.[116] In contrast, adventitial cells stained with a fluorescent dye are not detected in the media or the neointima but are found exclusively in the adventitia after balloon angioplasty in the same animal model.[127] Therefore, whether myofibroblasts migrate from the adventitia to the subendothelial layer to participate in neointimal formation remains unclear.

Finally, accumulated evidence strongly suggests that neointimal SMCs originate, at least in part, from circulating progenitor cells. Hematopoietic stem cells rapidly and constitutively migrate through the blood.[128] Bone marrow cells migrate to the infarcted lesion of the heart, replicate, differentiate, and ultimately promote myocardial repair.[129] Blood cells contain progenitors that have the potential to differentiate into SMCs or endothelial cells in vitro.[130] In addition, neointimal SMCs express a number of hematopoietic lineage markers.[105,131,132] In transplant vasculopathy observed in the murine heterotopic cardiac allograft, most neointimal cells derive from the recipient.[133] Neointimal cells developed in the murine aortic transplant allograft derive almost exclusively from the recipient, and at least a subset originates

from recipient bone marrow cells.[134] Recently, it has been discovered that purified hematopoietic stem cells differentiate into SMCs in vitro and in vivo and that bone marrow cells engender most SMCs and endothelial cells that contribute to neointimal formation in mouse models of atherosclerosis, transplant vasculopathy, and postangioplasty restenosis.[135] These different origins of neointimal SMCs are most likely not mutually exclusive but participate together in creating the cell population in the neointima after arterial injury.

### Smooth Muscle Cell Proliferation

Cell proliferation is ultimately dependent on key cell-cycle events (Fig. 25-2). A number of positive and negative regulatory molecules play crucial roles in proper progression of the cell cycle, including cyclins, cyclin-dependent kinases (cdks), and cyclin-dependent kinase inhibitors (cdkis). Cyclins form a complex with cdks to initiate the cell cycle, whereas cdkis maintain the quiescent status by inhibiting cyclin/cdk complexes. The cdkis are structurally divided into two families: the Ink4 family (p14, $p15^{Ink4B}$, $p16^{Ink4A}$, $p18^{Ink4C}$, $p19^{Ink4D}$) and the Kip/Cip family ($p21^{Cip1}$, $p27^{Kip1}$, $p57^{Kip2}$). The Ink4 family controls the $G_1$ phase through inhibition of cyclin D/$cdk_4$ and cyclin D/$cdk_6$ complexes, whereas the Kip/Cip family is induced by a tumor suppressor protein p53 and controls all phases of the cell cycle.[136,137] Among the cdkis, $p27^{Kip1}$ is the pivotal molecule that regulates the transition from the $G_1$ to S phase. Growth factors activate early cyclins ($D_{1,2,3}$), which form a complex with early cdks ($cdk_{4,5,6}$) and proliferating cell nuclear antigen (PCNA), a cofactor of DNA polymerase δ.[138] The activated cyclin D/$cdk_4$/PCNA complexes reduce $p27^{Kip1}$, which

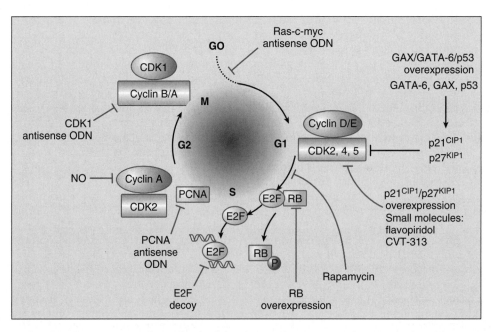

**FIGURE 25-2.** Cell cycle. Cell-cycle progression is dependent on the orchestrated expression and activation of specific enzymes (cdks) that form holoenzymes with their regulatory subunits, the cyclins. The cdkis ($p27^{Kip1}$ and $p21^{Cip1}$) bind to and inhibit the activation of cyclin–cdk complexes. *(From Dzau VJ, Braun-Dullaeus RC, Sedding DG: Vascular proliferation and atherosclerosis: New perspectives and therapeutic strategies. Nat Med 2002;8:124956. Copyright ©2002 Nature Publishing Group. Reprinted with permission from Nature and Dzau VJ.)*

maintained the cell in $G_1$ by inhibiting these complexes, and the cell enters the S phase.[139] Ablation of p27[Kip1] gene leads to overproliferation of cells in most organs because of uncontrolled cell-cycle regulation.[140-142] Another negative regulator that maintains the quiescent status is the retinoblastoma gene product RB.[143,144] The active form of RB binds to a family of transcription factors E2F and maintains the cell cycle in $G_1$. Upregulated $G_1$ cyclin/cdk complexes phosphorylate and deactivate RB, which then releases E2Fs that interact with chromosomal DNA and RB-related proteins, upregulating genes required for the transition from the $G_1$ to S phase.[145-150]

SMCs in the adult artery normally exist in the $G_{0-1}$ phase of the cell cycle and do not proliferate. The quiescent state of SMCs may also be regulated by surrounding polymerized type I collagen fibrils via integrin signaling pathways.[151] A growth arrest homeobox gene *gax,* mainly expressed in cardiovascular tissues, is downregulated within hours after angioplasty.[152] Within 24 hours after balloon injury, the expression of p27[Kip1] is rapidly downregulated, whereas both p21[Cip1] and p53 protein levels are increased in the neointima within 7 days.[153-155] p21[Cip1] is believed to provide a counterbalance to the increased accumulation and enzymatic activity of cyclin/cdk complexes.[139] Balloon angioplasty also induces upregulation of PCNA, cdk2, cyclin E, and cyclin A within 48 hours.[153,156-159] The expression of these molecules is increased in the media at 36 to 60 hours and in the neointima within 2 weeks.[159]

In light of multiple potential origins of neointimal cells, the extent of contribution of SMC proliferation in the subendothelial layer to neointimal formation is not clear. Atherectomy tissues from human restenosis lesions contain a small number of proliferating cells, and the number of SMCs decreases over time as extracellular matrix increases.[15,159-164] However, these tissues are mostly obtained at the chronic phase, and only fugacious proliferation immediately after injury may generate a sufficient number of cells to produce the extracellular matrix of neointimal lesions. In addition, approaches aimed at cell-cycle inhibition have been successful in preventing neointimal formation in various animal models. These include the rapamycin (sirolimus)-eluting stent (Fig. 25-3A) (see the section on prevention of restenosis), antisense ODN-mediated inhibition of the positive regulators (PCNA, cdk1, cdk2, cyclin B1), viral vector-mediated overexpression of the negative regulators (RB, RB2/p130, p27[Kip1], p21[Cip1], p53, Gax), and E2F-decoy ODN.[156,157,165-173] The efficacy of E2F-decoy ODN, which binds to and inactivates E2F, was evaluated in a clinical trial, and fewer graft occlusions, revisions, or critical stenoses were observed in the E2F-decoy group than in the untreated group[172] (Fig. 25-3B). Furthermore, the antiproliferation approaches used in cancer therapy have also been shown to be effective. Overexpression of cytosine deaminase, thymidine kinase, or Fas ligand in combination with parenteral drugs are the classic examples, and all of them significantly reduce neointimal formation.[174-177] Therefore, SMC proliferation still appears to be one of the major components of neointimal formation, regardless of the origin of such cells.

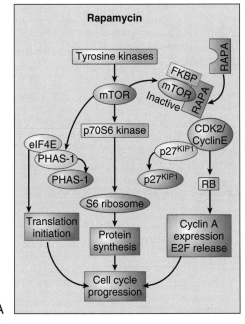
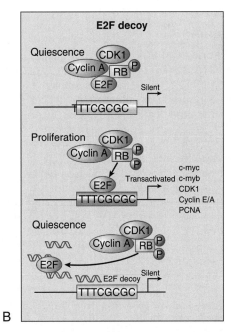

A    B

**FIGURE 25-3.** Mechanisms of action of rapamycin and E2F decoy. *A,* The mTOR–p70 S6 kinase signaling pathway. Rapamycin (RAPA) interferes with mTOR and its downstream signaling cascades, involving p70 S6 kinase and eIF4E, leading to a reduction in protein synthesis and concomitant cell cycle arrest. FKBP, FK-binding protein; PHAS-1, the EIF4E-binding protein. *B,* Principle of E2F decoy therapy. *Top,* The transcription factor E2F is inactivated by its binding to hypophosphorylated (P in circle; represents monophosphate) RB. *Middle,* Hyperphosphorylation of RB by G1-phase cyclin–CDK complexes liberates E2F, which binds to the *cis* element of cell cycle–regulatory genes and induces their transactivation. *Bottom,* Double-stranded decoy *cis* element binds to free E2F and prevents E2F-dependent gene transactivation. *(From Dzau VJ, Braun-Dullaeus RC, Sedding DG: Vascular proliferation and atherosclerosis: New perspectives and therapeutic strategies. Nat Med 2002;8:1249–56 Copyright ©2002 Nature Publishing Group. Reprinted with permission from Nature Publishing Group and Dzau VJ.)*

## Extracellular Matrix

The architectural integrity of the vascular layers is largely dependent on the equilibrium between MMPs and TIMPs. MMPs degrade extracellular matrix components and facilitate cell migration across the layers. The expressions of MMPs and TIMPs are very low in uninjured vessels but increase 2 hours after balloon injury. By 3 days after injury, gelatinases (MMP2 and MMP9) are highly expressed in the adventitial myofibroblasts surrounding the injury site, which are subsequently localized to the developing neointima.[117,178] Expression of MMP2 and MMP9 is more intense and sustained in stent implantation than in balloon angioplasty.[179] MMP inhibitors dramatically suppress SMC migration into the intima, but resultant neointimal formation is not affected, mainly because MMP inhibitors result in accelerated proliferation of SMCs that contributes to compensatory growth of the neointima.[180-183] Adenoviral gene transfer of TIMP-1 reduced SMC migration after balloon injury in rats.[184] Tenascin is another extracellular matrix protein associated with cell migration and the breaking of focal adhesions holding cells in place.[117] Tenascin is upregulated early after vascular injury by angiotensin II (AngII) and PDGF-BB and mainly expressed by adventitial myofibroblasts. Tenascin expression shifts toward the luminal surface and reaches the developing neointima by 1 week, implying active migration from the adventitia to the neointima.[185] In addition to active breakdown of extracellular components mediated by MMPs, balloon injury induces significant increase in synthesis of extracellular matrix components, including collagen, elastin, and proteoglycan, suggesting that there is a compensatory mechanism to maintain vascular structure.[186]

## Protooncogenes

Growth factors and cytokines appear to regulate the cell cycle through activation of proto-oncogenes in response to various stimuli induced by vascular injury.[187] Within 30 minutes to 2 hours after balloon injury, growth factors induce a series of protooncogene expressions in SMCs, such as c-*myc*, c-*fos*, c-*jun,* and thrombospondin.[188-190] The proto-oncogene c-*myc* is crucial for the progression from $G_0$ to $G_1$ in the cell cycle, which promptly activates cyclin E/cdk2 and cyclin D/cdk4 complexes in quiescent cells.[191-193] Disruption of the c-*myc* gene delays the expression of cyclin E and cyclin A, but the expression of cyclin Ds and cdk2 is unaffected.[194] The c-*myc* or c-*myb* antisense ODNs reduces neointimal formation in animal models of artery injury, but the recently completed ITALICS trial failed to prove any benefit in humans.[195-197] The upregulation of c-*myc* and c-*fos* in response to balloon injury mirrors the downregulation of *gax.* The protooncogene products induce the expression of cell-cycle regulator genes (cyclin Ds, cdk4, cyclin E) and growth factors (PDGF-A, TGF-β1, bFGF receptor), resulting in SMC proliferation in an autocrine fashion.[198,199] A number of signal transduction cascades induced by growth regulatory signals (EGF, PDGF, bFGF, and IGF-1) converge on a membrane-associated GTPase *ras,* which activates cytoplasmic second-messenger pathways leading to cell prolifera-tion.[200-204] The cooperative action of *ras* and *myc* controls the activation of cyclin E/cdk2 and E2F.[205] Overexpression of *ras* protein increases cyclin $D_1$ and shortens the $G_1$ phase, resulting in cellular transformation, whereas antibodies against *ras* inhibit entry of cells into the S phase.[206,207] Adenoviral gene transfer of a dominant negative form of *ras* in animal angioplasty models results in a marked reduction in neointimal formation, whereas a constitutively active form results in significant augmentation of neointimal formation.[208,209]

## Mitogen-Activated Protein Kinases

Through phosphorylation cascades, *ras* regulates the downstream mitogen-activated protein kinases (MAPKs), such as c-*jun* N-terminal kinases (JNKs) extracellular signal-regulated kinases (ERKs), and p38.[210] JNKs appear to contribute to SMC hypertrophy and hyperplasia.[211] ERKs regulate SMC proliferation in response to various growth stimuli.[212,213] Balloon injury of the rat carotid artery dramatically enhances JNK and ERK activities, which are followed by an increase in the DNA binding activity of transcription factor activator protein-1 (AP-1) that contains Jun and Fos proteins.[214] JNK activation is remarkably suppressed by ACE inhibitors and AngII type 1 receptor (AT1) antagonists. AT1 receptor antagonists also prevent activation of ERKs by suppressing their tyrosine phosphorylation, although ACE inhibitors fail to prevent such activation. The increased AP-1 DNA binding activity was significantly inhibited by both ACE inhibitors and AT1 receptor antagonists.[214] Activated by growth factors (PDGF, TGF-1β, bFGF) and cytokines (TNF-α, and IL-1) that are increased in balloon-injured vessels, the level of p38 increases as early as 15 minutes after balloon injury.[215-217] In balloon-injured vessels, the distribution of p38 roughly corresponds to that of dedifferentiated α-SMA positive cells, and inhibition of p38 reduces neointimal formation.[218]

## Angiotensin II

Arterial injury by angioplasty induces local expression of ACE, and ACE level is increased in the subsequently developed neointimal lesions.[219,220] AngII enhances neointimal proliferation *in vivo* after vascular injury, whereas ACE inhibitors prevent this process by inhibiting PDGF-AB synthesis in SMCs.[221-224] In addition, AT1 receptor antagonists reduce neointimal formation by inhibiting activation of PDGF α- and β-receptors and by downregulating PDGF-A and PDGF-B chains in injured arteries.[225] AngII also appears to stimulate SMC proliferation through MAPK pathways. However, high-dose and long-term ACE inhibition did not prevent restenosis and did not favorably influence the overall clinical and angiographic outcome after coronary angioplasty in a large-scale clinical trial.[226]

The ACE gene exhibits an insertion/deletion (I/D) polymorphism depending on the insertion (I) or deletion (D) of 287 base pairs in intron 16, and the DD phenotype is associated with high plasma and tissue ACE levels. Therefore, it has been speculated that the DD phenotype has a higher rate of neointimal formation.

However, the results from a number of clinical studies are inconsistent, and the causal relationship between the ACE I/D polymorphism and restenosis remains unproven.[227]

## Nitric Oxide

Endothelial denudation by angioplasty also results in loss of NO, an endogenous proapoptotic substance. Overexpression of inducible NO synthase (iNOS) in SMCs leads to marked apoptosis, suggesting a counteractive role of NO against neointimal proliferation.[228] NO inhibits platelet aggregation and SMC mitogenesis and proliferation via a cGMP-dependent pathway.[229,230] Dietary administration of L-arginine, an NO precursor, reduces neointimal formation and substantially inhibits the accumulation of macrophages in the injured vessels of hypercholesterolemic rabbits.[231] Overexpression of NOS, either endothelial (eNOS) or inducible (iNOS), has been shown to reduce neointimal formation in various animal models. In addition, endothelial progenitor cells isolated from peripheral blood, amplified *ex vivo*, and seeded on decellularized vessel grafts were found to produce NO and remain patent for 150 days, whereas the control grafts occluded within 15 days.[130] These results indicate the significance of NO in neointimal formation and provide the basis for a novel therapy for restenosis.

## Endothelin

Endothelin-1 (ET-1) augments neointimal formation *in vivo,* and its level is elevated in the human coronary sinus after coronary balloon angioplasty. Endothelin converting enzyme (ECE-1) is also increased in neointimal SMCs in both rat balloon-injured arteries and in human coronary atherosclerotic lesions. Blockade of ET receptor or ECE-1 reduces neointimal formation after balloon injury in experimental models.[232,233]

## INFECTION AND RESTENOSIS

Over the past decade, infectious agents have attracted attention as a potential culprit of the pathogenesis of coronary restenosis. Approximately 33% of restenosis lesions contain sequences of cytomegalovirus (CMV) DNA, and SMCs grown from the restenosis lesions express CMV protein IE84 and high amounts of p53. Because IE84 binds to and inhibits p53, a hypothesis has been formed that CMV may enhance SMC proliferation via cell-cycle regulation.[234] A prospective study of 75 patients undergoing directional atherectomy showed that CMV-seropositive patients had a greater reduction in the luminal diameter, resulting in a significantly higher rate of restenosis at 6 months than seronegative patients.[235] Other epidemiologic studies have shown an increased prevalence of seropositivity of *Chlamydia pneumoniae* and *Helicobacter pylori* in patients with coronary artery disease. However, larger clinical studies failed to establish an association between the risk of restenosis and the serologic status of CMV, *C. pneumoniae,* or *H. pylori.*[234,236-238] Therefore, it remains unclear whether these infectious agents contribute to pathogenesis of coronary restenosis.

## PREVENTION OF RESTENOSIS

Although the need to overcome coronary restenosis resulted in an aggressive pursuit for novel therapies, more than 100 drugs and devices have failed to show any benefits.[239-242] Recently, elucidation of molecular mechanism of neointimal formation has contributed to the emergence of potent antirestenosis therapies that yield consistently positive results.

## Heparin-Coated Stents

Because subacute stent thrombosis was a major issue with early stent devices, various stent surface coatings were developed to reduce protein deposition and platelet adhesion. In early clinical studies, heparin-coated stents appeared to reduce subacute stent thrombosis in comparison with historical controls, but they did not significantly decrease the long-term restenosis rate.[8,243] Heparin-coating of the stent was subsequently shown to have no impact on subacute stent thrombosis or on restenosis in direct comparison with bare metal stents.[244,245]

## Intravascular Brachytherapy

Ionizing radiation nonspecifically destroys DNA double strands and, thus blocks cell proliferation.[246] In response to DNA damage elicited by radiation, a tumor suppressor protein p53 upregulates p21[Cip1] that directly inhibits PCNA, thereby allowing DNA repair and arresting cells in the $G_1$ phase.[247-251] In addition to inhibiting neointimal cell proliferation, intracoronary radiation therapy *(brachytherapy)* appears to prevent remodeling of the angioplastied vessel by inhibiting myofibroblast proliferation in the tunica adventitia, thereby attenuating adventitial scar formation and subsequent vascular remodeling.[252,253] Two sources of radiation have been tested for brachytherapy: γ (photons) and β (electrons). γ-radiation penetrates beyond the vessel wall and requires extensive radiation protection of the operating personnel, whereas β-radiation is absorbed in living tissue by more than 99% within 5 mm from the source. Intracoronary brachytherapy with both γ and β radiation has been shown to be effective in preventing ISR in randomized clinical trials, reducing the rate of angiographic restenosis and repeat revascularization within the first year.[254-257] In the SCRIPPS study, reduction of the rate of restenosis was still observed at 3-year follow-up, despite progressive decrease in lumen diameter between 6 months and 3 years.[258,259]

The initial excitement with intracoronary brachytherapy was dampened by several serious complications. *Late stent thrombosis,* manifesting as acute target vessel closure leading to acute myocardial infarction, occurs 1 to 9 months after brachytherapy in as many as 6% to 7% of the patients.[260] The risk of late stent thrombosis appears low in the absence of new stent placement and with extended antiplatelet therapy after intracoronary radiation. The FDA, therefore, recommends that antiplatelet therapy with aspirin and a theinopyridine derivative (clopidogrel or ticlopidine) be prescribed for a minimum of 6 months, and for at least 12 months if a new stent is implanted. The FDA also suggests that implantation of new stents be avoided after brachytherapy. *Edge restenosis,* or renarrowing at the proximal and distal edges of the irradiated lesions, occurs often in patients who develop postbrachytherapy restenosis. Radioactive stent implantation is often associated with edge restenosis, or *candy-wrapper effect.* Therefore, radioactive stents perhaps delay but do not prevent neointimal proliferation.[261] Edge restenosis may be due to a progressive attenuation of radiation dose from the radiation source to the edges or from *geographical miss* resulting from technical issues or errors during the procedure. Development of *coronary aneurysms* within 6 months of brachytherapy has also been reported.[262,263] The very long-term outcomes and complications of brachytherapy remain to be defined.[264]

## Drug-Eluting Stents

Antineoplastic or immunosuppressive drugs with antiproliferative activity have been shown to be effective in preventing neointimal formation in various animal models of vascular injury. However, these drugs have a high toxicity profile with systemic administration. Consequently, the previously developed surface-coating technology was applied to produce drug-eluting stents, which elute antiproliferative agents in the injured vessels. The advantage of drug-eluting stents is the achievement of highly concentrated drug delivery for a prolonged period of time with minimal systemic exposure. A variety of drug-eluting stents are currently under investigation, and some of them have yielded promising results.

### Sirolimus (Rapamycin)

Sirolimus belongs to the class of macrocyclic immunosuppressive agents that bind to specific cytosolic proteins called immunophilins.[265] Cyclosporin A and tacrolimus (FK506) are two other members of this class. Although sirolimus and its analog tacrolimus share the same family of immunophilins (FKBP), sirolimus acts at a later stage in T-cell cycle progression by blocking cytokine-mediated signal transduction pathways.[265] $FKBP_{12}$, a sirolimus receptor, has been found to be up-regulated in neointimal SMCs in human atherectomy specimens from ISR lesions.[105] Sirolimus/FKBP complex ceases the cell cycle in transition from the $G_1$ to S phase by inhibiting a specific cytosolic protein, the mammalian target of rapamycin (mTOR). mTOR is a key regulatory kinase that plays a major role in the mammalian cell cycle, and the inhibition of mTOR results in manifold effects to cease cell-cycle progression: downregulation of PCNA that is essential for DNA replication, inactivation of p70 S6 kinase and eukaryotic initiation factor 4E (eIF4E) that are crucial components of increasing protein synthesis in preparation for cell division, and inhibi-

tion of kinase activity of the cyclin D/cdk4 and cyclin E/cdk2 complexes via activation of p27$^{Kip1}$ and RB (Fig. 25-3A).[266] Sirolimus blocks both proliferation and migration of SMCs *in vitro,*[267,268] inhibits arterial neointimal thickening, and reduces restenosis after angioplasty in various animal models of arterial injury.[269-273]

A small preliminary clinical trial demonstrated little neointimal formation at 12 month in patients with sirolimus-eluting stents.[274,275] Subsequently, a multicenter, randomized clinical trial (RAVEL) reported significant reduction in angiographic restenosis in the sirolimus-eluting stent group compared with the bare metal stents group at 6 month (0% vs. 26.6%, P < 0.0001). There were no episodes of stent thrombosis, and the overall rate of major cardiac events was significantly lower in the sirolimus-stent group than in the standard-stent group during a follow-up period of up to 1 year (5.8% vs. 28.8%, P < 0.001).[276] Clinical benefits of sirolimus-eluting stents have consistently been demonstrated in larger double-blind clinical trials in patients with more challenging and complex lesions.[277,278]

### Paclitaxel

Paclitaxel is an anticancer agent active against a broad range of cancers including breast, ovarian, and lung cancer. Paclitaxel promotes the polymerization of microtubules, which are extraordinarily stable and dysfunctional, thereby causing the death of the cell by disrupting the normal microtubule dynamics required for cell division and vital interphase processes.[279,280] SMC proliferation and migration are inhibited by paclitaxel in both cell culture and a carotid artery balloon-injury model in rats.[281] In atherosclerotic rabbits, locally administered paclitaxel by a microporous balloon catheter prevented neointimal formation after balloon angioplasty.[282,283] In a pig coronary angioplasty model, paclitaxel-coated stents produced a significant dose-dependent inhibition of neointimal formation and luminal encroachment 28 days after implantation.[284]

A randomized, double-blind, multicenter feasibility trial to evaluate the safety of the paclitaxel-coated stents (TAXUS I) demonstrated significant reductions in angiographic and intravascular ultrasound measures of restenosis for the paclitaxel-coated stents with no adverse events compared with bare metal stents.[285] Subsequently, the ASPECT trial reported a dose-dependent reduction in angiographic percent-diameter stenosis at 6 months,[286] and the TAXUS II trial demonstrated significant reductions in MACE at 12 months in patients treated with the paclitaxel-coated stents with focal *de novo* native coronary lesions.[287]

## Biodegradable Stents

Because coronary stents counteract elastic recoil and negative remodeling within a relatively short period of time, biodegradable stents may be ideal to minimize long-term complications. The Igaki-Tamai stent is made of a poly-l-lactic (PLLA) monofilament, which has been used in orthopedic surgery. The stent takes 18 to 24 months to completely degrade. A small clinical study to evaluate safety and feasibility of the PLLA Igaki-Tamai stent has revealed no stent thrombosis and no major cardiac event within 6 months.[288] Drug-eluting stents made of biodegradable materials are also under investigation. In animal studies, biodegradable stents coated with a tyrosine kinase inhibitor or recombinant polyethylene glycol (r-PEG)-hirudin and the prostacyclin analog iloprost significantly reduced angiographic restenosis.[289,290]

# FUTURE DIRECTIONS

Restenosis has been resistant to the technologic advances of PCIs for the last 3 decades, frustrating both patients and cardiologists. As noted previously, the complexity of the molecular and cellular mechanisms leading to restenosis is beginning to be deciphered. Drug-eluting stents are one of the excellent examples of clinical application of basic cardiovascular science; elucidation of molecular and cellular pathogenesis at the bench has been brought back to the bedside in the form of a novel therapeutic modality. The emerging popularity of drug-eluting stents, no matter what pharmacologic agents are selected, is firmly supported by the promising data from clinical trials, the simple delivery system, and the minimal systemic toxicity profile. Nevertheless, the enthusiasm for a cure should not cloud critical and objective attitudes toward new technologies or limit other potential options. Whether a therapeutic modality turns out to be the answer to the longstanding predicament of restenosis remains to be clarified by long-term clinical trials.

# REFERENCES

1. Smith SC, Dove JT, Jacobs AK, et al: ACC/AHA guidelines for percutaneous coronary intervention (revision of the 1993 PTCA guidelines): A report of the American College of Cardiology/American Heart Association Task Force on practice guidelines endorsed by the Society for Cardiac Angiography and Interventions. J Am Coll Cardiol 2001;37:221-239.
2. Serruys PW, Unger F, Sousa JE, et al: Comparison of coronary-artery bypass surgery and stenting for the treatment of multivessel disease. N Engl J Med 2001;344:1117-1124.
3. Detre K, Holubkov R, Kelsey S, et al: Percutaneous transluminal coronary angioplasty in 1985-1986 and 1977-1981: The National Heart, Lung, and Blood Institute Registry. N Engl J Med 1988;318:265-270.
4. Bengtson JR, Mark DB, Honan MB, et al: Detection of restenosis after elective percutaneous transluminal coronary angioplasty using the exercise treadmill test. Am J Cardiol 1990;65:28-34.
5. Anderson HV, Shaw RE, Brindis RG, et al: A contemporary overview of percutaneous coronary interventions. J Am Coll Cardiol 2002;39:1096-1103.
6. Fischman DL, Leon MB, Baim DS, et al: A randomized comparison of coronary-stent placement and balloon angioplasty in the treatment of coronary artery disease: Stent Restenosis Study Investigators. N Engl J Med 1994;331:496-501.
7. Serruys PW, de Jaegere P, Kiemeneij F, et al: A comparison of balloon-expandable-stent implantation with balloon angioplasty in patients with coronary artery disease: Benestent Study Group. N Engl J Med 1994;331:489-495.
8. Serruys PW, van Hout B, Bonnier H, et al: Randomised comparison of implantation of heparin-coated stents with balloon angioplasty in selected patients with coronary artery disease (Benestent II). Lancet 1998;352:673-681.
9. Elezi S, Kastrati A, Neumann FJ, et al: Vessel size and long-term outcome after coronary stent placement. Circulation 1998;98:1875-1880.
10. Hoffmann R, Mintz GS, Dussaillant GR, et al: Patterns and mechanisms of in-stent restenosis. A serial intravascular ultrasound study. Circulation 1996;94:1247-1254.
11. Mudra H, Regar E, Klauss V, et al: Serial follow-up after optimized ultrasound-guided deployment of Palmaz-Schatz stents: In-stent neointimal proliferation without significant reference segment response. Circulation 1997;95:363-370.
12. Mach F: Toward new therapeutic strategies against neointimal formation in restenosis. Arterioscler Thromb Vasc Biol 2000;20:1699-1700.
13. Liu MW, Roubin GS, and King SB 3rd: Restenosis after coronary angioplasty: Potential biologic determinants and role of intimal hyperplasia. Circulation 1989;79:1374-1387.
14. Kearney M, Pieczek A, Haley L, et al: Histopathology of in-stent restenosis in patients with peripheral artery disease. Circulation 1997;95:1998-2002.
15. Grewe PH, Deneke T, Machraoui A, et al: Acute and chronic tissue response to coronary stent implantation: Pathologic findings in human specimen. J Am Coll Cardiol 2000;35:157-163.
16. Glover C, O'Brien ER: Pathophysiological insights from studies of retrieved coronary atherectomy tissue. Semin Interv Cardiol 2000;5:167-173.
17. Karas SP, Gravanis MB, Santoian EC, et al: Coronary intimal proliferation after balloon injury and stenting in swine: An animal model of restenosis. J Am Coll Cardiol 1992;20:467-474.
18. den Heijer P, Foley DP, Escaned J, et al: Angioscopic versus angiographic detection of intimal dissection and intracoronary thrombus. J Am Coll Cardiol 1994;24:649-654.
19. Wilensky RL, March KL, Gradus-Pizlo I, et al: Vascular injury, repair, and restenosis after percutaneous transluminal angioplasty in the atherosclerotic rabbit. Circulation 1995;92:2995-3005.
20. Deitch JS, Williams JK, Adams MR, et al: Effects of beta3-integrin blockade (c7E3) on the response to angioplasty and intra-arterial stenting in atherosclerotic nonhuman primates. Arterioscler Thromb Vasc Biol 1998;18:1730-1737.
21. Walsh K, Smith RC, Kim HS: Vascular cell apoptosis in remodeling, restenosis, and plaque rupture. Circ Res 2000;87:184-188.
22. Angelini GD, Newby AC: The future of saphenous vein as a coronary artery bypass conduit. Eur Heart J 1989;10:273-280.
23. Salomon RN, Hughes CC, Schoen FJ, et al: Human coronary transplantation-associated arteriosclerosis: Evidence for a chronic immune reaction to activated graft endothelial cells. Am J Pathol 1991;138:791-798.
24. Dilley RJ, McGeachie JK, Prendergast FJ: A review of the histologic changes in vein-to-artery grafts, with particular reference to intimal hyperplasia. Arch Surg 1988;123:691-696.
25. Ip JH, Fuster V, Badimon L, et al: Syndromes of accelerated atherosclerosis: Role of vascular injury and smooth muscle cell proliferation. J Am Coll Cardiol 1990;15:1667-1687.
26. Miller AM, McPhaden AR, Wadsworth RM, et al: Inhibition by leukocyte depletion of neointima formation after balloon angioplasty in a rabbit model of restenosis. Cardiovasc Res 2001;49:838-850.
27. Tanaka H, Sukhova GK, Swanson SJ, et al: Sustained activation of vascular cells and leukocytes in the rabbit aorta after balloon injury. Circulation 1993;88:1788-1803.
28. Kennedy S, McPhaden AR, Wadsworth RM, et al: Correlation of leukocyte adhesiveness, adhesion molecule expression and leukocyte-induced contraction following balloon angioplasty. Br J Pharmacol 2000;130:95-103.
29. Springer TA: Traffic signals for lymphocyte recirculation and leukocyte emigration: The multistep paradigm. Cell 1994;76:301-314.
30. Gahmberg CG, Valmu L, Fagerholm S, et al: Leukocyte integrins and inflammation. Cell Mol Life Sci 1998;54:549-555.
31. Kumar A, Hoover JL, Simmons CA, et al: Remodeling and neointimal formation in the carotid artery of normal and P-selectin-deficient mice. Circulation 1997;96:4333-4342.
32. Bienvenu JG, Tanguay JF, Theoret JF, et al: Recombinant soluble p-selectin glycoprotein ligand-1-Ig reduces restenosis through inhibition of platelet-neutrophil adhesion after double angioplasty in swine. Circulation 2001;103:1128-1134.

33. Hayashi S, Watanabe N, Nakazawa K, et al: Roles of P-selectin in inflammation, neointimal formation, and vascular remodeling in balloon-injured rat carotid arteries. Circulation 2000;102: 1710–1717.

34. Barron MK, Lake RS, Buda AJ, et al: Intimal hyperplasia after balloon injury is attenuated by blocking selectins. Circulation 1997;96:3587–3592.

35. Merhi Y, Provost P, Chauvet P, et al: Selectin blockade reduces neutrophil interaction with platelets at the site of deep arterial injury by angioplasty in pigs. Arterioscler Thromb Vasc Biol 1999; 19:372–377.

36. Inoue T, Sakai Y, Hoshi K, et al: Lower expression of neutrophil adhesion molecule indicates less vessel wall injury and might explain lower restenosis rate after cutting balloon angioplasty. Circulation 1998;97:2511–2518.

37. Inoue T, Sohma R, Miyazaki T, et al: Comparison of activation process of platelets and neutrophils after coronary stent implantation versus balloon angioplasty for stable angina pectoris. Am J Cardiol 2000;86:1057–1062.

38. Yasukawa H, Imaizumi T, Matsuoka H, et al: Inhibition of intimal hyperplasia after balloon injury by antibodies to intercellular adhesion molecule-1 and lymphocyte function-associated antigen-1. Circulation 1997;95:1515–1522.

39. Zou Y, Hu Y, Mayr M, et al: Reduced neointima hyperplasia of vein bypass grafts in intercellular adhesion molecule-1-deficient mice. Circ Res 2000;86:434–440.

40. Simon DI, Dhen Z, Seifert P, et al: Decreased neointimal formation in Mac-1(-/-) mice reveals a role for inflammation in vascular repair after angioplasty. J Clin Invest 2000;105:293–300.

41. Welt FG, Edelman ER, Simon DI, et al: Neutrophil, not macrophage, infiltration precedes neointimal thickening in balloon-injured arteries. Arterioscler Thromb Vasc Biol 2000;20: 2553–2558.

42. Koch W, Bottiger C, Mehilli J, et al: Association of a CD18 gene polymorphism with a reduced risk of restenosis after coronary stenting. Am J Cardiol 2001;88:1120–1124.

43. Rao GN, Corson MA, Berk BC: Uric acid stimulates vascular smooth muscle cell proliferation by increasing platelet-derived growth factor A-chain expression. J Biol Chem 1991;266: 8604–8608.

44. Rao GN, Berk BC: Active oxygen species stimulate vascular smooth muscle cell growth and proto-oncogene expression. Circ Res 1992;70:593–599.

45. Miller DD, Craig FE, Dressler FA, et al: Immunohistochemical characterization of immune cell composition and cytokine receptor expression in human coronary atherectomy tissue. Coron Artery Dis 1995;6:965–972.

46. Furukawa Y, Matsumori A, Ohashi N, et al: Anti-monocyte chemoattractant protein-1/monocyte chemotactic and activating factor antibody inhibits neointimal hyperplasia in injured rat carotid arteries. Circ Res 1999;84:306–314.

47. Feldman LJ, Aguirre L, Ziol M, et al: Interleukin-10 inhibits intimal hyperplasia after angioplasty or stent implantation in hypercholesterolemic rabbits. Circulation 2000;101:908–916.

48. Labinaz M, Hoffert C, Pels K, et al: Infusion of an antialpha4 integrin antibody is associated with less neoadventitial formation after balloon injury of porcine coronary arteries. Can J Cardiol 2000;16:187–196.

49. Osada M, Takeda S, Ogawa R, et al: T lymphocyte activation and restenosis after percutaneous transluminal coronary angioplasty. J Interferon Cytokine Res 2001;21:219–221.

50. Bevilacqua MP, Pober JS, Wheeler ME, et al: Interleukin 1 acts on cultured human vascular endothelium to increase the adhesion of polymorphonuclear leukocytes, monocytes, and related leukocyte cell lines. J Clin Invest 1985;76:2003–2011.

51. Moser R, Schleiffenbaum B, Groscurth P, et al: Interleukin 1 and tumor necrosis factor stimulate human vascular endothelial cells to promote transendothelial neutrophil passage. J Clin Invest 1989;83:444–455.

52. Furie MB, McHugh DD: Migration of neutrophils across endothelial monolayers is stimulated by treatment of the monolayers with interleukin-1 or tumor necrosis factor-alpha. J Immunol 1989;143:3309–3317.

53. Ikeda U, Ikeda M, Oohara T, et al: Mitogenic action of interleukin-1 alpha on vascular smooth muscle cells mediated by PDGF. Atherosclerosis 1990;84:183–188.

54. Hajjar KA, Hajjar DP, Silverstein RL, et al: Tumor necrosis factor-mediated release of platelet-derived growth factor from cultured endothelial cells. J Exp Med 1987;166:235–245.

55. Selzman CH, Shames BD, Reznikov LL, et al: Liposomal delivery of purified inhibitory-kappaBalpha inhibits tumor necrosis factor-alpha-induced human vascular smooth muscle proliferation. Circ Res 1999;84:867–875.

56. Fukumoto Y, Shimokawa H, Ito A, et al: Inflammatory cytokines cause coronary arteriosclerosis-like changes and alterations in the smooth-muscle phenotypes in pigs. J Cardiovasc Pharmacol 1997;29:222–231.

57. Wainwright CL, Miller AM, Wadsworth RM: Inflammation as a key event in the development of neointima following vascular balloon injury. Clin Exp Pharmacol Physiol 2001;28:891–895.

58. Suzuki T, Ishiwata S, Hasegawa K, et al: Raised interleukin 6 concentrations as a predictor of postangioplasty restenosis. Heart 2000;83:578.

59. Buffon A, Liuzzo G, Biasucci LM, et al: Preprocedural serum levels of C-reactive protein predict early complications and late restenosis after coronary angioplasty. J Am Coll Cardiol 1999; 34:1512–1521.

60. Fingerle J, Johnson R, Clowes AW, et al: Role of platelets in smooth muscle cell proliferation and migration after vascular injury in rat carotid artery. Proc Natl Acad Sci USA 1989;86:8412–8416.

61. Komatsu R, Ueda M, Naruko T, et al: Neointimal tissue response at sites of coronary stenting in humans: Macroscopic, histological, and immunohistochemical analyses. Circulation 1998;98: 224–233.

62. Farb A, Sangiorgi G, Carter AJ, et al: Pathology of acute and chronic coronary stenting in humans. Circulation 1999;99:44–52.

63. Taubman MB: Gene induction in vessel wall injury. Thromb Haemost 1993;70:180–183.

64. Speidel CM, Eisenberg PR, Ruf W, et al: Tissue factor mediates prolonged procoagulant activity on the luminal surface of balloon-injured aortas in rabbits. Circulation 1995;92:3323–3330.

65. Okazaki H, Majesky MW, Harker LA, et al: Regulation of platelet-derived growth factor ligand and receptor gene expression by alpha-thrombin in vascular smooth muscle cells. Circ Res 1992;71:1285–1293.

66. Graham DJ, Alexander JJ: The effects of thrombin on bovine aortic endothelial and smooth muscle cells. J Vasc Surg 1990;11: 307–312; discussion 312–313.

67. Gertz SD, Fallon JT, Gallo R, et al: Hirudin reduces tissue factor expression in neointima after balloon injury in rabbit femoral and porcine coronary arteries. Circulation 1998;98:580–587.

68. Asada Y, Hara S, Tsuneyoshi A, et al: Fibrin-rich and platelet-rich thrombus formation on neointima: Recombinant tissue factor pathway inhibitor prevents fibrin formation and neointimal development following repeated balloon injury of rabbit aorta. Thromb Haemost 1998;80:506–511.

69. Abendschein DR, Recchia D, Meng YY, et al: Inhibition of thrombin attenuates stenosis after arterial injury in minipigs. J Am Coll Cardiol 1996;28:1849–1855.

70. Serruys PW, Herrman JP, Simon R, et al: A comparison of hirudin with heparin in the prevention of restenosis after coronary angioplasty: Helvetica Investigators. N Engl J Med 1995;333: 757–763.

71. Ellis SG, Effron MB, Gold HK, et al: Acute platelet inhibition with abciximab does not reduce in-stent restenosis (ERASER study). Circulation 1999;100:799–806.

72. Herrman JP, Hermans WR, Vos J, et al: Pharmacological approaches to the prevention of restenosis following angioplasty: The search for the Holy Grail? (Part I). Drugs 1993;46:18–52.

73. Jawien A, Bowen-Pope DF, Lindner V, et al: Platelet-derived growth factor promotes smooth muscle migration and intimal thickening in a rat model of balloon angioplasty. J Clin Invest 1992;89:507–511.

74. Nabel EG, Yang Z, Liptay S, et al: Recombinant platelet-derived growth factor B gene expression in porcine arteries induce intimal hyperplasia in vivo. J Clin Invest 1993;91:1822–1829.

75. Sirois MG, Simons M, Edelman ER: Antisense oligonucleotide inhibition of PDGFR-beta receptor subunit expression directs suppression of intimal thickening. Circulation 1997;95:669–676.

76. Hart CE, Kraiss LW, Vergel S, et al: PDGFbeta receptor blockade inhibits intimal hyperplasia in the baboon. Circulation 1999;99: 564–569.

77. Ferns GA, Raines EW, Sprugel KH, et al: Inhibition of neointimal smooth muscle accumulation after angioplasty by an antibody to PDGF. Science 1991;253:1129–1132.

78. Maresta A, Balducelli M, Cantini L, et al: Trapidil (triazolopyrimidine), a platelet-derived growth factor antagonist, reduces restenosis after percutaneous transluminal coronary angioplasty: Results of the randomized, double-blind STARC study—Studio Trapidil versus Aspirin nella Restenosi Coronarica. Circulation 1994;90:2710–2715.

79. Cuevas P, Gonzalez AM, Carceller F, et al: Vascular response to basic fibroblast growth factor when infused onto the normal adventitia or into the injured media of the rat carotid artery. Circ Res 1991;69:360–369.

80. Nabel EG, Yang ZY, Plautz G, et al: Recombinant fibroblast growth factor-1 promotes intimal hyperplasia and angiogenesis in arteries in vivo. Nature 1993;362:844–846.

81. Lindner V, Reidy MA: Proliferation of smooth muscle cells after vascular injury is inhibited by an antibody against basic fibroblast growth factor. Proc Natl Acad Sci USA 1991;88:3739–3743.

82. Reidy MA, Fingerle J, Lindner V: Factors controlling the development of arterial lesions after injury. Circulation 1992;86:III43–46.

83. Chen JK, Hoshi H, McKeehan WL: Transforming growth factor type beta specifically stimulates synthesis of proteoglycan in human adult arterial smooth muscle cells. Proc Natl Acad Sci USA 1987;84:5287–5291.

84. Nabel EG, Shum L, Pompili VJ, et al: Direct transfer of transforming growth factor beta 1 gene into arteries stimulates fibrocellular hyperplasia. Proc Natl Acad Sci USA 1993;90:10759–10763.

85. Yamamoto K, Morishita R, Tomita N, et al: Ribozyme oligonucleotides against transforming growth factor-beta inhibited neointimal formation after vascular injury in rat model: Potential application of ribozyme strategy to treat cardiovascular disease. Circulation 2000;102:1308–1314.

86. Grant MB, Wargovich TJ, Ellis EA, et al: Expression of IGF-I, IGF-I receptor and IGF binding proteins-1, -2, -3, -4 and -5 in human atherectomy specimens. Regul Pept 1996;67:137–144.

87. Stiles CD, Capone GT, Scher CD, et al: Dual control of cell growth by somatomedins and platelet-derived growth factor. Proc Natl Acad Sci USA 1979;76:1279–1283.

88. Delafontaine P, Lou H, Alexander RW: Regulation of insulin-like growth factor I messenger RNA levels in vascular smooth muscle cells. Hypertension 1991;18:742–747.

89. Clemmons DR: Variables controlling the secretion of a somatomedin-like peptide by cultured porcine smooth muscle cells. Circ Res 1985;56:418–426.

90. Grant MB, Wargovich TJ, Ellis EA, et al: Localization of insulin-like growth factor I and inhibition of coronary smooth muscle cell growth by somatostatin analogues in human coronary smooth muscle cells: A potential treatment for restenosis? Circulation 1994;89:1511–1517.

91. Baserga R, Rubin R: Cell cycle and growth control. Crit Rev Eukaryot Gene Expr 1993;3:47–61.

92. Banskota NK, Taub R, Zellner K, et al: Insulin, insulin-like growth factor I and platelet-derived growth factor interact additively in the induction of the protooncogene c-myc and cellular proliferation in cultured bovine aortic smooth muscle cells. Mol Endocrinol 1989;3:1183–1190.

93. Wang J, Niu W, Nikiforov Y, et al: Targeted overexpression of IGF-I evokes distinct patterns of organ remodeling in smooth muscle cell tissue beds of transgenic mice. J Clin Invest 1997;100:1425–1439.

94. Carrozza JP, Jr, Kuntz RE, Fishman RF, et al: Restenosis after arterial injury caused by coronary stenting in patients with diabetes mellitus. Ann Intern Med 1993;118:344–349.

95. Bornfeldt KE, Arnqvist HJ, Capron L: In vivo proliferation of rat vascular smooth muscle in relation to diabetes mellitus insulin-like growth factor I and insulin. Diabetologia 1992;35:104–108.

96. Serri O, Brazeau P, Kachra Z, et al: Octreotide inhibits insulin-like growth factor-I hepatic gene expression in the hypophysectomized rat: Evidence for a direct and indirect mechanism of action. Endocrinology 1992;130:1816–1821.

97. Lundergan C, Foegh ML, Vargas R, et al: Inhibition of myointimal proliferation of the rat carotid artery by the peptides, angiopeptin and BIM 23034. Atherosclerosis 1989;80:49–55.

98. Santoian ED, Schneider JE, Gravanis MB, et al: Angiopeptin inhibits intimal hyperplasia after angioplasty in porcine coronary arteries. Circulation 1993;88:11–14.

99. Bauters C, Van Belle E, Wernert N, et al: Angiopeptin inhibits oncogene induction in rabbit aorta after balloon denudation. Circulation 1994;89:2327–2331.

100. Eriksen UH, Amtorp O, Bagger JP, et al: Randomized double-blind Scandinavian trial of angiopeptin versus placebo for the prevention of clinical events and restenosis after coronary balloon angioplasty. Am Heart J 1995;130:1–8.

101. von Essen R, Ostermaier R, Grube E, et al: Effects of octreotide treatment on restenosis after coronary angioplasty: Results of the VERAS study. VErringerung der Restenoserate nach Angioplastie durch ein Somatostatin-analogon. Circulation 1997;96:1482–1487.

102. Emanuelsson H, Beatt KJ, Bagger JP, et al: Long-term effects of angiopeptin treatment in coronary angioplasty: Reduction of clinical events but not angiographic restenosis—European Angiopeptin Study Group. Circulation 1995;91:1689–1696.

103. Ross R: The pathogenesis of atherosclerosis: A perspective for the 1990s. Nature 1993;362:801–809.

104. Ross R: Atherosclerosis: An inflammatory disease. N Engl J Med 1999;340:115–126.

105. Zohlnhofer D, Klein CA, Richter T, et al: Gene expression profiling of human stent-induced neointima by cDNA array analysis of microscopic specimens retrieved by helix cutter atherectomy: Detection of FK506-binding protein 12 upregulation. Circulation 2001;103:1396–1402.

106. Lemire JM, Covin CW, White S, et al: Characterization of cloned aortic smooth muscle cells from young rats. Am J Pathol 1994;144:1068–1081.

107. Bochaton-Piallat ML, Ropraz P, Gabbiani F, et al: Phenotypic heterogeneity of rat arterial smooth muscle cell clones: Implications for the development of experimental intimal thickening. Arterioscler Thromb Vasc Biol 1996;16:815–820.

108. Majesky MW, Giachelli CM, Reidy MA, et al: Rat carotid neointimal smooth muscle cells reexpress a developmentally regulated mRNA phenotype during repair of arterial injury. Circ Res 1992;71:759–768.

109. Thyberg J, Blomgren K, Roy J, et al: Phenotypic modulation of smooth muscle cells after arterial injury is associated with changes in the distribution of laminin and fibronectin. J Histochem Cytochem 1997;45:837–846.

110. Thyberg J: Phenotypic modulation of smooth muscle cells during formation of neointimal thickenings following vascular injury. Histol Histopathol 1998;13:871–891.

111. Campbell GR, Campbell JH: Smooth muscle phenotypic changes in arterial wall homeostasis: Implications for the pathogenesis of atherosclerosis. Exp Mol Pathol 1985;42:139–162.

112. Schwartz SM, Heimark RL, Majesky MW: Developmental mechanisms underlying pathology of arteries. Physiol Rev 1990;70:1177–1209.

113. Schmitt-Graff A, Desmouliere A, Gabbiani G: Heterogeneity of myofibroblast phenotypic features: An example of fibroblastic cell plasticity. Virchows Arch 1994;425:3–24.

114. Zalewski A, Shi Y: Vascular myofibroblasts: Lessons from coronary repair and remodeling. Arterioscler Thromb Vasc Biol 1997;17:417–422.

115. Faggin E, Puato M, Zardo L, et al: Smooth muscle-specific SM22 protein is expressed in the adventitial cells of balloon-injured rabbit carotid artery. Arterioscler Thromb Vasc Biol 1999;19:1393–1404.

116. Li G, Chen SJ, Oparil S, et al: Direct in vivo evidence demonstrating neointimal migration of adventitial fibroblasts after balloon injury of rat carotid arteries. Circulation 2000;101:1362–1365.

117. Wilcox JN, Okamoto EI, Nakahara KI, et al: Perivascular responses after angioplasty which may contribute to postangioplasty restenosis: A role for circulating myofibroblast precursors? Ann N Y Acad Sci 2001;947:68–90; discussion 90–92.

118. Ronnov-Jessen L, Petersen OW, Bissell MJ: Cellular changes involved in conversion of normal to malignant breast: Importance of the stromal reaction. Physiol Rev 1996;76:69–125.

119. Gabbiani G: Evolution and clinical implications of the myofibroblast concept. Cardiovasc Res 1998;38:545–548.

120. Serini G, Gabbiani G: Mechanisms of myofibroblast activity and phenotypic modulation. Exp Cell Res 1999;250:273-283.

121. Powell DW, Mifflin RC, Valentich JD, et al: Myofibroblasts. I. Paracrine cells important in health and disease. Am J Physiol 1999;277:C1-9.

122. Dettman RW, Denetclaw W Jr, Ordahl CP, et al: Common epicardial origin of coronary vascular smooth muscle, perivascular fibroblasts, and intermyocardial fibroblasts in the avian heart. Dev Biol 1998;193:169-181.

123. Desmouliere A, Geinoz A, Gabbiani F, et al: Transforming growth factor-beta 1 induces alpha-smooth muscle actin expression in granulation tissue myofibroblasts and in quiescent and growing cultured fibroblasts. J Cell Biol 1993;122:103-111.

124. Desmouliere A, Rubbia-Brandt L, Abdiu A, et al: Alpha-smooth muscle actin is expressed in a subpopulation of cultured and cloned fibroblasts and is modulated by gamma-interferon. Exp Cell Res 1992;201:64-73.

125. Desmouliere A, Rubbia-Brandt L, Grau G, et al: Heparin induces alpha-smooth muscle actin expression in cultured fibroblasts and in granulation tissue myofibroblasts. Lab Invest 1992;67: 716-726.

126. Smith JD, Bryant SR, Couper LL, et al: Soluble transforming growth factor-beta type II receptor inhibits negative remodeling, fibroblast transdifferentiation, and intimal lesion formation but not endothelial growth. Circ Res 1999;84:1212-1222.

127. De Leon H, Ollerenshaw JD, Griendling KK, et al: Adventitial cells do not contribute to neointimal mass after balloon angioplasty of the rat common carotid artery. Circulation 2001;104:1591-1593.

128. Wright DE, Wagers AJ, Gulati AP, et al: Physiological migration of hematopoietic stem and progenitor cells. Science 2001;294: 1933-196.

129. Orlic D, Kajstura J, Chimenti S, et al: Mobilized bone marrow cells repair the infarcted heart, improving function and survival. Proc Natl Acad Sci USA 2001;98:10344-10349.

130. Kaushal S, Amiel GE, Guleserian KJ, et al: Functional small-diameter neovessels created using endothelial progenitor cells expanded ex vivo. Nat Med 2001;7:1035-1040.

131. Zohlnhofer D, Richter T, Neumann F, et al: Transcriptome analysis reveals a role of interferon-gamma in human neointima formation. Mol Cell 2001;7:1059-1069.

132. Miyamoto T, Sasaguri Y, Sasaguri T, et al: Expression of stem cell factor in human aortic endothelial and smooth muscle cells. Atherosclerosis 1997;129:207-213.

133. Saiura A, Sata M, Hirata Y, et al: Circulating smooth muscle progenitor cells contribute to atherosclerosis. Nat Med 2001;7: 382-383.

134. Shimizu K, Sugiyama S, Aikawa M, et al: Host bone-marrow cells are a source of donor intimal smooth-muscle-like cells in murine aortic transplant arteriopathy. Nat Med 2001;7:738-741.

135. Sata M, Saiura A, Kunisato A, et al: Hematopoietic stem cells differentiate into vascular cells that participate in the pathogenesis of atherosclerosis. Nat Med 2002;8:403-409.

136. Vidal A, Koff A: Cell-cycle inhibitors: Three families united by a common cause. Gene 2000;247:1-15.

137. Pines J: Cyclin-dependent kinase inhibitors: The age of crystals. Biochim Biophys Acta 1997;1332:M39-42.

138. Sherr CJ: G1 phase progression: Cycling on cue. Cell 1994;79: 551-555.

139. Sherr CJ, Roberts JM: Inhibitors of mammalian G1 cyclin-dependent kinases. Genes Dev 1995;9:1149-1163.

140. Nakayama K, Ishida N, Shirane M, et al: Mice lacking p27(Kip1) display increased body size, multiple organ hyperplasia, retinal dysplasia, and pituitary tumors. Cell 1996;85:707-720.

141. Kiyokawa H, Kineman RD, Manova-Todorova KO, et al: Enhanced growth of mice lacking the cyclin-dependent kinase inhibitor function of p27(Kip1). Cell 1996;85:721-732.

142. Fero ML, Rivkin M, Tasch M, et al: A syndrome of multiorgan hyperplasia with features of gigantism, tumorigenesis, and female sterility in p27(Kip1)-deficient mice. Cell 1996;85:733-744.

143. Taya Y: RB kinases and RB-binding proteins: New points of view. Trends Biochem Sci 1997;22:14-17.

144. Weinberg RA: The retinoblastoma protein and cell cycle control. Cell 1995;81:323-330.

145. Nevins JR: E2F: A link between the Rb tumor suppressor protein and viral oncoproteins. Science 1992;258:424-429.

146. Dynlacht BD, Moberg K, Lees JA, et al: Specific regulation of E2F family members by cyclin-dependent kinases. Mol Cell Biol 1997;17:3867-3875.

147. Fan J, Bertino JR: Functional roles of E2F in cell cycle regulation. Oncogene 1997;14:1191-1200.

148. Harbour JW, Dean DC: The Rb/E2F pathway: Expanding roles and emerging paradigms. Genes Dev 2000;14:2393-2409.

149. DeGregori J, Kowalik T, Nevins JR: Cellular targets for activation by the E2F1 transcription factor include DNA synthesis- and G1/S-regulatory-genes. Mol Cell Biol 1995;15:4215-4224.

150. Fry CJ, Slansky JE, Farnham PJ: Position-dependent transcriptional regulation of the murine dihydrofolate reductase promoter by the E2F transactivation domain. Mol Cell Biol 1997; 17:1966-1976.

151. Koyama H, Raines EW, Bornfeldt KE, et al: Fibrillar collagen inhibits arterial smooth muscle proliferation through regulation of Cdk2 inhibitors. Cell 1996;87:1069-1078.

152. Weir L, Chen D, Pastore C, et al: Expression of gax, a growth arrest homeobox gene, is rapidly down-regulated in the rat carotid artery during the proliferative response to balloon injury. J Biol Chem 1995;270:5457-5461.

153. Braun-Dullaeus RC, Mann MJ, Seay U, et al: Cell cycle protein expression in vascular smooth muscle cells in vitro and in vivo is regulated through phosphatidylinositol 3-kinase and mammalian target of rapamycin. Arterioscler Thromb Vasc Biol 2001; 21:1152-1158.

154. Yang ZY, Simari RD, Perkins ND, et al: Role of the p21 cyclin-dependent kinase inhibitor in limiting intimal cell proliferation in response to arterial injury. Proc Natl Acad Sci USA 1996; 93:7905-7910.

155. Aoyagi M, Yamamoto M, Azuma H, et al: Expression of p53 protein and p53 gene transcripts in rabbit carotid arteries after balloon denudation. Histochem Cell Biol 1997;107:365-370.

156. Morishita R, Gibbons GH, Ellison KE, et al: Intimal hyperplasia after vascular injury is inhibited by antisense cdk 2 kinase oligonucleotides. J Clin Invest 1994;93:1458-1464.

157. Morishita R, Gibbons GH, Ellison KE, et al: Single intraluminal delivery of antisense cdc2 kinase and proliferating-cell nuclear antigen oligonucleotides results in chronic inhibition of neointimal hyperplasia. Proc Natl Acad Sci USA 1993;90: 8474-8478.

158. Abe J, Zhou W, Taguchi J, et al: Suppression of neointimal smooth muscle cell accumulation in vivo by antisense cdc2 and cdk2 oligonucleotides in rat carotid artery. Biochem Biophys Res Commun 1994;198:16-24.

159. Wei GL, Krasinski K, Kearney M, et al: Temporally and spatially coordinated expression of cell cycle regulatory factors after angioplasty. Circ Res 1997;80:418-426.

160. O'Brien ER, Alpers CE, Stewart DK, et al: Proliferation in primary and restenotic coronary atherectomy tissue: Implications for antiproliferative therapy. Circ Res 1993;73:223-231.

161. Gordon D, Reidy MA, Benditt EP, et al: Cell proliferation in human coronary arteries. Proc Natl Acad Sci USA 1990;87: 4600-4604.

162. Ciezki JP, Hafeli UO, Song P, et al: Parenchymal cell proliferation in coronary arteries after percutaneous transluminal coronary angioplasty: A human tissue bank study. Int J Radiat Oncol Biol Phys 1999;45:963-968.

163. Moreno PR, Palacios IF, Leon MN, et al: Histopathologic comparison of human coronary in-stent and post-balloon angioplasty restenotic tissue. Am J Cardiol 1999;84:462-466, A9.

164. O'Brien ER, Urieli-Shoval S, Garvin MR, et al: Replication in restenotic atherectomy tissue. Atherosclerosis 2000;152:117-126.

165. Simons M, Edelman ER, Rosenberg RD: Antisense proliferating cell nuclear antigen oligonucleotides inhibit intimal hyperplasia in a rat carotid artery injury model. J Clin Invest 1994;93: 2351-2356.

166. Morishita R, Gibbons GH, Kaneda Y, et al: Pharmacokinetics of antisense oligodeoxyribonucleotides (cyclin B1 and CDC 2 kinase) in the vessel wall in vivo: Enhanced therapeutic utility for restenosis by HVJ-liposome delivery. Gene 1994;149:13-19.

167. Chang MW, Barr E, Seltzer J, et al: Cytostatic gene therapy for vascular proliferative disorders with a constitutively active form of the retinoblastoma gene product. Science 1995;267: 518-522.

168. Claudio PP, Fratta L, Farina F, et al: Adenoviral RB2/p130 gene transfer inhibits smooth muscle cell proliferation and prevents restenosis after angioplasty. Circ Res 1999;85:1032-1039.

169. Chang MW, Barr E, Lu MM, et al: Adenovirus-mediated over-expression of the cyclin/cyclin-dependent kinase inhibitor, p21 inhibits vascular smooth muscle cell proliferation and neointima formation in the rat carotid artery model of balloon angioplasty. J Clin Invest 1995;96:2260-2268.

170. Chen D, Krasinski K, Sylvester A, et al: Downregulation of cyclin-dependent kinase 2 activity and cyclin A promoter activity in vascular smooth muscle cells by p27(KIP1), an inhibitor of neointima formation in the rat carotid artery. J Clin Invest 1997;99:2334-2341.

171. Yonemitsu Y, Kaneda Y, Tanaka S, et al: Transfer of wild-type p53 gene effectively inhibits vascular smooth muscle cell proliferation in vitro and in vivo. Circ Res 1998;82:147-156.

172. Mann MJ, Whittemore AD, Donaldson MC, et al: Ex-vivo gene therapy of human vascular bypass grafts with E2F decoy: The PREVENT single-centre, randomised, controlled, trial. Lancet 1999;354:1493-1498.

173. Maillard L, Van Belle E, Tio FO, et al: Effect of percutaneous adenovirus-mediated Gax gene delivery to the arterial wall in double-injured atheromatous stented rabbit iliac arteries. Gene Ther 2000;7:1353-1361.

174. Harrell RL, Rajanayagam S, Doanes AM, et al: Inhibition of vascular smooth muscle cell proliferation and neointimal accumulation by adenovirus-mediated gene transfer of cytosine deaminase. Circulation 1997;96:621-627.

175. Steg PG, Tahlil O, Aubailly N, et al: Reduction of restenosis after angioplasty in an atheromatous rabbit model by suicide gene therapy. Circulation 1997;96:408-411.

176. Luo Z, Sata M, Nguyen T, et al: Adenovirus-mediated delivery of fas ligand inhibits intimal hyperplasia after balloon injury in immunologically primed animals. Circulation 1999;99:1776-1779.

177. Luo Z, Garron T, Palasis M, et al: Enhancement of Fas ligand-induced inhibition of neointimal formation in rabbit femoral and iliac arteries by coexpression of p35. Hum Gene Ther 2001;12:2191-2202.

178. Jenkins GM, Crow MT, Bilato C, et al: Increased expression of membrane-type matrix metalloproteinase and preferential localization of matrix metalloproteinase-2 to the neointima of balloon-injured rat carotid arteries. Circulation 1998;97:82-90.

179. Feldman LJ, Mazighi M, Scheuble A, et al: Differential expression of matrix metalloproteinases after stent implantation and balloon angioplasty in the hypercholesterolemic rabbit. Circulation 2001;103:3117-3122.

180. Bendeck MP, Irvin C, Reidy MA: Inhibition of matrix metalloproteinase activity inhibits smooth muscle cell migration but not neointimal thickening after arterial injury. Circ Res 1996; 78:38-43.

181. Bendeck MP, Zempo N, Clowes AW, et al: Smooth muscle cell migration and matrix metalloproteinase expression after arterial injury in the rat. Circ Res 1994;75:539-545.

182. de Smet BJ, de Kleijn D, Hanemaaijer R, et al: Metalloproteinase inhibition reduces constrictive arterial remodeling after balloon angioplasty: A study in the atherosclerotic Yucatan micropig. Circulation 2000;101:2962-2967.

183. Sierevogel MJ, Pasterkamp G, Velema E, et al: Oral matrix metalloproteinase inhibition and arterial remodeling after balloon dilation: An intravascular ultrasound study in the pig. Circulation 2001;103:302-307.

184. Dollery CM, Humphries SE, McClelland A, et al: In vivo adenoviral gene transfer of TIMP-1 after vascular injury reduces neointimal formation. Ann NY Acad Sci 1999;878:742-743.

185. Wallner K, Sharifi BG, Shah PK, et al: Adventitial remodeling after angioplasty is associated with expression of tenascin mRNA by adventitial myofibroblasts. J Am Coll Cardiol 2001;37:655-661.

186. Strauss BH, Chisholm RJ, Keeley FW, et al: Extracellular matrix remodeling after balloon angioplasty injury in a rabbit model of restenosis. Circ Res 1994;75:650-658.

187. Hunter T: Oncoprotein networks. Cell 1997;88:333-346.

188. Kelly K, Cochran BH, Stiles CD, et al: Cell-specific regulation of the c-myc gene by lymphocyte mitogens and platelet-derived growth factor. Cell 1983;35:603-610.

189. Miano JM, Tota RR, Vlasic N, et al: Early proto-oncogene expression in rat aortic smooth muscle cells following endothelial removal. Am J Pathol 1990;137:761-765.

190. Bauters C, de Groote P, Adamantidis M, et al: Proto-oncogene expression in rabbit aorta after wall injury: First marker of the cellular process leading to restenosis after angioplasty? Eur Heart J 1992;13:556-559.

191. Shichiri M, Hanson KD, Sedivy JM: Effects of c-myc expression on proliferation, quiescence, and the G0 to G1 transition in non-transformed cells. Cell Growth Differ 1993;4:93-104.

192. Steiner P, Philipp A, Lukas J, et al: Identification of a Myc-dependent step during the formation of active G1 cyclin-cdk complexes. EMBO J 1995;14:4814-4826.

193. Daksis JI, Lu RY, Facchini LM, et al: Myc induces cyclin D1 expression in the absence of de novo protein synthesis and links mitogen-stimulated signal transduction to the cell cycle. Oncogene 1994;9:3635-3645.

194. Hanson KD, Shichiri M, Follansbee MR, et al: Effects of c-myc expression on cell cycle progression. Mol Cell Biol 1994;14:5748-5755.

195. Shi Y, Fard A, Galeo A, et al: Transcatheter delivery of c-myc antisense oligomers reduces neointimal formation in a porcine model of coronary artery balloon injury. Circulation 1994;90:944-951.

196. Simons M, Edelman ER, DeKeyser JL, et al: Antisense c-myb oligonucleotides inhibit intimal arterial smooth muscle cell accumulation in vivo. Nature 1992;359:67-70.

197. Kutryk MJ, Foley DP, van den Brand M, et al: Local intracoronary administration of antisense oligonucleotide against c-myc for the prevention of in-stent restenosis: Results of the randomized investigation by the Thoraxcenter of antisense DNA using local delivery and IVUS after coronary stenting (ITALICS) trial. J Am Coll Cardiol 2002;39:281-287.

198. Phuchareon J, Tokuhisa T: Deregulated c-Fos/AP-1 modulates expression of the cyclin and the cdk gene in splenic B cells stimulated with lipopolysaccharide. Cancer Lett 1995;92:203-208.

199. Miano JM, Vlasic N, Tota RR, et al: Smooth muscle cell immediate-early gene and growth factor activation follows vascular injury: A putative in vivo mechanism for autocrine growth. Arterioscler Thromb 1993;13:211-219.

200. Bourne HR, Sanders DA, McCormick F: The GTPase superfamily: Conserved structure and molecular mechanism. Nature 1991;349:117-127.

201. Boguski MS, McCormick F: Proteins regulating Ras and its relatives. Nature 1993;366:643-654.

202. Feramisco JR, Gross M, Kamata T, et al: Microinjection of the oncogene form of the human H-ras (T-24) protein results in rapid proliferation of quiescent cells. Cell 1984;38:109-117.

203. Stacey DW, Kung HF: Transformation of NIH 3T3 cells by microinjection of Ha-ras p21 protein. Nature 1984;310:508-511.

204. Thomas SM, DeMarco M, D'Arcangelo G, et al: Ras is essential for nerve growth factor- and phorbol ester-induced tyrosine phosphorylation of MAP kinases. Cell 1992;68:1031-1040.

205. Leone G, DeGregori J, Sears R, et al: Myc and Ras collaborate in inducing accumulation of active cyclin E/Cdk2 and E2F. Nature 1997;387:422-426.

206. Liu JJ, Chao JR, Jiang MC, et al: Ras transformation results in an elevated level of cyclin D1 and acceleration of G1 progression in NIH 3T3 cells. Mol Cell Biol 1995;15:3654-3663.

207. Dobrowolski S, Harter M, Stacey DW: Cellular ras activity is required for passage through multiple points of the G0/G1 phase in BALB/c 3T3 cells. Mol Cell Biol 1994;14:5441-5449.

208. Jin G, Chieh-Hsi Wu J, Li YS, et al: Effects of active and negative mutants of Ras on rat arterial neointima formation. J Surg Res 2000;94:124-132.

209. Wu CH, Lin CS, Hung JS, et al: Inhibition of neointimal formation in porcine coronary artery by a Ras mutant. J Surg Res 2001;99:100-106.

210. Hill CS, Treisman R: Transcriptional regulation by extracellular signals: Mechanisms and specificity. Cell 1995;80:199-211.

211. Xu Q, Liu Y, Gorospe M, et al: Acute hypertension activates mitogen-activated protein kinases in arterial wall. J Clin Invest 1996;97:508-514.

212. Mii S, Khalil RA, Morgan KG, et al: Mitogen-activated protein kinase and proliferation of human vascular smooth muscle cells. Am J Physiol 1996;270:H142-150.

213. Davis RJ: The mitogen-activated protein kinase signal transduction pathway. J Biol Chem 1993;268:14553-14556.

214. Kim S, Izumi Y, Yano M, et al: Angiotensin blockade inhibits activation of mitogen-activated protein kinases in rat balloon-injured artery. Circulation 1998;97:1731-1737.

215. Ferns GA, Avades TY: The mechanisms of coronary restenosis: Insights from experimental models. Int J Exp Pathol 2000;81:63-88.

216. Chamberlain J, Gunn J, Francis SE, et al: TGFbeta is active, and correlates with activators of TGFbeta, following porcine coronary angioplasty. Cardiovasc Res 2001;50:125-136.

217. Chin BY, Mohsenin A, Li SX, et al: Stimulation of pro-alpha(1)(I) collagen by TGF-beta(1) in mesangial cells: Role of the p38 MAPK pathway. Am J Physiol Renal Physiol 2001;280:F495-504.

218. Ju H, Nerurkar S, Sauermelch CF, et al: Sustained activation of p38 mitogen-activated protein kinase contributes to the vascular response to injury. J Pharmacol Exp Ther 2002;301:15-20.

219. Rakugi H, Kim DK, Krieger JE, et al: Induction of angiotensin converting enzyme in the neointima after vascular injury. Possible role in restenosis. J Clin Invest 1994;93:339-346.

220. Ohishi M, Ueda M, Rakugi H, et al: Upregulation of angiotensin-converting enzyme during the healing process after injury at the site of percutaneous transluminal coronary angioplasty in humans. Circulation 1997;96:3328-3337.

221. Daemen MJ, Lombardi DM, Bosman FT, et al: Angiotensin II induces smooth muscle cell proliferation in the normal and injured rat arterial wall. Circ Res 1991;68:450-456.

222. Dzau VJ, Gibbons GH, Pratt RE: Molecular mechanisms of vascular renin-angiotensin system in myointimal hyperplasia. Hypertension 1991;18:II100-105.

223. Powell JS, Clozel JP, Muller RK, et al: Inhibitors of angiotensin-converting enzyme prevent myointimal proliferation after vascular injury. Science 1989;245:186-188.

224. Wong J, Rauhoft C, Dilley RJ, et al: Angiotensin-converting enzyme inhibition abolishes medial smooth muscle PDGF-AB biosynthesis and attenuates cell proliferation in injured carotid arteries: Relationships to neointima formation. Circulation 1997;96:1631-1640.

225. Abe J, Deguchi J, Matsumoto T, et al: Stimulated activation of platelet-derived growth factor receptor in vivo in balloon-injured arteries: A link between angiotensin II and intimal thickening. Circulation 1997;96:1906-1913.

226. Faxon DP: Effect of high dose angiotensin-converting enzyme inhibition on restenosis: Final results of the MARCATOR Study, a multicenter, double-blind, placebo-controlled trial of cilazapril. The Multicenter American Research Trial With Cilazapril After Angioplasty to Prevent Transluminal Coronary Obstruction and Restenosis (MARCATOR) Study Group. J Am Coll Cardiol 1995;25:362-369.

227. Jorgensen E, Kelbaek H, Helqvist S, et al: Predictors of coronary in-stent restenosis: Importance of angiotensin-converting enzyme gene polymorphism and treatment with angiotensin-converting enzyme inhibitors. J Am Coll Cardiol 2001;38:1434-1439.

228. Iwashina M, Shichiri M, Marumo F, et al: Transfection of inducible nitric oxide synthase gene causes apoptosis in vascular smooth muscle cells. Circulation 1998;98:1212-1218.

229. Garg UC, Hassid A: Nitric oxide-generating vasodilators and 8-bromo-cyclic guanosine monophosphate inhibit mitogenesis and proliferation of cultured rat vascular smooth muscle cells. J Clin Invest 1989;83:1774-1777.

230. Yao SK, Ober JC, Krishnaswami A, et al: Endogenous nitric oxide protects against platelet aggregation and cyclic flow variations in stenosed and endothelium-injured arteries. Circulation 1992;86:1302-1309.

231. Wang BY, Candipan RC, Arjomandi M, et al: Arginine restores nitric oxide activity and inhibits monocyte accumulation after vascular injury in hypercholesterolemic rabbits. J Am Coll Cardiol 1996; 28:1573-1579.

232. Douglas SA, Louden C, Vickery-Clark LM, et al: A role for endogenous endothelin-1 in neointimal formation after rat carotid artery balloon angioplasty: Protective effects of the novel nonpeptide endothelin receptor antagonist SB 209670. Circ Res 1994;75:190-197.

233. Minamino T, Kurihara H, Takahashi M, et al: Endothelin-converting enzyme expression in the rat vascular injury model and human coronary atherosclerosis. Circulation 1997;95:221-230.

234. Speir E, Modali R, Huang ES, et al: Potential role of human cytomegalovirus and p53 interaction in coronary restenosis. Science 1994;265:391-394.

235. Zhou YF, Leon MB, Waclawiw MA, et al: Association between prior cytomegalovirus infection and the risk of restenosis after coronary atherectomy. N Engl J Med 1996;335:624-630.

236. Schiele F, Batur MK, Seronde MF, et al: Cytomegalovirus, Chlamydia pneumoniae, and Helicobacter pylori IgG antibodies and restenosis after stent implantation: An angiographic and intravascular ultrasound study. Heart 2001;85:304-311.

237. Carlsson J, Miketic S, Brom J, et al: Prior cytomegalovirus, Chlamydia pneumoniae or Helicobacter pylori infection and the risk of restenosis after percutaneous transluminal coronary angioplasty. Int J Cardiol 2000;73:165-171.

238. Manegold C, Alwazzeh M, Jablonowski H, et al: Prior cytomegalovirus infection and the risk of restenosis after percutaneous transluminal coronary balloon angioplasty. Circulation 1999;99:1290-1294.

239. Casterella PJ, Teirstein PS: Prevention of coronary restenosis. Cardiol Rev 1999;7:219-231.

240. Tardif JC, Cote G, Lesperance J, et al: Probucol and multivitamins in the prevention of restenosis after coronary angioplasty: Multivitamins and Probucol Study Group. N Engl J Med 1997;337:365-372.

241. Takagi T, Akasaka T, Yamamuro A, et al: Troglitazone reduces neointimal tissue proliferation after coronary stent implantation in patients with non-insulin dependent diabetes mellitus: A serial intravascular ultrasound study. J Am Coll Cardiol 2000;36:1529-1535.

242. Tamai H, Katoh K, Yamaguchi T, et al: The impact of tranilast on restenosis after coronary angioplasty: The Second Tranilast Restenosis Following Angioplasty Trial (TREAT-2). Am Heart J 2002;143:506-513.

243. Vrolix MC, Legrand VM, Reiber JH, et al: Heparin-coated Wiktor stents in human coronary arteries (MENTOR trial). MENTOR Trial Investigators. Am J Cardiol 2000;86:385-389.

244. Wohrle J, Al-Khayer E, Grotzinger U, et al: Comparison of the heparin coated vs the uncoated Jostent: No influence on restenosis or clinical outcome. Eur Heart J 2001;22:1808-1816.

245. Haude M, Konorza TF, Kalnins U, et al: Heparin-coated stent placement for the treatment of stenoses in small coronary arteries of symptomatic patients. Circulation 2003;107:1265-1270.

246. Rubin P, Soni A, Williams JP: The molecular and cellular biologic basis for the radiation treatment of benign proliferative diseases. Semin Radiat Oncol 1999;9:203-214.

247. Levine AJ: p53, the cellular gatekeeper for growth and division. Cell 1997;88:323-331.

248. el-Deiry WS, Tokino T, Velculescu VE, et al: WAF1, a potential mediator of p53 tumor suppression. Cell 1993;75:817-825.

249. Luo Y, Hurwitz J, Massague J: Cell-cycle inhibition by independent CDK and PCNA binding domains in p21Cip1. Nature 1995;375:159-161.

250. Knibiehler M, Goubin F, Escalas N, et al: Interaction studies between the p21Cip1/Waf1 cyclin-dependent kinase inhibitor and proliferating cell nuclear antigen (PCNA) by surface plasmon resonance. FEBS Lett 1996;391:66-70.

251. Waga S, Hannon GJ, Beach D, et al: The p21 inhibitor of cyclin-dependent kinases controls DNA replication by interaction with PCNA. Nature 1994;369:574-578.

252. King SB 3rd, Williams DO, Chougule P, et al: Endovascular beta-radiation to reduce restenosis after coronary balloon angioplasty: Results of the beta energy restenosis trial (BERT). Circulation 1998;97:2025-2030.

253. Waksman R, Rodriguez JC, Robinson KA, et al: Effect of intravascular irradiation on cell proliferation, apoptosis, and vascular remodeling after balloon overstretch injury of porcine coronary arteries. Circulation 1997;96:1944-1952.

254. Leon MB, Teirstein PS, Moses JW, et al: Localized intracoronary gamma-radiation therapy to inhibit the recurrence of restenosis after stenting. N Engl J Med 2001;344:250-256.

255. Waksman R, White RL, Chan RC, et al: Intracoronary gamma-radiation therapy after angioplasty inhibits recurrence in patients with in-stent restenosis. Circulation 2000;101: 2165-2171.

256. Waksman R, Bhargava B, White L, et al: Intracoronary beta-radiation therapy inhibits recurrence of in-stent restenosis. Circulation 2000;101:1895-1898.

257. Waksman R, Raizner AE, Yeung AC, et al: Use of localised intracoronary beta radiation in treatment of in-stent restenosis: The INHIBIT randomised controlled trial. Lancet 2002;359:551-557.

258. Teirstein PS, Massullo V, Jani S, et al: Catheter-based radiotherapy to inhibit restenosis after coronary stenting. N Engl J Med 1997;336:1697-1703.

259. Teirstein PS, Massullo V, Jani S, et al: Three-year clinical and angiographic follow-up after intracoronary radiation: Results of a randomized clinical trial. Circulation 2000;101:360-365.

260. Kuntz RE, Baim DS: Prevention of coronary restenosis: The evolving evidence base for radiation therapy. Circulation 2000;101: 2130-2133.

261. Kay IP, Wardeh AJ, Kozuma K, et al: Radioactive stents delay but do not prevent in-stent neointimal hyperplasia. Circulation 2001; 103:14-17.

262. Condado JA, Waksman R, Gurdiel O, et al: Long-term angiographic and clinical outcome after percutaneous transluminal coronary angioplasty and intracoronary radiation therapy in humans. Circulation 1997;96:727-732.

263. Vandergoten P, Brosens M, Benit E: Coronary aneurysm five months after intracoronary beta-irradiation. Acta Cardiol 2000;55:313-315.

264. Sheppard R, Eisenberg MJ: Intracoronary radiotherapy for restenosis. N Engl J Med 2001;344:295-297.

265. Sehgal SN: Rapamune (Sirolimus, rapamycin): An overview and mechanism of action. Ther Drug Monit 1995;17:660-665.

266. Regar E, Sianos G, Serruys PW: Stent development and local drug delivery. Br Med Bull 2001;59:227-248.

267. Marx SO, Jayaraman T, Go LO, et al: Rapamycin-FKBP inhibits cell cycle regulators of proliferation in vascular smooth muscle cells. Circ Res 1995;76:412-417.

268. Poon M, Marx SO, Gallo R, et al: Rapamycin inhibits vascular smooth muscle cell migration. J Clin Invest 1996;98:2277-2283.

269. Gregory CR, Huie P, Billingham ME, et al: Rapamycin inhibits arterial intimal thickening caused by both alloimmune and mechanical injury: Its effect on cellular, growth factor, and cytokine response in injured vessels. Transplantation 1993;55:1409-1418.

270. Gregory CR, Huang X, Pratt RE, et al: Treatment with rapamycin and mycophenolic acid reduces arterial intimal thickening produced by mechanical injury and allows endothelial replacement. Transplantation 1995;59:655-661.

271. Poston RS, Billingham M, Hoyt EG, et al: Rapamycin reverses chronic graft vascular disease in a novel cardiac allograft model. Circulation 1999;100:67-74.

272. Gallo R, Padurean A, Jayaraman T, et al: Inhibition of intimal thickening after balloon angioplasty in porcine coronary arteries by targeting regulators of the cell cycle. Circulation 1999;99: 2164-2170.

273. Suzuki T, Kopia G, Hayashi S, et al: Stent-based delivery of sirolimus reduces neointimal formation in a porcine coronary model. Circulation 2001;104:1188-1193.

274. Sousa JE, Costa MA, Abizaid A, et al: Lack of neointimal proliferation after implantation of sirolimus-coated stents in human coronary arteries: A quantitative coronary angiography and three-dimensional intravascular ultrasound study. Circulation 2001; 103:192-195.

275. Sousa JE, Costa MA, Abizaid AC, et al: Sustained suppression of neointimal proliferation by sirolimus-eluting stents: One-year angiographic and intravascular ultrasound follow-up. Circulation 2001;104:2007-2011.

276. Morice MC, Serruys PW, Sousa JE, et al: A randomized comparison of a sirolimus-eluting stent with a standard stent for coronary revascularization. N Engl J Med 2002;346:1773-1780.

277. Moses JW, Leon MB, Popma JJ, et al: Sirolimus-eluting stents versus standard stents in patients with stenosis in a native coronary artery (SIRIUS). N Engl J Med 2003;349:1315-23.

278. Schofer J, Schluter M, Gershlick AH, et al: Sirolimus-eluting stents for treatment of patients with long atherosclerotic lesions in small coronary arteries: double-blind, randomised controlled trial (E-SIRIUS). Lancet 2003;362:1093-1099.

279. Schiff PB, Fant J, Horwitz SB: Promotion of microtubule assembly in vitro by Taxol. Nature 1979;277:665-667.

280. Rowinsky EK, Donehower RC: Paclitaxel (Taxol). N Engl J Med 1995;332:1004-1014.

281. Sollott SJ, Cheng L, Pauly RR, et al: Taxol inhibits neointimal smooth muscle cell accumulation after angioplasty in the rat. J Clin Invest 1995;95:1869-1876.

282. Axel DI, Kunert W, Goggelmann C, et al: Paclitaxel inhibits arterial smooth muscle cell proliferation and migration in vitro and in vivo using local drug delivery. Circulation 1997;96:636-645.

283. Herdeg C, Oberhoff M, Baumbach A, et al: Local paclitaxel delivery for the prevention of restenosis: Biological effects and efficacy in vivo. J Am Coll Cardiol 2000;35:1969-1976.

284. Heldman AW, Cheng L, Jenkins GM, et al: Paclitaxel stent coating inhibits neointimal hyperplasia at 4 weeks in a porcine model of coronary restenosis. Circulation 2001;103:2289-2295.

285. Grube E, Silber S, Hauptmann KE, et al: TAXUS I: six- and twelve-month results from a randomized, double-blind trial on a slow-release paclitaxel-eluting stent for de novo coronary lesions. Circulation 2003;107:38-42.

286. Park SJ, Shim WH, Ho DS, et al: A paclitaxel-eluting stent for the prevention of coronary restenosis. N Engl J Med 2003;348: 1537-1545.

287. Colombo A, Drzewiecki J, Banning A, et al: Randomized study to assess the effectiveness of slow- and moderate-release polymer-based paclitaxel-eluting stents for coronary artery lesions. Circulation 2003;108:788.

288. Tamai H, Igaki K, Kyo E, et al: Initial and 6-month results of biodegradable poly-l-lactic acid coronary stents in humans. Circulation 2000;102:399-404.

289. Yamawaki T, Shimokawa H, Kozai T, et al: Intramural delivery of a specific tyrosine kinase inhibitor with biodegradable stent suppresses the restenotic changes of the coronary artery in pigs in vivo. J Am Coll Cardiol 1998;32:780-786.

290. Alt E, Haehnel I, Beilharz C, et al: Inhibition of neointima formation after experimental coronary artery stenting: A new biodegradable stent coating releasing hirudin and the prostacyclin analogue iloprost. Circulation 2000;101:1453-1458.

## EDITOR'S CHOICE

Indolfi C, Mongiardo A, Curcio A, Torella D: Molecular mechanisms of in-stent restenosis and approach to therapy with eluting stents. Trends Cardiovasc Med 2003;13:142-148.

*Nice review of a rapidly expanding area at the intersection of biologics and devices.*

Morice MC, Serruys PW, Sousa JE, et al: A randomized comparison of a sirolimus-eluting stent with a standard stent for coronary revascularization. N Engl J Med 2002;346:1773-1780.

*Coated stents show promise, suggest that crossover into drug elution for conditions aside from in-stent restenosis maybe in the offing.*

Park SJ, Shim WH, Ho DS, et al: A paclitaxel-eluting stent for the prevention of coronary restenosis. N Engl J Med 2003;348:1537-1545.

*Second generation stents on the horizon, likely to be a wide variety in the coming years, raises the prospects of head-to-head clinical evaluations down the road.*

# Molecular Basis for the Potential Use of NMDA Receptor Open-Channel Blockers in the Treatment of Cerebral Ischemia and Other Brain Insults

*Stuart A. Lipton*
*Stephen F. Heinemann*

Cerebral ischemia (stroke) is the third leading cause of death in the United States. Excitotoxicity (excessive exposure to the neurotransmitter glutamate) has been implicated as one of the factors contributing to neuronal injury and death during the ischemic process. This type of excitotoxic cell death is due, at least in part, to excessive activation of $N$-methyl-D-aspartate (NMDA)-type glutamate receptors and hence excessive $Ca^{2+}$ influx through the receptor's associated ion channel. Physiologic NMDA receptor activity, however, is also essential for normal neuronal function. This means that potential neuroprotective agents that block virtually all NMDA receptor activity will very likely have unacceptable clinical side effects. For this reason many NMDA receptor antagonists have disappointingly failed advanced clinical trials for stroke. In contrast, studies in our laboratory have shown that the adamantine derivative, memantine, blocks only excessive NMDA receptor activity without disrupting normal activity. Memantine does this through its action as an open-channel blocker; it increasingly enters the receptor-associated ion channel when it is excessively open, and, most importantly, its off-rate from the channel is relatively fast so that it does not substantially interfere with normal synaptic transmission. Past clinical use for other indications has demonstrated that memantine is safe, and it has recently been approved in Europe for the treatment of Alzheimer's disease and vascular dementia, and for Alzheimer's disease in the U.S. Clinical studies of the safety and efficacy of memantine for other neurologic disorders, including cerebral ischemia, are currently underway. A series of second-generation memantine derivatives are currently in development and may prove to have even greater neuroprotective properties than does memantine. The NMDA receptor has other modulatory sites in addition to its ion channel that potentially could also be used for clinical intervention in the future.

The focus of stroke therapy today is on "clot busting" with the FDA-approved tissue plasminogen activator (t-PA). This is a proven method for treating and potentially ameliorating stroke damage. It is well known, however, that stroke is also a neurodegenerative disease in which neurons die. Glutamate is the major excitatory neurotransmitter in the brain. There are three classes of glutamate-gated ion channels, known as AMPA, kainate, and NMDA receptors. The ion channels coupled to classical NMDA receptors are the most permeable to $Ca^{2+}$. Excessive activation of any of these receptors, but the NMDA receptor in particular, leads to production of damaging free radicals and other enzymatic processes that contribute to cell death.[1,2] With the disruption of energy metabolism during a stroke, glutamate is not cleared properly and may even be inappropriately released. During periods of ischemia and in many neurodegenerative diseases, excessive stimulation of glutamate receptors is thought to occur because of increasing levels of glutamate that leak from damaged cells or because of neuronal membrane depolarization as cells become injured, thus relieving the usual voltage-dependent block of NMDA receptors by magnesium ions. These neurodegenerative diseases, including Alzheimer's disease, Parkinson's disease, Huntington's disease, HIV-associated dementia, multiple sclerosis, amyotrophic lateral sclerosis, and glaucoma, are caused by different mechanisms but may share a final common pathway to neuronal injury because of the overstimulation of glutamate receptors, especially of the NMDA subtype.[1] Hence, NMDA receptor antagonists could potentially be of therapeutic benefit in a number of neurologic disorders, including stroke and dementia. NMDA receptors are made up of different subunits: NR1 (whose presence is mandatory), NR2A-D, and in some cases NR3A or B subunits. The receptor is probably composed of a tetramer of these subunits. The subunit composition determines the pharmacology and other parameters of the receptor-ion channel complex. Alternative splicing of some subunits, such as NR1, further contributes to the pharmacologic properties of the receptor. The subunits are differentially expressed both regionally in the brain and temporally during development. For this reason some authorities have suggested developing antagonists selective for particular subunits such as NR2B, which is present in the forebrain.[3]

# THE QUEST FOR NMDA RECEPTOR ANTAGONISTS

Excitotoxicity is a particularly attractive target for neuroprotective efforts because it is implicated in the pathophysiology of a wide variety of acute and chronic neurodegenerative disorders.[1] The challenge facing those who are trying to devise strategies for combating excitotoxicity is that the same processes that, in excess, lead to excitotoxic cell death are, at lower levels, absolutely critical for normal neuronal function. Until recently, all of the drugs that showed the most promise as excitotoxicity blockers also blocked normal neural function and consequently had severe and unacceptable side effects, so clinical trials for stroke and traumatic brain injury failed.[4-6]

Recently, however, the well-tolerated, but under-appreciated drug memantine has been rediscovered to be not only capable of blocking excitotoxic cell death[7] but, most importantly, also capable of doing it in a safe, nontoxic manner.[8-11] Memantine is currently being used in Europe for the treatment of Parkinson's disease and spasticity, was recently approved in Europe for the treatment of Alzheimer's disease and vascular dementia, and in the U.S. for the treatment of moderate to severe Alzheimer's disease.[12,13] It is also under investigation as a potential treatment for stroke, glaucoma, and other neurodegenerative disorders, including HIV-associated dementia and neuropathic pain.

This chapter provides a brief primer on excitotoxicity as a promising target of neuroprotective strategies and presents a scientific and clinical overview of the excitotoxicity blocker memantine. Some preliminary information on second-generation memantine derivatives, termed NitroMemantines, is also provided.

# EXCITOTOXICITY

## Definition and Clinical Relevance

The ability of the nervous system to rapidly convey sensory information and complex motor commands from one part of the body to another and to form thoughts and memories is largely dependent on glutamate, a powerful excitatory neurotransmitter. There are other excitatory neurotransmitters in the brain, but glutamate is the most common and widely distributed. Most neurons contain high concentrations of glutamate ($\sim 10$ mM)[1]; after sequestration inside synaptic vesicles, glutamate is released for a very brief time (milliseconds) to communicate with other neurons via synaptic endings. Because glutamate is so powerful, however, its presence in excessive amounts or for excessive periods of time can literally excite cells to death.

This phenomenon was first documented when Lucas and Newhouse[14] observed that subcutaneously injected glutamate selectively damaged the inner layer of the retina (primarily representing the retinal ganglion cells). John Olney later coined the term "excitotoxicity" to describe this phenomenon.[15,16]

Unfortunately, a variety of naturally occurring conditions can lead to the excessive release of glutamate within the nervous system and, thus, excitotoxic cell death. When the nervous system suffers a severe mechanical insult, as in head or spinal cord injury, large amounts of glutamate are released from injured cells. These high levels of glutamate wash over thousands of nearby cells that had survived the original trauma, causing them to depolarize, swell, lyse, and die. The lysing cells release more glutamate leading to a cascade of autodestructive events and progressive cell death that can continue for hours or even days after the original injury. A similar phenomenon occurs in stroke; the ischemic event deprives many neurons of the energy they need to maintain ionic homeostasis, causing them to depolarize, lyse, die, and propagate the same type of autodestructive events that are seen in traumatic injury.[1,17] This acute form of cell death occurs by a necrotic-like mechanism, although a slower component leading to an apoptotic-like death can also be present (see later).

A slower, more subtle form of excitotoxicity is implicated in a variety of slowly progressing neurodegenerative disorders and in the penumbra (outskirts) of stroke damage. In disorders such as Huntington's disease, Parkinson's disease, Alzheimer's disease, multiple sclerosis, HIV-associated dementia, amyotrophic lateral sclerosis (ALS or Lou Gehrig's disease), and glaucoma it is hypothesized that chronic exposure to moderately elevated glutamate concentrations or glutamate receptor hyperactivity for longer periods than occur during normal neurotransmission trigger cellular processes in neurons that eventually lead to apoptotic-like cell death, a form of cell death related to the programmed cell death that occurs during normal development.[2,18-24]

Importantly, elevations in extracellular glutamate are not necessary to invoke an excitotoxic mechanism. Excitotoxicity can come into play even with normal levels of glutamate if NMDA receptor activity is increased, for example, when neurons are injured and, thus, become depolarized (more positively charged); this condition relieves the normal block of the ion channel by $Mg^{2+}$ and, thus, abnormally increases NMDA receptor activity.[25]

Increased activity of the enzyme nitric oxide synthase (NOS) is associated with excitotoxic cell death. The neuronal isoform of the enzyme is physically tethered to the NMDA receptor and activated by $Ca^{2+}$ influx via the receptor-associated ion channel, and increased levels of nitric oxide (NO) have also been detected in animal models of stroke and neurodegenerative diseases.

## Pathophysiology of Excitotoxicity: Role of the NMDA Receptor

Apoptotic-like excitotoxicity is caused at least in part by excessive stimulation of the NMDA subtype of glutamate receptor (Fig. 26-1). When activated, the NMDA receptor opens a channel that allows $Ca^{2+}$ (and other cations) to move into the cell. In some areas of the brain, this activity is important for long-term potentiation, which is thought to be a cellular and electrophysiologic correlate of learning and memory formation. Under normal conditions of synaptic transmission, the NMDA-receptor channel is blocked by $Mg^{2+}$ sitting in the channel and only activated for brief periods. Under pathologic conditions,

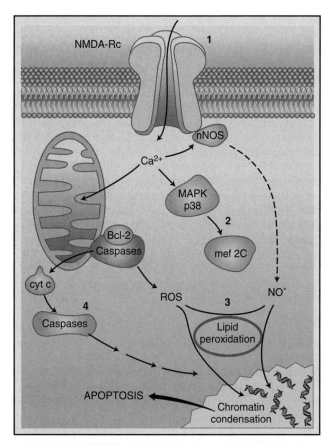

**FIGURE 26-1.** Schematic model of the link of excessive NMDA receptor activity to apoptotic pathways. Steps to cell death include: (1) NMDA receptor (NMDA-Rc) hyperactivation; (2) activation of the p38 MAPK—MEF2C (transcription factor) pathway. MEF2 is subsequently cleaved by caspases to form an endogenous dominant-interfering form that contributes to neuronal cell death; (3) toxic effects of free radicals such as NO and reactive oxygen species (ROS); and (4) activation of apoptosis-inducing enzymes including caspases. Cyt c, cytochrome c; nNOS, nitric oxide synthase. (See color plate.) *(From Okamoto S-i, Li Z, Ju C, Schölzke MN, et al: Dominant-interfering forms of MEF2 generated by caspase cleavage contribute to NMDA-induced neuronal apoptosis. Proc Natl Acad Sci USA 2002;99:3974-3979.)*

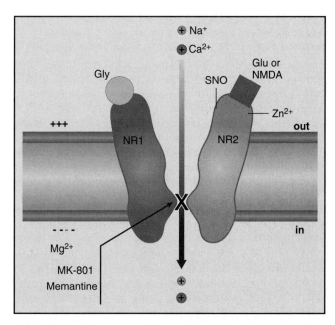

**FIGURE 26-2.** Model of the NMDA receptor with important binding and modulatory sites. Glu or NMDA, glutamate or NMDA binding site; Gly, glycine binding site; NR1, NMDA receptor subunit 1; NR2, NMDA receptor subunit 2A; SNO, cysteine sulfhydryl group with which NO species reacts; X, $Mg^{2+}$, MK-801, and memantine binding sites within the ion channel; $Zn^{2+}$, zinc binding site.

however, overactivation of the receptor causes an excessive amount of $Ca^{2+}$ influx into the nerve cell, which then triggers a variety of processes that can lead to necrosis or apoptosis. The latter processes include $Ca^{2+}$ overload of mitochondria, resulting in oxygen free radical formation and activation of caspases; $Ca^{2+}$-dependent activation of neuronal NOS, leading to increased NO production and formation of toxic peroxynitrite ($ONOO^-$); and stimulation of mitogen-activated protein kinase p38 (MAPK p38), which activates transcription factors that can go into the nucleus and influence neuronal injury and apoptosis.[18,26-32]

As mentioned previously, conventional NMDA receptors consist of two subunits (NR1 and NR2A-D) and more rarely NR3A or B subunits. There are binding sites for glutamate, the endogenous agonist, and glycine, which is required as a coagonist for receptor activation[33] (Fig. 26-2). NMDA is not thought to be an endogenous substance in the body; it is an experimental tool that is highly selective for this subtype of glutamate receptors

and, therefore, these receptors were named after NMDA. When glutamate and glycine bind, the NMDA-receptor channel opens and, if the cell is depolarized to remove $Mg^{2+}$ block, there is an influx of $Ca^{2+}$ and $Na^+$ into the cell, the amount of which can be altered by higher levels of agonists and by substances binding to one of the modulatory sites on the receptor. The two modulatory sites that are most relevant to this review are the $Mg^{2+}$ site within the ion channel and an S-nitrosylation site located toward the N-terminus (and hence extracellular region) of the receptor. (One should note that S-nitrosylation reactions represent transfer of NO to a thiol or sulfhydryl group [-SH] of a critical cysteine residue. This reaction modulates protein function, in this case a decrease in the activity of the NMDA receptor.) Each of these sites can be considered as targets for therapeutic intervention to block excitotoxicity, as explained later. Moreover, other modulatory sites also exist on the NMDA receptor and may prove to be of therapeutic value. These include binding sites for $Zn^{2+}$, polyamines, the drug ifenprodil (the endogenous ligand remains unknown), and a pH (i.e., proton)-sensitive site.[34] In addition, three pairs of cysteine residues can modulate channel function by virtue of their redox sensitivity.[35]

To be clinically acceptable, an antiexcitotoxicity therapy must block excessive activation of the NMDA receptor while leaving normal function relatively intact. Drugs that simply compete with glutamate or glycine at the agonist binding sites block normal function and, therefore, do not meet this requirement. These drugs failed in clinical trials because of side effects (drowsiness, hallucinations, and even coma).[1,8,12,36-40] Competitive antagonists compete one-to-one with the agonist (glutamate or glycine) and block healthy areas of the brain (where lower, more physiologic levels of these agonists exist) before they can affect pathologic areas (where agonist levels are rising). Thus, such drugs preferentially block normal activity and most likely would be displaced from the receptor by the high concentrations of glutamate that can exist under excitotoxic conditions.

The NMDA receptor can be thought of like a television set. The agonist sites are like the on and off switch of the television. Drugs that block these sites cut off all normal NMDA receptor function. Investigators need to find the equivalent of the volume control (or in biophysical terms, the gain) of the NMDA receptor. Then, when excessive $Ca^{2+}$ fluxes through the NMDA receptor-associated ion channel, one could simply turn down the "volume" of the $Ca^{2+}$ flux toward normal. A blocker that acts at the $Mg^{2+}$ site within the channel would act in such a manner. However, in the case of $Mg^{2+}$ itself, the block is too ephemeral, a so-called flickery block, and the cell continues to depolarize until the $Mg^{2+}$ block is totally relieved. Hence, in most cases $Mg^{2+}$ does not effectively block excessive $Ca^{2+}$ influx to the degree needed to prevent neurotoxicity. If a channel blocker binds too tightly or works too well at low levels of receptor activation, it will block normal and excessive activation and be clinically unacceptable. Following the television set analogy, turning the volume all the way down is as bad as turning off the on and off switch in terms of normal functioning of the television. This is the case with MK-801; it is a very good excitotoxicity blocker, but because its "dwell time" in the ion channel is so long (reflecting its slow off rate) because of its high affinity for the $Mg^{2+}$ site, it also blocks critical normal functions. A human taking MK-801 not only would become drowsy but also would lapse into a coma. Drugs with slightly shorter but still excessively long dwell times (off rates) make patients hallucinate (e.g., phencyclidine, also known as Angel Dust) or so drowsy that they are anesthetics (e.g., ketamine).

A clinically tolerated NMDA receptor antagonist would not make a patient drowsy, hallucinate, or comatose and should spare normal neurotransmission while blocking the ravages of excessive NMDA receptor activation. One type of drug that would do this and would block preferentially higher (pathologic) levels of glutamate over normal (physiologic) levels would be an uncompetitive antagonist. An uncompetitive antagonist is distinct from a noncompetitive antagonist (which simply acts allosterically at a noncompetitive site, i.e., a site other than the agonist-binding site). An uncompetitive antagonist is defined as an inhibitor whose action is contingent on prior activation of the receptor by the agonist. Hence, the same amount of antagonist blocks higher concentrations of agonist better than lower concentrations of agonist. This uncompetitive mechanism of action coupled with a longer dwell time in the channel (and consequently a slower off rate from the channel) than $Mg^{2+}$ but a substantially shorter dwell time (faster off rate) than MK-801 would yield a drug that blocks NMDA receptor-operated channels only when they are excessively open while relatively sparing normal neurotransmission. Evidence suggests that memantine is such a drug (see later).

Note that the dwell time in (or off rate from) the channel is the major determinant of the clinical tolerability of an open-channel blocker because excessive dwell time (associated with a slow off rate) causes accumulation of the drug in the channels, and hence unacceptable adverse effects (as is the case with MK-801), whereas too short a dwell time (too fast an off rate) yields a relatively ineffectual blockade especially with membrane depolarization that relieves the block of positively charged molecules (such as seen with $Mg^{2+}$). The apparent affinity of a positively charged channel blocker at a particular membrane voltage is related to its off rate divided by its on rate (Table 26-1). The on rate not only is a property of the drug but also is affected by the drug's concentration, whereas the off rate is an intrinsic property of the drug interaction with the ion channel, unrelated to the concentration.[9]

The memantine class of drugs represents a relatively low-affinity, open-channel blocker, that is, these drugs enter the channel only when it is already opened by agonist. In the case of memantine, at concentrations administered to patients, the drug appears to enter the channel increasingly when it is (pathologically) activated for long periods (e.g., under conditions of excessive glutamate exposure). As shown previously,[9] memantine has nearly ideal kinetics in the channel to provide neuroprotection while displaying minimal adverse effects (occasional restlessness or, in rare cases, slight dizziness at higher dosages).[1,8]

# MEMANTINE

## Background and Pharmacology

Memantine was first synthesized by Eli Lilly and Company and patented in 1968, as documented in the Merck Index. It has a three-ring (adamantane) structure with a bridgehead amine ($-NH_2$) that under physiologic conditions carries a positive charge ($-NH_3^+$) and binds at or near the $Mg^{2+}$ site in the NMDA receptor-associated channel (Fig. 26-3).[8-11,41,42] Memantine is a derivative of amantadine, which lacks the two methyl ($-CH_3$) side groups and is an antiinfluenza compound that is also somewhat effective in the treatment of Parkinson's disease. The efficacy of amantadine and memantine in Parkinson's disease led people to believe that these compounds were dopaminergic or possibly anticholinergic drugs. It was not until the late 1980s that memantine was found to be neither dopaminergic nor anticholinergic at its clinically used dosage but instead an NMDA receptor antagonist.[43] Work in one of our laboratories (S.A.L.) first showed why memantine could be clinically tolerated as an NMDA receptor antagonist; namely, that it was an uncompetitive open-channel blocker with a short dwell time because of its relatively fast off rate from the channel that limited pathologic activity of the NMDA receptor while sparing normal synaptic activity.[9-11] These findings led to a number of U.S. and world-wide patents on the use of memantine for NMDA receptor-mediated disorders and spurred on several successful clinical trials with the drug, as discussed later. (The Lipton laboratory was then at Harvard Medical School, so these patents are assigned to Harvard-affiliated institutions, including Children's Hospital of Boston.)

**TABLE 26-1** CHANNEL KINETICS OF THE UNCOMPETITIVE OPEN-CHANNEL NMPA RECEPTOR ANTAGONIST, MEMANTINE

| Channel + MEM ↔ Channel-MEM (Blocked channel) | (Eq 1) |

This simple bimolecular scheme predicts that the macroscopic blocking and unblocking actions of memantine (MEM) proceeds with exponential relaxation, the macroscopic pseudo-first-order rate constant of blocking (kon) depends linearly on memantine concentration (and constant A), and the macroscopic unblocking rate (koff) is independent of memantine concentration ([MEM]).

$$kon = A \cdot [MEM] \qquad \text{(Eq 2)}$$

$$koff: [MEM] \text{ independent} \qquad \text{(Eq 3)}$$

These predictions were borne out experimentally.[9] Both the macroscopic blocking and unblocking processes could be well fitted by a single exponential function. The macroscopic on-rate constant is the reciprocal of the measured time constant for onset ($\tau_{on}$) and is the sum of the pseudo-first-order blocking rate constant (kon) and unblocking constant (koff). The unblocking rate constant (koff) is the reciprocal of the measured macroscopic unblocking time constant ($\tau_{off}$). These transformations lead to Equations (4) and (5):

$$kon = 1/\tau_{on} - 1/\tau_{off} \qquad \text{(Eq 4)}$$

$$koff = 1/\tau_{off} \qquad \text{(Eq 5)}$$

The kon calculated from Equation (4) increased linearly with memantine concentration with a slope factor of $0.4 \pm 0.03 \ 10^6 \ M^{-1}s^{-1}$ (mean ± SD), whereas the koff from Equation (5) remained relatively constant with a Y-axis intercept of $0.44 \pm 0.1 \ s^{-1}$.[9] A rapid method to validate this result was obtained by estimating the equilibrium apparent dissociation constant (Ki) for memantine action from the following equation:

$$Ki = koff/(kon/[MEM]) \qquad \text{(Eq 6)}$$

Here we found empirically that memantine was a relatively low-affinity (apparent affinity ~1 μM) open-channel blocker of the NMDA receptor-coupled ion channel, and a major component of the affinity was determined by koff at clinically relevant concentrations in the low micromolar range.

Figure 26-4 illustrates the efficacy of memantine in blocking NMDA-induced ionic currents when the membrane voltage of the neuron is held at the resting potential (approximately −50 to −60 mV). The concentration of memantine used in this experiment is similar to those levels that can be achieved in human brain and retina when the drug is used clinically. At such concentrations, memantine greatly reduces pathologically high levels of NMDA-induced current to near zero within approximately 1 second. Once the memantine application stops, the NMDA response returns to previous levels over a period of about 5 seconds. This indicates that memantine is an effective, but temporary, NMDA receptor blocker.

Perhaps the most astonishing property of memantine is illustrated in Figure 26-5.[8,10] In this experiment, the concentration of memantine was held constant (at the clinically achievable level of 1 μM) while the concentration of NMDA was increased over a wide range. It was found that the degree to which this fixed concentration of memantine blocked NMDA receptor activity actually increased as the NMDA concentration was increased to pathologic levels. Memantine was relatively ineffective at

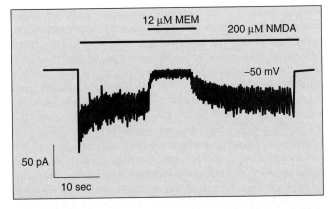

**FIGURE 26-4.** Memantine blockade of NMDA current. At a holding potential of −50 mV, whole-cell recording of NMDA-evoked current from a solitary neuron revealed that the on time (time until peak blockade) of micromolar memantine was approximately 1 sec, whereas the off time (recovery time) from the effect was ~5.5 sec. Memantine was effective only during NMDA receptor activation, consistent with the notion that its mechanism of action is open-channel block. (*Modified from Chen H-SV, Pellegrini JW, Aggarwal SK, et al: Open-channel block of NMDA responses by memantine: Therapeutic advantage against NMDA receptor-mediated neurotoxicity. J Neurosci 1992;12: 4427–4436.*)

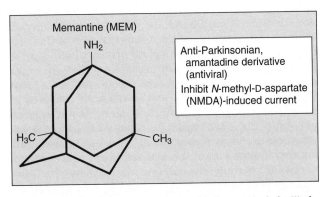

**FIGURE 26-3.** Memantine structure. Notable features include (1) the three-ring structure and the bridgehead amine (−NH₂ group), which is charged at the physiologic pH of the body ($-NH_3^+$) and represents the region of memantine that binds at or near the $Mg^{2+}$ binding site in the NMDA receptor-associated ion channel and (2) the methyl group ($-CH_3$) side chains (unlike amantadine), which serve to stabilize memantine's interaction in the channel region of the NMDA receptor.

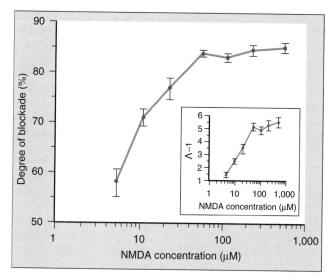

**FIGURE 26-5.** Effect of NMDA concentration on memantine blockade of NMDA current. The effect of increasing concentrations of NMDA is blocked to a higher degree than lower concentrations by a fixed dose of the antagonist memantine (1 μM in this case). This finding is characteristic of an uncompetitive antagonist. *(Modified from Chen H-SV, Pellegrini JW, Aggarwal SK, et al: Open-channel block of NMDA responses by memantine: Therapeutic advantage against NMDA receptor-mediated neurotoxicity. J Neurosci 1992;12:4427–4436.)*

blocking the low levels of receptor activity associated with normal neurologic function but became exceptionally effective at higher concentrations. This is classical uncompetitive antagonist behavior.

Further studies indicated that memantine exerts its effect on NMDA receptor activity by binding at or near the $Mg^{2+}$ site within the ion channel.[8-11,41] This information and the pharmacologic data presented previously suggests that memantine can act to block NMDA receptor activity only if the ion channel is already open and remains open long enough for memantine to get inside the channel. During normal synaptic activity, the channel is open only for a few milliseconds and memantine is unable to act; hence, synaptic activity continues essentially unabated. Moreover, because of its relatively rapid off rate, memantine does not accumulate in the channels like MK–801 and hence does not progressively block neurotransmission. In technical terms, the component of the excitatory postsynaptic current resulting from activation of NMDA receptors is inhibited by only 10% or less.[11] During prolonged activation of the receptor, however, as occurs under excitotoxic conditions, memantine is a very effective blocker. In essence, memantine acts only under pathologic conditions without much affecting normal function, thus relatively sparing synaptic transmission, preserving long-term potentiation, and maintaining physiologic function on behavioral tests such as the Morris Watermaze.[11] This explains the favorable clinical safety profile that has been seen with memantine treatment.

## Neuroprotective Efficacy

The neuroprotective properties of memantine have been studied in a large number of *in vitro* and *in vivo* animal models by several laboratories.[44] Among neurons protected in this manner both in culture and *in vivo* are cerebrocortical neurons, cerebellar neurons, and retinal neurons.[8-11,21,42,45-47] In addition, in a rat model of stroke, memantine, given as long as 2 hours after the ischemic event, reduces the amount of brain damage by approximately 50%.[10,11]

A series of human clinical trials have been launched to investigate the efficacy of memantine for the treatment of Alzheimer's disease, vascular dementia, HIV-associated dementia, diabetic neuropathic pain, and glaucoma. Several of these studies have been recently completed and remain unpublished at this time except in abstract form; however, the results of the European and U.S. phase III (final) clinical dementia studies of Alzheimer's disease and vascular dementia were sufficiently positive to prompt the European Union to approve memantine for the treatment of dementia, and very recently, the FDA approved memantine for the treatment of moderate to severe Alzheimer's disease in the U.S.[12] Two full-length publications of multicenter, randomized controlled trials have reported that memantine was beneficial in moderately to severely demented patients.[48,49] Another recent publication of a randomized, placebo-controlled clinical trial described significant benefit from memantine therapy (20 mg/day) in mild to moderate vascular dementia.[13] Most trials have reported minimal adverse effects of memantine. In those trials reporting adverse effects, the only memantine-induced side effects encountered were rare dizziness and occasional restlessness and agitation at higher doses (40 mg/day), but these effects were mild and dose related.

As promising as the results with memantine are, we are continuing to pursue ways to use additional modulatory sites (the volume controls) on the NMDA receptor to safely block excitotoxicity even more effectively and safely than with memantine alone.

## NITROMEMANTINES

NitroMemantines are second-generation memantine derivatives that were designed to have enhanced neuroprotective efficacy without sacrificing clinical testability. As mentioned earlier, a nitrosylation site is located on the N-terminus or extracellular domain of the NMDA receptor, and S-nitrosylation of this site (NO reaction with the sulfhydryl group of the cysteine residue) downregulates receptor activity (Fig. 26-2). The drug nitroglycerin, which generates NO-related species, can act at this site to limit excessive NMDA receptor activity. In rodent models, nitroglycerin can limit ischemic damage,[50] and there is some evidence that patients taking nitroglycerin for other medical reasons may be resistant to glaucomatous visual field loss.[51]

From crystal structure models and electrophysiologic experiments, we have found that NO binding to the NMDA receptor at the major S-nitrosylation site apparently induces a conformational change in the receptor protein that makes glutamate and $Zn^{2+}$ bind more tightly to the receptor. The enhanced binding of glutamate and $Zn^{2+}$ in turn cause the receptor to desensitize and, consequently, the ion channel to close.[35] Electrophysiologic studies have demonstrated this effect of NO on the NMDA channel.[28,52,53]

Unfortunately, nitroglycerin is not very attractive as a neuroprotective agent. The same cardiovascular vasodilator effect that make it useful in the treatment of angina could cause dangerously large drops in blood pressure in stroke, traumatic injury, or glaucoma patients. Consequently, we carefully characterized S-nitrosylation sites on the NMDA receptor to determine if we could design a nitroglycerin-like drug that would more specifically target the NMDA receptor.

In brief, five different cysteine residues on the NMDA receptor were found that could interact with NO. One of these, located at cysteine residue 399 on the NR2A subunit of the NMDA receptor, mediates approximately 90% of the effect of NO. Using this kind of information, we created modified memantine molecules called NitroMemantines that will interact with both the memantine site within the NMDA receptor-associated ion channel and the predominant nitrosylation site. Two sites of modulation are analogous to having two volume controls on a television set for fine tuning the audio signal.

Preliminary studies have shown NitroMemantines to be highly neuroprotective in both *in vitro* and *in vivo* animal models. It appears to be substantially more effective than memantine. Moreover, because the memantine portion makes these drugs specific for the NMDA receptor, NitroMemantines appear to lack the blood pressure lowering effect typical of nitroglycerin.

More research still must be performed on Nitro-Memantine drugs, but that fact that they chemically combine two clinically tolerated drugs (memantine and nitroglycerin) enhances their promise as second-generation memantine derivatives that are clinically safe and neuroprotective.

## SUMMARY

Necrosis- and apoptosis-mediated excitotoxic cell death is implicated in the pathophysiology of many cerebral diseases, including stroke. This type of excitotoxicity is caused, at least in part, by excessive activation of NMDA-type glutamate receptors. Intense insults, such as that occurring in the ischemic core after a stroke, lead to massive stimulation of NMDA receptors because of increased glutamate and energy failure leading to membrane depolarization, relief of $Mg^{2+}$ block of NMDA channels, and disruption of ionic homeostasis. The fulminant buildup of ions results in neuronal cell swelling and lysis (necrosis). In contrast, more moderate NMDA-receptor hyperactivity, such as that occurring in the ischemic penumbra of a stroke or in many slow-onset neurodegenerative diseases, results in moderately excessive influx of calcium ions into nerve cells that, in turn, triggers free radical formation and multiple pathways leading to the initiation of apoptosis.[18,54] Blockade of NMDA receptor activity prevents necrosis- and apoptosis-related excitotoxicity. However, NMDA receptor activity is also required for normal neural function, so only those NMDA blockers that selectively reduce excessive receptor activation without affecting normal function will be clinically acceptable. Memantine is such a drug. It has been shown in laboratory tests to block only excessive NMDA receptor activation but not normal, low-level activation. Importantly, one of us (S.A.L.) with Vincent Chen (a graduate student at the time) reported that memantine had a relatively short dwell time in (and hence fast off rate from) the NMDA-associated ion channel, in part explaining the drug's relatively low apparent affinity as an antagonist.[8-10] We realized that the relatively short dwell time and rapid off rate from the channel was the predominant factor in determining the drug's clinical tolerability and its neuroprotective profile.[8] Most importantly, this mode of action meant that memantine blocked high (pathologic) levels of glutamate at the NMDA receptor while relatively sparing the effects of low (physiologic) levels of glutamate seen during normal neurotransmission. The discovery that memantine, a low-affinity but still highly selective agent with a mechanism of uncompetitive antagonism, is neuroprotective yet clinically tolerated triggered a paradigm shift in the history of drug development by the pharmaceutical industry.[8-11] Before that discovery, low-affinity drugs were thought to be inferior and not clinically useful. In particular, the relatively rapid off rate from the NMDA receptor-associated ion channel of the memantine class of drugs largely accounts for its clinical tolerability and its low affinity. Clinical studies have borne out our hypothesis that the low-affinity and relatively fast off rate memantine is a safe NMDA receptor antagonist in humans and is beneficial in the treatment of a variety of neurologic disorders mediated, at least in part, by excitotoxicity.

The NitroMemantines are another class of low-affinity and fast off rate NMDA receptor antagonists that may work even better than memantine by using the memantine binding site for the targeted delivery of NO to a second modulatory site on the NMDA receptor. Work is progressing rapidly in this area of investigation.

Clinical studies of the efficacy of memantine in the treatment of stroke, Alzheimer's disease, vascular dementia, HIV-associated dementia, glaucoma, and neuropathic pain are currently underway, and there is every reason to expect the results to be positive, although this is, of course, not yet proven except in the case of Alzheimer's disease and vascular dementia in which phase III (final) clinical trials have proven successful. The efficacy of memantine in these neurodegenerative diseases and the ability of memantine to protect neurons in animal models of stroke suggest that memantine or drugs acting in a similar manner could become a very important new weapon in the fight against the damage caused by cerebral ischemia.

## REFERENCES

1. Lipton SA, Rosenberg RA: Mechanisms of disease: Excitatory amino acids as a final common pathway in neurologic disorders. N Engl J Med 1994;330:613–622.
2. Lipton SA, Nicotera P: Calcium, free radicals and excitotoxins in neuronal apoptosis. Cell Calcium 1998;23:165–171.

3. Kemp JA, McKernan RM: NMDA receptor pathways as drug targets. Nat Neurosci 2002;5(Suppl):1039–1042.

4. Kemp JA, Kew JN, Gill R: Ionotropic Glutamate receptors in the CNS, In Jonas P, Monyer H (eds): Handbook of Experimental Pharmacology, vol 141. Berlin, Springer, 1999, pp 495–527.

5. Lees KR, Asplund K, Carolei A, et al: Glycine antagonist (gavestinel) in neuroprotection (GAIN International) in patients with acute stroke: A randomized controlled trial. GAIN International Investigators. Lancet 2000;355:1949–1954.

6. Sacco RL, DeRosa JT, Haley EC Jr, et al: Glycine antagonist in neuroprotection for patients with acute stroke: GAIN Americas: a randomized controlled trial. JAMA 2001;28:1719–1728.

7. Seif el Nasr M, Peruche B, Rossberg C, et al: Neuroprotective effect of memantine demonstrated in vivo and in vitro. Eur J Pharmacol 1990;185:19–24.

8. Lipton SA: Prospects for clinically-tolerated NMDA antagonists: Open-channel blockers and alternative redox states of nitric oxide. Trends Neurosci 1993;16:527–532.

9. Chen H-SV, Lipton SA: Mechanism of memantine block of NMDA-activated channels in rat retinal ganglion cells: Uncompetitive antagonism. J Physiol (Lond) 1997;499:27–46.

10. Chen H-SV, Pellegrini JW, Aggarwal SK, et al: Open-channel block of NMDA responses by memantine: Therapeutic advantage against NMDA receptor-mediated neurotoxicity. J Neurosci 1992;12:4427–4436.

11. Chen H-SV, Wang YF, Rayudu PV, et al: Neuroprotective concentration of the NMDA open-channel blocker memantine are effective without cytoplasmic vacuolization following post-ischemic administration and do not block maze learning or LTP. Neuroscience 1998;86:1121–1132.

12. Le DA, Lipton SA: Potential and current use of N-methyl-D-aspartate (NMDA) receptor antagonists in diseases of aging. Drugs Aging 2001;18:717–724.

13. Orgogozo JM, Rigaud AS, Stoffler A, et al: Efficacy and safety of memantine in patients with mild to moderate vascular dementia: A randomized, placebo-controlled trial (MMM 300). Stroke 2002;33:1834–1839.

14. Lucas DR, Newhouse JP: The toxic effect of sodium L-glutamate on the inner layers of the retina. Arch Ophthalmol 1957;58:193–201.

15. Olney JW: Glutamate-induced retinal degeneration in neonatal mice: Electron microscopy of the acutely evolving lesion. J Neuropath Exp Neurol 1969;28:455–474.

16. Olney JW, Ho OL: Brain damage in infant mice following oral intake of glutamate, aspartate or cysteine. Nature 1970;227:609–611.

17. Lipton SA: Molecular mechanisms of trauma-induced neuronal degeneration. Curr Opin Neurol Neurosurg 1993;6:588–596.

18. Bonfoco E, Krainc D, Ankarcrona M, et al: Apoptosis and necrosis: Two distinct events induced respectively by mild and intense insults with NMDA or nitric oxide/superoxide in cortical cell cultures. Proc Natl Acad Sci USA 1995;92:7162–7166.

19. Dreyer EB, Zhang D, Lipton SA: Transcriptional or translational inhibition blocks low dose NMDA-mediated cell death. Neuroreport 1995;6:942–944.

20. Quigley HA, Nickells RW, Kerrigan LA, et al: Retinal ganglion cell death in experimental glaucoma and after axotomy occurs by apoptosis. Invest Ophthalmol Vis Sci 1995;36:774–786.

21. Vorwerk CK, Lipton SA, Zurakowski D, et al: Chronic low dose glutamate is toxic to retinal ganglion cells: Toxicity blocked by memantine. Invest Ophthalmol Vis Sci 1996;37:1618–1624.

22. Dreyer EB, Grosskreutz CL: Excitatory mechanisms in retinal ganglion cell death in primary open angle glaucoma (POAG). Clin Neurosci 1997;4:270–273.

23. Dreyer EB, Lipton SA: New perspectives on glaucoma. JAMA 1999;281:306–308.

24. Naskar R, Vorwerk CK, Dreyer EB: Saving the nerve from glaucoma: Memantine to caspases. Semin Ophthalmol 1999;4:152–158

25. Zeevalk GD, Nicklas WJ: Evidence that the loss of the voltage-dependent $Mg^{2+}$ block of the N-methyl-D-aspartate receptor underlies receptor activation during inhibition of neuronal metabolism. J Neurochem 1992;59:1211–1220.

26. Dawson VL, Dawson TM, London ED, et al: Nitric oxide mediates glutamate neurotoxicity in primary cortical cultures. Proc Natl Acad Sci USA 1991;88:6368–6371.

27. Dawson VL, Dawson TM, Bartley, DA et al: Mechanisms of nitric oxide-mediated neurotoxicity in primary brain cultures. J Neurosci 1993;13:2651–2661.

28. Lipton SA, Choi Y-B, Pan Z-H, et al: A redox-based mechanism for the neuroprotective and neurodestructive effects of nitric oxide and related nitroso-compounds. Nature 1993;364:626–632.

29. Tenneti L, D'Emilia DM, Troy CM, Lipton SA: Role of caspases in N-methyl-D-aspartate-induced apoptosis in cerebrocortical neurons. J Neurochem 1998;71:946–959.

30. Yun HY, Gonzalez-Zulueta M, Dawson VL et al: Nitric oxide mediates N-methyl-D-aspartate receptor-induced activation of p21ras. Proc Natl Acad Sci USA 1998;95:5773–5778.

31. Budd SL, Tenneti L, Lishnak T, Lipton SA: Mitochondrial and extramitochondrial apoptotic signaling pathways in cerebrocortical neurons. Proc Natl Acad Sci USA 2000;97:6161–6166.

32. Okamoto S-i, Li Z, Ju C, Schölzke MN, et al: Dominant-interfering forms of MEF2 generated by caspase cleavage contribute to NMDA-induced neuronal apoptosis. Proc Natl Acad Sci USA 2002;99:3974–3979.

33. Johnson J, Ascher P: Glycine potentiates the NMDA response in cultured mouse brain neurons. Nature 1987;325:529–531.

34. McBain CJ, Mayer ML: N-Methyl-D-aspartic acid receptor structure and function. Physiol Rev 1994;74:723–760.

35. Lipton SA, Choi Y-B, Takahashi T, et al: Cysteine regulation of protein function—as exemplified by NMDA-receptor modulation. Trends Neurosci 2002;25:474–490.

36. Koroshetz WJ, Moskowitz MA: Emerging treatments for stroke in humans. Trends Pharmacol Sci 1996;17:227–233.

37. Hickenbottom SL, Grotta J: Neuroprotective therapy. Semin Neurol 1998;18:485–492.

38. Lutsep HL, Clark WM: Neuroprotection in acute ischaemic stroke: Current status and future potential. Drug Res Dev 1999;1:3–8.

39. Rogawski MA: Low affinity channel blocking (uncompetitive) NMDA receptor antagonists as therapeutic agents: Toward an understanding of their favorable tolerability. Amino Acids 2000;19:133–149.

40. Palmer GC: Neuroprotection by NMDA receptor antagonists in a variety of neuropathologies. Curr Drug Targ 2001;2:241–271.

41. Chen H-SV, Rastogi, Lipton SA: Q/R/N site mutations in the M2 region of NMDAR1/NMDAR2A receptors reveal a nonspecific site for memantine action. Soc Neurosci Abstr 1998;24:342.

42. Lipton SA: Memantine prevents HIV coat protein-induced neuronal injury in vitro. Neurology 1992;42:1403–1405.

43. Bormann J: Memantine is a potent blocker of N-methyl-D-aspartate (NMDA) receptor channels. Eur J Pharm 1989;166:591–592.

44. Parsons CG, Danysz W, Quack G: Memantine is a clinically well tolerated N-methyl-D-aspartate (NMDA) receptor antagonist-a review of preclinical data. Neuropharmacology 1999;38:735–767.

45. Pellegrini JW, Lipton SA: Delayed administration of memantine prevents NMDA receptor-mediated neurotoxicity. Ann Neurol 1993;33:403–407.

46. Sucher NJ, Lipton SA, Dreyer EB: Molecular basis of glutamate toxicity in retinal ganglion cells. Vis Res 1997;37:3483–3493.

47. Osborne NN: Memantine reduces alterations to the mammalian retina, in situ, induced by ischemia. Vis Neurosci 1999;16:45–52.

48. Winblad B, Poritis N: Memantine in severe dementia: results of the 9M-Best Study (benefit and efficacy in severely demented patients during treatment with memantine). Int J Geriatr Psychiatry 1999;14:135–146.

49. Reisberg B, Doody R, Stöffler A, et al: Memantine in moderate to severe Alzheimer's disease. N Engl J Med 2003;348:1333–1341.

50. Lipton SA, Wang YF: NO-related species can protect from focal cerebral ischemia/reperfusion. In Krieglstein J, Oberpichler-Schwenk H (eds): Pharmacology of Cerebral Ischemia. Stuttgart, Germany Wissenschaftliche Verlagsgesellschaft mbH, 1996, pp 183–191.

51. Zurakowski D, Vorerk CK, Gorla M, et al: Nitrate therapy may retard glaucomatous optic neuropathy, perhaps through modulation of glutamate receptors. Vis Res 1998;38:1489–1494.

52. Lipton SA, Rayudu, PV, Choi Y-B, et al: Redox modulation of the NMDA receptor by NO-related species. Progr Brain Res 1998;118:73-82.

53. Choi Y-B, Tenneti L, Le DA, et al: Molecular basis of NMDA receptor-coupled ion channel modulation by S-nitrosylation. Nat Neurosci 2000;3:15-21.

54. Ankarcrona M, Dypbukt JM, Bonfoco E, et al: Glutamate-induced neuronal death: A succession of necrosis or apoptosis depending on mitochondrial integrity. Neuron 1995;15:961-973.

■ ■ ■ chapter 2 7

# Platelets and Antiplatelet Therapy in Cardiovascular Disease: Molecular Mechanisms

*Ori Ben-Yehuda*

Platelets, a necessary and primary component in hemostasis and wound healing, also play a key pathologic role in ischemic heart disease, the major cardiovascular disease afflicting humans. Platelet plugs occur at sites of pathologic vascular injury such as during plaque rupture, and platelets form an essential and primary component of the white thrombus that is thought to mediate most ACSs including st segment-elevation MI. Platelets also cause abrupt vessel closure in the setting of percutaneous coronary intervention (PCI) and participate in the pathogenesis of stroke syndromes. Thus, platelet function has profound implications in many aspects of vascular disease, and platelet function must be interpreted in the context of events that occur in the vessel wall at both the endothelial and the subendothelial matrix levels. Recently, along with a greater understanding of the complexity of platelet signaling and interactions, their role in atherosclerosis and restenosis has gained attention. The expression and release of various mediators from platelets, such as thrombin, CD-40 ligand (CD40L), serotonin, and ADP, have significant effects on events in the vessel wall. Platelets and their products provide an important connection between the two main disease processes involved in ischemic heart disease and stroke, namely atherosclerosis and thrombosis. Thus, the understanding of platelet function in health and disease and of antiplatelet therapy is fundamental to the modern practice of cardiology.

Although platelets are only nonnucleated cell fragments, they are complex entities that respond to changes in their environment through multiple often redundant and intricate signaling pathways. The past few years have seen a marked advance in the understanding of these complex pathways. These advances have occurred despite the challenges of studying a non-nucleated system that is, therefore, not amenable to the usual direct molecular biology techniques.

Understanding the molecular basis of platelet function has led to the development of novel antiplatelet therapies, particularly the thienopyridines (ticlopidine and clopidogrel) and the glycoprotein IIb/IIIa inhibitors. Based on large-scale clinical trials, these newer therapies

along with ASA have gained an important role in coronary care in general and interventional cardiology in particular. The identification of novel targets involved in platelet function and particularly platelet-vessel wall interaction promise to yield new therapies for ACSs, stroke, PCI, and atherosclerosis. More precise control of platelet function will undoubtedly result in even greater clinical benefit with enhanced safety. This chapter reviews the molecular basis of platelet function and antiplatelet therapies, as well as the monitoring of antiplatelet therapies.

## RESTING PLATELET STRUCTURE AND FUNCTION

Platelets are fragments of megakaryocytes that are shed in the process of megakaryocyte maturation from elongated structures termed proplatelets.[1,2] Platelets are not simple, random cell fragments; they are actually highly organized and complex. They are notable for a receptor-rich membrane that includes serpentine receptors for thrombin, ADP, thromboxane $A_2$ ($TXA_2$), and epinephrine; glycoprotein receptors for von Willebrand factor (vWF); integrin receptors for collagen, fibrinogen, and vWF; and immunoglobulin receptors such as the Fc receptor and GP VI. The membrane compartment is organized into a complex system including the open canalicular system (OCS) and the dense tubular system (DTS). A cytoskeletal system includes a spectrin submembrane layer, a marginal microtubule coil, and an extensive actin-based filament structure. Platelet storage granules ($\alpha$ granules and dense granules) secrete a host of adhesion proteins, enzymes, growth factors, and activating agents. Finally, platelets also contain mitochondria, lysosomes, and peroxisomes.

In a nonactivated state, the platelets circulate as small nonnucleated discs, with diameters varying both between and within individuals and ranging from 1.5 to 5 $\mu$m, about one-fourth to one-third the diameter of an erythrocyte.[3,4] The surface appears flat except for pits that identify entrances into to the OCS, which is a com-

■ ■ ■

**TABLE 27-1**    MAJOR PLATELET MEMBRANE RECEPTORS

| Protein | Type | No. of Receptors/ Platelet | Ligand | Function |
|---|---|---|---|---|
| GP Ibαβ-IX-V (CD42) | Leucine-rich glycoprotein | 25,000 | vWF Thrombin | Adhesion |
| GP Ia-IIa ($\alpha_2\beta_1$) (CD49b-CD29) | Integrin | 1000 | Collagen | Adhesion |
| GP IIb-IIIa ($\alpha_{IIb}\beta_3$) | Integrin | 80,000 | Fibrinogen vWF Fibronectin | Aggregation Vitronectin |
| GP IV (GP IIIb,CD 36) | Transmembrane glycoprotein | 12,000–25,000 | Thrombospondin Collagen | Adhesion |
| GP VI | Immunoglobulin superfamily | 1000 | Collagen | Adhesion |
| GP Ic-IIa ($\alpha_5\beta_1$) | Integrin | 1000 | Fibronectin | Adhesion |
| PAR-1 | G-protein coupled seven-transmembrane domain | 1000–2000 | Thrombin | Adhesion |
| PAR-4 | G-protein coupled seven-transmembrane domain | 1000–2000 | Thrombin | Adhesion |
| $P2Y_{12}$ | G-protein coupled seven-transmembrane domain | 1000 | ADP | Activation |
| $P2Y_1$ | G-protein coupled seven-transmembrane domain | 1000 | ADP | Activation |
| $P2X_1$ | Ionotropic | ? | ADP | ? |
| GP Ic-IIa ($\alpha_6\beta_1$) (CD49f-CD29) | Integrin | 1000 | Laminin | Adhesion |
| $\alpha_v\beta_3$ | Integrin | 50–100 | Vitronectin | Adhesion |
| P-selectin (CD62) | Selectin family | 12,000 (after platelet activation) | Neutrophils/ monocytes | Platelet attachment to neutrophils/monocytes (platelet-leukocyte interactions) |
| Thromboxane $A_2$ receptor | G-protein coupled seven-transmembrane domain | 1000 | Thromboxane $A_2$ | Activation |

Additional receptors exist for serotonin, epinephrine, vasopressin, platelet activating factor (PAF), immune complexes, LDL, and fatty acids. Estrogen and prostaglandins ($PGI_2$, $PGD_2$, $PGE_2$) are inhibitory.

plex system of membrane invaginations forming channels within the cell. Despite its smooth appearance the membrane is actually rich in receptors, covering approximately one fourth of its surface area. The GP IIb/IIIa ($\alpha_{IIb}\beta_{IIIa}$) receptor is the most abundant, followed by the GPI bαβ-IX-V complex (vWF receptor) followed by the GP Ia/IIa ($\alpha_2\beta_1$) collagen receptor (Table 27-1). The OCS functions as a conduit for granule content release, as a storage site for membrane receptors, and as a source of membrane for the formation of platelet extension during activation.

Platelet granules are in close association with the OCS, which provides a pathway of tubes for the release of mediators into the surroundings.[2] Because of the extensive actin cytoskeleton (which is enhanced in the platelet cortex following activation of platelets) platelet granules are otherwise prevented from efficiently reaching the plasma membrane for exocytosis. The fusion and release of granules with the OCS is dependent on an increase in cytosolic calcium concentration to the micromolar range. There are two types of storage granules (Table 27-2): the more abundant α granules, which contain adhesion molecules such as fibrinogen and vWF along with growth factors and P-selectin, and dense granules, so named because on electron microscopy they display an electron-dense

core. Dense granules recruit additional platelets through the release of platelet agonists, primarily ADP and serotonin.

The DTS is another membranous compartment, which is present throughout the cytoplasm and serves as a source of $Ca^{2+}$ during platelet activation. The DTS is also the site of $TXA_2$ synthesis.

Platelet shape is maintained by three elements—an actin and tubulin cytoskeleton, a layer of spectrin, and a cell membrane. An extensive actin and tubulin cytoskeleton connects to a layer of spectrin that is adherent to the cell membrane. The tubulin component is arranged as a microtubule coil around the periphery of the platelet and is associated with motor proteins such as dynein and kinesins. The microtubule coil plays a key role in the shedding of platelets from megakaryocytes and helps maintain the discoid shape of the resting platelet. β1 Tubulin isoform knockout mice have irregularly shaped platelets and low platelet counts.[5]

Actin filaments are in equilibrium with actin monomers, which make up the majority of the 0.5 mM of actin in the resting platelet.[5-9] The filaments have a barbed end associated with myosin subfragments. The monomeric actin is complexed with β4-thymosin, a small protein.[10,11] Although the affinity of monomeric actin to β4-thymosin is less than that of monomeric actin to the

■ ■ ■

## TABLE 27-2  PLATELET GRANULES CONTENT

**α-Granules**

Fibrinogen
Fibronectin
Thrombospondin
von Willebrand factor
Plasminogen
Factor V
PF4
Platelet-derived growth factor
RANTES
TGF-α
TGF-β
Endothelial cell growth factor (ECGF)
P-selectin

**Dense Granules**

ADP
ATP
Serotonin

barbed end of the protein, the presence of sequestering proteins capZ or capping protein and gelsolin prevent binding to the barbed end in the resting state.[12]

Actin filaments compose about 10% of the resting platelets and are cross linked by filamins, large dimeric proteins, and the smaller α-actinin.[13,14] Filamins not only cross link actin but also attach the lattice to the cell membrane by binding to the cytoplasmic tail of the α-chain of GP Ib. This binding to the vWF receptor has the effect of aligning the receptors in linear rows. Patients with the Bernard-Soulier syndrome (BSS), phenotypically characterized by large fragile platelets, lack this connection because of mutations in the vWF components.

The spectrin molecules form a support structure for the membrane. Actin filaments connect spectrin tetramers. Moreover, through the binding of actin to vWF (occurring through pores in the spectrin skeleton) the spectrin submembrane is fixed to the submembrane area and is prevented from expanding. BSS platelets, despite having an intact spectrin layer, loose their shape because of failure of the filamin-vWFR linkage.

## PLATELETS AND FLOW

Historically, the study of platelet function has been conducted in suspension.[15-19] Such systems have only limited relevance to *in vivo* systems, particularly on the arterial side where events occur under flow conditions. Despite constant recirculation and possible physical interaction with the vessel wall, in the absence of vessel wall damage with resultant release of mediators, there is no activation of platelets. Conversely, in the presence of vascular damage, platelets rapidly adhere, activate, and aggregate, thereby forming the nidus of clot formation. During the formation of a thrombus under flow conditions, however, only a fraction of the platelets interact with the endothelium and even a smaller percentage are actually incorporated into the forming aggregate.

When blood flows, adjacent layers move at different speeds, much slower at the vessel wall and faster toward the center of the vessel, thereby creating a parabolic velocity profile.[15] This parallel motion between adjacent fluid layers creates shear, which is characterized by two parameters, shear rate ($s^{-1}$) and shear stress (dynes/cm²). Shear rate refers to the rapidity of movement of the fluid layers and is zero at the axis of the flow and maximal at the vessel wall. It varies directly with the flow velocity of the blood and inversely with the diameter of the vessel. Thus, it is lowest in large veins (<50 $s^{-1}$), higher in arteries (~1500 $s^{-1}$), and maximal in areas of severe stenoses (up to 40,000 $s^{-1(20)}$).[20] Shear stress is the measure of the force exerted by the flowing fluid on adjacent lamina and, in analogy with shear rate, is minimal in large veins (1 dyn/cm²) and maximal at areas of arterial stenoses (up to 1000 dyn/cm²). With increasing shear rate, erythrocytes concentrate at the axis of flow; platelets, being smaller, are pushed against the vessel wall.[21] Platelet adhesion to the vessel wall also increases with increasing shear up to 1800 $s^{-1}$, decreasing at very high shear rates, whereas aggregation continues to increase at least up to a wall shear rate of 10,500 $s^{-1}$.[22] Thus, although venous thrombosis is characterized by a platelet-poor and fibrin- and erythrocyte-rich clot (red clot), arterial thrombosis, particularly at the high shear rate associated atherosclerotic stenoses, is characterized by the formation of platelet-rich white clot, with red clot at both the proximal and distal portions of the artery.[23]

## STRUCTURE OF ACTIVATED PLATELETS

When platelets are activated, key structural changes occur.[24,25] As noted previously, platelets in suspension and *in vivo* under flow conditions are discoid in shape when not activated. In suspension, activated platelets lose their discoid form and become irregular, with the granules concentrated in the center and enclosed within a ring of microtubules. The OCS appears more prominent and is occasionally filled with granule content, and the α granules merge with the OCS. In contrast, when platelets activate on surfaces under flow conditions there is a continuous layer of platelets that are oriented in the direction of flow. The organelles are usually lost and the OCS maximally externalizes on the platelets, thereby increasing their surface area more than fourfold. Spiny formations termed filopods and lamellipodia form; this process depends on new actin filament formation.

Platelet structural changes that occur during activation are dependent on a rise in the calcium concentration in the cytoplasm, which occurs because of the activation of phospholipase C (PLC).[26,27] PLC in turn is activated during agonist binding, such as thrombin (PLC-β) and collagen (PLC-γ2). The rise in calcium activates gelsolin, one of three capping proteins on the actin filament barbed end. Gelsolin, an 80-kd protein present at a concentration of 5 μmol, undergoes a conformational change on calcium binding.[28] Activated gelsolin binds to the actin filament, cleaves it, and remains bound to the new barbed filament end.[29] The result is a marked increase in the number of actin filaments, which are now appreciably shorter. This has the effect of removing the constraint on the spectrin layer. The cell membrane can now flow outward, resulting in a round larger platelet.

The exposure of the newly formed barbed ends of the actin filament results in binding of monomeric actin and the formation of filopods and lamellipodia, which markedly increases platelet surface area. The association of gelsolin with actin is very rapid, occurring within 5 seconds after platelets are stimulated with thrombin. Gelsolin knockout mice demonstrate a 50% to 75% reduction in actin filament formation after platelet activation. Once new actin filaments are created gelsolin dissociates rapidly.

Adducin, an additional capping protein, is found in concentrations of more than 3 μmol in the resting platelet where it caps the barbed end of the actin filament. On exposure to calcium-calmodulin or phosphorylation by PKC, adducin dissociates from actin, thereby allowing barbed end exposure and cleavage by gelsolin. Rho-associated protein kinase (ROCK) has the opposite effect and increases the binding to actin.[30]

Cap Z, the third major capping protein, becomes attached after gelsolin and adducin dissociate.[31] Cap Z appears to prevent gelsolin from attaching to actin barbed ends in the resting state and to terminate new filament formation by capturing newly formed barbed ends when activation has occurred. Therefore, it acts as a braking mechanism to limit platelet activation.

Once new actin filaments are formed by cleavage they undergo elongation by incorporation of actin monomers. Two actin-related proteins, Arp2 and Arp3, in a complex with five associated actin-related complex (arc) proteins promote the polymerization of the filaments.

## PLATELET-PLATELET INTERACTIONS: FORMATION OF A PLATELET PLUG

Based primarily on *in vitro* studies, the formation of a platelet plug has traditionally been divided into three phases: adhesion, activation, and aggregation. This division is somewhat artificial, because the three phases occur concurrently on a growing thrombus. However, these conceptual phases provide a useful framework for understanding platelet function.

## Adhesion and Activation: Multiple Mediators and Receptors

Intact healthy endothelium does not favor platelet adhesion because of both physical and biochemical considerations. Both the endothelium and platelets are negatively charged.[23] Prostacyclin (PGI$_2$) and NO are produced by healthy endothelial cells. Blood flow generates physical forces that act to dislodge adherent platelets. Platelets also produce inhibitors of adhesion, namely PGI$_2$, PGE$_2$, and NO. PGI$_2$ and PGE$_2$, through their binding to IP and EP receptors on the platelet surface, activate Gs proteins, resulting in elevated cAMP within the platelet. NO, after diffusing into the platelet, interacts with guanylate cyclase to increase conversion of GTP to cGMP. Elevated cGMP and cAMP in turn stimulate PKG and PKA respectively, leading to phosphorylation of platelet agonist receptors, thereby maintaining the platelet in a nonactivated (quiescent) state. Additional platelet antagonists include the constitutively expressed membrane enzyme CD39, an ADPase, and PDGF.

Conversely, once the integrity of the endothelium is violated, multiple pathways lead to platelet adhesion and aggregation. Initial platelet adhesion is mediated by membrane glycoproteins, both integrin and nonintegrins (Table 27-1). The primary platelet agonists (ADP, thrombin, vWF, collagen) act through redundant agonist receptors; this may reflect an evolutionary mechanism aimed at preventing blood loss.

Acute coronary events are precipitated in most cases by plaque rupture. In a minority of cases, particularly in smokers, endothelial erosion without plaque rupture may also occur.[32] In both situations, exposure of the subendothelial layer brings platelets in contact with various extracellular matrix components that are normally not in contact with flowing blood. Deeper injuries and more complex plaque ruptures expose different extracellular components, usually with increased thrombogenic potential. Ultimately platelet-derived agonists [ADP, thrombin, thrombospondin (TSP), serotonin, and vWF] play an important role in recruitment of additional platelets into the growing platelet plug. The same mediator may be present in the vessel wall and in the platelet, as has been demonstrated for TSP, which is found in both the subendothelial matrix and the platelet α granule and is secreted during platelet activation. In addition, circulating components such as thrombinogen are activated during vascular injury and contribute significantly to platelet activation. In the case of some mediators such as vWF, the mediator circulates in the bloodstream, is found in the vessel wall, and is secreted by platelets.

### Subendothelial Matrix Proteins

The subendothelial basement membrane contains proteoglycans,[33] collagen type IV,[34] laminin,[35,36] fibulin,[37] and entactin.[36] Collagen type IV, although not as thrombogenic as collagens found in deeper layers, is capable of initiating platelet adhesion and activation. Associated with collagen type IV in a tight assembly are entactin (nidogen) and the glycoprotein laminins. Fibulins, both tissue bound and circulating, can assemble with fibrinogen and fibronectin and may enhance platelet adhesion.

Deeper vessel wall injury, as occurs in complex plaque rupture, exposes fibronectins[38]; collagen types I, III, and VI; and vWF that can bind to the platelet. Circulating fibrinogen (and its cleavage product fibrin) and TSP, when immobilized in an area of injury, can also serve as substrates for platelet adhesive receptors.[39] TSP-induced platelet activation occurs through a five trans-membrane-spanning receptor called integrin-associated protein (IAP). IAP is associated not only with integrins but also with the large G-protein G$_{\alpha i}$ through which IAP appears to activate the IIb/IIIa receptor. Fibronectins, modular macromolecules that are found in the vessel wall and in plasma and that contain the Arg-Gly-Asp (RGD) sequence, bind to the IIb/IIIa, the Ic/IIa, and the vitronectin receptors.[38]

Collagen types I, III, and VI interact with vWF; type VI mediates thrombosis under slow flow conditions, whereas types I and III are involved in thrombosis under high flow rates, with its attendant high shear rate.[40]

Collagen can directly activate platelets through glycoprotein VI and the $\alpha_2\beta_1$ (GP Ia/IIa) integrin receptor. Collagen binding to $\alpha_2\beta_1$ is dependent on $Mg^{2+}$ and is inhibited by $Ca^{2+}$ and is considered secondary in importance to binding to GP VI.[41] A member of the immunoglobulin superfamily of proteins, GP VI is coupled to an Fc receptor $\gamma$ chain (FcR$\gamma$). FcR$\gamma$ functions as an immunoreceptor tyrosine-based activation motif (ITAM). It is dephosphorylated by the tyrosine kinase *src* and ultimately activates PLC$\gamma$.

## Thrombin

In terms of potency thrombin is the most powerful platelet agonist identified.[42] It is produced during humoral coagulation from the zymogen prothrombin and serves as an important link between cellular (platelet) hemostasis and the humoral coagulation system. Moreover, thrombin release during thrombolytic therapy leads to important platelet activation.

Thrombin acts through protease-activated receptors (PARs).[43] PAR-1, PAR-3, and PAR-4 are seven-domain transmembrane-spanning G-protein-coupled receptors that are expressed on platelets and other cells. G-protein activation leads to PLC activation. Several isoforms of PLC have been identified in platelets: PLC$\beta$2 and PLC$\gamma$ predominate; PLC$\beta$2 is activated by G$\alpha$q and Gi$\beta\gamma$, whereas PLC$\gamma$ is phosphorylated by nonreceptor protein tyrosine kinases. The existence of multiple PARs allows for redundancy in the system, so that PAR-1 knockout mice respond normally to thrombin (in mice the predominant PAR pathways involves PAR-3 and PAR-4 vs. PAR-1 and PAR-4 in human platelets).[44,45] The PLC$\beta$ pathway is not dependent on IIb/IIIa activation and is, therefore, active in platelets from patients with Glanzmann's thrombasthenia (thrombasthenic platelets).

Thrombin cleaves a 41-residue amino-terminal peptide in its PAR receptors, leaving a tethered ligand. Both the tethered ligand and the cleaved amino-terminal peptide are potent platelet agonists. Once PLC$\beta$ is phosphorylated, it hydrolyses the membrane-associated phosphatidylinositol 4,5P2, leading to formation of second messengers such as IP3 and diglyceride. IP3 leads to calcium mobilization, whereas diglyceride activates PKC. $Ca^{2+}$ increases activated PLA2, which hydrolyzes membrane phospholipids and gives rise to arachidonic acid (AA) and thromboxane.

## ADP

ADP plays a central role in platelet activation.[46-52] It is present in high concentrations and is secreted from dense bodies on platelet adhesion and when other agonists, such as thrombin, are present, thereby amplifying the platelet response. It acts through several pathways: an ATP ligand-gated ion channel and three purinoreceptors, $P2Y_1$, $P2Y_{12}$, and $P2X_i$. The most important is $P2Y_1$, a $G_q$-coupled receptor that activates PLC$\beta$ and leads to a rise in $Ca^{2+}$. $P2Y_{12}$, the target of the thienopyridines ticlopidine and clopidogrel, is coupled to $G_i$ and inhibits adenylyl cyclase. $P2X_i$, on binding of ligand, undergoes

receptor clustering, thereby creating a transmembrane pore that allows $Ca^{2+}$ influx.

## Thromboxane $A_2$

Platelet membrane phospholipids provide substrate for the generation of prostaglandin mediators. Under the action of phospholipase $A_2$ both AA and platelet-activating factor (PAF) are released. AA undergoes further metabolism through the cyclooxygenase (COX) and lipoxygenase pathways, generating various mediators including $TXA_2$, which is the most potent mediator.[53] Platelets contain the constitutive enzyme COX-1 but not the inducible COX-2 enzyme. COX-2 selective antiinflammatory drugs, therefore, have no direct effect on platelets. ASA, the most widely used antiplatelet agent inhibits the COX-1 enzyme.

$TXA_2$ acts through specific G-protein-coupled seven-transmembrane receptors on the platelet membrane. The $\alpha$ isoform (termed TP$\alpha$) with 343 amino acids appears to be the active receptor on platelets.[53,54] Coupled to G-proteins,[55] binding of $TXA_2$ leads to PLC$\beta$ activation. Phosphorylation of TP$\alpha$ turns off the receptor.

## von Willebrand Factor

The vWF plays a central role in platelet adhesion[56] and is found in various compartments, with different degrees of polymerization. It circulates freely in the plasma as small polymers, whereas larger polymers are released from platelet $\alpha$ granules after activation and are also found in the subendothelium. Plasma vWF is particularly important in adhesion because it rapidly binds, through its A3 domain, to exposed collagen and possibly other proteoglycans. Because of the rapid immobilization of plasma vWF on collagen, binding of platelets to immobilized collagen type I and III is essentially instantaneous. This interaction between vWF and collagen is of particular relevance in the setting of plaque rupture where exposure of the subendothelium to blood occurs.

Platelet binding to vWF occurs initially through the binding of the vWF A1 domain to the GP Ib$\alpha$-Ib$\beta$-IX-X receptor (vWFR). In the high-shear situations likely present in the arterial tree, particularly in areas of plaque rupture, initial platelet adhesion to vWF is a prerequisite of thrombus formation, because only the A1 domain is capable of capturing fast-flowing platelets.[57] In contrast fibrinogen and fibrin are only capable of directly binding to platelets under low-shear conditions, through the IIB/IIIA receptor (Fig. 27-1). This ability of vWF is predicated on its multimeric nature because there are multiple active A1 domains available for interaction with the platelet receptor. Therefore, binding of vWF to the receptor occurs with high efficiency even in the high-sheer stress conditions prevalent in arteries. The binding of the vWF A1 domains to the GP Ib$\alpha$ receptor is characterized, however, by fast dissociation, and is, therefore, reversible. Therefore, platelets continue to move with flowing blood. However, they are slowed sufficiently so that subsequently, through platelet activation, activated

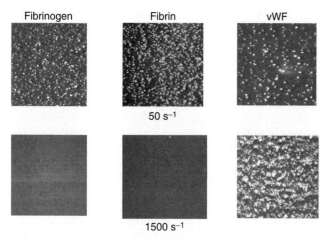

**FIGURE 27-1.** Platelet adhesion to fibrinogen, fibrin, and vWF under different shear stress conditions. Platelet adhesion to fibrinogen and fibrin occurs only in low shear rate *(upper panel)* conditions because of the slow association with the nonactivated IIb/IIIa receptor. Conversely, adhesion to immobilized vWF through the vWF receptor can occur at both high and low shear rates. Notably, platelet adhesion to vWF appears to be more efficient at high shear rate, probably because of the delivery of platelets to the wall under high flow. *(From Savage B, Salvidar E, Ruggeri CM: Initiation of platelet adhesion by arrest onto fibrinogen or translocation on von Willebrand factor. Cell 1996;84:289-297).*

GP IIb/IIIa becomes capable of binding to vWF. Thereafter, a more stable platelet thrombus can be formed (Fig. 27-2).

On the platelet side, GP Ib forms a complex with GP IX and GP V, with about 25,000 copies of the complex per platelet. The receptor site for vWF is located in the α subunit of GP Ib. GP IX is thought to stabilize the

bonds between the α and β subunits of GP Ib. GP V may act as a thrombin receptor, in addition to its stabilizing function. GP Ib is connected to actin-binding protein across the membrane to the submembrane actin cytoskeleton. Clinical situations in which there may be alterations in GP Ib (in either number or function) include diabetes (with an increase in the number of GP Ib receptors) and dialysis, uremia, and aortocoronary bypass (with a decrease in GP Ib expression). Following platelet activation, an inward movement of the vWFR occurs, with ultimately about 80% of the receptor being internalized (centralized) through remnants of the OCS.[58]

### Other Platelet Agonists

Although vWF, TXA$_2$, collagen, and ADP are physiologically the most important platelet agonists, various mediators, some with their own receptors, are capable of activating platelets. Thus, α$_2$-adrenergic receptors that are coupled to G$_i$ and bound to epinephrine have been described.[59] Platelet receptors for serotonin (released from dense granules) are also G-protein coupled.[60] Receptors are present for vasopressin[61] and PAF.[62] Platelets can also be activated by immune complexes,[63] cytokines,[64] and even LDL.[65]

### Platelet Antagonists

Prostacyclin, produced by endothelial cells, binds to a specific seven-transmembrane protein receptor (IP) on the platelet. Activation of the IP receptor activates adenylyl cyclase and increases cAMP levels, thereby inhibiting platelet aggregation.[66]

## Dual Step Platelet Adhesion to von Willebrand Factor

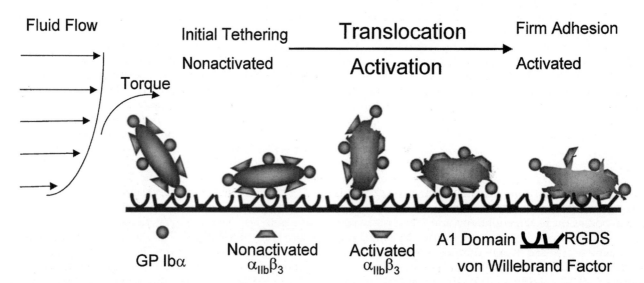

**FIGURE 27-2.** Schematic representation of platelet adhesion to vWF. Platelets are able to bind to immobilized vWF in high shear rate conditions through the GP Ibα component of the vWF receptor on the platelet. Although this binding is very efficient and can occur despite high shear, it is also characterized by fast dissociation and is, therefore, reversible. Particularly at the trailing edge, under the influence of flowing blood, platelets will tend to detach. Firm adhesion results once the GP IIb/IIIa receptor is activated. The activated receptor can then bind to vWF through the RGD sequence in the vWF C1 carboxyl terminal domain. *(From Ruggeri ZM: von Willebrand Factor. J Clin Invest 1997;99:559-564, with permission.)*

# Platelet Aggregation: Central Role of IIb/IIIa Receptor

The glycoprotein IIb/IIIa receptor, which is absent or defective in patients with Glanzmann's thrombasthenia, is central to the normal hemostatic function of platelets.[67] The recognition that platelets in Glanzmann's thrombasthenia have no aggregation in response to all known platelet agonists led to the discovery that these platelets lacked two glycoproteins, GP IIb and GP IIIa. Subsequently it was shown that these two glycoproteins form a $Ca^{2+}$-dependent complex on the platelet membrane.[68-70]

The GP IIb/IIIa ($\alpha_{IIb}\beta_3$) receptor belongs to the ubiquitous family of integrin adhesion receptors, but essentially it is found only in platelets (and their megakaryocyte precursors). It is also the most abundant protein on the platelet surface (~80,000 copies per resting platelet), with an additional 40,000 copies in reserve in $\alpha$ granules that are expressed after platelet activation.[69] The complex serves as a receptor for fibrinogen, fibronectin, vWF, and TSP. In addition to participating in platelet adhesion, the receptor mediates platelet aggregation and, thus, is central to thrombus formation.

The IIb/IIIa receptor (Fig. 27-3), like all integrins, is composed of two noncovalently linked $\alpha$ (the IIb component) and $\beta$ (the IIIa component) heterodimers, with each subunit coded by a separate gene.[71,72] Both genes are located on the long arm of chromosome 17q21.32. In both subunits, the carboxyl terminals are part of a short cytoplasmic domain, and the amino terminal is part of a large extracellular domain. The $\alpha_{IIb}$ precursor polypeptide is cleaved into a transmembrane light chain (25 kd) and an extracellular heavy chain (105 kd), which are disulfide linked. The $\alpha$ chain confers specificity of the integrin complex, while the $\beta$ chain is also present on other integrins, such as the vitronectin receptor (CD51). The $\beta$ chain is a single 762 amino acid chain with extracellular, transmembrane, and intracellular domains.

The IIb/IIIa receptor has a total of five calcium binding sites, four on the $\alpha$ chain and one on the $\beta$ chain. At 1 mmol Ca concentration (physiologic) the sites are fully occupied, but in the presence of lowered concentration, as in the presence of the anticoagulant sodium citrate, the occupancy is lower and its binding to fibrinogen is impaired. At extremely low levels of calcium (<1μmol) the two subunits dissociate.

The ligand-binding domain of the receptor is a pocket formed in the amino-terminal components of both chains. One of the key sequences in ligand binding is an RGD site found on the $\beta_{IIIa}$ subunit,[72] which corresponds to the RGD sequence on fibrinogen. This motif is also found on other integrins. Therefore, other sites on both the $\beta_{IIIa}$ and the $\alpha_{IIb}$ chain provide specificity. The other key binding sites recognize Lys-Glu-Ala-Gly-Asp-Val (KQAGDV motif) and the Lys-Gly-Asp (KGD motifs) (Fig. 27-3).

In addition to their adhesion function, integrins, including the IIb/IIIa receptor, have important signaling functions. Following initial platelet adhesion to immobilized vWF, collagen, ADP, or thrombin (the primary platelet agonists), a series of signaling events initiates

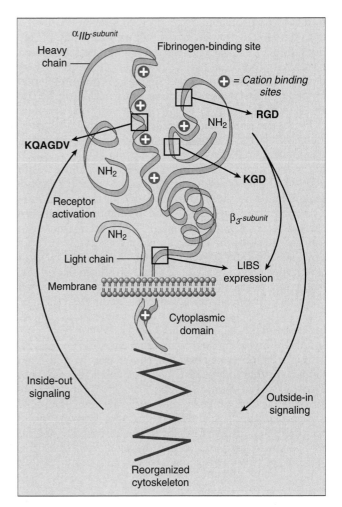

**FIGURE 27-3.** The GP IIb/IIIa receptor. The receptor is composed of noncovalently linked $\alpha$ (IIb component) and $\beta$ (IIIa component) heterodimer. The receptor has a total of five calcium-binding sites. Also illustrated are the RGD, KQAGDV, and KGD binding sites. Inside-out signaling leads to receptor activation, whereas outside-in signaling leads to secretion of platelet agonists as detailed in the text. *(From Chew DP, Moliterno DJ: A critical appraisal of platelet glycoprotein IIb/IIIa inhibition. J Am Coll Cardiol 2000;36:2028–2035.)*

cross-linking of the multivalent vWF and fibrinogen, thus leading to formation of a platelet aggregate. The cytoplasmic tails of the receptor subunits, although lacking enzymatic activity, provide anchor sites for signaling proteins and for cytoskeletal protein attachment, thereby linking the receptor to the platelet cytoskeleton.

## Glycoprotein IIb/IIIa Signaling Mechanisms

Signaling may occur in two distinct and complementary mechanisms: *inside-out* and *outside-in*.[73-75] In inside-out signaling, ligand binding to the IIb/IIIa receptor is regulated by the translation of intracellular signals to the cell-surface and extracellular environment. A conformational change occurs in the presence of platelet agonists (e.g., ADP, collagen, thrombin, or immobilized vWF) that transforms the IIb/IIIa receptor from a default low-affinity state to a high-affinity state for the soluble adhesive proteins, fibrinogen and vWF. Binding of intracellular proteins such as β3 endonexin to the β3 cytoplasmic tail may be involved in this signaling phase. In addition, receptor clustering occurs. The multivalent nature of vWF and fibrinogen then allows for cross-linking of platelets. Inside-out signaling is downregulated by NO and PGI$_2$ and is mediated, at least partly, by the PKC pathway.

In outside-in signaling biochemical signals are generated within the cell as a result of ligand occupation (fibrinogen, vWF, and synthetic compounds) and clustering of the receptor. Conformational changes in the ligand lead to the expression of neoepitopes called ligand-induced binding sites (LIBS). Outside-in signaling involves tyrosine phosphorylation of the β3 subunit within the integrin cytoplasmic tyrosine (ICY) domain. Outside-in signaling leads to the expression and secretion of secondary platelet products such as CD40L and platelet factor 4 (PF4) (involved in inflammation), prothrombinase and factor Xase (involved in coagulation), TXA$_2$ and serotonin (involved in vascular tone), and PDGF and other mitogens (involved in cell proliferation). α Granule proteins (including P-selectin, PDGF, TGFβ, and PF4) and dense body constituents (including serotonin and ADP) are secreted. These secreted platelet products function in autocrine loops to further induce platelet adhesion and aggregation. Thus, inside-out signaling is the primary event that initiates aggregation, whereas outside-in signaling is crucial for propagation, consolidation, and stabilization of the platelet plug and the vascular effects of platelets. Figure 27-4 summarizes the effects of inside-out and outside-in signaling.

## Aggregation

Although the IIb/IIIa receptor can bind to various adhesive proteins, its main importance is in platelet aggregation, which occurs when multivalent fibrinogen and vWF are bound to the receptor. The result is cross-linking of platelets and, hence, the formation of a platelet aggregate. Thus, although platelet adhesion can be initiated through multiple pathways involving a myriad of receptors binding multiple agonists, platelet aggregation occurs exclusively through the activation of the IIb/IIIa receptor. As such, activation of the receptor and the binding of fibrinogen and vWF represent the final common pathway of platelet thrombus formation.

Binding of vWF to the IIb/IIIa receptor occurs through the RGD sequence, which is also shared by other ligands, including fibronectin, vitronectin, and fibrinogen. The main binding site on fibrinogen, however, appears to be the KQAGDV sequence found in the carboxyl terminal of the γ chain of fibrinogen. The RGD motif also appears to contribute to binding of fibrinogen, because peptides containing this motif inhibit the binding of fibrinogen to the GP receptor.

As alluded to in the discussion on vWF, under high-shear conditions present in the arterial tree, initial platelet adhesion is mediated through GP Ibα to vWF (A1 domain). After platelet tethering to GP Ibα and activation, the GP IIb/IIIa receptor also binds to vWF, through binding to the Arg-Gly-Asp-Ser (RGDS) sequence on the C1 domain. Before activation, the IIB/IIIA receptor can only bind to immobilized fibrinogen and fibrin. Because this binding occurs relatively slowly, under

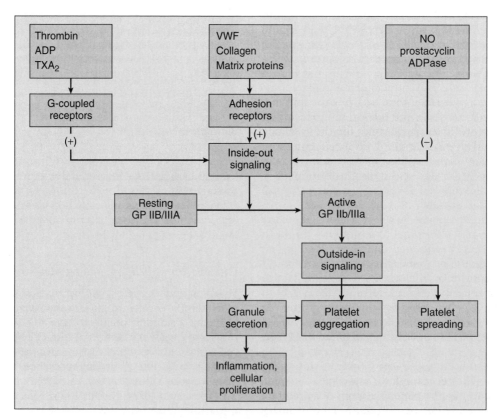

**FIGURE 27-4.** Inside-out and outside-in signaling.

high-shear and high-flow conditions initial binding to vWF is essential for platelet activation (Fig. 27-2). Thus, although aggregation ultimately requires IIb/IIIa activation, in high-shear conditions relevant in the arterial circulation, initial binding to vWF is a prerequisite to aggregation.

During activation there is an increase in the number of GP IIb/IIIa receptors on the platelet membrane because of the release of stored receptors from $\alpha$ granules. As with the vWFr (GP Ib$\alpha$-Ib$\beta$-IX-V) receptor, the GP IIb/IIIa receptor also redistributes on the surface of the platelet during activation. The redistribution occurs because of a conformational change, which not only allows for binding to fibrinogen but also links the receptor to the actin cytoskeleton, thereby stabilizing the ligand-receptor complex. Initially the receptor-ligand complexes are concentrated at the cell cortex, but subsequently a process of centralization occurs along linear tracks, most probably actin filaments. This redistribution may play a role in clot retraction.

## PLATELET GLYCOPROTEIN RECEPTOR POLYMORPHISMS

Inherited defects in platelet function include both the clinically obvious absent or defective glycoprotein receptor (e.g., Glanzmann's thrombasthenia) and subtle polymorphisms. Inherited polymorphisms in platelet glycoproteins have been implicated in platelet antigenicity with immunologic implications in such conditions as posttransfusion purpura, alloimmune thrombocytopenia, and refractoriness to platelet transfusions.[76] Whether platelet GP polymorphisms affect risk for thrombosis and ischemic events has generated great interest and controversy. Interestingly, venous thrombosis has not been associated with any integrin polymorphisms, reinforcing the role of platelets in arterial but not venous thrombosis.

Polymorphisms of the IIb/IIIa receptor involving both the $\alpha$IIb and $\beta$3 subunit have been described. Three alleles involving two residues are known for the $\alpha$IIb and eight different alleles differing in seven positions for the $\beta$3 subunit; two of the alleles (Leu40 and Arg40) are serologically indistinguishable. Similarly five alleles of GP Ib$\alpha$ have been described, differing in residue 145 (Thr/Met) and in size, depending on the number of tandem 13-amino-acid repeats in the macroglycopeptide portion of the molecule along with two alleles for the Ib$\beta$ subunit. The collagen receptor $\alpha$2$\beta$1 (GP Ia-IIa) has four allelic variants dependent on positions 505 (Glu, Lys) and 799 (Thr/Met); the different alleles determine receptor density that in turn correlates with adhesion to collagen I and III.

Given the central role of platelet integrins in adhesion and aggregation, platelet integrin polymorphisms have been the subject of intense scrutiny for a possible association with risk for vascular disease. The greatest data, with both positive and negative studies, involves the $\beta_3$PI$^{A2}$ allele found in approximately 15% of the population.[76] A cytosine to thymidine substitution on exon 2 of the GP IIIa($\beta$3) gene leads to a leucine to proline substi-

tution at position 33, with resultant change in the conformation of the amino terminus. This polymorphism has been associated in some but not all studies with increased risk of arterial thrombosis. Platelet function tests, including binding to fibrinogen, have also yielded contradictory results. One possible explanation is that elevated fibrinogen levels are also requisite for enhanced aggregability with the PlA1/A1 polymorphism.

The PlA2 genotype has also been associated with aspirin resistance. *In vitro* combination inhibition or higher aspirin doses appear to overcome aspirin resistance. Absence of vWFR (GP Ib-IX) results in BSS characterized by giant platelets, thrombocytopenia, and mild bleeding. BSS may occur from nonsense mutations or deletions in GP Ib$\alpha$, GP Ib$\beta$, or GP IX. Three main polymorphisms have been described for the vWFR, all involving GP Ib$\alpha$: the Kozak polymorphism in position 5 (thymine for cytosine), HPA 2 polymorphism at position 145 (threonine for methionine), and variability in the number of 13-amino-acid tandem repeats (VNTR) in the mucin-like macroglycopeptide stalk of the receptor. Studies linking these polymorphisms to clinical events have been conflicting. Polymorphisms in the collagen receptor GP Ia/IIa •$\alpha_2\beta_1$) that involve the $\alpha_2$ chain have been described. However, clinical relevance is unclear. Given the polygenic nature of the system along with changing environmental influences, it is not surprising that these relatively subtle polymorphisms produce variable clinical outcomes in different populations.

## POTENTIAL ROLE OF PLATELETS IN ATHEROSCLEROSIS

Platelets have been postulated to participate in the response to injury model of atherosclerosis. The appreciation of the platelets' ability to occasionally adhere to dysfunctional but intact endothelial cells, along with the presence of various proinflammatory mediators (such as TGF-$\beta$, PF4, RANTES, and P-selectin) in platelet $\alpha$ granules, has helped implicate platelets in atherosclerosis.

P-selectin (CD62) is found in platelets and stored in $\alpha$ granules. On platelet activation it is rapidly detectable on the surface, with about 12,000 molecules per platelet.[77,78] P-selectin is a cysteine-rich glycosylated transmembrane protein, with a domain similar to the repeated motifs of epidermal growth factor and nine sushi domains. P-selectin mediates platelet attachment to neutrophils and monocytes. Conversely, P-selectin on endothelial cells may also bind to platelets[79] through the GP Ib receptor, thereby leading to platelet adhesion. Given the role of P-selectin in mediating platelet-endothelial and platelet-inflammatory cell interactions, it may play a role in atherosclerosis.[80] Platelet activation leads to expression and release of P-selectin, and increased blood levels have been used to document platelet activation. The prognostic implications in coronary disease are uncertain.[81]

Platelets are also a major source of circulating CD40L, a trimeric transmembrane protein of the tumor necrosis family. Originally described as an important signal involved in B-cell maturation, it was subsequently shown that both the ligand and its receptor (CD40) are found on platelets. Following platelet stimulation CD40L is expressed on the platelet surface, where a soluble trimeric fragment termed sCD40L is released through cleavage. Increased sCD40L levels have been documented in patients with ACSs,[82] those undergoing PCI or cardiopulmonary bypass, and those with peripheral arterial occlusive disease. The sCD40L fragment appears to retain much of the multifunctionality of the parent compound, which can bind and activate both the IIb/IIIa receptor and the CD40 receptor. The IIb/IIIa receptor in turn appears to contribute to sCD40L release. Both prothrombic and proinflammatory effects, such as the expression of various adhesion molecules, have been attributed to activation of CD40 by its ligand. Interestingly, recent data suggests that patients with ACSs and elevated sCD40L derive benefit from GP IIb/IIIa blockade.[82]

Given the central role of inflammation in atherosclerosis, the potential role of platelets and the CD40 system has received growing attention. In the LDL receptor deficient mouse, blocking of the CD40 system prevented the progression of atherosclerotic lesions.[83] Similar results have been described in the ApoE-deficient mouse.[84] Recent data has also implicated thrombus-derived sCD40L in restenosis after PCI.[85]

## TESTS OF PLATELET AGGREGATION

Presently, there is no accepted, standardized platelet aggregation test. Consequently, different pharmacodynamic studies have used different tests, making comparisons across studies difficult. The need for point-of-care testing, particularly in the catheterization laboratory has led to the development of rapid platelet function tests, and there are increasing amounts of data generated by these tests.

The Ivy template bleeding time, long used to screen patients for bleeding diatheses before surgery, has not been shown to be of prognostic use in the absence of antiplatelet therapy (surgical and medical patients)[86] and in the setting of IIb/IIIa inhibition.[87] Thus, it has no role in the current evaluation of antiplatelet therapy.

The most common method for assessing platelet function in vitro is light transmission aggregometry (LTA), or turbidimetry. Agonist is added to platelet-rich plasma (PRP), resulting in increased light transmission as the platelet aggregates sediment to the bottom of the tube. The presence of IIb/IIIa antagonist results in reduced aggregation and, hence, reduced light transmission. Unfortunately, there is no accepted standardization of agonist use and concentration, and it is not known whether a normalization to the platelet count must be performed.

LTA is time consuming and operator dependent and, therefore, not readily applicable to routine clinical situations. An alternative approach that is rapidly gaining popularity is the automated rapid platelet function assay (RFPA) (Ultegra, Accumetrics, Inc, San Diego, CA).[88] The assay relies on the agglutination of fibrinogen-coated beads added to whole blood anticoagulated with either citrate or PPACK. The assay uses iso-TRAP (modified thrombin-receptor activating peptide) instead of 20-μmol ADP agonist. The results of RFPA using the Ultegra machine do not correlate precisely with LTA results; the Ultegra machine gives somewhat higher values.

Another approach, independent of the choice of agonist or the presence of non-IIb/IIIa antiplatelet agents, assesses IIb/IIIa receptor occupancy.[89] With abciximab, radiolabeled antibody is added to blood treated with the unlabeled antibody, and percent binding is calculated, reflecting unoccupied receptors. With small-molecule IIb/IIIa inhibitors, the induction of LIBS allows the use of specific antibodies, such as D3, to detect receptor occupancy using flow cytometry. Receptor occupancy correlates better with plasma drug levels than LTA does, but it requires special equipment and proficiency to perform and, therefore, is not widely used clinically.

Alternative approaches to platelet aggregation assays include thromboelastography, shear-induced platelet aggregation, and whole-blood electric-impedance aggregometry. In thromboelastographic assays, blood clotting is measured by the reduction in the movement of a rotary bar and reflects both the platelet and humoral coagulation cascade. In shear-induced platelet aggregation, various chambers have been developed in which platelets are subjected to both shear stress and agonists, and the induction of a platelet plug leads to closure of an aperture. Impedance aggregometry takes advantage of an increase in electrical impedance when platelets aggregate in solution.

## Choice of Platelet Agonists in Aggregation Tests

The estimated efficacy of antiplatelet agents such as the IIb/IIIa antagonists varies depending on the type of agonist used and its concentration. A more potent agonist used at a higher concentration will result in greater mobilization of IIb/IIIa receptors and hence will result in lesser inhibition of platelet aggregation in the presence of a given antagonist. The choice of platelet agonist for in vitro testing remains controversial. Historically, ADP has been widely used, at both 5 μmol/L (used in the initial dose-finding studies with tirofiban) and 20 μmol/L (used in the initial dose-finding studies with eptifibatide and abciximab). Recently TRAPs, iso-TRAP, and collagen, which is physiologically relevant to plaque rupture, have gained acceptance.[90] TRAPs are 6- to 14-amino-acid peptides and mimic the portion of the thrombin receptor, which on binding of thrombin is cleaved and then acts as a tethered PAR-1 ligand, promoting platelet activation. TRAP-induced platelet aggregation is more resistant to the effect of IIb/IIIa inhibitors. The use of non-ADP agonists also allows the assessment of antiplatelet activity in patients treated with ticlopidine and clopidogrel. Because these drugs are often administered before PCI, the use of non-ADP agonists allows for clinically relevant monitoring in the catheterization laboratory, as is the case with the use of the Ultegra machine.

## Choice of Anticoagulant in Platelet Assays

The choice of anticoagulant used in platelet assays is also of importance. Both EDTA and citrate chelate calcium ions, thereby adversely affecting the function of the IIB/IIIA receptor, which has five calcium-binding sites. EDTA cannot be used in platelet assays because of its potent calcium-chelating effect, whereas citrate has been shown to reduce free calcium concentration in plasma samples from 1 mmol/L to 40 to 50 μmol/L. This decrease in calcium concentration results in an antiaggregatory effect and hence leads to an overestimation of the effect of anti-IIb/IIIa agents. This effect was first recognized with eptifibatide: the platelet aggregation IC50 was found to be fourfold higher if the anticoagulant PPACK was used instead of citrate (PPACK does not chelate calcium).[91] Similar, but somewhat less profound findings, have been found with tirofiban and abciximab. The implication is that dose-ranging studies using citrated samples may have led to underdosing, through overestimation of the degree of platelet inhibition.

## ANTIPLATELET THERAPY

### Aspirin

Although its use as an analgesic (in the form of the willow bark) dates back centuries and its antipyretic effects date from the 18th century, the antiplatelet effects of aspirin were first recognized in the 1960s.[92] Aspirin is now prescribed almost universally to patients with coronary disease and is also widely used for primary prevention of MI.

Aspirin, in doses of 30 to 1500 mg per day, inhibits the production of cyclic prostanoids such as $TXA_2$ and $PGI_2$. ASA, by acetylating ser529 of COX-1 and ser516 of COX-2, inhibits both isoforms; however, ASA is more than 150 times more potent as a COX-1 inhibitor. By inhibiting platelet production of $TXA_2$, platelet aggregation is markedly reduced. The negative impact on prostacyclin production appears not to have major clinical impact, because of the reserve of the prostacyclin system.[93] This may partly be due to the ability of endothelial cells to generate new COX enzyme, which is unmatched in the platelet because it does not have a nuclear apparatus. Aspirin may also have antioxidant effects and may increase NO production in endothelial cells and platelets.

Aspirin is rapidly absorbed from the upper GI tract but has a very short half-life of only 20 minutes in the plasma. Because platelets cannot regenerate COX-1 and aspirin binds covalently to ser529, platelets are inhibited for their entire lifespan of 10 days. Hemostasis may recover in a matter of 2 to 3 days, however, because of the availability of new platelets.

The benefit of ASA in the setting of acute MI was firmly established in the ISIS-2 trial, in which aspirin alone produced a 23% reduction in vascular mortality, equal to that achieved by streptokinase; the two treatments in combination yielded a 42% risk reduction.[94] Similarly, aspirin has been shown to be of benefit in patients with unstable angina and non-ST-segment elevation MI, with a 49% to 72% reduction in nonfatal MI or death. Benefits were also demonstrated in long-term use of aspirin for secondary prevention in a meta-analysis of over 140 trials, although each individual trial did not demonstrate statistical reductions in mortality.[95] In high-risk secondary prevention patients the meta-analysis revealed an 18% reduction in vascular mortality.[95] Primary prevention with aspirin has also been shown to be beneficial in preventing nonfatal MI in the Physicians' Health Study (PHS), with a 44% reduction in this all-male study.[96,97] This effect was limited to those older than 50 years and was not accompanied by a mortality benefit, whereas a trend toward increased hemorrhagic stroke was noted. In the similar but smaller British Physicians' Study (5139 subjects vs. 22,071 subjects in the U.S. PHS), there was no reduction in MI risk and there was a troubling increase in disabling stroke.[98] In the higher risk patients enrolled in the Thrombosis Prevention Trial, there was a 20% reduction in ischemic heart disease events (fatal and nonfatal MI, other cardiac death) but again no mortality reduction.[99] Similarly, in patients with hypertension enrolled in the Hypertension Optimal Treatment (HOT) randomized trial, low-dose aspirin (75 mg/day) reduced major CV events by 15% (P = 0.03) and MI by 36% (P = 0.002).[100] There was no effect on stoke and no increase in fatal bleeds, but major nonfatal bleeds were twice as common in the aspirin arm. Patients with stable chronic angina have been shown to have marked benefit. Importantly, no randomized data on the efficacy of aspirin is available for women (the role of aspirin in women is being evaluated in the ongoing Women's Health Study). Thus, it appears that the use of aspirin for primary prevention is predicated on the underlying risk of MI (see reference 99 for a recent analysis of risk vs. benefit for aspirin in primary prevention).

Besides the well-known GI side effects of aspirin, antiplatelet therapy with aspirin is limited by the phenomenon of aspirin resistance, with up to 40% demonstrating resistance even at higher doses.[101-103] Moreover, aspirin does not completely inhibit the production of $TXA_2$, and other agonists may bypass the $TXA_2$ pathway of platelet activation. Indeed, in the IIb/IIIa trials of upstream use in UA/NSTEMI, prior aspirin use predicted benefit of the IIb/IIIa agent, most probably because it identified patients with aspirin resistance who were having thrombotic events despite the use of aspirin.

### Aspirin, NSAIDs, and COX-2 Selective Agents

The identification of two isoforms of COX–COX-1 and COX-2–has allowed the development of COX-2 selective agents.[104] COX-2 expression occurs at sites of inflammation, whereas COX-1 is constitutively expressed throughout the body, including the gastric mucosa where constitutive COX-1expression produces protective prostaglandins. Nonselective NSAID use is estimated to cause more than 100,000 hospitalizations and 16,500 deaths in the United States per year. Selective COX-2 inhibitors hold the promise of providing anti-inflammatory effects that are equal to nonselective agents, while avoiding the side effects of nonselective NSAIDs, particularly the GI side effects thought to be induced by COX-1 inhibition of the gastric mucosa. The COX-2 hypothesis has been confirmed in the VIGOR study, which randomized 8076 patients with rheumatoid arthritis to double the standard dose of rofecoxib (50 mg/day) or to the standard dose of naproxen (500 mg twice daily).[86] Despite the higher rofecoxib dose, there was a 54% reduction in the primary GI endpoint, a composite of perforations, ulcers, and bleeds.

The VIGOR study, while demonstrating the greater GI safety of rofecoxib, was also noteworthy for raising CV safety issues relating to the use of selective COX-2 agents, particularly the highly selective agent rofecoxib. In VIGOR, there was a significantly higher nonfatal MI rate in the rofecoxib arm compared with the naproxen arm (0.5% vs. 0.1%), with no significant difference in total mortality. Given that selective COX-2 agents inhibit prostacyclin ($PGI_2$) production in endothelial cells, the concern has been raised that COX-2 agents may lead to a prothrombic state. The prostacyclin system is noteworthy for its reserve, so that in normal subjects even full-dose COX-2 inhibition, which leads to a 60% to 70% decrease in prostacyclin metabolite excretion, does not lead to any measurable increase in platelet activity. However, an effect in patients at risk for CV events, who may have diminished prostacyclin reserve, has not been ruled out by such studies in normal subjects. Because the VIGOR study did not contain a placebo arm, it is not clear whether the difference between the two arms was the result of a lowered event rate with naproxen, an increased event rate with rofecoxib, or a combination of the two. Reassuringly, data from two placebo-controlled trials in elderly patients with multiple CV factors found no increase in thrombotic complications in the rofecoxib arms.[86]

Depending on their level of COX-1 inhibition on platelets, nonselective NSAIDs may have significant antiplatelet effects. Naproxen has been shown to inhibit platelet activation to a similar extent as 81 mg of aspirin throughout its dosing interval. Ibuprofen, on the other hand, inhibits platelets immediately postdosage, but this effect is markedly attenuated at the end of the dosing interval. Despite its antiplatelet effects, naproxen is not an ideal antiplatelet agent because its binding to COX is noncovalent, and, therefore, the antiplatelet effect lasts only as long as the agent is taken without interruption. A single dose of aspirin, given the covalent nature of aspirin binding to COX, confers an antiplatelet effect for up to 10 days.

Nonselective NSAID binding to COX-1 on platelets has been shown to prevent access of aspirin to Ser-529, acetylation of which is necessary for the antiplatelet effect of aspirin. A recent study has shown that prior dosing with ibuprofen reduced the antiplatelet effect of aspirin.[87] In contrast prior dosing with either acetaminophen or rofecoxib, both of which do not have significant binding to platelet COX, did not alter the efficacy of aspirin.

## GP IIb/IIIa Inhibitors

The identification of the GP IIb/IIIa receptor has led to the development of both intravenous and oral inhibitors of the receptor. Three intravenous inhibitors—the antibody abciximab and the small molecules eptifibatide and tirofiban—have now been studied in patients in randomized clinical trials. Although all three agents effectively inhibit the IIb/IIIa receptors, there are marked differences among them in receptor specificity, pharmacokinetics, and pharmacodynamics, with clinical implications.

Abciximab,[105-111] a chimeric murine monoclonal antibody, binds to the IIb/IIIa receptor in a site distinct from the RGD sequence as evidenced by binding despite occupation of the binding pocket by RGD peptides. Interference with receptor function may, therefore, depend on steric hindrance by the large (47.6 kd) antibody molecule. Abciximab appears to bind to the IIIa subunit ($\beta3$ integrin). It also binds to the vitronectin receptor ($\alpha v\beta3$) that shares the $\beta3$ integrin subunit with the IIb/IIIa receptor and to the Mac-1 ($\alpha M\beta2$) integrin, although with lower affinity.

Abciximab is rapidly and uniformly bound to the IIb/IIIa receptor after an intravenous bolus, and the free drug in plasma is rapidly eliminated. The plasma half-life is only 26 minutes, but platelet-bound abciximab has been detected for up to 14 days after cessation of the infusion. The dissociation constant (KD) is approximately 5 nmol/L consistent with very high affinity for the IIb/IIIa receptor. A bolus of 0.25 mg/kg followed by a 12-hour infusion of 10 µg/minute has been shown to provide more than 80% receptor occupancy and more than 80% inhibition of platelet aggregation as measured by turbidimetric assay using 20-µmol/L ADP as agonist during the infusion period. Significantly, receptor occupancy dropped to approximately 70% within 12 hours after discontinuing the infusion, and platelet aggregation increased to 60% of baseline within 6 hours. Abciximab and other IIb/IIIa agents demonstrate a steep dose-response curve, with greater than 80% receptor occupancy necessary for significant inhibition of platelet aggregation. Moreover, clinical data suggests that this threshold is also prerequisite for prevention of clinical events.

Abciximab redistributes to new, unoccupied platelets; if no additional dose is delivered, this results in a reduction in receptor occupancy, which, if below threshold, would be accompanied by a return of platelet aggregation. This provides for a mechanism to reverse bleeding complications with platelet transfusions.

Eptifibatide (Integrilin, Millenium Pharmaceuticals) is a synthetic cyclic heptapeptide (832 d) based on the structure of barbourin, a 73-amino-acid peptide derived from the venom of *Sistrurus m. barbouri,* a southeastern pigmy rattlesnake.[112] Barbourin is one of many snake venoms that comprise the disintegrin family, so named because of their ability to bind and block various integrins. Barbourin is highly specific for the GP IIb/IIIa receptor but is rapidly degraded by proteases, thereby limiting its clinical usefulness. By modifying its structure into a cyclic heptapeptide, resistance to plasma proteases is conferred. Antigenic potential is also reduced by the compact cyclic structure.

Eptifibatide like barbourin binds to the GP IIb/IIIa receptor through a KGD sequence, in contrast to physiologic ligands that bind through an RGD sequence.

Binding of eptifibatide requires the presence of calcium and intact receptor structures. Binding is reversible, so that, after discontinuation of the infusion, platelet function returns to normal within 6 hours. Eptifibatide has a lower affinity to the receptor than abciximab, so that the majority of the drug circulates unbound. Excretion is primarily renal, and reduced dosing should be used in patients with moderate renal insufficiency. Use in severe renal failure is associated with a marked increase in drug levels.

Tirofiban (Aggrastat, Merck & Co), the smallest of the GP IIb/IIIa inhibitors (495 d), is a nonantigenic tyrosine analog that mimics the RGD motif.[113] It has a high affinity and very high specificity to the IIb/IIIa receptor. Renal clearance mandates reduction of the dose in severe renal failure (creatinine clearance <30 mL/minute).

### Pharmacodynamics of IIb/IIIa inhibitors: Dose Selection

The dosing of IIb/IIIa inhibitors has been an area of continued investigation and controversy for many years. Several factors have contributed to the difficulties in determining the optimal dosing of these agents:

1. The exact degree of platelet inhibition requisite for optimal clinical outcome varies depending on the clinical condition (ACS vs. elective; upstream use vs. catheterization laboratory use).
2. Given the myriad of platelet agonists (ADP, thrombin, collagen, etc.) available, the ideal *in vitro* agonist and its dosage is yet to be determined.
3. Platelet aggregation has traditionally been measured in suspension, with limited applicability to *in vivo* flow conditions; no gold standard test of aggregation has been identified.
4. Preparation of blood samples with the anticoagulant citrate reduces the availability of free calcium, thereby decreasing platelet aggregation and leading to overestimation of antiplatelet effect, particularly in the setting of eptifibatide use. Recently, anticoagulants that do not chelate (e.g., PPACK) have replaced citrate.

Historical animal studies using LTA assays have identified a target of more than 80% inhibition of platelet aggregation as necessary and sufficient to prevent thrombus formation. This goal was, therefore, accepted as the target for dose identification in the development of IIb/IIIa inhibitors as discussed in the section on GP IIb/IIIa inhibitors.

Using citrated blood, abciximab dosing was selected in phase II studies in patients with PCI. The dose selected was 0.25 mg/kg bolus, followed by a 12-hour infusion of 10 µg/kg. In this regimen, 95% of the total dose is given as a bolus, achieving greater than 80% platelet inhibition.

The clinical efficacy of the intravenous GP IIb/IIIa inhibitors (abciximab, tirofiban, and eptifibatide) has been extensively evaluated in a large number of clinical trials, enrolling in aggregate more than 100,000 patients. Three main areas of clinical use have been identified: PCI, non-ST elevation ACS, and ST-segment elevation MI.

The greatest clinical use and the most robust data from clinical trials has been in the catheterization laboratory setting. PCI, whether with balloon angioplasty, atherectomy, or with stenting, results in significant disruption of the endothelial layer and, thus, creates the condition for platelet activation and aggregation. In this regard PCI mimics and provides a model for ACS and plaque rupture, the very disease it is designed to treat. Ischemic complications, the major complications of PCI, have been consistently reduced; a pooled analysis demonstrated a 34% relative and a 2.9% absolute reduction in death and MI (Fig. 27-5).

Abciximab use for PCI (evaluated vs. placebo) has been studied in EPIC,[114] EPILOG, CAPTURE,[115] and EPISTENT,[116] the latter demonstrating a benefit in the setting of stenting. Notably, in EPISTENT, balloon angioplasty with abciximab was superior to stenting without abciximab and equivalent to stenting with abciximab, demonstrating the importance of IIb/IIIa inhibition in the acute PCI setting; the benefit of stenting was long term with a reduction in restenosis.

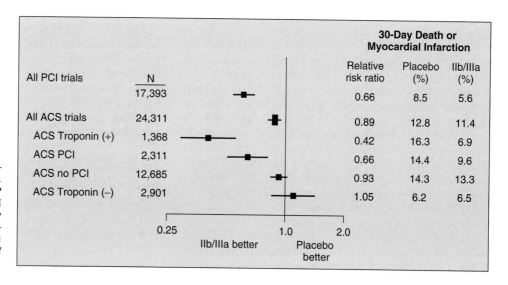

**FIGURE 27-5.** GP IIb/IIIa receptor antagonists in clinical practice. Pooled analysis of intravenous GP IIb/IIIa receptor antagonists in PCI trials and ACS trials. *(From Chew DP, Moliterno DJ: A critical appraisal of platelet glycoprotein IIb/IIIa inhibition. J Am Coll Cardiol 2000;36: 2028–2035.)*

|  | N | | 30-Day Death or Myocardial Infarction | | |
|---|---|---|---|---|---|
|  |  |  | Relative risk ratio | Placebo (%) | IIb/IIIa (%) |
| All PCI trials | 17,393 |  | 0.66 | 8.5 | 5.6 |
| All ACS trials | 24,311 |  | 0.89 | 12.8 | 11.4 |
| ACS Troponin (+) | 1,368 |  | 0.42 | 16.3 | 6.9 |
| ACS PCI | 2,311 |  | 0.66 | 14.4 | 9.6 |
| ACS no PCI | 12,685 |  | 0.93 | 14.3 | 13.3 |
| ACS Troponin (−) | 2,901 |  | 1.05 | 6.2 | 6.5 |

0.25     1.0     2.0
IIb/IIIa better     Placebo better

The use of abciximab for ST-segment elevation MI (STEMI) with PCI has been studied in the RAPPORT[117] trial using angioplasty and in the ISAR 2,[118] ADMIRAL,[119] and CADILLAC[120,121] studies using stenting. Although ISAR-2 and ADMIRAL demonstrated a benefit of abciximab in the setting of STEMI treated with primary stenting, the CADILLAC trial did not show a benefit of abciximab in the setting of stenting nor was the postprocedural TIMI grade 3 flow improved with abciximab. The relatively low-risk population enrolled in this study, as reflected by the much lower mortality rate when compared with other primary PCI trials, may have accounted for this surprising lack of benefit.

Eptifibatide was initially evaluated for use in PCI in the IMPACT-II study.[122] Eptifibatide was infused at a 135 µg/kg bolus followed by either a 0.5 or 0.75 µg/kg/minute infusion for 20 to 24 hours postprocedure. Although there was a trend toward reduction of events at 30 days, it was not statistically significant. Moreover, there was actually less benefit seen with the higher dose. When the effect of citrate anticoagulation (which increases the apparent inhibitory effect of eptifibatide) on the dosing of eptifibatide was appreciated, it became apparent that the IMPACT-II dose was suboptimal. The subsequent ESPRIT[123,124] trial used a higher loading dose (two 180 µg/kg boluses given 10 minutes apart, followed by a continuous infusion of 2.0 µg/kg/minute) versus placebo in stable patients. The trial showed a 35% risk reduction at 30 days (3.7% absolute risk reduction; P = 0.0034), which was sustained at 6 months with a 22% relative risk reduction (4.1% absolute risk reduction; P = 0.0083). In ESPRIT, the anticoagulation regimen used was identical in the two arms, the eptifibatide arm and the placebo arm, with a targeted activated clotting time (ACT) of 250 seconds. A meta-analysis of the placebo arms of six trials with abciximab, has identified a U-shaped relationship; an ACT range of 350 to 375 seconds provides the lowest ischemic event rate (34% lower than the rate observed between 171 and 295 seconds).[125] In the presence of abciximab, the U-shaped relationship no longer held, with a plateau in event rates across ACT values between 275 to 375 seconds. The implication of this meta-analysis is that the benefit seen in recent IIB/IIIa trials using lower ACT targets in the placebo arm, such as in ESPRIT, may be overstated.

The use of tirofiban for PCI was evaluated in the RESTORE[126] trial, using a dose of 10 µg/kg bolus plus a 0.15 µg/kg/minute infusion. The treated group had a relative risk reduction of 24% in the 30-day composite endpoint of death, MI, and urgent target-vessel revascularization (10.5% vs. 8.0%), but this difference did not reach statistical significance. The lack of routine CK monitoring and administration of the drug only after the lesion was crossed with a wire was postulated to have led to a somewhat diminished result. The TARGET trial,[127] the only head-to-head large-scale evaluation of two different IIb/IIIa agents, randomized patients undergoing both emergent (ACS) and elective PCI procedures to tirofiban and abciximab. The primary endpoint (death, MI, and target-vessel revascularization) at the predefined 30 days was 7.55% versus 6.01%, demonstrating

superiority of abciximab to tirofiban with the benefit being driven by patients with ACS. At 6 months, moreover, results in the two treatment arms were not significantly different.

The availability of point-of-care (POC) testing for platelet inhibition has allowed for better determination of IIb/IIIa dosing for both efficacy and safety. The GOLD study,[128] using the Ultegra RPA assessed the level of platelet inhibition at 10 minutes, 1 hour, 8 hours, and 24 hours in 500 patients undergoing PCI. The incidence of MACE (death, MI, and urgent target-vessel revascularization) correlated with the level of IIb/IIIa inhibition measured by the RFPA at all time points. RFPA inhibition of 95% or more at 10 minutes was associated with a markedly decreased incidence of MACE (8.1%), whereas platelet inhibition of less than 70% at 8 hours was associated with a MACE rate of 25%. The importance of achieving very high levels of platelet inhibition, particularly during the initial minutes of an intervention, may at least partly explain the results of the TARGET trial. A recent study using LTA in 17 patients treated with tirofiban versus abciximab (using the TARGET dosage) found that in the time period of 15 to 60 minutes postbolus the abciximab dose provided greater platelet inhibition.[129] This time period is considered critical in the setting of PCI, because iatrogenic vessel injury occurs during this time period. Given that 70% of the dose of abciximab is delivered in the loading dose, the results of this trial are consistent with the pharmacologic characteristics of the two agents. Conceivably, adjusting the dosage of tirofiban may overcome this limitation, but this requires validation in a large outcome study.

The benefit of IIb/IIIa inhibitors for ACS (NSTEMI/Unstable Angina [UA]) has been demonstrated with the small molecules eptifibatide (PURSUIT[130]) and tirofiban (PRISM[131], PRISM-PLUS[132]). Moreover, the TACTICS trial (TIMI-18)[133] demonstrated the superiority of an invasive catheterization based approach in patients with ACS in the setting of tirofiban use. Previous studies, before the era of IIb/IIIa inhibitors and widespread stent use, were unable to substantiate a benefit of the invasive approach.[134-136] Particular benefit was demonstrated for patients with ST-segment depression and troponin elevations.

Abciximab has been evaluated in the medical therapy of ACS patients (NSTEMI/UA) in the large GUSTO IV-ACS trial.[137] Surprisingly, in stark contrast to the benefit of abciximab when given for PCI, there was no benefit demonstrated. Possibly a lack of sustained platelet inhibition over the 48 to 72 hours of abciximab infusion (because most of the administered dose is in the initial bolus) may explain the lack of benefit.

## GP IIb/IIIa Inhibitors in ST-Segment Elevation Myocardial Infarction

Although the role of GP IIb/IIIa inhibition in the setting of UA/NSTEMI and PCI has been firmly established, its use in the setting of ST elevation is less well established. Lytic therapy, although effective in reestablishing vessel patency, achieves TIMI III flow rates in only 60%

of patients, and persistent normal tissue perfusion is probably achieved in only 25% of patients. Lytic therapy, partly because of the release of thrombin, is associated with platelet activation. Coupled with the central role of platelet aggregation in coronary thrombosis and the efficacy of aspirin as shown in the ISIS-2 study,[92] IIb/IIIa inhibition appears theoretically attractive.

Multiple dose-ranging studies, particularly with abciximab but also with eptifibatide and to a lesser extent with tirofiban, have evaluated the role of these agents alone and in combination with lytic therapy. Without lytic therapy, IIb/IIIa inhibition leads only to minimally increased flow compared with placebo. Combination therapy with half-dose lytic therapy and full-dose IIb/IIIa inhibition does lead to increased rates of TIMI 3 flow at 90 minutes, but this improvement has not been accompanied by significant reductions in mortality. Moreover, in the large GUSTO-V trial,[138] combination therapy was associated with an increased risk of bleeding, including intracranial hemorrhage, in patients older than 75 years; all patients showed an increase in major nonintracranial and minor bleeding.

### Oral IIB/IIIAs

The efficacy of intravenous IIB/IIIA agents to reduce CV events in patients with UA/NSTEMI and in those undergoing PCI has led to the development of oral agents in the hope of extending the benefit to outpatient chronic use. Trials with agents such as orbofiban, sibrafiban, and xemilofiban have demonstrated either no long-term benefit or an actual increase in event-rate.[139] A potential mechanism for this disappointing and initially surprising findings is that the relatively short-acting oral agents actually lead to a prothrombic state on dissociating from the receptor, whereupon the receptor is left in an activated state and is able to bind soluble fibrinogen. A study in which low-dose abciximab was added and washed from platelets demonstrated just such increased fibrinogen binding. In the OPUS/TIMI-16 trial[140] with orbofiban, increased fibrinogen binding was demonstrated, along with increased P-selectin levels (a marker of platelet activation). Thus, a leading hypothesis is that trough levels of inhibition are associated with increased platelet aggregation. Whether oral agents with longer half-lives would be of greater benefit remains to be seen.

## Thienopyridine ADP Receptor Blockers

Ticlopidine and clopidogrel inhibit platelet aggregation by blocking the ADP receptor $P2Y_{12}$ on platelets. The short-term (30 day) use of these agents, in conjunction with ASA, has been shown to markedly reduce the risk of stent thrombosis. Ticlopidine, which is administered twice daily, has been associated with neutropenia, usually within the first 2 months of therapy. Aplastic anemia has also been associated with the use of ticlopidine. Although both agents have been associated with thrombotic thrombocytopenic purpura (TTP),[141,142] the incidence appears to be lower with clopidogrel. The CLASSICS trial[143] demonstrated similar protection from stent thrombosis with the use of both agents in conjunction with ASA; clopidogrel was better tolerated, and, thus, it has largely supplanted ticlopidine in clinical practice.

Long-term use of clopidogrel in both medically and mechanically treated patients has been evaluated in several large trails. In 19,185 patients with a history of previous MI, stroke, or peripheral vascular disease (PVD) enrolled in the CAPRIE trial.[144] Those treated with clopidogrel had an annual 5.32% risk of ischemic stroke, MI, or vascular death compared with 5.83% with aspirin for a relative risk reduction of 8.7% in favor of clopidogrel (95% CI 0.3 to 16.5). Notably, the benefit appeared driven by the patients with PVD. The CURE trial[145] randomized 12,562 patients with unstable angina to clopidogrel plus aspirin versus aspirin alone for 3 to 12 months, with a median duration of 9 months. Clopidogrel was administered within 24 hours of presentation at a dose of 75 mg/day following a loading dose of 300 mg, and aspirin was administered at a dose of 75 to 325 mg daily. There was a 20% reduction in the primary composite endpoint of CV death, nonfatal MI, or stroke (9.3% vs. 11.4%; RR 0.80 with 95% CI 0.72 to 0.90; P < 0.001) and also a reduction in significant, but not life-threatening, bleeding (3.7% vs. 2.7%; RR 1.38; P = 0.001). In the subgroup of patients (n = 2658) undergoing PCI (who received clopidogrel for 6 days on average before their procedure), there was a 30% reduction in the 30-day composite of death, MI, or urgent target-vessel revascularization.[146] Long-term administration was also associated with a significant event reduction, for a total 31% reduction in death or MI. Whether clopidogrel should be continued post-PCI beyond 30 days was also evaluated in the CREDO trial.[147] Patients (n = 2116) undergoing elective PCI were given a loading dose of 300 mg clopidogrel followed by 75 mg/day for 12 months versus a placebo loading dose and 75 mg/day for 30 days followed by placebo. There was a 27% relative risk reduction in the combined endpoint of death, MI, or stroke (absolute risk reduction of 3%). Pretreatment was not associated with reduced risk overall, but in a predefined subgroup given clopidogrel more than 6 hours before their procedure there was a 38% risk reduction in the primary composite endpoint at 28 days.

## Phosphodiesterase Inhibitors

Although thienopyridines inhibit platelet aggregation by increasing platelet adenylyl cyclase activity, phosphodiesterase inhibitors, such as dipyridamole, increase the level of the enzyme by inhibiting its degradation. At the plasma concentrations achieved *in vivo*, dipyridamole does not provide sufficient platelet inhibition for sustained clinical benefit. Cilostazol (Pletal) inhibits phosphodiesterase 3 (the most abundant phosphodiesterase in platelets). Cilostazol has both antiplatelet and vasodilating effects and has been approved for the treatment of intermittent claudication. However, it does not appear to have sufficient platelet inhibition for post-PCI use.

## CONCLUSION

Understanding the central role of platelets in CV disease has led to new therapies that have profoundly affected treatment. Antiplatelet therapy has made stenting possible and has become the mainstay of pharmacologic therapy in the catheterization laboratory. Future insights into the workings of platelets will further knowledge about CV disease and lead to the development of better therapies.

## Acknowledgments

I would like to thank Katherine Schmidt for her editorial assistance.

## REFERENCES

1. Italiano JLP Jr, Lecine P, Shivdasani RA, et al: Blood platelets are assembled principally at the ends of proplatelet processes produced by differentiated megakaryocytes. J Cell Biol 1999; 147:1299–1312.
2. Zucker-Franklin D: The ultrastructure of megakaryocytes and platelets. In Gordon A (ed): Regulation of Hematopoiesis. New York, Appleton-Century-Crofts, 1970, pp 1553–1586.
3. Nachmias VT, Sullender J, Fallon J, Asch A: Observations on the "cytoskeleton" of human platelets. Thromb Haemost 1980;42: 1661–1666.
4. Nachmias VT: Cytoskeleton of human platelets at rest and after spreading. J Cell Biol 1980;86:795–802.
5. Schwer HD, Lecine P, Tiwari S, et al: A lineage-restricted and divergent beta-tubulin isoform is essential for the biogenesis, structure and function of blood platelets. Curr Biol 2001;11:579–586.
6. Carlier MF, Jean C, Rieger KJ, et al: Modulation of the interaction between G-actin and thymosin beta 4 by the ATP/ADP ratio: Possible implication in the regulation of actin dynamics. Proc Natl Acad Sci USA 1993;90:5034–5038.
7. Pantaloni D, Carlier MF: How profilin promotes actin filament assembly in the presence of thymosin beta 4. Cell 1993; 75:1007–1014.
8. Markey F, Persson T, Lindberg U: Characterization of platelet extracts before and after stimulation with respect to the possible role of profilactin as microfilament precursor. Cell 1981; 23:145–153.
9. Huxley H: Electron microscopic studies on the structure of natural and synthetic proteins filaments from striated muscle. J Mol Biol 1963;3:281–308.
10. Nachmias VT, Cassimeris L, Golla R, Safer D: Thymosin beta 4 (T beta 4) in activated platelets. Eur J Cell Biol 1993;61:314–320.
11. Nachmias VT: Small actin-binding proteins: The beta-thymosin family. Curr Opin Cell Biol 1993;5:56–62.
12. Yin H: Calcium and polyphosphoinositide regulation of actin network structure by gelsolin. Adv Exp Med Biol 1989;255:31:5–23.
13. Hartwig JH, DeSisto M: The cytoskeleton of the resting human blood platelet: Structure of the membrane skeleton and its attachment to actin filaments. J Cell Biol 1991;112:407–425.
14. Stossel TP, Condeelis J, Cooley L, et al: Filamins as integrators of cell mechanics and signalling. Nat Rev Mol Cell Biol 2001;2: 138–145.
15. Goldsmith HL, Turitto VT: Rheological aspects of thrombosis and haemostasis: Basic principles and applications. ICTH-Report—Subcommittee on Rheology of the International Committee on Thrombosis and Haemostasis. Thromb Haemost 1986;55: 415–435.
16. Goldsmith HL: The Microcirculatory Society Eugene M. Landis Award lecture: The microrheology of human blood. Microvasc Res 1986;31:121–142.
17. Goldsmith HL: Poiseuille Gold Medal award ceremony: Laudatio: Poiseuille Awardee Yuan-Cheng Fung. Biorheology 1986;23: 567–569, 571.
18. Sakariassen KS, Hanson SR, Cadroy Y: Methods and models to evaluate shear-dependent and surface reactivity-dependent antithrombotic efficacy. Thromb Res 2001;104:149–174.
19. Turitto V: Blood viscosity, mass transport, and thrombogenesis. In Spaet TM (ed): Progress in Hemostasis and Thrombosis. New York, Grune & Stratton, 1981, pp 139–174.
20. Strony J, Beaudoin A, Brands D, Adelman B: Analysis of shear stress and hemodynamic factors in a model of coronary artery stenosis and thrombosis. Am J Physiol 1993;265:H1787–796.
21. Aarts PA, van den Broek SA, Prins GW, et al: Blood platelets are concentrated near the wall and red blood cells, in the center in flowing blood. Arteriosclerosis 1988;8:819–824.
22. Roux SP, Sakariassen KS, Turitto VT, Baumgartner HR: Effect of aspirin and epinephrine on experimentally induced thrombogenesis in dogs: A parallelism between in vivo and ex vivo thrombosis models. Arterioscler Thromb 1991;11:1182–1191.
23. Ware JA, Heistad DD: Seminars in medicine of the Beth Israel Hospital, Boston: Platelet-endothelium interactions. N Engl J Med 1993;328:628–635.
24. Carlsson L, Markey F, Blikstad I, et al: Reorganization of actin in platelets stimulated by thrombin as measured by the DNase I inhibition assay. Proc Natl Acad Sci USA 1979;76:6376–6380.
25. Karlsson R, Lassing I, Hoglund AS, Lindberg U: The organization of microfilaments in spreading platelets: A comparison with fibroblasts and glial cells. J Cell Physiol 1984;121:96–113.
26. Imamura M, Endo T, Kuroda M, et al: Substructure and higher structure of chicken smooth muscle alpha-actinin molecule. J Biol Chem 1988;263:7800–7805.
27. Brass LF, Manning DR, Cichowski K, Abrams CS: Signaling through G proteins in platelets: To the integrins and beyond. Thromb Haemost 1997;78:581–589.
28. Yin HL: Gelsolin: A calcium and polyphosphoinositide-regulated actin-modulating protein. BioEssays 1987;7:176–179.
29. Yin HL, Stossel TP: Control of cytoplasmic actin gel-sol transformation by gelsolin, a calcium-dependent regulatory protein. Nature 1979;281:583–586.
30. Kimura K, Fukata Y, Matsuoka Y, et al: Regulation of the association of adducin with actin filaments by Rho-associated kinase (Rho-kinase) and myosin phosphatase. J Biol Chem 1998;273: 5542–5548.
31. Nachmias VT, Golla R, Casella JF, Barron-Casella E: Cap Z: A calcium insensitive capping protein in resting and activated platelets. FEBS Lett 1996;378:258–262.
32. Burke AP, Farb A, Malcom GT, et al: Coronary risk factors and plaque morphology in men with coronary disease who died suddenly. N Engl J Med 1997;336:1276–1282.
33. Iozzo RV, Murdoch AD: Proteoglycans of the extracellular environment: Clues from the gene and protein side offer novel perspectives in molecular diversity and function. FASEB J 1996;10:598–614.
34. Olsen B: Basement membrane collagens (type IV). In Kreis TVR (ed): Guidebook to the Extracellular Matrix and Adhesion Proteins. Oxford, Oxford University Press, 1993.[AU2]
35. Timpl R, Brown JC: The laminins. Matrix Biol 1994;14:275–281.
36. Timpl R: Nidogen/Entactin. In Kreis TVR (ed) Guidebook to the Extracellular Matrix and Adhesion Proteins. Oxford, [AU3]Oxford University Press, 1993, pp 75–76.
37. Argraves WS, Tran H, Burgess WH, Dickerson K: Fibulin is an extracellular matrix and plasma glycoprotein with repeated domain structure. J Cell Biol 1990;111:3155–3164.
38. Hynes RO: Fibronectins. New York, Springer-Verlag, 1990.
39. Lawler J, Duquette M, Whittaker CA, et al: Identification and characterization of thrombospondin-4, a new member of the thrombospondin gene family. J Cell Biol 1993;120:1059–1067.
40. Ross JM, McIntire LV, Moake JL, Rand JH: Platelet adhesion and aggregation on human type VI collagen surfaces under physiological flow conditions. Blood 1995;85:1826–1835.
41. Nieswandt B, Brakebusch C, Bergmeier W, et al: Glycoprotein VI but not alpha2beta1 integrin is essential for platelet interaction with collagen. EMBO J 2001;20:2120–2130.
42. De Candia E, Hall SW, Rutella S, et al: Binding of thrombin to glycoprotein Ib accelerates the hydrolysis of Par-1 on intact platelets. J Biol Chem 2001;276:4692–4698.
43. Shapiro MJ, Weiss EJ, Faruqi TR, Coughlin SR: Protease-activated receptors 1 and 4 are shut off with distinct kinetics after activation by thrombin. J Biol Chem 2000;275:25216–25221.

44. Kahn ML, Zheng YW, Huang W, et al: A dual thrombin receptor system for platelet activation. Nature 1998;394:690-694.

45. Kahn ML, Nakanishi-Matsui M, Shapiro MJ, et al: Protease-activated receptors 1 and 4 mediate activation of human platelets by thrombin. J Clin Invest 1999;103:879-887.

46. Mills DC: ADP receptors on platelets. Thromb Haemost 1996;76:835-856.

47. Jin J, Daniel JL, Kunapuli SP: Molecular basis for ADP-induced platelet activation. II. The P2Y1 receptor mediates ADP-induced intracellular calcium mobilization and shape change in platelets. J Biol Chem 1998;273:2030-2034.

48. Hollopeter G, Jantzen HM, Vincent D, et al: Identification of the platelet ADP receptor targeted by antithrombotic drugs. Nature 2001;409:202-207.

49. Foster CJ, Prosser DM, Agans JM, et al: Molecular identification and characterization of the platelet ADP receptor targeted by thienopyridine antithrombotic drugs. J Clin Invest 2001;107:1591-1598.

50. MacKenzie AB, Mahaut-Smith MP: Chloride channels in excised membrane patches from human platelets: Effect of intracellular calcium. Biochim Biophys Acta 1996;1278:131-136.

51. Rolf MG, Brearley CA, Mahaut-Smith MP: Platelet shape change evoked by selective activation of P2X1 purinoceptors with alpha,beta-methylene ATP. Thromb Haemost 2001;85:303-308.

52. Leon C, Hechler B, Freund M, et al: Defective platelet aggregation and increased resistance to thrombosis in purinergic P2Y(1) receptor-null mice. J Clin Invest 1999;104:1731-1737.

53. Habib A, FitzGerald GA, Maclouf J: Phosphorylation of the thromboxane receptor alpha, the predominant isoform expressed in human platelets. J Biol Chem 1999;274:2645-2651.

54. Hirata T, Ushikubi F, Kakizuka A, et al: Two thromboxane A2 receptor isoforms in human platelets: Opposite coupling to adenylyl cyclase with different sensitivity to Arg60 to Leu mutation. J Clin Invest 1996;97:949-956.

55. Walsh M-T, Foley JF, Kinsella BT: The alpha, but not the beta, isoform of the human thromboxane A2 receptor is a target for prostacyclin-mediated desensitization. J Biol Chem 2000;275:20412-20423.

56. Ruggeri ZM, Ware J: von Willebrand factor. FASEB J 1993;7:308-316.

57. Savage B, Saldivar E, Ruggeri ZM: Initiation of platelet adhesion by arrest onto fibrinogen or translocation on von Willebrand factor. Cell 1996;84:289-297.

58. Nurden AT, Jallu V, Hourdille P: GP Ib and Bernard-Soulier platelets. Blood 1989;73:2225-2227.

59. Kobilka BK, Matsui H, Kobilka TS, et al: Cloning, sequencing, and expression of the gene coding for the human platelet alpha 2-adrenergic receptor. Science 1987;238:650-656.

60. Saltzman AG, Morse B, Whitman MM, et al: Cloning of the human serotonin 5-HT2 and 5-HT1C receptor subtypes. Biochem Biophys Res Commun 1991;181:1469-1478.

61. Thibonnier M, Chehade N, Hinko A: A V1-vascular vasopressin antagonist suitable for radioiodination and photoaffinity labeling. Am J Hypertens 1990;3:471-475.

62. Saeed SA, Rasheed H: Calcium-dependent synergistic interaction of platelet activating factor and epinephrine in human platelet aggregation. Acta Pharmacol Sin 2003;24:31-36.

63. Gratacap MP, Herault JP, Viala C, et al: FcgammaRIIA requires a Gi-dependent pathway for an efficient stimulation of phosphoinositide 3-kinase, calcium mobilization, and platelet aggregation. Blood 2000;96:3439-3446.

64. Oda A, Miyakawa Y, Druker BJ, et al: Thrombopoietin primes human platelet aggregation induced by shear stress and by multiple agonists. Blood 1996;87:4664-4670.

65. Pedreno J, Hurt-Camejo E, Wiklund O, et al: Low-density lipoprotein (LDL) binds to a G-protein coupled receptor in human platelets: Evidence that the proaggregatory effect induced by LDL is modulated by down-regulation of binding sites and desensitization of its mediated signaling. Atherosclerosis 2001;155:99-112.

66. Paul BZ, Ashby B, Sheth SB: Distribution of prostaglandin IP and EP receptor subtypes and isoforms in platelets and human umbilical artery smooth muscle cells. Br J Haematol 1998;102:1204-1211.

67. Nurden AT, Caen JP: An abnormal platelet glycoprotein pattern in three cases of Glanzmann's thrombasthenia. Br J Haematol 1974;28:253-260.

68. Phillips DR, Charo IF, Parise LV, Fitzgerald LA: The platelet membrane glycoprotein IIb-IIIa complex. Blood 1988;71:831-843.

69. Wagner CL, Mascelli MA, Neblock DS, et al: Analysis of GPIIb/IIIa receptor number by quantification of 7E3 binding to human platelets. Blood 1996;88:907-914.

70. Jennings LK, Phillips DR: Purification of glycoproteins IIb and III from human platelet plasma membranes and characterization of a calcium-dependent glycoprotein IIb-III complex. J Biol Chem 1982;257:10458-10466.

71. Thornton MA, Poncz M, Korostishevsky M, et al: The human platelet alphaIIb gene is not closely linked to its integrin partner beta3. Blood 1999;94:2039-2047.

72. D'Souza SE, Ginsberg MH, Plow EF: Arginyl-glycyl-aspartic acid (RGD): A cell adhesion motif. Trends Biochem Sci 1991;16:246-250.

73. Shattil SJ, Ginsberg MH: Integrin signaling in vascular biology. J Clin Invest 1997;100:S91-95.

74. Casserly IP, Topol EJ: Glycoprotein IIb/IIIa antagonists–from bench to practice. Cell Mol Life Sci 2002;59:478-500.

75. Shattil SJ: Signaling through platelet integrin alpha IIb beta 3: Inside-out, outside-in, and sideways. Thromb Haemost 1999;82:318-325.

76. Price DT, Loscalzo J: Cellular adhesion molecules and atherogenesis. Am J Med 1999;107:85-97.

77. Barkalow FJ, Barkalow KL, Mayadas TN: Dimerization of P-selectin in platelets and endothelial cells. Blood 2000;96:3070-3077.

78. Frenette PS, Wagner DD: Adhesion molecules: Blood vessels and blood cells—second of two parts. N Engl J Med 1996;335:43-45.

79. Vestweber D, Blanks JE: Mechanisms that regulate the function of the selectins and their ligands. Physiol Rev 1999;79:181-213.

80. Huo Y, Schober A, Forlow SB, et al: Circulating activated platelets exacerbate atherosclerosis in mice deficient in apolipoprotein E. Nat Med 2003;9:61-67.

81. Lindmark E, Wallentin L, Siegbahn A: Blood cell activation, coagulation, and inflammation in men and women with coronary artery disease. Thromb Res 2001;103:249-259.

82. Heeschen C, Dimmeler S, Hamm CW, et al: Soluble CD40 ligand in acute coronary syndromes. N Engl J Med 2003;348:1104-1111.

83. Mach F, Schonbeck U, Sukhova GK, et al: Reduction of atherosclerosis in mice by inhibition of CD40 signalling. Nature 1998;394:200-203.

84. Lutgens E, Gorelik L, Daemen MJ, et al: Requirement for CD154 in the progression of atherosclerosis. Nat Med 1999;5:1313-1316.

85. Urbich C, Dernbach E, Aicher A, et al: CD40 ligand inhibits endothelial cell migration by increasing production of endothelial reactive oxygen species. Circulation 2002;106:981-986.

86. Bombardier C, Laine L, Reicin A, et al: Comparison of upper gastrointestinal toxicity of rofecoxib and naproxen in patients with rheumatoid arthritis: VIGOR Study Group. N Engl J Med 2000;343:1520-1528,1530.

87. Catella-Lawson F, Reilly MP, Kapoor SC, et al: Cyclooxygenase inhibitors and the antiplatelet effects of aspirin. N Engl J Med 2001;345:1809-1817.

88. Coller BS, Lang D, Scudder LE: Rapid and simple platelet function assay to assess glycoprotein IIb/IIIa receptor blockade. Circulation 1997;95:860-867.

89. Jennings LK, White MM: Expression of ligand-induced binding sites on glycoprotein IIb/IIIa complexes and the effect of various inhibitors. Am Heart J 1998;135:S179-183.

90. Coller BS, Springer KT, Scudder LE, et al: Substituting isoserine for serine in the thrombin receptor activation peptide SFLLRN confers resistance to aminopeptidase M-induced cleavage and inactivation. J Biol Chem 1993;268:20741-20743.

91. Phillips DR, Teng W, Arfsten A, et al: Effect of Ca2+ on GP IIb-IIIa interactions with integrilin: Enhanced GP IIb-IIIa binding and inhibition of platelet aggregation by reductions in the concentration of ionized calcium in plasma anticoagulated with citrate. Circulation 1997;96:1488-1494.

92. Awtry EH, Loscalzo J: Aspirin. Circulation 2000;101:1206-1218.

93. Jaffe EA, Weksler BB: Recovery of endothelial cell prostacyclin production after inhibition by low doses of aspirin. J Clin Invest 1979;63:532-535.

94. Randomised trial of intravenous streptokinase, oral aspirin, both, or neither among 17,187 cases of suspected acute myocardial infarction: ISIS-2—ISIS-2 (Second International Study of Infarct Survival) Collaborative Group. Lancet 1988;2:349-360.

95. Collaborative overview of randomised trials of antiplatelet therapy. I. Prevention of death, myocardial infarction, and stroke by prolonged antiplatelet therapy in various categories of patients: Antiplatelet Trialists' Collaboration. BMJ 1994;308:81–106.

96. Physician's Health Study: Aspirin and primary prevention of coronary heart disease. N Engl J Med 1989;321:1825–1828.

97. Final report on the aspirin component of the ongoing Physicians' Health Study: Steering Committee of the Physicians' Health Study Research Group. N Engl J Med 1989;321:129–135.

98. Peto R, Gray R, Collins R, et al: Randomised trial of prophylactic daily aspirin in British male doctors. BMJ (Clin Res Educ) 1988;296:313–316.

99. Thrombosis Prevention Trial: Randomised trial of low-intensity oral anticoagulation with warfarin and low-dose aspirin in the primary prevention of ischaemic heart disease in men at increased risk: The Medical Research Council's General Practice Research Framework. Lancet 1998;351:233–41.

100. Hansson L, Zanchetti A, Carruthers SG, et al: Effects of intensive blood-pressure lowering and low-dose aspirin in patients with hypertension: Principal results of the Hypertension Optimal Treatment (HOT) randomised trial. HOT Study Group. Lancet 1998;351:1755–1762.

101. Andersen K, Hurlen M, Arnesen H, Seljeflot I: Aspirin non-responsiveness as measured by PFA-100 in patients with coronary artery disease. Thromb Res 2002;108:37–42.

102. Buchanan MR, Schwartz L, Bourassa M, et al: Results of the BRAT study: A pilot study investigating the possible significance of ASA nonresponsiveness on the benefits and risks of ASA on thrombosis in patients undergoing coronary artery bypass surgery. Can J Cardiol 2000;16:1385–1390.

103. Buchanan MR, Brister SJ: Individual variation in the effects of ASA on platelet function: Implications for the use of ASA clinically. Can J Cardiol 1995;11:221–227.

104. Mitchell J, Akarasereenont P, Thiemermann C, et al: Selectivity of nonsteroidal antiinflammatory drugs as inhibitors of constitutive and inducible cyclooxygenase. PNAS 1993;90:11693–11697.

105. Coller BS: A new murine monoclonal antibody reports an activation-dependent change in the conformation and/or microenvironment of the platelet glycoprotein IIb/IIIa complex. J Clin Invest 1985;76:101–108.

106. Coller BS, Scudder LE: Inhibition of dog platelet function by in vivo infusion of F(ab')2 fragments of a monoclonal antibody to the platelet glycoprotein IIb/IIIa receptor. Blood 1985; 66:1456–1459.

107. Coller BS, Folts JD, Scudder LE, Smith SR: Antithrombotic effect of a monoclonal antibody to the platelet glycoprotein IIb/IIIa receptor in an experimental animal model. Blood 1986;68: 783–786.

108. Coller BS, Peerschke EI, Seligsohn U, et al: Studies on the binding of an alloimmune and two murine monoclonal antibodies to the platelet glycoprotein IIb-IIIa complex receptor. J Lab Clin Med 1986;107:384–392.

109. Coller BS, Scudder LE, Beer J, et al: Monoclonal antibodies to platelet glycoprotein IIb/IIIa as antithrombotic agents. Ann NY Acad Sci 1991;614:193–213.

110. Coller BS, Anderson K, Weisman HF: New antiplatelet agents: Platelet GPIIb/IIIa antagonists. Thromb Haemost 1995;74: 302–308.

111. Coller BS, Anderson KM, Weisman HF: The anti-GPIIb-IIIa agents: Fundamental and clinical aspects. Haemostasis 1996;26(Suppl 4):285–293.

112. Phillips DR, Scarborough RM: Clinical pharmacology of eptifibatide. Am J Cardiol 1997;80:11B–20B.

113. Lynch JJ Jr, Cook JJ, Sitko GR, et al: Nonpeptide glycoprotein IIb/IIIa inhibitors. 5. Antithrombotic effects of MK-0383. J Pharmacol Exp Ther 1995;272:20–32.

114. Use of a monoclonal antibody directed against the platelet glycoprotein IIb/IIIa receptor in high-risk coronary angioplasty. The EPIC Investigation. N Engl J Med 1994;330:956–961.

115. Randomised placebo-controlled trial of abciximab before and during coronary intervention in refractory unstable angina: The CAPTURE Study. Lancet 1997;349:1429–1435.

116. Randomised placebo-controlled and balloon-angioplasty-controlled trial to assess safety of coronary stenting with use of platelet glycoprotein-IIb/IIIa blockade: The EPISTENT Investigators—Evaluation of Platelet IIb/IIIa Inhibitor for Stenting. Lancet 1998;352:87–92.

117. Brener SJ, Barr LA, Burchenal JE, et al: Randomized, placebo-controlled trial of platelet glycoprotein IIb/IIIa blockade with primary angioplasty for acute myocardial infarction: ReoPro and Primary PTCA Organization and Randomized Trial (RAPPORT) Investigators. Circulation 1998;98:734–741.

118. Neumann FJ, Kastrati A, Schmitt C, et al: Effect of glycoprotein IIb/IIIa receptor blockade with abciximab on clinical and angiographic restenosis rate after the placement of coronary stents following acute myocardial infarction. J Am Coll Cardiol 2000;35:915–921.

119. Montalescot G, Barragan P, Wittenberg O, et al: Platelet glycoprotein IIb/IIIa inhibition with coronary stenting for acute myocardial infarction. N Engl J Med 2001;344:1895–1903.

120. Simoons ML: Effect of glycoprotein IIb/IIIa receptor blocker abciximab on outcome in patients with acute coronary syndromes without early coronary revascularisation: The GUSTO IV-ACS randomised trial. Lancet 2001;357:1915–1924.

121. Stone GW, Grines CL, Cox DA, et al: Comparison of angioplasty with stenting, with or without abciximab, in acute myocardial infarction. N Engl J Med 2002;346:957–966.

122. Randomised placebo-controlled trial of effect of eptifibatide on complications of percutaneous coronary intervention: IMPACT-II: Integrilin to Minimise Platelet Aggregation and Coronary Thrombosis-II. Lancet 1997;349:1422–1428.

123. O'Shea JC, Buller CE, Cantor WJ, et al: Long-term efficacy of platelet glycoprotein IIb/IIIa integrin blockade with eptifibatide in coronary stent intervention. JAMA 2002;287:618–621.

124. O'Shea JC, Hafley GE, Greenberg S, et al: Platelet glycoprotein IIb/IIIa integrin blockade with eptifibatide in coronary stent intervention: The ESPRIT trial: A randomized controlled trial. JAMA 2001;285:2468–2473.

125. Chew DP, Bhatt DL, Lincoff AM, et al: Defining the optimal activated clotting time during percutaneous coronary intervention: Aggregate results from 6 randomized, controlled trials. Circulation 2001;103:961–966.

126. Effects of platelet glycoprotein IIb/IIIa blockade with tirofiban on adverse cardiac events in patients with unstable angina or acute myocardial infarction undergoing coronary angioplasty: The RESTORE Investigators: Randomized Efficacy Study of Tirofiban for Outcomes and REstenosis. Circulation 1997;96:1445–1453.

127. Topol EJ, Moliterno DJ, Herrmann HC, et al: Comparison of two platelet glycoprotein IIb/IIIa inhibitors, tirofiban and abciximab, for the prevention of ischemic events with percutaneous coronary revascularization. N Engl J Med 2001;344:1888–1894.

128. Steinhubl SR, Moliterno DJ: Glycoprotein IIb/IIIa receptor antagonists for the treatment of unstable angina. Heart Vessels 1997;(Suppl 12):148–155.

129. Kabbani SS, Aggarwal A, Terrien EF, et al: Suboptimal early inhibition of platelets by treatment with tirofiban and implications for coronary interventions. Am J Cardiol 2002;89:647–650.

130. Inhibition of platelet glycoprotein IIb/IIIa with eptifibatide in patients with acute coronary syndromes: The PURSUIT Trial Investigators—Platelet Glycoprotein IIb/IIIa in Unstable Angina: Receptor Suppression Using Integrilin Therapy. N Engl J Med 1998;339:436–443.

131. A comparison of aspirin plus tirofiban with aspirin plus heparin for unstable angina: Platelet Receptor Inhibition in Ischemic Syndrome Management (PRISM) Study Investigators. N Engl J Med 1998;338:1498–1505.

132. Inhibition of the platelet glycoprotein IIb/IIIa receptor with tirofiban in unstable angina and non-Q-wave myocardial infarction: Platelet Receptor Inhibition in Ischemic Syndrome Management in Patients Limited by Unstable Signs and Symptoms (PRISM-PLUS) Study Investigators. N Engl J Med 1998;338: 1488–1497.

133. Cannon CP, Weintraub WS, Demopoulos LA, et al: Comparison of early invasive and conservative strategies in patients with unstable coronary syndromes treated with the glycoprotein IIb/IIIa inhibitor tirofiban. N Engl J Med 2001;344:1879–1887.

134. Heggunje PS, Wade MJ, O'Rourke RA, et al: Early invasive versus ischaemia-guided strategies in the management of non-Q wave myocardial infarction patients with and without prior myocardial infarction: Results of Veterans Affairs Non-Q Wave Infarction

Strategies in Hospital (VANQWISH) trial. Eur Heart J 2000;21: 2014-2025.

135. Boden WE, O'Rourke RA, Crawford MH, et al: Outcomes in patients with acute non-Q-wave myocardial infarction randomly assigned to an invasive as compared with a conservative management strategy: Veterans Affairs Non-Q-Wave Infarction Strategies in Hospital (VANQWISH) Trial Investigators. N Engl J Med 1998;338:1785-1792.

136. Cannon CP, Weintraub WS, Demopoulos LA, et al: Invasive versus conservative strategies in unstable angina and non-Q-wave myocardial infarction following treatment with tirofiban: Rationale and study design of the international TACTICS-TIMI 18 Trial: Treat Angina with Aggrastat and determine Cost of Therapy with an Invasive or Conservative Strategy. Thrombolysis in Myocardial Infarction. Am J Cardiol 1998;82:731-736.

137. Cohen M: Glycoprotein IIb/IIIa receptor blockers in acute coronary syndromes: Gusto IV-ACS. Lancet 2001;357:1899-1900.

138. Topol EJ: Reperfusion therapy for acute myocardial infarction with fibrinolytic therapy or combination reduced fibrinolytic therapy and platelet glycoprotein IIb/IIIa inhibition: The GUSTO V randomised trial. Lancet 2001;357:1905-1914.

139. Cannon CP: Learning from the recently completed oral glycoprotein IIb/IIIa receptor antagonist trials. Clin Cardiol 2000;(23 Suppl 6):VI-14-17.

140. Cannon CP, McCabe CH, Wilcox RG, et al: Oral glycoprotein IIb/IIIa inhibition with orbofiban in patients with unstable coronary syndromes (OPUS-TIMI 16) trial. Circulation 2000; 102:149-156.

141. Bennett CL, Connors JM, Carwile JM, et al: Thrombotic thrombocytopenic purpura associated with clopidogrel. N Engl J Med 2000;342:1773-1777.

142. Bennett CL, Davidson CJ, Raisch DW, et al: Thrombotic thrombocytopenic purpura associated with ticlopidine in the setting of coronary artery stents and stroke prevention. Arch Intern Med 1999;159:2524-2528.

143. Bertrand ME, Rupprecht HJ, Urban P, et al: Double-blind study of the safety of clopidogrel with and without a loading dose in combination with aspirin compared with ticlopidine in combination with aspirin after coronary stenting: The Clopidogrel Aspirin Stent International Cooperative Study (CLASSICS). Circulation 2000;102:624-629.

144. A randomised, blinded, trial of clopidogrel versus aspirin in patients at risk of ischaemic events (CAPRIE): CAPRIE Steering Committee. Lancet 1996;348:1329-1339.

145. The Clopidogrel in Unstable Angina to Prevent Recurrent Events Trial Investigators: Effects of clopidogrel in addition to aspirin in patients with acute coronary syndromes without ST-segment elevation. N Engl J Med 2001;345:494-502.

146. Mehta SR, Yusuf S, Peters RJ, et al: Effects of pretreatment with clopidogrel and aspirin followed by long-term therapy in patients undergoing percutaneous coronary intervention: The PCI-CURE study. Lancet 2001;358:527-533.

147. Steinhubl SR, Berger PB, Mann JT 3rd, et al: Early and sustained dual oral antiplatelet therapy following percutaneous coronary intervention: A randomized controlled trial. JAMA 2002;288: 2411-2420.

# Blood Coagulation and Atherothrombosis

*Hiroshi Ashikaga*
*Kenneth R. Chien*

Atherothrombosis, or thrombosis at atherosclerotic sites, is the main culprit in the pathogenesis of myocardial infarction and stroke. Therefore, it is also the major factor responsible for atherosclerosis-related morbidity and mortality. Coagulation pathways play a crucial role in the pathogenesis of atherothrombosis by facilitating the generation of occlusive thrombotic plugs at sites of ruptured atherosclerotic plaques. Although the major contribution of the extrinsic pathway of coagulation to the initiation of atherothrombosis is well established, recent observations have indicated involvement of the intrinsic coagulation pathway as well. However, the understanding of biochemical mechanisms involved in activation of these pathways at atherosclerotic lesions is still incomplete.

## NORMAL COAGULATION PATHWAYS

Coagulation pathways are dependent on a group of proteins termed coagulation factors that are normally present in inactive proenzyme forms (Table 28-1).[1-3] The sequential activation of coagulation factors forms a coagulation cascade that eventually results in fibrin clot formation. The blood coagulation system includes two pathways composed of distinct groups of coagulation factors: the extrinsic or tissue factor-dependent pathway and the intrinsic pathway. The final step in both the extrinsic and the intrinsic pathways is the activation of factor X (fX) to factor Xa (fXa). Generation of fXa merges both pathways in a common pathway that leads to the production of the multifunctional molecule thrombin (Fig. 28-1). In addition, several mechanisms to counteract the coagulation cascade exist to maintain intact blood circulation and prevent clotting. These mechanisms, including antithrombin, the protein C/protein S/thrombomodulin system, and tissue factor pathway inhibitor (TFPI), regulate the coagulation cascade at different levels to mitigate clot formation under physiologic circumstances (Fig. 28-2).

Activation of the extrinsic pathway begins with binding of tissue factor (TF), a cell-surface glycoprotein, to an activated serine protease fVIIa. Exposure of TF to circulating blood is caused by disruption of the endothelial layer as in vascular injury or by heterotropic TF expression in different cell types in response to various stimuli. Small amounts of fVIIa are present (1% to 2%) and circulate in the blood.[4] TF on the cell surface binds to free fVIIa in the plasma to form the TF/fVIIa complex.[5-7] Both proteins possess low enzymatic activity in their free forms, but the TF/fVIIa complex acts as a potent enzyme to further activate free fVII to generate fVIIa, producing more TF/fVIIa complexes to amplify the initial trigger (*TF-mediated fVII autoactivation*). The TF/fVIIa complex then activates fX to yield fXa, either directly or indirectly by initially converting fIX to fIXa, which subsequently activates fX in the presence of fVIIIa.

The intrinsic pathway is triggered by the autoactivation of fXII to fXIIa, which subsequently initiates the cascade of sequential activation of fXI and fIX to generate fIXa. Then fIXa catalyzes the conversion of fX to fXa, but this reaction requires an activated form of another coagulation factor fVIIIa, which is generated by thrombin-mediated activation of fVIII.

Factor Xa, the end product of both the extrinsic and intrinsic pathways, triggers the common pathway of coagulation by converting prothrombin to thrombin, which in turn initiates formation of fibrin from fibrinogen. The conversion of prothrombin to thrombin requires a cofactor fVa, which is produced by thrombin-mediated activation of fV. Thrombin also activates fXIII to form fXIIIa, which catalyzes the formation of cross-linked fibrin polymer.

Antithrombin (antithrombin III) is a plasma protease inhibitor that inactivates thrombin and other activated coagulation factors in the intrinsic and common pathways by binding to the active site of these enzymes. The anticoagulant heparin's major mechanism of action is to accelerate the formation of these neutralizing complexes.

Protein C is a plasma glycoprotein that is activated by thrombin, and activated protein C (APC) is a potent anticoagulant that inactivates fVa and fVIIIa through the thrombin-thrombomodulin complex. The thrombin-induced activation of protein C occurs physiologically on thrombomodulin, a transmembrane proteoglycan-binding site for thrombin on endothelial cell surfaces. The rate of this reaction is increased by a cofactor, protein S, which increases the affinity of APC for phospholipids in the formation of the membrane-bound protein Case complex (Fig. 28-3).

TFPI is the endogenous inhibitor of the TF/fVIIa complex (Fig. 28-4). TFPI is a multivalent Kunitz-type serine protease inhibitor, consisting of three tandem Kunitz domains, which exerts inhibitory effects against the TF/fVIIa complex and fXa, thereby regulating the extrinsic pathway of coagulation.[8] Endothelial cells are the principal source of plasma TFPI.[9-11]

■ ■ ■

## TABLE 28-1   BLOOD CLOTTING FACTORS AND INHIBITORS

| Protein | Chromosome | Gene (kb) | mRNA (kb) | Plasma (Half-Life) | Concentration (nm) | Clinical Manifestation H | T |
|---|---|---|---|---|---|---|---|
| Prothrombin | 11 | 21 | 2 | 2.5 | 1400 | + | − |
| Factor V | 1q 21–25 | 80 | 7 | 0.5 | 20 | + | + |
| Factor VIII | Xq 28 | 186 | 9 | 0.3–0.5 | 0.7 | + | − |
| Factor VII | 13 | 12.8 | 2.5 | 0.25 | 10 | + | +/− |
| Factor IX | X | 34 | 2.8 | 1 | 90 | + | |
| Factor X | 13q 32-qter | 27 | 1.5 | 1.25 | 170 | + | |
| Factor XI | 4q 35 | 23 | 2.1 | 2.5–3.3 | 30 | +/− | |
| Factor XII | 5q 33-qter | 12 | 2.6 | 2–3 | 375 | − | |
| High molecular weight kininogen | 3q 26-qter | 27 | 2.015 | 5 | 600 | − | |
| Prekallikrein | 4q34-q35 | 22 | 2.4 | NA | 450 | | |
| Factor XIIIa | 6 p-24-25 | >160 | 3.8 | 9–10 | 70 | + | +/− |
| Factor XIIIb | 1 q31-q32.1 | 28 | 2.3 | NA | | | |
| Tissue factor | 1 | 12.4 | 2.3 | — | | | |
| Protein C | 2q 14–21 | 11 | 1.7 | 0.25 | 60 | | + |
| Protein S | 3 | 80 | 3.5 | 1.75 | 300 | | + |
| Thrombomodulin | 20p 12-cen | 3.7 | 3.7 | — | | | |
| Fibrinogen | 4q 23-q 32 | 50 | | 3–5 | 8800 | + | +/− |
| α chain | | 5.4 | 2.2 | | | | |
| β chain | | 8 | 1.9 | | | | |
| γ chain | | 8.5 | 1.6 | | 2500 | + | + |
| Antithrombin III | 1 q 22–25 | 14 | 1.4 | 2.5–4 | | | |
| Heparin cofactor II | 22q 11 | 16 | 2.3 | 2.5 | 1200 | + | +/− |
| Tissue factor pathway inhibitor | 2q 31–32.1 | | 1.4, 4 | NA | 2.5 | | |
| Thrombin activated fibrinolysis inhibition | 13 | | 1.8 | NA | 73 | | |

H, Hemorrhagic disease/hemophilia; NA, not available; T, thrombotic disease/thrombophilia.

It has recently been recognized that the coagulation mechanism involves the assembly of multiprotein complexes on the phospholipid cellular membrane, including the extrinsic and intrinsic Xase (tenase) complex, prothrombinase complex, and protein Case complex (Fig. 28-3, Table 28-2). Each complex consists of an enzyme, its zymogen substrate, and its cofactor on the phospholipid membrane surface. The formation of these complexes on the cell membrane surface promotes the reactions in the coagulation and anticoagulation pathways.

## COAGULATION PATHWAYS IN ATHEROSCLEROSIS

### Extrinsic Pathway

#### Tissue Factor

The initiation of the coagulation cascade in the pathogenesis of the atherothrombosis has largely been ascribed to the extrinsic, TF-dependent pathway.[12] TF is a 263 amino acid, membrane-bound glycoprotein consisting of three domains: the extracellular (residues 1 to 219), transmembrane (residues 220 to 242), and cytoplasmic (residues 243 to 263) domains. The extracellular domain is responsible for the binding to the fVIIa, thereby initiating the extrinsic pathway of the coagulation cascade.[13-15] Normal arteries and veins lack TF mRNA and protein, except for a small amount present in vascular smooth muscle cells (SMCs) in the tunica media and fibroblasts in

the adventitia.[16,17] Under normal conditions, TF is not expressed in peripheral blood cells or endothelial cells. TF is, therefore, physically separated from the bloodstream. In contrast, extensive evidence demonstrates abundant TF expression in all stages of human atherosclerotic lesions.[18] Both TF content and activity are significantly higher in plaques from patients with acute coronary syndrome compared with those with stable angina.[19-22] Abnormal TF expression and activity are also implicated in postischemic reperfusion injury.[23]

The concept that the extrinsic pathway plays a major role in the initiation of atherothrombosis is strongly supported by the finding that disruption of human atherosclerotic plaques containing high levels of TF results in platelet deposition, which positively correlates with the TF content.[24] In patients with acute coronary syndrome, thrombosis is seen only in TF-positive atherosclerotic plaques,[25] and fibrin deposition occurs mainly around macrophages expressing TF.[26] Inhibition of TF activity in atherosclerotic plaques with recombinant TFPI (rTFPI), antihuman TF antibodies, or adenoviral gene transfer of human TFPI significantly reduces plaque thrombogenicity, inhibiting both platelet and fibrinogen deposition without affecting systemic coagulation status.[27,28]

The source of this heterotropically expressed TF in atherosclerotic lesions is a number of different cell types that occupy approximately 60% of the cell population in the atherosclerotic plaque: endothelial cells, SMCs, monocytes, macrophages, foam cells, and mesenchymal-appearing intimal cells.[16,18,25,29-33] Heterotropic TF is

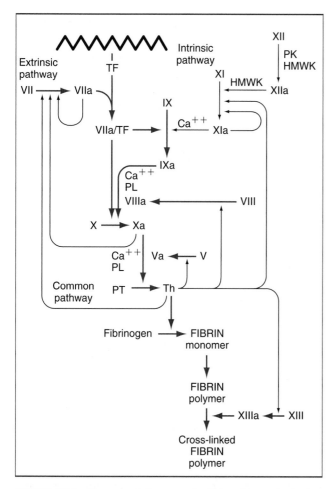

**FIGURE 28-1.** The coagulation cascade. This scheme emphasizes recent understanding of the importance of the TF pathway in initiating clotting *in vivo*, the interactions between pathways, and the pivotal role of thrombin in sustaining the cascade by feedback activation of coagulation factors. HMWK, high molecular weight kininogen; PK, prekallikrein; PL, phospholipid; PT, prothrombin; TF, tissue factor; Th, thrombin. *(From Braunwald E, Zipes D, Libby P: Heart Disease, 6 ed. WB Saunders, Philadelphia, 2001, p. 2101.)*

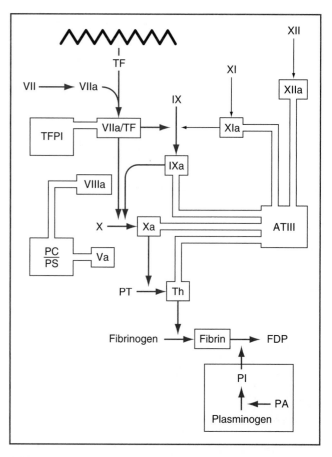

**FIGURE 28-2.** Sites of action of the four major physiologic antithrombotic pathways: antithrombin (AT); protein C/protein S (PC/PS); tissue factor pathway inhibitor (TFPI); and the fibrinolytic system, consisting of plasminogen, plasminogen activator (PA), and plasmin (PI). *(From Braunwald E, Zipes D, Libby P: Heart Disease, 6 ed. WB Saunders, Philadelphia, 2001, p. 2103.)*

also found in the extracellular matrix surrounding TF-producing foam cells, macrophages, and SMCs, adjacent to the cholesterol clefts and within the necrotic cores of the plaques.[16,18,25,30,31] Significant platelet deposition is found on the lipid-rich atheromatous core, which also exhibits the most intense TF staining compared with other arterial components.[24]

In addition to a membrane-bound form, significantly high levels of circulating soluble form of TF are found in patients with acute coronary syndrome.[34,35] The soluble TF levels in the blood are an important predictor of clinical outcome that reflects the hypercoagulable state of these patients, and the levels return to normal values after successful treatment with anticoagulation or antiplatelet agents.[36-38] The blood-borne TF may trigger thrombus formation independent of procoagulants in atherosclerotic plaques, contributing to propagation of thrombus formation at the site of vascular injury. However, the source of the circulating TF is not clear; it may originate from membrane-bound TF at the site of atherosclerosis or from circulating neutrophils and monocytes.[39] It was also discovered that TF is transferred from monocytes and polymorphonuclear leukocytes to platelets, through the interaction

of CD15 and TF with platelets. This transfer phenomenon enables platelets to initiate and propagate thrombosis.[40] These findings have added new insights to the original premise that vessel wall injury and exposure of TF within the vasculature to blood is required for arterial thrombosis.

A number of polymorphisms of TF have been identified, but none has been found to alter the susceptibility to atherothrombosis. For example, patients homozygous for the I1208D polymorphism in the 5′ regulatory region have reduced plasma TF levels and are at a decreased risk of venous thromboembolism, but there is no significant difference in risk for coronary thrombosis between these patients and healthy controls.[41]

### Factor VII

The fVII gene (12.8 kb) is encoded on chromosome 13 and yields mRNA of 2.5 kb.[42,43] Factor VII (50 kd) is a vitamin K-dependent coagulation factor that circulates in plasma predominantly as a single-chain inactive zymogen.[44] It is activated by fIXa, fXIIa, fXa, f VIIa, and thrombin through a single peptide bond cleavage at Arg152-Ile153. The activated form of fVII, fVIIa, contains a light chain (20 kd) and a heavy chain (30 kd) that are covalently linked by a disulfide bond.

High levels of fVII in the plasma are associated with increased risk of ischemic events,[45] whereas low plasma

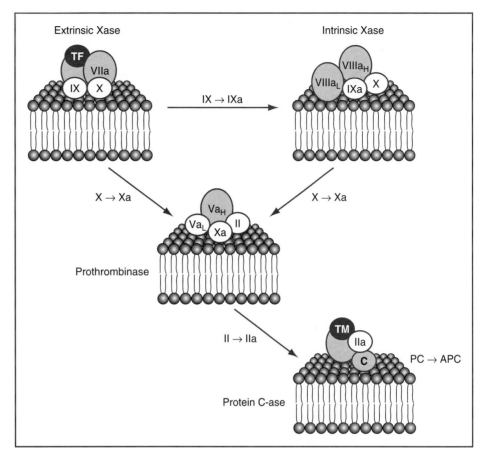

**FIGURE 28-3.** Schematic representation of the phospholipid membrane-associated enzyme complexes of coagulation. Each vitamin-K-dependent serine protease [(factors VIIa, IXa, and Xa and alpha-thrombin [IIa]) is shown in association with its cofactor protein (TF, factors VIIIa and Va, and thrombomodulin [TM]) and zymogen substrate(s) (factors IX and X, prothrombin [II] and protein C [C]) on the membrane surface. The cofactor proteins factor VIIIa and factor Va, are characterized by a two-domain structure and consist of heavy (H) and light (L) chains that are bridged together by Ca$^{2+}$ ions. Both domains are required for cofactor-membrane association and cofactor-protease binding. *(From Braunwald E, Zipes D, Libby P: Heart Disease, 6 ed. WB Saunders, Philadelphia, 2001, p. 2102.)*

fVII levels appear to attenuate the risk. In a study of an arginine-glutamine mutation at amino acid 353 (R353Q) and an H7H7 polymorphism in the hypervariable region 4 of intron 7 of fVII, patients with the QQ or H7H7 genotype had significantly lower levels of both fVII antigen and clotting activity and a lower risk of myocardial infarction than those with the RR or H6H6 genotype.[46] Another polymorphism in intron 1a of the fVII gene was identified; it is caused by the nucleotide change G to A at position +73 (G73A), which may be in a strong linkage disequilibrium with the Q353 allele. Patients with both 73A and Q353 alleles had lower fVII levels and lower risk of myocardial infarction than individuals without the mutation.[47] These findings suggest that polymorphisms of the fVII gene may attenuate the risk of atherothrombosis, presumably through alterations in the plasma fVII levels.

## Intrinsic Pathway

### Factor XII

The fXII gene, consisting of 14 exons and 13 introns on chromosome 5, gives rise to an mRNA of 2.4 kb. The

mature fXII protein is composed of 596 amino acid residues (80 kd) in a single polypeptide chain.[48] Factor XII, or Hageman factor, is the first coagulation factor of the intrinsic pathway and is activated by plasma kallikrein to form fXIIa. This activation process is facilitated by high molecular weight kininogen (HMWK) and by contact with negatively charged surfaces such as glass or collagen. Factor XIIa converts fXI to fXI and prekallikrein to kallikrein. However, patients with fXII deficiency do not develop a bleeding diathesis, and fXIIa does not appear to play a significant role in the coagulation cascade *in vivo*.

### Factor XI

The fXI gene (23 kb) is located on chromosome 4 and contains 15 exons and 14 introns.[49] The fXI protein (160 kd) consists of two identical polypeptide chains linked by a disulfide bond.[50] These identical polypeptide chains are cleaved by fXIIa at Arg369-Ile370 in the presence of HMWK and a negatively charged surface and by α-thrombin to yield active sites in each of the polypeptide chains.

A deficiency of fXI is associated with bleeding, whereas high levels of plasma fXI are a risk factor for venous thromboembolism.[51] No polymorphism of fXI that is associated with increased or decreased incidence of arterial thrombosis has been reported, and the role of fXI in the pathogenesis of acute coronary syndrome remains unclear.

**TFPI**
**34,000**

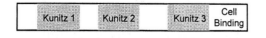

**FIGURE 28-4.** Schematic representation of the TFPI molecule; the Kunitz domains and cell-binding domains are identified.

**TABLE 28-2**   COAGULATION FACTOR ENZYME COMPLEXES

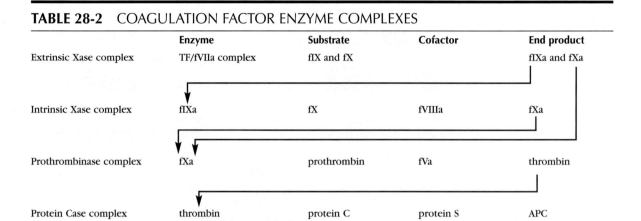

| | Enzyme | Substrate | Cofactor | End product |
|---|---|---|---|---|
| Extrinsic Xase complex | TF/fVIIa complex | fIX and fX | | fIXa and fXa |
| Intrinsic Xase complex | fIXa | fX | fVIIIa | fXa |
| Prothrombinase complex | fXa | prothrombin | fVa | thrombin |
| Protein Case complex | thrombin | protein C | protein S | APC |

### Factor IX

Factor IX is one of the critical components of the intrinsic pathway, and its deficiency leads to hemophilia B. The fIX gene (34 kb), located on X chromosome, gives rise to an mRNA of 2.8 kb.[52] The mature protein (56 kd) requires vitamin K for its synthesis. Factor IX can be activated by the TF/fVIIa complex in the extrinsic pathway or fXIa in the intrinsic pathway. Conversion of fIX to fIXa results in the expression of the fVIII-binding site and the active enzyme site with maximal procoagulant activity. The significance of alterations in fIX in arterial and venous thrombosis has not been established.

### Factor VIII

Factor VIII (187 kb) is encoded on the X chromosome, and is divided into 26 exons.[53,54] It is synthesized as a single-chain protein consisting of more than 2200 amino acids, which undergoes post-translational modifications. The mature, circulating form of fVIII is a heterodimer (330 kd) consisting of a heavy chain and light chain. Thrombin cleaves at least four peptide bonds in fVIII, and the cleavage of the peptide bonds at Arg 372-373 and Arg 1686-1689 are required for fVIII activation.[55] The activation process generates fragments A1 and A2 from the heavy chain and A3-C1-C2 from the light chain, resulting in the heterotrimer fVIIIa molecule.[56] Functional or absolute fVIII deficiency results in hemophilia A, the most common hereditary bleeding disorder.

A number of epidemiologic observations in hemophilia patients, who have a bleeding tendency because of perturbation of the intrinsic pathway, support the involvement of the intrinsic pathway in atherothrombosis. In a cohort study of 919 males with either hemophilia A or B over a period of 20 years, a fivefold reduction in mortality from myocardial infarction was reported compared with that of the general male population.[57] The risk ratio based on the atherosclerosis risk factor profile of hemophilia patients compared with healthy controls was 0.78, which accounts for only a part of the significant risk reduction of coronary artery disease-related mortality.[58] Although these epidemiologic studies strongly support the protective effects of hemophilia on ischemic heart disease, the evidence for pro-

tective effects on atherogenesis is conflicting.[59,60] However, high plasma fVIII levels are an important predictor of unfavorable outcome in patients with acute coronary syndrome, and they correlate with coronary artery disease, carotid atherosclerosis, and venous thromboembolism.[61-64] Elevated fVIII may well be a consequence of active thrombin formation, and whether fVIII participates in atherogenesis independent of the extrinsic pathway is still uncertain.

## Common Pathway

### Factor X

Factor X, one of the vitamin K-dependent serine proteases, plays a crucial role in the coagulation cascade as the first enzyme in the common pathway of thrombus formation. The fX gene (27 kb), located on chromosome 13, is composed of eight exons, each of which encodes a specific functional domain within the protein.[65] The mature protein (59 kDa) is comprised of a covalently linked heavy chain (42 kd) and a light chain (16.5 kd). The cleavage of the heavy chain at Arg194-195 yields its active form fXa. Factor X is at the confluence of the extrinsic pathway and the intrinsic pathway and can be activated by the TF/fVIIa complex or the fIXa/fVIIIa complex.

A deficiency of fX, which is one of the rarest of the hereditary bleeding disorders, exhibits an autosomal recessive inheritance. Homozygous fX deficiency has an incidence of 1:1,000,000 in the general population. Heterozygotes are often clinically asymptomatic. A deficiency of fX may also be acquired, usually in association with amyloidosis.[66]

A number of novel anticoagulant strategies to target fXa have been investigated, and some of them have been proven effective in preventing thrombosis in clinical settings (see the section on anticoagulation therapies).

### Factor V

The fV gene (80 kb), located on chromosome 1, encodes a 6.8-kb mRNA.[67,68] Factor V is a glycoprotein that circulates in blood in the plasma and in platelets.[69]

The activated form of fV, or fVa, is a critical component of the coagulation cascade; it acts as a cofactor for fXa in the prothrombinase complex to convert prothrombin to thrombin and as a cofactor for APC to degrade fVIIIa.

The factor V Leiden, first described in 1993[70] and present in approximately 5% of Caucasians, is the most studied mutation in fV and is related to an increased risk of thrombosis. It is the result of a point mutation in the fV gene on chromosome 1 (1691GA), resulting in an arginine-glutamine substitution at amino acid 506 (R506Q), the site where APC cleaves fVa.[71] This mutation confers APC resistance on fVa, resulting in continued activation of thrombin in the prothrombinase complex. The factor V Leiden mutation is seen in up to 50% of patients with venous thromboembolism,[71] and heterozygotes and homozygotes have approximately an 8-fold and an 80-fold increased risk for venous thrombosis, respectively.[72] However, the association between factor V Leiden and arterial thrombosis is not clear.

### Prothrombin

The prothrombin gene (21 kb) is encoded on chromosome 11 and consists of 14 exons.[73,74] The fXa/fVa complex formed on membranes in the presence of $Ca^{2+}$ is known as the prothrombinase complex, which facilitates conversion of prothrombin to thrombin.

Prothrombin deficiency is a rare form of coagulation disease with hemorrhagic manifestations that is inherited in an autosomal recessive manner. Conversely, a common mutation of the prothrombin gene is associated with elevated prothrombin levels in blood and an increased risk of both arterial and venous thrombosis. A G-to-A transition at position 20210 (20210GA) in the sequence of the 3′-UT region of the prothrombin gene was identified, which is present in 1% to 2% of the general population. The 20210GA mutation is associated with elevated plasma levels of prothrombin, thrombin-antithrombin complex, and prothrombin fragment 1+2. Patients with the prothrombin 20210GA mutation are at an increased risk of myocardial infarction,[75] ischemic stroke,[76,77] and venous thromboembolism.[78] The thrombophilic tendency of the 20210GA mutation is also reflected by a significantly increased endogenous thrombin potential (ETP) found in heterozygotes of the 20210GA mutation; homozygotes have an even higher ETP compared with controls.[79]

### Fibrinogen

Fibrinogen is encoded by three separate genes, and each gene encodes one of the three subunits of fibrinogen ($\alpha$, $\beta$, and $\gamma$). These three genes are closely linked in a 50-kb region of chromosome 4: the $\alpha$ gene in the middle flanked by the $\beta$-gene on one side and the $\gamma$ gene on the other.[80] The regulation of these genes is coordinated at the transcriptional level to yield simultaneous production of the three fibrinogen polypeptide chains.[81] The $\alpha$, $\beta$, and $\gamma$ chains are highly homologous in their amino acid sequence, which suggests that they evolved from a common ancestral gene.[82-85] The mature form of fibrinogen is a glycoprotein (340 kDa) that consists of three pairs of polypeptide chains: two A$\alpha$ chains, two B$\beta$ chains and two $\gamma$ chains.[86] Fibrinogen circulates in blood as a biologically inactive form. Thrombin converts fibrinogen to its active form, fibrin, by cleaving both A$\alpha$ and B$\beta$ chains. The fibrin monomers noncovalently homopolymerize to form two-stranded protofibrils.

High levels of plasma fibrinogen are an independent predictor of cardiovascular disease and are strongly associated with arterial thrombosis including myocardial infarction and stroke.[45,87] A large number of mutations in the fibrinogen gene have been described that lead to variable bleeding and thrombotic tendencies. Fibrinogen Oslo I has a short thrombin time, fast polymerization, and increased platelet aggregation. Fibrinogen New York I has a B$\beta$9-72 deletion that has defective t-PA binding to fibrin with decreased potentiation of plasminogen activation.[88] Fibrinogen Dusart (Paris V), or Chapel Hill III, has a single base change that results in the substitution R554C in the A$\alpha$ chain, conferring resistance against plasmin degradation; patients who are heterozygous for this substitution suffer from recurrent thrombotic disorders.[89] The $\alpha$ fibrinogen T312A polymorphism is associated with an increased poststroke mortality in patients with atrial fibrillation.[90] Another polymorphism at nucleotide 148 in the $\beta$ fibrinogen promoter region is associated with an increased risk of carotid atherosclerosis despite normal fibrinogen levels in the plasma.[91]

### Factor XIII

Factor XIII is a zymogen of a cysteine transglutaminase, consisting of two peptide subunits, the $\alpha$ chain (75 kDa) and the $\beta$ chain (80 kDa). The $\alpha$ gene and $\beta$ gene are encoded on chromosome 6 and 1, respectively.[92,93] Factor XIII (320 kDa) is a tetramer of two $\beta$ chains and two $\beta$ chains. Thrombin activates fXIII into fVIIIa by cleaving the $\alpha$ chain at Arg37-38. The two-stranded protofibrils consist of noncovalently linked fibrin monomers; therefore, the strands are unstable. Activated factor XIII (fXIIIa), a transglutaminase, catalyzes the condensation of lysine residues on one chain and glutamic acid residue on the second chain, giving rise to a stable, cross-liked fibrin polymer.[94]

Several point mutations in the $\alpha$ gene result in fXIII deficiency, which presents as a rare autosomal recessive bleeding disorder. A C-to-T transition at Arg661 in exon 14 creates a premature stop codon, resulting in a 10- to 30-fold reduction in fXIII mRNA levels. Another mutation, the T-to-C transition in exon 6, results in a substitution of threonine242 for methionine, but this does not appear to affect the level of mRNA. Both mutations lead to an absence of a functional and immunodetectable fXIII protein, presumably because of an altered conformation of the mutant polypeptide, resulting in early degradation of the defective protein.[95] Factor XIII-V34L, a common point mutation (G/T) in exon 2 of the $\alpha$ gene, may protect against myocardial infarction and venous thromboembolism but predispose to intracranial hemorrhage.[96-98]

# Natural Anticoagulant Mechanisms

## Protein C Pathway

The protein C pathway is a highly coordinated anticoagulation mechanism that converts the coagulation signal generated by thrombin into an anticoagulant response through the activation of protein C by the thrombin-thrombomodulin complex (Fig. 28-2). Protein C and thrombin assemble on the three epidermal growth factor (EGF) repeats of thrombomodulin on the endothelial cell, and thrombin rapidly cleaves the Arg169-Leu170 bond in its heavy, chain yielding APC. APC then interacts with protein S to inactivate two critical coagulation cofactors, fVa and fVIIIa, thereby blocking further thrombin generation. Protein S appears to alter the cleavage site preferences of APC in fVa, presumably by changing the distance of the active site of APC relative to the membrane surface.[99]

Protein C (34 kDa) is a vitamin K-dependent zymogen comprised of a heavy chain and a light chain linked by a disulfide bond.[100] The protein C gene (12 kb), containing 9 exons, is encoded on chromosome 2, and yields an mRNA of 1.5 kb. Thrombomodulin, a thrombin receptor on the luminal surface of endothelial cells, serves as a critical cofactor for the protein C anticoagulation pathway. The thrombomodulin gene is encoded on chromosome 20. No introns are present within the coding region; therefore, the EGF type B repeats and a membrane-spanning region are not isolated within discrete exons. The overall genetic structure of thrombomodulin exhibits homology to the human LDL receptor.[101] Thrombomodulin gene expression is downregulated at the transcriptional level by TNF-α through a signaling cascade that involves binding to a member of the Ets nuclear factor family.[102] Protein S (60 kDa) is another vitamin K dependent plasma protein encoded by the gene (80 kb) on chromosome 3 that contains 15 exons.[103] Endothelial cell protein C receptor (EPCR) is a member of the CD1/major histocompatibility complex superfamily that binds to both inert protein C and APC in a $Ca^{2+}$-dependent fashion. Both the function and expression of EPCR are attenuated by exposure of endothelium to TNF-α. EPCR is likely to enhance efficient transfer of protein C to thrombomodulin on endothelial cell surfaces.[104]

Patients with congenital deficiencies in the protein C pathway are at increased risk for both arterial and venous thrombosis.[105-109] Acute inflammatory disease such as sepsis can result in acquired deficiencies in the protein C pathway with resultant increase in the plasma TNF-α levels, whereas administration of APC decreases the circulating levels of TNF-α.[110] Reduction in plasma protein C levels is associated with poor clinical outcomes in patients with septic shock, and treatment with recombinant APC significantly reduces mortality in patients with severe sepsis.[111] Therefore, the protein C pathway appears to modulate inflammatory response as well as coagulation cascades.

Natural phospholipids including phosphatidyletethanolamine and cardiolipin appear to stimulate the anticoagulant protein C pathway by increasing the affinity of phospholipid surfaces for the protein C complex to enhance enzymatic degradation of fVa. Antiphospholipid or anticardiolipin antibodies inhibit this enhancement of protein C pathway, resulting in a clinical thrombophilic tendency.[112,113] Neutral glycolipids, glucosylceramide, lactosylceramide, and globotriaosylceramide can enhance anticoagulant activity of the protein C pathway by mechanisms distinctly different from those of phospholipids alone, and the deficiency of these glycolipids may be a risk factor for venous thrombosis.[114,115]

The C allele in a C/T dimorphism at nucleotide 1418 in the thrombomodulin gene is associated with premature myocardial infarction.[116] This polymorphism results in an A455V substitution in the sixth EGF-like domain. Because no association between the C/T dimorphism and the plasma levels of thrombomodulin is observed, the C/T dimorphism may mitigate the function of thrombomodulin as a cofactor for APC.[117]

## Antithrombin

Antithrombin, or antithrombin III, is an endogenous anticoagulant that inhibits thrombin and fXa to block the coagulation cascade. Antithrombin also inactivates fXIa, fXIIa, and VIIa but to a lesser extent (Fig. 28-2). The antithrombin gene (15 kb), consisting of 7 exons, is located on chromosome 1, and encodes for a 1.8-kb mRNA that yields the single-chain glycoprotein protease inhibitor antithrombin (68 kd).[118,119] Antithrombin belongs to the serine protease inhibitor (serpin) superfamily and inactivates thrombin and other activated coagulation factors by forming a complex between the active site of the enzyme and the reactive center (Arg393-Ser394) of antithrombin. Antithrombin contains a C-terminal arginine-serine reactive site that interacts with coagulation factors and two positively charged regions that bind to the sulfated polysaccharides, heparin and heparan sulfate.[120]

Coagulation factors slowly interact with antithrombin in the absence of heparin or heparan sulfate, but the addition of these polysaccharides significantly accelerates the rate of reactions by a factor of several thousand to inactivate coagulation factors. Heparin-bound antithrombin undergoes a conformational change in the reactive sites. Arginine reactive centers of antithrombin bind to the enzyme active center serines of thrombin and other serine protease coagulation factors, thereby neutralizing their activities. Heparin then dissociates from these complexes and can be reused to bind to other antithrombin molecules. Heparin, thus, acts as a catalyst in accelerating the neutralization of thrombin and other activated clotting factors by antithrombin.[1] Patients with quantitative or qualitative deficiencies of antithrombin manifest recurrent thrombotic complications.[121,122]

## Tissue Factor Pathway Inhibitor

TFPI, an endogenous inhibitor of TF (Fig. 28-2), is a plasma protein (34 kd) that exhibits an acidic amino-terminal region, three tandem repeated serine protease inhibitor domains homologous in structure to Kunitz trypsin inhibitor, and a basic carboxyl-terminal sequence (Fig. 28-4).[123,124] The first Kunitz domain (Kunitz 1) binds to the TF/fVIIa complex, whereas the Kunitz 2 domain forms a complex with fXa with assistance from other portions of the molecule. The function of the Kunitz 3 domain remains unknown. The TFPI gene is located on chromosome 2 and contains nine exons and eight introns.

In all types of atherosclerotic lesions of coronary arteries (type I, II, III, and IV), TFPI is increased in the endothelial cells and macrophages[125] and appears to attenuate the TF activity in atherosclerotic plaques.[126] This may reflect a physiologic response to counteract thrombogenic tendency in atherothrombosis.

Plasma levels of total and free TFPI, possibly originating from endothelial cells and monocytes, are also increased in patients with acute coronary syndrome,[127] and a positive correlation is observed between TF and TFPI plasma levels.[128] The plasma TFPI levels are higher in patients with unstable angina than those with stable angina and myocardial infarction, and high TFPI levels are associated with unfavorable clinical outcomes.[37] Intravenous unfractionated heparin (UFH) administration does not affect TFPI levels but markedly lowers the TF levels, which supports the clinical efficacy of anticoagulation therapy in patients with acute coronary syndrome.[36] TFPI is also implicated in a rebound increase in thrombophilic potential after abrupt cessation of intravenous UFH among patients with non-ST segment elevation acute coronary syndrome. After UFH cessation, the plasma level of TFPI decreases while thrombin generation progressively increases. This heparin rebound phenomenon can be attenuated by an abbreviated intravenous weaning strategy.[129] Fibrinolytic therapy in patients with acute myocardial infarction significantly decreases plasma TFPI levels and surface-associated TFPI on circulating monocytes. This reduction in TFPI level, presumably resulting from enzymatic inactivation of TFPI by plasmin, may contribute to thrombotic complications after fibrinolytic therapy.[130]

Some patients heterozygous for V264M polymorphism in exon 9 of the TFPI gene exhibit significantly lower plasma TFPI levels than those with the most common genotype. However, no increased incidence of acute coronary syndromes is observed among these heterozygotes.[131]

## PROCOAGULANT FACTORS IN ATHEROTHROMBOSIS

### Lipoproteins

LDL, particularly oxidized LDL, contributes to activation of both the extrinsic and intrinsic pathways of coagulation in atherosclerotic lesions, whereas HDL is a potent stimulator of the anticoagulant protein C pathway.[132] Oxidized LDL is atherogenic, and it provides an important mechanistic basis that links atherosclerosis with atherothrombosis. Oxidized LDL induces atherosclerosis by stimulating monocyte infiltration and SMC migration and proliferation. Oxidized LDL contributes to

atherothrombosis through several mechanisms: induction of plaque erosion by endothelial cell apoptosis, impairment of the anticoagulant balance in endothelium, stimulation of TF production on SMCs and induction of apoptosis in macrophages.[133] Oxidized LDL also provides a phospholipid surface to support the assembly of the prothrombinase complex and the extrinsic and intrinsic Xase complex, thereby contributing to thrombin generation.[132,134,135] Therefore, oxidized LDL accumulated in atherosclerotic lesions is likely to play a major role in enhancing the procoagulant activity.

LDL increases synthesis and activity of TF in atherosclerotic lesions, but the presence of oxidation appears to be critical. Native LDL increases TF synthesis in human SMCs, while oxidants, some of which exist in atherosclerotic plaques, activate the TF pathway on the cell surface.[136] Oxidized LDL increases both TF synthesis and surface TF pathway activity in SMCs, whereas native LDL, which does induce TF mRNA, does not increase TF activity.[137-140] Oxidized LDL also upregulates TF expression in endothelial cells and macrophages[141-143] and significantly potentiates the procoagulant activity of the extrinsic pathway in these cells.[137,144-146]

Macrophages and SMCs can promote the intrinsic, fVIIIa/IXa-dependent activation of fX by supporting the assembly of the intrinsic Xase complex, but the rate of fX activation is much lower than that of activated platelets.[147] Oxidized LDL enhances the ability of these cells to support the activity of the intrinsic Xase complex and prothrombinase complex, resulting in a significant increase in thrombin formation. The intrinsic pathway may, thus, contribute to the procoagulant activity of atherosclerotic lesions on denudation of the endothelial layer and exposure of macrophages and SMCs to blood. The contribution of the intrinsic, fVIII-dependent pathway is also supported by the finding on human atherectomy specimens that fVIII is present adjacent to macrophages and SMCs in atheromatous areas with large deposits of oxidized LDL.[148] In endothelial cells, oxidized LDL does not facilitate the intrinsic pathway, but it increases the thrombogenicity in the extrinsic pathway by stimulating TF expression and by reducing protein C activation.[146]

Endocytosed oxidized LDL induces severe impairment of lysosomal degradation mechanisms in macrophages not only by partially inactivating lysosomal enzymes but also by destabilizing the acidic vacuolar compartment, leading to relocation of lysosomal enzymes to the cytosol.[149] This may result in incomplete scavenger clearance of apoptotic microparticles, which are thrombogenic and contribute to atherothrombosis.

LDL receptor-related protein (LRP) is a multifunctional cell-surface receptor that binds and mediates the endocytosis of several structurally and functionally distinct ligands. LRP is involved in a variety of biologic processes, including the regulation of the coagulation-fibrinolysis balance, lipoprotein metabolism, cellular migration, proliferative processes, and degenerative diseases, thus implicated in the development of atherosclerosis. There is a significant correlation between increased LRP mRNA levels and atherosclerotic plaque progression.[150] LRP is essential for macrophage-mediated LDL oxidation by the enzyme 12/15-lipoxygenase,[151] which was shown to contribute significantly to the initiation and propagation of atherosclerotic lesions in apolipoprotein E deficient mice.[152] LRP also participates in inactivation of both the extrinsic and intrinsic coagulation pathways. LRP inactivates the extrinsic pathway by downregulating TF expression through TFPI-dependent internalization of TF/fVIIa complex.[153] LRP also attenuates the intrinsic pathway by binding and internalizing fVIIIa and fIXa.[154]

Lipoprotein (a), through its apolipoprotein (a) moiety, binds and inactivates TFPI in a dose-dependent fashion *in vitro*. Because apolipoprotein (a) and TFPI coexist in SMC-rich areas of the intima in human atherosclerotic plaques, TFPI in the plaques, at least in part, may be dysfunctional because of inactivation by apolipoprotein (a).[155]

## Apoptosis

Apoptosis may also play a major role in increasing thrombogenicity in atherosclerotic lesions, and it appears to affect both the extrinsic and intrinsic pathways of coagulation. Apoptosis is virtually absent in nonatherosclerotic regions, whereas abundant apoptotic cells, originating from SMCs, macrophages, and T lymphocytes, are observed in atherosclerotic lesions. Oxidized LDL induces apoptosis in SMCs,[156] endothelial cells,[157] and macrophages,[158] possibly through induction of a proapoptotic protein in these cells.[159] Apoptotic cells are seen subendothelially, in the fibrous cap, and in the underlying media and may, thus, destabilize the plaque and promote rupture. Marked TF expression in atherosclerotic plaques is detected in proximity to apoptotic cells and debris within the lipid core, suggesting a potential causal relationship between the apoptotic cell surfaces and procoagulant activity of plaque extracts.[160] These apoptotic microparticles are present in and out of phagocytic macrophages in atherosclerotic lesions,[161] and they are also found at high levels in the blood of patients with acute coronary syndrome.[162] These shed membrane apoptotic microparticles, mainly originating from monocytes, lymphocytes, and SMCs, contain a large amount of phosphatidylserine (PS), which contributes to procoagulant activity. PS is an anionic phospholipid that is redistributed on the cell surface during apoptotic death, conferring a potent procoagulant activity to the apoptotic cell. The cell membranes containing PS not only facilitate the assembly of enzymatic complexes of both extrinsic and intrinsic pathways but also significantly increase the efficiency of the intrinsic Xase enzyme complex to produce fXa.[163] These apoptotic microparticles are also a major source of TF that is activated by PS,[164] which may explain the abundant TF present in the acellular lipid-rich core of atherosclerotic plaques.[24] Apoptosis of endothelial cells increases thrombogenicity by increased expression of PS and decreased activities of thrombomodulin, heparan sulfate, and TFPI. Luminal endothelial cell apoptosis may be responsible for thrombus formation on eroded plaques without rupture.[162]

## Diabetes

Diabetes is a significant risk factor for cardiovascular morbidity and mortality through at least three separate mechanisms: accelerated atherosclerosis, development of rupture-prone plaques, and a procoagulant state. Coronary tissue from patients with diabetes exhibits a larger content of lipid-rich atheromas, macrophage infiltration, and subsequent thrombosis than tissue from patients without diabetes.[165] Thrombophilic state and subsequent development of atherothrombosis in patients with diabetes or insulin resistance are ascribed to defective fibrinolytic activities. Diabetic patients have increased plasma levels of fibrinogen and PAI-1 that favor both thrombosis and defective dissolution of clots once formed.[166,167] Animal studies have shown that both acute hyperglycemia and acute hyperinsulinemia can decrease plasma fibrinolytic potential by increasing plasma PAI-1 and decreasing free t-PA activities.[168] High levels of PAI-1 have been associated with both arterial and venous thrombosis, including myocardial infarction,[169,170] ischemic stroke,[171] and deep venous thrombosis.[172] Treatment of diabetic patients with thiazolidinediones causes reduction of plasma PAI-1 levels, which may recover the fibrinolytic activity and potentially reduce the risk of acute coronary events.[173]

## Obesity

Obesity is associated with procoagulant tendency and increased risks of both arterial and venous thrombosis. In obese patients, higher plasma concentrations of fibrinogen, PAI-1, von Willebrand factor, and fVII are observed as compared with nonobese controls. The plasma levels of fibrinogen, von Willebrand factor, and fVII correlate with central fat, whereas the plasma levels of PAI-1 correlate with visceral fat. Obesity is also associated with increased plasma levels of t-PA and protein C, which may account for the physiologic response to counteract thrombophilia. Secretion of IL-6 by adipose tissue, combined with the actions of adipose tissue expressed TNF-α in obesity, may underlie the association of insulin resistance with endothelial dysfunction, coagulopathy, and coronary artery disease.[174]

Not only diet and exercise but also pharmacologic therapy appear to be effective in improving the obesity-associated procoagulant profile.[174] Thiazolidinediones have an antiinflammatory action that may be beneficial for obese nondiabetics as well as diabetics in reducing the risk of atherothrombosis.[175] Administration of troglitazone in obese, nondiabetic subjects results in significant reduction of plasma levels of insulin without significant change in plasma glucose levels. The proinflammatory transcription factor NF-κB in mononuclear cells is downregulated, and the levels of NF-κB-regulated inflammatory mediators—TNF-α, soluble intercellular adhesion molecule (sICAM)-1, monocyte chemoattractant protein (MCP)-1, and PAI-1—significantly decrease. Plasma C reactive protein (CRP) concentration also decreases, whereas the plasma level of IL-10, an antiinflammatory cytokine, significantly increases. Reduction in PAI-1 levels in troglitazone-treated obese nondiabetic patients is mainly affected by weight loss.[176]

## Homocysteine

Elevated plasma homocysteine levels are associated with arterial and venous thrombosis as well as atherosclerosis. Inherited forms of hyperhomocysteinemia, including mutations or polymorphisms that lead to functional deficiency of cystathionine-β-synthase, methylenetetrahydrofolate reductase, or methionine synthase, often result in marked elevation of homocysteine in the plasma, whereas acquired forms usually present with intermediate to mild increase in plasma homocysteine levels. These acquired forms of hyperhomocysteinemia include vitamin deficiencies (B$_{12}$, folate, and B$_6$), renal insufficiency, hypothyroidism, psoriasis, inflammatory bowel disease, and rheumatoid arthritis.[177]

Homocysteine is a potent procoagulant amino acid that exerts different effects on practically all the pathways involved in the coagulation system. In endothelial cells, homocysteine activates fV and subsequent formation of the intrinsic Xase complex to promote fX activation.[178] Homocysteine also irreversibly inhibits thrombomodulin (TM) surface expression on endothelial cells, thus inactivating the protein C pathway.[179,180] Homocysteine binds to fVa to confer APC resistance by modification of free cysteine(s) on fVa.[181] This functional APC resistance as a result of fVa homocysteinylation may account for the high levels of plasma APC in hyperhomocysteinemic patients with a history of venous thromboembolism.[182] Homocysteine enhances both TF expression and activity in endothelial cells and monocytes in a dose-dependent fashion, thereby activating the extrinsic pathway.[183,184] Homocysteine reduces the antithrombin protein level on the endothelial cell surface in a dose-dependent fashion, and homocysteine-treated endothelial cells exhibit a substantial reduction in antithrombin binding capacity of heparan sulfate that is mediated by the generation of hydrogen peroxide through alteration of the redox potential.[185] Furthermore, homocysteine inhibits the fibrinolytic pathway by directly blocking the t-PA binding domain of annexin II, a phospholipid-binding protein that mediates binding of t-PA to endothelial cells.[186] Hyperhomocysteinemia is also a significant predictor of elevated plasma levels of asymmetric dimethylarginine (ADMA), an endogenous inhibitor of NO synthase, which is associated with atherosclerotic disease and ischemic stroke.[187]

## Angiotensin II

Angiotensin II induces an increase of both synthesis and activity of TF and PAI-1 in endothelial cells, which are effectively inhibited by ACE inhibitors,[188] type I angiotensin II receptor (AT1) antagonists,[189] natriuretic peptides,[190,191] or adrenomodulin.[192] The angiotensin II-induced TF gene transcription is mediated by NF-κB, activator protein-1 (AP-1) and at least in part by endothelin receptors (A/B).[193,194] The significant role of angiotensin II in activating the TF pathway is supported by a recent discovery that autoantibodies directed at the AT1 receptor found in the serum of preeclamptic patients, whose placentas are often infarcted and express TF, stimulate the AT1 receptor and initiate a signaling cascade resulting in TF expression.[195] The angiotensin-II-mediated induction of TF may account for the potency of the inhibition of the renin-angiotensin system in preventing acute coronary syndromes, in addition to its antihypertensive and antihypertrophic effects.

## Growth Factors

PDGF-BB stimulates SMCs to produce MCP-1[196]; both are potent chemotactic and activating factors that can separately induce a dose-dependent TF expression on human SMCs and monocytes.[197-199] Active TF on the surface of SMCs induced by PDGF represents only approximately 20% of total TF in the cell, and the remaining TF is present as encrypted surface TF and also in an intracellular pool. This may be an important mechanism to limit the thrombophilic potential of viable SMCs exposed to growth factor stimulation, whereas the encrypted surface TF and intracellular pools may provide a rich source of TF on disruption of cellular architecture of SMC during atherosclerotic plaque rupture or balloon arterial injury.[199] TF expression is also induced by VEGF on the surface of endothelial cells in the presence of TNF-α. VEGF and TNF-α synergistically increases TF mRNA, protein, and total activity.[200]

## C Reactive Protein

CRP is an acute-phase reactant, and clinical studies have shown that high levels of CRP positively correlate with poor outcome in patients with acute coronary syndrome.[201] CRP promotes atherogenesis through effects on monocytes and endothelial cells, and recent evidence suggests that CRP also contributes to atherothrombosis, especially in diabetics. CRP induces the production of TF in monocytes, increasing thrombogenicity in the extrinsic pathway.[202] CRP also induces PAI-1 expression and activity in a time- and dose-dependent fashion in endothelial cells, and the induction is pronounced under hyperglycemic conditions.[167] Observational studies have shown a strong association between a family history of type 2 diabetes and high plasma CRP concentrations in nonsmoking healthy adult women.[203]

## CD40/CD40 Ligand

The induction of TF protein and activity is also caused by ligation of CD40 receptor by T cells, activated platelets, or CD40 ligand (CD40L).[204,205] CD40L is an immunoregulatory signaling molecule expressed by human vascular endothelial cells, SMCs, human macrophages, and CD4+ T cells. CD40L and its receptor CD40 are coexpressed on these cell types in human atherosclerotic lesions.[206] Stimulation of human monocytes, macrophages, or SMCs through CD40 by CD40L induces active TF expression on these cells.[207-209] Recent clinical studies have underscored the major role of CD40L in atherothrombosis. Patients with unstable coronary artery disease who have elevated serum levels of soluble CD40L are at an increased risk of cardiovascular events, and the risk is significantly reduced by antiplatelet treatment with abciximab.[210]

## Cytokines

A number of inflammatory cytokines present in atherosclerotic lesions are found to induce TF expression, thereby contributing to thrombophilia in the extrinsic pathway of coagulation. Th1-derived cytokines, including IFN-γ induce TF production in human monocytes in the presence of activated T cells, whereas Th2-derived cytokines (IL-4, IL-13, and IL-10) inhibit TF production.[211,212] In human endothelial cells, TF expression is also induced by IL-1[213] and TNF-α.[214-216]

## ANTICOAGULATION THERAPIES

## Conventional Agents

### Unfractionated/Low Molecular Weight Heparin

UFH has been widely used to treat cardiovascular disease because of its immediate onset of action. A meta-analysis showed a trend toward benefit of heparin plus aspirin compared with aspirin alone in reducing risk of myocardial infarction or death in patients with unstable angina.[217] However, UFH has several unfavorable properties as an anticoagulant: unpredictable pharmacokinetics, narrow therapeutic range, and short serum half-life. These critical disadvantages of UFH led to the development of low molecular weight heparin (LMWH), a new generation of heparin. LMWH results from chemical or enzymatic depolymerization of approximately 50 residues (15 kd) of UFH. LMWH contains oligosaccha-

rides of less than 18 residues (<5.4 kDa), which bind to antithrombin and specifically inhibit fXa, and oligosaccharides of greater than 18 residues (>5 to 7 kd), which neutralize both fXa and thrombin (Fig. 28-5).[1] LMWH exhibits less interaction with endothelial cells and plasma proteins, which leads to higher predictability of anticoagulant effect and prolonged half-life in the plasma.[218] LMWH exhibits first-order kinetics with a plasma half-life approximately twofold to fourfold longer than UFH and minimal interpatient variability in effective drug levels. These properties reduce the need for continuous administration and frequent laboratory monitoring for proper dosing, resulting in a reduction of bleeding complications. LMWH also exhibits significantly fewer interactions with platelets compared with UFH. Clinical trials have shown that the incidence of heparin-induced thrombocytopenia, associated thrombotic events, and heparin-dependent IgG antibodies are significantly less common in patients treated with LMWH than in those treated with UFH.[219]

In addition to stimulating antithrombin activity, both UFH and LMWH provide an additional antithrombotic effect through mitigation of the TF pathway activity. Both UFH and LMWH decrease TF expression on the monocyte and endothelial cell surface, dampening the cellular procoagulant potential.[220,221] In humans, both heparin preparations (intravenously or subcutaneously administered) also release TFPI from endothelial cells into the blood circulation.[10,222] These agents appear to displace TFPI from endothelial cell surface glycosaminoglycans with subsequent release into the circulation and formation of heparin-TFPI complexes.[223,224] Repeated or continued intravenous heparin administration depletes intravascular pools of TFPI, resulting in attenuation of the antithrombotic actions of heparin.[225]

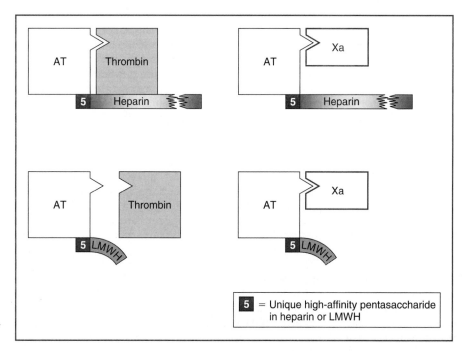

**FIGURE 28-5.** Mechanisms of inhibitory action of unfractionated heparin (heparin) and low molecular weight heparin (LMWH) on thrombin and factor Xa. Both unfractionated heparin and LMWH bind to antithrombin (AT) through a high-affinity pentasaccharide sequence (5) that both types of heparin contain. Inhibition of thrombin *(left side of figure)* requires formation of a ternary complex of heparin with both antithrombin (AT) and thrombin. Unfractionated heparins have sufficient length to accomplish this but LMWHs do not. In contrast, inhibition of factor Xa *(right side of figure)* requires that heparin bind only to AT, which unfractionated heparin and LMWH can catalyze equally effectively through their common pentasaccharide sequences. Thus, LMWH (but not unfractionated heparin) inactivates factor Xa selectively relative to thrombin. *(From Braunwald E, Zipes D, Libby P: Heart Disease, 6 ed. WB Saunders, Philadelphia, 2001, p. 2109.)*

5 = Unique high-affinity pentasaccharide in heparin or LMWH

The antithrombotic efficacy of LMWH is equal or superior to UFH. Fibrinogen, prothrombin fragment 1+2 (F1+2), thrombin antithrombin complex, von Willebrand factor, TF, and TFPI manifest a similar response to UFH and LMWH among patients admitted for acute coronary syndrome.[226] In a meta-analysis comparing LMWH with UFH in non-ST elevation acute coronary syndrome, no difference was found in the risk of myocardial infarction and death.[227] The pooled data extracted from the ESSENCE and TIMI11B studies revealed that LMWH is superior to UFH in reducing myocardial infarction and emergency revascularization in patients with acute coronary syndrome without increasing the risk of major bleeding. LMWH was associated with a 20% reduction in death and serious cardiac ischemic events compared with UFH.[228] In patients with ST-elevation myocardial infarction, the combination of LMWH and tenecteplase was superior to that of UFH and tenecteplase in reducing the frequency of ischemic complications.[229]

### Warfarin

Warfarin inhibits the synthesis of six vitamin K-dependent proteins involved in regulation of blood coagulation: prothrombin, fIX, fVII, fX, protein C, and protein S. These proteins contain 9 to 12 residues of γ-carboxyglutamic acid within the first 45 residues of their NH$_2$-termini.[230,231] γ-Carboxylation of glutamic acids is a result of post-translational modification by a membrane-bound γ-carboxylase, and this enzyme requires the reduced form of vitamin K (KH$_2$) as a cofactor. γ-Carboxyglutamic acid residues in the NH$_2$-terminal of these proteins are required to bind to Ca$^{2+}$ and form stable vitamin K-dependent enzyme complexes on cellular phospholipid surfaces.[232,233] Warfarin inhibits reductase enzymes that are required to recycle vitamin K epoxide to vitamin KH$_2$ after γ-carboxylation, thereby depleting the active vitamin K cofactor (Fig. 28-6). Warfarin rarely causes skin necrosis in the first few days of administration, especially in patients with decreased levels of protein C or protein S. This is caused by mitigation of the protein C pathway resulting from rapid decrease of protein C levels compared with other vitamin K-dependent coagulation factors.

Warfarin is the most common oral anticoagulant and is used in a variety of clinical conditions, including atrial arrhythmias, ischemic heart disease, heart failure, and stroke. In a randomized clinical trial, warfarin, in combination with aspirin or given alone, was superior to aspirin alone in reducing the incidence of composite events after an acute myocardial infarction but was associated with a higher risk of bleeding.[234]

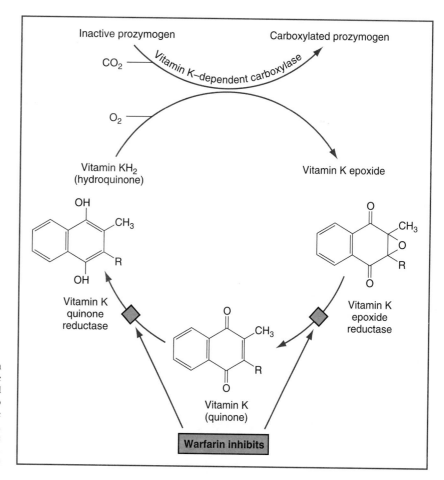

**FIGURE 28-6.** Vitamin K cycle and its inhibition by warfarin. Warfarin inhibits vitamin K epoxide reductase and vitamin K quinone reductase and so blocks the conversion of vitamin K epoxide to vitamin KH$_2$. Vitamin KH$_2$ is a cofactor for the carboxylation of inactive proenzymes (factors II, VII, IX, and X) to their active forms. *(From Braunwald E, Zipes D, Libby P: Heart Disease, 6 ed. WB Saunders, Philadelphia, 2001, p. 2111.)*

## Lipid-Lowering Agents

HMG-CoA reductase inhibitors (statins) have been proven effective in both primary and secondary prevention of coronary artery disease. In addition to their lipid-lowering effects, statins appear to reduce the propensity for atherothrombosis by attenuating the extrinsic pathway of coagulation in patients with atherosclerosis. Statins reduce TF expression and activity through inhibition of Rho/Rho-kinase and activation of Akt in human macrophages and endothelial cells.[221,235,236] Statins also inhibit cytokine-stimulated CD40 expression on these cells, further reducing TF upregulation.[237]

High-resolution MRI has enabled long-term, noninvasive observation of atherosclerotic plaques in human patients. Prolonged statin therapy causes significant regression of established atherosclerotic lesions with markedly decreased lipid content.[238,239] Observational studies reported that early initiation of statin therapy in patients with acute myocardial infarction is associated with a significant risk reduction in mortality, and discontinuation of statins after onset of symptoms completely abrogates this beneficial effect.[240,241] However, a recent randomized clinical trial showed that early initiation of aggressive statin therapy for patients with acute coronary syndrome did not reduce the risk of major cardiac events compared with the placebo group, despite significant reduction in recurrent ischemic events in the first 16 weeks.[242]

## Angiotensin-Converting Enzyme Inhibitors/Angiotensin II Receptor Blockers

The efficacy of ACE inhibitors and AT1 receptor antagonists in reducing cardiovascular mortality may partially derive from inhibition of angiotensin II-mediated activation of the extrinsic pathway of coagulation. ACE inhibitors and AT1 receptor antagonists downregulate TF expression and the resultant thrombin generation in atherosclerotic plaques and monocytes.[221,243,244] ACE inhibitors also decrease plasma TF levels and MCP-1 in patients with acute myocardial infarction, suggesting that both reduction in TF expression and inhibition of the accumulation of monocytes and macrophages may contribute to the antithrombotic effects of ACE inhibitors and AT1 receptor antagonists.[245]

# Novel Agents

## Active Site Inactivated Recombinant Factor VIIa

Several types of recombinant fVIIa with inactivation of the active site have been engineered. Active site inactivated fVIIa (fVIIai) inhibits the TF/fVIIa complex-mediated fXa production by competing with endogenous fVIIa for TF, resulting in cessation of the extrinsic pathway of coagulation. However, fVIIai may not be as potent as TFPI. TFPI inhibits the fXa generation already in progress, whereas fVIIai does not.[246] Administration of fVIIai abolishes thrombus formation at sites of vascular injury, increases vessel patency, and inhibits cyclic flow variations caused by recurrent thrombus formation in animal models. Remarkably,

antithrombotic effects of fVIIai are not complicated by bleeding.[247-249] Treatment with fVIIai in rabbit balloon-injury models inhibits fibrin deposition, reduces loss of lumen, and decreases neointimal hyperplasia at the sites of vessel injury.[250,251] A phase II clinical trial showed that fVIIai also significantly reduced thrombin generation and fibrin deposition in blood obtained from a human who received fVIIai.[252]

## Anti-Tissue Factor Monoclonal Antibodies

Antibodies against TF markedly reduce plaque thrombogenicity in human arterial segments.[27] Animal studies have shown that anti-TF monoclonal antibodies prevent thrombosis and decrease occlusion of the eversion femoral artery graft,[253] successfully block thrombus formation in carotid arteries,[254] and significantly shorten lysis time and decrease reocclusion rates following fibrinolytic therapy in a carotid thrombosis model.[255] Anti-TF monoclonal antibodies also attenuate myocardial ischemia/reperfusion injury resulting in reduced infarct size.[256] These promising preclinical studies led to the development of a humanized monoclonal antibody against human TF, which is under investigation. These humanized antibodies display potent inhibition of plasma clotting and TF *in vitro,* and completely prevent fibrin deposition in a human *ex vivo* thrombosis model under venous blood flow conditions.[257]

## Mutant Human Tissue Factor

The substrate recognition region of TF contains two residues, Lys165 and Lys166, which are important for macromolecular substrate activation by the TF/fVIIa complex. Replacement of these two residues with alanine (K165A:K166A) in a soluble version of human TF (sTF, residues 1 to 219) results in a mutant hTFAA, which binds fVIIa with kinetics and affinity equivalent to wild-type sTF. However, the hTFAA/fVIIa complex shows a 34-fold reduction in catalytic efficiency for fX activation compared with the activity measured for sTF/VIIa. A significant antithrombotic effect is displayed in arterial thrombosis when hTFAA is compared with heparin.[258,259] Phage display technology allowed affinity maturation of hTFAA to fVIIa leading to development of an hTFAA variant with an improved antithrombotic activity that is currently under preclinical investigation.[260]

## Recombinant Tissue Factor Pathway Inhibitor

Recombinant TFPI (rTFPI) is one of the most extensively studied anticoagulants. This anticoagulant significantly reduces both platelet and fibrinogen deposition on human atherosclerotic arterial segments.[27] Animal studies, however, showed conflicting results on its effect in preventing reocclusion in models of acute arterial thrombosis.[261-263] In clinical studies, rTFPI has shown favorable effects in patients with severe sepsis,[264] but rTFPI has not been investigated in patients with acute coronary syndrome.

## Nematode Anticoagulant Protein c2

Recombinant nematode anticoagulant protein c2 (rNAPc2) is a potent small protein anticoagulant isolated from the hookworm *Ancylostoma caninum*. It exerts its anticoagulant effect by fX-dependent inhibition of the TF/fVIIa complex. The anticoagulant rNAPc2 forms a binary complex with fX at a site on the fXa that is distinct from the catalytic center (exo-site) and inhibits the catalytic activity of the TF/fVIIa complex to activate fX.[265] The formation of the binary complex with circulating fX determines the pharmacokinetic profile of rNAPc2 in humans, resulting in a prolonged elimination half-life of longer than 50 hours. A phase II clinical trial has shown that subcutaneous injections of rNAPc2 were safe and effective in patients undergoing elective, unilateral total knee replacement, and the overall incidence of deep venous thrombosis was reduced by more than 50% compared with historic controls with LMWH.[266] Another phase IIa trial demonstrated the safety of rNAPc2 and the significant suppression of thrombin generation in patients undergoing elective percutaneous coronary intervention treated with standard anticoagulant and antiplatelet therapies.[267]

## Active Site Blocked Factor IXa

Active site blocked fIXa (fIXai) is a competitive inhibitor of fIXa assembly into the intrinsic Xase activation complex. Animal studies have shown that fIXai blocks intravascular thrombosis without substantially disturbing normal hemostasis.[259,268,269] In a human *ex vivo* blood flow system, fIXai inhibits fibrin deposition.[270] It accomplishes long-term patency and decreased aneurysmal dilation in polytetrafluoroethylene (PTFE) vascular repair, while eliminating the intraoperative morbidity of needle-hole bleeding.[271] In addition, fIXai appears to be an effective alternative anticoagulant strategy in cardiopulmonary bypass when heparin is contraindicated, affording inhibition of intravascular and extracorporeal circuit thrombosis with enhanced hemostasis in the surgical wound.[272] Active site blocked fIXa limited fibrin deposition within the extracorporeal circuit, comparable with the antithrombotic effect seen with heparin. In contrast to heparin, effective antithrombotic doses of fIXai significantly diminished blood loss in the thoracic cavity and in an abdominal incisional bleeding model.[273] The efficacy of fIXai in atherothrombosis remains unknown.

## Factor Xa Inhibitors

Naturally occurring fXa inhibitors include tick anticoagulant peptide (TAP) and antistatin.[274,275] Both are potent and specific factor Xa inhibitors and are available in recombinant forms. Synthetic fXa inhibitors include fondaparinux, DX-9065a, and ZK-807834. A pentasaccharide, fondaparinux is an indirect fXa inhibitor that exerts its antithrombotic effects by binding to and neutralizing antithrombin. Randomized control studies have shown that fondaparinux is superior to LMWH in preventing venous thromboembolism in patients undergoing hip fracture surgery,[276] hip-replacement surgery,[277] and elec-

tive major knee surgery.[278] A meta-analysis of these trials have shown a major benefit of fondaparinux over LMWH in patients undergoing major orthopedic surgery, achieving an overall risk reduction of venous thromboembolism greater than 50% without increasing the risk of clinically relevant bleeding.[279] A randomized clinical trial has demonstrated that fondaparinux is as safe and effective as UFH in restoring coronary artery patency in patients with ST-elevation acute myocardial infarction undergoing fibrinolytic therapy.[280] An oral, small-molecule fXa inhibitor, DX-9065a, that directly and reversibly inhibits fXa with high specificity is currently under investigation in human clinical trials.[281] In animal studies, ZK-807834 and recombinant TAP decrease reocclusion and improve patency of recanalized arteries without increasing bleeding complications compared with heparin and aspirin.[282]

## Thrombin Inhibitors

Direct thrombin inhibitors interact with thrombin and block its catalytic activity on a wide range of substrates. Hirudin, originally isolated from the saliva of a medicinal leech, *Hirudo medicinalis,* is a 65 amino acid polypeptide that forms a reversible, 1:1 stoichiometric complex with thrombin. Despite important pharmacokinetic and theoretical advantages over heparin, early randomized trials failed to demonstrate a net clinical benefit of recombinant hirudin because of an excess of hemorrhagic stroke and only modest efficacy gains compared with heparin.[283] Recently, however, clinical efficacy of hirudin and its derivatives has been re-evaluated by a number of clinical studies.[284] In patients with acute coronary syndrome, hirudin is associated with less thrombin activity and slower increases in thrombin formation after discontinuation than heparin, although hirudin does not prevent generation of new thrombin.[285] In the HERO-2 trial, bivalirudin significantly reduced the rate of adjudicated reinfarction, despite no mortality benefit, compared with UFH in patients with acute myocardial infarction treated with streptokinase. Small absolute increases were seen in mild and moderate bleeding in patients given bivalirudin.[286] In patients with non-ST-elevation acute coronary syndrome undergoing early percutaneous coronary intervention, hirudin was shown to be more effective than heparin in reducing the incidence of death or myocardial infarction.[287]

In addition to hirudin and bivalirudin, another class of direct thrombin inhibitors is emerging as antithrombotic drugs with a wide range of indications. These synthetic, small-molecule direct thrombin inhibitors include argatroban, efegatran, inogatran, napsagatran, and melagatran/ximelagatran. The tripeptide type or peptidomimetic compounds, including argatroban, efegatran, inogatran, and napsagatran, represent a first generation of thrombin inhibitors that are pharmacokinetically characterized by relatively rapid hepatobiliary clearance and short half-lives necessitating their administration as an intravenous infusion.[288] Ximelagatran is an oral form of direct thrombin inhibitor. After oral administration, ximelagatran is rapidly absorbed and converted to its active form, melagatran, which can also be administered subcutaneously. Ximelagatran or melagatran does not require routine coagulation monitoring. Randomized clinical studies revealed equivalent or superior effects of ximelagatran/melagatran compared with LMWH in reducing the risk of venous thromboembolism after major elective orthopedic surgery and no significant difference in clinically important bleeding events.[289,290]

## REFERENCES

1. Schafer AI, Ali NM, Levine GN: Hemostasis, thrombosis, fibrinolysis, and cardiovascular disease. In Libby P (ed): Heart Disease: A Textbook of Cardiovascular Medicine. Philadelphia, WB Saunders, 2001, pp 2099-2132.
2. Khrenov AV, Ananyeva NM, Griffin JH, et al: Coagulation pathways in atherothrombosis. Trends Cardiovasc Med 2002;12:317-324.
3. Mann KG: Biochemistry and physiology of blood coagulation. Thromb Haemost 1999;82:165-174.
4. Mann KG, Bovill EG, Krishnaswamy S: Surface-dependent reactions in the propagation phase of blood coagulation. Ann NY Acad Sci 1991;614:63-75.
5. Nemerson Y: The tissue factor pathway of blood coagulation. Semin Hematol 1992;29:170-176.
6. Edgington TS, Mackman N, Brand K, et al: The structural biology of expression and function of tissue factor. Thromb Haemost 1991;66:67-79.
7. Ruf W, Edgington TS: Structural biology of tissue factor, the initiator of thrombogenesis in vivo. FASEB J 1994;8:385-390.
8. Girard TJ, Warren LA, Novotny WF, et al: Functional significance of the Kunitz-type inhibitory domains of lipoprotein-associated coagulation inhibitor. Nature 1989;338:518-520.
9. Bajaj MS, Kuppuswamy MN, Saito H, et al: Cultured normal human hepatocytes do not synthesize lipoprotein-associated coagulation inhibitor: Evidence that endothelium is the principal site of its synthesis. Proc Natl Acad Sci USA 1990;87:8869-8873.
10. Sandset PM, Abildgaard U, Larsen ML: Heparin induces release of extrinsic coagulation pathway inhibitor (EPI). Thromb Res 1988;50:803-813.
11. Novotny WF, Brown SG, Miletich JP, et al: Plasma antigen levels of the lipoprotein-associated coagulation inhibitor in patient samples. Blood 1991;78:387-393.
12. Moons AH, Levi M, Peters RJ: Tissue factor and coronary artery disease. Cardiovasc Res 2002;53:313-325.
13. Morrissey JH, Fakhrai H, Edgington TS: Molecular cloning of the cDNA for tissue factor, the cellular receptor for the initiation of the coagulation protease cascade. Cell 1987;50:129-135.
14. Scarpati EM, Wen D, Broze GJ Jr, et al: Human tissue factor: cDNA sequence and chromosome localization of the gene. Biochemistry 1987;26:5234-5238.
15. Mackman N, Morrissey JH, Fowler B, et al: Complete sequence of the human tissue factor gene, a highly regulated cellular receptor that initiates the coagulation protease cascade. Biochemistry 1989;28:1755-1762.
16. Wilcox JN, Smith KM, Schwartz SM, et al: Localization of tissue factor in the normal vessel wall and in the atherosclerotic plaque. Proc Natl Acad Sci USA 1989;86:2839-2843.
17. Osterud B, Bajaj MS, Bajaj SP: Sites of tissue factor pathway inhibitor (TFPI) and tissue factor expression under physiologic and pathologic conditions: On behalf of the Subcommittee on Tissue factor Pathway Inhibitor (TFPI) of the Scientific and Standardization Committee of the ISTH. Thromb Haemost 1995;73:873-875.
18. Hatakeyama K, Asada Y, Marutsuka K, et al: Localization and activity of tissue factor in human aortic atherosclerotic lesions. Atherosclerosis 1997;133:213-219.
19. Moreno PR, Bernardi VH, Lopez-Cuellar J, et al: Macrophages, smooth muscle cells, and tissue factor in unstable angina: Implications for cell-mediated thrombogenicity in acute coronary syndromes. Circulation 1996;94:3090-3097.
20. Ardissino D, Merlini PA, Ariens R, et al: Tissue-factor antigen and activity in human coronary atherosclerotic plaques. Lancet 1997;349:769-771.
21. Serneri GG, Abbate R, Gori AM, et al: Transient intermittent lymphocyte activation is responsible for the instability of angina. Circulation 1992;86:790-797.
22. Annex BH, Denning SM, Channon KM, et al: Differential expression of tissue factor protein in directional atherectomy specimens from patients with stable and unstable coronary syndromes. Circulation 1995;91:619-622.
23. Golino P, Ragni M, Cirillo P, et al: Effects of tissue factor induced by oxygen free radicals on coronary flow during reperfusion. Nat Med 1996;2:35-40.
24. Toschi V, Gallo R, Lettino M, et al: Tissue factor modulates the thrombogenicity of human atherosclerotic plaques. Circulation 1997;95:594-599.
25. Marmur JD, Thiruvikraman SV, Fyfe BS, et al: Identification of active tissue factor in human coronary atheroma. Circulation 1996;94:1226-1232.
26. Kaikita K, Ogawa H, Yasue H, et al: Tissue factor expression on macrophages in coronary plaques in patients with unstable angina. Arterioscler Thromb Vasc Biol 1997;17:2232-2237.
27. Badimon JJ, Lettino M, Toschi V, et al: Local inhibition of tissue factor reduces the thrombogenicity of disrupted human atherosclerotic plaques: Effects of tissue factor pathway inhibitor on plaque thrombogenicity under flow conditions. Circulation 1999;99:1780-1787.
28. Nishida T, Ueno H, Atsuchi N, et al: Adenovirus-mediated local expression of human tissue factor pathway inhibitor eliminates shear stress-induced recurrent thrombosis in the injured carotid artery of the rabbit. Circ Res 1999;84:1446-1452.
29. Landers SC, Gupta M, Lewis JC: Ultrastructural localization of tissue factor on monocyte-derived macrophages and macrophage foam cells associated with atherosclerotic lesions. Virchows Arch 1994;425:49-54.
30. Thiruvikraman SV, Guha A, Roboz J, et al: In situ localization of tissue factor in human atherosclerotic plaques by binding of digoxigenin-labeled factors VIIa and X. Lab Invest 1996;75:451-461.
31. Ichikawa K, Nakagawa K, Hirano K, et al: The localization of tissue factor and apolipoprotein(a) in atherosclerotic lesions of the human aorta and their relation to fibrinogen-fibrin transition. Pathol Res Pract 1996;192:224-232.
32. Muhlfelder TW, Teodorescu V, Rand J, et al: Human atheromatous plaque extracts induce tissue factor activity (TFa) in monocytes and also express constitutive TFa. Thromb Haemost 1999;81:146-150.
33. Jonasson L, Holm J, Skalli O, et al: Regional accumulations of T cells, macrophages, and smooth muscle cells in the human atherosclerotic plaque. Arteriosclerosis 1986;6:131-138.
34. Suefuji H, Ogawa H, Yasue H, et al: Increased plasma tissue factor levels in acute myocardial infarction. Am Heart J 1997;134:253-259.
35. Misumi K, Ogawa H, Yasue H, et al: Comparison of plasma tissue factor levels in unstable and stable angina pectoris. Am J Cardiol 1998;81:22-26.
36. Yamamoto N, Ogawa H, Oshima S, et al: The effect of heparin on tissue factor and tissue factor pathway inhibitor in patients with acute myocardial infarction. Int J Cardiol 2000;75:267-274.
37. Soejima H, Ogawa H, Yasue H, et al: Heightened tissue factor associated with tissue factor pathway inhibitor and prognosis in patients with unstable angina. Circulation 1999;99:2908-2913.
38. Marco J, Ariens RA, Fajadet J, et al: Effect of aspirin and ticlopidine on plasma tissue factor levels in stable and unstable angina pectoris. Am J Cardiol 2000;85:527-531.
39. Giesen PL, Rauch U, Bohrmann B, et al: Blood-borne tissue factor: Another view of thrombosis. Proc Natl Acad Sci USA 1999;96:2311-2315.
40. Rauch U, Bonderman D, Bohrmann B, et al: Transfer of tissue factor from leukocytes to platelets is mediated by CD15 and tissue factor. Blood 2000;96:170-175.
41. Arnaud E, Barbalat V, Nicaud V, et al: Polymorphisms in the 5' regulatory region of the tissue factor gene and the risk of myocardial infarction and venous thromboembolism: The ECTIM and PATHROS studies. Etude Cas-Temoins de l'Infarctus du Myocarde. Paris thrombosis case-control study. Arterioscler Thromb Vasc Biol 2000;20:892-898.

42. Hagen FS, Gray CL, O'Hara P, et al: Characterization of a cDNA coding for human factor VII. Proc Natl Acad Sci USA 1986;83:2412–2416.

43. O'Hara PJ, Grant FJ, Haldeman BA, et al: Nucleotide sequence of the gene coding for human factor VII, a vitamin K-dependent protein participating in blood coagulation. Proc Natl Acad Sci USA 1987;84:5158–5162.

44. Broze GJ Jr, Majerus PW: Purification and properties of human coagulation factor VII. J Biol Chem 1980;255:1242–1247.

45. Meade TW, Mellows S, Brozovic M, et al: Haemostatic function and ischaemic heart disease: Principal results of the Northwick Park Heart Study. Lancet 1986;2:533–537.

46. Iacoviello L, Di Castelnuovo A, De Knijff P, et al: Polymorphisms in the coagulation factor VII gene and the risk of myocardial infarction. N Engl J Med 1998;338:79–85.

47. Peyvandi F, Mannucci PM, Bucciarelli P, et al: A novel polymorphism in intron 1a of the human factor VII gene (G73A): Study of a healthy Italian population and of 190 young survivors of myocardial infarction. Br J Haematol 2000;108:247–253.

48. Cool DE, MacGillivray RT: Characterization of the human blood coagulation factor XII gene: Intron/exon gene organization and analysis of the 5′-flanking region. J Biol Chem 1987;262:13662–13673.

49. Asakai R, Davie EW, Chung DW: Organization of the gene for human factor XI. Biochemistry 1987;26:7221–7228.

50. Fujikawa K, Chung DW, Hendrickson LE, et al: Amino acid sequence of human factor XI, a blood coagulation factor with four tandem repeats that are highly homologous with plasma prekallikrein. Biochemistry 1986;25:2417–2424.

51. Meijers JC, Tekelenburg WL, Bouma BN, et al: High levels of coagulation factor XI as a risk factor for venous thrombosis. N Engl J Med 2000;342:696–701.

52. Yoshitake S, Schach BG, Foster DC, et al: Nucleotide sequence of the gene for human factor IX (antihemophilic factor B). Biochemistry 1985;24:3736–3750.

53. Vehar GA, Keyt B, Eaton D, et al: Structure of human factor VIII. Nature 1984;312:337–342.

54. Toole JJ, Knopf JL, Wozney JM, et al: Molecular cloning of a cDNA encoding human antihaemophilic factor. Nature 1984;312:342–347.

55. Pittman DD, Kaufman RJ: Proteolytic requirements for thrombin activation of anti-hemophilic factor (factor VIII). Proc Natl Acad Sci USA 1988;85:2429–2433.

56. Fay PJ, Haidaris PJ, Smudzin TM: Human factor VIIIa subunit structure: Reconstruction of factor VIIIa from the isolated A1/A3-C1-C2 dimer and A2 subunit. J Biol Chem 1991;266:8957–8962.

57. Triemstra M, Rosendaal FR, Smit C, et al: Mortality in patients with hemophilia: Changes in a Dutch population from 1986 to 1992 and 1973 to 1986. Ann Intern Med 1995;123:823–827.

58. Rosendaal FR, Briet E, Stibbe J, et al: Haemophilia protects against ischaemic heart disease: A study of risk factors. Br J Haematol 1990;75:525–530.

59. Sramek A, Reiber JH, Gerrits WB, et al: Decreased coagulability has no clinically relevant effect on atherogenesis: Observations in individuals with a hereditary bleeding tendency. Circulation 2001;104:762–767.

60. Bilora F, Boccioletti V, Zanon E, et al: Hemophilia A, von Willebrand disease, and atherosclerosis of abdominal aorta and leg arteries: Factor VIII and von Willebrand factor defects appear to protect abdominal aorta and leg arteries from atherosclerosis. Clin Appl Thromb Hemost 2001;7:311–313.

61. Kraaijenhagen RA, in't Anker PS, Koopman MM, et al: High plasma concentration of factor VIIIc is a major risk factor for venous thromboembolism. Thromb Haemost 2000;83:5–9.

62. Rosendaal FR: Factor VIII and coronary heart disease. Eur J Epidemiol 1992;8(Suppl 1):71–75.

63. Pan WH, Bai CH, Chen JR, et al: Associations between carotid atherosclerosis and high factor VIII activity, dyslipidemia, and hypertension. Stroke 1997;28:88–94.

64. Koster T, Blann AD, Briet E, et al: Role of clotting factor VIII in effect of von Willebrand factor on occurrence of deep-vein thrombosis. Lancet 1995;345:152–155.

65. Leytus SP, Foster DC, Kurachi K, et al: Gene for human factor X: A blood coagulation factor whose gene organization is essentially identical with that of factor IX and protein C. Biochemistry 1986;25:5098–5102.

66. Uprichard J, Perry DJ: Factor X deficiency. Blood Rev 2002;16:97–110.

67. Cripe LD, Moore KD, Kane WH: Structure of the gene for human coagulation factor V. Biochemistry 1992;31:3777–3785.

68. Jenny RJ, Pittman DD, Toole JJ, et al: Complete cDNA and derived amino acid sequence of human factor V. Proc Natl Acad Sci USA 1987;84:4846–4850.

69. Tracy PB, Eide LL, Bowie EJ, et al: Radioimmunoassay of factor V in human plasma and platelets. Blood 1982;60:59–63.

70. Dahlback B, Carlsson M, Svensson PJ: Familial thrombophilia due to a previously unrecognized mechanism characterized by poor anticoagulant response to activated protein C: Prediction of a cofactor to activated protein C. Proc Natl Acad Sci USA 1993;90:1004–1008.

71. Bertina RM, Koeleman BP, Koster T, et al: Mutation in blood coagulation factor V associated with resistance to activated protein C. Nature 1994;369:64–67.

72. Bertina RM: Molecular risk factors for thrombosis. Thromb Haemost 1999;82:601–609.

73. Royle NJ, Irwin DM, Koschinsky ML, et al: Human genes encoding prothrombin and ceruloplasmin map to 11p11-q12 and 3q21-24, respectively. Somat Cell Mol Genet 1987;13:285–292.

74. Degen SJ, Davie EW: Nucleotide sequence of the gene for human prothrombin. Biochemistry 1987;26:6165–6177.

75. Rosendaal FR, Siscovick DS, Schwartz SM, et al: A common prothrombin variant (20210 G to A) increases the risk of myocardial infarction in young women. Blood 1997;90:1747–1750.

76. De Stefano V, Chiusolo P, Paciaroni K, et al: Prothrombin G20210A mutant genotype is a risk factor for cerebrovascular ischemic disease in young patients. Blood 1998;91:3562–3565.

77. Franco RF, Trip MD, ten Cate H, et al: The 20210 G->A mutation in the 3′-untranslated region of the prothrombin gene and the risk for arterial thrombotic disease. Br J Haematol 1999;104:50–54.

78. Poort SR, Rosendaal FR, Reitsma PH, et al: A common genetic variation in the 3′-untranslated region of the prothrombin gene is associated with elevated plasma prothrombin levels and an increase in venous thrombosis. Blood 1996;88:3698–3703.

79. Kyrle PA, Mannhalter C, Beguin S, et al: Clinical studies and thrombin generation in patients homozygous or heterozygous for the G20210A mutation in the prothrombin gene. Arterioscler Thromb Vasc Biol 1998;18:1287–1291.

80. Kant JA, Fornace AJ Jr, Saxe D, et al: Evolution and organization of the fibrinogen locus on chromosome 4: Gene duplication accompanied by transposition and inversion. Proc Natl Acad Sci USA 1985;82:2344–2348.

81. Crabtree GR, Kant JA: Coordinate accumulation of the mRNAs for the alpha, beta, and gamma chains of rat fibrinogen following defibrination. J Biol Chem 1982;257:7277–7279.

82. Crabtree GR, Kant JA: Molecular cloning of cDNA for the alpha, beta, and gamma chains of rat fibrinogen: A family of coordinately regulated genes. J Biol Chem 1981;256:9718–9723.

83. Chung DW, Chan WY, Davie EW: Characterization of a complementary deoxyribonucleic acid coding for the gamma chain of human fibrinogen. Biochemistry 1983;22:3250–3256.

84. Rixon MW, Chan WY, Davie EW, et al: Characterization of a complementary deoxyribonucleic acid coding for the alpha chain of human fibrinogen. Biochemistry 1983;22:3237–3244.

85. Chung DW, Que BG, Rixon MW, et al: Characterization of complementary deoxyribonucleic acid and genomic deoxyribonucleic acid for the beta chain of human fibrinogen. Biochemistry 1983;22:3244–3250.

86. McKee PA, Mattock P, Hill RL: Subunit structure of human fibrinogen, soluble fibrin, and cross-linked insoluble fibrin. Proc Natl Acad Sci USA 1970;66:738–744.

87. Kannel WB, Wolf PA, Castelli WP, et al: Fibrinogen and risk of cardiovascular disease: The Framingham Study. JAMA 1987;258:1183–1186.

88. Al-Mondhiry H, Bilezikian SB, Nossel HL: Fibrinogen "New York": An abnormal fibrinogen associated with thromboembolism: Functional evaluation. Blood 1975;45:607–619.

89. Wada Y, Lord ST: A correlation between thrombotic disease and a specific fibrinogen abnormality (A alpha 554 Arg->Cys) in two unrelated kindred, Dusart and Chapel Hill III. Blood 1994;84: 3709-3714.

90. Carter AM, Catto AJ, Bamford JM, et al: Gender-specific associations of the fibrinogen B beta 448 polymorphism, fibrinogen levels, and acute cerebrovascular disease. Arterioscler Thromb Vasc Biol 1997;17:589-594.

91. Schmidt H, Schmidt R, Niederkorn K, et al: Beta-fibrinogen gene polymorphism (C148->T) is associated with carotid atherosclerosis: Results of the Austrian Stroke Prevention Study. Arterioscler Thromb Vasc Biol 1998;18:487-492.

92. Ichinose A, Davie EW: Characterization of the gene for the a subunit of human factor XIII (plasma transglutaminase), a blood coagulation factor. Proc Natl Acad Sci USA 1988;85:5829-5833.

93. Ichinose A, Davie EW: Primary structure of human coagulation factor XIII. Adv Exp Med Biol 1988;231:15-27.

94. Folk JE, Finlayson JS: The epsilon-(gamma-glutamyl)lysine crosslink and the catalytic role of transglutaminases. Adv Protein Chem 1977;31:1-133.

95. Mikkola H, Syrjala M, Rasi V, et al: Deficiency in the A-subunit of coagulation factor XIII: Two novel point mutations demonstrate different effects on transcript levels. Blood 1994;84:517-525.

96. Kohler HP, Stickland MH, Ossei-Gerning N, et al: Association of a common polymorphism in the factor XIII gene with myocardial infarction. Thromb Haemost 1998;79:8-13.

97. Catto AJ, Kohler HP, Coore J, et al: Association of a common polymorphism in the factor XIII gene with venous thrombosis. Blood 1999;93:906-908.

98. Franco RF, Reitsma PH, Lourenco D, et al: Factor XIII Val34Leu is a genetic factor involved in the etiology of venous thrombosis. Thromb Haemost 1999;81:676-679.

99. Esmon CT: Regulation of blood coagulation. Biochim Biophys Acta 2000;1477:349-360.

100. Kisiel W: Human plasma protein C: Isolation, characterization, and mechanism of activation by alpha-thrombin. J Clin Invest 1979;64:761-769.

101. Jackman RW, Beeler DL, Fritze L, et al: Human thrombomodulin gene is intron depleted: Nucleic acid sequences of the cDNA and gene predict protein structure and suggest sites of regulatory control. Proc Natl Acad Sci USA 1987;84:6425-6429.

102. von der Ahe D, Nischan C, Kunz C, et al: Ets transcription factor binding site is required for positive and TNF alpha-induced negative promoter regulation. Nucleic Acids Res 1993;21: 5636-5643.

103. Long GL, Marshall A, Gardner JC, et al: Genes for human vitamin K-dependent plasma proteins C and S are located on chromosomes 2 and 3, respectively. Somat Cell Mol Genet 1988;14:93-98.

104. Fukudome K, Esmon CT: Identification, cloning, and regulation of a novel endothelial cell protein C/activated protein C receptor. J Biol Chem 1994;269:26486-26491.

105. Griffin JH, Evatt B, Zimmerman TS, et al: Deficiency of protein C in congenital thrombotic disease. J Clin Invest 1981;68: 1370-1373.

106. Engesser L, Broekmans AW, Briet E, et al: Hereditary protein S deficiency: Clinical manifestations. Ann Intern Med 1987;106: 677-682.

107. Amitrano L, Guardascione MA, Ames PR, et al: Thrombophilic genotypes, natural anticoagulants, and plasma homocysteine in myeloproliferative disorders: Relationship with splanchnic vein thrombosis and arterial disease. Am J Hematol 2003;72:75-81.

108. Tiong IY, Alkotob ML, Ghaffari S: Protein C deficiency manifesting as an acute myocardial infarction and ischaemic stroke. Heart 2003;89:E7.

109. Cakir O, Ayyildiz O, Oruc A, et al: A young adult with coronary artery and jugular vein thrombosis: A case report of combined protein S and protein C deficiency. Heart Vessels 2002; 17:74-76.

110. Esmon CT, Fukudome K: Cellular regulation of the protein C pathway. Semin Cell Biol 1995;6:259-268.

111. Bernard GR, Vincent JL, Laterre PF, et al: Efficacy and safety of recombinant human activated protein C for severe sepsis. N Engl J Med 2001;344:699-709.

112. Fernandez JA, Kojima K, Petaja J, et al: Cardiolipin enhances protein C pathway anticoagulant activity. Blood Cells Mol Dis 2000;26:115-123.

113. Safa O, Hensley K, Smirnov MD, et al: Lipid oxidation enhances the function of activated protein C. J Biol Chem 2001;276: 1829-1836.

114. Deguchi H, Fernandez JA, Pabinger I, et al: Plasma glucosylceramide deficiency as potential risk factor for venous thrombosis and modulator of anticoagulant protein C pathway. Blood 2001;97:1907-1914.

115. Deguchi H, Fernandez JA, Griffin JH: Neutral glycosphingolipid-dependent inactivation of coagulation factor Va by activated protein C and protein S. J Biol Chem 2002;277:8861-8865.

116. Ohlin AK, Norlund L, Marlar RA: Thrombomodulin gene variations and thromboembolic disease. Thromb Haemost 1997;78: 396-400.

117. Norlund L, Holm J, Zoller B, et al: A common thrombomodulin amino acid dimorphism is associated with myocardial infarction. Thromb Haemost 1997;77:248-251.

118. Winter JH, Bennett B, Watt JL, et al: Confirmation of linkage between antithrombin III and Duffy blood group and assignment of AT3 to 1q22 lead to q25. Ann Hum Genet 1982;46: 29-34.

119. Prochownik EV: Relationship between an enhancer element in the human antithrombin III gene and an immunoglobulin light-chain gene enhancer. Nature 1985;316:845-848.

120. Stephens AW, Siddiqui A, Hirs CH: Site-directed mutagenesis of the reactive center (serine 394) of antithrombin III. J Biol Chem 1988;263:15849-15852.

121. Rosenberg RD, Aird WC: Vascular-bed–specific hemostasis and hypercoagulable states. N Engl J Med 1999;340:1555-1564.

122. Okajima K, Ueyama H, Hashimoto Y, et al: Homozygous variant of antithrombin III that lacks affinity for heparin, AT III Kumamoto. Thromb Haemost 1989;61:20-24.

123. Broze GJ Jr, Miletich JP: Isolation of the tissue factor inhibitor produced by HepG2 hepatoma cells. Proc Natl Acad Sci USA 1987;84:1886-1890.

124. Wun TC, Kretzmer KK, Girard TJ, et al: Cloning and characterization of a cDNA coding for the lipoprotein-associated coagulation inhibitor shows that it consists of three tandem Kunitz-type inhibitory domains. J Biol Chem 1988;263:6001-6004.

125. Kaikita K, Takeya M, Ogawa H, et al: Co-localization of tissue factor and tissue factor pathway inhibitor in coronary atherosclerosis. J Pathol 1999;188:180-188.

126. Caplice NM, Mueske CS, Kleppe LS, et al: Presence of tissue factor pathway inhibitor in human atherosclerotic plaques is associated with reduced tissue factor activity. Circulation 1998;98: 1051-1057.

127. Kamikura Y, Wada H, Yamada A, et al: Increased tissue factor pathway inhibitor in patients with acute myocardial infarction. Am J Hematol 1997;55:183-187.

128. Falciani M, Gori AM, Fedi S, et al: Elevated tissue factor and tissue factor pathway inhibitor circulating levels in ischaemic heart disease patients. Thromb Haemost 1998;79:495-499.

129. Becker RC, Spencer FA, Li Y, et al: Thrombin generation after the abrupt cessation of intravenous unfractionated heparin among patients with acute coronary syndromes: Potential mechanisms for heightened prothrombotic potential. J Am Coll Cardiol 1999;34:1020-1027.

130. Ott I, Malcouvier V, Schomig A, et al: Proteolysis of tissue factor pathway inhibitor-1 by thrombolysis in acute myocardial infarction. Circulation 2002;105:279-281.

131. Moatti D, Seknadji P, Galand C, et al: Polymorphisms of the tissue factor pathway inhibitor (TFPI) gene in patients with acute coronary syndromes and in healthy subjects: Impact of the V264M substitution on plasma levels of TFPI. Arterioscler Thromb Vasc Biol 1999;19:862-869.

132. Griffin JH, Kojima K, Banka CL, et al: High-density lipoprotein enhancement of anticoagulant activities of plasma protein S and activated protein C. J Clin Invest 1999;103:219-227.

133. Mertens A, Holvoet P: Oxidized LDL and HDL: Antagonists in atherothrombosis. FASEB J 2001;15:2073-2084.

134. Moyer MP, Tracy RP, Tracy PB, et al: Plasma lipoproteins support prothrombinase and other procoagulant enzymatic complexes. Arterioscler Thromb Vasc Biol 1998;18:458-465.

135. Khrenov A, Sarafanov A, Ananyeva N, et al: Molecular basis for different ability of low-density and high-density lipoproteins to support activity of the intrinsic Xase complex. Thromb Res 2002;105:87-93.

136. Penn MS, Patel CV, Cui MZ, et al: LDL increases inactive tissue factor on vascular smooth muscle cell surfaces: Hydrogen peroxide activates latent cell surface tissue factor. Circulation 1999;99:1753-1759.

137. Penn MS, Cui MZ, Winokur AL, et al: Smooth muscle cell surface tissue factor pathway activation by oxidized low-density lipoprotein requires cellular lipid peroxidation. Blood 2000;96:3056-3063.

138. Drake TA, Morrissey JH, Edgington TS: Selective cellular expression of tissue factor in human tissues. Implications for disorders of hemostasis and thrombosis. Am J Pathol 1989;134:1087-1097.

139. Drake TA, Hannani K, Fei HH, et al: Minimally oxidized low-density lipoprotein induces tissue factor expression in cultured human endothelial cells. Am J Pathol 1991;138:601-607.

140. Lewis JC, Bennett-Cain AL, DeMars CS, et al: Procoagulant activity after exposure of monocyte-derived macrophages to minimally oxidized low density lipoprotein: Co-localization of tissue factor antigen and nascent fibrin fibers at the cell surface. Am J Pathol 1995;147:1029-1040.

141. Wada H, Kaneko T, Wakita Y, et al: Effect of lipoproteins on tissue factor activity and PAI-II antigen in human monocytes and macrophages. Int J Cardiol 1994;47:S21-25.

142. Fei H, Berliner JA, Parhami F, et al: Regulation of endothelial cell tissue factor expression by minimally oxidized LDL and lipopolysaccharide. Arterioscler Thromb 1993;13:1711-1717.

143. Brand K, Banka CL, Mackman N, et al: Oxidized LDL enhances lipopolysaccharide-induced tissue factor expression in human adherent monocytes. Arterioscler Thromb 1994;14:790-797.

144. Schuff-Werner P, Claus G, Armstrong VW, et al: Enhanced procoagulatory activity (PCA) of human monocytes/macrophages after in vitro stimulation with chemically modified LDL. Atherosclerosis 1989;78:109-112.

145. Tipping PG, Malliaros J, Holdsworth SR: Procoagulant activity expression by macrophages from atheromatous vascular plaques. Atherosclerosis 1989;79:237-243.

146. Weis JR, Pitas RE, Wilson BD, et al: Oxidized low-density lipoprotein increases cultured human endothelial cell tissue factor activity and reduces protein C activation. FASEB J 1991;5:2459-2465.

147. Brinkman HJ, Mertens K, Holthuis J, et al: The activation of human blood coagulation factor X on the surface of endothelial cells: A comparison with various vascular cells, platelets and monocytes. Br J Haematol 1994;87:332-342.

148. Ananyeva NM, Kouiavskaia DV, Shima M, et al: Intrinsic pathway of blood coagulation contributes to thrombogenicity of atherosclerotic plaque. Blood 2002;99:4475-4485.

149. Li W, Yuan XM, Olsson AG, et al: Uptake of oxidized LDL by macrophages results in partial lysosomal enzyme inactivation and relocation. Arterioscler Thromb Vasc Biol 1998;18:177-184.

150. Handschug K, Schulz S, Schnurer C, et al: Low-density lipoprotein receptor-related protein in atherosclerosis development: Up-regulation of gene expression in patients with coronary obstruction. J Mol Med 1998;76:596-600.

151. Xu W, Takahashi Y, Sakashita T, et al: Low density lipoprotein receptor-related protein is required for macrophage-mediated oxidation of low density lipoprotein by 12/15-lipoxygenase. J Biol Chem 2001;276:36454-36459.

152. Cyrus T, Pratico D, Zhao L, et al: Absence of 12/15-lipoxygenase expression decreases lipid peroxidation and atherogenesis in apolipoprotein e-deficient mice. Circulation 2001;103:2277-2282.

153. Hamik A, Setiadi H, Bu G, et al: Down-regulation of monocyte tissue factor mediated by tissue factor pathway inhibitor and the low density lipoprotein receptor-related protein. J Biol Chem 1999;274:4962-4969.

154. Neels JG, Bovenschen N, van Zonneveld AJ, et al: Interaction between factor VIII and LDL receptor-related protein: Modulation of coagulation? Trends Cardiovasc Med 2000;10:8-14.

155. Caplice NM, Panetta C, Peterson TE, et al: Lipoprotein (a) binds and inactivates tissue factor pathway inhibitor: A novel link between lipoproteins and thrombosis. Blood 2001;98:2980-2987.

156. Bachem MG, Wendelin D, Schneiderhan W, et al: Depending on their concentration oxidized low density lipoproteins stimulate extracellular matrix synthesis or induce apoptosis in human

157. Sata M, Walsh K: Endothelial cell apoptosis induced by oxidized LDL is associated with the down-regulation of the cellular caspase inhibitor FLIP. J Biol Chem 1998;273:33103-33106.

158. Wintergerst ES, Jelk J, Rahner C, et al: Apoptosis induced by oxidized low density lipoprotein in human monocyte-derived macrophages involves CD36 and activation of caspase-3. Eur J Biochem 2000;267:6050-6059.

159. Okura Y, Brink M, Itabe H, et al: Oxidized low-density lipoprotein is associated with apoptosis of vascular smooth muscle cells in human atherosclerotic plaques. Circulation 2000;102:2680-2686.

160. Mallat Z, Hugel B, Ohan J, et al: Shed membrane microparticles with procoagulant potential in human atherosclerotic plaques: A role for apoptosis in plaque thrombogenicity. Circulation 1999;99:348-353.

161. Bjorkerud S, Bjorkerud B: Apoptosis is abundant in human atherosclerotic lesions, especially in inflammatory cells (macrophages and T cells), and may contribute to the accumulation of gruel and plaque instability. Am J Pathol 1996;149:367-380.

162. Tedgui A, Mallat Z: Apoptosis as a determinant of atherothrombosis. Thromb Haemost 2001;86:420-426.

163. Gilbert GE, Arena AA: Activation of the factor VIIIa-factor IXa enzyme complex of blood coagulation by membranes containing phosphatidyl-L-serine. J Biol Chem 1996;271:11120-11125.

164. Bombeli T, Karsan A, Tait JF, et al: Apoptotic vascular endothelial cells become procoagulant. Blood 1997;89:2429-2442.

165. Moreno PR, Murcia AM, Palacios IF, et al: Coronary composition and macrophage infiltration in atherectomy specimens from patients with diabetes mellitus. Circulation 2000;102:2180-2184.

166. Vinik AI, Erbas T, Park TS, et al: Platelet dysfunction in type 2 diabetes. Diabetes Care 2001;24:1476-1485.

167. Devaraj S, Xu DY, Jialal I: C-reactive protein increases plasminogen activator inhibitor-1 expression and activity in human aortic endothelial cells: Implications for the metabolic syndrome and atherothrombosis. Circulation 2003;107:398-404.

168. Pandolfi A, Giaccari A, Cilli C, et al: Acute hyperglycemia and acute hyperinsulinemia decrease plasma fibrinolytic activity and increase plasminogen activator inhibitor type 1 in the rat. Acta Diabetol 2001;38:71-76.

169. Hamsten A, de Faire U, Walldius G, et al: Plasminogen activator inhibitor in plasma: Risk factor for recurrent myocardial infarction. Lancet 1987;2:3-9.

170. Thogersen AM, Jansson JH, Boman K, et al: High plasminogen activator inhibitor and tissue plasminogen activator levels in plasma precede a first acute myocardial infarction in both men and women: Evidence for the fibrinolytic system as an independent primary risk factor. Circulation 1998;98:2241-2247.

171. Margaglione M, Di Minno G, Grandone E, et al: Abnormally high circulation levels of tissue plasminogen activator and plasminogen activator inhibitor-1 in patients with a history of ischemic stroke. Arterioscler Thromb 1994;14:1741-1745.

172. Wiman B, Ljungberg B, Chmielewska J, et al: The role of the fibrinolytic system in deep vein thrombosis. J Lab Clin Med 1985;105:265-270.

173. Plutzky J, Viberti G, Haffner S: Atherosclerosis in type 2 diabetes mellitus and insulin resistance: Mechanistic links and therapeutic targets. J Diabet Complications 2002;16:401-415.

174. De Pergola G, Pannacciulli N: Coagulation and fibrinolysis abnormalities in obesity. J Endocrinol Invest 2002;25:899-904.

175. Ghanim H, Garg R, Aljada A, et al: Suppression of nuclear factor-kappaB and stimulation of inhibitor kappaB by troglitazone: Evidence for an anti-inflammatory effect and a potential antiatherosclerotic effect in the obese. J Clin Endocrinol Metab 2001;86:1306-1312.

176. Charles MA, Morange P, Eschwege E, et al: Effect of weight change and metformin on fibrinolysis and the von Willebrand factor in obese nondiabetic subjects: The BIGPRO1 Study—Biguanides and the Prevention of the Risk of Obesity. Diabetes Care 1998;21:1967-1972.

177. Key NS, McGlennen RC: Hyperhomocyst(e)inemia and thrombophilia. Arch Pathol Lab Med 2002;126:1367-1375.

178. Rodgers GM, Kane WH: Activation of endogenous factor V by a homocysteine-induced vascular endothelial cell activator. J Clin Invest 1986;77:1909-1916.

coronary artery smooth muscle cells. Clin Chem Lab Med 1999;37:319-326.

179. Lentz SR, Sadler JE: Inhibition of thrombomodulin surface expression and protein C activation by the thrombogenic agent homocysteine. J Clin Invest 1991;88:1906–1914.

180. Rodgers GM, Conn MT: Homocysteine, an atherogenic stimulus, reduces protein C activation by arterial and venous endothelial cells. Blood 1990;75:895–901.

181. Undas A, Williams EB, Butenas S, et al: Homocysteine inhibits inactivation of factor Va by activated protein C. J Biol Chem 2001;276:4389–4397.

182. Cattaneo M, Franchi F, Zighetti ML, et al: Plasma levels of activated protein C in healthy subjects and patients with previous venous thromboembolism: Relationships with plasma homocysteine levels. Arterioscler Thromb Vasc Biol 1998;18:1371–1375.

183. Fryer RH, Wilson BD, Gubler DB, et al: Homocysteine, a risk factor for premature vascular disease and thrombosis, induces tissue factor activity in endothelial cells. Arterioscler Thromb 1993;13:1327–1333.

184. Khajuria A, Houston DS: Induction of monocyte tissue factor expression by homocysteine: A possible mechanism for thrombosis. Blood 2000;96:966–972.

185. Nishinaga M, Ozawa T, Shimada K: Homocysteine, a thrombogenic agent, suppresses anticoagulant heparan sulfate expression in cultured porcine aortic endothelial cells. J Clin Invest 1993;92:1381–1386.

186. Hajjar KA, Mauri L, Jacovina AT, et al: Tissue plasminogen activator binding to the annexin II tail domain: Direct modulation by homocysteine. J Biol Chem 1998;273:9987–9993.

187. Yoo JH, Lee SC: Elevated levels of plasma homocyst(e)ine and asymmetric dimethylarginine in elderly patients with stroke. Atherosclerosis 2001;158:425–430.

188. Nagata K, Ishibashi T, Sakamoto T, et al: Effects of blockade of the renin-angiotensin system on tissue factor and plasminogen activator inhibitor-1 synthesis in human cultured monocytes. J Hypertens 2001;19:775–783.

189. Nishimura H, Tsuji H, Masuda H, et al: Angiotensin II increases plasminogen activator inhibitor-1 and tissue factor mRNA expression without changing that of tissue type plasminogen activator or tissue factor pathway inhibitor in cultured rat aortic endothelial cells. Thromb Haemost 1997;77:1189–1195.

190. Yoshizumi M, Tsuji H, Nishimura H, et al: Atrial natriuretic peptide inhibits the expression of tissue factor and plasminogen activator inhibitor 1 induced by angiotensin II in cultured rat aortic endothelial cells. Thromb Haemost 1998;79:631–634.

191. Yoshizumi M, Tsuji H, Nishimura H, et al: Natriuretic peptides regulate the expression of tissue factor and PAI-1 in endothelial cells. Thromb Haemost 1999;82:1497–1503.

192. Sugano T, Tsuji H, Masuda H, et al: Adrenomedullin inhibits angiotensin II-induced expression of tissue factor and plasminogen activator inhibitor-1 in cultured rat aortic endothelial cells. Arterioscler Thromb Vasc Biol 2001;21:1078–1083.

193. Muller DN, Mervaala EM, Dechend R, et al: Angiotensin II (AT(1)) receptor blockade reduces vascular tissue factor in angiotensin II-induced cardiac vasculopathy. Am J Pathol 2000;157:111–122.

194. Muller DN, Mervaala EM, Schmidt F, et al: Effect of bosentan on NF-kappaB, inflammation, and tissue factor in angiotensin II-induced end-organ damage. Hypertension 2000;36:282–290.

195. Dechend R, Homuth V, Wallukat G, et al: AT(1) receptor agonistic antibodies from preeclamptic patients cause vascular cells to express tissue factor. Circulation 2000;101:2382–2387.

196. Poon M, Hsu WC, Bogadanov VY, et al: Secretion of monocyte chemotactic activity by cultured rat aortic smooth muscle cells in response to PDGF is due predominantly to the induction of JE/MCP-1. Am J Pathol 1996;149:307–317.

197. Taubman MB, Marmur JD, Rosenfield CL, et al: Agonist-mediated tissue factor expression in cultured vascular smooth muscle cells. Role of Ca$^{2+}$ mobilization and protein kinase C activation. J Clin Invest 1993;91:547–552.

198. Ernofsson M, Siegbahn A: Platelet-derived growth factor-BB and monocyte chemotactic protein-1 induce human peripheral blood monocytes to express tissue factor. Thromb Res 1996;83:307–320.

199. Schecter AD, Giesen PL, Taby O, et al: Tissue factor expression in human arterial smooth muscle cells: TF is present in three cellular pools after growth factor stimulation. J Clin Invest 1997;100:2276–2285.

200. Camera M, Giesen PL, Fallon J, et al: Cooperation between VEGF and TNF-alpha is necessary for exposure of active tissue factor on the surface of human endothelial cells. Arterioscler Thromb Vasc Biol 1999;19:531–537.

201. Liuzzo G, Biasucci LM, Gallimore JR, et al: The prognostic value of C-reactive protein and serum amyloid a protein in severe unstable angina. N Engl J Med 1994;331:417–424.

202. Cermak J, Key NS, Bach RR, et al: C-reactive protein induces human peripheral blood monocytes to synthesize tissue factor. Blood 1993;82:513–520.

203. Pannacciulli N, De Pergola G, Giorgino F, et al: A family history of Type 2 diabetes is associated with increased plasma levels of C-reactive protein in non-smoking healthy adult women. Diabet Med 2002;19:689–692.

204. Slupsky JR, Kalbas M, Willuweit A, et al: Activated platelets induce tissue factor expression on human umbilical vein endothelial cells by ligation of CD40. Thromb Haemost 1998;80:1008–1014.

205. Miller DL, Yaron R, Yellin MJ: CD40L-CD40 interactions regulate endothelial cell surface tissue factor and thrombomodulin expression. J Leukoc Biol 1998;63:373–379.

206. Mach F, Schonbeck U, Sukhova GK, et al: Functional CD40 ligand is expressed on human vascular endothelial cells, smooth muscle cells, and macrophages: Implications for CD40-CD40 ligand signaling in atherosclerosis. Proc Natl Acad Sci USA 1997;94:1931–1936.

207. Mach F, Schonbeck U, Bonnefoy JY, et al: Activation of monocyte/macrophage functions related to acute atheroma complication by ligation of CD40: Induction of collagenase, stromelysin, and tissue factor. Circulation 1997;96:396–399.

208. Pradier O, Willems F, Abramowicz D, et al: CD40 engagement induces monocyte procoagulant activity through an interleukin-10 resistant pathway. Eur J Immunol 1996;26:3048–3054.

209. Schonbeck U, Mach F, Sukhova GK, et al: CD40 ligation induces tissue factor expression in human vascular smooth muscle cells. Am J Pathol 2000;156:7–14.

210. Heeschen C, Dimmeler S, Hamm CW, et al: Soluble CD40 ligand in acute coronary syndromes. N Engl J Med 2003;348:1104–1111.

211. Del Prete G, De Carli M, Lammel RM, et al: Th1 and Th2 T-helper cells exert opposite regulatory effects on procoagulant activity and tissue factor production by human monocytes. Blood 1995;86:250–257.

212. Osnes LT, Westvik AB, Joo GB, et al: Inhibition of IL-1 induced tissue factor (TF) synthesis and procoagulant activity (PCA) in purified human monocytes by IL-4, IL-10 and IL-13. Cytokine 1996;8:822–827.

213. Bevilacqua MP, Pober JS, Majeau GR, et al: Interleukin 1 (IL-1) induces biosynthesis and cell surface expression of procoagulant activity in human vascular endothelial cells. J Exp Med 1984;160:618–623.

214. Bevilacqua MP, Pober JS, Majeau GR, et al: Recombinant tumor necrosis factor induces procoagulant activity in cultured human vascular endothelium: Characterization and comparison with the actions of interleukin 1. Proc Natl Acad Sci USA 1986;83:4533–4537.

215. Conway EM, Bach R, Rosenberg RD, et al: Tumor necrosis factor enhances expression of tissue factor mRNA in endothelial cells. Thromb Res 1989;53:231–241.

216. Mulder AB, Hegge-Paping KS, Magielse CP, et al: Tumor necrosis factor alpha-induced endothelial tissue factor is located on the cell surface rather than in the subendothelial matrix. Blood 1994;84:1559–1566.

217. Oler A, Whooley MA, Oler J, et al: Adding heparin to aspirin reduces the incidence of myocardial infarction and death in patients with unstable angina: A meta-analysis. JAMA 1996;276:811–815.

218. Miller GJ, Bauer KA, Barzegar S, et al: Increased activation of the haemostatic system in men at high risk of fatal coronary heart disease. Thromb Haemost 1996;75:767–771.

219. Warkentin TE, Levine MN, Hirsh J, et al: Heparin-induced thrombocytopenia in patients treated with low-molecular-weight heparin or unfractionated heparin. N Engl J Med 1995;332:1330–1335.

220. Abbate R, Gori AM, Modesti PA, et al: Heparin, monocytes, and procoagulant activity. Haemostasis 1990;20(Suppl 1):98–100.

221. Lindmark E, Siegbahn A: Tissue factor regulation and cytokine expression in monocyte-endothelial cell co-cultures: Effects of a statin, an ACE-inhibitor and a low-molecular-weight heparin. Thromb Res 2002;108:77-84.

222. Hoppensteadt DA, Walenga JM, Fasanella A, et al: TFPI antigen levels in normal human volunteers after intravenous and subcutaneous administration of unfractionated heparin and a low molecular weight heparin. Thromb Res 1995;77:175-185.

223. Valentin S, Nordfang O, Bregengard C, et al: Evidence that the C-terminus of tissue factor pathway inhibitor (TFPI) is essential for its in vitro and in vivo interaction with lipoproteins. Blood Coagul Fibrinol 1993;4:713-720.

224. Valentin S, Larnkjer A, Ostergaard P, et al: Characterization of the binding between tissue factor pathway inhibitor and glycosaminoglycans. Thromb Res 1994;75:173-183.

225. Hansen JB, Sandset PM, Huseby KR, et al: Depletion of intravascular pools of tissue factor pathway inhibitor (TFPI) during repeated or continuous intravenous infusion of heparin in man. Thromb Haemost 1996;76:703-709.

226. Vila V, Martinez-Sales V, Reganon E, et al: Effects of unfractionated and low molecular weight heparins on plasma levels of hemostatic factors in patients with acute coronary syndromes. Haematologica 2001;86:729-734.

227. Eikelboom JW, Anand SS, Malmberg K, et al: Unfractionated heparin and low-molecular-weight heparin in acute coronary syndrome without ST elevation: A meta-analysis. Lancet 2000;355:1936-1942.

228. Antman EM, Cohen M, Radley D, et al: Assessment of the treatment effect of enoxaparin for unstable angina/non-Q-wave myocardial infarction. TIMI 11B-ESSENCE meta-analysis. Circulation 1999;100:1602-1608.

229. ASSENT-3: Efficacy and safety of tenecteplase in combination with enoxaparin, abciximab, or unfractionated heparin: The ASSENT-3 randomised trial in acute myocardial infarction. Lancet 2001;358:605-613.

230. Stenflo J, Fernlund P, Egan W, et al: Vitamin K dependent modifications of glutamic acid residues in prothrombin. Proc Natl Acad Sci USA 1974;71:2730-2733.

231. Nelsestuen GL, Zytkovicz TH, Howard JB: The mode of action of vitamin K. Identification of gamma-carboxyglutamic acid as a component of prothrombin. J Biol Chem 1974;249:6347-6350.

232. Prendergast FG, Mann KG: Differentiation of metal ion-induced transitions of prothrombin fragment 1. J Biol Chem 1977;252:840-850.

233. Soriano-Garcia M, Park CH, Tulinsky A, et al: Structure of $Ca^{2+}$ prothrombin fragment 1 including the conformation of the Gla domain. Biochemistry 1989;28:6805-6810.

234. Hurlen M, Abdelnoor M, Smith P, et al: Warfarin, aspirin, or both after myocardial infarction. N Engl J Med 2002;347:969-974.

235. Colli S, Eligini S, Lalli M, et al: Vastatins inhibit tissue factor in cultured human macrophages: A novel mechanism of protection against atherothrombosis. Arterioscler Thromb Vasc Biol 1997;17:265-272.

236. Eto M, Kozai T, Cosentino F, et al: Statin prevents tissue factor expression in human endothelial cells: Role of Rho/Rho-kinase and Akt pathways. Circulation 2002;105:1756-1759.

237. Wagner AH, Gebauer M, Guldenzoph B, et al: 3-hydroxy-3-methylglutaryl coenzyme A reductase-independent inhibition of CD40 expression by atorvastatin in human endothelial cells. Arterioscler Thromb Vasc Biol 2002;22:1784-1789.

238. Corti R, Fuster V, Fayad ZA, et al: Lipid lowering by simvastatin induces regression of human atherosclerotic lesions: Two years' follow-up by high-resolution noninvasive magnetic resonance imaging. Circulation 2002;106:2884-2887.

239. Zhao XQ, Yuan C, Hatsukami TS, et al: Effects of prolonged intensive lipid-lowering therapy on the characteristics of carotid atherosclerotic plaques in vivo by MRI: A case-control study. Arterioscler Thromb Vasc Biol 2001;21:1623-1629.

240. Stenestrand U, Wallentin L: Early statin treatment following acute myocardial infarction and 1-year survival. JAMA 2001;285:430-436.

241. Heeschen C, Hamm CW, Laufs U, et al: Withdrawal of statins increases event rates in patients with acute coronary syndromes. Circulation 2002;105:1446-1452.

242. Schwartz GG, Olsson AG, Ezekowitz MD, et al: Effects of atorvastatin on early recurrent ischemic events in acute coronary syndromes: The MIRACL study: A randomized controlled trial. JAMA 2001;285:1711-1718.

243. Kubo-Inoue M, Egashira K, Usui M, et al: Long-term inhibition of nitric oxide synthesis increases arterial thrombogenecity in rat carotid artery. Am J Physiol Heart Circ Physiol 2002;282:H1478-484.

244. Napoleone E, Di Santo A, Camera M, et al: Angiotensin-converting enzyme inhibitors downregulate tissue factor synthesis in monocytes. Circ Res 2000;86:139-143.

245. Soejima H, Ogawa H, Yasue H, et al: Angiotensin-converting enzyme inhibition reduces monocyte chemoattractant protein-1 and tissue factor levels in patients with myocardial infarction. J Am Coll Cardiol 1999;34:983-988.

246. Valentin S, Reutlingsperger CP, Nordfang O, et al: Inhibition of factor X activation at extracellular matrix of fibroblasts during flow conditions: A comparison between tissue factor pathway inhibitor and inactive factor VIIa. Thromb Haemost 1995;74:1478-1485.

247. Harker LA, Hanson SR, Wilcox JN, et al: Antithrombotic and antilesion benefits without hemorrhagic risks by inhibiting tissue factor pathway. Haemostasis 1996;26(Suppl 1):76-82.

248. Arnljots B, Ezban M, Hedner U: Prevention of experimental arterial thrombosis by topical administration of active site-inactivated factor VIIa. J Vasc Surg 1997;25:341-346.

249. Golino P, Ragni M, Cirillo P, et al: Antithrombotic effects of recombinant human, active site-blocked factor VIIa in a rabbit model of recurrent arterial thrombosis. Circ Res 1998;82:39-46.

250. Jang Y, Guzman LA, Lincoff AM, et al: Influence of blockade at specific levels of the coagulation cascade on restenosis in a rabbit atherosclerotic femoral artery injury model. Circulation 1995;92:3041-3050.

251. Courtman DW, Schwartz SM, Hart CE: Sequential injury of the rabbit abdominal aorta induces intramural coagulation and luminal narrowing independent of intimal mass: Extrinsic pathway inhibition eliminates luminal narrowing. Circ Res 1998;82:996-1006.

252. Lev EI, Marmur JD, Zdravkovic M, et al: Antithrombotic effect of tissue factor inhibition by inactivated factor VIIa: An ex vivo human study. Arterioscler Thromb Vasc Biol 2002;22:1036-1041.

253. Jang IK, Gold HK, Leinbach RC, et al: Antithrombotic effect of a monoclonal antibody against tissue factor in a rabbit model of platelet-mediated arterial thrombosis. Arterioscler Thromb 1992;12:948-954.

254. Pawashe AB, Golino P, Ambrosio G, et al: A monoclonal antibody against rabbit tissue factor inhibits thrombus formation in stenotic injured rabbit carotid arteries. Circ Res 1994;74:56-63.

255. Ragni M, Cirillo P, Pascucci I, et al: Monoclonal antibody against tissue factor shortens tissue plasminogen activator lysis time and prevents reocclusion in a rabbit model of carotid artery thrombosis. Circulation 1996;93:1913-1918.

256. Erlich JH, Boyle EM, Labriola J, et al: Inhibition of the tissue factor-thrombin pathway limits infarct size after myocardial ischemia-reperfusion injury by reducing inflammation. Am J Pathol 2000;157:1849-1862.

257. Presta L, Sims P, Meng YG, et al: Generation of a humanized, high affinity anti-tissue factor antibody for use as a novel antithrombotic therapeutic. Thromb Haemost 2001;85:379-389.

258. Kelley RF, Refino CJ, O'Connell MP, et al: A soluble tissue factor mutant is a selective anticoagulant and antithrombotic agent. Blood 1997;89:3219-3227.

259. Himber J, Refino CJ, Burcklen L, et al: Inhibition of arterial thrombosis by a soluble tissue factor mutant and active site-blocked factors IXa and Xa in the guinea pig. Thromb Haemost 2001;85:475-481.

260. Yang J, Lee GF, Riederer MA, et al: Enhancing the anticoagulant potency of soluble tissue factor mutants by increasing their affinity to factor VIIa. Thromb Haemost 2002;87:450-458.

261. Abendschein DR, Meng YY, Torr-Brown S, et al: Maintenance of coronary patency after fibrinolysis with tissue factor pathway inhibitor. Circulation 1995;92:944-949.

262. Haskel EJ, Torr SR, Day KC, et al: Prevention of arterial reocclusion after thrombolysis with recombinant lipoprotein-associated coagulation inhibitor. Circulation 1991;84:821-827.

263. Lefkovits J, Malycky JL, Rao JS, et al: Selective inhibition of factor Xa is more efficient than factor VIIa-tissue factor complex block-

ade at facilitating coronary thrombolysis in the canine model. J Am Coll Cardiol 1996;28:1858-1865.

264. Abraham E, Reinhart K, Svoboda P, et al: Assessment of the safety of recombinant tissue factor pathway inhibitor in patients with severe sepsis: A multicenter, randomized, placebo-controlled, single-blind, dose escalation study. Crit Care Med 2001;29:2081-2089.

265. Stassens P, Bergum PW, Gansemans Y, et al: Anticoagulant repertoire of the hookworm Ancylostoma caninum. Proc Natl Acad Sci USA 1996;93:2149-2154.

266. Lee A, Agnelli G, Buller H, et al: Dose-response study of recombinant factor VIIa/tissue factor inhibitor recombinant nematode anticoagulant protein c2 in prevention of postoperative venous thromboembolism in patients undergoing total knee replacement. Circulation 2001;104:74-78.

267. Vlasuk GP, Rote WE: Inhibition of factor VIIa/tissue factor with nematode anticoagulant protein c2. From unique mechanism to a promising new clinical anticoagulant. Trends Cardiovasc Med 2002;12:325-331.

268. Benedict CR, Ryan J, Wolitzky B, et al: Active site-blocked factor IXa prevents intravascular thrombus formation in the coronary vasculature without inhibiting extravascular coagulation in a canine thrombosis model. J Clin Invest 1991;88:1760-1765.

269. Wong AG, Gunn AC, Ku P, et al: Relative efficacy of active site-blocked factors IXa, Xa in models of rabbit venous and arteriovenous thrombosis. Thromb Haemost 1997;77:1143-1147.

270. Kirchhofer D, Tschopp TB, Baumgartner HR: Active site-blocked factors VIIa and IXa differentially inhibit fibrin formation in a human ex vivo thrombosis model. Arterioscler Thromb Vasc Biol 1995;15:1098-1106.

271. Spanier TB, Oz MC, Madigan JD, et al: Selective anticoagulation with active site blocked factor IXa in synthetic patch vascular repair results in decreased blood loss and operative time. ASAIO J 1997;43:M526-30.

272. Spanier TB, Chen JM, Oz MC, et al: Selective anticoagulation with active site-blocked factor IXA suggests separate roles for intrinsic and extrinsic coagulation pathways in cardiopulmonary bypass. J Thorac Cardiovasc Surg 1998;116:860-869.

273. Spanier TB, Oz MC, Minanov OP, et al: Heparinless cardiopulmonary bypass with active-site blocked factor IXa: A preliminary study on the dog. J Thorac Cardiovasc Surg 1998;115:1179-1188.

274. Tuszynski GP, Gasic TB, Gasic GJ: Isolation and characterization of antistasin: An inhibitor of metastasis and coagulation. J Biol Chem 1987;262:9718-9723.

275. Hauptmann J, Sturzebecher J: Synthetic inhibitors of thrombin and factor Xa: From bench to bedside. Thromb Res 1999;93:203-241.

276. Eriksson BI, Bauer KA, Lassen MR, et al: Fondaparinux compared with enoxaparin for the prevention of venous thromboembolism after hip-fracture surgery. N Engl J Med 2001;345:1298-1304.

277. Lassen MR, Bauer KA, Eriksson BI, et al: Postoperative fondaparinux versus preoperative enoxaparin for prevention of venous thromboembolism in elective hip-replacement surgery: A randomised double-blind comparison. Lancet 2002;359:1715-1720.

278. Bauer KA, Eriksson BI, Lassen MR, et al: Fondaparinux compared with enoxaparin for the prevention of venous thromboembolism after elective major knee surgery. N Engl J Med 2001;345:1305-1310.

279. Turpie AG, Bauer KA, Eriksson BI, et al: Fondaparinux vs enoxaparin for the prevention of venous thromboembolism in major orthopedic surgery: A meta-analysis of 4 randomized double-blind studies. Arch Intern Med 2002;162:1833-1840.

280. Coussement PK, Bassand JP, Convens C, et al: A synthetic factor-Xa inhibitor (ORG31540/SR9017A) as an adjunct to fibrinolysis in acute myocardial infarction: The PENTALYSE study. Eur Heart J 2001;22:1716-1724.

281. Dyke CK, Becker RC, Kleiman NS, et al: First experience with direct factor Xa inhibition in patients with stable coronary disease: A pharmacokinetic and pharmacodynamic evaluation. Circulation 2002;105:2385-2391.

282. Abendschein DR, Baum PK, Verhallen P, et al: A novel synthetic inhibitor of factor Xa decreases early reocclusion and improves 24-h patency after coronary fibrinolysis in dogs. J Pharmacol Exp Ther 2001;296:567-572.

283. GUSTOIIa: Randomized trial of intravenous heparin versus recombinant hirudin for acute coronary syndromes. The Global Use of Strategies to Open Occluded Coronary Arteries (GUSTO) IIa Investigators. Circulation 1994;90:1631-1637.

284. Eikelboom JW, French J: Management of patients with acute coronary syndromes: What is the clinical role of direct thrombin inhibitors? Drugs 2002;62:1839-1852.

285. Kottke-Marchant K, Bahit MC, Granger CB, et al: Effect of hirudin vs heparin on haemostatic activity in patients with acute coronary syndromes: the GUSTO-IIb haemostasis substudy. Eur Heart J 2002;23:1202-1212.

286. White H: Thrombin-specific anticoagulation with bivalirudin versus heparin in patients receiving fibrinolytic therapy for acute myocardial infarction: The HERO-2 randomised trial. Lancet 2001;358:1855-1863.

287. Mehta SR, Eikelboom JW, Rupprecht HJ, et al: Efficacy of hirudin in reducing cardiovascular events in patients with acute coronary syndrome undergoing early percutaneous coronary intervention. Eur Heart J 2002;23:117-123.

288. Hauptmann J: Pharmacokinetics of an emerging new class of anticoagulant/antithrombotic drugs: A review of small-molecule thrombin inhibitors. Eur J Clin Pharmacol 2002;57:751-758.

289. Heit JA, Colwell CW, Francis CW, et al: Comparison of the oral direct thrombin inhibitor ximelagatran with enoxaparin as prophylaxis against venous thromboembolism after total knee replacement: A phase 2 dose-finding study. Arch Intern Med 2001;161:2215-2221.

290. Glynn O: The express study: Preliminary results. Int J Clin Pract 2003;57:57-59.

# chapter 29

# Thrombosis and Thrombolytic Therapy

*H.R. Lijnen*
*H. Pannekoek*
*J. Vermylen*

Integrity of the vascular wall is a prerequisite for normal functioning blood vessels and for the maintenance of a nonthrombotic state. When the continuity of the vascular endothelium is disrupted, platelets and fibrin seal off the defect, and the fibrinolytic system then dissolves the blood clot. The endothelial cells, which form a monolayer lining the inner surface of blood vessels, synthesize and release activators and inhibitors of platelet aggregation, blood coagulation, and fibrinolysis and, thus, play an active role in the regulation of these systems by providing both procoagulant and anticoagulant substances.

Blood coagulation has classically been divided into an extrinsic and an intrinsic pathway. This model, although valuable for laboratory diagnosis of coagulation abnormalities, has now been revised.[1] The main basis for this revision was the discovery of tissue factor pathway inhibitor (TFPI) and the finding that fXI can be activated by thrombin. In the current model, the extrinsic Xase reaction initiates coagulation. Once critical amounts of fXa (required for the initiation of thrombin generation) are formed, the extrinsic Xase reaction is efficiently turned off by TFPI, and further formation of thrombin is maintained via positive feedback mechanisms involving thrombin-induced activation of fV, fVIII, and fXI. Excess thrombin is efficiently inhibited by its physiologic inhibitor antithrombin and downregulates its own generation via stimulation of the protein C pathway (Fig. 29-1). Some of the properties of procoagulant and anticoagulant molecules are summarized in Table 29-1.

The fibrinolytic system plays an important role in the dissolution of blood clots and in the maintenance of a patent vascular system. The fibrinolytic system (Fig. 29-2) comprises an inactive proenzyme plasminogen that can be converted to the active enzyme plasmin, which degrades fibrin into soluble fibrin degradation products. Two immunologically distinct physiologic plasminogen activators have been identified in blood: t-PA and urokinase-type plasminogen activator (u-PA). Inhibition of the fibrinolytic system may occur either at the level of the plasminogen activators, by specific plasminogen activator inhibitors (PAI-1 and PAI-2), or at the level of plasmin, mainly by $\alpha_2$-antiplasmin. Some of the main properties of the components of the fibrinolytic system are summarized in Table 29-2. Plasminogen activation mediated by t-PA is primarily involved in the dissolution of fibrin in the circulation.[2] Enhanced activation of cell-bound plasminogen results when u-PA binds to a specific cellular receptor (u-PAR). The main role of u-PA appears to be in the induction of pericellular proteolysis.[3] The physiologic relevance of the fibrinolytic system is inferred from the associations between impaired fibrinolysis and thrombosis and between excessive fibrinolysis and bleeding. This chapter deals with molecular mechanisms contributing to thrombosis and with current concepts of thrombolytic therapy.

## BIOCHEMICAL PROPERITES OF COMPONENTS OF THE FIBRINOLYTIC SYSTEMF

### Plasminogen

Human plasminogen is a single-chain glycoprotein with $M_r$ of 92,000, which is present in plasma at a concentration of 1.5 to 2 μM. It consists of 791 amino acids and contains five homologous triple-loop structures or "kringles."[4] These kringles contain lysine-binding sites and aminohexyl-binding sites, which mediate the specific binding of plasminogen to fibrin and the interaction of plasmin with $\alpha_2$-antiplasmin and, thereby, play a crucial role in the regulation of fibrinolysis.[5]

Native plasminogen, with $NH_2$-terminal glutamic acid (Glu-plasminogen), is converted by limited plasmic digestion of the Arg68-Met69, Lys77-Lys78, or Lys78-Val79 peptide bonds to modified forms, designated Lys-plasminogen. Plasminogen is converted to plasmin by cleavage of the Arg561-Val562 peptide bond.[6] The plasmin molecule is a two-chain trypsin-like serine proteinase with an active site composed of His603, Asp646, and Ser741.[4]

### Tissue-Type Plasminogen Activator (t-PA)

Human t-PA was first isolated as a single-chain serine proteinase with $M_r$ of 70,000, consisting of 527 amino acids with Ser as the $NH_2$-terminal amino acid (Fig. 29-3).[7] It was subsequently shown that native t-PA contains an $NH_2$-terminal extension of three amino acids, but in general the initial numbering system has been maintained. The plasma concentration of t-PA antigen is about 5 ng/mL, whereas the concentration of free t-PA is probably less than 1 ng/mL. Limited plasmic hydrolysis of the Arg275-Ile276 peptide bond converts t-PA to a

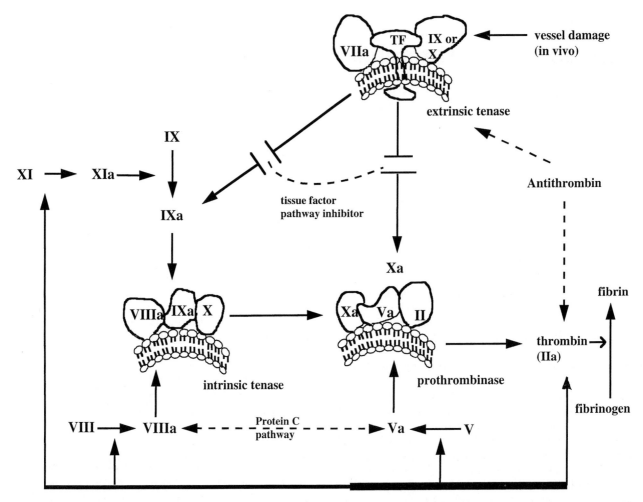

**FIGURE 29-1.** Simplified scheme of procoagulant and anticoagulant pathways of coagulation. On vascular injury, blood coagulation is initiated by the extrinsic Xase reaction. Once critical amounts of fXa (required for the initiation of coagulation) are generated, the extrinsic Xase reaction is efficiently turned off by TFPI and probably by antithrombin; further formation of thrombin is maintained via positive feedback mechanisms involving thrombin-induced activation of fV, fVIII, and fXI. Thrombin is efficiently inhibited by its physiologic inhibitor antithrombin and downregulates its own generation via stimulation of the protein C pathway. *(From Lijnen HR, Arnout J, Collen D: Vascular endothelial cell function and thrombosis. In Willerson JT, Cohn JN (eds): Cardiovascular Medicine, 2nd ed. Philadelphia, Churchill Livingstone, 2000.)*

two-chain molecule held together by one interchain disulfide bond. The t-PA molecule contains four domains: (1) an NH₂-terminal region of 47 residues (residues 4 to 50) (F-domain), which is homologous with the finger domains mediating the fibrin affinity of fibronectin; (2) residues 50 to 87 (E-domain), which are homologous with epidermal growth factor; (3) two regions comprising residues 87 to 176 and 176 to 262 (K₁ and K₂ domains), which share a high degree of homology with the five kringles of plasminogen; and (4) a serine proteinase domain (P, residues 276 to 527) with the active site residues His322, Asp371 and Ser478.[7] The t-PA molecule comprises three potential N-glycosylation sites, at Asn117 (K₁), Asn184 (K₂), and Asn448 (P). In contrast to the single-chain precursor form of most serine proteinases, single-chain t-PA is enzymatically active. Lys156 appears to contribute directly to the enzymatic activity of single-chain t-PA, by forming a salt bridge with Asp194 that selectively stabilizes the active conformation.[8,9]

## Urokinase-Type Plasminogen Activator (u-PA)

The urokinase-type plasminogen activator is secreted as a single-chain serine proteinase of 411 amino acids, with active-site triad His204, Asp255, and Ser356 [single-chain urokinase (scu)-PA, pro-urokinase].[10] It contains an NH₂-terminal growth factor domain and one kringle structure homologous to the five kringles found in plasminogen and the two kringles in t-PA.[11] It contains only one N-glycosylation site (at Asn302) and contains a fucosylated threonine residue at position 18. Conversion of scu-PA to two-chain urokinase (tcu)-PA occurs after proteolytic cleavage at position Lys158-Ile159 by plasmin but also occurs by kallikrein, trypsin, cathepsin B, human T-cell-associated serine proteinase-1, and thermolysin. A fully active tcu-PA derivative is obtained after additional proteolysis by plasmin at position Lys135-Lys136. A low molecular weight form of scu-PA (32 kd) can be obtained by selective cleavage at position Glu143-Leu144.[12] In contrast, scu-PA is converted to an inactive two-chain

**TABLE 29-1    OVERVIEW OF THE MAIN PROCOAGULANT AND ANTICOAGULANT PROTEINS WITH SOME OF THEIR PROPERTIES**

| | Function or Main Substrate of the Active Form | $M_r$ (kD) | Chain Composition | Plasma Concentration (μg/mL) | $T\{1/2\}$ (hr) | DOMAINS | | | | |
|---|---|---|---|---|---|---|---|---|---|---|
| | | | | | | Gla | EGF | Kringle | Catalytic | Other |
| *Zymogens* | | | | | | | | | | |
| Prothrombin | Fibrinogen, factor XIII | 72 | sc, 581 AA | 100 | 72 | 10 AA | None | 2 | Ser proteinase | |
| Factor VII | Factor X, factor IX | 50 | sc, 406 AA | 0.5 | 5 | 10 AA | 2 | None | Ser proteinase | |
| Factor X | Prothrombin | 59 | tc, 254 AA, 139 AA | 8 | 32 | 11 AA | 2 | None | Ser proteinase | |
| Factor IX | Factor X | 56 | sc, 415 AA | 5 | 24 | 12 AA | 2 | None | Ser proteinase | |
| Factor XI | Factor IX | 160 | tc, 607 AA each | 5 | 72 | None | None | None | Ser proteinase | |
| Factor XII | Factor XI | 80 | sc, 596 AA | 30 | 60 | None | 2 | 1 | Ser proteinase | |
| Protein C | Factor Va, factor VIIIa | 62 | tc, 262 AA, 155 AA | 3–5 | 7 | 9 AA | 2 | None | Ser proteinase | |
| *Cofactors* | | | | | | | | | | |
| Tissue factor | Extrinsic Xase cofactor | 45 | sc, 263 AA | Cell-bound | — | None | None | None | — | Two barrel-like structures; Transmembrane module; Cytoplasmic tail |
| Factor V | Prothrombinase cofactor | 330 | sc, 2196 AA | 7–10 | 12 | None | None | None | — | A1,A2,B,A3,C1,C2 |
| Factor VIII | Intrinsic Xase cofactor | 280 | tc, 1313 AA, 684 AA | 0.2 | 12 | None | None | None | — | A1,A2,B,A3,C1,C2 |
| Protein S | Cofactor for activated Protein C | 75 | sc, 635 AA | 20 | 42 | 11 AA | 4 | None | — | Sex hormone-binding globulin-like module |
| Thrombomodulin | Cofactor for protein C activation | 60 | sc, 557 AA | Cell-bound | — | None | 6 | None | — | Lectin-like module; Hydrophobic region; Transmembrane module; Cytoplasmic tail |
| *Inhibitors* | | | | | | | | | | |
| Antithrombin | Inhibitor of thrombin and factor Xa | 58 | sc, 432 AA | 125 | 48 | None | None | None | — | |
| Tissue factor Pathway inhibitor | Inhibitor of extrinsic tenase and factor Xa | 42 | sc, 276 AA | 0.1 | — | — | — | — | — | Kunitz domains 1, 2, and 3 |

AA, number of amino acids; sc, single chain; tc, two chain.
From Lijnen HR, Arnout J, Collen D: Vascular endothelial cell function and thrombosis. In Willerson JT, Cohn JN (eds): Cardiovascular Medicine, 2nd ed. Philadelphia, Churchill Livingstone, 2000, p 1317.

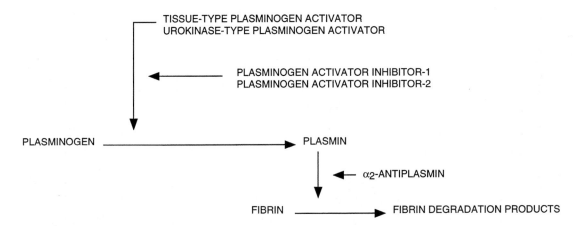

**FIGURE 29-2.** Schematic representation of the fibrinolytic system. The zymogen plasminogen is converted to the active serine proteinase plasmin, which degrades fibrin into soluble degradation products by t-PA or u-PA. Inhibition may occur at the level of plasminogen activators by PAI-1 or PAI-2 or at the level of plasmin mainly by $\alpha_2$-antiplasmin.

### TABLE 29-2    BIOCHEMICAL PROPERTIES OF THE MAIN COMPONENTS OF THE FIBRINOLYTIC SYSTEM

| | $M_r$ (kD) | Carbohydrate Content (%) | Amino Acids (n) | Catalytic Triad or Reactive Site | Plasma Concentration (mg/L) |
|---|---|---|---|---|---|
| Plasminogen | 92 | 2 | 791 | His603, Asp646, Ser741 | 200 |
| Plasmin | 85 | 2 | ±715 | His603, Asp646, Ser741 | — |
| t-PA | 68 | 7 | 527 | His322, Asp371, Ser478 | 0.005 |
| scu-PA | 54 | 7 | 411 | His204, Asp255, Ser356 | 0.008 |
| $\alpha_2$-Antiplasmin | 67 | 13 | 452 (464) | Arg364-Met365 | 70 |
| PAI-1 | 52 | ND | 379 | Arg346-Met347 | 0.05 |
| PAI-2 | 47 | ND | 393 | Arg358-Thr359 | <0.005 |

ND, not determined; PAI-1, plasminogen activator inhibitor-1; PAI-2, plasminogen activator inhibitor-2; scu-PA, single-chain urokinase-type plasminogen activator (prourokinase); t-PA, tissue-type plasminogen activator.
Modified from Collen D, Lijnen HR: Fibrinolysis and the control of hemostasis. In Stamatoyannopoulos G, Nienhuis AW, Majerus PW, Varmus H (eds): Molecular Basis of Blood Diseases, 2nd ed. Philadelphia, WB Saunders, 1993, p 725.

molecule by thrombin after proteolytic cleavage at position Arg156-Phe157. This inactivation is strongly enhanced in the presence of thrombomodulin and is dependent on the 0-linked glycosaminoglycan of thrombomodulin.[13]

## Alpha$_2$-Antiplasmin

$\alpha_2$-Antiplasmin is the main physiologic plasmin inhibitor in human plasma, whereas plasmin formed in excess of $\alpha_2$-antiplasmin may be neutralized by $\alpha_2$-macroglobulin. $\alpha_2$-Antiplasmin, a $M_r$ 67,000 single-chain glycoprotein containing 464 amino acids and 13% carbohydrate, is present in plasma at a concentration of about 1 $\mu$M. The reactive site of the inhibitor is the Arg376-Met377 peptide bond. $\alpha_2$-Antiplasmin is unique among serpins (serine proteinase inhibitors) by having a COOH-terminal extension of 51 amino acid residues.[14] This extension contains a secondary binding site that reacts with the lysine-binding sites of plasminogen and plasmin. The plasminogen-binding form of $\alpha_2$-antiplasmin becomes partly converted in the circulating blood to a nonplasminogen binding, less reactive form (about 30% of the total), which lacks the 26 COOH-terminal residues.[15] Two forms of $\alpha_2$-antiplasmin were detected in about equal amounts in purified preparations of the inhibitor: a native 464 residues long inhibitor with NH$_2$-terminal methionine and a shorter form (12 amino acids less) with NH$_2$-terminal asparagine.[16] It is not known whether the latter is present in the circulating blood or whether it is generated *in vitro*. The NH$_2$-terminal Gln14-residue of $\alpha_2$-antiplasmin can crosslink to A$\alpha$ chains of fibrin in a process that requires Ca$^{2+}$ and that is catalyzed by activated fXIII.[17]

## Plasminogen Activator Inhibitor-1

Rapid inhibition of both t-PA and u-PA in normal human plasma occurs primarily by PAI-1.[18] In healthy individuals, highly variable plasma levels of both PAI activity and PAI-1 antigen have been observed. PAI activity ranges from 0.5 to 47 U/mL (t-PA neutralizing units, 1 mg active PAI-1 corresponds to 700,000 units) with 80% of the values less than 6 U/mL. PAI-1 antigen ranges between 6 and 85 ng/mL (geometric mean: 24 ng/mL). PAI-1 levels are strongly elevated in several thromboembolic disease states (see later). PAI-1 is a single-chain glycoprotein with $M_r$ of about 52,000 and consisting of 379 amino acids. It is a member of the serpin family with a reactive site peptide bond Arg346-Met347.[19-22]

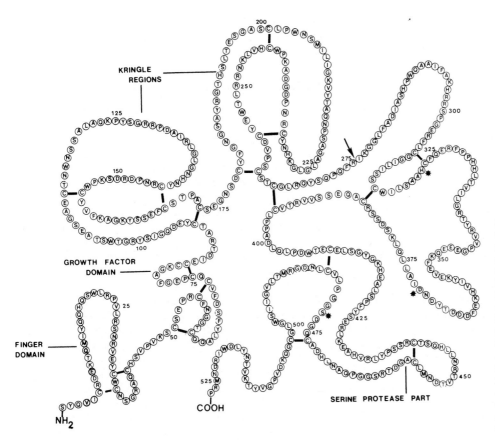

**FIGURE 29-3.** Schematic representation of the primary structure of t-PA. The amino acids are represented by their single letter symbols, and black bars indicate disulfide bonds. The active site residues His322, Asp371, and Ser478 are indicated with an asterisk. The arrow indicates the plasmin cleavage site for conversion of single-chain t-PA to two-chain t-PA. *(From Collen D, Lijnen HR: Fibrinolysis and the control of fibrinolysis. In Stamatoyannopoulos G, Nienhuis HW, Majerus PW, Varmus H (eds): Molecular Basis of Blood Diseases, 2nd edition. Philadelphia, WB Saunders, 1993.)*

PAI-1 is stabilized by binding to S-protein or vitronectin.[23] The PAI-1 binding motif is localized at residues 12 to 30 of the somatomedin B domain of vitronectin; this motif is anchored in the active conformation by disulfide bonds.[24] In the presence of vitronectin, PAI-1 displays a 200-fold accelerated thrombin inhibition, which may result from a conformational effect of vitronectin binding on the reactive site loop of PAI-1.[25,26] As a result of its high-affinity binding to vitronectin, PAI-1 may play a role in cell adhesion and migration by competing with u-PA receptor- or integrin-dependent binding of cells to the extracellular matrix.

## Plasminogen Activator Inhibitor-2 (PAI-2)

PAI-2 is a serpin of 393 amino acids with reactive site peptide bond Arg358-Thr359. PAI-2 levels in plasma are very low, but they are drastically elevated during pregnancy.[27] PAI-2 exists in two different forms with comparable inhibitory properties that are derived from a single mRNA: an intracellular nonglycosylated form with $M_r$ 47,000 and pI 5.0 and a secreted glycosylated form with $M_r$ 60,000 and pI 4.4. PAI-2 extracted from placenta is essentially nonglycosylated, whereas circulating PAI-2 observed during pregnancy is glycosylated. The function of intracellular PAI-2 is unclear because its main target enzyme (u-PA) is found extracellularly. It may constitute a storage pool from which PAI-2 can be secreted on cell injury.[28] The precise physiologic and pathophysiologic roles of PAI-2 remain to be determined. PAI-2 inhibits two-chain u-PA about 10-fold slower than PAI-1 does. It also efficiently inhibits two-chain t-PA, less efficiently inhibits single-chain t-PA, and does not inhibit single-chain u-PA.

## REGULATION OF PHYSIOLOGIC FIBRINOLYSIS

The fibrinolytic system is regulated by controlled activation and inhibition. Activation of plasminogen by t-PA is enhanced in the presence of fibrin or at the endothelial cell surface. Inhibition of fibrinolysis occurs at the level of plasminogen activation or at the level of plasmin. Fibrinolysis may also be regulated as a result of increased or decreased synthesis and/or secretion of t-PA and of PAI-1, primarily from the vessel wall. The mechanisms involved in synthesis and secretion of t-PA and PAI-1 have been reviewed elsewhere.[29] Molecular mechanisms involved in the regulation of physiologic fibrinolysis are discussed later.

## Inhibition of Plasmin by α₂-Antiplasmin

α₂-Antiplasmin forms an inactive 1:1 stoichiometric complex with plasmin. The inhibition of plasmin (P) by α₂-antiplasmin (A) can be represented by two consecutive reactions: a fast, second-order reaction producing a reversible inactive complex (PA), which is followed by a slower first-order transition resulting in an irreversible complex (PA′). This model can be represented by: P + A ⇔ PA → PA′. The second-order rate constant of inhibition is very high (2 to $4 \times 10^7$ M$^{-1}$s$^{-1}$), but this high inhibition rate is dependent on the presence of a free lysine-binding site and active site in the plasmin molecule and on the availability of a plasminogen-binding site and reactive site peptide bond in the inhibitor.[30,31] The half-life of plasmin molecules on the fibrin surface, which have both their lysine-binding sites and active sites occupied, is estimated to be two to three orders of magnitude longer than that of free plasmin.[31]

## Clearance of Plasminogen Activators

Cellular receptors play a role in the rapid clearance of t-PA from the circulation. Circulating t-PA (half-life of 5 to 6 minutes in humans) may interact with several receptor systems in the liver. Liver endothelial cells have a mannose receptor that recognizes the high mannose-type carbohydrate antenna on $K_1$, whereas parenchymal cells contain a calcium-dependent receptor that interacts with the F-and/or E-domains of t-PA.[32] Parenchymal cells also contain a high-affinity receptor for the uptake and degradation of t-PA/PAI-1 complexes, which also binds free t-PA albeit with lower affinity; this receptor, termed LDL receptor-related protein (LRP), is identical to the $\alpha_2$-macroglobulin receptor.[33] The domains involved in rapid clearance of u-PA (half-life of about 6 minutes in humans) are within the 32-kd u-PA moiety and are independent of glycosylation.[34]

## Inhibition of Plasminogen Activators by PAI-1

PAI-1 reacts very rapidly with single-chain and two-chain t-PA and with two-chain u-PA, with second-order inhibition rate constants on the order of $10^7$ M$^{-1}$s$^{-1}$, and it does not react with scu-PA.[35,36] Like other serpins, PAI-1 inhibits its target proteinases by formation of a 1:1 stoichiometric reversible complex, followed by covalent binding between the hydroxyl group of the active site serine residue of the proteinase and the carboxyl group of the P1 residue at the reactive center ("bait region") of the serpin. The rapid inhibition of both t-PA and u-PA by PAI-1 involves a reversible high-affinity second-site interaction, which does not depend on a functional active site.[37] Residues 350 to 355 of PAI-1, which contain three negatively charged amino acids, interact with highly positively charged regions in t-PA (residues 296 to 304)[38] or in u-PA (residues 179 to 184).[39]

PAI-1 occurs as an active inhibitory form that spontaneously converts to a latent form that can be partially reactivated by denaturing agents.[40] The latency of PAI-1 is due to insertion of part of the reactive center loop in the major β-sheet of PAI-1, which is thereby not accessible to the target enzyme. Reactivation of latent PAI-1 by denaturants results from partial elimination of this insertion.[41] Another molecular form of intact PAI-1 has been isolated that does not form stable complexes with t-PA but is cleaved at the P1-P1′ peptide bond ("substrate PAI-1").[42] The x-ray structure of the cleaved substrate variant shows that it has a new β-strand (s4A) formed by insertion of the NH$_2$-terminal portion of the reactive site loop into β-sheet A subsequent to cleavage.[43] Thus, inhibitory PAI-1 may not only convert to

latent PAI-1, which can be reactivated, but also convert to substrate PAI-1, which is irreversibly degraded by its target proteinases.

## Plasminogen Activation by t-PA

In the absence of fibrin, t-PA is a poor enzyme, but the presence of fibrin strikingly enhances the activation rate of plasminogen. Kinetic data supports a mechanism in which fibrin provides a surface to which t-PA and plasminogen adsorb in a sequential and ordered way yielding a cyclic ternary complex.[44] Plasminogen binding to fibrin involves the lysine-binding sites in the kringle structures, whereas binding of t-PA to fibrin is mediated via the finger and kringle 2 domains. Formation of this complex results in an enhanced affinity of t-PA for plasminogen, yielding up to three orders of magnitude higher efficiencies for plasminogen activation. Plasmin formed at the fibrin surface has both its lysine-binding sites and active site occupied and is, thus, only slowly inactivated by $\alpha_2$-antiplasmin (half-life of about 10 to 100 seconds); in contrast, free plasmin, when formed, is rapidly inhibited by $\alpha_2$-antiplasmin (half-life of about 0.1 second).[31] In agreement with this mechanism, the increase in stimulation by fibrin after formation of fibrin X-polymers is associated with an enhanced binding of t-PA and plasminogen. This increased and altered binding of both enzyme and substrate to fibrin is mediated in part by COOH-terminal lysine residues generated by plasmin cleavage. Interaction of these COOH-terminal lysines with lysine-binding sites on t-PA and plasminogen may allow an improved alignment and allosteric changes of the t-PA and plasminogen moieties, thus enhancing the rate of plasminogen activation.[45]

Consequently, proteins that remove COOH-terminal lysine residues from the fibrin surface, such as the thrombin activatable fibrinolysis inhibitor (TAFI) may have an antifibrinolytic action. TAFI is a $M_r$ 60,000 single-chain protein, identical to plasma procarboxypeptidase B, that occurs at a concentration of 75 nM.[46-48] Thrombin, trypsin, or plasmin convert the protein to an active carboxypeptidase B.

## Plasminogen Activation by u-PA

In contrast to tcu-PA, scu-PA displays very low activity toward low molecular weight chromogenic substrates, but it appears to have some intrinsic plasminogen activating potential, which represents 0.5% or less of the catalytic efficiency of tcu-PA.[49,50] Other investigators, however, have claimed that scu-PA has no measurable intrinsic amidolytic or plasminogen activator activities.[51] The occurrence of a transitional state of scu-PA with a higher catalytic efficiency for native plasminogen than tcu-PA has also been postulated.[52] A charge interaction between Ile159 and Asp355 was shown to be the primary force stabilizing the active conformation of tcu-PA and determining the intrinsic catalytic activity of scu-PA.[53] In plasma, in the absence of fibrin, scu-PA is stable and does not activate plasminogen; in the presence of a fibrin clot, scu-PA, but not tcu-PA, induces fibrin-specific clot lysis.[49] Although scu-PA does not bind to a significant extent to fibrin, its intrinsic activity toward fibrin-bound plasminogen may contribute to its fibrin specificity. In addition, plasma $\alpha_2$-antiplasmin prevents conversion of scu-PA to tcu-PA outside the clot and, thus, preserves fibrin specificity.[54] Fibrin fragment E-2 selectively promotes the activation of plasminogen by scu-PA, mainly by enhancing the catalytic rate constant of the activation.[55] Although scu-PA is an inefficient activator of plasminogen bound to internal lysine residues on intact fibrin, it has a higher activity toward plasminogen bound to newly generated COOH-terminal lysine residues on partially degraded fibrin.[56] Thus, the fibrin-specificity of scu-PA does not require its conversion to tcu-PA but is mediated by enhanced binding of plasminogen to partially digested fibrin.[57]

## RELATIONSHIP BETWEEN DEFECTIVE FIBRINOLYSIS AND THROMBOSIS

The physiologic importance of the fibrinolytic system is demonstrated by the association between abnormal fibrinolysis and a tendency toward bleeding or thrombosis. Excessive fibrinolysis resulting from increased levels of t-PA, or to $\alpha_2$-antiplasmin or PAI-1 deficiency, may result in a bleeding tendency.[58] Impairment of fibrinolysis represents a commonly observed hemostatic abnormality associated with thrombosis. It may be due to a defective synthesis and/or release of t-PA from the vessel wall, to a deficiency or functional defect in the plasminogen molecule, or to increased levels of inhibitors of t-PA or plasmin. The relationships between defective fibrinolysis and thrombosis are discussed later.

## Plasminogen Activator Inhibitor-1 and Thrombosis

Increased levels of plasma PAI-1 have been associated with thrombosis. This has been inferred from follow-up studies of men who survived an acute myocardial infarction before the age of 45.[59,60] These studies indicated that a high PAI-1 activity is independently related to a reinfarction within 3 years of the primary event. However, to unambiguously establish PAI-1 as a risk factor in the epidemiologic sense, its relationship to myocardial infarction and angina pectoris should be demonstrated in prospective studies with healthy individuals. So far, only a prospective multicenter analysis of patients suffering from angina pectoris, the European Concerted Action on Thrombosis and Disabilities (ECAT) study, has been performed, which showed that higher baseline concentrations of PAI-1 are associated with an increased incidence of cardiovascular events.[61] However, the association was insignificant after adjustment for parameters reflecting insulin resistance.[62] From these clinical studies one may conclude that the relevance of PAI-1 as an independent risk factor in myocardial infarction, angina pectoris, and arterial and venous thromboembolism remains controversial.

Studies with transgenic mice, overexpressing human PAI-1, indicate that an excess of PAI-1 causes thrombosis.[63] These mice transiently developed necrotic tail tips and swollen hind legs, because of venous occlusions. These observations are explained by the occurrence of thrombosis as a result of hypofibrinolysis.

## Plasminogen Activator Deficiency and Thrombosis

A deficient fibrinolytic response may be caused by a deficient release of t-PA from the vessel wall and also by an increased rate of neutralization.[64,65] Defective release of t-PA from the vessel wall during venous occlusion and/or a decreased t-PA content in walls of superficial veins is found in about 70% of patients with idiopathic recurrent venous thrombosis.[66]

To date, genetic deficiencies of t-PA or u-PA have not been reported in humans. Thus, inactivation of the t-PA or u-PA genes in mice might have been anticipated to result in a lethal phenotype. However, single- and double-deficient mice are normal at birth, suggesting that neither t-PA nor u-PA, individually or in combination, is required for normal embryonic development.[67] The role of plasminogen activators in clearing fibrin deposits is confirmed by the observation that t-PA-deficient and t-PA:u-PA-deficient mice have virtually no endogenous spontaneous thrombolytic potential and that u-PA-deficient and t-PA:u-PA-deficient mice suffer occasional or extensive spontaneous fibrin deposition, respectively.[67]

## Plasminogen Deficiency and Thrombosis

In the few patients with plasminogen deficiency (activity and antigen levels between 30% and 50% of normal) that have been reported, recurrent thrombotic events were observed.[58,68] A correlation between the plasminogen deficiency and the occurrence of thrombosis is, however, not always obvious. Acquired plasminogen deficiencies, with activity levels between 25% and 45% of normal, as a result of reduced hepatic synthesis or of increased consumption, have been observed in patients with liver disease and sepsis. Abnormalities in the plasminogen molecule (dysplasminogenemia) resulting in defective conversion to plasmin have been described in a small number of patients.[58,68] In some cases, a normal antigen level but impaired activity has been explained by a single amino acid substitution near the active site residues.[69] The propositus was always identified after thrombotic complications, whereas other family members with the same dysplasminogenemia often were not affected. In other cases of dysplasminogenemia, observed in males with a history of recurrent deep venous thrombosis, the abnormality consists in an activation defect as a result of different catalytic efficiencies for activation of plasminogen to plasmin.[58]

Homozygous plasminogen deficiency has recently been described in patients with ligneous conjunctivitis, a rare and unusual form of chronic pseudomembranous conjunctivitis caused by massive fibrin deposition within the extravascular space of mucous membranes.[70] In several patients a homozygous point mutation was identified as a probable cause of the deficiency.[71,72] Replacement therapy with Lys-plasminogen was found to be successful.[72] The finding that plasminogen-deficient mice also develop ligneous conjunctivitis supports a causal role of plasminogen in the disease.[73]

Two independent studies have shown that disruption of the plasminogen gene in mice causes a severe thrombotic phenotype but is compatible with development and reproduction.[74,75] Homozygous plasminogen-deficient mice display a greatly reduced spontaneous lysis of pulmonary plasma clots, and young animals develop multiple spontaneous thrombotic lesions.[74,75] Restoration of normal plasminogen levels in these mice by bolus administration of plasminogen resulted in normalization of the thrombolytic potential toward experimentally induced pulmonary emboli and in removal of endogenous fibrin deposits in the liver, thus establishing conclusively that in vivo fibrin dissolution is critically dependent on the plasminogen-plasmin system.[76] Interestingly, removal of fibrin or fibrinogen from the extracellular environment (mice with combined deficiency of plasminogen and fibrinogen) alleviates the diverse spontaneous pathologies associated with plasminogen deficiency.[77]

## Dysfibrinogenemia and Thrombosis

In most cases, dysfibrinogenemia is clinically asymptomatic, whereas in a small number of families it is associated with thrombosis.[78] This thrombotic tendency may be explained by disturbed interactions of plasminogen and/or t-PA with fibrin or fibrinogen at several levels. In fibrinogen New York I (deletion of amino acids 9 to 72 of the Bβ chain), stimulation of plasminogen activation by t-PA in the presence of fibrin was impaired, apparently because of reduced binding of t-PA to fibrin.[79] In fibrinogen Dusard, abnormal fibrin monomer polymerization resulted in decreased binding of plasminogen and reduced capacity of fibrin to stimulate plasminogen activation by t-PA.[80,81] These cases of dysfibrinogenemia, thus, confirm the physiologic relevance of the model for plasminogen activation by t-PA in the presence of fibrin, which was discussed previously. Interference with the ternary complex formation between fibrin, t-PA, and plasminogen resulting from decreased fibrin binding of either the substrate or the enzyme may result in defective fibrinolysis and cause thrombotic complications. Alternatively, cases of dysfibrinogenemia were reported in patients with recurrent venous thrombosis associated with formation of extremely rigid fibrin gels, which are resistant to degradation by plasmin.[82] A comprehensive overview of the relationships between dysfibrinogenemia and thrombosis was recently published.[83] An index with more than 200 molecular abnormalities of fibrinogen is available on the Internet (http://www.geht.org/pages/database_ang.html).

## RELATIONSHIP BETWEEN ENHANCED FIBRINOLYSIS AND BLEEDING

## Plasminogen Activator Inhibitor-1 Deficiency and Bleeding

Hyperfibrinolysis resulting from deficiency of PAI-1 has been reported in a 9-year-old girl with a moderate bleed-

ing tendency and subsequently for a large number of her family members, spanning different generations.[84,85] The deficiency is caused by a homozygous frameshift within the PAI-1 gene, resulting in a premature stop codon and presumably a truncated PAI-1 protein. These individuals exhibit no developmental abnormalities and suffer from excessive bleeding only on trauma or surgery, supporting the notion that PAI-1 primarily serves to regulate fibrinolysis.

This conclusion is also drawn from studies using homozygous PAI-1 deficient mice.[86] Analogous to the patients described previously, PAI-1 deficiency in mice also has no effect on viability, fertility, and development. These animals exhibit no overt bleeding tendency but show a faster lysis of pulmonary clots and develop venous thrombi less often after endotoxin administration than their wild-type counterparts.[87] Collectively, these studies provide support for the notion that PAI-1 is a major regulator of fibrinolysis in mice and humans. Its absence causes a bleeding tendency in humans, in contrast to mice that do not display spontaneous bleeding.

## $\alpha_2$-Antiplasmin Deficiency and Bleeding

The first case of congenital homozygous $\alpha_2$-antiplasmin deficiency was described in a patient who presented with a hemorrhagic diathesis.[88] Several cases of heterozygosity have been described with no or only mild bleeding symptoms.[58] The $\alpha_2$-antiplasmin levels in all heterozygotes described thus far are consistently between 40% and 60% of normal. Antigen and activity levels usually correspond well, suggesting that the deficiency is due to decreased synthesis of a normal $\alpha_2$-antiplasmin molecule. The bleeding tendency in these patients may be due to premature lysis of hemostatic plugs, because in the absence of $\alpha_2$-antiplasmin, the half-life of plasmin molecules generated on the fibrin surface may be considerably prolonged.

The molecular defect in $\alpha_2$-antiplasmin Okinawa was identified as a trinucleotide deletion in exon 7 leading to deletion of Glu137 in the protein.[89] $\alpha_2$-Antiplasmin Nara insertion of a cytidine nucleotide in exon 10 leads to a shift in the reading frame of the mRNA, resulting in deletion of the COOH-terminal 12 amino acids of native $\alpha_2$-antiplasmin and replacement with 178 unrelated amino acids.[90] These mutations may lead to the deficiency by affecting the folding of the protein into the native configuration and thereby blocking its intracellular transport from the endoplasmic reticulum to the Golgi complex.[89]

Acquired $\alpha_2$-antiplasmin deficiency associated with enhanced fibrinolysis has been reported in some conditions, including liver disease,[91] disseminated intravascular coagulation and/or fibrinolysis, and acute promyelocytic leukemia.[92] $\alpha_2$-Antiplasmin levels may be significantly reduced in patients undergoing thrombolytic therapy, as a result of systemic activation of the fibrinolytic system.[93]

A dysfunctional $\alpha_2$-antiplasmin molecule ($\alpha_2$-antiplasmin Enschede), associated with a serious bleeding tendency, has been found in two siblings in a Dutch family. The ability of the protein to bind reversibly to plasminogen was not affected, but it was converted from an inhibitor of plasmin into a substrate. The molecular defect of $\alpha_2$-antiplasmin Enschede consists of the insertion of an extra alanine residue (GCG insertion) somewhere between amino acid residues 365 and 359 (four Ala residues), 7 to 10 positions on the $NH_2$-terminal side of the P1 residue (Arg376) in the reactive site of $\alpha_2$-antiplasmin.[94]

## Enhanced Plasminogen Activator Activity and Bleeding

Excessive fibrinolysis resulting from increased t-PA activity levels may be associated with a bleeding tendency, but life-long hemorrhagic disorders, resulting from increased levels of circulating plasminogen activator, have been described in only a few patients.[95,96]

## THE CELLULAR BASIS OF THROMBOSIS

A thrombus consists of cellular elements (platelets, leukocytes, and red cells) held together by fibrin. This section discusses how activated platelets and leukocytes act in concert to form the fibrin network that protects the thrombus from disruption by flow.

## Blood Coagulation as a Surface-Catalyzed Process

With the exception of fibrinogen, the clotting factors are trace proteins that must be concentrated on a surface for efficient interactions. The main physiologic catalytic surface is a layer of phospholipid containing negatively charged phospholipids such as phosphatidylserine. Phosphatidylserine normally is sequestered in the inner leaflet of a cellular phospholipid bilayer. On activation of cells, particularly platelets, phospholipid scrambling occurs.[97] Cell surface-exposed phosphatidylserine following scrambling serves as a ligand for the vitamin K-dependent coagulation factors and for fV and fVIII. The vitamin K-dependent coagulation factors are prothrombin, fVII, fIX, and fX. Glutamic acid (glu) residues at the aminoterminal ends of these proteins are carboxylated to gammacarboxyglutamic acid (gla) residues in a vitamin K-dependent reaction.[98] This gla-domain anchors these proenzymes to the negatively charged phospholipid membrane in a $Ca^{2+}$-dependent manner. Factors V and VIII are protein cofactors that facilitate the interaction of the vitamin K-dependent (pro)enzymes. Their sequence contains six sequential domains arranged in the order $A_1$-$A_2$-B-$A_3$-$C_1$-$C_2$. They bind to phospholipid through the $C_2$ domain by the burial of hydrophobic residues within the phospholipid bilayer; these hydrophobic residues are surrounded by positively charged residues that interact with the negatively charged phospholipid head groups.[99] Factor V(a) is secreted from the alpha granules of activated platelets and binds with high affinity to the phospholipid surface. Factor VIII is concentrated on activated platelets via its carrier protein, von Willebrand factor.[100] The latter, submitted to shear stress, binds to activated platelets

through their membrane GP Ib/IX/V and GP IIb/IIIa complexes.[101] Finally, the proenzyme fXI also binds to the platelet GP Ib/IX/V complex.[102]

## The Origin of Intravascular Tissue Factor

On adhesion to and spreading on collagen, activated platelets assemble on their surface a number of proenzymes and protein cofactors that could interact efficiently through lateral diffusion on the phospholipid surface. What triggers their interaction? It is now generally accepted that the physiologic trigger of blood coagulation is tissue factor.[103] Tissue factor is an integral membrane protein that is normally present on the surface of most cells outside the vasculature.[104] Vascular injury results in exposure of tissue factor to the blood. It, therefore, is clear that tissue-factor-initiated coagulation limits the extravasation of blood from a transected vessel.

How can tissue factor contribute to thrombus formation within a vessel? Endothelial cells can be induced to express tissue factor in vitro, but whether this phenomenon occurs in pathologic conditions in vivo is doubtful.[105] Atheromatous plaques are rich in tissue factor, which mainly originates from macrophages.[106] However, recent work by Hathcock and Nemerson[107] indicates that platelets adhering to the ruptured plaque effectively prevent contact between the plaque tissue factor and the blood. Previously, this group made the following striking observation: when native human blood is allowed to flow over a glass coverslip at high shear, platelets adhere to the coverslip and tissue factor containing microparticles adhere to the platelet layer; the adherent tissue factor is biologically active, as evidenced by fibrin formation.[108] Until that moment, tissue factor had essentially been located extravascularly; now blood-borne tissue factor has emerged. In further work, the same group showed that monocytes and possibly polymorphonuclear leukocytes are the source of the tissue-factor-positive microparticles, which are transferred to the adhering platelets.[109] The membrane of platelet $\alpha$ granules contains P-selectin (CD62P).[110] In activated platelets, the $\alpha$ granule membranes fuse with the plasma membrane, which becomes decorated with P-selectin. Surface P-selectin then can interact with CD15 (a leukocyte membrane-bound carbohydrate known as sialyl Lewis X) or with P-selectin glycoprotein ligand-1,[111] also on leukocytes. This interaction results in conjugate formation between activated platelets and leukocytes or leukocyte microparticles. The origin of the leukocyte microparticles requires further study: Are they circulating physiologically and looking for activated platelets (or activated endothelial cells) to land on? Or are they remnants of reversible interactions between a layer of activated platelets and leukocytes flowing over this layer?

Under normal conditions, most cell-surface tissue factor is encrypted, which means that the tissue factor binds fVIIa but is not capable of initiating coagulation. Encrypted tissue factor allows circulating tissue-factor-positive monocytes to be present in the circulation without generalized coagulation ensuing.[112] However, when the phospholipids in the monocyte plasma membrane are scrambled by calcium ionophore, which would allow binding of clotting factors as described previously, tissue factor becomes de-encrypted and coagulation ensues.[113] The transfer of tissue-factor-positive microparticles to the surface of a spread platelet that has bound clotting factors, therefore, allows fibrin formation to take place.

## The Process of Coagulation and Thrombus Formation

The process of coagulation can be separated into an initiation phase and a propagation phase. Tissue factor is a transmembrane protein cofactor not an enzyme. Blood always contains small amounts of fVIIa. Tissue factor binds both fVII and fVIIa and promotes the autocatalytic activation of fVII. This reaction requires that the tissue factor-fVIIa and tissue factor-fVII complexes encounter each other by lateral diffusion in the plane of the membrane.[114] Tissue factor-fVIIa on cells activates both fX and fIX.[115] Factor X activation is responsible for the initiation phase. Factor Xa activates prothrombin on the phospholipid surface with fV provided by the platelet $\alpha$ granules as surface-bound cofactor. The cleavage of prothrombin is sequential. In the first stage, meizothrombin is generated[116]; this active enzyme remains attached to the phospholipid surface. Subsequent removal of fragments including the gla-domain of prothrombin results in soluble thrombin, which diffuses away from the catalytic phospholipid surface.

Both meizothrombin and thrombin are responsible for the propagation phase of blood coagulation. Meizothrombin, by lateral diffusion on the phospholipid surface, effectively activates fV[117] and fXI.[118] Thrombin causes further platelet activation and dissociates fVIII from von Willebrand factor and activates it.[119] Activated fVIII binds to the phospholipid surface through its $C_2$ domain. Factor VIIIa is a protein cofactor for fIXa; it is required for the propagation phase induced by fIXa. The propagation phase consists of a new burst of fX activation by the fIXa-fVIIIa complex; this in turn leads to an explosive generation of thrombin. Factor IX is activated not only by tissue factor-fVIIa but also by fXIa; this explains why some patients with fXI deficiency have a bleeding tendency.[120]

At the site of adherent platelets, additional platelets accumulate while the coagulation process is ongoing. These platelets are attracted and activated by products released by the adhering platelets, such as ADP, synthesized by the activated platelet, such as thromboxane $A_2$, or generated on the surface of the activated platelet, such as thrombin. The activated platelets are held together by protein bridges consisting of fibrinogen or von Willebrand factor. These proteins are anchored on the GP IIb/IIIa complexes of adjacent activated platelets. Thrombin escaping from the platelet surface rapidly converts fibrinogen into fibrin threads. The platelet thrombus is, thus, captured within a fibrin network.

The colocalization of platelets, blood-borne tissue factor, and fibrin in blood flowing over an *ex vivo* surface has recently been visualized in real time.[121] Furie et al.[122] used intravital confocal microscopy of the microcirculation of living mice to study thrombosis induced by laser injury. Colocalization of platelets, leukocytes, and fibrin was observed. Their preliminary experiments have shown that thrombus formation is significantly reduced in mice either deficient in P-selectin or in P-selectin glycoprotein ligand-1.

## Stasis and Thrombus Development

The previous section describes the formation of a thrombus when blood flows over exposed collagen, to which platelets adhere, spread, and become activated. This process indicates how a thrombus forms in a damaged vessel. Can it also explain thrombus formation induced by stasis, for instance in a fibrillating left atrium? Kawasaki et al.[123] studied fibrin formation within the mouse common carotid artery that had simply been ligated proximal to the bifurcation, thereby resulting in a column of stagnant blood. After 1 day, platelet-leukocyte conjugates started to line the endothelium. They were associated with the appearance of tissue-factor-positive fibrin deposits. This intravascular fibrin formed the structure used for the invasion of the lumen by vessel wall cells. Neointima formation was reduced in mice in which the platelet count or the fibrinogen level had been lowered or in which the fVIII gene was deficient; it was enhanced in mice in which the u-PA gene was deficient. This model had originally been developed by Kumar and Lindner.[124] They showed that P-selectin gene deficiency in this model leads to dramatic reduction in lesion thickness.[125] Therefore, it is possible that in areas of stasis mutual activation of platelets and leukocytes occurs[126] and that cellular conjugates form involving P-selectin. These conjugates bind clotting factors, express tissue factor, and provide a nidus for thrombin formation. In view of the presence of stasis, thrombin is not rapidly diluted or swept away; as a result, a fibrin-rich thrombus forms. This process may be responsible for thrombus development in a fibrillating left atrium or in the veins of an immobilized limb.

## Pharmacologic Interference with Thrombosis

In 1992, Palabrica et al.[127] noted that leukocyte accumulation promotes fibrin deposition, that it is mediated *in vivo* by P-selectin on adherent platelets, and that an anti-P-selectin antibody inhibits the deposition of fibrin within a thrombus. If platelet-leukocyte interaction via P-selectin is the cellular basis for intravascular thrombus formation, then inhibition of P-selectin function seems an attractive therapeutic strategy, which currently is actively pursued. Either anti-P-selectin antibodies[127,128] or recombinant soluble P-selectin glycoprotein ligand 1[129] are being evaluated. In primate models, pretreatment with a blocking monoclonal antibody to P-selectin accelerated pharmacologic thrombolysis of arterial thrombosis[130] or reduced stasis-induced venous thrombosis.[128] Recombinant PSGL-Ig has also been shown to accelerate thrombolysis and prevent reocclusion in a porcine model[131] or to inhibit stasis-induced venous thrombosis.[132,133]

Antithrombotic agents include substances impeding thrombin generation and action (the anticoagulants), aspirin that irreversibly blocks the synthesis of thromboxane $A_2$ by platelets, and ticlopidine and clopidogrel that block platelet activation by ADP through the $P_2Y_{12}$ receptor.[134] All these agents have shown activity in long-term prevention of thrombosis. Short-term administration of anti-GP IIb/IIIa drugs, usually in combination with aspirin and heparin, markedly improves the outcome in patients undergoing percutaneous coronary interventions or suffering from acute coronary syndromes.[135] The results of long-term secondary prevention trials with oral GP IIb/IIIa antagonists were, however, unexpected and perplexing. In a meta-analysis of phase III multicenter randomized studies, Chew et al.[136] found a significantly increased rather than a decreased mortality with oral platelet GP IIb/IIIa antagonists. Although this observation is unexplained, a possible hint may be given by the *in vitro* observations of Li et al.[126] When platelets are activated with collagen in hirudinized whole blood in the presence of a GP IIb/IIIa antagonist, more platelet-leukocyte conjugates are formed. Presumably because of the inhibition of platelet-platelet aggregation by GP IIb/IIIa antagonists, more activated platelets would be available for heterotypic conjugation with leukocytes. Such platelet-leukocyte conjugates not only express tissue factor activity, as discussed previously, but also facilitate the adhesion of leukocytes to the vessel wall in areas of high shear stress.[137] They, therefore, may enhance inflammation in atherosclerotic plaques and thereby promote plaque destabilization. If such mechanisms also operate *in vivo*, they may help to explain the striking therapeutic paradox with GP IIb/IIIa antagonists.

# THROMBOPHILIA

Thrombophilia refers to a tendency to develop thrombosis. More specifically, it relates to hematologic disorders that predispose to thrombosis. Atrial fibrillation, for instance, is not considered under the heading of thrombophilia.

Hematologic disorders that predispose to thrombosis are classified as inherited or acquired, although sometimes it is not possible to decide whether the abnormality is hereditary. Elevated levels of fVIII, for instance, predispose to venous thrombosis[138]; a genetic basis for such rise has not been found.

## Inherited Thrombophilia

### Antithrombin Deficiency

The first thrombophilic state to be described was congenital antithrombin deficiency, found in 1965 in a Norwegian family.[139] Affected patients were heterozygotes, with antithrombin activities of approximately 50%. Antithrombin is a proteinase inhibitor that not only blocks thrombin but also fXa and other clotting enzymes. Antithrombin is a slow inhibitor *in vitro*. Its efficiency is increased more than 1000-fold following binding to heparan-containing proteoglycans on healthy endothelium or following injection of heparin as

a anticoagulant. Heparan and heparins induce a conformational change in antithrombin that allows efficient interaction with the target proteinase. Antithrombin complexed to endothelial cell proteoglycan is a first example of mechanisms that protect healthy endothelium against extension of thrombosis. Congenital antithrombin deficiency is rare and is found in about 1% of consecutive patients with a history of thrombosis.[140]

### Protein C-Protein S System

The protein C-protein S pathway is another example of how healthy endothelium protects itself against thrombosis. Healthy endothelium carries a transmembrane thrombin-binding protein called thrombomodulin. Thrombomodulin binds thrombin; thrombin then loses its procoagulant properties. It no longer can cleave fibrinogen or activate fV, fVIII, or platelets; instead, thrombin becomes an anticoagulant by selectively activating protein C.[141] Protein C is a vitamin K-dependent proenzyme; it has a gla-domain and effectively binds to negatively charged phospholipid. As mentioned in the previous section, healthy cells, including endothelium, do not expose phosphatidylserine. However, endothelial cells have a specific protein C receptor, allowing reversible binding of protein C to normal endothelium.[142] Once activated by thrombin, activated protein C would translocate to the phosphatidylserine-containing phospholipid bilayers where the complexes fIXa-fVIIIa and fXa-fVa, leading to thrombin generation, are assembled. Activated protein C cleaves and inactivates the cofactors fVIIIa and fVa, thereby turning down further thrombin generation. To efficiently cleave these cofactors within the complexes, activated protein C requires a cofactor, protein S.[143] Protein S also is a vitamin K-dependent protein that binds to phosphatidylserine-containing surfaces through its gla-domain, but it is not an enzyme.[144] Factor Va is inactivated in part by cleavage at Arg506. The protein C-protein S pathway again illustrates how extension of thrombin generation into a healthy vessel, distant from vascular damage, is prevented.

Mutations in thrombomodulin or in the endothelial cell protein C receptor have not yet been clearly associated with thrombosis. On the other hand, heterozygous protein C and protein S deficiencies have definitely been linked to thrombophilia.[145,146] However, one should remember that thrombophilia refers to a tendency to develop thrombosis. Not all persons with heterozygous protein C deficiency actually develop thrombosis; this was elegantly stressed by the population study of Miletich et al.[147] The prevalence of heterozygous protein C or protein S deficiency in consecutive patients with a history of thrombosis is 3.2% and 2.2%, respectively,[140] whereas the prevalence of heterozygous protein C deficiency in the general population is 0.3%. On the other hand, homozygous protein C or S deficiency presents with purpura fulminans in the neonate, because of widespread thrombosis in cutaneous vessels and skin necrosis.[148]

In 1993, Dahlbäck et al.[149] linked familial thrombosis to insufficient prolongation of clotting times following addition of activated protein C to plasma. A year later, Bertina et al.[150] showed that this resistance to activated protein C is due to substitution of Arg506 for Glu in fV. This mutation has been called the fV Leiden mutation. Its prevalence in consecutive patients with a history of thrombosis is 21%.[151]

### Prothrombin

In 1996, Poort et al.[152] described a G-to-A substitution in the 3′ untranslated portion of the prothrombin gene, which is associated with an increased risk to develop venous thrombosis; the prevalence of this substitution in consecutive patients with a history of thrombosis is 6.2%. The only phenotypic manifestation is a moderate increase in the plasma concentration of prothrombin (to 130%); presumably this could lead to enhanced thrombin generation.

These various inherited thrombophilic states, leading to enhanced local thrombin activity, are mainly associated with venous thrombosis. Presumably, a high local thrombin concentration is more important for the development of a fibrin-rich thrombus than for the growth of a platelet-rich thrombus. These thrombophilic states are also associated with an increased frequency of fetal loss, linked to thrombotic complications within the placental circulation.[153,154]

The high frequency of the fV Leiden and prothrombin mutations in the general white population, 4.8% and 2.7%, respectively,[155] accounts for the fact that patients occasionally suffer from combined defects; the resulting thrombotic risk is considerably enhanced.[156,157] The risk is also increased by nongenetic factors such as the use of oral contraceptives.[158]

### Hyperhomocysteinemia

Hyperhomocysteinemia is a risk factor for thrombosis and can be either inherited or acquired. A rare example of excessive hyperhomocysteinemia is homozygous homocystinuria resulting from cystathionine β-synthase deficiency; 50% of affected individuals present with venous or arterial thrombosis by the age of 29 years.[159] Homozygosity for the C677T mutation in the methylenetetrahydrofolate reductase gene is a cause of mild hyperhomocysteinemia in 5% to 15% of white populations, but its relation to venous thrombosis is controversial.[160] Hyperhomocysteinemia is also a consequence of folic acid, vitamin $B_{12}$, or vitamin $B_6$ deficiency; of hypothyroidism; or of renal failure. Hyperhomocysteinemia has been suggested to interfere with normal endothelial function; induction of tissue factor activity[161] or inhibition of protein C activation[162] have been suggested as pathogenetic mechanisms that would explain thrombosis.

## Acquired Thrombophilia

### Heparin-induced Thrombocytopenia

Among acquired causes of thrombophilia, much interest has recently been provoked by antibody-mediated thrombosis.[163] Heparin-induced thrombocytopenia and thrombosis is the best studied.[164] In patients treated with heparin for more than 5 days, an abrupt fall of the platelet count may occur, which then often is associated with massive thrombosis. Remarkably, arterial thrombosis mainly occurs when heparin is given for an arterial problem (e.g., following arterial surgery), and venous thrombosis occurs when heparin is administered to prevent or treat venous thromboembolism. It has become obvious that the antibody that is elicited in this condition is not directed against heparin as such but against the complex of heparin with PF4.[165] PF4 is a very basic protein that is stored in platelet α granules and is released on platelet activation. PF4 has a binding site on the platelet surface. It also binds to the highly acidic heparin glycosaminoglycan chain. The PF4-glycosaminoglycan complex is immunogenic. This complex binds to the platelet surface via the PF4 binding site; antibodies to this complex also bind on the platelet surface. When attached to the complex by their $F(ab)_2$ part, the antibodies engage the Fc receptor on the platelet membrane FcγRIIa (CD32) through their Fc part. Engagement leads to tyrosine phosphorylation of the cytoplasmic tail of FcγRIIa, resulting in a cascade of signaling processes, platelet aggregation, platelet secretion, exposure of P-selectin on the platelet surface, and the release of microparticles. Activated platelets and platelet microparticles exposing P-selectin form platelet-leukocyte aggregates,[166] which are highly thrombogenic, as discussed in the previous section. Released PF4 also binds to heparan-containing proteoglycans on the surface of endothelial cells[167]; antibody can bind to those complexes, presumably followed by complement activation. Activated complement leads to endothelial damage, including cell lysis or retraction, exposing subendothelial collagen and von Willebrand factor. In addition, the activated endothelial cells secrete the contents of their Weibel-Palade bodies, leading to surface expression of von Willebrand factor and P-selectin, resulting in platelet and leukocyte adhesion and fibrin formation. From this description it is obvious how the antibody amplifies an incipient thrombotic process that releases PF4. This explains how heparin-induced thrombocytopenia is linked to arterial thrombosis following arterial damage and to venous thrombosis following venous irritation.

### Antiphospholipid Syndrome

The antiphospholipid syndrome is another acquired thrombophilic state that resembles heparin-induced thrombocytopenia and thrombosis.[168] It consists of recurrent arterial and/or venous thrombosis (recurrent fetal loss occurs in women) associated with the presence of anticardiolipin antibodies and/or the lupus anticoagulant. These antibodies were originally considered to interact directly with negatively charged phospholipid. Anticardiolipin antibodies were subsequently shown not to bind to cardiolipin directly but to the serum protein $β_2$-glycoprotein I, which binds cardiolipin. Likewise, the immunoglobins with lupus anticoagulant properties do not bind directly to the coagulation-promoting phospholipid phosphatidylserine but bind to $β_2$-glycoprotein I or prothrombin on the negatively charged phospholipid surface. $\beta_2$-Glycoprotein I has a weak affinity for coagulant phospholipids, but the affinity increases markedly when two $\beta_2$-glycoprotein I molecules are linked by bivalent antibody.[169] In *in vitro* clotting tests, the phospholipid catalytic surface is occupied by these complexes; these impede the assembly of clotting factors on this surface and, therefore, act as an anticoagulant. How can an antibody that is anticoagulant *in vitro* becomes procoagulant *in vivo*? It has been proposed that the antibody may interfere with physiologic antithrombotic mechanisms, such as with generation of antiaggregant prostacyclin in response to injury,[170] with the inactivation of fVa or fVIIIa by the protein Ca-protein S complex on the phospholipid surface,[171,172] or with the activity of annexin V, a vascular protein with high affinity for phosphatidylserine.[173] By binding to phosphatidylserine, annexin V prevents its interaction with coagulation factors and thus is a potent anticoagulant *in vitro*. Vermylen et al.[163] have suggested that these antibodies are procoagulant *in vivo* in the same manner as the antibodies in heparin-induced thrombocytopenia. In the patient, both $\beta_2$-glycoprotein I or prothrombin and low affinity antibodies to $\beta_2$-glycoprotein I or prothrombin are simultaneously present in blood. The levels of $\beta_2$-glycoprotein I and of prothrombin are usually (but not always) normal in the antiphospholipid syndrome. When platelets are activated locally, negatively charged phospholipid appears. Positive cooperation results in deposition of $\beta_2$-glycoprotein I- or prothrombin-antibody complexes on the platelet surface; the complexes would engage the FcyRIIa, and platelet aggregation, microparticle formation, P-selectin exposure, leukocyte-platelet conjugation, thrombin generation, and thrombosis ensue. Therefore, the antibody would markedly amplify an incipient thrombotic process.

### Antibodies to Protein S

Children recovering from varicella can occasionally develop severe protein S deficiency because of the appearance of IgG and IgM antibodies to protein S; they present with a clinical picture of purpura fulminans and laboratory results indicating disseminated intravascular coagulation. The disease often is complicated by impaired perfusion of limbs and digits, resulting in amputations; the hardly detectable protein S levels fail to respond to infusions of fresh frozen plasma, implying accelerated clearance of the infused protein by immune complex formation. Within 3 months, the antibodies to protein S disappeared in the five patients studied by Levin et al.[174]; decline of the anti-protein S IgG antibody was associated with normalization of the plasma protein S levels and recovery.

### Acquired Thrombophilia Not Related to Antibodies

Acquired thrombophilia not related to antibodies includes paroxysmal nocturnal hemoglobinuria and malignancy. Paroxysmal nocturnal hemoglobinuria is an acquired clonal hematopoietic stem cell disorder. It is characterized by hemolysis that is caused by complement activation, an associated predisposition to bone marrow failure, and a predilection to thrombosis. The red cell vulnerability to lysis stems from absent complement-regulatory proteins CD59 and decay accelerating factor.[175] The pathogenesis of the thrombotic tendency in paroxysmal nocturnal hemoglobinuria may be related to complement-induced vesiculation, exposure of phosphatidylserine, and assembly of clotting factors on the platelet membrane.[176] Elevated levels of circulating procoagulant microparticles have been observed in patients with paroxysmal nocturnal hemoglobinuria.[177]

The association between thrombosis and malignancy dates to 1865, when Trousseau[178] recognized the occurrence of deep venous thrombosis in patients with visceral cancer, especially in patients with gastric malignancy. Many tumors express tissue factor,[179] and some express an enzyme directly activating fX.[180] Furthermore, tumor cells or microparticles derived from tumor cells often present with exposed phosphatidylserine, allowing assembly of coagulation factors on their surface.[181]

## THROMBOLYTIC THERAPY

### Current Thrombolytic Therapy

Acute myocardial infarction and ischemic stroke are two main causes of death and disability in Western societies. The modern era of thrombolytic therapy started around 1980 with the demonstration by De Wood et al.[182] that myocardial infarction in its early stage was invariably associated with thrombotic coronary artery occlusion and the demonstration by Rentrop et al.[183] that infusion of streptokinase within the infarct-related coronary artery early after symptom onset induced rapid recanalization. At present, several thrombolytic agents are either approved or under clinical investigation, including streptokinase; recombinant tissue-type plasminogen activator (rt-PA or alteplase); rt-PA derivatives such as reteplase, lanoteplase, and tenecteplase; anisoylated plasminogen-streptokinase activator complex (APSAC or anistreplase); tcu-PA (urokinase); recombinant scu-PA (pro-u-PA, or prourokinase); and recombinant staphylokinase and derivatives. Fibrin-selective agents (rt-PA and derivatives, staphylokinase and derivatives, and to a lesser extent scu-PA) that digest the clot in the absence of systemic plasminogen activation are distinguished from non-fibrin-selective agents (streptokinase, tcu-PA, and APSAC) that activate systemic and fibrin-bound plasminogen relatively indiscriminately (Fig. 29-4). Non-fibrin-selective agents are less efficient for clot dissolution and cause a systemic generation of plasmin, depletion of $\alpha_2$-antiplasmin, and degradation of coagulation factors, which, however, protect against reocclusion of the infarct-related artery.[2] In contrast, fibrin-selective agents require conjunctive use of heparin anticoagulation, as established in several mechanistic studies in experimental animals and patients[184] and confirmed by meta-analysis of mortality in more than 100,000 patients.[185]

The beneficial effects of thrombolytic therapy in acute myocardial infarction have been well established in placebo-controlled clinical trials, and thrombolytic

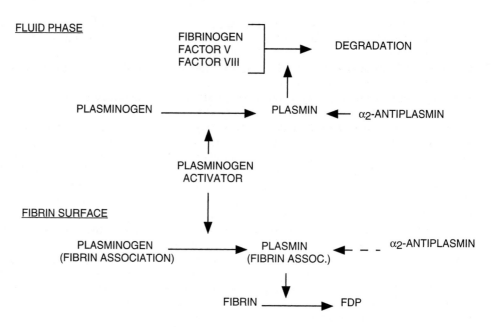

**FIGURE 29-4.** Schematic representation of the concept of fibrin selectivity. Non-fibrin-selective plasminogen activators (e.g., streptokinase, urokinase, APSAC) activate both plasminogen in the fluid phase and fibrin-associated plasminogen relatively indiscriminately. Systemic plasminogen activation leads to exhaustion of the substrate (reduced thrombolytic efficacy) and depletion of $\alpha_2$-antiplasmin (systemic fibrinolytic state with fibrinogen break-down). Fibrin-specific plasminogen activators (t-PA, scu-PA, staphylokinase) preferentially activate fibrin-associated plasminogen. Fibrin-selective agents preserve plasminogen and spare fibrinogen.

therapy has become routine treatment. It is given to more than 750,000 patients per year worldwide, and at least three times that number could potentially benefit from this treatment. The current indications and contraindications to thrombolytic therapy in patients with acute myocardial infarction have been reviewed elsewhere.[186,187]

Initially two coronary patency studies (TIMI-1 and ECSG-1) supported the higher efficacy of fibrin-selective rt-PA over non-fibrin-selective streptokinase. Similar results were obtained in several mechanistic trials of the TIMI, ECSG, and TAMI organizations.[188] However, two subsequent megatrials (GISSI-2 and ISIS-3) could not confirm that this translated into a mortality benefit. Unfortunately, these latter two studies omitted the required conjunctive use of heparin anticoagulation. Finally, the Global Utilization of Streptokinase and rt-PA for Occluded coronary arteries (GUSTO) trial[189] and its angiographic substudy[190] revisited the "open artery hypothesis" and conclusively demonstrated that brisk (TIMI 3 flow), early, and persistent coronary artery recanalization is the primary determinant of clinical benefit.[191] A follow-up analysis of the GUSTO results revealed that the difference in mortality persisted after 1 year[192] and that patients who were at higher risk derived a greater absolute benefit from treatment with rt-PA with intravenous heparin than with streptokinase.[193] The beneficial effect of fibrin selectivity with respect to bleeding is less convincing. Although stroke-free survival was significantly higher with alteplase than with streptokinase, the rate of intracranial hemorrhage was also slightly but significantly higher.

All these available thrombolytic agents suffer significant shortcomings including large therapeutic doses, limited efficacy, reocclusion, and bleeding complications. Thus, rt-PA, the most effective agent presently available, produces functional recanalization of the occluded coronary artery in approximately 55% of patients; recanalization requires 45 minutes or more. Reocclusion occurs in

5% to 10%, and cerebral bleeding occurs in 0.5% to 1.0% of patients. Therefore, there is a need for more efficient and safe thrombolytic agents and regimens.

## Toward Improved Thrombolytic Therapy

Thrombolytic therapy could be improved by earlier and accelerated treatment to reduce the duration of ischemia; by the use of plasminogen activators with increased thrombolytic potency to enhance coronary thrombolysis, which can be administered by bolus injection; and by the use of more specific and potent anticoagulant and antiplatelet agents to accelerate recanalization and prevent reocclusion.[194]

Patients should receive thrombolytic therapy as soon after the onset of symptoms as possible. In GUSTO, the mortality was 4.3% in patients receiving alteplase within 2 hours after the onset of symptoms, 5.5% for those treated 2 to 4 hours after the onset, and 8.9% in those treated 4 to 6 hours after the onset of symptoms. The mortality of patients treated with streptokinase in the same time intervals was 5.4%, 6.7%, and 9.3%, respectively.[189,190] Therefore, early recanalization must remain the main objective of pharmacologic coronary thrombolysis. Variants of rt-PA have been constructed with altered pharmacokinetic or functional properties, including reduced clearance, altered binding to fibrin and stimulation by fibrin, and resistance to plasma protease inhibitors. In addition, the fibrin-specific bacterial plasminogen activator staphylokinase is under clinical evaluation (see later discussion).

Improved adjunctive therapy may also contribute to improved thrombolysis. Aspirin and heparin have a limited impact on the speed of coronary thrombolysis and on the resistance to lysis and do not consistently prevent reocclusion. This could have been anticipated on the basis of the unselective inhibition by aspirin of the synthesis of both proaggregatory and antiaggregatory prostaglandins and of the relative inefficacy of heparin for the inhibition of clot-associated thrombin. Several more specific approaches to reduction of platelet aggregation including monoclonal antibodies against the platelet GP IIb/IIIa receptor and small synthetic arginine-glycine-aspartic acid (RGD)-containing peptides are presently being explored.[195] The concomitant administration of potent platelet GP IIb/IIIa antagonists with aspirin, heparin, and thrombolytic therapy has been shown to be safe and feasible, and phase II studies have been sufficiently encouraging to warrant larger clinical trials such as TIMI 14, SPEED, and GUSTO IV.[196] Another approach consists of the use of selective thrombin inhibitors, including hirudin and its derivatives, or synthetic thrombin inhibitors. Some of these agents have indeed been shown to be more effective than aspirin and/or heparin for the acceleration of arterial recanalization and for the prevention of reocclusion, but several clinical trials with thrombolytic agents were terminated prematurely because of excess (cerebral) bleeding.[197] Alternatively, specific inhibitors of fXa and of the fVIIa/tissue factor pathway are being explored for conjunctive use with thrombolytic agents.

## Mutants and Variants of Fibrin-Specific Agents

### Mutants and Variants of t-PA

By deletion or substitution of functional domains, by site-specific point mutations, and/or by altering the carbohydrate composition, mutants of rt-PA have been produced with higher fibrin specificity, more zymogenicity, slower clearance from the circulation, and resistance to plasma proteinase inhibitors.[198,199] During thrombolytic therapy there is a vast excess of t-PA over PAI-1 in the circulation, but critical lysis occurs at the surface of an arterial thrombus where the local PAI-1 concentration can be very high.[200] Therefore, mutants with resistance to PAI-1 may be useful to reduce reocclusion. In addition, mutants with prolonged half-life may allow efficient thrombolysis by bolus administration at a reduced dose. Several mutants and variants of t-PA are presently being evaluated at the preclinical level in animal models of venous and arterial thrombosis and in pilot studies, mainly in patients with acute myocardial infarction.

Reteplase (Rapilysin or Ecokinase) is a single-chain nonglycosylated deletion variant consisting only of the kringle 2 and the proteinase domain of human t-PA; it contains amino acids 1 to 3 and 176 to 527 of rt-PA (deletion of Val4-Glu175); the Arg275-Ile276 plasmin cleave site is maintained. The plasminogenolytic activity of reteplase and of t-PA in the absence of a stimulator does not differ, but the activity of reteplase in the presence of a fibrin or fibrinogen stimulator was fourfold lower as compared with t-PA, and its binding to fibrin was fivefold lower. Reteplase and rt-PA are inhibited by PAI-1 to a similar degree. In patients, an initial half-life of 14 to 18 minutes was observed for reteplase, as compared with about 4 minutes for wild-type rt-PA. In the GUSTO-III trial, about 15,000 patients with acute myocardial infarction were randomly assigned to receive reteplase (two

boluses of 10 MU given 30 minutes apart) or 100 mg alteplase over 90 minutes. No clinical benefit of reteplase over alteplase could be demonstrated, in terms of 30-day mortality or frequency of hemorrhagic stroke, leading to the conclusion that both agents are equivalent.[201]

In TNK-rt-PA (tenecteplase), replacement of Asn117 with Gln (N117Q) deletes the glycosylation site in kringle 1, whereas substitution of Thr103 by Asn (T103N) reintroduces a glycosylation site in kringle 1 but at a different locus. These modifications substantially decrease the plasma clearance rate. In addition, the amino acids Lys296-His297-Arg298-Arg299 were each replaced with Ala, which confers resistance to inhibition by PAI-1. TNK-rt-PA has a similar ability as wild-type rt-PA to bind to fibrin and lyses fibrin clots in a plasma milieu with enhanced fibrin specificity. In patients with acute myocardial infarction, TNK-rt-PA has a half-life of about 20 minutes.[202] In the TIMI-10B trial, a phase II efficacy trial, a single bolus of 40 mg TNK-t-PA yielded similar TIMI-3 flow rates at 90 minutes as accelerated t-PA, with faster and more complete reperfusion.[203] In the ASSENT-2 study (about 17,000 patients with acute myocardial infarction of less than 6 hours) 0.5 mg/kg bolus tenecteplase yielded similar 30-day mortality and rate of intracranial bleeding as front-loaded alteplase (100 mg over 90 minutes).[204]

Different molecular forms of the Desmodus salivary plasminogen activator (DSPA) have been purified, characterized, cloned, and expressed. Two high molecular weight forms, DSPAα1 (43 kd) and DSPAα2 (39 kd) exhibit about 85% homology to human t-PA but contain neither a kringle 2 domain nor a plasmin-sensitive cleavage site. DSPAβ lacks the finger domain, and DSPAγ lacks the finger and epidermal growth factor domains. DSPAα1 and DSPAα2 exhibit a specific activity *in vitro* that is equal to or higher than that of rt-PA, a relative PAI-1 resistance, and a greatly enhanced fibrin specificity with a strict requirement for polymeric fibrin as a cofactor. In several animal models of thrombolysis, DSPAα1 has a 2.5 times higher potency and four- to eightfold slower clearance than rt-PA.[198,199] Patient data has so far not been reported.

Lanoteplase is a deletion mutant of rt-PA (without the finger and growth factor domains) in which glycosylation at Asn117 is lacking. Given as a single bolus of 120 U/kg in the Intravenous n-PA for Treating Infarcting Myocardium Early (InTIME-2) trial (about 15,000 patients), the 30-day mortality was very similar to that obtained with front-loaded alteplase, but the extent of intracerebral hemorrhage was significantly increased in the lanoteplase group.[205]

Monteplase, with a single amino acid substitution in the growth factor domain (Cys84 to Ser) has a prolonged half-life of 23 minutes following bolus injection of 0.22 mg/kg.[206] Pamiteplase, with deletion of the kringle 1 domain and substitution of Arg275 to Glu (rendering it resistant to conversion to a two-chain molecule by plasmin) has a half-life of more than 30 minutes following bolus injection.[207] Both agents were investigated in dose-finding studies in patients with acute myocardial infarction,[208,209] but no large scale trials on safety or mortality were reported.

## Mutants and Variants of Staphylokinase

The *staphylokinase* gene encodes a protein of 163 amino acids that is processed to a mature protein of 136 amino acids, consisting of a single polypeptide chain without disulfide bridges.[210-212] Staphylokinase is not an enzyme, but it forms a 1:1 stoichiometric complex with plasmin and plasminogen that activates other plasminogen molecules. When staphylokinase is added to human plasma containing a fibrin clot, it reacts poorly with plasminogen in plasma but reacts with high affinity with traces of plasmin at the clot surface and converts into plasmin-staphylokinase complex that, at the clot surface, efficiently activates plasminogen to plasmin. Plasmin-staphylokinase and plasmin bound to fibrin are protected from inhibition by $\alpha_2$-antiplasmin, whereas once liberated from the clot or generated in plasma, they are rapidly inhibited. Thereby the process of plasminogen activation is confined to the thrombus, preventing excessive plasmin generation, $\alpha_2$-antiplasmin depletion, and fibrinogen degradation in plasma.[210-212]

Intravenous staphylokinase (SakSTAR), combined with heparin and aspirin, was shown to be a potent, rapidly acting, and highly fibrin-selective thrombolytic agent in patients with acute myocardial infarction[213-215] and peripheral arterial occlusion.[216,217] However, most patients develop high titers of neutralizing specific IgG after infusion of staphylokinase, which would predict therapeutic refractoriness on repeated administration.

In an effort to optimize the activity-to-antigenicity ratio, a comprehensive site-directed mutagenesis study was carried out, yielding SakSTAR mutants with a maintained fibrinolytic potency and fibrin selectivity in a human plasma milieu and a markedly reduced reactivity with anti-SakSTAR antibodies in pooled immunized patient plasma. Furthermore, a recombinant staphylok-inase variant with reduced immunogenicity (in which Ser in position 3 of the protein sequence was mutated into Cys) (S3C,K35A, E65Q,K74R,E80A,D82A,T90A,E99D,T101S,E108A, K109A,K130T,K135R) was derivatized with maleimide-substituted polyethylene glycol (P) with molecular weights of 5000 (P5), 10,000 (P10), or 20,000 (P20) and characterized *in vitro* and *in vivo*.[218,219] SakSTAR-related antigen following bolus injection disappeared from plasma with an initial half-life of 15, 30, and 120 minutes and was cleared at a rate of 75, 43, and 8 mL/minute for variants substituted with P5, P10, and P20, respectively, as compared with an initial half-life of 3 minutes and a clearance of 360 mL/minute for wild-type staphylokinase.[219] Intravenous bolus injection of 5 mg of the P5 variant in 18 patients with acute myocardial infarction, restored TIMI-3 flow at 60 minutes in 14 patients. On the basis of these results, this staphylokinase mutant, substituted with a single polyethylene glycol molecule with a molecular weight of 5000, has been selected for clinical development as a single intravenous bolus agent for thrombolytic therapy of acute myocardial infarction.

## REFERENCES

1. Broze GJ Jr: Tissue factor pathway inhibitor and the revised theory of coagulation. Annu Rev Med 1995;46:103.

2. Collen D, Lijnen HR: Basic and clinical aspects of fibrinolysis and thrombolysis. Blood 1991;78:3114.

3. Blasi F: Urokinase and urokinase receptor: A paracrine/autocrine system regulating cell migration and invasiveness. BioEssays 1993;15:105.

4. Forsgren M, Raden B, Israelsson M, et al: Molecular cloning and characterization of a full-length cDNA clone for human plasminogen. FEBS Lett 1987;213:254.

5. Collen D: On the regulation and control of fibrinolysis. Thromb Haemost 1980;43:77.

6. Robbins KC, Summaria L, Hsieh B, et al: The peptide chains of human plasmin: Mechanism of activation of human plasminogen to plasmin. J Biol Chem 1967;242:2333.

7. Pennica D, Holmes WE, Kohr WJ, et al: Cloning and expression of human tissue-type plasminogen activator cDNA in E. coli. Nature 1983;301:214.

8. Tachias K, Madison EL: Converting tissue type plasminogen activator into a zymogen. J Biol Chem 1997;272:28.

9. Renatus M, Engh RA, Stubbs MT, et al: Lysine 156 promotes the anomalous proenzyme activity of tPA: X-ray crystal structure of single-chain human tPA. EMBO J 1997;16:4797.

10. Günzler WA, Steffens GJ, Otting F, et al: The primary structure of high molecular mass urokinase from human urine: The complete amino acid sequence of the A chain. Hoppe-Seyler Z Physiol Chem 1982;363:1155.

11. Holmes WE, Pennica D, Blaber M, et al: Cloning and expression of the gene for pro-urokinase in Escherichia coli. Biotechnology 1985;3:923.

12. Stump DC, Lijnen HR, Collen D: Purification and characterization of a novel low molecular weight form of single-chain urokinase-type plasminogen activator. J Biol Chem 1986;261:17120.

13. de Munk GA, Parkinson JF, Groeneveld E, et al: Role of the glycosaminoglycan component of thrombomodulin in its acceleration of the inactivation of single-chain urokinase-type plasminogen activator by thrombin. Biochem J 1993;290:655.

14. Holmes WE, Nelles L, Lijnen HR, et al: Primary structure of human $\alpha_2$-antiplasmin, a serine protease inhibitor (serpin). J Biol Chem 1987;262:1659.

15. Sugiyama N, Sasaki T, Iwamoto M, et al: Binding site of $\alpha_2$-plasmin inhibitor to plasminogen. Biochim Biophys Acta 1988;952:1.

16. Bangert K, Johnsen AH, Christensen U, et al: Different N-terminal forms of $\alpha_2$-plasmin inhibitor in human plasma. Biochem J 1993;291:623.

17. Kimura S, Aoki N: Cross-linking site in fibrinogen for $\alpha_2$-plasmin inhibitor. J Biol Chem 1986;261:15591.

18. Kruithof EKO, Tran-Thang C, Ransijn A, et al: Demonstration of a fast-acting inhibitor of plasminogen activators in human plasma. Blood 1984;64:907.

19. Ny T, Sawdey M, Lawrence D, et al: Cloning and sequence of a cDNA coding for the human ß-migrating endothelial-cell-type plasminogen activator inhibitor. Proc Natl Acad Sci USA 1986;83:6776.

20. Pannekoek H, Veerman H, Lambers H, et al: Endothelial plasminogen activator inhibitor (PAI): A new member of the serpin gene family. EMBO J 1986;5:2539.

21. Ginsburg D, Zeheb R, Yang AY, et al: cDNA cloning of human plasminogen activator-inhibitor from endothelial cells. J Clin Invest 1986;78:1673.

22. Andreasen PA, Riccio A, Welinder KG, et al: Plasminogen activator inhibitor type-1: Reactive center and amino-terminal heterogeneity determined by protein and cDNA sequencing. FEBS Lett 1986;209:213.

23. Declerck PJ, De Mol M, Alessi MC, et al: Purification and characterization of a plasminogen activator inhibitor-1 binding protein from human plasma: Identification as a multimeric form of S protein (Vitronectin). J Biol Chem 1988;263:15454.

24. Deng G, Royle G, Wang S, et al: Structural and functional analysis of the plasminogen activator inhibitor-1 binding motif in the somatomedin B domain of vitronectin. J Biol Chem 1996; 271:12716.

25. Ehrlich HJ, Klein Gebbink R, Preissner KT, et al: Thrombin neutralizes plasminogen activator inhibitor 1 (PAI-1) that is complexed with vitronectin in the endothelial cell matrix. J Cell Biol 1991;115:1773.

26. Gibson A, Baburaj K, Day DE, et al: The use of fluorescent probes to characterize conformational changes in the interaction

between vitronectin and plasminogen activator inhibitor-1. J Biol Chem 1997;272:5112.

27. Kruithof EKO, Gudinchet A, Bachmann F: Plasminogen activator inhibitor 1 and plasminogen activator inhibitor 2 in various disease states. Thromb Haemost 1988;59:7.

28. Belin D: Biology and facultative secretion of plasminogen activator inhibitor-2. Thromb Haemost 1993;70:144.

29. Lijnen HR, Arnout J, Collen D: Vascular endothelial cell function and thrombosis. In Willerson JT, Cohn JN (eds): Cardiovascular Medicine, 2nd ed. New York, Churchill Livingstone, 2000, p 1311.

30. Wiman B, Collen D: On the mechanism of the reaction between human $\alpha_2$-antiplasmin and plasmin. J Biol Chem 1979;254:9291.

31. Wiman B, Collen D: On the kinetics of the reaction between human antiplasmin and plasmin. Eur J Biochem 1978;84:573.

32. Otter M, Zocková P, Kuiper J, et al: Isolation and characterization of the mannose receptor from human liver potentially involved in the plasma clearance of tissue-type plasminogen activator. Hepatology 1992;16:54.

33. Strickland DK, Kounnas MZ, Williams SE, et al: LDL receptor-related protein (LRP): A multiligand receptor. Fibrinolysis 1994;8(Suppl 1):204.

34. Lijnen HR, Stump DC, Collen D: Single-chain urokinase-type plasminogen activator (prourokinase). In Messerli FH (ed): Cardiovascular Drug Therapy. Philadelphia, WB Saunders, 1996, p 1578.

35. Kruithof EKO: Plasminogen activator inhibitors: A review. Enzyme 1988;40:113.

36. Thorsen S, Philips M, Selmer J, et al: Kinetics of inhibition of tissue-type and urokinase-type plasminogen activator by plasminogen-activator inhibitor type 1 and type 2. Eur J Biochem 1988; 175:33.

37. Chmielewska J, Ranby M, Wiman B: Kinetics of the inhibition of plasminogen activators by the plasminogen-activator inhibitor. Evidence for 'second site' interactions. Biochem J 1988;251:327.

38. Madison EL, Goldsmith EJ, Gerard RD, et al: Serpin-resistant mutants of human tissue-type plasminogen activator. Nature 1989;339:721.

39. Adams DS, Griffin LA, Nachajko WR, et al: A synthetic DNA encoding a modified human urokinase resistant to inhibition by serum plasminogen activator inhibitor. J Biol Chem 1991;266:8476.

40. Hekman CM, Loskutoff DJ: Endothelial cells produce a latent inhibitor of plasminogen activators that can be activated by denaturants. J Biol Chem 1985;260:11581.

41. Mottonen J, Strand A, Symersky J, et al: Structural basis of latency in plasminogen activator inhibitor-1. Nature 1992;355:270.

42. Declerck PJ, De Mol M, Vaughan DE, et al: Identification of a conformationally distinct form of plasminogen activator inhibitor-1, acting as a non-inhibitory substrate for tissue-type plasminogen activator. J Biol Chem 1992;267:11693.

43. Aertgeerts K, De Bondt HL, De Ranter CJ, et al: Mechanisms contributing to the conformational and functional flexibility of plasminogen activator inhibitor-1. Nat Struct Biol 1995;2:891.

44. Hoylaerts M, Rijken DC, Lijnen HR, et al: Kinetics of the activation of plasminogen by human tissue plasminogen activator: Role of fibrin. J Biol Chem 1982;257:2912.

45. Thorsen S: The mechanism of plasminogen activation and the variability of the fibrin effector during tissue-type plasminogen activator-mediated fibrinolysis. Ann N Y Acad Sci 1992;667:52.

46. Bajzar L, Manuel R, Nesheim ME: Purification and characterization of TAFI, a thrombin-activable fibrinolysis inhibitor. J Biol Chem 1995;270:14477.

47. Eaton DL, Malloy BE, Tsai SP, et al: Isolation, molecular cloning, and partial characterization of a novel carboxypeptidase B from human plasma. J Biol Chem 1991;266:21833.

48. Nesheim M, Wang W, Boffa M, et al: Thrombin, thrombomodulin and TAFI in the molecular link between coagulation and fibrinolysis. Thromb Haemost 1997;78:386.

49. Gurewich V, Pannell R, Louie S, et al: Effective and fibrin-specific clot lysis by a zymogen precursor form of urokinase (pro-urokinase): A study in vitro and in two animal species. J Clin Invest 1984;73:1731.

50. Lijnen HR, Van Hoef B, Nelles L, et al: Plasminogen activation with single-chain urokinase-type plasminogen activator (scu-PA). Studies with active site mutagenized plasminogen (Ser740→Ala) and plasmin-resistant scu-PA (Lys158→Glu). J Biol Chem 1990; 265:5232.

51. Husain SS: Single-chain urokinase-type plasminogen activator does not possess measurable intrinsic amidolytic or plasminogen activator activities. Biochemistry 1991;30:5797.

52. Liu JN, Pannell R, Gurewich V: A transitional state of pro-urokinase that has a higher catalytic efficiency against Glu-plasminogen than urokinase. J Biol Chem 1992;267:15289.

53. Sun Z, Liu BF, Chen Y, et al: Analysis of the forces which stabilize the active conformation of urokinase-type plasminogen activator. Biochemistry 1998;37:2935.

54. Declerck PJ, Lijnen HR, Verstreken M, et al: Role of alpha 2-antiplasmin in fibrin-specific clot lysis with single-chain urokinase-type plasminogen activator in human plasma. Thromb Haemost 1991;65:394.

55. Liu JN, Gurewich V: Fragment E-2 from fibrin substantially enhances pro-urokinase-induced Glu-plasminogen activation: A kinetic study using the plasmin-resistant mutant pro-urokinase Ala-158-rpro-UK. Biochemistry 1992;31:6311.

56. Fleury V, Gurewich V, Anglés-Cano E: A study of the activation of fibrin-bound plasminogen by tissue-type plasminogen activator, single chain urokinase and sequential combinations of the activators. Fibrinolysis 1993;7:87.

57. Fleury V, Lijnen HR, Angles Cano E: Mechanism of the enhanced intrinsic activity of single-chain urokinase-type plasminogen activator during ongoing fibrinolysis. J Biol Chem 1993;268:18554.

58. Lijnen HR, Collen D: Congenital and acquired deficiencies of components of the fibrinolytic system and their relation to bleeding or thrombosis. Fibrinolysis 1989;3:67.

59. Hamsten A, Wiman B, de Faire U, et al: Increased plasma levels of a rapid inhibitor of tissue plasminogen activator in young survivors of myocardial infarction. N Engl J Med 1985;313:1557.

60. Hamsten A, de Faire U, Walldius G, et al: Plasminogen activator inhibitor in plasma: Risk factor for recurrent myocardial infarction. Lancet 1987;2:3.

61. Haverkate F, Thompson SG, Duckert F: Haemostatic factors in angina pectoris: Relation to gender, age and acute-phase reaction. Results of the ECAT Angina Pectoris Study Group. Thromb Haemost 1995;73:561.

62. Juhan-Vague I, Pyke SD, Alessi MC, et al: Fibrinolytic factors and the risk of myocardial infarction or sudden death in patients with angina pectoris: ECAT Study Group. European Concerted Action on Thrombosis and Disabilities. Circulation 1996;94:2057.

63. Erickson LA, Fici GJ, Lund JE, et al: Development of venous occlusions in mice transgenic for the plasminogen activator inhibitor-1 gene. Nature 1990;346:74.

64. Nilsson IM, Ljungner H, Tengborn L: Two different mechanisms in patients with venous thrombosis and defective fibrinolysis: Low concentration of plasminogen activator or increased concentration of plasminogen activator inhibitor. BMJ 1985;290:1453.

65. Juhan-Vague I, Valadier J, Alessi MC, et al: Deficient t-PA release and elevated PA inhibitor levels in patients with spontaneous or recurrent deep venous thrombosis. Thromb Haemost 1987; 57:67.

66. Isacson S, Nilsson IM: Defective fibrinolysis in blood and vein walls in recurrent "idiopathic" venous thrombosis. Acta Chir Scand 1972;138:813.

67. Carmeliet P, Schoonjans L, Kieckens L, et al: Physiological consequences of loss of plasminogen activator gene function in mice. Nature 1994;368:419.

68. Wiman B, Hamsten A: The fibrinolytic enzyme system and its role in the etiology of thromboembolic disease. Semin Thromb Hemost 1990;16:207.

69. Azuma H, Uno Y, Shigekiyo T, et al: Congenital plasminogen deficiency caused by Ser[672] to Pro mutation. Blood 1993;82:475.

70. Mingers AM, Heimburger N, Zeitler P, et al: Homozygous type I plasminogen deficiency. Semin Thromb Hemost 1997;23:259.

71. Schuster V, Mingers AM, Seidenspinner S, et al: Homozygous mutations in the plasminogen gene of two unrelated girls with ligneous conjunctivitis. Blood 1997;90:958.

72. Schott D, Dempfle CE, Beck P, et al: Successful therapy with Lys-plasminogen in homozygous type 1 plasminogen deficiency. Fibrinolysis Proteolysis 1997;11(Suppl 3):20.

73. Drew AF, Kaufman AH, Kombrinck KW, et al: Ligneous conjunctivitis in plasminogen-deficient mice. Blood 1998;91:1616.

74. Ploplis VA, Carmeliet P, Vazirzadeh S, et al: Effects of disruption of the plasminogen gene on thrombosis, growth, and health in mice. Circulation 1995;92:2585.

75. Bugge TH, Flick MJ, Daugherty CC, et al: Plasminogen deficiency causes severe thrombosis but is compatible with development and reproduction. Genes Dev 1995;9:794.

76. Lijnen HR, Carmeliet P, Bouché A, et al: Restoration of thrombolytic potential in plasminogen-deficient mice by bolus administration of plasminogen. Blood 1996;88:870.

77. Bugge TH, Kombrinck KW, Flick MJ, et al: Loss of fibrinogen rescues mice from the pleiotropic effects of plasminogen deficiency. Cell 1996;87:709.

78. Haverkate F, Samama M: Familial dysfibrinogenemia and thrombophilia: Report on a study of the SSC subcommittee on fibrinogen. Thromb Haemost 1995;73:151.

79. Liu CY, Koehn JA, Morgan FJ: Characterization of fibrinogen New York 1: A dysfunctional fibrinogen with a deletion of Bβ (9-72) corresponding exactly to exon 2 of the gene. J Biol Chem 1985;260:4390.

80. Lijnen HR, Soria J, Soria C, et al: Dysfibrinogenemia (fibrinogen Dusard) associated with impaired fibrin-enhanced plasminogen activation. Thromb Haemost 1984;51:108.

81. Collet JP, Soria J, Mirshahi M, et al: Dusard syndrome: A new concept of the relationship between fibrin clot architecture and fibrin clot degradability: Hypofibrinolysis related to an abnormal clot structure. Blood 1993;82:2462.

82. Carrell N, Gabriel DA, Blatt PM, et al: Hereditary dysfibrinogenemia in a patient with thrombotic disease. Blood 1983;62:439.

83. Mosesson MW: Dysfibrinogenemia and thrombosis. Sem Thromb Haemost 1999;3:311.

84. Fay WP, Shapiro AD, Shih JL, et al: Brief report: Complete deficiency of plasminogen activator inhibitor type 1 due to a frameshift mutation. N Engl J Med 1992;327:1729.

85. Fay WP, Parker AC, Condrey LR, et al: Human plasminogen activator inhibitor-1 (PAI-1) deficiency: Characterization of a large kindred with a null mutation in the PAI-1 gene. Blood 1997;90:204.

86. Carmeliet P, Kiekens L, Schoonjans L, et al: Plasminogen activator inhibitor-1 gene deficient mice. I. Generation by homologous recombination and characterization. J Clin Invest 1993;92:2746.

87. Carmeliet P, Stassen JM, Schoonjans L, et al: Plasminogen activator inhibitor-1 gene deficient mice. II. Effects on haemostasis, thrombosis and thrombolysis. J Clin Invest 1993;92:2756.

88. Koie K, Ogata K, Kamiya T, et al: $\alpha_2$-Plasmin inhibitor deficiency (Miyasato disease). Lancet 1978;2:1334.

89. Miura O, Sugahara Y, Aoki N: Hereditary $\alpha_2$-plasmin inhibitor deficiency caused by a transport-deficient mutation ($\alpha_2$-PI-Okinawa): Deletion of Glu137 by a trinucleotide deletion blocks intracellular transport. J Biol Chem 1989;264:18213.

90. Miura O, Hirosawa S, Kato A, Aoki N: Molecular basis for congenital deficiency of $\alpha_2$-plasmin inhibitor: A frameshift mutation leading to elongation of the deduced amino acid sequence. J Clin Invest 1989;83:1598.

91. Aoki N, Yamanaka T: The $\alpha_2$-plasmin inhibitor levels in liver diseases. Clin Chim Acta 1978;84:99.

92. Avvisati G, ten Cate JW, Sturk A, et al: Acquired alpha-2-antiplasmin deficiency in acute promyelocytic leukaemia. Br J Haematol 1988;70:43.

93. Collen D, Bounameaux H, De Cock F, et al: Analysis of coagulation and fibrinolysis during intravenous infusion of recombinant human tissue-type plasminogen activator in patients with acute myocardial infarction. Circulation 1986;73:511.

94. Holmes WE, Lijnen HR, Nelles L, et al: An alanine insertion in $\alpha_2$-antiplasmin 'Enschede' abolishes its plasmin inhibitory activity. Science 1987;238:209.

95. Booth NA, Bennett B, Wijngaards G, Grieve JHK: A new life-long hemorrhagic disorder due to excess plasminogen activator. Blood 1983;61:267.

96. Aznar J, Estellés A, Vila V, et al: Inherited fibrinolytic disorder due to an enhanced plasminogen activator level. Thromb Haemost 1984;52:196.

97. Sims PJ, Wiedmer T: Unraveling the mysteries of phospholipid scrambling. Thromb Haemost 2001;86:266.

98. Stenflo J, Fernlund P, Egan W, et al: Vitamin K dependent modification of glutamic acid residues in prothrombin. Proc Natl Acad Sci USA 1974;71:2730.

99. Pratt KP, Shen BW, Takeshima K, et al: Structure of the C2 domain of human factor VIII at 1.5 Å resolution. Nature 1999;402:439.

100. Kawasaki T, Kaida T, Arnout J, et al: A new animal model of thrombophilia confirms that high plasma factor VIII levels are thrombogenic. Thromb Haemost 1999;81:306.

101. Ruggeri ZM: Mechanisms initiating platelet thrombus formation. Thromb Haemost 1997;78:611.

102. Baglia FA, Badellino KO, Lopez JA, et al: Factor XI binding to the platelet glycoprotein Ib/IX/V complex promotes factor XI activation by thrombin [abstract]. Thromb Haemost Suppl July 2001, OC 2388.

103. Mann KG: Biochemistry and physiology of blood coagulation. Thromb Haemost 1999;82:165.

104. Drake TA, Morrissey JH, Edgington TS: Selective cellular expression of tissue factor in human tissues: Implication for disorders of hemostasis and thrombosis. Am J Pathol 1988;86:1087.

105. Osterud B, Rao LVM, Olsen JO: Induction of tissue factor expression in whole blood: Lack of evidence for the presence of tissue factor expression in granulocytes. Thromb Haemost 2000;83:861.

106. Fuster V, Fallon JT, Badimon JJ, et al: The unstable atherosclerotic plaque: Clinical significance and therapeutic intervention. Thromb Haemost 1997;78:247.

107. Hathcock JJ, Nemerson Y: Adherent platelets block surface-bound tissue factor activity: A blood-borne source of procoagulant activity is essential to thrombus growth [abstract]. Thromb Haemost Suppl July 2001, OC 2404.

108. Giesen PLA, Rauch U, Bohrmann B, et al: Blood-borne tissue factor: Another view of thrombosis. Proc Natl Acad Sci USA 1999;96:2311.

109. Rauch U, Bonderman D, Borhman B, et al: Transfer of tissue factor from leukocytes to platelets is mediated by CD15 and tissue factor. Blood 2000;96:170.

110. Johnston GI, Cook RG, McEver RP: Cloning of GMP-140, a granule membrane protein of platelets and endothelium: Sequence similarity to proteins involved in cell adhesion and inflammation. Cell 1989;56:1033.

111. Sako D, Chang XJ, Barone KM, et al: Expression cloning of a functional glycoprotein ligand for P-selectin. Cell 1993;75:1179.

112. Maynard JR, Heckman CA, Pitlick FA, et al: Association of tissue factor activity with the surface of cultured cells. J Clin Invest 1975;55:814.

113. Bach R, Rifkin DB: Expression of tissue factor procoagulant activity: Regulation by cytosolic calcium. Proc Natl Acad Sci USA 1990;87:6995.

114. Neuenschwander PF, Fiore MM, Morrissey JH: Factor VII autoactivation proceeds via interaction of distinct protease-cofactor and zymogen-cofactor complexes: Implications of a two-dimensional enzyme kinetic mechanism. J Biol Chem 1993;268:21489.

115. Almus FE, Rao LVM, Rapaport SI: Functional properties of factor VIIa/tissue factor formed with purified tissue factor and with tissue factor expressed on cultured endothelial cells. Thromb Haemost 1989;62:1067.

116. Krishnaswamy S, Mann KG, Nesheim ME: The prothrombinase-catalyzed activation of prothrombin proceeds through the intermediate meizothrombin in an ordered, sequential reaction. J Biol Chem 1986;261:8977.

117. Tans G, Nicolaes GA, Thomassen MC, et al: Activation of factor V by meizothrombin. J Biol Chem 1994;269:15969.

118. von dem Borne PAK, Mosnier LO, Tans G, et al: Factor XI activation by meizothrombin: Stimulation by phospholipid vesicles containing both phosphatidylserine and phosphatidylethanolamine. Thromb Haemost 1997;78:834.

119. Vlot AJ: Factor VIII and von Willebrand factor. Thromb Haemost 1998;79:456.

120. Walsh PN: Roles of platelets and factor XI in the initiation of blood coagulation by thrombin. Thromb Haemost 2001;86:75.

121. Balasubramanian V, Bini A, Grabowski E, et al: Co-localization of platelets, blood-borne tissue factor, and fibrin in ex-vivo thrombi visualized in real-time [abstract]. Thromb Haemost Suppl July 2001, OC 1025.

122. Furie B, Furie BC, Flaumenhaft R: A journey with platelet P-selectin: The molecular basis of granule secretion, signalling and cell adhesion. Thromb Haemost 2001;86:214.

123. Kawasaki T, Dewerchin M, Lijnen HR, et al: Mouse carotid artery ligation induces platelet-leukocyte-dependent luminal fibrin, required for neointima development. Circ Res 2001;88:159.

124. Kumar A, Lindner V: Remodeling with neointima formation in the mouse carotid artery after cessation of blood flow. Arterioscler Thromb Vasc Biol 1997;17:2238.

125. Kumar A, Hoover JL, Simmons CA, et al: Remodeling and neointimal formation in the carotid artery of normal and P-selectin-deficient mice. Circulation 1997;96:4333.

126. Li N, Hu H, Lindquist M, et al: Platelet-leukocyte cross talk in whole blood. Arterioscler Thromb Vasc Biol 2000;20:2702.

127. Palabrica T, Lobb R, Furie BC, et al: Leukocyte accumulation promoting fibrin deposition is mediated in vivo by P-selectin on adherent platelets. Nature 1992;359:948.

128. Downing LJ, Wakefield TW, Strieter RM, et al: Anti-P-selectin antibody decreases inflammation and thrombus formation in venous thrombosis. J Vasc Surg 1997;25:816.

129. Khor SP, McCarthy K, Dupont M, et al: Pharmacokinetics, pharmacodynamics, allometry, and dose selection for rPSGL-Ig for phase I trial. J Pharm Exp Ther 2000;293:618.

130. Toombs CF, DeGraef GL, Martin JP, et al: Pretreatment with a blocking monoclonal antibody to P-selectin accelerates pharmacological thrombolysis in a primate model of arterial thrombosis. J Pharm Exp Ther 1995;275:941.

131. Kumar A, Villami MP, Patel UK, et al: Recombinant soluble form of PSGL-1 accelerates thrombolysis and prevents reocclusion in a porcine model. Circulation 1999;99:1363.

132. Eppihimer MJ, Schaub RG: P-selectin-dependent inhibition of thrombosis during venous stasis. Arterioscler Thromb Vasc Biol 2000;20:2483.

133. Myers DD, Schaub R, Wrobleski SK, et al: P-selectin antagonism causes dose-dependent venous thrombosis inhibition. Thromb Haemost 2001;85:423.

134. Gachet C: ADP receptors of platelets and their inhibition. Thromb Haemost 2001;86:222.

135. Coller BS: Anti GPIIb/IIIa drugs: Current strategies and future directions. Thromb Haemost 2001;86:427.

136. Chew DP, Bhatt DL, Sapp S, et al: Increased mortality with oral platelet glycoprotein IIb/IIIa antagonists: A meta-analysis of phase III multicenter randomized trials. Circulation 2001;103:201.

137. Theilmeier G, Lenaerts T, Remacle C, et al: Circulating activated platelets assist THP-1 monocytoid/endothelial cell interaction under shear stress. Blood 1999;94:2725.

138. Koster T, Blann AD, Briet E, et al: Role of clotting factor VIII in effect of von Willebrand factor on occurrence of deep-vein thrombosis. Lancet 1995;345:152.

139. Egeberg O: Inherited antithrombin III deficiency causing thrombophilia. Thromb Diath Haemorrh 1965;13:516.

140. Heijboer H, Brandjes DP, Buller HR, et al: Deficiencies of coagulation-inhibiting and fibrinolytic proteins in outpatients with deep-vein thrombosis. N Engl J Med 1990;323:1512.

141. Esmon CT: Thrombomodulin as a model of molecular mechanisms that modulate protease specificity and function at the vessel surface. FASEB J 1995;9:946.

142. Fukudome K, Esmon CT: Identification, cloning and regulation of a novel endothelial cell protein C/activated protein C receptor. J Biol Chem 1994;269:26486.

143. Rosing J, Hoekema L, Nicolaes GAF, et al: Effects of protein S and factor Xa on peptide bond cleavages during inactivation of factor Va and factor Va R506Q by activated protein C. J Biol Chem 1995;270:27852.

144. Dahlbäck B: Purification of human vitamin K-dependent protein S and its limited proteolysis by thrombin. Biochem J 1983;209:837.

145. Griffin JH, Evatt B, Zimmerman TS, et al: Deficiency of protein C in congenital thrombotic disease. J Clin Invest 1981;68:1370.

146. Comp PC, Esmon CT: Recurrent venous thromboembolism in patients with a partial deficiency of protein S. N Engl J Med 1984;311:1525.

147. Miletich J, Sherman J, Broze G Jr: Absence of thrombosis in subjects with heterozygous protein C deficiency. N Engl J Med 1987;317:991.

148. Marlar RA, Neumann A: Neonatal purpura fulminans due to homozygous protein C or protein S deficiencies. Semin Thromb Haemost 1990;16:299.

149. Dahlbäck B, Carlsson M, Svensson PJ: Familial thrombophilia due to a previously unrecognized mechanism characterized by poor anticoagulant response to activated protein C: Prediction of a cofactor to activated protein C. Proc Natl Acad Sci USA 1993; 90:1004.

150. Bertina RM, Koeleman BPC, Koster T, et al: Mutation in blood coagulation factor V associated with resistance to activated protein C. Nature 1994;369:64.

151. Koster T, Rosendaal FR, de Ronde H, et al: Venous thrombosis due to poor anticoagulant response to activated protein C: Leiden Thrombophilia Study. Lancet 1993;342:1503.

152. Poort SR, Rosendaal FR, Reitsma PH, et al: A common genetic variation in the 3′ untranslated region of the prothrombin gene is associated with elevated plasma prothrombin levels and an increase in venous thrombosis. Blood 1996;88:3698.

153. Preston FE, Rosendaal FR, Walker ID, et al: Increased fetal loss in women with heritable thrombophilia. Lancet 1996;348:913.

154. Martinelli I, Taioli E, Cetin I, et al: Mutations in coagulation factors in women with unexplained late fetal loss. N Engl J Med 2000;343:1015.

155. Seligsohn U, Lubetsky A: Genetic susceptibility to venous thrombosis. N Engl J Med 2001;344:1222.

156. Koeleman BPC, Reitsma PH, Allaart CF, et al: Activated protein C resistance as an additional risk factor for thrombosis in protein C-deficient families. Blood 1994;84:1031.

157. DeStefano V, Martinelli I, Mannucci PM, et al: The risk of recurrent deep venous thrombosis among heterozygous carriers of both factor V Leiden and the G20210A prothrombin mutation. N Engl J Med 1999;341:801.

158. Vandenbroucke JP, Koster T, Briet J, et al: Increased risk of venous thrombosis in oral-contraceptive users who are carriers of factor V Leiden mutation. Lancet 1994;344:1453.

159. Mudd SH, Skovby F, Levy HL, et al: The natural history of homocystinuria due to cystathionine beta-synthase deficiency. Am J Hum Genet 1985;37:1.

160. Alhenc-Gelas M, Arnaud E, Nicaud V, et al: Venous thromboembolic disease and the prothrombin, methylene tetrahydrofolate reductase and factor V genes. Thromb Haemost 1999;81:506.

161. Fryer R, Wilson B, Gubler D, et al: Homocysteine, a risk factor for premature vascular disease and thrombosis, induces tissue factor activity in endothelial cells. Arterioscler Thromb Vasc Biol 1993;13:405.

162. Lentz S, Sadler J: Inhibition of thrombomodulin surface expression and protein C activation by the thrombogenic agent homocysteine. J Clin Invest 1991;88:1906.

163. Vermylen J, Hoylaerts MF, Arnout J: Antibody-mediated thrombosis. Thromb Haemost 1997;78:420.

164. Warkentin TE, Chong BH, Greinacher A: Heparin-induced thrombocytopenia; towards consensus. Thromb Haemost 1998;79:1.

165. Amiral J, Bridey F, Dreyfus M, et al: Platelet factor 4 complexed to heparin is the target for antibodies generated in heparin-induced thrombocytopenia. Thromb Haemost 1992;68:95.

166. Khairy M, Lasne D, Brohard-Bohn B, et al: A new approach in the study of the molecular and cellular events implicated in heparin-induced thrombocytopenia: Formation of leukocyte-platelet aggregates. Thromb Haemost 2001;85:1090.

167. Visentin GP, Ford SE, Scott JP, et al: Antibodies from patients with heparin-induced thrombocytopenia/thrombosis are specific for platelet factor 4 complexed with heparin or bound to endothelial cells. J Clin Invest 1994;93:81.

168. Arnout J: The pathogenesis of the antiphospholipid syndrome: A hypothesis based on parallelisms with heparin-induced thrombocytopenia. Thromb Haemost 1996;75:536.

169. Arnout J, Wittevrongel C, Vanrusselt M, et al: Beta-2-glycoprotein I dependent lupus anticoagulants form stable bivalent antibody-beta-2-glycoprotein I complexes on phospholipid surfaces. Thromb Haemost 1998;79:79.

170. Carreras LO, Machin SJ, Deman R, et al: Arterial thrombosis, intrauterine death and "lupus" anticoagulant: Detection of immunoglobulin interfering with prostacyclin formation. Lancet 1981;i:244.

171. Malia RG, Kitchen S, Greaves M, et al: Inhibition of activated protein C and its cofactor protein S by antiphospholipid antibodies. Br J Haematol 1990;76:101.

172. Marciniak E, Romond EH: Impaired catalytic function of activated protein C: A new in vitro manifestation of lupus anticoagulant. Blood 1989;74:2426.

173. Rand JH, Wu X-X, Andree HAM, et al: Antiphospholipid antibodies accelerate plasma coagulation by inhibiting annexin-V binding to phospholipids: A "lupus anticoagulant" phenomenon. Blood 1998;92:1652.

174. Levin M, Elay BS, Louis J, et al: Postinfectious purpura fulminans caused by an auto-antibody directed against protein S. J Pediatr 1995;127:355.

175. Nicholson-Weller A, Spicer DB, Austen KF: Deficiency of the complement regulatory protein, "decay-accelerating factor", on membranes of granulocytes, monocytes and platelets in paroxysmal nocturnal hemoglobinuria. N Engl J Med 1985;312:1091.

176. Wiedmer T, Hall SE, Ortel TL, et al: Complement-induced vesiculation and exposure of membrane prothrombinase sites in platelets of paroxysmal nocturnal hemoglobinuria. Blood 1993;82:1447.

177. Hugel B, Socie G, Vu T, et al: Elevated levels of circulating procoagulant microparticles in patients with paroxysmal nocturnal hemoglobinuria and aplastic anemia. Blood 1999;93:3451.

178. Trousseau A: Phlegmasia alba dolens. In Clinique Médicale de l'Hôtel-Dieu de Paris. Paris, JB Baillière et fils, 1865;3:654.

179. Rickles FR, Levine MN, Dvorak HF: Abnormalities of hemostasis in malignancy. In Colman RW, Hirsh J, Marder VJ, et al. (eds): Hemostasis and Thrombosis: Basic Principles and Clinical Practice. Lippincott Williams & Wilkins, 2001, p 1131.

180. Falanga A, Gordon SG: Isolation and characterization of cancer procoagulant A: A cysteine protease from malignant tissue. Biochemistry 1985;24:5558.

181. Van De Water L, Tracy PB, Aronson D, et al: Tumor cell generation of thrombin via functional prothrombinase assembly. Cancer Res 1985;45:5521.

182. De Wood MA, Spores J, Notske R, et al: Prevalence of total coronary occlusion during the early hours of transmural myocardial infarction. N Engl J Med 1980;303:897.

183. Rentrop KP, Feit F, Blanke H, et al: Effects of intracoronary streptokinase and intracoronary nitroglycerin injection on coronary angiographic patterns and mortality in patients with acute myocardial infarction. N Engl J Med 1984;311:1457.

184. Collen D: Trials comparing the available thrombolytic agents. Coron Art Dis 1992;3:117.

185. Grünewald M, Seifried E: Meta-analysis of all available published clinical trials (1958–1990) on thrombolytic therapy for AMI: Relative efficacy of different therapeutic strategies. Fibrinolysis 1994;8:67.

186. Collen D: The plasminogen (fibrinolytic) system. Thromb Haemost 1999;82:259.

187. Schlandt RC: Reperfusion in acute myocardial infarction. Circulation 1994;90:2091.

188. Becker RC (ed): The Modern Era of Coronary Thrombolysis. Boston, Kluwer Academic Publisher, 1994.

189. The GUSTO Investigators: An international randomized trial comparing four thrombolytic strategies for acute myocardial infarction. N Engl J Med 1993;329:673.

190. The GUSTO Angiographic Investigators: The effects of tissue plasminogen activator, streptokinase, or both on coronary-artery patency, ventricular function, and survival after acute myocardial infarction. N Engl J Med 1993;329:1615.

191. Braunwald E: The open-artery theory is alive and well-again. N Engl J Med 1993;329:1650.

192. Califf RM, White HD, Van de Werf F, et al: One-year results from the Global Utilization of Streptokinase and t-PA for Occluded Coronary Arteries (GUSTO-I) trial. Circulation 1996;94:1233.

193. Califf RM, Woodlief LH, Harrell FE Jr, et al: Selection of thrombolytic therapy for individual patients: Development of a clinical model. Am Heart J 1997;133:630.

194. Collen D: Towards improved thrombolytic therapy. Lancet 1993;342:34.

195. Moliterno DJ, Topol EJ: Conjunctive use of platelet glycoprotein IIb/IIIa antagonists and thrombolytic therapy for acute myocardial infarction. Thromb Haemost 1997;78:214.

196. Cannon CP: Bridging the gap with new strategies in acute ST elevation myocardial infarction: Bolus thrombolysis, glycoprotein IIb/IIIa inhibitors, combination therapy, percutaneous coronary intervention, and "facilitated" PCI. J Thromb Thrombolysis 2000;9:235.

197. Verstraete M, Zoldhelyi P, Willerson JT: Specific thrombin inhibitors. In Verstraete M, Fuster V, Topol EJ (eds): Cardiovascular

Thrombosis: Thrombocardiology and Thromboneurology, 2nd ed. Philadelphia, Lippincott-Raven Publishers, 1998, p 141.

198. Lijnen HR, Collen D: Strategies for the improvement of thrombolytic agents. Thromb Haemost 1991;66:88.

199. Lijnen HR, Collen D: Tissue-type plasminogen activator. In Barrett AJ, Rawlings ND, Woessner JF (eds): Handbook of Proteolytic Enzymes. London, Academic Press, 1998, p 184.

200. Stringer HAR, van Swieten P, Heijnen HFG, et al: Plasminogen activator inhibitor 1 (PAI-1) released from activated platelets plays a key role in thrombolysis resistance: Studies generated in the Chandler loop. Arterioscler Thromb 1994;14:1452.

201. The GUSTO-III investigators: A comparison of reteplase with alteplase for acute myocardial infarction. N Engl J Med 1997; 337:1118.

202. Cannon CP, McCabe CH, Gibson CM, et al: TNK-tissue plasminogen activator in acute myocardial infarction: Results of the Thrombolysis in Myocardial Infarction (TIMI) 10A dose-ranging trial. Circulation 1997;95:351.

203. Cannon CP, McCabe CH, Gibson MC, et al: TNK-tissue plasminogen activator compared with front-loaded tissue plasminogen activator in acute myocardial infarction: Primary results of the TIMI-10B trial. Circulation 1997;96(Suppl I):206.

204. Assessment of the Safety and Efficacy of a New Thrombolytic (ASSENT-2) Investigators: Single-bolus tenecteplase compared with front-loaded alteplase in acute myocardial infarction: The ASSENT-2 double-blind randomised trial. Lancet 1999;354:716.

205. Antman EM, Wilcox RG, Giugliano RP, et al: Long term comparison of lanoteplase and alteplase in ST elevation myocardial infarction: 6 month follow-up in InTIME II trial. Circulation 1999;100:498.

206. Kawai C, Hosada S, Kimata S, et al: Coronary thrombolysis in acute myocardial infarction of E6010 (novel modified t-PA): A multicenter, double-blind dose-finding study. Jpn Pharmacol Ther 1994; 22:3925.

207. Hashimoto K, Oikawa K, Miyamoto I, et al: Phase I study of a novel modified t-PA. Jpn J Med Pharm Sci 1996;36:623.

208. Kawai C, Yui Y, Hosada S, et al: A prospective, randomized, double-blind multicenter trial of a single bolus injection of the novel modified t-PA E6010 in the treatment of acute myocardial infarction: Comparison with native t-PA. J Am Coll Cardiol 1997; 29:1447.

209. Yui Y, Haze K, Kawai C, et al: Randomized, double-blind multicenter trial of YM866 (modified t-PA) by intravenous bolus injection in patients with acute myocardial infarction in comparison with tisokinase (native t-PA). J New Remedies Clin 1996;45:2175.

210. Collen D, Lijnen HR: Staphylokinase, a fibrin-specific plasminogen activator with therapeutic potential? Blood 1994;84:680.

211. Lijnen HR, Collen D: Staphylokinase, a fibrin-specific bacterial plasminogen activator. Fibrinolysis 1996;10:119.

212. Collen D: Staphylokinase: A potent, uniquely fibrin-selective thrombolytic agent. Nat Med 1998;4:279.

213. Vanderschueren S, Barrios L, Kerdsinchai P, et al: A randomized trial of recombinant staphylokinase versus alteplase for coronary artery patency in acute myocardial infarction. Circulation 1995;92:2044.

214. Vanderschueren S, Collen D, Van de Werf F: A pilot study on bolus administration of recombinant staphylokinase for coronary artery thrombolysis. Thromb Haemost 1996;76:541.

215. Armstrong P, Burton J, Palisaitis D, et al: Collaborative angiographic patency trial of recombinant staphylokinase (CAPTORS). Am Heart J 2000;139:820.

216. Vanderschueren S, Stockx L, Wilms G, et al: Thrombolytic therapy of peripheral arterial occlusion with recombinant staphylokinase. Circulation 1995;92:2050.

217. Heymans S, Vanderschueren S, Verhaeghe R, et al: Outcome and one year follow-up of intra-arterial staphylokinase in 191 patients with peripheral arterial occlusion. Thromb Haemost 2000; 83:666.

218. Vanwetswinkel S, Plaisance S, Zhi-Yong Z, et al: Pharmacokinetic and thrombolytic properties of cysteine-linked polyethylene glycol derivatives of staphylokinase. Blood 2000;95:936.

219. Collen D, Sinnaeve P, Demarsin E, et al: Polyethylene glycol-derivatized cysteine-substitution variants of recombinant staphylokinase for single-bolus treatment of acute myocardial infarction. Circulation 2000;102:1766.

■ ■ ■ chapter 3 0

# Molecular Targets of Antihypertensive Drug Therapy

*Edwin W. Willems*
*Ahsan Husain*
*Robert M. Graham*

Hypertension has been recognized for many years as a major risk factor for important cardiovascular disorders, such as coronary artery disease, heart failure, stroke, peripheral vascular disease, and renal failure. The relationship between blood pressure and cardiovascular risk is positive and continuous and applies independently to systolic, diastolic, and pulse pressure.[1,2] Approximately 25% of the adult population in industrialized countries is afflicted by hypertension; therefore, it represents a very significant public health problem and is a major contributor to premature morbidity and mortality. On the plus side, benefits of pharmacologic treatment of hypertension have been amply documented, with large, randomized trials showing benefits from even modest reductions in arterial pressure. For example, data from the Hypertension Optimal Treatment (HOT) trial, involving 18,790 patients from 26 countries, showed that reductions in systolic and diastolic pressure averaging 4.0 mm Hg resulted in a 28% reduction in the risk of myocardial infarction.[3] These benefits extend also to the elderly, with the combined data from several large trials showing that 12 to 14 mm Hg reductions in systolic blood pressure result in 34%, 19%, and 23% reductions in the risk of stroke, coronary heart disease, and vascular death, respectively.[4] Since 1947, there has been evidence that pharmacologic treatment could induce a remission in some of the signs and symptoms of malignant hypertension—a condition that, if left untreated, causes death in 50% of affected individuals within 6 months.[5] Since that time a large armamentarium of antihypertensive agents have been developed that not only effectively lower arterial pressure but also are well tolerated. Nevertheless, given that the pathophysiology of essential hypertension has not been defined, almost all agents are aimed at targets and pathways involved in the physiologic regulation of blood pressure. Recent groundbreaking elucidation of the molecular defects underlying several monogenetic causes of hypertension have not only confirmed the primacy of the kidney in blood pressure regulation but also have revealed that several widely used antihypertensive agents do indeed target patho-

physiologic mechanisms. Furthermore, in these individuals the absence of phenotypic effects outside the kidney suggests that pharmacologic agents targeting the genetically altered pathway should not produce adverse effects in other organ systems. These studies of monogenetic causes of hypertension have also highlighted the need for continued drug development to allow more effective blockade of pathogenetic targets, such as the epithelial sodium channel, because in some cases currently available drugs only weakly inhibit these targets.[6]

Because of these advances in the understanding of the molecular mechanisms regulating blood pressure control, this chapter does not consider antihypertensive therapy from the point of view of the drugs, per se, because many such monographs are already available. Instead, it focuses on the molecular targets and signaling pathways for antihypertensive drugs, because a comprehensive consideration of such data is currently not available. In general, these considerations have been restricted to the targets and pathways used by drugs already available for clinical use (Table 30-1), although in some instances those used by experimental agents (Table 30-2)[7-30] are also considered. It is surprising that the exact antihypertensive drug targets are completely unknown for some drugs (e.g., hydralazine) or are only very poorly understood (e.g., α–methyldopa, β-blockers), although these agents have been used widely and effectively in the management of hypertension. This clearly reflects the past empiricism of antihypertensive drug development, which one can only hope will yield to more rational drug design as the molecular pathways of hypertension are revealed and as the key players in these pathways are elucidated at the molecular level.

## SYMPATHETIC NERVOUS SYSTEM TARGETS

The autonomic nervous system, also called the visceral, vegetative, or involuntary system, consists of the peripheral nerves, ganglia, and plexuses that innervate the

■ ▦ ■

**TABLE 30-1**   CLASSIFICATION OF ANTIHYPERTENSIVE DRUGS, THEIR PRIMARY TARGET SITES, AND MECHANISM OF ACTION

| Drugs | Target | Mechanism of Action |
|---|---|---|
| *Sympatholytics* | | |
| Centrally acting agents (methyldopa, clonidine, guanabenz, guanfacine) | Central $\alpha_2$-adrenergic receptors (activation) | Inhibition of sympathetic outflow |
| Ganglionic blockers (trimethaphan) | Ganglionic nicotinic receptors | Inhibition of ganglionic transmission |
| Catecholamine biosynthesis inhibitors (metyrosine) | Catecholamine biosynthesizing enzymes | Reduction in sympathetic transmission |
| Adrenergic neuronal blockers (guanethidine, guanadrel, reserpine) | Sympathetic nerve terminal storage vesicles | Neurotransmitter depletion |
| β-Adrenergic receptor antagonists (propranolol, metoprolol, etc.) | β-Adrenergic receptors | Inhibition of prejunctional neurotransmitter release; inhibition of renin release |
| α-Adrenergic receptor antagonists (prazosin, terazosin, doxazosin, phenoxybenzamine, phentolamine) | $\alpha_1$-Adrenergic receptors | Inhibition of sympathetically mediated vasoconstriction |
| Mixed adrenergic antagonists (labetalol) | α- and β-Adrenergic receptors | Inhibition of sympathetically mediated vasoconstriction |
| Dopamine receptor agonists (fenoldopam) | Dopamine DA1 receptor | Vasodilation |
| *Renin Angiotensin System Inhibitors* | | |
| ACE inhibitors (captopril, enalapril, lisinopril, quinapril, ramipril, etc.) | ACE | Reduction in peripheral resistance |
| Angiotensin II receptor antagonists (losartan, irbesartan, candesartan, etc.) | Angiotensin $AT_1$ receptor | Reduction in peripheral resistance |
| *Vasodilators* | | |
| $Ca^{2+}$ channel blockers (verapamil, diltiazem, nifedipine, nimodipine) | $Ca^{2+}$ channels | Vasodilation |
| *Direct-Acting Vasodilators* | | |
| Hydralazine | Unknown | Vasodilation |
| Minoxidil, diazoxide | ATP-sensitive $K^+$ channel (activation) | Vasodilation |
| Sodium nitroprusside | Guanylate cyclase (activation) | Vasodilation |
| *Diuretics* | | |
| Thiazides and related agents (hydrochlorothiazide, chlorthalidone, indapamide, etc.) | Thiazide-sensitive electroneural<br><br>$Na^+$-Cl-cotransporter (inhibition) | Extracellular volume (ECV) depletion; reduction in peripheral resistance |
| Loop diuretics (furosemide, bumetanide, ethacrynic acid) | Bumetanide-sensitive electroneutral $Na^+$-$K^+$-$2Cl^-$ cotransporter (inhibition) | ECV depletion; reduction in peripheral resistance |
| *Potassium-Sparing Agents* | | |
| Amiloride, triamterene | Epithelial $Na^+$ channel (inhibition) | ECV depletion; reduction in peripheral resistance |
| Spironolactone | Mineralocorticoid receptor (inhibition) | ECV depletion; reduction in peripheral resistance |

heart, blood vessels, glands, other visceral organs, and vascular smooth muscle. Skeletal muscle is innervated by myelinated, somatic nerves. Autonomic nerves are widely distributed throughout the body and regulate functions that occur without conscious control.[31] On the efferent side, the autonomic nervous system consists of two main anatomic divisions: (1) the parasympathetic or craniosacral outflow and (2) the sympathetic nervous system or thoracolumbar outflow. The enteric nervous system consisting of neurons lying in the intramural plexuses of the gastrointestinal tract forms a third division, although it is closely interconnected with the sympathetic and parasympathetic systems.

Sympathetic tone in organs (e.g., heart or blood vessels) is controlled by sympathetic outflow. Thus, norepinephrine released from nerve terminals activates adrenergic receptors. As described in the section on cat-

echolamine biosynthesizing enzymes, norepinephrine is synthesized in sympathetic nerve terminals from its precursors (tyrosine, DOPA, and dopamine) (Fig. 30-1). This process involves several enzymes; tyrosine hydroxylase is rate limiting. On release into the synaptic cleft, about 90% of norepinephrine reenters the prejunctional (i.e., presynaptic in central nervous system) nerve terminals via the uptake I transporter, which constitutes an important regulator of released norepinephrine and, thus, sympathetic tone; the uptake II norepinephrine transporter, on the other hand, is located in the postjunctional plasma membrane. Released norepinephrine either stimulates receptors or is metabolized by the enzymes monoamine oxidase (MAO) and catecholamine-*O*-methyltransferase (COMT). The circulating hormone epinephrine (released from the adrenal medulla) also activates receptors or is taken up by prejunctional nerve

■ ■ ■

## TABLE 30-2   RECEPTOR-, ENZYME-, AND ION-CHANNEL-SELECTIVE COMPOUNDS

| Molecular Target | Agonists | Antagonists |
|---|---|---|
| *Receptors and Enzymes* | | |
| $\alpha_1$-*Adrenergic Receptors* | | |
| $\alpha_{1A}$ | A61603 | KMD3213, (+)-niguldipine, SNAP5089, RS17053, SNAP5272, SB216469 |
| $\alpha_{1B}$ | — | L-765,314 |
| $\alpha_{1D}$ | — | BMY7378 |
| $\alpha_{1A, B, or D}$ | Phenylephrine, methoxamine, cirazoline | Prazosin, terazosin, doxazosin, corynanthine |
| $\alpha_2$-*Adrenergic Receptors* | | |
| $\alpha_{2A}$ | Monoxidine, oxymetazoline | BRL 44408 |
| $\alpha_{2B}$ | — | ARC239, prazosin, imiloxan |
| $\alpha_{2C}$ | — | ARC239, prazosin, MK912 |
| $\alpha_{2A, B, or C}$ | Clonidine, BHT933, UK14304 | Rauwolscine, yohimbine |
| $\beta$-*Adrenergic Receptors* | | |
| $\beta_1$ | Denopamine, RO363 | CGP20712A, betaxolol, atenolol |
| $\beta_2$ | Procaterol, zinterol, salmeterol, formoterol, terbutaline, femoterol | ICI118551 |
| $\beta_3$ | BRL3744, L742791, SB251023 | L748328 |
| $\beta_{1, 2, or 3}$ | Isoprenaline | Propranolol |
| *Dopamine Receptors* | | |
| $D_1$ | Fenoldopam, R (+)SKF38393, R (+)SKF81297 | SCH23390, SKF83566, SCH39166 |
| $D_2$ | (+)PHNO | Raclopride |
| $D_3$ | PD128907 | S33084, nafadotride, (+)S14297, SB277011 |
| $D_4$ | PD168077 | L745870, L741742 |
| $D_5$ | Fenoldopam, SKF38393, SKF81297, SKF75670 | SCH23390 |
| *Endothelin Receptors* | | |
| $ET_A$ | — | Darusentan, J-0413, EMD-94246, LU-208075, BQ123, A127722, LU135252, SB234551, PD156707, FR139317 |
| $ET_B$ | [ALA[1,3,11,15]]ET-1, BQ3020, IRL1620, sarafotoxin S6c, BQ3020 | IRL2500, RES7011, BQ788, Ro468443, A192621 |
| $ET_{A or B}$ | ET-1, ET-2, ET-3 | Bosentan, TAK044, SB 234551 |
| *RAS Enzymes* | | |
| Renin | — | 3z, CGP60536B, SPP100, enalkiren |
| ACE | — | Captopril, enalapril, lisinopril, quinapril, ramipril |
| Chymase | — | BCEAB, NK3201 |
| ACE/NEP | — | Omapatrilat, SQ 28603, CGS 25115, Sch 39370, Sch 32615, CGS 26303 |
| *Angiotensin (AT) Receptors* | | |
| $AT_1$ | L163491 | EXP3174, eprosartan, valsartan, irbesartan, losartan |
| $AT_2$ | [p-NH$_2$-Phe[6]]-Ang II | PD123319, PD123177 |
| *Ion channels* | | |
| *Calcium (Ca2+) Channels* | | |
| L-type (Ca$_v$1.1-Ca$_v$1.4) | (−)-(S)-BAY8644, FPL64176, SDZ (+)-(S)-202791 | Nifedipine, diltiazem, verapamil, calciseptine |
| P-/Q-type (Ca$_v$2.1) | — | ω-Agatoxin IVA, ω-Agatoxin IVB |
| N-type (Ca$_v$2.2) | — | ω-Conotoxin GVIA, ω-Conotoxin MVIIC |
| T-type (Ca$_v$3.1-Ca$_v$ 3.3) | — | Ni$^{2+}$, flunarizine, kurtoxin, SB209712 |
| R-type (Ca$_v$2.3) | — | SNX482, Ni$^{2+}$ |
| *Potassium (K+) Channels* | | |
| $K_V$ | cAMP, NO | 4-AP, charybdotoxin, imperator toxin, 3,4-DAP, margatoxin |
| $BK_{Ca}$ | 17β-Estradiol, NS004, NS1619, DHS1, hydrochlorothiazide | Iberiotoxin, charybdotoxin, noxiustoxin, penitrem-A, TEA (triethylamine) |
| $K_{IR}$ | — | Gaboon viper venom, tetriapin, Mg$^{2+}$, Sr$^{2+}$, Ba$^{2+}$, Cs$^+$ |
| $K_{ATP}$ | Cromakalim, diazoxide, aprikalim, pinacidil, calcitonin gene-related peptide, norepinephrine, prostacyclin, (−)-MJ-451, minoxidil | Glibenclamide, tolbutamide, phentolamine, ciclazindol |

Data from references 7 to 30.

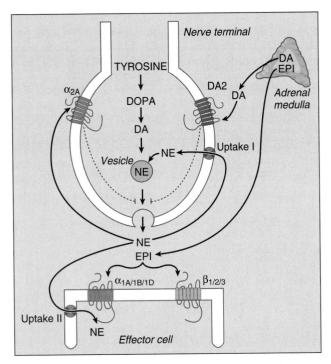

**FIGURE 30-1.** Sympathetic prejunctional and postjunctional neuroeffector events. Cytoplasmic enzymes mediating catecholamine biosynthesis (detailed in Fig. 30-2) catalyze the conversion of tyrosine to DOPA and dopamine (DA) and finally to the sympathetic neurotransmitter norepinephrine (NE), which is stored in vesicles. Arrival of an action potential at the sympathetic nerve terminal triggers fusion of the vesicle with the plasma membrane, resulting in exocytosis of NE (and other cotransmitters such as ATP and NPY; not shown). Most of the released NE, however, is taken back up into the prejunctional nerve terminal (via Uptake I) and either catabolized by MAO or restored in vesicles. Released NE activates postjunctional $\alpha_{1A/1B/1D}$- or $\beta_{1/2/3}$-adrenergic receptors on effector cells and prejunctional $\alpha_{2A}$-adrenergic receptors that negatively regulate exocytotic NE release *(dashed line)*. Some NE is taken up by the postjunctional effector cell (via Uptake II) and is rapidly metabolized by COMT to normetanephrine (not shown). Epinephrine (EPI) and dopamine released from the adrenal medulla activate postjunctional $\alpha_{1A/1B/1D}$-/$\beta_{1/2/3}$-adrenergic receptors at effector cells and prejunctional DA2 receptors, respectively; the latter inhibits the release of NE *(dashed line)*. (See color plate.)

terminals (via the uptake I transporter) and costored in vesicles with norepinephrine.[32]

Autonomic tone is determined by the balance between sympathetic and parasympathetic outflow via efferent nerves and is modulated by the nucleus tractus solitarius (in brainstem) in an integrated and reciprocal manner; inhibitory input from mechanoreceptors in the heart and aorta and carotid baroreceptors travel via afferent vagal nerves back to the central nervous system. Functional responses mediated by the sympathetic (e.g., vasoconstriction by $\alpha_1$-adrenergic receptors) and the parasympathetic nervous system (e.g., vasodilation by muscarinic $M_2$ receptors) in most cases are opposing (so-called physiologic or functional antagonists). Sympathetic nerve terminals express several distinct receptors subtypes, both prejunctionally and postjunctionally. Because these receptors often display opposite functional effects, differences in their distribution and sensitivity to circulating catecholamines allows regional modifications of

autonomic tone in specific organs and vascular beds and, thereby, a wide range of physiologic responses.

As detailed later, activation of vascular postjunctional $\alpha_1$-adrenergic receptors by locally released norepinephrine causes vasoconstriction.[7,33] By contrast, activation of $\alpha_2$-adrenergic receptors causes a biphasic blood pressure response, that is, an initial hypertensive response, mediated by postjunctional vascular $\alpha_2$-adrenergic receptors and followed by a decrease in blood pressure resulting from prejunctional $\alpha_2$-adrenergic receptor-mediated inhibition of norepinephrine release. Postjunctional $\beta_1$-adrenergic receptors are mainly located in the heart (ventricles and atria) and regulate moment-to-moment changes in heart rate and contractility, whereas activation of $\beta_2$- or $\beta_3$-adrenergic receptors on resistance vessels causes vasodilation.[7,33] Another $\beta$-adrenergic receptor subtype ($\beta_4$) has been identified but remains poorly characterized.

Because of these considerations and the central role of the sympathetic nervous system in blood pressure control and, possibly, in the pathogenesis of hypertension, it is not surprising that catecholamine synthesizing enzymes, uptake proteins, and receptors have been exploited as potential antihypertensive drug targets. Drugs acting at other sympathetically relevant targets, including ganglion-blocking agents (acetylcholine $N_1$ receptor antagonists, e.g., hexamethonium), adrenergic-neuronal blocking agents (e.g., guanethidine), and monoamine depletors (e.g., reserpine), have also been developed and are effective blood-pressure-lowering agents but are rarely used chronically because they not infrequently cause side effects.

## Enzymes

The enzymes involved in catecholamine biosynthesis are detailed in Figure 30-2. For a detailed consideration of the processes involved in the synthesis, storage, and release of catecholamines, the reader is referred to *Goodman & Gilman's: The Pharmacological Basis of Therapeutics.*[31]

Tyrosine hydroxylase, is a nonheme iron, tetrahydrobiopterin-dependent protein. It is the rate-limited enzyme in catecholamine biosynthesis and is found only in catecholamine-containing cells, where it is localized mainly in the cytoplasm.[34] Its activity is regulated by a wide variety of short- and long-term regulatory mechanisms, including dynamic changes in phosphorylation state,[35] and negative feedback mechanisms mediated by the catecholamine products. An early loss of tyrosine hydroxylase activity followed by a decline in protein expression is thought to contribute to the catecholamine (i.e., dopamine) deficiency and manifestations of Parkinson's disease.[36] Tyrosine hydroxylase has also been implicated in the pathophysiology of hypertension.[37] For example, its mRNA[38] and activity[39] are increased in the adrenal medulla and in distinct brain regions of different strains of hypertensive rats, particularly the medulla oblongata, an area important for blood pressure regulation and synthesis of catecholamines. Also, in cyclosporine-induced hypertensive rats, increased plasma and adrenal medullary levels of epinephrine and

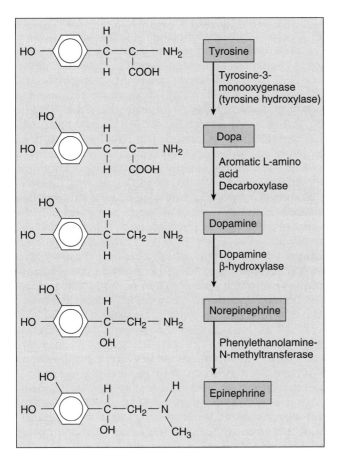

**FIGURE 30-2.** Enzymes involved in catecholamine biosynthesis. Note, tyrosine hydroxylase is rate limiting and is reciprocally regulated by norepinephrine, whereas phenylethanolamine-N-methyltransferase is present only in the adrenal medulla and central nervous system, the sites of epinephrine biosynthesis.

norepinephrine and increased tyrosine hydroxylase activity are normalized by administration of the specific tyrosine hydroxylase inhibitor α-methyl-p-tyrosine (metyrosine).[40,41] This agent is also of use in the management of refractory hypertension resulting from a malignant pheochromocytoma. Tyrosine hydroxylase antisense gene therapy has also been shown to lower blood pressure in spontaneously hypertensive rats.[42] However, there is no association between tyrosine hydroxylase polymorphisms (tetranucleotide TCAT and Val181-Met) and essential hypertension in humans.[34]

Although little is known about the role of the enzyme DOPA decarboxylase (aromatic L-amino acid decarboxylase) in the pathogenesis of hypertension,[43] selective inhibitors of the enzyme have been suggested to be effective in the treatment of essential hypertension.[44] In addition, this enzyme metabolizes the antihypertensive drug α-methyldopa to α-methyldopamine, which is then converted to α-methylnorepinephrine by dopamine β-oxidase. The latter metabolite lowers blood pressure by stimulating central α2-adrenergic receptors and thereby decreases adrenergic neuronal outflow from the brainstem. Oral administration of dopamine β-hydroxylase inhibitors, such as Nepicastat (RS-25560-197) and SK&F 102698, lowers plasma levels of norepinephrine (and

increases dopamine levels) and correspondingly lowers blood pressure in dogs and rats.[44,45] In humans, however, the therapeutic utility of dopamine β-hydroxylase inhibitors (disulfiram, FLA-63, SCH 10595, fusaric acid, BRL 8242, and SK&F 102698) has been hampered by low potency, lack of selectivity for dopamine β-hydroxylase, and toxic effects. Nevertheless, Nepicastat, which shows oral efficacy in heart failure patients,[44,45] may be useful for the treatment of hypertension.

The conversion of norepinephrine into epinephrine is mediated by phenylethanolamine N-methyltransferase (Fig. 30-2), which is predominantly found in chromaffin cells of the adrenal medulla and in certain hypothalamic and brainstem regions (e.g., rostral ventrolateral medulla), areas that play an important role in blood pressure homeostasis. At present, little is know about the role of this enzyme in hypertension. However, significant increases in its activity and epinephrine content have been observed in several hypertensive animal models.[46] Selective phenylethanolamine N-methyltransferase inhibitors (e.g., CGS 19281A, SK&F 64139) reduce enzyme activity and lower blood pressure in spontaneously hypertensive rats and deoxycorticosterone acetate-salt rat models of hypertension, suggesting it may be involved in the development and maintenance of hypertension.[46,47] However, further studies are required to validate this effect in humans.

Although nonselective inhibitors of MAO enzymes lower blood pressure, their use is limited by the risk of severe increase in blood pressure that occurs when treated patients ingest tyramine-containing foods.[48,49] Acute administration of selective MAO inhibitors, particularly those that are specific for the MAO-A enzyme, results in N-acetylation of pineal serotonin into N-acetylserotonin, which lowers blood pressure in spontaneously hypertensive rats.[49] Whether such agents will prove to be useful for the long-term treatment of essential hypertension remains unclear.

## Receptors

### α₁-Adrenergic Receptors

α₁-Adrenergic receptors have been one of the most widely studied of receptor families, because of their major importance in the control of blood pressure, blood flow, and a variety of other physiologic responses.[7,8,33] Although side effects have limited the use of nonselective α-blockers, selective α₁-adrenergic receptor antagonists (e.g., prazosin) have been widely used in the treatment of hypertension for several decades.[7]

#### *Molecular Characteristics of α₁-Adrenergic Receptor Subtypes*

Human $\alpha_{1A}$-, $\alpha_{1B}$-, and $\alpha_{1D}$-adrenergic receptors are encoded by distinct genes located on chromosomes 8, 5, and 20, respectively.[7,8] In addition, there is evidence, currently based entirely on pharmacologic criteria (low affinity for prazosin and other antagonists), for a fourth α₁-subtype designated as the $\alpha_{1L}$-receptor.[50] The cloned subtypes are all members of the biogenic amine family of

G-protein-coupled receptors. Like the light-activated photoreceptor rhodopsin,[51] $\alpha_1$-adrenergic receptors are single polypeptides (466, 515, and 561 amino acids in length, respectively) that contain seven transmembrane (TM)-spanning $\alpha$-helical domains linked by three intracellular and three extracellular loops.[52,53] Their N-termini are located extracellularly and their C-termini, intracellularly. Structure-function studies indicate that their $\alpha$-helical bundles cluster to form the ligand-binding pocket, whereas amino acids in the intracellular regions, particularly in the third intracellular loop, mediate interactions of the receptors with their cognate G-proteins and, thus, with signaling and regulatory pathways.[54] All three subtypes couple to phospholipase C and, thus, to $Ca^{2+}$-activation via members of the $G\alpha_{q/11}$ G-protein family. The $\alpha_{1B}$ and $\alpha_{1D}$ subtypes, but not the $\alpha_{1A}$ subtype, may also couple to phospholipase $\delta_1$ activation via $G_h$. In addition, $\alpha_1$-adrenergic receptors may increase intracellular $Ca^{2+}$ levels by enhancing $Ca^{2+}$ influx via both voltage-dependent and voltage-independent $Ca^{2+}$ channels and may augment arachidonic acid release and phospholipase D, MAP kinase, and rho kinase activation. None of these pathways downstream of the receptors have been targeted for antihypertensive drug development so far, although preliminary studies of rho kinase inhibition suggest that targeting this enzyme may result in effective blood pressure reduction.[55]

Binding of catecholamines to $\alpha_1$-adrenergic receptors involves an ionic interaction between the basic aliphatic nitrogen atom common to all sympathomimetic amines and an aspartate (Asp125 in the hamster $\alpha_{1B}$-adrenergic receptor) in the third TM-spanning segment (TMIII).[56,57] In the ground state, this TMIII aspartate forms a salt bridge with a lysine residue (Lys331 in the $\alpha_{1B}$-adrenergic receptor) in TMVII. Activation of $\alpha_1$-adrenergic receptors, as for rhodopsin, likely involves disruption of this ionic interaction. With $\alpha_1$-adrenergic receptors, this is due to competition between the catechol protonated amine and the TMVII lysine, which is just favored by the slightly more basic $pK_a$ of the protonated amine ($pK_a$ 11.0) versus the lysine ($pK_a$ 10.5) Thus, the TMIII aspartate serves as a counter ion and most likely is important for agonist binding and activation of all adrenergic receptors.[53] Agonist binding to $\alpha_1$-adrenergic receptors also involves H-bond interactions between the catechol *meta* hydroxyl moiety and a serine residues (Ser188, $\alpha_{1A}$-receptor numbering) in TMV, whereas an interaction between the *para* hydroxyl and another TMV serine (Ser192) contributes only minimally to receptor activation.[58] These interactions differ somewhat with those of $\beta_2$-adrenergic receptors, where binding of both hydroxyl groups to two TMV serines (Ser203 and Ser207) is required for receptor activation.[58,59] Moreover, because the interacting serines in the $\alpha_{1A}$-adrenergic receptor are separated by three residues, whereas those in the $\beta_2$-adrenergic receptor are separated by only two residues, docking of the catecholamine ring is in a more planar orientation in the former, being orientated by about 120 degrees to that in the $\beta_2$-adrenergic receptor.

This altered ring orientation may also contribute to other docking differences between these two classes of adrenergic receptors. For example, the well-characterized stereoselectivity of catecholamine binding and activation has been attributed, in part, to a hydrogen bond interaction between the chiral benzylic hydroxyl group attached to the $\beta$-carbon atom of catecholamines, and Asn293 in TMVI of the $\beta_2$-adrenergic receptor.[59,60] Although stereoselectivity of catecholamine binding and activation is preserved with $\alpha_1$-adrenergic receptors, the determinants of stereoselectivity have not been defined, and the Asn293 equivalent is replaced by a residue (leucine or methionine) lacking H-bonding potential.

A further important interaction, for both binding and activation, involves an aromatic bond between the catechol ring and a phenylalanine (Phe310 for the $\alpha_{1B}$-adrenergic receptor) in TMVI.[61] Aromatic bond interactions between two phenylalanines (Phe163 and Phe187) in TMIV and TMV, respectively, and the catechol ring have also been suggested to be important for agonist binding but not for activation, although binding with Phe163 may be indirect because this residue is replaced by a leucine in the $\alpha_{1B}$- and $\alpha_{1D}$-adrenergic receptors.

Residues critical for subtype-selective agonist recognition have been evaluated and, importantly, just two of the approximately 172 residues in the TM domains (Ala204 in TMV and Leu314 in TMVI, and Val185 in TMV and Met293 in TMVI of the $\alpha_{1B}$- and $\alpha_{1A}$-receptors, respectively) have been shown to account entirely for the selective agonist-binding profiles of the $\alpha_{1A}$- and $\alpha_{1B}$-subtypes.[60] In addition to the TMIII-TMVII salt bridge disruption mentioned previously, $\alpha_1$-adrenergic receptor activation involves movement of TMVI that is likely critical for the interaction between the intracellular third loop and the G-protein.[62]

Interactions between antagonists and $\alpha_1$-adrenergic receptors are less well defined, although recent elegant studies by Perez et al. have shown that the subtype selectivity of two $\alpha_{1A}$-antagonists, phentolamine and WB4101, results from interactions with three consecutive residues (Gly196, Val197 and Thr198) in the second extracellular loop.[53,63] Evidence from these investigators also indicates that antagonists are docked high in the binding pocket, close to the extracellular surface, and that two residues, Phe308 and Phe312, are critical for antagonist binding but not for the binding of phenethylamine agonists.[64] Furthermore, these residues are involved in the binding of all imidazoline agonists, and, thus, this class of ligands interacts differently with $\alpha_1$-adrenergic receptors than with native catecholamines or their derivatives—a finding that also explains the partial agonist activity of imidazoline compounds.

$\alpha_1$-Adrenergic receptors are subject to agonist-induced regulation that results in both short- and long-term desensitization of signaling.[65] These regulatory responses are mediated by agonist-induced conformational changes that lead to C-terminal tail receptor-phosphorylation, both by receptor-linked PKC and by G-protein-coupled receptor kinases, followed by the binding of arrestins and internalization by the clathrin pathway. These responses have been studied in most detail for the $\alpha_{1A}$- and $\alpha_{1B}$-receptors, whereas there is less information available for the $\alpha_{1D}$-subtype.[66,67] A coding region polymorphism has been identified for the $\alpha_{1A}$-adrenergic receptor that involves an arginine to cysteine change (Arg492-Cys) in an arginine-rich region of the C-terminal tail.[68] This polymorphic receptor is found with higher frequency in African Americans, but it is not associated with the phenotype of essential hypertension.[68] In addition, it is unclear if it alters receptor regulation or produces any other functional effects. Thus, currently there is no evidence to suggest that alteration in receptor regulation impacts either from a pathogenetic or from a pharmacodynamic point of view on the selection of $\alpha_{1A}$-adrenergic receptors as antihypertensive targets.

### Role of $\alpha_1$-Adrenergic Receptors in Hypertension

The major rationale for targeting $\alpha_1$-adrenergic receptors in the treatment of hypertension is their important role in mediating postjunctional sympathetic vasoconstrictor responses and, thus, in regulating peripheral resistance.[69] In this regard, it would be of interest to know which $\alpha_1$-subtype is the major regulator of blood pressure, because selective targeting of this subtype may lead to more specific therapies with fewer attendant side effects. To date, however, such efforts have been largely confined to animal studies, which may have limited applicability to humans and/or have produced conflicting results.[7,33] For example, consistent with findings in rodents,[47] clinical trials of $\alpha_{1A}$-selective blockers have implicated this subtype as a major regulator of blood pressure.[71,72] In contrast, Berkowitz et al.[73] have recently identified a factor in the plasma of a patient with sympathotonic orthostatic hypotension that selectively and irreversibly inhibits only the $\alpha_{1B}$-subtype, suggesting that this may be a major regulator of resistance in humans.[74] In addition, expression of the $\alpha_{1B}$-adrenergic receptor increases in the elderly at a time when hypertension is commonly manifested.[75] Thus, there is evidence for $\alpha_{1A}$- and $\alpha_{1B}$-adrenergic receptor involvement in blood pressure control in humans. Moreover, studies in the rat and in mouse knockout models indicate that the $\alpha_{1D}$-subtype can also play a role in blood pressure regulation.[53,66,76]

Studies of transgenic and knockout mouse models suggest that sympathetic regulation of vascular tone by the various $\alpha_1$-subtypes is complex and may involve cross-regulation of their contractile effects and/or of their expression. For example, inactivation of the $\alpha_{1A}$-adrenergic receptor resulted in a small but significant decrease in basal blood pressure and in pressor responses to the $\alpha_1$-agonist phenylephrine.[53] Inactivation of the $\alpha_{1D}$-adrenergic receptor, on the other hand, also partially impairs vasoconstrictor responses but without a change in basal blood pressure. Taken together with the findings that overexpression of the $\alpha_{1B}$-adrenergic receptor in transgenic mice does not increase systemic arterial blood pressure and that inactivation of this subtype results in only a very small attenuation of phenylephrine pressor responses with no change in basal blood pressure,[53] it could reasonably be suggested that the $\alpha_{1A}$- and $\alpha_{1D}$-receptors, but not the

$\alpha_{1B}$-receptor, are the mediators of contractile function in blood vessels. However, mice lacking either both the $\alpha_{1A}$- and $\alpha_{1B}$-receptors or both the $\alpha_{1B}$- and $\alpha_{1D}$-receptors show profound attenuation of phenylephrine pressor responses. Thus, the contribution of the $\alpha_{1B}$-subtype to vasoconstrictor mechanisms is complex but can be unmasked under appropriate circumstances. Clearly, further studies are required to fully elucidate the mechanisms involved, but if also relevant to humans, these findings bear importantly on the issue of exactly which individual subtypes, or which combinations of subtypes, should best be targeted to optimize antihypertensive activity.

### $\alpha_2$-Adrenergic Receptors and $I_1$ Imidazoline-Binding Sites

Drugs that activate $\alpha_2$-adrenergic receptors are effective antihypertensive agents.[33,77] However, their clinical use has waned considerably in recent years because of a high incidence of side effects, including drowsiness, dry mouth, and rebound hypertension with abrupt discontinuation of therapy. $\alpha_2$-Adrenergic agonists (e.g., clonidine) lower blood pressure predominantly by activating central nervous system sympathoinhibitory pathways to decrease sympathetic outflow and, thus, to reduce peripheral vascular resistance.

### Molecular Characteristics of $\alpha_2$-Adrenergic Receptors

Three distinct $\alpha_2$-adrenergic receptor subtypes have been cloned, and in humans the genes coding for $\alpha_{2A}$-, $\alpha_{2B}$- and $\alpha_{2C}$-adrenergic receptors are located on chromosomes 10, 2, and 4, respectively.[8,52] The $\alpha_{2A}$-adrenergic receptor mediates platelet aggregation, pancreatic β-cell insulin release, inhibition of lipolysis, and inhibition of neurotransmitter release from prejunctional nerve terminals, whereas the $\alpha_{2B}$-subtype mediates postjunctional smooth muscle vasoconstrictor responses. Physiologic functions mediated by the $\alpha_{2C}$-adrenergic receptor remain poorly characterized, although this subtype may also contribute to postjunctional regulation of vascular tone and prejunctional control of neurotransmitter release from cardiac sympathetic nerves and central neurons and to a variety of neurophysiologic effects.[7,33,78] Unlike $\alpha_1$-adrenergic receptor subtypes, which show no interspecies differences in ligand recognition, the human and porcine $\alpha_{2A}$-adrenergic receptors recognize some compounds, such as yohimbine and UK14,304, with higher affinity than their rodent (rat, mouse, and guinea pig) orthologs (also referred to as the $\alpha_{2D}$-adrenergic subtype, although for simplicity referred to here merely as the $\alpha_{2A}$-subtype).[79] This difference in ligand binding has been localized to a single cysteine residue (Cys201) in TMV, as compared with the rodent orthologs that contain a serine at the 201 position. Interspecies differences in ligand recognition, however, are not observed for the $\alpha_{2B}$- or $\alpha_{2C}$-subtypes. The molecular structure,[8,51] bonding interactions with catecholamines, and activation mechanisms of $\alpha_2$-adrenergic receptors likely resemble those of the $\alpha_1$-receptors.[56] Stereoselective binding of catecholamines may involve a serine in TMII (Ser90) and/or TMVII (Ser419) but not the TMVI residue equivalent to Asn293 that subserves this function in the $\beta_2$-adrenergic receptor.[80]

Activation of $\alpha_2$-adrenergic receptors results in inhibition of adenylyl cyclase activity and, thus, in reduced cAMP generation.[7,8] In addition, stimulation of $\alpha_2$-adrenergic receptors activates $K^+$ channels and inhibits voltage-gated $Ca^{2+}$ channels. These responses are mediated by receptor coupling to the heterotrimeric G-proteins, $G_i$ and $G_o$. Mutation of an aspartate in TMII (Asp79) to an asparagine (D79N point mutation) uncouples the $\alpha_{2A}$-adrenergic receptor from $K^+$ channel activation without altering its ability to inhibit cAMP generation or $Ca^{2+}$ channels.[81,82] $\alpha_{2A}$-Adrenergic receptors also activate MAP kinase; $Na^+$-$H^+$ exchange; and the $A_2$, D, and C isoforms of phospholipase. In vascular smooth muscle, these receptors induce contraction by activation of $Ca^{2+}$ channels, which enhances $Ca^{2+}$ entry into the cell.[33] Like $\alpha_1$-adrenergic receptors, the three $\alpha_2$-subtypes are differentially regulated by G-protein-coupled receptor kinase and arrestin mechanisms. Interestingly, in contrast to the $\alpha_{2A}$- and $\alpha_{2B}$-subtypes, the $\alpha_{2C}$-receptor is resistant to agonist-stimulated desensitization[83]; an effect that is most likely due to the lack of a serine-rich motif in its C-terminal tail. Polymorphisms of all three $\alpha_2$-subtypes have been identified.[84] One involving the noncoding region of the $\alpha_{2A}$-receptor has been reported to be associated with salt-sensitive hypertension in African Americans, although a functional mechanism explaining this association has yet to be defined. Coding region polymorphisms of $\alpha_{2A}$-, $\alpha_{2B}$-, and $\alpha_{2C}$-receptors have been functionally characterized following overexpression of the polymorphic receptors in heterologous cell systems.[33,84] They produce increased agonist-promoted receptor functioning, impaired phosphorylation and desensitization, and increased agonist sensitivity, respectively. Although these polymorphisms occur with increased frequency in African Americans, they are not associated with hypertension. Nevertheless, given their functional consequences, one can speculate that individuals harboring the $\alpha_{2A}$ polymorphism would be uniquely sensitive to the antihypertensive effects of centrally acting $\alpha_2$-agonists (e.g., clonidine), whereas those with the $\alpha_{2B}$ polymorphism would potentially be susceptible to severe rebound hypertension following abrupt cessation of such agents. Although these postulates require direct confirmation from clinical studies, they potentially represent important pharmacogenomic considerations in the management of hypertension.

### Role of $\alpha_2$-Adrenergic Receptors in Hypertension

In addition to central nervous system sympathoinhibition resulting from activation of $\alpha_2$-adrenergic receptors in the cardiovascular centers of the medulla oblongata, there is evidence that $\alpha_2$-agonists lower blood pressure by a peripheral mechanism involving prejunctional inhibition of neurotransmitter release.[9] Also, activation of endothelial $\alpha_2$-adrenergic receptors may oppose vascular smooth muscle $\alpha_2$-receptor constrictor responses by a nitric oxide (NO)-dependent mechanism.[85] The subtypes responsible for these and the many other physio-

logic effects of $\alpha_2$-adrenergic receptors have been difficult to determine because of the lack of highly subtype-selective agonists and antagonists. Nevertheless, the development of genetically engineered mouse lines that are deficient in a specific subtype have provided major insights. These receptor knockout models have confirmed that the major subtype mediating inhibition of sympathetic outflow is the $\alpha_{2A}$-adrenergic receptor, whereas that mediating vasoconstrictor response is the $\alpha_{2B}$-receptor.[33] Interestingly, cardiovascular responses to $\alpha_2$-agonists are largely unaltered in $\alpha_{2C}$ null mice.

### Potential Involvement of Imidazoline-Binding Sites

Several centrally acting antihypertensive drugs have been developed that are recognized with high affinity by the $I_1$ imidazoline receptor.[9,86] This receptor, whose structure has not been definitively identified, is expressed in the rostroventrolateral part of the brainstem.[9] It has been suggested that activation of $I_1$ imidazoline receptors lowers blood pressure by a mechanism independent of $\alpha_2$-adrenergic receptors. However, mice lacking the $\alpha_{2A}$-adrenergic receptor show no blood pressure reduction when treated with imidazoline-type agonists that also bind $\alpha_2$-receptors.[87] This suggests that drugs that have been developed to specifically target $I_1$ imidazoline receptors, lower blood pressure merely because they are nonselective and, thus, activate $\alpha_2$-mediated sympathoinhibitory pathways.[86]

### β-Adrenergic Receptors

Drugs that block β-adrenergic receptors have been used widely as first-line antihypertensive agents since the 1960s.[88,89] Their efficacy in this regard, however, was entirely unexpected, given that β-adrenergic receptors are major physiologic mediators of sympathetic vasodilator responses.[7,69,90] The mechanisms whereby they lower blood pressure are still poorly understood, and initiation of therapy increases peripheral vascular resistance, although this falls to, or below, normal with sustained treatment. Although inhibition of renin release and cardiac output resulting from blockade of β-adrenergic receptors in the kidney and heart[88,89,91] may contribute to their antihypertensive effect, blockade of prejunctional β-receptors that facilitate neurotransmitter release may also be importantly involved.[89]

### Molecular Characteristics of β-Adrenergic Receptors

Three distinct β-adrenergic receptor subtypes have been cloned: $\beta_1$-, $\beta_2$-, and $\beta_3$-adrenergic receptor; they are encoded by distinct genes located on human chromosomes 10, 5, and 8, respectively.[7,33,90,92] A fourth subtype has been suggested based on pharmacologic studies, but it has not yet been cloned and could represent a particular state of one of the known subtypes. The molecular structure, bonding interactions with catecholamines, and activation mechanisms of β-adrenergic receptors have been extensively studied and resemble those of the $\alpha_1$-adrenergic receptors and other members of the biogenic amine family of G-protein-coupled receptors.[92]

Like $\alpha_1$-adrenergic receptors, bonding with catecholamine ligands involves a salt-bridge interaction between the protonated amine of the ligand and an aspartate (Asp113, $\beta_2$-receptor numbering) in TMIII, H-bond interactions between the *meta* and *para* hydroxyl groups of catecholamines and serines (Ser204 and Ser207) in TMV, and interactions between the catechol ring and phenylalanine residues (Phe289 and Phe290) in TMVI.[53,59] Stereoselectivity of binding is due to an H-bond interaction between the chiral hydroxyl and Asn293 in TMVI. Although the interaction with the TMIII aspartate is preserved with $\beta$-antagonists, other interactions are not. Instead, they may interact with Asn312 in TMVII. Interestingly, $\beta$-adrenergic receptor agonists have been developed that produce prolonged receptor activation, by either being sequestered into a plasma membrane pool (because of the drug's marked hydrophobicity) that acts as a depot for their sustained slow release and receptor activation (e.g., formoterol) or by their hydrophobic tail targeting an additional specific binding site deep within the receptors' TM domains (e.g., salmeterol).[93] All $\beta$-adrenergic receptor subtypes activate adenylyl cyclase to generate cAMP via coupling to the G-protein $G_s$, although in certain tissues (e.g., human ventricle) the $\beta_3$-receptor can also couple to other effectors, such as $K^+$ channels, via $G_i$.[90,92] In the heart, cAMP generated by $\beta_1$- and, to a lesser extent, by $\beta_2$-adrenergic receptor activation results in enhanced protein kinase A activity. This augments $Ca^{2+}$ entry via phosphorylation of L-type $Ca^{2+}$ channels that, together with increased phosphorylation of troponin I, enhances contractility. In addition, protein kinase A mediated phosphorylation of phospholamban disinhibits the sarcoendoplasmic reticular $Na^+$-$K^+$-ATPase, resulting in enhanced $Ca^{2+}$ uptake into the sacroplasmic reticulum and, thus, in the lusitropic effects characteristic of cardiac $\beta$-receptor stimulation.[90] In vascular smooth muscle, $\beta$-receptor activation causes vasodilation via protein kinase A mediated phosphorylation of contractile proteins and by activation of $Ca^{2+}$-dependent $K^+$ channels. $\beta_3$-Adrenergic receptors, on the other hand, classically mediate lipolysis in brown adipose tissue.[90,92] As with other G-protein-coupled receptors, $\beta_1$- and $\beta_2$-adrenergic receptor expression and signaling is highly regulated, resulting in agonist-stimulated desensitization resulting from receptor-G-protein uncoupling, protein kinase A and G-protein-coupled receptor kinase-mediated receptor phosphorylation, arrestin binding, and sequestration via clathrin-coated pits.[92,94] In contrast, the absence of G-protein-coupled receptor kinase phosphorylation sites on $\beta_3$-receptors renders them resistant to desensitization. These subtype-specific physiologic responses and effects have been confirmed with the development and characterization of mouse knockout models.[92,95]

### The Role of β-Adrenergic Receptors in Hypertension

Despite the efficacy of $\beta$-antagonists in hypertension, evidence for the involvement of $\beta$-adrenergic receptors in the pathogenesis on essential hypertension is still scanty. It has been suggested that $\beta$-adrenergic receptor signaling is attenuated in cardiovascular tissues of hypertensive individuals and animals.[88,89] Similarly, the finding that isometric exercise increases peripheral resistance in hypertensive but not in normotensive subjects has been interpreted to suggest that $\beta$-receptor-mediated vasodilator responses are desensitized in hypertensive subjects.[69] This desensitization could be due to enhanced sympathetic tone and increased neurotransmitter release and/or to increased expression of G-protein-coupled receptor kinases that phosphorylate and desensitize $\beta$-adrenergic receptors.[69] Enhanced sympathetic activity in hypertensive patients may also contribute to $\beta$-adrenergic receptor desensitization by inducing oxidative stress.

Polymorphisms of all three $\beta$-adrenergic receptor subtypes have been reported, and some of these have been linked to essential hypertension.[96-99] However, in most instances these findings are merely associative and, thus far, provide little insight either into the potential mechanisms involved, or into the potential for these polymorphisms to attenuate or augment antihypertensive responses to drugs targeting $\beta$-adrenergic receptors.

### Dopamine Receptors

Dopamine receptors, particularly those expressed in peripheral tissues, are potentially attractive antihypertensive drug targets.[43,100] They mediate vasodilation (either by direct effects on vascular smooth muscle or by inhibition of neurotransmitter release from sympathetic nerve terminals) and promote natriuresis and diuresis by actions at the level of the renal tubules. In addition, peripheral dopamine receptors have been implicated in the pathogenesis of essential hypertension.[43] Nevertheless, the pharmacology of dopamine is complex. Low doses lower diastolic blood pressure and increase renal perfusion by activating peripheral dopamine D-A1 receptors. Intermediate doses increase heart rate and cardiac contractility by activation of $\beta$-adrenergic receptors. Higher doses cause $\alpha$-adrenergic receptor-mediated vasoconstriction and hypertension. Moreover, dopamine is a substrate for catabolism by both MAO and COMT and, thus, is ineffective orally.[101] Not surprisingly, therefore, no orally active agents that target dopamine receptors have been developed for the treatment of hypertension, although recently a dopamine D-A1 agonist, fenoldopam, has been approved for in-hospital, short-term management of severe hypertension.[102] For this reason, dopamine receptors are not considered here in detail. For detailed considerations of fenoldopam and dopamine receptors, the reader is referred to several excellent recent reviews.[43,100,103]

## ENDOTHELIN RECEPTORS

Endothelin (ET) is a potent vasoconstrictor that was initially isolated from cultured porcine aortic endothelial cells but is now known to be produced in most tissues.[10] ET plasma levels are elevated in hypertension, suggesting that ET plays a role in the pathogenesis of this disease.

## Molecular Characteristics of Endothelin Receptor

ET occurs as three related isopeptides (ET-1, ET-2, and ET-3).[10] These peptides are produced within the cells from a 212-amino-acid human precursor preproendothelin, which undergoes multiple proteolytic cleavage-processing events to form a 38-amino-acid intermediate-inactive big ET. The conversion of big ET-1 into the biologically active 21-amino-acid ET-1 is catalyzed by one or more unique type II zinc-binding metalloproteinases, known as endothelin-converting enzymes (ECE). Two isoforms of ECE exist: ECE-1 and ECE–2. The former occurs as four splice variants.[10] Although both proteases are implicated in big ET-1 processing, ECE-1 is the major enzyme responsible for this prohormone activation in vascular endothelial cells.[104]

In mammals, two distinct ET receptor subtypes have been cloned: $ET_A$ and $ET_B$ receptors. Their genes are located on chromosome 4 and 13, respectively. $ET_A$ (ET-1 = ET-2 > ET-3) and $ET_B$ (ET-1 = ET-2 = ET-3) receptors display differential binding profiles toward the three different ETs. The overall identity between the two mature proteins (with 427 and 442 residues, respectively) is between 55% and 64%, depending on the species studied.[105] Both $ET_A$ and $ET_B$ receptors belong to the superfamily of seven TM-spanning G-protein-coupled receptors.[51,106] The TM domains and cytoplasmic loops of $ET_A$ and $ET_B$ receptors have highly conserved regions. The N-terminal and extracellular domains exhibit differences in both length and amino acid sequence.[105] $ET_A$ receptors are mainly expressed in vascular smooth muscle, whereas $ET_B$ receptor mRNAs are abundant in endothelial cells; Naicker and Bhoola[105] provide a detailed mapping of their distribution in the kidneys and other tissues. ET-1 peptides activate complex, tightly regulated pathways of signal transduction that result in short-term (e.g., contraction, secretion) and long-term (e.g., mitogenesis) biologic actions. In Chinese hamster ovary cells, both $ET_A$ and $ET_B$ receptors are linked to the pertussis-toxin-insensitive $G_{\alpha q}$ pathways that stimulate phosphatidylinositol phosphate turnover and 1,2-diacylglycerol production and increase intracellular $Ca^{2+}$ concentrations.[107] They differ in their effects on the adenylyl-cyclase-dependent pathway: $ET_A$ receptor signals through $G_{\alpha s}$, to increase cAMP formation, whereas the $ET_B$ receptor attenuates forskolin-stimulated cAMP production, via $G_{\alpha i}$.[107] In turn, elevated levels of $Ca^{2+}$ and 1,2-diacylglycerol activate PKC. PKC mediates both short- and long-term events of ET.[105] ET can enhance phospholipase A activity, resulting in increased arachidonic acid derived mediators, such as prostaglandins and thromboxane, and it can activate the electroneutral $Na^+$-$K^+$ antiporter. Sarcolemmal $Na^+$-$K^+$ exchange has been demonstrated to sensitize cardiac myofilaments and to elevate intracellular $Ca^{2+}$ concentrations, thereby contributing to the inotropic activity of ET. Studies on chimeric $ET_A$ and $ET_B$ receptors aimed at elucidating the molecular basis of subtype-selective ligand binding has shown that TM regions I to IV and the first extracellular loop comprise a subdomain for $ET_A$ receptor antagonists, and critical binding determinants for $ET_B$ receptor agonists appear to reside in TM regions IV to VI. For example, Tyr129, located in the second TM region of the $ET_A$ receptor is a critical component for subtype-selectivity of ligands.[11] The extracellular N-terminus of $ET_A$ and $ET_B$ are not important for subtype specificity, but they are crucial for ET-1 binding. With regard to its mitogenic signaling, in addition to activating the serine/threonine-specific PKC, ET also activates S6 kinase that phosphorylates the sixth protein of the small ribosomal subunit.[105] The signaling capacity of ET receptors is fine-tuned by post-translational modifications that affect their structure and activity.[107] Moreover, palmitoylation of conserved cysteine residues in the cytosolic tail region of ET receptors is an absolute requirement for ET-1 promoted mitogenic activity in various cell types. The cytoplasmic tails of both ET receptors play decisive roles in the intracellular receptor internalization and recycling of these receptors.[109]

## Role of Endothelin and Its Receptors in Hypertension

ET peptides influence cardiac, renal, and endocrine functions and also cause cell proliferation and differentiation.[105] Several studies support the role of the ET system in the pathogenesis of hypertension.[10,106,109,110] Tissue and plasma ET-1 is increased in a number of cardiovascular disorders, including vasospasm and hypertension.[10] These findings suggest a therapeutic potential for compounds that antagonize ET receptors. In recent years, several peptide and nonpeptide antagonists, subtype selective or nonselective, have been developed.[10] One of such compounds is the nonpeptide mixed $ET_A$/$ET_B$ receptor antagonist, Ro 47-0203, later named bosentan.[106] Several *in vitro* and *in vivo* studies have demonstrated that bosentan inhibits vasoconstriction produced by ET-1, with a long duration of action.[106] In healthy individuals, administration of mixed $ET_A$/$ET_B$ receptor antagonists causes an increase in forearm blood flow and a small decrease in blood pressure, providing evidence that ET-1 is involved in regulating vascular tone.[10] However, chronic administration of bosentan has little effect on blood pressure in various animal models of hypertension.[106] The efficacy of bosentan (monotherapy) in experimental hypertension seems more apparent in the alleviation of the complications associated with hypertension, rather than in the (moderate) decrease in blood pressure. The beneficial effects of ET-receptor antagonists in experimental hypertension may be due to their role in the associated remodeling (e.g., decreased cardiac hypertrophy and fibrosis). In spontaneously hypertensive and normotensive rats, bosentan inhibits angiotensin-induced hypertension and renal structural alterations, the sympathetic nervous system, and secretor activity of adrenocortical cells.[106] In contrast to these findings from experimental animal studies, a clinical trial in essential hypertension demonstrated that bosentan reduced diastolic blood pressure to levels observed with the ACE inhibitor enalapril, although the dose of bosentan required was large (500 mg).

ET-receptor antagonism may be useful therapy in patients with salt-sensitive hypertension who have high circulating levels of ET-1.[111] Systemic infusion of ET-1 produces sustained renal vasoconstriction, which is often preceded by a transient vasodilator response possibly resulting from $ET_B$ receptor-mediated release of NO.[109] ET-1 also modulates ATP-sensitive $K^+$ channels and calcium-activated $K^+$ channels to produce vasodilation in certain vascular beds.[112] $ET_A$ receptors mediate vasoconstriction, proliferation, hypertrophy of cardiac myocytes, and positive inotropic and chronotropic effects.[11,106] Therefore, selective $ET_A$ receptor antagonists may be superior vasodilators,[113] because NO stimulation and vasodilation by $ET_B$ receptors remains unblocked. A wide range of selective, peptide and nonpeptide $ET_A$ receptor antagonists have been developed in recent years,[10,11] and clinical trials of such agents (e.g., darusentan, J-0413, EMD-94246, LU-208075) are ongoing in the treatment of hypertension.[10] On the other hand, $ET_B$ receptors, which are predominantly found in the brain, endothelium, and smooth muscle cells, mainly mediate endothelium-dependent vasodilation through the release of NO, prostacyclin, and adrenomedullin.[106,114] Adult $ET_B$-deficient mice exhibit elevated blood pressure. Furthermore, tonic activation of NO-coupled $ET_B$ receptors in the renal medulla causes natriuresis and diuresis and decreases blood pressure.[109] On the basis of the *in vitro* effects of $ET_B$ receptor agonists (S6c, IRL-1620), a number of studies have suggested the presence of two $ET_B$-receptor subtypes,[12] designated $ET_{B1}$ and $ET_{B2}$. $ET_{B1}$ receptors mediate vasodilation and can be regarded as "beneficial" in the treatment of hypertension, whereas stimulation of the putative $ET_{B2}$ receptor produces undesired effects, such as smooth muscle contraction.[114] *In vitro* and *in vivo* pharmacologic studies using the novel $ET_A/ET_{B2}$ receptor antagonist SB 234551 substantiated this hypothesis.[12] Because the $ET_B$ receptor may be an important target for hypertension therapy, it would also be of interest to determine the functional roles of the other two ET peptides (i.e., ET-2 and ET-3) and their role in blood pressure regulation. A preliminary search for candidate genes for hypertension has provided genetic and epidemiologic evidence supporting roles for ET-2 and ET-3 in perturbations of blood pressure homeostasis.[115] Finally, there could be therapeutic possibilities for ECE-inhibitors in hypertension, particularly those targeting ECE-1.

## MINERALOCORTICOID RECEPTORS

Aldosterone is a mineralocorticoid hormone that acts via cytoplasmically located mineralocorticoid receptors in epithelial cells (kidney, colon, and sweat glands) and in the central nervous system, on mononuclear leukocytes, on large blood vessels, and in the heart, to maintain electrolyte and blood pressure homeostasis.[116] Although aldosterone-sensitive sites in the distal nephron regulate only a small fraction of the filtered sodium load reabsorbed by the kidney, this final step in the sodium reabsorption process is a critical regulator of net salt balance. Not surprisingly, therefore, blockade of sodium reabsorption at this nephron site by mineralocorticoid receptor antagonists produces clinically

useful natriuretic and antihypertensive effects.[117,118] Drugs acting on this receptor pathway are, thus, widely used as adjuncts to blood pressure control and to the treatment of fluid retention states, such as congestive heart failure.

## Molecular Characteristics of Mineralocorticoid Receptors

Mineralocorticoid receptors, together with glucocorticoid receptors, belong to the steroid hormone receptor family of ligand-dependent transcription factors.[119] Both receptors bind cortisol (or corticosterone in rodents) with high affinity, whereas only the mineralocorticoid receptor binds aldosterone with high affinity.[119] Specificity is conferred by the enzyme 11β-hydroxysteroid dehydrogenase type 2 isoform, which converts cortisol to the less active cortisone, thus allowing aldosterone, which is present at much lower concentrations in the circulation, to bind to mineralocorticoid receptors.[120] The human mineralocorticoid receptor consists of (1) an N-terminal domain required for transcriptional activation, (2) a DNA-binding domain that binds to specific DNA sequences on target genes, and (3) a C-terminal ligand-binding domain.[120] The unbound receptor is inactive and is complexed with heat-shock proteins such as HSP70 and HSP90.[121,122] These are displaced as a result of a conformational change induced by the binding of aldosterone to the cytoplasmically located receptor. The activated receptor-complex then migrates to the nucleus, where it binds to target genes to initiate transcription. In addition to these genomic responses, aldosterone also triggers cellular responses that occur rapidly. These include changes in intracellular electrolytes and increases in intracellular calcium via the inositol 1,4,5 trisphosphate-signaling pathway, followed by intracellular alkalinization resulting from direct stimulation of plasma membrane $Na^+$-$H^+$ exchange.[121,122] Aldosterone and glucocorticoid hormones also regulate the expression of the α and β subunits of the $Na^+$-$K^+$-ATPase genes.[123] Aldosterone directly stimulates the activity of the $PKC_\alpha$ (but not $PKC_\delta$, $PKC_\varepsilon$, or $PKC_\zeta$), promoting PKC-dependent $Ca^{2+}$ entry through L-type $Ca^{2+}$ channels.[124] Intracellular alkalinization upregulates an ATP-dependent $K^+$ channel, which is involved in $K^+$ recycling to maintain the electrical driving force for $Na^+$ absorption, while inhibiting a $Ca^{2+}$-dependent $K^+$ channel that generates the charge balance for $Cl^-$ secretion.[124] Mice overexpressing human mineralocorticoid receptors show both renal (e.g., enlarged kidneys) and cardiac abnormalities (e.g., dilated cardiomyopathy, increased heart rate), although their blood pressure is normal.[125] Nevertheless, the physiologic relevance of these early nongenomic responses is still not completely understood.

## Role of Mineralocorticoid Receptors in Hypertension

The incident of mineralocorticoid excess hypertension is low, accounting for no more than 1% of hypertensive patients and occurring only rarely in the absence of hypokalaemia.[126] Nevertheless, essential hypertension patients often respond to treatments that interfere with mineralocorticoid actions, even though circulating levels of these steroids are within the normal range.[117] Increased circulating levels of aldosterone causes a wide variety of adverse cardiovascular responses, independent of the effects on blood pressure,[126] including left ventricle hypertrophy, impaired diastolic and systolic function, and salt and water retention, which can aggravate congestion in patients with established heart failure. In neonatal cardiomyocytes, aldosterone (but not corticosterone) can cause hypertrophy by mineralocorticoid receptor activation.[118] Continuous intracerebroventricular infusion of aldosterone, at doses devoid of pressor effects when administered systemically, increases resting blood pressure; an effect that is blocked by intracerebroventricular infusion of a mineralocorticoid receptor antagonist (RU28318).[117]

## RENIN ANGIOTENSIN SYSTEM

Drugs that interfere with the renin angiotensin system (RAS) are important in the treatment of several cardiovascular diseases, including hypertension and heart failure.[13,127] The active component of RAS is the octapeptide hormone angiotensin II (AngII), which elicits a variety of effects including vasoconstriction; dipsogenesis; increased cardiac contractility; and the release of catecholamines from nerve endings, aldosterone from the adrenal gland, and vasopressin from the posterior pituitary resulting in renal sodium and water reabsorption.[13,14]

AngII is produced systemically via the classical or renal RAS and locally via the tissue RAS. In the circulatory system, renal-derived renin cleaves hepatic-derived angiotensinogen at its N-terminus to form the inactive decapeptide angiotensin I (AngI). (Fig. 30-3). AngI is subsequently converted to AngII by endothelial and circulating ACE. Most known effects of AngII are due to an action on specific angiotensin receptors (AT receptors) (Fig. 30-3). Ninety percent of total ACE is localized in tissues and ACE-dependent conversion of AngI into AngII is thought to occur locally within tissues and their blood vessels.[15] In addition to ACE-dependent AngII generation, non-ACE pathways have also been identified (e.g., by the chymotrypsin-like serine protease, chymase [Fig. 30-3], which has been identified in various human tissues).[13,127,128] Conceptually, antihypertensive drugs targeting the RAS could be developed that (1) inhibit renin, (2) inhibit ACE and chymase, or (3) block the AT$_1$ receptor.[129] Inhibition of renin should afford effective suppression of the RAS, because this enzyme initiates the RAS cascade. Moreover, following AngI production, multiple pathways are used to generate AngII, and AngII has multiple receptor targets.[16] Despite the established clinical efficacy of renin inhibitors, almost all renin inhibitor-development projects have been discontinued because of low oral bioavailability, rapid biliary elimination, and the expense of making complex renin inhibitor molecules. Neutral endopeptidase (NEP 24.11) is an endothelial cell surface metalloprotease similar to ACE that

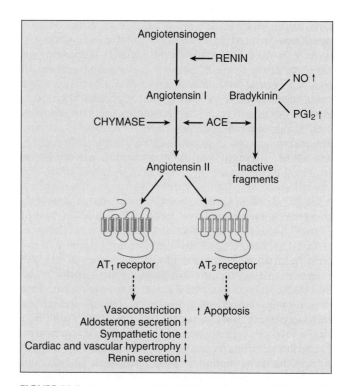

**FIGURE 30-3.** Components of the RAS and their main effects on the cardiovascular system. Renin catalyzes the cleavage of the hepatic-derived $\alpha_2$-macroglobulin angiotensinogen, into inactive angiotensin I, which is subsequently converted to active hormone angiotensin II by both ACE and chymase. ACE also degrades bradykinin into inactive fragments, thereby preventing bradykinin-induced increases in the vasodilators NO and prostacyclin (PGI$_2$). Most known effects of angiotensin II are due to activation of specific AT receptors, namely AT$_1$ and AT$_2$ receptors.

mediates the degradation of atrial natriuretic peptides. Therefore, combined ACE/NEP inhibitors, also called vasopeptidase inhibitors (e.g., omapatrilat), decrease the production of AngII and in parallel enhance the levels of vasodilator natriuretic peptides, thus producing vasodilation and natriuresis.

The following sections discuss the molecular aspects and potential therapeutic role of the RAS-based molecular targets (i.e., both enzymes and receptors) that are involved in the potential pathophysiologic role of AngII in hypertension. Because of the development of combined ACE/NEP inhibitors as a novel class of antihypertensive agents, we have included NEP as a molecular target in this section on RAS.

## Enzymes

### Renin

Renin (EC 3.4.23.15), elaborated by the juxtaglomerular cell of the kidney, catalyzes the first and rate-limiting step in the RAS cascade to produce AngI, which is then further processed by ACE and chymase to generate AngII[129] (Fig. 30-3). Renin is an aspartic proteinase and contains two aspartates (Asp32 and Asp215) that are essential for catalytic activity.[130] The gene and cDNA encoding human renin has been cloned.[131] Sequence analysis of the human renin precursor cDNA predicts a

406-residue polypeptide containing a 20- and 46-residue presegment and prosegment, respectively. Renin orthologs are found in all mammals studied. Renin efficiently cleaves the Leu10-Val11 bond in angiotensinogen at neutral pH; this action of renin is atypical because other aspartic proteinases are optimal at acidic pH. Although there is a high degree of complementarity in the renin-angiotensinogen reaction in a given species, renin from one species is often unable to hydrolyze angiotensinogen from another species. Thus, renin inhibitors show an unusually high level of species specificity.

The x-ray crystal structure of recombinant human renin has been solved.[132,133] Human renin consists of two mainly β-sheet domains related by an approximately twofold axis passing between the catalytic aspartates. The active-site cleft is located between these two domains and extends over eight to nine residues of the respective substrate.[130] In aspartic proteinases, the common catalytic mechanism involves substrate hydrolysis in which water stereospecifically attacks the carbonyl of the scissile amide bond and the aspartate moieties act as anchors, mediating the appropriate proton transfer.[129] A prominent structural feature of aspartic proteinases is the β-hairpin ("flap") in the N-terminal lobe that partially covers the active site and plays an important role in substrate-inhibitor binding and substrate catalysis. In inhibitor-bound renins, each subunit provides and equivalent flap that closes down on top of the inhibitor. Specificity determining residues in human and mouse renins are used to recognize P4 to P3′ substrate and inhibitor residues, and these P-S and P′-S′ interactions are the basis for the high degree of observed specificity. Use of these extended specificity-determining interactions have lead to the development of large and complex renin inhibitors, which are highly specific, but have added to their manufacturing costs. A study of renin-inhibitor complexes shows that even minor alterations in the positions of secondary structural elements can lead to major changes in ligand-binding. Therefore, understanding active-site organization has allowed the development of small, nonpeptidic renin inhibitors with high oral efficacy.[129] To date, the most potent human renin inhibitor has an $IC_{50}$ of 10 pM.[129] Sarma et al.[134] recently described cyclic peptides with renin inhibitor activity; however, their oral efficacy has not yet been tested.

Nonpeptidic renin inhibitors (e.g., 3z, CGP60536B, SPP100[16-18]), which produce potent and long-lasting reductions in blood pressure after oral administration to animals and humans, may ultimately prove to be useful antihypertensive agents. Human renal vasodilator response to the renin inhibitor enalkiren exceeded results observed with ACE inhibitors,[129] suggesting that such agents may be useful for treating in cardiovascular diseases. The outcomes of larger clinical trials of these compounds in humans are awaited with great interest.

## ACE

In mammals, ACE has two isoforms. These isoforms arise from a common gene because of alternate transla-

tion initiation sites.[135] Somatic ACE (sACE), an isoform that is also referred to as pulmonary ACE (ACE-P), is found in endothelial, epithelial, and neuronal cells and has a molecular weight of 170 kd. The other isoform, known as germinal ACE (gACE) or testicular ACE (ACE-T), has a molecular weight of 70 kd.

ACE is a type I membrane protein with a large extracellular domain, a single TM domain, and a small cytoplasmic tail domain (Fig. 30-4). In sACE, the extracellular domain consists of two homologous independently active catalytic domains, N and C, that are likely to have arisen from an ancient gene duplication event.[15] In contrast, germinal ACE has a single catalytic domain that is identical to the C-terminal catalytic domain of somatic ACE. The N- and C-domains contain a zinc-binding motif, HEXXH, that is a characteristic of gluzincin metalloproteases. Two glutamate residues, Glu389 and Glu987, in the N- and C-domains, respectively, form the third zinc-coordinating residue of each domain. The enzyme transition state is stabilized by an interaction between the substrate or inhibitor and the coordinated zinc and between the substrate or inhibitor and two histidine residues, His491 and His1089, of the N- and C-domains, respectively.[136] These interactions that stabilize the transition state are critical for catalysis and for high-affinity binding of sulfhydryl-, carboxyl-, or phosphinyl-group containing transition-state inhibitors.

ACE cleaves dipeptides from the C-terminus of polypeptide substrates with a free C-terminal carboxyl group. However, both tripeptides and dipeptides are usually cleaved from peptide substrates with an aminated C-terminus. Both the N- and C-domains of ACE convert AngI to AngII (although the C-domain is somewhat more efficient in this reaction) and degrade bradykinin into inactive fragments.[137] There are more notable differences in substrate specificity between domains, as recently illustrated by the finding of a much

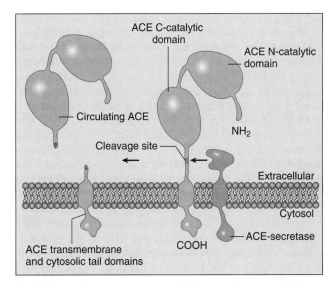

**FIGURE 30-4.** Schematic showing the cleavage of the somatic form of ACE by ACE-secretase. Both ACE-secretase and its substrate ACE are embedded in the same lipid bilayer. ACE-secretase cleaves ACE in its membrane-proximal stalk region, generating the soluble, circulating form of ACE. (See color plate.)

higher specificity of the N-domain, compared with the C-domain, for the inactivation of AcSDKP, an inhibitor of hematopoietic stem cell proliferation.[138] Such differences in domain specificity have been exploited to produce an N-domain-specific inhibitor.[139]

Activation by monovalent anions, particularly chloride, is a property of ACE that is unique among metalloproteases.[140] The effect of chloride on catalysis is substrate-, domain-, and species-dependent. Chloride binding, which is associated with an increase in substrate hydrolysis, is generally of higher affinity with larger substrates, and with substrates with a P2′ basic residue.[141] However, the mechanisms that determine why the hydrolysis of some substrates is greatly enhanced by chloride, whereas those of others are minimally affected, remain unknown. Site-directed mutagenesis studies have shown that a conserved arginine in the ACE C-domain (Arg1098) and the N-domain (Arg500) is critical for the chloride-enzyme interaction that leads to enzyme activation.[141] It is postulated that chloride disrupts the intramolecular interaction involving Arg1098 that keeps the enzyme in a low-affinity state and that chloride-substrate interactions are more important for the hydrolysis of short substrates than for the larger AngI.

The occurrence of two catalytic domains in somatic ACE was not appreciated before the development of several clinically used ACE inhibitors. Notable differences in affinity of ACE inhibitors for the N- and C-domain are now apparent, particularly with more highly optimized inhibitors such as quinaprilat. However, the importance of these differences in therapeutics remains to be delineated and exploited. Physical properties, such as lipophilicity, also appear to be important in increasing the half-life of the inhibitor at its membrane site of action in tissues; this physical property is likely to be the basis of the "tissue selectivity" that has been claimed by several manufacturers for certain ACE inhibitors.[142] Because most ACE is found associated with the plasma membrane, tissue selectivity in ACE inhibition is naturally important to achieve sustained inhibition, but it does not necessarily imply that the primary high affinity of an ACE inhibitor for ACE is different depending on whether the ACE is membrane anchored or in the circulation, following cleavage secretion by the membrane bound ACE secretase (Fig. 30-4).

ACE inhibition is a well-established treatment for hypertension and heart failure.[144-146] The mechanisms involved in the vasculoprotective effects of ACE inhibitors appear in large part to be related to their effects on endothelial function. The endothelium is a source of paracrine mediators such as NO, endothelium-derived hyperpolarizing factor, and ET. Many circulatory mediators, including AngII, regulate the release of these substances. On the other hand, the natriuretic peptide system, consisting of atrial and brain natriuretic peptides, counteracts the responses to activation of RAS and ET, by producing a wide range of responses, particularly vasodilation. ACE degrades bradykinin, a known stimulator of the L-arginine (NO-donor) and cyclo-oxygenase pathways.[146] Therefore, ACE inhibitors not only decrease the production of the potent vasoconstrictor AngII (which also has proliferative properties) but also diminish the degradation of bradykinin and, in turn, increase the production of NO and prostacyclin.[147] In normal and hypertensive rats and in several human isolated blood vessels, improved endothelial function has been observed with ACE inhibitors, in part because of decreased degradation of bradykinin and enhanced NO production.[146] Also, in the human forearm circulation, ACE inhibition enhances arterial vasodilation in healthy volunteers and in patients with hypertension.[143-145] A wide range of large, randomized clinical trials for hypertension have confirmed the favorable effect of ACE inhibitors (e.g., lowering of systemic vascular resistance without a compensatory tachycardia and enhanced natriuresis).[144-146,148] However, interestingly, a substantial number of hypertensive patients are not adequately controlled with ACE inhibitors alone and need combined therapy with diuretics or β-blockers and/or $Ca^{2+}$ channel blockers.

## Chymase

The inability of ACE inhibitors to chronically suppress plasma AngII levels and to completely inhibit AngI to AngII conversion in isolated human and dog tissue preparations led to a search for an AngII-forming enzyme other than ACE.[149] This resulted in the identification of chymase as the major AngII-forming enzyme in the human heart and blood vessels.[150] Chymase, a 30-kd chymotrypsin-like serine protease, is found in all mammals studied. It is chiefly elaborated by mast cells where it is stored in secretory granules that also contain heparin proteoglycans, histamine, and tryptases. Chymase is synthesized as a zymogen but is stored in an active form after proteolytic activation by dipeptidylpeptidase I. Not all mast cells in humans contain chymase; thus, chymase is a marker for a subset of mast cells known as $MC_{TC}$ cells.[151]

In humans, there is a single chymase gene that encodes α-chymase. Human α-chymase orthologs are found in all mammals. Some mammals, particularly rodents, also contain one or more chymases that are phylogenetically distinct from α-chymases and are known as β-chymase. β-Chymase encoding genes could simply be paralogous with no distinct counterpart in rodents or, alternatively, could be orthologous genes.[149] Human chymase has several structural similarities with other mammalian chymases, for example, a conserved acidic two-residue propeptide and the presence of a catalytic triad (Ser184, His47, Asp91) that is found in all members the trypsin superfamily of serine proteases.

All chymases show a preference for a $P_1$-Tyr, $P_1$-Phe, or $P_1$-Trp.[152,153] Because AngI has two hydrophobic aromatic residues, one (Phe8) serves as a specificity-determining residue for chymase-dependent formation of AngII, whereas the other (Tyr4) serves as a specificity determining residue for chymase-dependent AngII degradation. Thus, the preference of a given chymase for one cleavage site over the other in AngI can determine if that chymase is an AngII-forming enzyme or an angiotensinase. Human chymase has an unusually high specificity for cleavage after the Phe8 residue in AngI, resulting in an approximately 1000-fold preference for AngII-forming activity over angiotensinase activity.[154] This high specificity is due to the extended substrate-binding site in human chymase that serves to favor $P_1$ hydrophobic aromatic residues within a sequence context. This context is found around the Phe8 residue in AngI. Primate and dog α-chymases are highly efficient AngII-forming enzymes with negligible angiotensinase activity. It remains to be determined if rodent α-chymases have a similar specificity to the primate enzymes. However, β-chymases discriminate much less (<20-fold) between the two cleavage sites in AngI, and some chymases (e.g., rat chymase-1) have high angiotensinase activity with negligible AngII-forming activity.[154] Recent studies suggest that chymases may also play a role in immune and inflammatory responses by hydrolyzing a variety of polypeptides—albeit at lower efficiencies than for AngII formation—including extracellular matrix proteins, vasoactive peptides, cytokines, metalloproteases, and lipoproteins.[151]

*In situ* hybridization and electron microscope immunohistochemical studies in the human heart indicate that chymase is mainly synthesized and stored in mast cells, but endothelial cells and other types of interstitial cells may also elaborate chymase.[128] Chymase activation in human cells other than mast cells has not been shown. In the human heart, chymase is mainly localized in the interstitial space associated with the interstitial matrix.[128] This association is proposed to be due to charge-charge interactions because chymase is highly basic and many matrix proteins are highly acidic. Microdialysis experiments in the dog not only support a physiologic role of the non-ACE pathway in AngII formation but also directly show that this pathway is compartmentalized in the heart such that circulating angiotensins cannot easily access the cardiac interstitial compartment.[155] Interestingly, acute ACE inhibition studies show that in the lumen of blood vessels, AngII formation is mainly due to ACE, whereas both ACE and non-ACE pathways are important in regulating AngII levels in the cardiac interstitial space. This implies that AngII-forming enzyme systems are compartment specific.

Chymase represents a novel drug target in the treatment of cardiovascular disease, particularly in situations in which interference with the RAS has yielded therapeutic advantage.[149] It has been shown that rat vascular chymase mRNA is increased in spontaneously hypertensive rats, compared with Wistar-Kyoto normotensive rats,[156] and chymase overexpression in blood vessels leads to hypertension.[157] Studies with human blood vessels *in vivo* further suggest that chymase is involved in generating AngII.[158,159] These findings seem very promising; however, studies with specific chymase inhibitors (BCEAB[19] or NK3201[20]) in hypertensive patients are required for proof. The role of chymase inhibition in cardiac remodeling associated with pressure and volume overload, and in coronary artery restenosis is, now being explored and could also prove to be important in the management of heart and vascular diseases. Chymase

inhibitors are now becoming available for preclinical studies, but, based on specificity differences between chymases, it is to be expected that these inhibitors will be species and subtype specific.

## Neutral Endopeptidase

Neutral endopeptidase (NEP 24.11; EC 3.4.24.11), also known as neprilysin, atriopeptidase, or enkephalinase, is an abundant, zinc-containing metalloendopeptidase.[21,160] Isolation and characterization of the human NEP gene shows that it consists of 24 exons spanning more than 80 kb. Roques et al.[161] provide a detailed consideration of the distribution of NEP in the central and peripheral nervous systems. Several studies have focused on the structure of the active site of NEP, and, strikingly, most of the active-site amino acids present in related zinc endopeptidases (such as thermolysin) have been preserved in NEP. These include three zinc-coordinating residues (His583, His587, and Glu646).[22] Other residues that stabilize the enzyme-substrate complex (e.g., Glu583) Asn542, Arg747, and Arg102 are also important for substrate binding. NEP preferentially cleaves peptide bonds on the amino side of hydrophobic residues such as Phe, and much of this specificity is due to interactions with a hydrophobic pocket.[22] These and other studies stimulated the development of selective NEP inhibitors, such as several dipeptides, sulfhydryl based inhibitors (e.g., SQ 28603, CGS 25115), carboxyl acid inhibitors (e.g., Sch 39370), hydroxamic acid inhibitors (Sch 32615), or phosphorus-based inhibitors (e.g., CGS 26303).[22]

A new treatment of hypertension has recently been introduced within the class of vasopeptidase inhibitors, of which omapatrilat (BMS-186176) is representative.[21,23] Omapatrilat potently inhibits ACE and NEP. Although ACE inhibitors are very effective in some animal models (e.g., renin-dependent and spontaneously hypertensive rat models), they are not effective in others (e.g., DOCA-salt hypertensive rats). NEP inhibitors are effective in DOCA-salt hypersensitive rats but not in spontaneously hypertensive rats.[21,23] These findings suggest that combination treatment would be more effective in the treatment of hypertensive patients. The synergism of such a combination of both ACE and NEP has been confirmed in several animal hypertension models and in hypertensive patients.[23,162,163] In patients with heart failure, it has been demonstrated that acute administration of omapatrilat, with or without a diuretic, results in more beneficial cardiorenal and humoral effects than does an ACE inhibitor with a diuretic; this difference may be due to the potentiation of natriuretic peptides by omapatrilat.[164] Although the underlying mechanisms of the beneficial effects are not completely understood, combined NEP/ACE inhibition may represent an important new approach in the treatment of hypertensive vascular diseases. Experience with omapatrilat, the most clinically advanced of these drugs, has shown it to be more effective than currently available ACE inhibitors or other widely used antihypertensive agents.[21]

## Angiotensin Receptors

The actions of AngII in cardiovascular and renal tissues are almost exclusively mediated by specific AT receptors. Therefore, approaches to the development of antihypertensive drugs have included AT receptor antagonism. A wide variety of potent nonpeptide angiotensin $AT_1$ receptors antagonists (e.g., losartan) have been developed and have proved to be highly effective in the treatment of hypertension.[13]

In mammals, AngII mediates its effects via at least two high-affinity plasma membrane receptors, $AT_1$ and $AT_2$. These receptors have been cloned and their genes ($at_1$ and $at_2$) are mapped to chromosome 3 and Xq22-q2, respectively.[13] In rats and mice, $AT_1$ receptors occur as two subtypes $AT_{1A}$ and $AT_{1B}$, which are highly homologous and have identical pharmacologic properties but have distinct patterns of tissue distribution. In rats, these genes are mapped to chromosome 17 and 2, respectively. $AT_1$ (359 amino acids) and $AT_2$ (363 amino acids) receptors are members of the seven TM-spanning G-protein-coupled receptor superfamily. $AT_1$ receptors occur in blood vessels, heart, kidney, adrenal gland, ovary, testis, liver, brain, and lungs. $AT_1$ receptor mediates virtually all of the known cardiovascular, renal, neuronal, endocrine, and hepatic actions of AngII, including vasoconstriction, aldosterone release, catecholamine release, and the positive inotropic effect.[13,14] Two other AT receptors, $AT_3$ and $AT_4$, have been described.[13,14] $AT_3$ was prematurely designated in the original classification and is not considered further here. $AT_4$, which binds AngII– (3-8), but not AngII, with high affinity was initially thought to be a receptor, but more recent studies indicate that it is an enzyme, namely insulin-regulated aminopeptidase (IRAP).[166] IRAP is a type II integral membrane protein with a large extracellular catalytic domain. The catalytic domain belongs to the metalloprotease family and contains a zinc-binding HEXXH motif. AngII– (3-8) likely functions by inhibiting the degradation of physiologic substrates of IRAP. Because AngII– (3-8) is an inhibitor for IRAP, the interaction cannot be considered as a typical hormone-receptor interaction and is not further considered here.

$AT_1$ receptors are primarily coupled through pertussis-toxin-insensitive $G_q$-protein to the activation of phospholipase C and $Ca^{2+}$ signaling.[13,14] Other effector systems coupled to the $AT_1$ receptor include phospholipase D; phospholipase $A_2$; adenylyl cyclase; and ion channels, such as L- and T-type voltage-sensitive $Ca^{2+}$ channels. As shown for other G-protein-coupled receptors, internalization of $AT_1$ receptors involves receptor phosphorylation by G-protein receptor kinases at specific serine (Ser338) and threonine residues (Thr332, Thr302, Thr312, Thr319, and Thr339) in cytoplasmic loops and the C-terminus.[166] Subsequent to internalization, the receptor is recycled back to the cell surface or degraded in lysosomes.[14]

$AT_2$ receptors are ubiquitously expressed in the developing fetus, and their expression decreases rapidly after birth.[14] A possible role for this receptor has been suggested in fetal development and organ morphogenesis, but the finding that development is unaltered in $AT_2$ null mice questions this view. There is no evidence

for $AT_2$ receptor subtypes, and there is little homology between $AT_2$ and either $AT_{1A}$ or $AT_{1B}$ receptors.[14] However, several $AT_1$ receptor residues that specifically interact with AngII are preserved in the $AT_2$ receptor. These include the C-terminal carboxylate-docking Lys ($AT_1$-Lys199 and its equivalent $AT_2$-Lys215), the AngII-Arg2-binding Asp ($AT_1$-Asp281 and its equivalent $AT_2$-Asp297), and the AngII-Tyr4 interacting Asn ($AT_1$-Asn111 and its equivalent $AT_2$-Asn127).[167,168] The AngII-Asp1-binding His183 in $AT_1$ is an Ala (Ala198) in the $AT_2$ receptor and could explain why the $AT_1$ receptor, but not the $AT_2$, can differentiate between AngII and des-Asp1-AngII (i.e., AngIII) binding.[167]

Inroads have recently been made in defining the signaling pathways and the functional role of $AT_2$ receptors; de Gasparo et al.[14] recently reviewed these topics. It has been reported that under physiologic conditions, $AT_2$ receptors antagonize $AT_1$-mediated proliferate responses by inhibiting cell growth and by inducing apoptosis (Fig. 30-3) and vasodilation (via NO and cGMP).[127,169] $AT_2$ receptor-specific agonists or antagonists have not yet been developed for clinical use.

Several studies have shown that vascular reactivity to AngII is enhanced in experimental and human hypertension.[13,170] Moreover, experimental and clinical studies demonstrate that ACE inhibitors and $AT_1$ receptor antagonists effectively lower blood pressure and associated cardiovascular effects involved in hypertension (e.g., cardiac and vascular remodeling). Enhanced mRNA expression for $AT_1$ and $AT_2$ receptors has been reported in aortic vessels from adult spontaneously hypertensive rats, compared with age-matched normotensive Wistar-Kyoto rats.[171] In contrast to the hypertension and impaired vascular responses observed in $AT_1$ receptor null mice, knockout of the $AT_2$ receptor leads to small elevation of blood pressure and increased vascular sensitivity to AngII.[172] Thus, the $AT_2$ receptor may exert a protective role in blood pressure regulation by opposing the function of the $AT_1$ receptor. The underlying mechanism of this $AT_2$-mediated response is poorly understood but could involve NO and cGMP pathways. As described by Touyz and Schiffrin,[13] the hyperresponsiveness of AngII in hypertension may be due to enhanced signaling (e.g., through a decrease in receptor desensitization) or to increased expression of G-protein-coupled receptor kinases (GRKs).

Signal transduction mechanisms mediating the pathophysiologic actions of AngII in hypertension have been reviewed.[13] Short-term signaling events include (1) increased AngII-induced stimulation of the phospholipase C-$IP_3$-diacylglycerol pathway, resulting in increased $Ca^{2+}$ levels and (2) an increased magnitude of AngII-induced reduction of vascular $[Mg^{2+}]$, and $[Na^+]_i$ resulting in increased $Na^+$-$Ca^{2+}$ exchanger activity, increased $Na^+$ influx, increased activation of the $Na^+$-$H^+$-exchanger (NHE), and alterations in the activity of $Na^+$-$K^+$-ATPase pump. Long-term signaling events include (1) AngII-induced production of reactive oxygen species (superoxide anions) that contribute to AngII-induced hypertrophy in hypertension. Treatment of AngII-induced hypertensive rats with liposome-encapsulated superoxide dismutase markedly decreased blood pressure and enhanced responses to vasodilators; (2) increased basal and AngII-induced activation of tyrosine kinases (JAK/STAT) and ERKs, which are involved in AngII-induced vascular and cardiac remodeling in hypertension; (3) increased AngII-mediated mitogen-activated protein kinase signaling, resulting in an enhanced growth of smooth muscle cells and increased vascular contractility in hypertension; and (4) regulation of other vasoconstrictor substances such as ET, growth factors TGF-$\beta_1$ and PDGF-A, or cytokines such as TNF-$\alpha$.

Clinical trials with $AT_1$ receptor blockers (e.g., losartan) have demonstrated improved morbidity and mortality in hypertension, congestive heart failure, and myocardial infarction.[13,173,174] However, as discussed by Csikos et al.,[175] this effect may not be entirely mediated by $AT_1$ receptor blockade, because the increased plasma levels of renin and angiotensins that occur after $AT_1$ blockade enhance $AT_2$ receptor-mediated vasodilation and other associated vascular structural and growth responses (see previous discussion).[175] In elderly patients with heart failure, treatment with losartan is also associated with a lower mortality rate than that found with the ACE inhibitor captopril.[176]

# ION CHANNELS AND TRANSPORTERS

Ion channels in the plasma membrane of vascular smooth muscle cells of resistance arteries and arterioles play an important role in the regulation of vascular tone.[177] Ion transporters of renal tubular cells, on the other hand, are important regulators of salt and water homeostasis, and point mutations in these proteins have been identified as the cause of monogenetic disorders of blood pressure and volume regulation. Moreover, ion channels and transporters are important targets for several widely used antihypertensive agents.

## Calcium Channels

Increases in intracellular $Ca^{2+}$ concentration ($[Ca^{2+}]_i$) that results in contraction of vascular smooth muscle cells, involves three distinct mechanisms: (1) $Ca^{2+}$ enters via voltage-sensitive $Ca^{2+}$ channels (L-, T-, N- or P-/Q-type) that open in response to depolarization of the membrane, (2) $Ca^{2+}$ is released from endoplasmic reticular stores in response to inositol-1,4,5-trisphosphate formed by receptor-mediated hydrolysis of membrane phosphatidylinositol-4,5-bisphosphate, and (3) ligand-mediated activation of receptor-operated $Ca^{2+}$ channels triggers entry of extracellular $Ca^{2+}$.[178] $Ca^{2+}$ currents produced by the L-type channel, which are the main $Ca^{2+}$ currents in smooth muscle and endocrine cells and are responsible for contraction and secretion, require strong depolarization for activation, are long-lasting, and are blocked by L-type $Ca^{2+}$ channel blockers.[179] $Ca^{2+}$ currents produced by N-type, P-/Q-type, and R-type $Ca^{2+}$ channels, which are observed in neurons where they initiate neurotransmission, also require strong depolarization to be activated but do not bind $Ca^{2+}$ channel blockers. Specific polypeptide toxins from snail and spider venoms block these $Ca^{2+}$ currents. $Ca^{2+}$ currents produced by T-type $Ca^{2+}$ channels, which are observed in a wide variety of cells controlling action potential development and patterns of repetitive firing, are activated by weak depolarization, are transient in nature, and are resistant to both organic L-type $Ca^{2+}$ channel blockers and snake and spider toxins. T-type and P-/Q-type $Ca^{2+}$ channels also contribute to arterial smooth muscle tone, but their exact contribution to this effect is unknown.[180] In addition to $Ca^{2+}$ entry via voltage-sensitive L-type channels, depletion of intracellular $Ca^{2+}$ stores activates $Ca^{2+}$ entry from the extracellular space via store depletion-activated channels (also called store-operated channels). This pathway also contributes to $Ca^{2+}$ entry in vascular smooth muscle cells.[180,181] However, its role in the regulation of blood pressure remains poorly understood, because drugs acting via these channels are not available.

The L-type $Ca^{2+}$ channel is the molecular target of all currently available $Ca^{2+}$ channel antagonists used in the treatment of hypertension and is discussed in detail later. Three structurally distinct classes of $Ca^{2+}$ channels blockers have been developed: 1,4-dihydropyridines, benzothiazepines, and phenylalkylamines. The therapeutic efficacy of these compounds in hypertension is comparable to other first-line antihypertensive agents, such as $\beta$-blockers, ACE inhibitors, diuretics, or $AT_1$ receptor antagonists.[182,183]

### Molecular Characteristics of L-Type $Ca^{2+}$ Channels

$Ca^{2+}$ channels are hetero-oligomeric proteins composed of four distinct subunits that are encoded by multiple genes.[179,184-186] The largest subunit $\alpha_1$ (~1800 amino acids; 190 to 250 kd) (Fig. 30-5) harbors the ion-conducting pore, voltage sensor, gating machinery, and drug-binding sites. This subunit is also targeted by intracellular signaling pathways. It consists of four homologous repeats (I to IV), each of which is composed of six TM helices (S1 to S6) (Fig. 30-5).[179] The different voltage-gated $Ca^{2+}$ channels can be classified based on their $\alpha$ subunits: (1) the $Ca_v1$ family ($Ca_v1.1$ through $Ca_v1.4$) includes $Ca^{2+}$ channels containing the $\alpha_1$ subunits $\alpha_{1S}$, $\alpha_{1C}$, $\alpha_{1D}$, and $\alpha_{1F}$, which mediate L-type $Ca^{2+}$ currents; (2) the $Ca_v2$ family ($Ca_v2.1$ through $Ca_v2.3$) includes channels containing $\alpha_{1A}$, $\alpha_{1B}$, and $\alpha_{1E}$ subunits, which mediate P/Q-type, N-type, and R-type $Ca^{2+}$ currents, respectively; and (3) the $Ca_v3$ family ($Ca_v3.1$ through $Ca_v3.3$) includes channels containing $\alpha_{1G}$, $\alpha_{1H}$, and $\alpha_{1I}$ subunits, which mediate T-type $Ca^{2+}$ currents.[184] Moreover, an intracellular $\beta$ subunit and a TM, disulfide-linked $\alpha_2\delta$ subunit complex are components of most types of $Ca^{2+}$ channels, whereas a $\gamma$ subunit has also been found in skeletal muscle $Ca^{2+}$ channels, and related subunits are expressed in the heart and brain. The $\beta$, $\alpha_2\delta$, and $\gamma$ subunits are accessory and modulate the function of the $\alpha_1$ subunit and increase its expression.[186]

The high-affinity $Ca^{2+}$ binding site is thought to be the $Ca^{2+}$ channel's selectivity filter. This biochemical filter can bind one $Ca^{2+}$ ion with high affinity to generate a nonpermeating state or can bind two $Ca^{2+}$ ions with lower affinity to generate a conformation that allows $Ca^{2+}$ permeation. The filter residues involved in $Ca^{2+}$

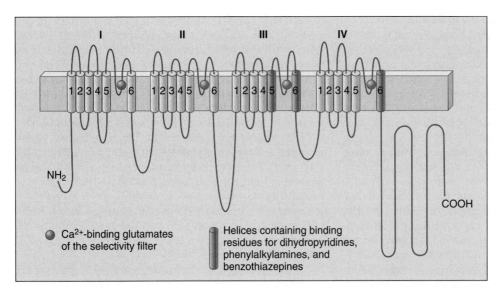

I    II    III    IV

1 2 3 4 5  6    1 2 3 4 5  6    1 2 3 4 5  6    1 2 3 4 5  6

NH₂

COOH

● Ca²⁺-binding glutamates
   of the selectivity filter

▮ Helices containing binding
   residues for dihydropyridines,
   phenylalkylamines, and
   benzothiazepines

**FIGURE 30-5.** Structure of L-type Ca²⁺ channel α₁-subunits. (See color plate.) *(Adapted from Striessnig J, Grabner M, Mitterdorfer J, et al: Structural basis of drug binding to L Ca²⁺ channels. Trends Pharmacol Sci 1998;19:108–115.)*

binding are four glutamates, each of which are located on the S5-S6 linkers of repeats I, II, III, or IV that are arranged in an asymmetric ring in the $\alpha_1$ subunit and are held in position by the pore-forming S5-S6 linkers (Fig. 30-5).

The binding pocket for antagonists in the $\alpha_1$ subunit is formed by IIIS5, IIIS6, and IVS6 TM helices.[179,185,187,188] Some residues in these $\alpha$-helices that are involved in dihydropyridine, phenylalkylamine, and benzothiazepine binding are common (e.g., Tyr1152 and Ile1153 in IIIS6 are required for high-affinity dihydropyridine and phenylalkylamine binding, and Tyr1463, Ala1467, and Ile1470 in IVS6 are required for high-affinity phenylalkylamine and benzothiazepine binding), whereas several others are distinct. Binding of one class of antagonists inhibits the binding of another class. The mechanism of this inhibition was initially thought to be allosteric, but, because the binding sites of different classes of antagonists overlap, steric hindrance may also be involved.[179] The glutamates of the Ca²⁺ filter and its coordinated Ca²⁺ ions are also involved in Ca²⁺ antagonist binding to the channel, but their influence on this binding is dependent on the nature of the Ca²⁺ antagonist. For example, one bound Ca²⁺ stabilizes high-affinity dihydropyridine binding to the channel, whereas two bound Ca²⁺ ions destabilize the binding of Ca²⁺ channel blockers from all three classes. There is no evidence for direct dihydropyridine binding to the glutamates of the Ca²⁺ filter; however, the basic nitrogen atoms of phenylalkylamines interact with the glutamates of the Ca²⁺ filter in repeats III and IV. Reciprocal steric and/or allosteric interactions between the channel-bound Ca²⁺ and the Ca²⁺ channel blocker could form the basis for the Ca²⁺ channel blocking effects of these drugs. Many critical Ca²⁺ antagonist-binding residues in the L-type Ca²⁺ channel are not present in other Ca²⁺ channels, and these differences are thought to underlie the inability of dihydropyridines, phenylalkylamines, and benzothiazepines to bind with high affinity to other classes of Ca²⁺ channels (Fig. 30-5).

N- and C-terminal sequences of L-type Ca²⁺ channels are intracellular and serve a regulatory function. Mutants with a truncated N-terminus are no longer sensitive to

regulation by PKC activators.[189] The C-terminus contains Ca²⁺ binding sites and a calmodulin-binding region that are involved in Ca²⁺-depedent inactivation, whereas Ser1928 in this domain is an important site for phosphorylation by cAMP-dependent protein kinase (PKA); a posttranslational modification that increases Ca$_v$1.2 channel activity.[190]

### Role of Voltage-Gated Ca²⁺ Channels in Hypertension

Voltage-gated Ca²⁺ channels play a very important role in the regulation of vascular tone: hyperpolarization closes the channel and leads to vasodilation, and depolarization opens them and causes vasoconstriction.[177] Nevertheless, although Ca²⁺ channel blockers are antihypertensive agents,[182,183,191] the role of L-type Ca²⁺ channels in the pathogenesis of hypertension remains unclear. The logic behind their therapeutic use comes from the understanding that hypertension is characterized by increased peripheral vascular resistance and increased $[Ca^{2+}]_i$.[192,193] Consistent with the elevated $[Ca^{2+}]_i$ levels, L-type voltage-dependent Ca²⁺ currents have also been reported to be enhanced in vascular smooth muscle of various animal models of hypertension.[193] Opening of Ca²⁺ channels increases local $[Ca^{2+}]_i$ resulting in enhanced binding of Ca²⁺ to the protein calmodulin, a process that activates myosin light-chain kinase, with resultant phosphorylation of myosin light chains. This promotes actin-myosin cross-bridge formation and contraction of smooth muscle.[178] The mechanisms underlying the increased levels of $[Ca^{2+}]_i^+$ that produce an increased peripheral resistance in hypertension could be due to either increased Ca²⁺ influx by Ca²⁺ channels or decreased Ca²⁺ extrusion by the plasma membrane Ca²⁺-ATPase. On the other hand, because vascular smooth muscle contraction is dependent on $[Ca^{2+}]_i$, inhibition of TM movement of Ca²⁺ should decrease the total amount of Ca²⁺ that reaches intracellular sites. Moreover, activity of L-type Ca²⁺ channels may be enhanced in hypertension,[193-195] and all L-type Ca²⁺ channel blockers (e.g., nifedipine, diltiazem, verapamil) lower blood pressure by relaxing arteriolar smooth muscle and decreasing peripheral vascular resistance.[192]

## Potassium Channels

K+ ion-specific channels are a diverse and ubiquitously expressed group of membrane-spanning proteins that selectively conduct K+ ions across the cell membrane along its electrochemical gradient.[24,112,196,197] They play an important role in the regulation of vascular tone and cell membrane potential ($E_m$) and in the regulation of many other physiologic processes. In vascular smooth muscle, K+ channel opening increases K+ efflux and thereby causes $E_m$ hyperpolarization. This results in closure of voltage-gated Ca2+ channels, a fall in $[Ca^{2+}]_i$, and, thus, vasodilation. Four distinct types of K+ channels have been identified: (1) the large conductance Ca2+-activated K+ channel ($BK_{Ca}$ or maxi K channel), which is activated by Ca2+ but is also voltage-dependent; (2) the voltage-dependent K+ channel ($K_v$); (3) the inwardly rectifying K+ channel ($K_{IR}$) that at physiologic $E_m$s paradoxically mediates K+ efflux when activated; and (4) the ATP-sensitive K+ channel ($K_{ATP}$) that is inhibited by intracellular ATP. Although only one ($K_{ATP}$) is currently a target of available antihypertensive drugs (e.g., minoxidil, diazoxide), they are all considered here, because vascular tone and its alterations in hypertension may involve all subtypes functioning in a coordinated manner.[24]

### Molecular Characteristics of K+ Channels

$BK_{Ca}$ channels are abundant in vascular smooth muscle and because of their large conductance are major regulators of $E_m$.[24,112,197] They are activated by agents that increase cAMP or cGMP levels and, importantly, by focal increases in intracellular Ca2+ released via ryanodine receptors from sarcoplasmic reticulum. $K_v$ channels are activated by membrane depolarization within the physiologic $E_m$ range and, thus, function to actively oppose vasoconstrictor influences. They can be activated by NO and cAMP and inhibited by PKC. $K_{IR}$ channels mediate K+ efflux in response to even small changes in extracellular [K+] and are likely open under basal physiologic conditions. In contrast, $K_{ATP}$ channels are inactive under physiologic conditions when ATP is replete within the cell. An important family of $K_{ATP}$ channel inhibitors is the sulfonylureas, such as glibenclamide.[197] In pancreatic β-cells, depolarization resulting from sulfonylurea-stimulated $K_{ATP}$ channel closure leads to insulin release.[198] By contrast, the antihypertensive agent diazoxide, although more selective for vascular smooth muscle $K_{ATP}$ channels, can, in large doses, induce hyperglycemia by activating pancreatic $K_{ATP}$ channels and, thus, inhibit insulin secretion. Other $K_{ATP}$ channel activators include endogenous vasodilators (e.g., hypoxia), acidosis, and mediators that increase cAMP (e.g. adenosine, prostacyclin, epinephrine).[24]

To allow the selective flux of K+ at rates of $10^6$ to $10^8$ ions/second, the structure of K+ channels has evolved to contain three principle features: (1) a water-filled permeation pathway or pore that allow K+ ions to flow freely across the cell membrane; (2) a selectivity filter

consisting of three residues [tripeptide motif: G (Y/F)G or GLG] located high in the pore toward the extracellular surface, which is required for the dissolution and selective permeation of K+ ions; and (3) a gating mechanism that switches the channel between its open and closed conformations.[24,197,199,200] These structural features are all inherent to the α subunits of K+ channels, which form the pore by four such subunits clustering together as homotetramers (Fig. 30-6). Each α-subunit is a single polypeptide chain with both N- and C-termini located intracellularly, with the different K+ channel subtypes variably containing six, four, or two TM segments (S), and either a single pore-forming loop between $S_4$ and $S_5$, or $S_1$ and $S_2$ for those with six or two TM segments, or two pore-forming units between $S_1$ and $S_2$, and $S_3$ and $S_4$ for those with four TM segments (Fig. 30-6). $K_v$ and $BK_{Ca}$ are members of the six-TM, one-pore family. The

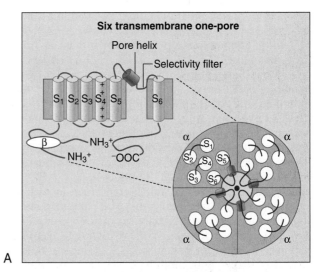

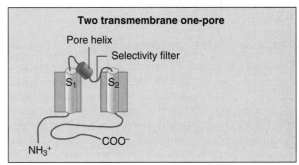

**FIGURE 30-6.** Schematic representation of six-TM (A) or two-TM (B) one-pore K+ channel α subunits, which cluster to form the K+ ion conducting pore. *A,* A six-TM, one-pore subunit. The voltage-gated K+ channels are composed of four segments each containing six TM segments (S1 to S6) and a pore helix between S5 and S6 with a voltage sensor (positively charged amino acids) located at S4. Some of the voltage-gated K+ channels include an auxiliary βsubunit that binds to the N-terminus of the αsubunit. The inset shows the general assembly of K+ channel α subunits to form the channel's conducting pore *B,* A two-TM, one-pore subunit. The inwardly rectifying K+ channels are members of this family, which are formed by the clustering of four subunits each containing two TM segments (S1 and S2) with a pore helix and selectivity filter in between. (See color plate.) *(Adapted from Shieh CC, Coghlan M, Sullivan JP, Gopalakrishnan M: Potassium channels: Molecular defects, diseases, and therapeutic opportunities. Pharmacol Rev 2000;52:557-594.)*

voltage dependence of these channels is due to another important structural feature—a voltage sensor consisting of five to seven positively charged residues regularly spaced along S4.[197,199] This sensor is responsible for the conformational change leading to channel opening with depolarization of the cell membrane. $K_{IR}$ and $K_{ATP}$, on the other hand, are members of the two-TM, one-pore family of $K^+$ channels. Gating of $K^+$ channels is complex. For the six-TM, one-pore family this involves both fast (N-type) and slow (C- and P-type) inactivation components resulting from movement of the N-terminal residues into the internal vestibule of the pore or rearrangements of the outer pore mouth, respectively. For the two-TM, one-pore channels, occlusion of the pore is by a gating mechanism involving intracellular $Mg^{2+}$ or polyamines (spermine, spermidine).

In addition to the $\alpha$ subunits that cluster to form the channel pore(s), auxiliary subunits have been identified that regulate channel activity (Fig. 30-6). These include cytoplasmic $\beta$ subunits for $K_v$ and sulfonylurea-binding proteins (also called sulfonylurea receptors, SURs) for $K_{ATP}$.[196,199] The latter are polytopic membrane-spanning proteins of the ATP-binding cassette (ABC) transporter family that bind and hydrolyze ATP. Two different genes encoding SUR variants (SUR1 and SUR2) have been identified. Alternate splicing adds further diversity to these regulatory proteins, and the different SUR isoforms account for tissue-specific differences in $K_{ATP}$ channels and, thus, as indicated previously, in their sensitivity to drugs. For example, SUR1 is the regulatory subunit for the channel in pancreatic $\beta$-cells, whereas SUR2B (a splice variant of SUR2) fulfills this role in vascular smooth muscle. Structurally the SUR subunits cluster together with the pore-forming tetrameric complex of Kir6.2 (a member of the inwardly rectifying $K^+$ channels) subunits to form an octameric $K_{ATP}$ complex. Binding sites for drugs and modulatory agents, particularly nucleotides, are found on both Kir6.2 and SURs.[199]

### Role of K+ Channels in Hypertension

Resting $E_m$ is increased in vascular smooth muscle cells harvested from several distinct rat models of hypertension.[24,201] This is associated with an increase in myogenic tone, which may be most pronounced in small arterioles that are the major determinants of peripheral vascular resistance. In addition, accumulating evidence suggests that these changes are due to alterations in the function and/or expression of $K^+$ channels. For example, pharmacologic inhibition of $BK_{Ca}$ channels produces more marked depolarization and more marked increases in arteriolar constriction in hypertensive animals than in their normotensive controls.[24] Persistent activation of this channel in chronic hypertensive states may be due to enhanced $Ca^{2+}$ entry secondary to increased sympathetic or other vasoconstrictor influences or may be a compensatory response to impaired $K^+$ conductance by the other three $K^+$ channel-subtypes and/or to increased pressure and vascular tone.[24,202] Impaired function of vascular smooth muscle $K_{ATP}$ and $K_v$ channels has been attributed to increases in $[Ca^{2+}]_i$ and to PKC activation, whereas decreased expression of $K_{IR}$ channels may fur-

ther contribute to enhanced depolarization and, thus, to increased peripheral resistance.[24,203,204] Given the central and significant role of $K^+$ channels in regulating vascular tone and peripheral resistance and the evidence implicating their involvement in the hypertensive process, it is not surprising that drugs targeting and activating these channels (e.g., minoxidil, diazoxide) are some of the most potent vasodilators known. Thus, they are extremely useful in the treatment of very severe hypertension.[23,205] Their clinical use, however, is currently limited, either because they have to be given parenterally or because of side effects (e.g., fluid retention, tachycardia, hirsutism). Nevertheless, it seems reasonable to anticipate that recent advances in the understanding of $K^+$ channel activity and expression will lead to new compounds [e.g., (−)-MJ-451[25]] that are more likely to be useful clinically because they selectively target $K^+$ channels only in specific vascular beds or only those channels that are directly mediating the increased resistance of chronic hypertension.

## Sodium Channels and Transporters

From a circulatory point of view, the kidney serves as a low-resistance conduit that normally receives approximately 20% of the cardiac output. For a 70- to 75-kg person with a cardiac output of 5 to 6 L/minute, this amounts to a renal blood flow of 1 to 1.2 L/minute. Coupled with the high hydrostatic pressure in glomerular capillaries, this large blood flow allows about 20% of plasma to be filtered, giving a glomerular filtration rate of 130 mL/minute or 180 L/day. Because the concentration of salt in plasma is about 135 mEq/L, the filtered salt load is 1.42 kg or 24.3 moles/day.[206] For salt homeostasis to be maintained on a dietary sodium intake of 100 mEq/day, this requires the kidneys to reabsorb almost 99.6% of filtered sodium. This is achieved by complex processes involving the integrated actions of several tubular ion transport proteins. These include (1) NHEs (also called countertransporters or antiporters), which are responsible for the proximal tubular reclamation of approximately 60% of filtered sodium; (2) the $Na^+$-$K^+$-$2Cl^-$ and $Na^+$-$Cl^-$ electroneutral cotransporters of the thick ascending limb (TAL) of the loop of Henle, and the cortical diluting segment of the distal convoluted tubule, respectively, which mediate reabsorption of 30% and 7% of filtered sodium; and (3) the epithelial $Na^+$ channel of the cortical collecting tubule that mediates passive reabsorption of the remaining 2% to 3% of filtered sodium down its electrochemical gradient.[6,207] Thus, it is not surprising that these $Na^+$ channels and transporters are the targets of a number of effective and widely used diuretic agents that also promote blood pressure lowering as a consequence of the fall in extracellular fluid volume and peripheral vascular resistance.[177,207-210] Paradoxically, however, the least efficacious of these agents are drugs that inhibit proximal $Na^+$ reabsorption. Despite the fact that the largest bulk of $Na^+$ is reclaimed at the proximal site, urinary sodium loss is minimized with the use of such agents, because the resulting enhanced distal delivery of $Na^+$ is largely compensated by more active reabsorption at distal sites. Moreover, although alterations in NHE activity have been linked to hypertension in several rat models,[211] these proteins are currently not the targets of any clinically used antihypertensive agents. For these reasons, NHEs are not further considered here.

### Cotransporters

Two important renal tubular cotransporters, expressed selectively in the cortical or medullary regions of the kidney, are the targets of two widely used classes of diuretic and antihypertensive agents, thiazides and loop diuretics, respectively.[6,211] Moreover, inactivating point mutations of these proteins results in rare but well-characterized monogenetic disorders of salt and water metabolism coupled with low or normal blood pressure. Although classified as cation-coupled Cl⁻ cotransporters (CCC), both mediate electroneutral cotransport of Na⁺; the CCC expressed in the cortical diluting segment of the distal tubule mediates Na⁺-Cl⁻ cotransport (NCC or the thiazide-sensitive cotransporter), and that in the TAL of the loop of Henle mediates Na⁺-K⁺-2Cl⁻ cotransport (NKCC or the bumetanide-sensitive cotransporter).[212]

Inhibition of NCC by thiazide diuretics produces effects that entirely mimic those observed in patients with Gitelman's syndrome, a rare genetic disorder resulting from inactivating point mutations on NCC.[6,211,213] This disorder is characterized by natriuresis, diuresis, hypovolemia, hypokalemic alkalosis, hyomagnesemia, increased plasma renin activity, and juxtaglomerular cell hyperplasia. Moreover, because of the associated volume contraction, calcium absorption at proximal nephron sites, particularly the TAL of the loop of Henle, is increased, resulting in diminished urinary calcium loss. In contrast, inhibition of NKCC by loop diuretics produces effects that mimic those observed in patients with Bartter's syndrome. This genetic disorder produces similar effects to those seen in Gitelman's, except that inactivation of NKCC also inhibits calcium reabsorption in the TAL. As a result urinary calcium loss is increased; a finding that critically distinguishes both Gitelman's and Bartter's syndromes and the actions of thiazide diuretics, as compared with loop diuretics.[212,214]

In addition to NKCC, per se, as a mediator of Na⁺ reabsorption, its function is critically dependent on the integrity of two TAL ion channels.[6,211] The first is the ATP-sensitive renal potassium channel (ROMK), which mediates K⁺ efflux from the tubular cell back into the lumen. This is required to prevent luminal fluid potassium depletion that would otherwise result from NKCC-mediated K⁺ influx and that would limit further Na⁺ resorption via NKCC, because it requires the cotransport of K⁺ and Na⁺ ions and Cl⁻ to be operative. The other is a Cl⁻ channel located on the tubular basolateral membrane that clears Cl⁻ from the cell to the blood, following its entry via NKCC. Not surprisingly, inactivating point mutations of either of these channels have also been reported to cause Bartter's syndrome variants. Another important feature of NKCC is its expression in distal tubular cells on the macula densa, which lie adjacent to the renin-producing smooth muscle cells of the juxtaglomerular apparatus. In this location, alterations in NKCC-mediated Cl⁻ transport contribute to two major renal homeostatic functions: tubuloglomerular feedback and renin secretion.[212]

NCC and NKCC are both large proteins (1021 and ~1200 amino acids, respectively) with similar topology involving 12 putative membrane-spanning domains connected by intracellular and extracellular loops and long cytoplasmically located N- and C-termini. Ion binding and transport and diuretic binding are likely localized to residues of the TM segments. In particular, TM2 of NKCC appears to be important for cation and diuretic binding. Chloride binding, however, appears to reside in TM4 and TM7.[215] Activity of NCC and NKCC are likely regulated by phosphorylation, because consensus phosphorylation sites are found in the highly conserved C-terminal domains. The exact mechanism of ion translocation from one side of the plasma membrane to the other, so-called *cis-trans* translocation, remains unclear but is electrically silent, because it is not driven by cellular TM voltage and does not directly generate a current (i.e., it is electroneutral).[212]

### Epithelial Na⁺ Channel

In contrast to the voltage-dependent Na⁺ channels underlying the influx of sodium ions that are responsible for action potentials in excitable cells, the epithelial Na⁺ channel (ENaC) is a member of the ENaC/degenerin family of voltage-independent ion channels.[207,216] This family mediates diverse functions including touch, pain, and other mechanosensory responses; memory; and regulation of extracellular Na⁺, volume, and blood pressure homeostasis via epithelial sodium reabsorption. In the kidney, ENaC is localized to the apical membrane of collecting duct cells, where its constitutively open state allows the passive flux of Na⁺ ions down their electrochemical gradient; sodium entry through the pore of ENaC is the rate-limiting step in Na⁺ reabsorption. At the basolateral membrane, Na⁺ is pumped out of the cell by Na⁺-K⁺-ATPase, resulting in net Na⁺ reclamation from the tubular fluid across the epithelial collecting duct cell and back into the blood.

ENaC is composed of three 65- to 70-kd subunits (α, β, and γENaC) that show 30% to 35% amino acid identity.[207] Although the β and γ subunits, alone or in combination, do not form functional channels, they markedly potentiate Na⁺ flux when coexpressed with αENaC, indicating that all three are required to produce a fully functional channel. All three subunits are single polypeptide chains with similar structural topology, involving two membrane-spanning domains (M₁ and M₂), cytoplasmic N- and C-termini, and a highly glycosylated extracellular loop. A fourth subunit δENaC can substitute functionally for αENaC, although its precise physiologic role remains unknown. ENaC consists of heteromultimers of four ($\alpha_2, \beta_1, \gamma_1$) or nine ($\alpha_3, \beta_3, \gamma_3$) subunits that cluster to form the channel pore.[207] Like K⁺ channels (see previous discussion), ENaC contains a selectivity filter involving residues (G/SXS) located in M₂ at the mouth of the pore. However, unlike K⁺ channels this allows the selective dissolution and permeation of Na⁺ as opposed to K⁺ ions. Residues involved in ENaC gating, located in the juxtamembranous region of the N-terminus and in the extracellular loop just before $M_2$, have also been identified, although gating of ENaC is very slow and, as indicated previously, physiologically the channel is constitutively open. Like the regulation of glucose entry into the cell by the GLUT transporters, regulation of $Na^+$ reabsorption by ENaC, therefore, is largely through alterations in the number of channels inserted into the cell membrane, rather than by conformational changes that alter its open-state probability.[207] The density of channels at the cell surface is the net result of membrane insertion (synthesis, vesicle trafficking, and exocytosis) and removal (Fig. 30-7). Membrane insertion is positively regulated by vasopressin via increased cAMP generation and by aldosterone via a variety of mediators, including serum- and glucocorticoid-regulated kinase (SGK) and K-ras2a, a small molecular weight G-protein involved in intracellular signaling.[207] Membrane removal, on the other hand, is regulated by the interaction of ENaC via a proline-rich region in the C-terminal tail of all three ENaC subunits with the modular adapter protein Nedd4. This targets ENaC for ubiquitylation of its N-terminal domain, which in turn triggers its internalization and degradation.[207]

ENaC is the target of three commonly used diuretics, amiloride, triamterene, and spironolactone.[216] With the first two diuretics, this is due to a direct interaction with residues in the pore (and possibly in the extracellular loop) that have been identified as forming the amiloride-binding site. In contrast, spironolactone blocks the membrane insertion and possibly the transcription of ENaC by an indirect action involving inhibition of aldosterones binding to the mineralocorticoid receptor and, thus, inhibition of aldosterone-activated gene transcription.[216] Importantly, ENaC-mediated $Na^+$ reabsorption results in an increased lumen negative potential, which provides the driving force for distal tubular $K^+$ and $H^+$ secretion. In contrast to other classes of diuretics, those inhibiting ENaC, therefore, produce enhanced urinary $Na^+$ loss without concomitant $K^+$ and $H^+$ ion wastage. Hence their designation as *K+-sparing* diuretics.

### Role of Na+ Channels and Transporters in Hypertension

$Na^+$ channels and transporters are the targets of diuretic and antihypertensive agents as indicated previously. In addition, point mutations of these proteins provide direct evidence for their involvement in blood pressure homeostasis, because they produce clinical syndromes characterized by dysregulation of salt and water metabolism.[6,207,216] Those involving NCC and NKCC have already been discussed. Mutations affecting ENaC-mediated $Na^+$ reabsorption have also been identified as monogenetic causes of disordered salt and water balance. For example, mutations of specific residues in the cytoplasmic N-terminus of ENaC subunits result in channels that are almost always closed and, thus, unable to support distal tubular $Na^+$ reabsorption.[217] This causes pseudohypoaldosteronism (PHA) type 1, a severe neonatal salt wasting disorder characterized by volume depletion and hypotension despite markedly elevated aldosterone levels, marked hyperkalemia, and metabolic acidosis. Alternatively, PHA may be due to heterozygous loss-of-function mutations of the mineralocorticoid receptor, which similarly impairs ENaC-mediated $Na^+$ reabsorption because membrane insertion of the channel is inhibited. In contrast to PHA, autosomal dominant mutations of the C-terminal domains of $\beta$ENaC and $\gamma$ENaC involved in their interaction with Nedd4 result in their sustained residence in the collecting duct-cell membrane. This produces Liddle's syndrome, a disorder characterized by constitutive ENaC-mediated $Na^+$ reabsorption, volume expansion, hypertension, hypokalemic alkalosis, suppressed plasma renin activity, and low plasma aldosterone levels.[6,216] These and other disorders of tubular $Na^+$ transport are considered in detail in Chapter 31.

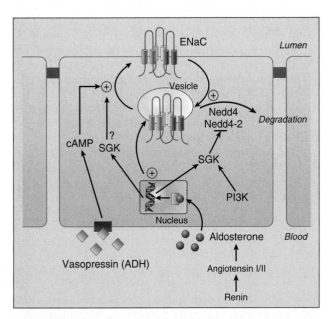

**FIGURE 30-7.** Regulation of ENaC membrane expression. $Na^+$ reabsorption via this channel is controlled by the number of channels at the cell surface. This is the net result of channel synthesis and exocytosis, which are stimulated by aldosterone and vasopressin, and endocytosis and degradation, which are modulated by Nedd4. PI3K phosphorylates SGK at two residues (Thr256 and Ser422). cAMP, cyclic adenosine monophosphate; SGK, serum and glucocorticoid-regulated kinase. *(From Snyder PM: The epithelial na(+) channel: Cell surface insertion and retrieval in Na+ homeostasis and hypertension. Endocr Rev 2002;23:258-275, with permission.)*

### REFERENCES

1. Kannel WB: Role of blood pressure in cardiovascular morbidity and mortality. Prog Cardiovasc Dis 1974;17:5-24.
2. Kannel WB: Fifty years of Framingham study contributions to understanding hypertension. J Hum Hypertens 2000;14:83-90.
3. Hansson L, Zanchetti A, Carruthers SG, et al: Effects of intensive blood-pressure lowering and low-dose aspirin in patients with hypertension: Principal results of the Hypertension Optimal Treatment (HOT) randomised trial. HOT Study Group. Lancet 1998;351:1755-1762.
4. MacMahon S, Rodgers A: The effects of blood pressure reduction in older patients: An overview of five randomized controlled trials in elderly hypertensives. Clin Exp Hypertens 1993;15: 967-978.

5. Freis ED: Studies in hemodynamics and hypertension. Hypertension 2001;38:1-5.

6. Lifton RP, Gharavi AG, Geller DS: Molecular mechanisms of human hypertension. Cell 2001;104:545-556.

7. Hieble JP: Adrenoceptor subclassification: An approach to improved cardiovascular therapeutics. Pharm Acta Helv 2000; 74:163-171.

8. Docherty JR: Subtypes of functional alpha1- and alpha2-adrenoceptors. Eur J Pharmacol 1998;361:1-15.

9. Szabo B: Imidazoline antihypertensive drugs: A critical review on their mechanism of action. Pharmacol Ther 2002;93:1-35 p232.

10. Ergul A: Endothelin-1 and endothelin receptor antagonists as potential cardiovascular therapeutic agents. Pharmacotherapy 2002;22:54-65.

11. Morimoto H, Shimadzu H, Kushiyama E, et al: Potent and selective ET-A antagonists. I. Syntheses and structure-activity relationships of N-(6-(2-(aryloxy)ethoxy)-4-pyrimidinyl)sulfonamide derivatives. J Med Chem 2001;44:3355-3368.

12. Ohlstein EH, Nambi P, Hay DW, et al: Nonpeptide endothelin receptor antagonists. XI. Pharmacological characterization of SB 234551, a high-affinity and selective nonpeptide ETA receptor antagonist. J Pharmacol Exp Ther 1998;286:650-656.

13. Touyz RM, Schiffrin EL: Signal transduction mechanisms mediating the physiological and pathophysiological actions of angiotensin II in vascular smooth muscle cells. Pharmacol Rev 2000;52:639-672.

14. de Gasparo M, Catt KJ, Inagami T, et al: International union of pharmacology. XXIII. The angiotensin II receptors. Pharmacol Rev 2000;52:415-472.

15. Dzau VJ, Bernstein K, Celermajer D, et al: The relevance of tissue angiotensin-converting enzyme: Manifestations in mechanistic and endpoint data. Am J Cardiol 2001;88:1L-20L.

16. Marki HP, Binggeli A, Bittner B, et al: Piperidine renin inhibitors: From leads to drug candidates. Farmaco 2001;56:21-27.

17. Guller R, Binggeli A, Breu V, et al: Piperidine-renin inhibitors compounds with improved physicochemical properties. Bioorg Med Chem Lett 1999;9:1403-1408.

18. Simoneau B, Lavallee P, Anderson PC, et al: Discovery of non-peptidic P2-P3 butanediamide renin inhibitors with high oral efficacy. Bioorg Med Chem 1999;7:489-508.

19. Jin D, Takai S, Yamada M, et al: Beneficial effects of cardiac chymase inhibition during the acute phase of myocardial infarction. Life Sci 2002;71:437-446.

20. Takai S, Jin D, Nishimoto M, et al: Oral administration of a specific chymase inhibitor, NK3201, inhibits vascular proliferation in grafted vein. Life Sci 2001;69:1725-1732.

21. Weber MA: Vasopeptidase inhibitors. Lancet 2001;358: 1525-1532.

22. Robl JA, Sun CQ, Stevenson J, et al: Dual metalloprotease inhibitors: Mercaptoacetyl-based fused heterocyclic dipeptide mimetics as inhibitors of angiotensin-converting enzyme and neutral endopeptidase. J Med Chem 1997;40:1570-1577.

23. Laurent S, Boutouyrie P, Azizi M, et al: Antihypertensive effects of fasidotril, a dual inhibitor of neprilysin and angiotensin-converting enzyme, in rats and humans. Hypertension 2000;35: 1148-1153.

24. Sobey CG: Potassium channel function in vascular disease. Arterioscler Thromb Vasc Biol 2001;21:28-38.

25. Lee YM, Yen MH, Peng YY, et al: The antihypertensive and cardioprotective effects of (−)-MJ-451, an ATP-sensitive K(+) channel opener. Eur J Pharmacol 2000;397:151-160.

26. Alexander P, Mathie A, Peters J, MacKenzie G: TiPS 2001 Nomenclature Supplement. London, Elsevier, 2001.

27. Aoyama Y, Uenaka M, Konoike T, et al: Synthesis and structure-activity relationships of a new class of 1-oxacephem-based human chymase inhibitors. Bioorg Med Chem Lett 2000;10: 2397-2401.

28. Calder JA, Schachter M, Sever PS: Potassium channel opening properties of thiazide diuretics in isolated guinea pig resistance arteries. J Cardiovasc Pharmacol 1994;24:158-164.

29. Ferrari P, Ferrandi M, Tripodi G, et al: PST 2238: A new antihypertensive compound that modulates Na,K-ATPase in genetic hypertension. J Pharmacol Exp Ther 1999;288:1074-1083.

30. Jose PA, Eisner GM, Felder RA: Renal dopamine receptors in health and hypertension. Pharmacol Ther 1998;80:149-182.

31. Hoffman BB, Lefkowitz RJ, Taylor P: Neurotransmission: The autonomic and somatic motor nervous system. In Hardman JG,

Goodman-Gilman A, Limbird LE (eds): Goodman & Gilman's: The Pharmacological Basis of Therapeutics. New York, McGraw-Hill, 1996, pp 105-139.

32. Amerena J, Julius S: Role of the nervous system in human hypertension. In Hollenberg NK (ed): Atlas of Heart Diseases. Philadelphia, Current Medicine, 2000, pp 34-58.

33. Guimaraes S, Moura D: Vascular adrenoceptors: An update. Pharmacol Rev 2001;53:319-356.

34. Jindra A, Jachymova M, Horky K, et al: Association analysis of two tyrosine hydroxylase gene polymorphisms in normotensive offspring from hypertensive families. Blood Press 2000;9:250-254.

35. Bevilaqua LR, Graham ME, Dunkley PR, et al: Phosphorylation of Ser(19) alters the conformation of tyrosine hydroxylase to increase the rate of phosphorylation of Ser(40). J Biol Chem 2001;276:40411-40416.

36. Blanchard-Fillion B, Souza JM, Friel T, et al: Nitration and inactivation of tyrosine hydroxylase by peroxynitrite. J Biol Chem 2001; 276:46017-46023.

37. Grattan-Smith PJ, Wevers RA, Steenbergen-Spanjers GC, et al: Tyrosine hydroxylase deficiency: Clinical manifestations of catecholamine insufficiency in infancy. Mov Disord 2002;17:354-359.

38. Kumai T, Tanaka M, Watanabe M, et al: Elevated tyrosine hydroxylase mRNA levels in medulla oblongata of spontaneously hypertensive rats. Brain Res Mol Brain Res 1996;36:197-199.

39. Lemberg A, Rubio M, Bengochea L, et al: Tyrosine hydroxilase activity in discrete brain regions from prehepatic portal hypertensive rats. Hepatogastroenterology 1998;45:547-550.

40. Kumai T, Asoh K, Tateishi T, et al: Involvement of tyrosine hydroxylase up regulation in dexamethasone-induced hypertension of rats. Life Sci 2000;67:1993-1999.

41. Shimizu H, Kumai T, Kobayashi S: Involvement of tyrosine hydroxylase upregulation in cyclosporine-induced hypertension. Jpn J Pharmacol 2001;85:306-312.

42. Kumai T, Tateishi T, Tanaka M, et al: Tyrosine hydroxylase antisense gene therapy causes hypotensive effects in the spontaneously hypertensive rats. J Hypertens 2001;19:1769-1773.

43. Jose PA, Eisner GM, Felder RA: Role of dopamine receptors in the kidney in the regulation of blood pressure. Curr Opin Nephrol Hypertens 2002;11:87-92.

44. Stanley WC, Lee K, Johnson LG, et al: Cardiovascular effects of nepicastat (RS-25560-197), a novel dopamine beta-hydroxylase inhibitor. J Cardiovasc Pharmacol 1998;31:963-970.

45. Stanley WC, Li B, Bonhaus DW, et al: Catecholamine modulatory effects of nepicastat (RS-25560-197), a novel, potent and selective inhibitor of dopamine-beta-hydroxylase. Br J Pharmacol 1997; 121:1803-1809.

46. Koike G, Jacob HJ, Krieger JE, et al: Investigation of the phenylethanolamine N-methyltransferase gene as a candidate gene for hypertension. Hypertension 1995;26:595-601.

47. Chatelain RE, Manniello MJ, Dardik BN, et al: Antihypertensive effects of CGS 19281A, an inhibitor of phenylethanolamine-N-methyltransferase. J Pharmacol Exp Ther 1990;252:117-125.

48. Mai A, Artico M, Esposito M, et al: 3-(1H-Pyrrol-1-yl)-2-oxazolidinones as reversible, highly potent, and selective inhibitors of monoamine oxidase type A. J Med Chem 2002;45:1180-1183.

49. Oxenkrug GF: Antidepressive and antihypertensive effects of MAO-A inhibition: Role of N-acetylserotonin: A review. Neurobiology 1999;7:213-224.

50. Muramatsu I, Murata S, Isaka M, et al: Alpha1-adrenoceptor subtypes and two receptor systems in vascular tissues. Life Sci 1998;62:1461-1465.

51. Ballesteros JA, Shi L, Javitch JA: Structural mimicry in G protein-coupled receptors: Implications of the high-resolution structure of rhodopsin for structure-function analysis of rhodopsin-like receptors. Mol Pharmacol 2001;60:1-19.

52. Graham RM, Neubig R, Lynch KR: Alpha 2-adrenoceptors take centre stage at Nashville meeting. Trends Pharmacol Sci 1996; 17:90-94.

53. Piascik MT, Perez DM: Alpha1-adrenergic receptors: New insights and directions. J Pharmacol Exp Ther 2001;298:403-410.

54. Zhong H, Neubig RR: Regulator of G protein signaling proteins: Novel multifunctional drug targets. J Pharmacol Exp Ther 2001; 297:837-845.

55. Kobayashi N, Nakano S, Mita S, et al: Involvement of Rho-kinase pathway for angiotensin II-induced plasminogen activator inhibitor-1 gene expression and cardiovascular remodeling in hypertensive rats. J Pharmacol Exp Ther 2002;301:459-466.

56. Graham RM, Perez DM, Hwa J, Piascik MT: Alpha 1-adrenergic receptor subtypes: Molecular structure, function, and signaling. Circ Res 1996;78:737-749.

57. Strader, Sigal IS, Register RB, et al: Identification of residues required for ligand binding to the beta-adrenergic receptor. Proc Natl Acad Sci USA 1987;84:4384-4388

58. Hwa J, Perez DM: The unique nature of the serine interactions for alpha 1-adrenergic receptor agonist binding and activation. J Biol Chem 1996;271:6322-6327.

59. Strader CD, Sigal IS, Dixon RA: Structural basis of beta-adrenergic receptor function. FASEB J 1989;3:1825-1832.

60. Chen S, Xu M, Lin F, et al: Phe310 in transmembrane VI of the alpha1B-adrenergic receptor is a key switch residue involved in activation and catecholamine ring aromatic bonding. J Biol Chem 1999;274:16320-16330.

61. Perez DM, Hwa J, Gaivin R, et al: Constitutive activation of a single effector pathway: Evidence for multiple activation states of a G protein-coupled receptor. Mol Pharmacol 1996;49:112-122.

62. Waugh DJ, Zhao MM, Zuscik MJ, Perez DM: Novel aromatic residues in transmembrane domains IV and V involved in agonist binding at alpha(1a)-adrenergic receptors. J Biol Chem 2000; 275:11698-11705.

63. Zhao MM, Hwa J, Perez DM: Identification of critical extra-cellular loop residues involved in alpha 1-adrenergic receptor subtype-selective antagonist binding. Mol Pharmacol 1996;50: 1118-1126.

64. Waugh DJ, Gaivin RJ, Zuscik MJ, et al: Phe-308 and Phe-312 in transmembrane domain 7 are major sites of alpha 1-adrenergic receptor antagonist binding: Imidazoline agonists bind like antagonists. J Biol Chem 2001;276:25366-25371.

65. Michelotti GA, Price DT, Schwinn DA: Alpha 1-adrenergic receptor regulation: Basic science and clinical implications. Pharmacol Ther 2000;88:281-309.

66. Garcia-Sainz JA, Vazquez-Cuevas FG, Romero-Avila MT: Phosphorylation and desensitization of alpha1d-adrenergic receptors. Biochem J 2001;353:603-610.

67. Garcia-Sainz JA, Vazquez-Prado J, del Carmen Medina L: Alpha 1-adrenoceptors: Function and phosphorylation. Eur J Pharmacol 2000;389:1-12.

68. Xie HG, Kim RB, Stein CM, et al: Alpha1A-adrenergic receptor polymorphism: Association with ethnicity but not essential hypertension. Pharmacogenetics 1999;9:651-656.

69. de Champlain J: Do most antihypertensive agents have a sympatholytic action? Curr Hypertens Rep 2001;3:305-313.

70. Vargas HM, Gorman AJ: Vascular alpha-1 adrenergic receptor subtypes in the regulation of arterial pressure. Life Sci 1995; 57:2291-2308.

71. Hieble JP, Kolpak DC, McCafferty GP, et al: Effects of alpha1-adrenoceptor antagonists on agonist and tilt-induced changes in blood pressure: Relationships to uroselectivity. Eur J Pharmacol 1999;373:51-62.

72. Pulito VL, Li X, Varga SS, et al: An investigation of the uroselective properties of four novel alpha(1a)-adrenergic receptor subtype-selective antagonists. J Pharmacol Exp Ther 2000;294:224-229.

73. Berkowitz BA, Arleth AJ, Sung CP, et al: Effects of the novel dopamine beta-hydroxylase inhibitor SK&F 102698 on catecholamines and blood pressure in spontaneously hypertensive rats. J Pharmacol Exp Ther 1988;245:850-857.

74. Shapiro RE, Winters B, Hales M, et al: Endogenous circulating sympatholytic factor in orthostatic intolerance. Hypertension 2000; 36:553-560.

75. Rudner XL, Berkowitz DE, Booth JV, et al: Subtype specific regulation of human vascular alpha(1)-adrenergic receptors by vessel bed and age. Circulation 1999;100:2336-2243.

76. Zhou L, Vargas HM: Vascular alpha 1D-adrenoceptors have a role in the pressor response to phenylephrine in the pithed rat. Eur J Pharmacol 19096;305:173-176.

77. Gavras I, Gavras H: Role of alpha2-adrenergic receptors in hypertension. Am J Hypertens 2001;14:171S-177S.

78. Willems EW, Valdivia LF, Villalon CM, Saxena PR: α-Adrenoceptors and acute migraine therapy. Drug News Perspect 2002;15: 140-146.

79. Cockcroft V, Frang H, Pihlavisto M, et al: Ligand recognition of serine-cysteine amino acid exchanges in transmembrane domain 5 of alpha2-adrenergic receptors by UK 14,304. J Neurochem 2000;74:1705-1710.

80. Hieble JP, Hehr A, Li YO, Ruffolo RR Jr: Molecular basis for the stereoselective interactions of catecholamines with alpha-adrenoceptors. Proc West Pharmacol Soc 1998;41:225-228.

81. Altman JD, Trendelenburg AU, MacMillan L, et al: Abnormal regulation of the sympathetic nervous system in alpha2A-adrenergic receptor knockout mice. Mol Pharmacol 1999; 56:154-161.

82. Kable JW, Murrin LC, Bylund DB: In vivo gene modification elucidates subtype-specific functions of alpha(2)-adrenergic receptors. J Pharmacol Exp Ther 2000;293:1-7.

83. Eason MG, Liggett SB: Subtype-selective desensitization of alpha 2-adrenergic receptors: Different mechanisms control short and long term agonist-promoted desensitization of alpha 2C10, alpha 2C4, and alpha 2C2. J Biol Chem 1992;267:25473-25479.

84. Small KM, Liggett SB: Identification and functional characterization of alpha(2)-adrenoceptor polymorphisms. Trends Pharmacol Sci 2001;22:471-477.

85. Figueroa XF, Poblete MI, Boric MP, et al: Clonidine-induced nitric oxide-dependent vasorelaxation mediated by endothelial alpha(2)-adrenoceptor activation. Br J Pharmacol 2001;134: 957-968.

86. Eglen RM, Hudson AL, Kendall DA, et al: 'Seeing through a glass darkly': Casting light on imidazoline 'I' sites. Trends Pharmacol Sci 1998;19:381-390.

87. MacMillan LB, Hein L, Smith MS, et al: Central hypotensive effects of the alpha2a-adrenergic receptor subtype. Science 1996;273: 801-803.

88. Hanes DS, Weir MR: The beta blockers: Are they as protective in hypertension as in other cardiovascular conditions? J Clin Hypertens (Greenwich) 2001;3:236-243.

89. Waeber B, Brunner HR: Antihypertensive agents: Mechanisms of drug action. In Hollenberg NK (ed): Atlas of Heart Diseases. Philadelphia, Current Medicine, 2000, pp 144-161.

90. Kaumann AJ, Molenaar P: Modulation of human cardiac function through 4 beta-adrenoceptor populations. Naunyn Schmiedebergs Arch Pharmacol 1997;355:667-681.

91. Blumenfeld JD, Sealey JE, Mann SJ, et al: Beta-adrenergic receptor blockade as a therapeutic approach for suppressing the renin-angiotensin-aldosterone system in normotensive and hypertensive subjects. Am J Hypertens 1999;12:451-459.

92. Dzimiri N: Regulation of beta-adrenoceptor signaling in cardiac function and disease. Pharmacol Rev 1999;51:465-501.

93. Anderson GP: Long acting inhaled beta-adrenoceptor agonists the comparative pharmacology of formoterol and salmeterol. Agents Actions Suppl 1993;43:253-269.

94. Noda K, Saad Y, Graham RM, Karnik SS: The high affinity state of the beta 2-adrenergic receptor requires unique interaction between conserved and non-conserved extracellular loop cysteines. J Biol Chem 1994;269:6743-6752.

95. Rohrer DK, Chruscinski A, Schauble EH, et al: Cardiovascular and metabolic alterations in mice lacking both beta1- and beta2-adrenergic receptors. J Biol Chem 1999;274:16701-16708.

96. Dishy V, Sofowora GG, Xie HG, et al: The effect of common polymorphisms of the beta2-adrenergic receptor on agonist-mediated vascular desensitization. N Engl J Med 2001;345: 1030-1035.

97. Herrmann SM, Nicaud V, Tiret L, et al: Polymorphisms of the beta2-adrenoceptor (ADRB2) gene and essential hypertension: The ECTIM and PEGASE studies. J Hypertens 2002;20:229-235.

98. Levin MC, Marullo S, Muntaner O, et al: The myocardium-protective Gly49 variant of the β1-adrenergic receptor exhibits constitutive activity and increased desensitiation and downregulation. J Biol Chem 2002;277:30429-30435.

99. Tonolo G, Melis MG, Secchi G, et al: Association of Trp64Arg beta 3-adrenergic-receptor gene polymorphism with essential hypertension in the Sardinian population. J Hypertens 1999;17:33-38.

100. Bek MJ, Eisner GM, Felder RA, Jose PA: Dopamine receptors in hypertension. Mt Sinai J Med 2001;68:362-369.

101. Hoffman BB, Lefkowitz RJ: Neurotransmission: The autonomic and somatic motor nervous system. In Hardman JG, Goodman-Gilman A, Limbird LE (eds): Goodman & Gilman's: The Pharmacological Basis of Therapeutics. New York, McGraw-Hill, 1996, pp 105-139.

102. Murphy MB, Murray C, Shorten GD: Fenoldopam: A selective peripheral dopamine-receptor agonist for the treatment of severe hypertension. N Engl J Med 2001;345:1548-1557.

103. Hussain T, Lokhandwala MF: Renal dopamine receptor function in hypertension. Hypertension 1998;32:187–197.

104. Lorenzo MN, Khan RY, Wang Y, et al: Human endothelin converting enzyme-2 (ECE2): Characterization of mRNA species and chromosomal localization. Biochim Biophys Acta 2001;1522:46–52.

105. Naicker S, Bhoola KD: Endothelins: Vasoactive modulators of renal function in health and disease. Pharmacol Ther 2001;90:61–88.

106. Roux S, Breu V, Ertel SI, Clozel M: Endothelin antagonism with bosentan: A review of potential applications. J Mol Med 1999;77:364–376.

107. Cramer H, Schmenger K, Heinrich K, et al: Coupling of endothelin receptors to the ERK/MAP kinase pathway. Roles of palmitoylation and G(alpha)q. Eur J Biochem 2001;268:5449–5459.

108. Paasche JD, Attramadal T, Sandberg C, et al: Mechanisms of endothelin receptor subtype-specific targeting to distinct intracellular trafficking pathways. J Biol Chem 2001;276:34041–34050.

109. Abassi ZA, Ellahham S, Winaver J, Hoffman A: The intrarenal endothelin system and hypertension. News Physiol Sci 2001;16:152–156.

110. Schiffrin EL: State-of-the-art lecture. Role of endothelin-1 in hypertension. Hypertension 1999;34:876–881.

111. Weber C, Schmitt R, Birnboeck H, et al: Pharmacokinetics and pharmacodynamics of the endothelin-receptor antagonist bosentan in healthy human subjects. Clin Pharmacol Ther 1996;60:124–137.

112. Lawson K: Potassium channel activation: A potential therapeutic approach? Pharmacol Ther 1996;70:39–63.

113. Verhaar MC, Strachan FE, Newby DE, et al: Endothelin-A receptor antagonist-mediated vasodilatation is attenuated by inhibition of nitric oxide synthesis and by endothelin-B receptor blockade. Circulation 1998;97:752–756.

114. Adner M, Shankley N, Edvinsson L: Evidence that ET-1, but not ET-3 and S6b, ET(A)-receptor mediated contractions in isolated rat mesenteric arteries are modulated by co-activation of ET(B) receptors. Br J Pharmacol 2001;133:927–935.

115. Deng AY, Dene H, Pravenec M, Rapp JP: Genetic mapping of two new blood pressure quantitative trait loci in the rat by genotyping endothelin system genes. J Clin Invest 1994;93:2701–2709.

116. Delyani JA, Rocha R, Cook CS, et al: Eplerenone: A selective aldosterone receptor antagonist (SARA). Cardiovasc Drug Rev 2001;19:185–200.

117. Gomez-Sanchez EP, Zhou M, Gomez-Sanchez CE: Mineralocorticoids, salt and high blood pressure. Steroids 1996;61:184–188.

118. Young MJ, Funder JW: Mineralocorticoids, salt, hypertension: Effects on the heart. Steroids 1996;61:233–235.

119. Rogerson FM, Dimopoulos N, Sluka P, et al: Structural determinants of aldosterone binding selectivity in the mineralocorticoid receptor. J Biol Chem 1999;274:36305–36311.

120. Zennaro MC, Borensztein P, Jeunemaitre X, et al: Molecular characterization of the mineralocorticoid receptor in pseudohypoaldosteronism. Steroids 1995;60:164–167.

121. Oberleithner H: Aldosterone and nuclear signaling in kidney. Steroids 1999;64:42–50.

122. Schafer C, Shahin V, Albermann L, et al: Aldosterone signaling pathway across the nuclear envelope. Proc Natl Acad Sci USA 2002;99:7154–7159.

123. Derfoul A, Robertson NM, Lingrel JB, et al: Regulation of the human Na/K-ATPase beta1 gene promoter by mineralocorticoid and glucocorticoid receptors. J Biol Chem 1998;273:20702–20711.

124. Harvey BJ, Doolan CM, Condliffe SB, et al: Non-genomic convergent and divergent signalling of rapid responses to aldosterone and estradiol in mammalian colon. Steroids 2002;67:483–491.

125. Le Menuet D, Isnard R, Bichara M, et al: Alteration of cardiac and renal functions in transgenic mice overexpressing human mineralocorticoid receptor. J Biol Chem 2001;276:38911–38920.

126. Stowasser M: New perspectives on the role of aldosterone excess in cardiovascular disease. Clin Exp Pharmacol Physiol 2001;28:783–791.

127. Kim S, Yoshiyama M, Izumi Y, et al: Effects of combination of ACE inhibitor and angiotensin receptor blocker on cardiac remodeling, cardiac function, and survival in rat heart failure. Circulation 2001;103:148–154.

128. Urata H, Boehm KD, Philip A, et al: Cellular localization and regional distribution of an angiotensin II-forming chymase in the heart. J Clin Invest 1993;91:1269–1281.

129. Fisher ND, Hollenberg NK: Is there a future for renin inhibitors? Expert Opin Invest Drugs 2001;10:417–426.

130. Dhanaraj V: Three-dimensional structure and substate specificity of Renin. In Husain A, Graham RM (eds): Drugs, Enzymes and Receptors of the Renin-Angiotensin System: Celebrating a Century of Discovery. Amsterdam, Harwood Academic Publishers, 2000, pp 283–301.

131. Sinn, PL, Sigmund CD: Understanding the regulation of Renin gene expression through in vitro and in vivo models. In Husain A, Graham RM (eds): Drugs, Enzymes and Receptors of the Renin-Angiotensin System: Celebrating a Century of Discovery. Amsterdam, Harwood Academic Publishers, 2000, pp 259–278.

132. Rahuel J, Rasetti V, Maibaum J, et al: Structure-based drug design: The discovery of novel nonpeptide orally active inhibitors of human renin. Chem Biol 2000;7:493–504.

133. Sielecki AR, Hayakawa K, Fujinaga M, et al: Structure of recombinant human renin, a target for cardiovascular-active drugs, at 2.5 A resolution. Science 1989;243:1346–1351.

134. Sarma AV, Ramana Rao MH, Sarma JA, Nagaraj R, Dutta AS, Kunwar AC: NMR study of cyclic peptides with renin inhibitor activity. J Biochem Biophys Methods 2002;51:27–45.

135. Kessler SP, Rowe TM, Gomos JB, et al: Physiological non-equivalence of the two isoforms of angiotensin-converting enzyme. J Biol Chem 2000;275:26259–26264.

136. Fernandez M, Liu X, Wouters MA, et al: Angiotensin I-converting enzyme transition state stabilization by HIS1089: Evidence for a catalytic mechanism distinct from other gluzincin metalloproteinases. J Biol Chem 2001;276:4998–5004.

137. Wei L, Clauser E, Alhenc-Gelas F, Corvol P: The two homologous domains of human angiotensin I-converting enzyme interact differently with competitive inhibitors. J Biol Chem 1992;267:13398–13405.

138. Azizi M, Rousseau A, Ezan E, et al: Acute angiotensin-converting enzyme inhibition increases the plasma level of the natural stem cell regulator N-acetyl-seryl-aspartyl-lysyl-proline. J Clin Invest 1996;97:839–844.

139. Dive V, Cotton J, Yiotakis A, et al: RXP 407, a phosphinic peptide, is a potent inhibitor of angiotensin I converting enzyme able to differentiate between its two active sites. Proc Natl Acad Sci USA 1999;96:4330–4335.

140. Vickers C, Hales P, Kaushik V, et al: Hydrolysis of biological peptides by human angiotensin-converting enzyme-related carboxypeptidase. J Biol Chem 2002;277:14838–14843.

141. Liu X, Fernandez M, Wouters MA, et al: Arg(1098) is critical for the chloride dependence of human angiotensin I-converting enzyme C-domain catalytic activity. J Biol Chem 2001;276:33518–33525.

142. Kinoshita E, Yamakoshi J, Kikuchi M: Purification and identification of an angiotensin I-converting enzyme inhibitor from soy sauce. Biosci Biotechnol Biochem 1993;57:1107–1110.

143. d'Uscio LV, Quaschning T, Burnett JC Jr, Luscher TF: Vasopeptidase inhibition prevents endothelial dysfunction of resistance arteries in salt-sensitive hypertension in comparison with single ACE inhibition. Hypertension 2001;37:28–33.

144. Quaschning T, d'Uscio LV, Shaw S, et al: Chronic vasopeptidase inhibition restores endothelin-converting enzyme activity and normalizes endothelin levels in salt-induced hypertension. Nephrol Dial Transplant 2001;16:1176–1182.

145. Quaschning T, d'Uscio LV, Shaw S, et al: Vasopeptidase inhibition restores renovascular endothelial dysfunction in salt-induced hypertension. J Am Soc Nephrol 2001;12;2280–2287.

146. Corti R, Burnett JC Jr, Rouleau JL, et al: Vasopeptidase inhibitors: A new therapeutic concept in cardiovascular disease? Circulation 2001;104;1856–1862.

147. Zhang X, Scicli GA, Xu X, et al: Role of endothelial kinins in control of coronary nitric oxide production. Hypertension 1997;30:1105–1111.

148. Burrell LM, Droogh J, Man in't Veld O, et al: Antihypertensive and antihypertrophic effects of omapatrilat in SHR. Am J Hypertens 2000;13:1110–1116.

149. Dell'Italia LJ, Husain A: Chymase: A critical evaluation of its role in AngiotensinII formation. In Husain A, Graham RM (eds): Drugs,

Enzymes and Receptors of the Renin-Angiotensin System: Celebrating a Century of Discovery. Amsterdam, Harwood Academic Publishers, 2000, pp 347-363.

150. Urata H, Kinoshita A, Misono KS, et al: Identification of a highly specific chymase as the major angiotensin II-forming enzyme in the human heart. J Biol Chem 1990;265;22348-22357.

151. Krishnaswamy G, Kelley J, Johnson D, et al: The human mast cell: Functions in physiology and disease. Front Biosci 2001;6: D1109-1127.

152. Kinoshita A, Urata H, Bumpus FM, Husain A: Multiple determinants for the high substrate specificity of an angiotensin II-forming chymase from the human heart. J Biol Chem 1991;266:19192-19197.

153. Powers JC, Tanaka T, Harper JW, et al: Mammalian chymotrypsin-like enzymes. Comparative reactivities of rat mast cell proteases, human and dog skin chymases, and human cathepsin G with peptide 4-nitroanilide substrates and with peptide chloromethyl ketone and sulfonyl fluoride inhibitors. Biochemistry 1985;24: 2048-2058.

154. Sanker S, Chandrasekharan UM, Wilk D, et al: Distinct multisite synergistic interactions determine substrate specificities of human chymase and rat chymase-1 for angiotensin II formation and degradation. J Biol Chem 1997;272:2963-2968.

155. Dell'italia LJ, Balcells E, Meng QC, et al: Volume-overload cardiac hypertrophy is unaffected by ACE inhibitor treatment in dogs. Am J Physiol 1997;273:H961-970.

156. Guo C, Ju H, Leung D, et al: A novel vascular smooth muscle chymase is upregulated in hypertensive rats. J Clin Invest 2001;107:703-715.

157. Ju H, Gros R, You X, et al: Conditional and targeted overexpression of vascular chymase causes hypertension in transgenic mice. Proc Natl Acad Sci USA 2001;98:7469-7474.

158. McDonald JE, Padmanabhan N, Petrie MC, et al: Vasoconstrictor effect of the angiotensin-converting enzyme-resistant, chymase-specific substrate [Pro(11)(D)-Ala(12)] angiotensin I in human dorsal hand veins: In vivo demonstration of non-ace production of angiotensin II in humans. Circulation 2001;104:1805-1808.

159. Richard V, Hurel-Merle S, Scalbert E, et al: Functional evidence for a role of vascular chymase in the production of angiotensin II in isolated human arteries. Circulation 2001;104:750-752.

160. Bonvouloir N, Lemieux N, Crine P, et al: Molecular cloning, tissue distribution, and chromosomal localization of MMEL2, a gene coding for a novel human member of the neutral endopeptidase-24.11 family. DNA Cell Biol 2001;20:493-498.

161. Roques BP, Noble F, Dauge V, et al: Neutral endopeptidase 24.11: Structure, inhibition, and experimental and clinical pharmacology. Pharmacol Rev 1993;45:87-146.

162. Campese VM, Lasseter KC, Ferrario CM, et al: Omapatrilat versus lisinopril: Efficacy and neurohormonal profile in salt-sensitive hypertensive patients. Hypertension 2001;38:1342-1348.

163. Intengan HD, Schiffrin EL: Vasopeptidase inhibition has potent effects on blood pressure and resistance arteries in stroke-prone spontaneously hypertensive rats. Hypertension 2000;35: 1221-1225.

164. Cataliotti A, Boerrigter G, Chen HH, et al: Differential actions of vasopeptidase inhibition versus angiotensin-converting enzyme inhibition on diuretic therapy in experimental congestive heart failure. Circulation 2002;105:639-644.

165. Albiston AL, McDowall SG, Matsacos D, et al: Evidence that the angiotensin IV (AT(4)) receptor is the enzyme insulin-regulated aminopeptidase. J Biol Chem 2001;276:48623-48626.

166. Berk BC, Corson MA: Angiotensin II signal transduction in vascular smooth muscle: Role of tyrosine kinases. Circ Res 1997;80: 607-616.

167. Feng YH, Noda K, Saad Y, et al: The docking of Arg2 of angiotensin II with Asp281 of AT1 receptor is essential for full agonism. J Biol Chem 1995;270:12846-12850.

168. Noda K, Saad Y, Karnik SS: Interaction of Phe8 of angiotensin II with Lys199 and His256 of AT1 receptor in agonist activation. J Biol Chem 1995;270:28511-28514.

169. Horiuchi M, Lehtonen JY, Daviet L: Signaling mechanism of the AT2 angiotensin II receptor: Crosstalk between AT1 and AT2 receptors in cell growth. Trends Endocrinol Metab 1999;10: 391-396.

170. van Geel PP, Pinto YM, Voors AA, et al: Angiotensin II type 1 receptor A1166C gene polymorphism is associated with an increased response to angiotensin II in human arteries. Hypertension 2000; 35:717-721.

171. Otsuka S, Sugano M, Makino N, et al: Interaction of mRNAs for angiotensin II type 1 and type 2 receptors to vascular remodeling in spontaneously hypertensive rats. Hypertension 1998;32: 467-472.

172. Hein L, Barsh GS, Pratt RE, et al: Behavioural and cardiovascular effects of disrupting the angiotensin II type-2 receptor in mice. Nature 1995;377:744-747.

173. Coats AJ: CAPRICORN: A story of alpha allocation and beta-blockers in left ventricular dysfunction post-MI. Int J Cardiol 2001;78:109-113.

174. Oparil S: Are there meaningful differences in blood pressure control with current antihypertensive agents? Am J Hypertens 2002;15:14S-21S.

175. Csikos T, Chung O, Unger T: Receptors and their classification: Focus on angiotensin II and the AT2 receptor. J Hum Hypertens 1998;12:311-318.

176. Pitt B, Segal R, Martinez FA, et al: Randomised trial of losartan versus captopril in patients over 65 with heart failure (Evaluation of Losartan in the Elderly Study, ELITE). Lancet 1997;349: 747-752.

177. Jackson WF: Ion channels and vascular tone. Hypertension 2000;35:173-178.

178. Robertson RM, Robertson D: Drugs used for the treatment of myocardial ischemia. In Hardman JG, Goodman-Gilman A, Limbird LE (eds): Goodman & Gilman's: The Pharmacological Basis of Therapeutics. New York, McGraw-Hill, 1996, pp 759-779.

179. Striessnig J, Grabner M, Mitterdorfer J, et al: Structural basis of drug binding to L $Ca^{2+}$ channels. Trends Pharmacol Sci 1998; 19:108-115.

180. Cribbs LL: Vascular smooth muscle calcium channels: Could "T" be a target? Circ Res 2001;89:560-562.

181. Ng LC, Gurney AM: Store-operated channels mediate Ca(2+) influx and contraction in rat pulmonary artery. Circ Res 2001;89:923-929.

182. Luft FC: Recent clinical trial highlights in hypertension. Curr Hypertens Rep 2001;3:133-138.

183. Opie LH: Calcium channel blockers in hypertension: Reappraisal after new trials and major meta-analyses. Am J Hypertens 2001; 14:1074-1081.

184. Ertel EA, Campbell KP, Harpold MM, et al: Nomenclature of volt-age-gated calcium channels. Neuron 2000;25:533-535.

185. Hering S, Berjukow S, Aczel S, Timin EN: $Ca^{2+}$ channel block and inactivation: Common molecular determinants. Trends Pharmacol Sci 1998;19:439-443.

186. Muth JN, Varadi G, Schwartz A: Use of transgenic mice to study voltage-dependent Ca2+ channels. Trends Pharmacol Sci 2001; 22:526-532.

187. Hockerman GH, Johnson BD, Abbott MR, et al: Molecular determinants of high affinity phenylalkylamine block of L-type calcium channels in transmembrane segment IIIS6 and the pore region of the alpha1 subunit. J Biol Chem 1997;272:18759-18765.

188. Hockerman GH, Peterson BZ, Johnson BD, Catterall WA: Molecular determinants of drug binding and action on L-type calcium channels. Annu Rev Pharmacol Toxicol 1997;37:361-396.

189. Shistik E, Keren-Raifman T, Idelson GH, et al: The N terminus of the cardiac L-type Ca(2+) channel alpha(1C) subunit. The initial segment is ubiquitous and crucial for protein kinase C modulation, but is not directly phosphorylated. J Biol Chem 1999;274: 31145-31149.

190. Gao L, Tripathy A, Lu X, Meissner G: Evidence for a role of C-terminal amino acid residues in skeletal muscle $Ca^{2+}$ release channel (ryanodine receptor) function. FEBS Lett 1997;412: 223-226.

191. Lambert GW, Ferrier C, Kaye DM, et al: Central nervous system norepinephrine turnover in essential hypertension. Ann NY Acad Sci 1995;763:679-694.

192. Oates JA: In Hardman JG, Goodman-Gilman A, Limbird LE (eds): Goodman & Gilman's: The Pharmacological Basis of Therapeutics. New York, McGraw-Hill, 1996, pp 780-808.

193. Wellman GC, Cartin L, Eckman DM, et al: Membrane depolarization, elevated Ca(2+) entry, and gene expression in cerebral arteries of hypertensive rats. Am J Physiol Heart Circ Physiol 2001;281:H2559-2567.

194. Kitazono T, Ago T, Kamouchi M, et al: Increased activity of calcium channels and Rho-associated kinase in the basilar artery during chronic hypertension in vivo. J Hypertens 2002;20:879-884.

195. Wilde DW, Furspan PB, Szocik JF: Calcium current in smooth muscle cells from normotensive and genetically hypertensive rats. Hypertension 1994;24:739-746.

196. Ashcroft FM, Gribble FM: New windows on the mechanism of action of K(ATP) channel openers. Trends Pharmacol Sci 2000;21:439-445.

197. Shieh CC, Coghlan M, Sullivan JP, Gopalakrishnan M: Potassium channels: Molecular defects, diseases, and therapeutic opportunities. Pharmacol Rev 2000;52:557-594.

198. Yokoshiki H, Sunagawa M, Seki T, Sperelakis N: ATP-sensitive K$^+$ channels in pancreatic, cardiac, and vascular smooth muscle cells. Am J Physiol 1998;274:C25-37.

199. Coetzee WA, Amarillo Y, Chiu J, et al: Molecular diversity of K$^+$ channels. Ann NY Acad Sci 1999;868:233-285.

200. Doyle DA, Morais Cabral J, Pfuetzner RA, et al: The structure of the potassium channel: Molecular basis of K$^+$ conduction and selectivity. Science 1998;280:69-77.

201. Rusch NJ, De Lucena RG, Wooldridge TA, et al: A Ca(2+)-dependent K$^+$ current is enhanced in arterial membranes of hypertensive rats. Hypertension 1992;19:301-307.

202. Grover GJ, Garlid KD: ATP-Sensitive potassium channels: A review of their cardioprotective pharmacology. J Mol Cell Cardiol 2000;32:677-695.

203. Martens JR, Gelband CH: Alterations in rat interlobar artery membrane potential and K$^+$ channels in genetic and nongenetic hypertension. Circ Res 1996;79:295-301.

204. Nelson MT, Quayle JM: Physiological roles and properties of potassium channels in arterial smooth muscle. Am J Physiol 1995;268:C799-822.

205. Lawson DL, Haught WH, Mehta P, Mehta JL: Studies of vascular tolerance to nitroglycerin: Effects of N-acetylcysteine, NG-monomethyl L-arginine, and endothelin-1. J Cardiovasc Pharmacol 1996;28:418-424.

206. Graham RM, Zisfein JB: In Fozzard HA, Jennings RB, Haber E, et al. (eds): The Heart and Cardiovascular System: Scientific Foundations. New York, Raven Press, 1986, pp 1559-1572.

207. Snyder PM: The epithelial na(+) channel: Cell surface insertion and retrieval in na(+) homeostasis and hypertension. Endocr Rev 2002;23:258-275.

208. Corvol P, Persu A, Gimenez-Roqueplo AP, Jeunemaitre X: Seven lessons from two candidate genes in human essential hypertension: Angiotensinogen and epithelial sodium channel. Hypertension 1999;33:1324-1331.

209. Goto A, Yamada K: An approach to the development of novel antihypertensive drugs: Potential role of sodium pump inhibitors. Trends Pharmacol Sci 1998;19:201-204.

210. Waeber B, Brunner HR: Clinical application and limitations in the use of AT$_1$-receptor antagonists. In Husain A, Graham RM: Drugs, Enzymes and Receptors of the Renin-Angiotensin System: Celebrating a Century of Discovery. Amsterdam, Harwood Academic Publishers, 2000, pp 159-170.

211. Orlov SN, Adragna NC, Adarichev VA, Hamet P: Genetic and biochemical determinants of abnormal monovalent ion transport in primary hypertension. Am J Physiol 1999;276:C511-536.

212. Russell JM: Sodium-potassium-chloride cotransport. Physiol Rev 2000;80:211-276.

213. Pollak MR, Delaney VB, Graham RM, Hebert SC: Gitelman's syndrome (Bartter's variant) maps to the thiazide-sensitive cotransporter gene locus on chromosome 16q13 in a large kindred. J Am Soc Nephrol 1996;7:2244-2248.

214. Bettinelli A, Bianchetti MG, Girardin E, et al: Use of calcium excretion values to distinguish two forms of primary renal tubular hypokalemic alkalosis: Bartter and Gitelman syndromes. J Pediatr 1992;120:38-43.

215. Isenring P, Jacoby SC, Payne JA, Forbush B 3rd: Comparison of Na-K-Cl cotransporters: NKCC1, NKCC2, and the HEK cell Na-L-Cl cotransporter. J Biol Chem 1998;273:11295-11301.

216. Alvarez de la Rosa D, Canessa CM, Fyfe GK, Zhang P: Structure and regulation of amiloride-sensitive sodium channels. Annu Rev Physiol 2000;62:573-594.

217. Chang SS, Grunder S, Hanukoglu A, et al: Mutations in subunits of the epithelial sodium channel cause salt wasting with hyperkalaemic acidosis, pseudohypoaldosteronism type 1. Nat Genet 1996;12:248-253.

# Mechanisms and Molecular Pathways in Hypertension

*Roger Brown*
*John Mullins*
*David J. Webb*

## OVERVIEW

This chapter explains the basis of blood pressure (BP) control and hypertension (HT) at the whole-body integrative level; then individual BP regulatory systems and finally the underlying molecular pathways, individual genes, and genomic loci are discussed. Working down from the whole-body level involves observations and studies from the clinical and classical physiology literature, which often involves clinical observations or more direct studies in animals. Building up from the molecular level there is a largely modern literature involving *in vitro* molecular and cellular work that extends upward to *in vivo* and more integrative physiologic levels through gene targeting and transgenic approaches in small animals especially mice. This chapter considers HT in which there is no recognized primary cause (i.e., human primary or essential HT), HT that is secondary to a number of causes (some much better defined and understood than others), and HT that often occurs in comorbid association with the complex disorders of obesity and insulin resistance.

There has been dramatic progress in the understanding of some forms of secondary HT in which single-gene disorders have been defined, mutated genes identified, and then genes targeted to reproduce these human disorders in mice. In the study of HT in association with obesity and insulin resistance there has been much progress in understanding. Many theories, with molecular and physiologic correlates, have been proposed, although often it is difficult to clarify a key issue in these comorbid states (i.e., which abnormalities simply coexist and which are the primary causes of others). Studies in gene-targeted mice and identification of the basis of usually rare, single-gene disorders that exhibit these comorbidities have assisted understanding. Nevertheless, the general applicability to most cases of HT remains unclear. In primary HT up to 50% of the variation in risk has a genetic basis, and it is now known that primary HT has a polygenic basis with no single gene having a huge proportionate effect (e.g., in contrast to type 1 diabetes mellitus [DM]). Many studies investigating human primary HT, however, were powered only to define genes having a large genetic effect, and consequently the identification of genes with a more modest effect is difficult. Nonetheless, evidence suggests several loci in the genome that may harbor genetic elements that contribute to HT. Some of these seem to be in areas of the

genome homologous to loci influencing BP in rodents. Although none of the causes underlying these loci are yet known, techniques allowing progression from loci identification to isolation of the causative genetic elements have recently been successful in other human polygenic disorders including type 2 DM. Similarly, some candidate genes, especially angiotensinogen and possibly the $\beta_2$-adrenergic receptor, appear to be involved. Thus, primary HT is not only a truly polygenic disorder but also a complex one with modulation of the influence of single-gene variations by interaction with other gene variations in the genetic background and with an individual's age and environment, especially as it affects body weight. In addition, ancestral genetic background also has a significant influence on which genetic loci are the source of major variation. Defining the genetic basis of human primary HT will not be a trivial task, but now it will be easier to design better powered and less noisy studies to provide more information about the genetic contribution in human primary HT.

New, and potentially new, BP control pathways have been discovered. In evaluating the importance of these pathways, there are many natural barriers to clinical investigation especially the aspects of human integrative physiology that cannot be easily monitored. In addition, clinically useful selective pharmacologic agents are often not available, and the effects of genetic variation on human BP regulatory systems is only rarely conclusively appreciable. Thus it is of great value when the bases of rare forms of familial secondary HT are discovered. Progress will be accelerated if animal modeling especially in gene-targeted mice is appropriately used to elucidate these aspects of human physiology and HT and to facilitate the identification of novel targets for treatment of HT in humans. Thus it is of critical importance when bridging between clinical and molecular levels to establish which aspects of human integrative physiology are reliably modeled by studies in mice or must be explored with other techniques.

## BLOOD PRESSURE MEASUREMENT AND DEFINITION OF HYPERTENSION

In a clinical context, BP generally refers to arterial pressure measured at the brachial artery in the relaxed patient who is seated for 5 minutes with the arm supported at the level of the heart. One listens over the brachial pulse while an appropriately sized cuff is inflated to more than 20 mm Hg above the point of disappearance of the audible pulse. Then, the cuff is deflated slowly (2 to 3 mm Hg/second). The systolic BP (SBP) is noted when the audible pulse reappears (Korotkoff phase I) and the diastolic BP (DBP) occurs when the audible pulse finally disappears again (Korotkoff phase V).[1] BP is then given as SBP/DBP (both in mm Hg), whereas pulse pressure is SBP-DBP. Mean arterial pressure (MAP) is derived as SBP + (pulse pressure)/3. In some people, especially children and pregnant women, DBP may be best estimated from the point at which the pulse sound suddenly muffles (Korotkoff phase IV). Phase V is unsuitable in these subjects because faint pulse sounds may continue to be audible nearly to zero.[1] Because of BP variability, to define HT one should take two BP readings separated by a few minutes on each of at least three such assessments interspaced by a minimum of 1 week.[2,3] If the BP seems high, measurements may be taken away from a medical/hospital setting (usually with a validated automatic cuff monitor) to identify people who have purely "white coat" or "office" HT with no evidence of end-organ damage. By monitoring BP according to guidelines,[2,3] BP represents a robust measurement of a physiologic variable with a normal distribution in populations. From large epidemiologic studies higher BP is known to be associated with higher cardiovascular morbidity (and mortality).[2-4] Thus, HT may be defined as sufficient elevation of BP that the benefits of BP reduction outweigh any risks.

Understandably, there is a degree of controversy over the exact point at which HT is defined in the continuous BP distribution.[2,3,5,6] Most current guidelines[2,3] indicate that for adults (age ≥18, both genders) moderate HT is 160/100 mm Hg or higher and mild HT is 140/90 mm Hg or higher. For those with high baseline cardiovascular risk (e.g., diabetics) it may be warranted to lower BP further. JNC VII guidelines from the United States[2] and the British HT Society guidelines from the U.K.,[3] respectively, define "prehypertensive" BP as 120 to 139/80 to 89 mm Hg[2] and a less radical "high normal" BP of 130 to 139/85 to 89 mm Hg[3] in which some lifestyle modification advice is minimally recommended. A substantial portion of the normal adult population will fall in this high normal category, and 60% of hypertensives (≥140/90 mm Hg) have DBP in the 90 to 100 mm Hg range. Hence such guidelines also have important public health implications for boundary line definition and for drug treatment. For those younger than age 18 and during pregnancy, BP is lower and separate normal ranges and guidelines for defining HT apply.[7,8]

Because BP rises with age in most populations, the implications of such definitions and guidelines is greatest for the elderly. Thus, more than 60% of those aged 65 to 74 have HT (BP ≥140/90 mm Hg), and 71% of ethnic Afro-Caribbeans have HT, especially isolated systolic HT (ISH).[9] However, it is important to remember that the absolute benefits in lowering BP in higher cardiovascular risk groups (elderly and diabetics) is greater because of the higher event rate they otherwise suffer.[9] Hence, defining such a large proportion of the elderly population as hypertensive seems appropriate.

## MECHANISMS IMPLICATED IN BLOOD PRESSURE CONTROL AND HYPERTENSION

### Physiologic Factors Generating Blood Pressure and Their Autoregulation

#### The Generation of Blood Pressure

Simplistically, the cardiac output (CO) drives blood across the total peripheral resistance (TPR) of the circulation by generating sufficient MAP. Because the circulating pressure returning to the heart at the right atrium is normally proportionately very small, the MAP approximates the net pressure gradient ($\Delta P$) across the systemic circulation. Thus, the simple equivalence applies: CO × TPR = MAP. Thus, factors that raise CO and/or TPR will predispose to HT. Figure 31-1 shows factors that influence the level of CO and TPR.

#### Factors Determining Cardiac Output

CO is the product of heart rate (HR) × stroke volume ejected per beat. The latter is influenced by the filling and ejection phases. Intrinsic cardiac properties of compliance (expandability: $\Delta V/\Delta P$) of the chambers facilitates filling. Contractility during ejection and normal valvular structures are important. Extrinsic factors also are important and derive from the coupling of the heart to the circulation and the influence of neural and humoral factors via the net "tone" that they exert on the heart. CO is coupled to the circulatory state because sufficient venous return (preload) to drive adequate filling and sufficient arterial distal run off is required, and compliance of the large arteries to permit ejection of the stroke volume against the afterload of the high pressure arterial system is necessary. Thus, preload and afterload are coupling factors by which the circulatory state influences CO. In the normal heart, increased preload couples via increased filling and myocardial fiber length to a greater contractile force ejecting the larger stroke volume. This coupling depends on the intrinsic myocardial length-force relationship, first described by Frank and

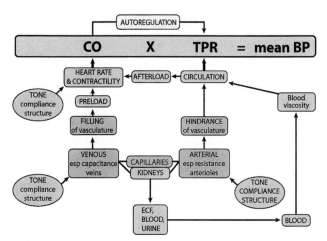

**FIGURE 31-1.** Factors generating BP. Aspects of the circulatory state and fluid balance influencing CO, TPR, and BP. ECF, extracellular fluid volume.

Starling. Neurohumoral effects on CO derive from several pathways, perhaps the most important is the sympathetic nervous system (SNS), which increases both HR and contractility. Neurohumoral and coupling factors can have a long-term significant influence on cardiac structure, which, when severe (e.g., marked hypertrophy, acquired cardiomyopathy, or valvular malfunction), can directly affect CO.

### Factors Determining Total Peripheral Resistance

The resistance (R) of flow (Q) of a liquid traversing a tube is dependent on the characteristics of the fluid and conduits and is described by Poiseuille's law, which can be expressed as $R = \Delta P/Q = 8\eta L/r^4$ (i.e., $R \propto L/r^4$), where $\eta$ is the fluid viscosity and L and r are the length and radius of the conduits. Hence, TPR is potentially powerfully affected by both blood viscosity ($\eta$) and hindrance (Z) to flow because of the structure of the vasculature, where $Z \propto L/r^4$. In particular TPR is profoundly influenced by the length and especially narrowness of the "bottleneck" in the vascular tree that comes at the level of the precapillary arterioles ("resistance vessels"), which have radii of approximately 25 to 100 μm and are relatively few in number compared with the branched capillary beds that follow. Factors affecting the compliance and especially the tone and structure of resistance vessels may change TPR and BP. Neural pathways, particularly the SNS, vasoactive mediators acting systemically (including adrenaline and AngII) or in a paracrine way (e.g., endothelin [ET]), NO, and products reflecting local tissue oxygenation and nutrition (e.g., ADP/ATP and lactic acid) are all able to affect resistance vessel tone. Increased luminal pressure stretches vascular muscle and stimulates calcium entry in a myogenic reflex promoting the maintenance of vessel caliber. Over longer periods (>30 minutes) in most tissues, if such pressure is maintained, the myogenic reflex in otherwise unstimulated vascular smooth muscle (VSM) fatigues giving way to a gradual stress-relaxation response whereby the smooth muscle fibrils "creep" back under the sustained pressure to a more relaxed, dilated position lowering the resistance and allowing the higher flow and pressure into the capillaries distally. The equivalent *afferent* arterioles in kidney have a strong myogenic reflex and specialized regulation allowing maintenance of similar blood flow across a wide range of arterial pressure. Again structural changes in the arterial tree, especially at the level of the resistance vessels, may play a very important role in determining long-term changes in TPR. Thus, chronic stimulation may lead to VSM hypertrophy, magnifying vasoconstrictor responses, attenuating vasodilator responses, and directly increasing the vascular hindrance by reducing the lumen radius. Similarly, atherosclerosis and other structural endothelial damage may impair vasodilation, and reduction of resistance vessel numbers (rarefaction) will hinder flow and increase TPR.

Thus, influences on small-vessel tone, structure, and compliance derive from a mixture of factors acting via neural, systemic humoral, and paracrine pathways, and mechanisms resulting from local metabolism and intrinsic to the vessel wall (the endothelial response to flow and VSM response to stretch). Distal to the resistance vessels, capillaries are much more numerous, and the venous vasculature is of larger diameter; thus, hindrance to flow is considerably less. Hydrostatic-osmotic (Starling) forces govern filtration and reabsorption between capillary beds and host tissues, thus partitioning blood and interstitial fluids. Similarly, the specialized glomerular and peritubular capillary beds in the kidney filter to and reabsorb from nephrons partitioning blood from tubular fluid and urine. Thus, in health the capillaries are less important in their influence on TPR than on ensuring normal tissue oxygenation and nutrition and facilitating normal fluid homeostasis and, thus, blood volume. The venous vascular tree has low resistance and high capacitance. Low-level venous sympathetic tone is surprisingly important in maintaining consistent venous return (preload) assisted by structural competence of venous valves and muscle and respiratory pump actions.

Blood viscosity plays an important role in determining TPR, but in practice it varies less than factors affecting vascular hindrance. Although there is no doubt that marked elevations in whole blood viscosity[10,11] (whether resulting from higher hematocrit, lower red cell deformability or higher plasma viscosity[11] involving globulins or fibrinogen levels) do increase BP and carry higher thrombotic risks especially risk of stroke,[12,13] the effects of lesser increases[14] are diminished by the non-newtonian characteristics of blood and may be difficult to distinguish from coexisting effects of hematocrit on tissue oxygenation.

### Systolic, Diastolic and Pulse Pressure

The previous discussion relates to MAP. Two factors that have little effect on MAP but do influence pulse pressure, raising SBP and lowering DBP, are slower HR (larger stroke volume ejected: SBP higher) and reduced large artery compliance (greater pressure rise on ejection: higher SBP). The latter is a major factor in the much increased frequency of ISH in the elderly. Increased speed of systolic ejection (as with increased contractility and force of ejection) would increase SBP, but it is often limited by the often-associated higher HR.

### The Autoregulation and Long-Term Interchange between $\Delta CO \leftrightarrow \Delta TPR$

In a number of animal models and in some observations on human HT, it seems that, although HT remains, there is *autoregulation* from a relatively elevated CO "hyperdynamic" state to a more chronic phase in which CO returns to normal but TPR is elevated. In some situations, including observations on young people at an early stage of HT, the TPR actually begins slightly low so that the hyperdynamic state is initially normotensive. The nature of the process causing such an autoregulatory or longer term interchange between early elevations of CO and later elevations of TPR remains obscure and somewhat contentious but is potentially of profound importance in understanding HT.

The involvement of different responses of heart and peripheral resistance vessels has led to the idea that differential neurohumoral stimulation is involved at these two sites. It is unclear whether this is initially coordinated by cardiovascular reflexes and/or by the CNS centers, such as the vasomotor center and hypothalamic nuclei, or peripherally as a consequence of altering tissue sensitivity to neurohumoral stimulation (e.g., by altered receptor expression). The basis of the rise in TPR remains obscure; it may relate to higher blood flow bringing in excess local mediators or excess washing out of local metabolites and thus triggering an intrinsic increase in tone. However, these theories come from old studies and have not been verified, and elucidating the true basis warrants modern studies of these issues. With increasing duration, age of the subject, or severity of HT these trends to normal or reduced CO and elevated TPR progress and are then seen increasingly as resulting from the end-organ effects of the high BP. Changes involving LVH and reduced compliance may, thus, limit CO, and hypertrophic VSM changes with elevated wall-to-lumen ratios and overlying endothelial dysfunction limiting NO-mediated vasodilation would contribute to TPR typically with associated increased VSM intracellular calcium and brisk responses to vasoconstrictor stimuli.

Considerable evidence indicates that persistence of HT implies impairment of renal $Na^+$ handling. If correct, it would follow that the autoregulatory rise of TPR is largely a consequence of the raised BP *unless* at an early stage it simultaneously disrupts normal pressure natriuresis.

## Power and Time Course of the Major Physiologic Mechanisms Regulating Blood Pressure

### Overview

Regulation of BP involves the coordinated action of several mechanisms (Fig. 31-2), each with distinct triggering, time course of action, and potency. Three powerful autonomic nervous system reflex mechanisms act very rapidly, within seconds or minutes: (1) the baroreceptor, (2) the chemoreceptor, and (3) the CNS ischemic response reflexes.

Three further mechanisms develop their major response over an intermediate time course of 30 minutes to a few hours: (1) the stress-relaxation response of resistance vessels, (2) the capillary fluid-shift response to BP transmitted to the capillary beds, and (3) the RAS triggered especially by pressure sensing at the specialized afferent (resistance) arterioles in kidneys. Finally, two slower-onset mechanisms are important when pressure changes persist for more than a few hours, and their responses continue to develop toward their full strength for more than 24 hours: (1) the powerful renal pressure natriuresis mechanism and (2) the regulation of aldosterone (downregulation if HT).

Much of the basis of this theory derives from pioneering studies of circulatory physiology in past decades[15] and, because the principles derived were accurate, it has stood the test of time with further expert insights guiding further developments.[16] Barriers to direct study of circulatory fundamentals in humans are clear. However,

with increasing sophistication of indirect monitoring, it is appropriate to consider whether it is now becoming possible to verify such overviews of the regulation of the short- and long-term control of BP in humans and compare findings to those originally derived from direct study in large animals such as dogs. Similarly it is of great benefit to focus on small animal models (e.g., mice) to comprehensively describe the gain and time course of major mechanisms controlling short- and long-term BP. Again, barriers to such study are diminishing with increasing miniaturization, and the advent of high-quality radiotelemetry permits at least some of the measurements required to monitor the intact conscious free-living mouse. If it were possible to analyze both human and mouse BP regulatory systems at a level equivalent to the analysis shown in Figure 31-2, one could potentially connect modern molecular and genetic studies with these physiologic fundamentals no longer isolated by a species divide of their basis. This would allow systems analysis in wild-type and hypertensive knockout mice to reveal which BP control systems had been perturbed and how their gain and time course had been affected. If the substantial difficulties in studying these BP control systems reliably and (largely) noninvasively in humans could be circumvented, then studies on normotensive and hypertensive family members could be compared to understand more clearly how these whole-body integrative processes are perturbed in causes of human secondary HT in which the genetic basis is known (e.g., Liddle's syndrome) and, for example, in twins discordant for essential HT. Finally, such a revisiting of these matters in humans and mice would allow the opportunity to place in context the role of other systems not currently integrated into the scheme shown in Figure 31-2 (e.g., the natriuretic peptide system [NPS]) in terms of gain and time course of effect. For the present, Figure 31-2 remains the best basis for description of these fundamentals, and because many aspects of these systems have been seen to perform similarly in humans, it appears this is probably a largely accurate account of the major principles governing BP control mechanisms in humans.

### The Rapidly Induced Reflexes

These reflexes all respond very rapidly (e.g., the baroceptor firing rate varies across the pressure swings during a heart beat). In response to a substantial change in BP, a maximal response develops in well under a minute.

### The Baroreceptor Reflex

The baroreceptors are high-pressure stretch-sensitive nerve endings in the carotid sinus (internal carotid near the common carotid bifurcation) and aortic arch that are stimulated by increased BP to trigger the BP-lowering reflex. Signals travel via the afferent fibers of the glossopharyngeal and vagus nerves, respectively, to the nucleus of the tractus solitarius, which then inhibits SNS outflow from the medullary vasoconstrictor (vasomotor) center and stimulates vagal tone, causing peripheral vasodilation and reduced CO (reduced HR and

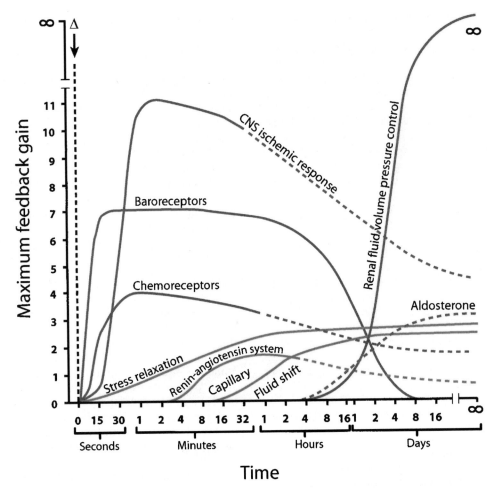

**FIGURE 31-2.** Major physiologic mechanisms regulating BP. Time course and strength (in terms of feedback gain) of BP corrective mechanisms after a sudden change in arterial pressure is applied (indicated by Δ) from time zero. Clearly the long-term control of BP is dominated by the renal fluid-volume pressure control (pressure natriuresis). *(Adapted from Guyton AC: Arterial Pressure and Hypertension. Philadelphia, WB Saunders, 1980, with permission.)*

contractility) that lowers BP. In health, the baroreceptor reflex normally ceases firing when BP falls to approximately 60 mm Hg and fires increasingly up to approximately 200 mm Hg maximum (more so if BP is rising rather than falling). This reflex is of key importance in short-term BP control, and through reflex adjustment in autonomic stimulation of heart and vasculature it dampens BP swings (e.g., with postural changes such as standing). Baroreflex denervation experiments in animals confirm an undamped much more labile BP, but the average MAP is not affected. As can be seen from Figure 31-2 a sustained rise in BP elicits a strong effect on the baroreceptor response, but this diminishes over several hours and resets and ceases after several days. The reflex, thus, probably contributes little to the defense against sustained HT.

### The Chemoreceptor Reflex

Normally the chemoreceptor reflex plays very little or no role in BP control. However, if $pO_2$ falls low enough to excite the chemoreceptors of the carotid and aortic

bodies, then this reflex stimulates respiration (with some ancillary augmentation on venous return, preload, and thus CO) and causes some stimulation of the vasomotor center increasing CO and TPR. Thus, its role in BP control is limited and would usually only become significant at times of hypotension (especially BP < 60 mm Hg) with coincident hypoxia as may occur in shock or hemorrhage. However, if hypoxia and HT were to coexist, the role played could be more significant. Local disease or abnormalities in chemoreceptor tissue could also potentially inappropriately excite this reflex.

### The CNS Ischemic Response Reflex

The CNS ischemic response reflex is excited by ischemic phenomena (raised $pCO_2$ and acidosis more than hypoxia) in the area of the medullary vasomotor center and normally represents a state with threatened brainstem damage because of local disease, systemic hypotension (BP < 50 mm Hg), and/or ischemia. The reflex is the most powerful stimulus of the SNS, causing considerably more profound vasoconstriction than full downregulation of the baroreceptor reflex. Because cerebrovascular, coronary, and renal blood flows are maintained by autoregulation, this reflex is not thought to play a role in control of BP at normal or high levels. It may be important if local disease in the brainstem altered the reflex or brainstem blood supply (e.g., by affecting local vasculature or raising intracranial pressure; such cases in humans have been reported[17-19]). What remains unclear is whether this reflex plays a role in chronic HT in larger groups of people (e.g., elderly people with cerebrovascular disease).[20]

### Responses of Intermediate Time Course

#### Stress-Relaxation and Capillary Fluid-Shift Mechanisms

The stress-relaxation response was mentioned previously (in the section about $\Delta CO$-$\Delta TPR$ autoregulation) and is due to the local effect of pressure causing otherwise unstimulated VSM fibers in resistance vessels to creep back to a more dilated state. This allows TPR to fall but at the expense of exposure of capillary beds to higher pressure. Such simple stress-relaxation is well developed within 30 minutes but does not occur at the same pressures in arterioles in the brain and kidney (afferent arterioles) in which there is autoregulation of blood flow. Stress-relaxation not only lowers TPR and thus BP but also facilitates the capillary fluid-shift mechanism that is due to the greater capillary bed hydrostatic pressure shifting the Starling force equilibrium to favor fluid movement from the circulation into interstitial fluid spaces. This reduces circulatory filling, preload, CO, and thus BP. The stress-relaxation and capillary fluid shift mechanisms are linked processes that begin within less than 30 minutes and are fully developed in approximately 12 hours. They help limit rapid BP rises. Such chronic peripheral tissue vasodilation may in the longer term give rise to harmful effects including vessel hypertrophic changes, thus increasing TPR again. This seems especially the case if the BP remains elevated despite the stress-relaxation fluid-shift response. If resistance vessels are simultaneously under vasoconstrictor influence, these will limit and slow relaxation and encourage more prominent vessel hypertrophy. In kidney the afferent arteriole autoregulates blood flow through to the glomerulus and integrates the stress-relaxation effect of increased BP with other stimuli affecting its contraction including those from SNS innervation, systemic neurohumoral mediators (e.g., ANP), and special localized influences deriving from the local juxtaglomerular (JG) apparatus (including adenosine and prostaglandins). As such, the aggregate response of the kidney afferent arterioles to pressure is to some extent involved in the remaining mechanisms.

#### Renin Angiotensin System

The wall of the afferent arteriole within the JG apparatus acts as an integrator of signals for activation of renin release—the rate-limiting factor in activation of the RAS. Thus, HT causes increased afferent pressure, reduced SNS stimulation (baroreceptor action), and inhibition of renin release (this also occurs when there is increased delivery of NaCl to the macula densa). Conversely, renin release is increased if BP and afferent pressure are low or with increased SNS stimulation (and with reduced NaCl delivery to the macula densa). The specialized smooth muscle cells and JG cells, lining the afferent arteriole, synthesize inert prorenin from which renin is produced by cleavage. Renin, a protease without vasoactive properties, has a half-life of approximately 30 minutes and cleaves a circulating renin substrate angiotensinogen made principally in the liver (but also elsewhere including in adipose tissue) that results in the formation of a 10 amino acid peptide angiotensin I (half-life of a few seconds) with only trivial vasoconstrictor properties. Angiotensin I is then cleaved by ACE (present especially in lung but also in renal epithelia and as a circulating enzyme) to an eight amino acid peptide AngII (circulating half-life ~2 minutes), a very potent vasoconstrictor of arteries (including renal arteries) which causes milder vasoconstriction of veins and causes some increase in tubular $Na^+$ reabsorption (especially in proximal tubule [PT] and to some extent in thick ascending limb [TAL]) and in tubuloglomerular feedback (TGF). AngII is also one of the strongest stimuli for aldosterone secretion from the adrenal. AngII is subject to cleavage; one of the products is a seven amino acid peptide AngIII, which circulates at around 20% of the concentration of AngII and is equipotent for stimulation of aldosterone release but a comparatively weak vasoconstrictor. Other enzymes further cleave AngII and AngIII to inert fragments.

The normal role of the RAS is twofold. First, release of renin in response to low BP leads to formation of AngII, which assists in raising BP via vasoconstriction and $Na^+$ retention. The RAS takes 20 to 30 minutes to significantly upregulate but can remain persistently activated. Second, at a local level the RAS assists in regulation of the nephron unit, raising renin levels if insufficient NaCl is reaching the distal nephron (sensed at the macula densa). In addition to the systemic RAS, there are some additional "tissue-based" renin angiotensin activities in other tissues including actions on the heart and some CNS effects including effects on thirst. In HT with normal blood flow to the kidney it would be expected that renin and AngII levels would be suppressed. This is often not the case, suggesting coexisting disease affecting renal blood flow or nephrons with reduced delivery of NaCl distally to macula densa. In aggregate, the RAS pathway has an important influence on long-term BP and interacts with the renal pressure-natriuresis system and the aldosterone-$Na^+$ retention pathway, which AngII plays a key role in stimulating.

Not only is the RAS involved in normal medium and long-term BP control but in several situations it appears to play an important role in the origin of raised BP by being inappropriately active in the face of elevated BP. This can occur if there is inappropriate elevation of SNS activity. It also seems to occur in two situations in which the kidney is affected in particular: (1) when there is arterial disease/narrowing afferent to glomeruli, in conjunction with normal or high BP this results in a population of nephrons with reduced perfusion, which elevates renin and triggers a further rise in BP; (2) when the BP is normal or high but the $Na^+$ delivery to the macula densa is reduced. This can occur with glomerular disease resulting in less filtration for normal afferent flow (reduced ultrafiltration coefficient $K_f$, for single nephrons: $K_f$ x N = $K_F$ for whole kidney, where N = nephron number). It can also occur if there is greater than normal proximal $Na^+$ reabsorption (as may occur in diabetes). In both situations less $Na^+$ reaches the macula densa and this stimulates renin release (and a rise in GFR of those nephrons via TGF) to restore adequate filtration but at the expense of somewhat elevated glomerular pressure (hyperfiltration, to bypass the glomerular filter disease or balance the high proximal reabsorption) and elevated renin despite normal BP, thus predisposing to HT. Thus, in two situations in which there is renal or renal arterial disease there may be inappropriate elevation of renin, predisposing to HT. These situations predispose to sustained HT because there is usually impairment of renal pressure natriuresis. Such chronic activation of the RAS, especially with imbalance between nephrons, may drive the hemodynamics of some to the point at which tubulointerstitial ischemia and nephron loss commence and a vicious cycle of renal decline may follow. It is in such situations that ACE inhibitors (or angiotensin receptors blockers) have been very promising in moderating these adverse intrarenal effects and in simultaneously lowering BP.

### Long-Term Mechanisms

Long-term mechanisms are "slow on slow off" responses that play no significant role in defense against BP swings over seconds to minutes but play major roles in long-term BP control developing over 1 day and strengthening further to dominate longer term BP control.

#### Renal Pressure-Natriuresis

The regulation of $Na^+$ homeostasis is of vital importance because this normally directly determines extracellular fluid (ECF) volume and BP. The renal pressure natriuresis mechanism plays a dominant role in long-term BP control, entraining $Na^+$ excretion to maintain normotension[15,16]; sustained HT occurs only if this pressure natriuresis is impaired. Despite the acknowledged importance of compensatory pressure natriuresis, understanding of the renal mechanisms involved is still incomplete. It seems clear, however, that in response to increased BP, a pressure rise is transmitted from the systemic circulation to the glomeruli of the nephrons across the afferent vascular resistance ($R_A$, i.e., between aorta and glomerulus). Effectiveness of the renal pressure natriuresis is impaired if transmission of pressure is limited by, for example, renal artery stenosis, an experimental narrowing applied to the renal artery (as in the clipped kidney in Goldblatt HT models), or servo controlling renal artery pressure to prevent the rise.[16] Increased pressure reaching the nephrons enables an increase in $Na^+$ and water filtration at the glomeruli with associated changes in renal $Na^+$ handling, which results in a reduced fractional reabsorption of $Na^+$ ($FR_{Na}$) and increased natriuresis. Pressure natriuresis is not merely a consequence of increased GFR and, although the molecular pathways underpinning it are not yet clear, it seems

that downregulation of $Na^+$ reabsorption pathways and blunting of feedback mechanisms that limit this in the nephron are involved. The reabsorption route for filtered $Na^+$ in the tubular fluid can either be transcellular (traversing apical and then basolateral membranes) or paracellular (traversing between cells at intercellular junctions). The understanding of transcellular $Na^+$ reabsorption has advanced rapidly; the cloning of transporters accounts for most $Na^+$ reabsorption across all nephron segments. Understanding of the paracellular route is more limited, and recent studies involving transgenic and knockout mice[21] suggest that it is not as quantitatively important as was thought previously and is substantially dependent on adjacent localization of transcellular transport. To downregulate $Na^+$ reabsorption and lower $FR_{Na}$ pressure natriuresis must, in part, involve alteration in the transcellular reabsorption of filtered $Na^+$. Although the basolateral $Na^+$-$K^+$-ATPase provides the driving force for transcellular $Na^+$ reabsorption across most of the nephron, $Na^+$ reabsorption is regarded as principally regulated at the point of apical entry, and the transport pathway involved is nephron segment specific. Approximately 60% of filtered $Na^+$ is reabsorbed in the PT, 30% in the TAL, 7% in the distal convoluted tubule/connecting tubule (DCT/CNT), and 1% to approximately 3% in the collecting duct (CD), especially the cortical CD (CCD), leaving no more than 2% and as little as 0.02% (usually <1%) finally passing in the urine. This normal 100-fold or so range in the fractional excretion of $Na^+$ ($FE_{Na}$) is of key importance in long-term $Na^+$ and ECF balance and is largely determined by the late DCT-CD and is responsive to aldosterone, the other late-onset mechanism (Fig. 31-2, and see later discussion).

Although PT is regarded as a relatively "leaky" epithelium, recent work indicates that most $Na^+$ reabsorption is transcellular and the significant minority that is paracellular is strongly facilitated indirectly by transcellular transport via generation of charge and concentration gradients. Several apical transporters are involved but the type 3 $Na^+$-$H^+$ exchanger (NHE3) dominates with 80% of all PT $Na^+$ reabsorption being attributable directly or indirectly to NHE3.[21] Thus, in homozygous NHE3 knockout ($-/-$) mice, PT $Na^+$ reabsorption is reduced by this order of magnitude. Much smaller contributions from the cotransport of $Na^+$ are due to the major apical glucose (SGLT2 and also SGLT1) and phosphate (Na/Pi-2) cotransporters, although it now seems that another $Na^+$ transport system, possibly the recently cloned NHE8, may account for more than half of the NHE3-independent $Na^+$ reabsorption.[21,22] More distally, 30% of filtered $Na^+$ is reabsorbed in TAL with almost all requiring the Na-K-Cl-Co-transporter type 2 (NKCC2 cotransporter). In DCT most (4% to 5% of filtered $Na^+$) of reabsorption is via TSC (the thiazide-sensitive cotransporter), the rest in the more distal DCT and CNT is via the amiloride-sensitive (epithelial) $Na^+$ channel ENaC that is also responsible for most CD $Na^+$ reabsorption (1% to approximately 3% filtered $Na^+$). NKCC2, TSC, and ENaC are all diuretic targets for the loop diuretics (such as frusemide), thiazides, and amiloride, respectively. NHE3 functions in association with a colocalized carbonic anhydrase, which is the target for another class of diuretics (carbonic anhydrase inhibitors, e.g., acetazolamide) acting on the PT.

An increase in filtered Na$^+$ load will normally be met by a series of compensatory mechanisms increasing its reabsorption: glomerulotubular balance (GTB) in PT, tubulo-tubular balance in TAL and DCT, TGF at the macula densa (end of TAL) feeding back to reduce GFR. Therefore, although 60% of Na$^+$ is reabsorbed in the PT, reductions in reabsorption at this level are normally met with a series of compensatory mechanisms (including TGF to reduce GFR) limiting the extent to which this unreabsorbed Na$^+$ ever reaches the urine. Consequently the relatively small 1% to approximately 3% Na$^+$ reabsorbed in CD is disproportionately very important, being the last nephron segment to influence the amount of Na$^+$ passed in urine.

Aldosterone is the principal regulator of Na$^+$ reabsorption in late DCT-CD and, thus, exerts a powerful effect on Na$^+$ balance as it regulates Na$^+$ reabsorption and hence tubular fluid Na$^+$ content just before it finally leaving the kidney as urine. The aldosterone-distal nephron Na$^+$ reabsorption mechanism is considered in detail later. However, there is much more to the regulation of pressure natriuresis than the role of aldosterone. First, other factors have some influence on Na$^+$ reabsorption in late DCT-CD. Both flow-dependent increase in reabsorption and ANP stimulated natriuresis in the medullary CD have some influence on Na$^+$ reabsorption in late DCT-CD. Other factors, such as insulin, TGF$\beta$, PGE2, and ET (via ET-B receptors) all may interact with aldosterone action to determine late DCT-CD Na$^+$ reabsorption. Second, in chronic aldosterone excess the increase in Na$^+$ retention and BP is eventually met by poorly understood compensatory mechanisms that appear to act more proximally in the nephron, increasing distal delivery to the point at which the Na$^+$ delivery overwhelms the limited capacity of late DCT-CD for Na$^+$ reabsorption. To bring about such an increase in Na$^+$ load (probably through a reduction in PT-TAL FR$_{Na}$ or possibly an increase in filtered Na$^+$ load) there must be blunting of the normal TGF response, which would downregulate GFR and stop the increased distal delivery. Third, if reabsorption in a proximal nephron segment is upregulated inappropriately (e.g., by greater surface expression and activation of NHE3), then distal delivery to the macula densa would be lower, TGF would increase GFR, and renin release would be increased. Accordingly, the tendency to high renin (and thus not fully suppressible aldosterone) and glomerular hyperfiltration with risks of nephron damage suggests that mechanisms regulating more proximal Na$^+$ reabsorption may also give rise to HT if dysregulated. Finally, the usefulness of loop diuretics and thiazides in treating HT indicate how TAL and DCT Na$^+$ reabsorption contribute importantly within the renal pressure natriuresis mechanism to influence BP. This is also emphasized by the lower BP[23,24] of patients with the corresponding Mendelian salt-wasting conditions of Bartter's syndrome[24-26] (defects in NKCC2 or channels working in concert with it, i.e., the apical K$^+$ channel ROMK or the 2 subunit basolateral Cl$^-$ channel composed of CLC-KB and Barttin[25,26]) and to a lesser extent Gitelman's syndrome (mutations in TSC[23]). These phenotypes are reproduced in mice with knockout of NKCC2,[21] ROMK,[27] or TSC.[21]

It is clear that the level of Na$^+$ reabsorption throughout the nephron can play a role in long-term BP control. Overall renal pressure natriuresis mechanisms are still incompletely understood, and it is beyond the scope of this chapter to consider the studies in further detail. Nonetheless, involvement of a range of mediators are proposed including adrenaline, noradrenaline, AngII, dopamine, ADH, NO, ET, prostaglandins, and others. There is no doubt that renal pressure natriuresis is a major determinant of long-term BP, and further understanding of the molecular pathways controlling this mechanism will give insight into the pathophysiology of HT and routes to its better treatment.

### Aldosterone-Distal Sodium Reabsorption

The aldosterone-distal Na$^+$ reabsorption pathway is the final pathway shown in Figure 31-2. The aldosterone-responsive distal nephron plays an important role in maintaining Na$^+$ balance. Normally it receives a relatively constant distal delivery of 2% to 3% of filtered Na$^+$, the reabsorption of which is regulated over a 100-fold range (usually 0.02% to >2% of filtered Na$^+$) to match requirements. Reduction in the upper limit of this range predisposes to Na$^+$ retention and HT and may result from inadequate distal delivery or distal reabsorption that does not shut off normally. The pathway by which aldosterone upregulates Na$^+$ reabsorption in kidney (shown in Fig. 31-3) is key in regulating Na$^+$ balance and highly implicated in BP control in humans. Thus, disturbances in the activity of this pathway at any stage (abnormal aldosterone levels or altered activity of any of the known genes participating in the pathway) cause BP abnormalities in humans.[28] Moreover, in gene targeted and knockout mice carrying the equivalent mutations in the corresponding mouse genes, it is striking how similar the renal and BP phenotype mirrors that in the equivalent human disorder. In the hypertensive conditions shown in Figure 31-3 and in low-renin HT more generally, Na$^+$ reabsorption does not shut off and remains inappropriately high. There are definitely gaps in this important pathway filled by as yet unidentified corticosteroid-regulated genes (CRG). Such CRGs are of great interest because, like other genes in these pathways, they participate in the control of BP and are candidate genes in the causation of HT. Recently, a kinase called sgk (serum and glucocorticoid kinase) has been identified as a strong renal CRG, because sgk is strongly upregulated in the distal nephron by aldosterone.[29,30] Very recently a sgk knockout mouse has been generated, which on a low-salt diet has low BP as expected.[31] Such genes are also of interest because they may also prove to be points of cross talk between aldosterone and other mediators proposed to influence distal nephron Na$^+$ reabsorption such as insulin, TGF$\beta$, and ET. Thus, for example, insulin exerts part of its Na$^+$-retaining influence via PI-3-kinase-dependent activation of sgk to upregulate ENaC activity[32] (Fig. 31-3). Finally, provocative findings that homozygous null CD-specific ENaC$\alpha$ knockout mice have no clear defects in electrolyte handling or BP even

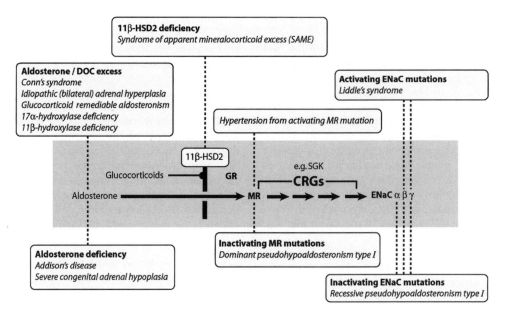

**FIGURE 31-3.** Corticosteroid regulation of sodium reabsorption and BP in the distal nephron. The known pathway of aldosterone-regulated sodium reabsorption in kidney collecting duct is illustrated. Corticosteroids (glucocorticoids and aldosterone) act via glucocorticoid and mineralocorticoid receptors (GR and MR), protected in distal nephron by the glucocorticoid inactivating enzyme 11β-HSD2, thus limiting their occupancy and ensuring that aldosterone determines MR binding. Bound receptors activate poorly understood pathways that require ongoing new gene transcription to increase sodium reabsorption via ENaC. There are as yet unidentified corticosteroid regulated genes (CRGs) mediating major upregulation of ENaC transport independent of transcription of ENaC subunits. The pathway from aldosterone to upregulation of sodium reabsorption via ENaC in the distal nephron is strongly implicated in BP control and causation of HT in humans. This is indicated by all the disorders directly disrupting this pathway causing hypotension *(bottom of diagram)* or HT *(top of diagram)*. The currently unidentified CRGs occupying the missing steps in this pathway are of key interest. The studies proposed involve assessment of the role of established and candidate CRGs in pathways controlling sodium handling and BP.

on low $Na^+$ diets[33] is leading to greatly renewed interest in amiloride-sensitive transport in connecting tubule and less distal nephron segments.

### Other Blood Pressure Control Mechanisms

In addition to the classical integrated overview of BP control represented in Figure 31-2, one must consider the indirect involvement of additional systems. Because of significant gaps in the present understanding, it is difficult to know how to incorporate such putative additional BP control systems as the natriuretic peptide, ET, and NO systems (and others mentioned in subsequent sections) into this classical overview (Fig. 31-2). Studies in gene-targeted mice show, for example, that mice with knockout of eNOS have chronic HT,[34] loss of atrial natriuretic peptide receptor causes marked HT,[35] and CD-specific loss of ET-1 causes salt-sensitive HT.[36] Moreover, the lack of global correlation of circulating markers of activation of other BP control systems with BP (e.g., in having both low- and high-renin HT) has never been taken as precluding systems such as the RAS from playing an important role in BP regulation. The natriuretic peptide and ET systems may be less critical than the RAS in normal BP control and may play most important roles in certain contexts such as the volume-expanded state (for ANP) or in renal ischemia (for ET) where their effects on long-term BP center on modulation of the renal-pressure natriuresis system. Nonetheless, in our view, these modern systems have their place alongside those established systems in an integrated view of the whole-body regulation of BP. With

renewed interest in integrative physiology, a revisiting of the basis of integrated control of BP in humans and in rodent models should seek to place these systems of more recent discovery alongside those in the classical view shown in Figure 31-2.

### Mechanisms Considered Especially Important in Long-Term Blood Pressure Control

Although all the previously discussed mechanisms play important roles in some contexts, it is clear that the renal pressure natriuresis mechanism plays a dominant role. Structural changes in the vessels afferent to the kidney, or intrarenally afferent to the glomeruli, can limit the extent to which the kidney can correctly sense systemic pressure; thus, at this level this afferent vasculature plays a key role. The RAS and aldosterone systems play important modulatory roles on pressure natriuresis and inappropriately high levels of one or both can force a long-term rise in BP from which escape by normal pressure natriuresis is impaired. Chronic inappropriately high levels of the RAS activation stimulates other phenomena still not fully understood, which promote hypertrophic responses in vasculature and the heart and alter renal hemodynamics to leave renal tissue more prone to ischemia and fibrotic change. All of these leave permanent adverse effects in a circulatory system already under stress from HT and in a kidney already coping with renal insufficiency. Similarly, chronic inappropriate aldosterone excess, especially in the face of continuing high BP and salt intake, appears to be accompanied by risks of adverse fibrotic changes in the heart, longer term greater arterial stiffness, and exacerbated proteinuric glomerular disease where it coexists because of hypervolemic hyperfiltration. Again these may leave long-term changes perpetuating HT.

## Candidate Biochemical and Molecular Pathways Regulating Blood Pressure

Many biochemical and molecular pathways have been implicated in the normal control of BP and as contributors to causation of HT. In the broadest terms HT can be directly caused or at least facilitated if a pathway capable of raising BP is dysregulated, by inappropriate upregulation or failure to switch off. Equally, a pathway capable of lowering BP may play a role in HT through inappropriate downregulated or failure to switch on. Useful evidence to implicate such pathways and mediators in HT come from several key sources including (1) theoretical involvement with BP control systems, (2) demonstration of inappropriate activity in HT and especially in the early or prehypertensive state, (3) pharmacologic intervention altering the pathway activity and BP as expected, (4) genetic defects or alternative alleles found in patients or "engineered" in animal models (especially transgenic or gene-targeted mice) altering the activity of the pathway and BP as expected, (5) linkage with BP or association studies at a sufficient level of statistical significance and in larger numbers of patients or populations (ideally of diverse geographical and racial mix) together with evidence that the genetic change is indicative of an alteration in pathway activity.

It is beyond the scope of this chapter to go into great detail on all these, although subsequent sections revisit many aspects and a relatively brief treatment follows immediately. Table 31-1 summarizes cardinal points under the five key sources outlined previously for pathways that have been widely studied and implicated in BP regulation and are, thus, regarded as candidates in contributing to causes of HT. Other possible such candidates that have been less studied are not included in Table 31-1 but are listed in Table 31-2. Table 31-1 deals with evidence supporting the case of the more important pathways seen as candidates determining interindividual variation in BP and affecting the risk of HT. There is long-established evidence for the RAS, adrenergic SNS, and aldosterone-ENaC pathway in regulating BP. However, a key issue here is not only whether systems regulate BP but also if they can attain inappropriate levels of activity and be involved in the origin of HT. These more important pathways are dealt with later in detail with discussion of the aldosterone-ENaC under mineralocorticoid HT. This and other renal $Na^+$ reabsorption pathways are also discussed in the section on long-term BP control mechanisms discussed previously.

### The Renin Angiotensin System

Evidence for a role of the RAS in HT is very strong. As a BP-elevating system it is certainly inappropriately active in high-renin HT and also in normal-renin HT. Moreover,

these states often show blunting or complete lack of modulation of renal blood flow or adrenal aldosterone secretion in response to AngII infusions[37,38] (infused or elicited by stepped changes in $Na^+$ intake). This "nonmodulation" intermediate phenotype in essential HT, thus, shows not only inappropriately high circulating renin for the raised BP but also abnormalities in the tissue responses of the RAS.[37] The effectiveness of ACE inhibitors (e.g., captopril and lisinopril) in achieving some reduction in BP and the similarly effective BP-lowering power of AT1 blockers (e.g., losartan) points to effects on the RAS rather than other ACE inhibitor effects (e.g., on bradykinin) being behind the BP reductions. In cases in which responses to the drug are large, there is an increased likelihood that the system blocked was actively contributing to the HT. Families with severe mutations of the RAS have not been reported, but where this has been achieved in animal models the long-term BP has always been altered as expected. Mice homozygous for knockout of angiotensinogen, ACE, and AT1A genes are all hypotensive[39] (mice have a second AT1B gene of relatively minor physiologic importance compared with the AT1A homolog of the single human AT1: complete AT1 knockout mice are also hypotensive). Similarly, complete knockout of renin in the mouse results in low BP[40,41]; depending on the mouse strain this would involve knockout of either 1[40] (ren1c) or 2[41] (ren1d and ren2) renin genes. Although homozygous knockout animals (−/−) of all these kinds have low BP the heterozygotes (+/−) have normal resting BP. Importantly, transgenic animals with overactivity of the RAS have HT often severe. The first of these to be established was a rat transgenic line carrying a murine (ren2) gene yielding a rat with an overactivated and not normally suppressible RAS and marked HT.[42] This TGR(mREN2)27 rat, the first transgenic hypertensive model, has been widely studied and both the original strain and its variants including one in which the transgene is inducible[43] have allowed insight into the RAS and its overactivation in causing HT, accelerated HT, and hypertensive tissue damage.[41,43,44] Other transgenic rodents overexpressing angiotensinogen or both renin and angiotensinogen are also hypertensive.[45] There has been a lot of attention paid to the components of the RAS in studies examining linkage and association to human primary HT, which have shown most positive findings for angiotensinogen (see tick/cross scoring in Table 31-1) and are summarized in detail later (see candidate genes sections). Although no genome scan reported has identified a component gene in the RAS as a major quantitative trait locus (QTL) in human primary HT, this system is without doubt involved in long-term regulation of BP and seems strongly implicated in abnormalities involved in this common human disorder.

### The Adrenergic Sympathetic Nervous System

The adrenergic SNS system has a role in short-term regulation of BP, but its role in sustaining long-term changes in BP has been less clear. However, the long-term BP lowering effects of β-blockers (e.g., atenolol), $\alpha_1$-blockers (e.g., doxazosin), and centrally acting $\alpha_2$-agonists (e.g.,

## TABLE 31-1  MAJOR BIOCHEMICAL/MOLECULAR PATHWAYS IMPLICATED IN REGULATING BLOOD PRESSURE

| System/Pathway | ΔBP | (i) Theory | (ii) Inappropriate Pathway Activity in Hypertension | (iii) Pharmacological Support | (iv) Support for Role in HT from Families, Animal Models — Families | Animal Models | (v) Genetic Link/Assoc with BP in Population — Association/Linkage | Overall |
|---|---|---|---|---|---|---|---|---|
| **Renin-Angiotensin System:** | ↑ | Long Established, Very Strong: ↑vasoconstriction, ↑aldosterone, ↑PCT Na$^+$ reabsorb, ↓NO vasodilation, ↑insulin resistance + renal decline, in CNS ↑ SNS, … | Yes: high renin HT, normal-renin HT, non-modulators. | Yes, very strong, ACE inhibitors AT1 blockers | ?No | Yes, Extensive: renin −/− BP↓ AGT−/− BP↓ ACE−/− BP↓ AT1−/− BP↓ (AT1A±B) + others | Extensive study:- AGT, M235T etc ✓✓✓✓✓✗✗ ACE, I/D ✓✓✗✗✗ AT1 ✓✗✗ Renin ?✗ | Strong |
| **Sympathetic Nervous System (SNS)** | ↑ | Long Established Clear short term BP, mechanism of long-term effect less clear. ↑CO, ↑vasocons-triction (α>β), ↑renin, ↑PCT Na$^+$ reabsorb etc | Yes phaeochromo-cytoma obesity diabetes more in young | Yes, very strong β-blockers (β1) α-blockers (α1B>rest) less strong for: central α2-agonists (~α2A) | Phaeochromo-cytoma Otherwise not for BP α2C and β1 in CCF β1 in HR α2b in BMR Not for BP | Yes, αADR action especially: α1A ADR −/− BP↓ α1D ADR −/− BP↓ α2A ADR −/− BP↑ α2B ADR required for salt loading BP↑, lost in −/− & +/− β2 ADR −/− resting BP = normal, exercise BP↑ | Extensive for: βADRs ✓✓✓✗✗ β2ADR ✓✗✗✗ β3ADR others, little β1 (✓for HR) ? for BP? α2A ?✓✗ | Good evidence: Phaeos, animal models and pharmacology Mechanism of long-term ΔBP not certain. |
| **Endothelin** | | Quite Recent Effects often local Some evidence effect on systemic long-term BP: ↑vasoconstriction, ETA/ETB balance Δ Na$^+$ reabsorb in collecting duct | ? Yes, renal disease ? Ischaemia | Yes, ET A bockers ET A/B joint blockers | ECE1 patient—labile BP and episodic HT, but multiple other pathology | Yes but complications if (−/−). ET-1 +/− BP↑. ET-B +/− BP↑. now collecting duct specific ET-1 −/− BP↑ | Very limited studies ET-1 ? ET-2 ? ET-A ? ET-B ? | Emerging, ?Role via intrarenal ET-B or ETB/ET-A balance |

| Mediator | | | | | | | | |
|---|---|---|---|---|---|---|---|---|
| **Nitric Oxide** → | Quite Recent Effects often local and associated with other mediators. Endothelium dependent vasodilatation, ↓Na+ reabsorb in TAL, ↓inotropic and vasoconstrictor effects of SNS, ± in CNS, NO ↓ SNS α outflow | Yes—Impaired endothelial dependent relaxation, NO↓ by lack of NOS activity (including via endothelial damage) or ↑NOS inhibitors e.g. ADMA, or ↑superoxide NO inactivation | Yes—L-NAME Nitroprusside soluble guanylate cyclase activators, also indirectly via ↑vasodilation with phosphodiesterases | No | Yes eNOS/- BP↑ | ✓××× ? ? | Quite extensive for eNOS, HT in pregnancy (more ✓) others limited nNOS iNOS | Reasonably strong. Some uncertainty over the extent other pathways compensate for lack if NO in long-term |
| **Dopaminergic** → | CVS roles still incompletely understood but include renal dopamergic mediated natriuresis, limit renin secretion and suppression of adrenal aldosterone secretion | Possibly, reduced in older and salt sensitive | Yes, both D-1 like and D2-like agonists cause hypotension | No except when malignant neuroblastoma phaeo chromocytocytomas causing BP↓ | Yes—very strong DRD1A −/− and +/− BP↑ DRD2−/− BP↑ DRD3−/− and +/− BP↑ DRD5 −/− BP↑ GRK4 (A420V) BP↑ | ? ? ? | Very limited study DRD1 DRD2 DRD3 | Knockout mouse findings suggest underestimated |
| **Arachadonic acid metabolite pathways** | Complex. Roles still incompletely resolved and controversial. Often seen as paracrine/local mediator. PGE2 and prostacyclin—vasodilator, ↓SNS terminal release, ↑natriuresis. TXA2/PGH2/PGF2α -vasoconstrictor, 12-HPETE/12-HETE roles in ANGII effects and 20-HETE in Na+ transport | Role in common HT not well established. Some evidence – prostacyclin ↓ in HT, some states with lowered vasoconstrictor sensitivity have PGE2↑ and PG/20HETE abnormalities in salt sensitive HT. | Some support, NSAIDs modest rise in SBP and from results of selective agents (e.g. TXA2/PGH2 –R blockers) in experimental HT | Rare cases of prostacyclin synthase mutations and HT | Both prostacyclin & TXA2 receptor −/− mice:BP = normal. PGE2-both EP2-R−/− and E P4-R −/−(males) have salt sensitive HT, low renin and on low Na+ diet BP may ↓ EP1-R −/− BP↓with renin↑ | ✓× | Very limited, studies Prostacyclin synthase | Complex: roles in natriuresis + salt sensitive HT via 20HETE and EP1-4. Interaction of prostacyclin and AngII in vessel tone in HT |

*Continued*

**TABLE 31-1** MAJOR BIOCHEMICAL/MOLECULAR PATHWAYS IMPLICATED IN REGULATING BLOOD PRESSURE—cont'd

| System/ Pathway | ΔBP | (i)Theory | (ii)Inappropriate Pathway Activity in Hypertension | (iii)Pharmacological Support | (iv)Support for Role Support in HT from Families, Animal Models | | (v)Genetic Link/Assoc with BP in Population | | Overall |
|---|---|---|---|---|---|---|---|---|---|
| | | | | | Families | Animal Models | Association/Linkage | ✓✗ | |
| **Natriuretic Peptide systems** | → | Role in hyper-volaemic responses, affecting natriuresis, afferent arteriolar resistance, and also vasopressin and myocardial responses | Evidence more of inadequate response or resistance to ANP or BNP. Local deficiency of ANP/BNP may be involved but no evidence of circulating ANP/BNP deficiency in HT. | Yes, but in humans long-term effects quite weak. | NO | Yes ANP −/− and +/− BP↑ (salt-sensitive) NPRA −/− and +/− BP↑ NPRC −/− BP↓ (ANP $t_{1/2}$↑) | Study mainly for ANP other-wise only limited study NPRA NPRC | ✓✗✗ ✓✗ ? | Clinical evidence weak. Clear HT from ANP/BNP resistance/ local deficiency in mice |
| **Bradykinin (BK)** | → | Vasodilator natriuretic and diuretic actions | Urinary kallikrein deficiency in primary/ salt sensitive HT. Role in impaired endothelium dependent vasodilatation. | Largely indirect evidence. Selective BK B2 agonists lower BP in animals. Fraction of vasopeptidase inhibitor action from BK is unclear. | Seeming against importance is finding of kininogen deficient families with ? normal BP. | Yes BK B2 −/− salt-sensitive BP↑ Mice over-expressing BK B2 or tissue kallikrein have BP↓ | Study very limited BK B2 | ? | Clinical evidence weak : kininogen deficiency reported normal Rodent findings suggest role in salt sensitive HT. |
| **Mineralocorticoid Aldosterone-ENaC pathway** (renal sodium reabsorption in late DCT/ collecting duct) | ↑ | Long established, major determinant of body sodium and extracellular fluid volume status | Yes, Primary aldosterone excess. Some low renin HT (with high aldosterone/ renin ratio) (Also secondarily active in high renin and non-modulating normal renin HT) | Yes spironolactone carbenoxolone amiloride (realization more BP↓ probably achievable with better ENaC blockers) | CYP11B2 defic BP↓ CYP 11B2 (GRH) BP↑ 11βOHase defic-BP↑ 17αOHase defic BP↑ 11βHSD2 defic BP↑ MR defic BP↓ MR[S810L] activ BP↑ ENaCαβγ defic BP↓ ENaCβγ Liddle's BP↑ | 11βHSD2 −/− BP↑ MR −/− BP↓ ENaCα −/− BP↓↓, ENaCβ −/−, BP↓↓, ENaCγ −/− BP↓↓ ENaCβ(Liddle's) BP↑ | Mainly ENaC + CYP11B2 CYP11B2 ENaCα ENaCβ ENaCγ 11βHSD2 In low renin HT CYP11B2 | ✓✓✗✗ ✓✗ ✗✗✗✓ ✗✓ ?✓✗ ?✓ | Established causes of secondary HT, probable role in low-renin primary HT |

| | | | | | | | |
|---|---|---|---|---|---|---|---|
| **Renal Sodium Re absorption in Proximal tubule: PT NHE3, (SGLT too)** ↑ | Site of 60% of Na⁺ reabsorption, theoretically crucial | Yes, Overactive PT reabsorption in diabetes and obesity associated HT? ouabain like factor effects (via affecting co-localized Na⁺ K⁺ ATPase pump) | Yes but weak, PT acting diuretics are surprisingly weak. However no drugs augmenting PT absorption | Weak, AQP1 –/– families have little change in BP. No NHE 3 mutations and no mutations increasing PT Na⁺ transport | NHE3 –/– modest BP↓. AQP1 –/– ? similar modest BP↓. No models with overactive PT transport | Almost no study NHE3 | ? | Only small role in down regulating to lower BP. Role in BP↑ if up regulated remains unclear |
| **Renal Sodium Re absorption in thick ascending limb: TAL NKCC2** ↑ | Site of 25% of Na⁺ reabsorption | Proposed to be involved in obesity ± insulin resistance related HT, and theoretically when medullary vasodilatation impaired—so ? when NO↓, vasodilator PG↓ peripherally and ? in elderly or in renal ischaemia | Yes, loop-diuretics | Bartter's syndrome BP↓ (defic of any of NKCC2, ROMK, CLC-KB, Barttin) | NKCC2 –/– BP↓↓ ROMK –/– BP↓↓ | Almost no study NKCC2 | ? | Role in down regulating BP. Unclear if upregulation causing HT but seems likely. Predict ± renin↑ on whether macula densa (in TAL) transport also ↑ |
| **Renal Sodium Re absorption in distal convoluted tubule: DCT. (ENaC considered above) TSC1 pathway WNK1/4 pathway** ↑ | Site of 7% of Na⁺ reabsorption | Thiazide diuretic success in treatment in elderly primary HT thought to indicate overactive | Yes, thiazide diuretics | Gitelman's syndrome BP↓ (TSC1 defic) Gordon's syndrome BP↑ (WNK1, WNK4 and third gene) | TSC1 –/– BP↓ | Almost no study TSC1 | ? | Roles in down regulating BP. Unclear if upregulation but seems likely—predicted to cause low renin HT without high aldosterone |

Information is presented under five general headings relating to the general roles of these systems in BP control and the extent that this is consistent with a possible involvement in the basis of HT. Aspects relevant to heading "Genetic Link/Association with BP in Population" are dealt with in detail in later sections on individual candidate genes and association of studies on human primary HT. An indication of the intensity and overall positive (✓)/negative (✗) balance of studies on individual candidate genes and association of their genetic variants with BP in human primary HT is given in a nonquantitative way, although in many cases the intensity of study is too low to allow any such indications (then indicated as ?). However, reference must be made to the sections dealing with these candidate genes in detail to allow the balance of these studies to be properly appreciated. BMR, basal metabolic rate; CCF, congestive cardiac failure; PCT, proximal convoluted tubule.

■ ■ ■

**TABLE 31-2**    OTHER SYSTEMS/PATHWAYS INVOLVED OR WITH SOME PUTATIVE ASSOCIATION WITH BLOOD PRESSURE CONTROL

| SYSTEM/PATHWAY | |
| --- | --- |
| **Endocrine (hormonal, hormone-like)** | **Others (locally acting/paracrine)** |
| Insulin | Hypoxic |
| Vasopressin | Cytokine/inflammatory |
| Leptin | Oxygen free radical/superoxide |
| Glucocorticoid | Heme oxygenase and carbon monoxide |
| Growth hormone | Vasodilator $K^+$ channels |
| Estrogens | Imidazoline |
| Thyroxine | Adenosine/purinergic receptor pathways |
| Parathyroid hormone/$Ca^{2+}$/$Ca^{2+}$-receptor | |
| MSH | |
| Erythropoietin | |
| Adrenomedullin | |
| Ouabain-like-factor (OAF) | |

The roles of these pathways in BP regulation are either less general or less well established and more controversial than those dealt with in Table 31-1. The entities listed cover a wide range from those in which a link with BP is not in doubt such as vasodilator $K^+$ channels (e.g., blocked by the powerful antihypertensive minoxidil but for which normal physiologic roles are not well elaborated) or glucocorticoids (in which clear excess [Cushing's syndrome] usually causes HT, yet pathways involved are not entirely clear) to much more nebulous locally acting phenomena, nonetheless, appearing associated with BP disturbances.

clonidine) and secondary HT in pheochromocytomas (with or without paroxysmal catecholamine release) support a long-term BP altering role of the adrenergic SNS. This then argues for such an effect contributing to HT in the milder SNS overactivity often accompanying other HT especially in obesity and diabetes and generally at an early stage in young subjects developing primary HT. Understanding of the adrenergic SNS has transformed with realization that there are nine adrenergic receptor (ADR) types, three $\alpha_1$ADRs ($\alpha_{1A}$, $\alpha_{1B}$, and $\alpha_{1D}$),[46,47] three $\alpha_2$ADRs ($\alpha_{2A}$, $\alpha_{2B}$, and $\alpha_{2C}$),[46] and three $\beta$ADRs ($\beta_1$, $\beta_2$, and $\beta_3$).[48] The $\alpha_1$ADRs are postsynaptic receptors and in most sites are the main mediators of adrenergic vasoconstriction.[47] All three $\alpha_1$ADRs contribute—$\alpha_{1D}$ is more important in aorta and larger branches[47]; $\alpha_{1A}$ is important in some branches such as renal artery, smaller branches, and resistance vessels;[47,49] and $\alpha_{1B}$ probably contributes to the vasoconstrictor response across the larger or whole arterial tree at a more modest level.[47,50] Consistent with these roles, knockout of either the $\alpha_{1A}$[51] or $\alpha_{1D}$ADRs[52] (but not $\alpha_{1B}$ADR[47,50]) causes resting hypotension in homozygotes; all three have reduced agonist-mediated vasoconstriction, and $\alpha_{1D}$ −/− mice have also been shown to have diminished salt-sensitive BP rise (in a reduced renal mass/high salt intake paradigm). It is $\alpha_{1A}$ that mediates the greatest vasoconstrictor effect on acute BP in most studies,[47,49,53] certainly in animal models, whereas in some human studies $\alpha_{1B}$ is an important contributor although the overall relative contribution of $\alpha_{1A}$ and $\alpha_{1B}$ remains uncertain because reports conflict.[49,53] It may be that overall $\alpha_{1A}$ predominates[49,53] and in certain vascular beds or contexts both contribute more equally, especially in the elderly.[53] The $\alpha_2$ADRs are largely presynaptic and distributed particularly in the CNS. Both $\alpha_{2A}$ and $\alpha_{2C}$ are required for normal modulation of SNS neurotransmitter release; $\alpha_{2a}$ at high frequencies

of firing and $\alpha_{2C}$ when frequencies are lower (typically having more influence on venous tone).[54] Mice without normal $\alpha_{2A}$ or $\alpha_{2C}$ have elevated noradrenaline and develop cardiac hypertrophy and reduced left-ventricular contractility.[54] Importantly, in the case of $\alpha_{2A}$ knockout (−/−) mice, the resting BP is raised. There are also postsynaptic $\alpha_{2A}$ in peripheral vessels that mediate the portion (30%) of $\alpha$-adrenergic pressor effect resulting from $\alpha_2$-receptors; this effect is lost in $\alpha_{2A}$ −/− mice. Thus, peripheral vascular $\alpha_{2A}$ mediates a BP-raising vasoconstriction, whereas centrally it exerts a tonic sympathoinhibitory tone lowering BP (the latter is responsible for the BP-lowering effects of clonidine). The central effect is predominant, and, thus, the net effect of $\alpha_{2A}$ −/− is HT with sympathetic overactivity. Although $\alpha_{2C}$ also exerts central sympathoinhibitory influence and $\alpha_{2C}$ −/− animals develop cardiac hypertrophy, it seems that $\alpha_{2C}$ receptors do not exert a hemodynamic influence and that resting BP appears unaffected in reports of $\alpha_{2C}$ −/− mice.[55] However, it may be that $\alpha_{2c}$ ADRs do play a role in arterial vasoconstriction response to cold exposure, at least in the cutaneous circulation. The third subtype $\alpha_{2B}$ seems to exert a central sympathoexcitatory effect in response to salt loading either as an acute (saline infusion[55]) or chronic (oral saline and reduced renal mass[56]) challenge and, thus, appears to have a link to the degree of predisposition to salt-sensitive HT. Certainly $\alpha_{2B}$ −/− mice lose this hypertensive effect of acute[55] or chronic salt loading,[56] and this is also true for heterozygotes. Thus, a full complement of $\alpha_{2B}$ seems to be required to develop this rise in BP induced by salt loading. Some reports indicate the presence of peripheral $\alpha_{2B}$ receptors, including within vasculature and kidney. However, there is controversy here and others indicate that there are no peripheral vascular $\alpha_{2B}$ receptors. It seems that the features of the hypertensive responses of salt loading are in keeping with a central $\alpha_{2B}$ effect on BP, although the pathway remains to be elucidated. There are some other CNS effects of $\alpha_2$ receptors reflected in some side effects of strong $\alpha_2$-agonist stimuli, for example, $\alpha_{2A}$ (sedation) and $\alpha_{2C}$ (alteration in intensity of some alarm and stress-startle responses).

Finally, the $\beta$-adrenergic receptors appear to be less vital and exhibit a greater ability to cross-compensate for one another than might have been expected. Certainly mice with single knockout of each $\beta$ADR appear, when reaching adulthood, to have normal resting HR and resting BP and no impairment in exercise tolerance (although abnormalities are manifest on exertion). From the understanding of the mechanism of $\beta$-blockers it is expected that loss of the $\beta_1$ADR would result in significant changes in cardiac function. Indeed there are some such changes in $\beta_1$ $-/-$ mice because the $\beta_1$ADR seems to be required for a full range of chronotropic and inotropic responses to $\beta$-agonists, noradrenaline, and exercise, but, surprisingly, resting HR, BP, and exercise tolerance are normal (despite reduced inotropic and chronotropic responses to exertion).[57] Although all three $\beta$-receptors contribute to vascular tone, recent findings indicate that $\beta_1$ADR may play a dominant role in mediating vasodilation in the mouse.[58] Nonetheless, although loss of $\beta_2$ADR leaves knockout animals with normal resting BP, they develop hypertensive BP levels on exertion,[59] which most likely is accounted for by an important $\beta_2$ADR vasodilatory deficit for which other systems including $\beta_1$ and $\beta_3$ADRs do not compensate.[57,59] $\beta_3$ADRs mediate lipolysis in adipose tissue, and their roles in the CVS are not yet well understood. In heart they appear able to couple to two G-protein pathways: $G_i$ leading to NO production and reduced inotropic state and probably also to Gs-adenyl cyclase and raised inotropic state. $\beta_3$ADR $-/-$ mice were initially reported to have no change in resting BP. Overall $\beta_3$ADRs are less positively inotropic than $\beta_1$ADRs, and $\beta_3$ADR $-/-$ mice have higher inotropic response to nonselective $\beta$-agonists (e.g., isoproterenol) reflecting the loss of $\beta_3$ "competition" for $\beta$-agonist and partly inhibitory signaling. The three $\beta$ADRs share a role in mediating changes in basal metabolic rate (BMR); thus, it is only when all three $\beta$ADRs are lost in mice (in so-called $\beta$-less mice) that a major effect on BMR and tendency to develop obesity become apparent.[60] There has been a considerable amount of work that looked at the linkage and association of genetic variation in the ADR genes with BP and HT (see later sections on primary HT). This study has focused disproportionately on the $\beta$ADRs especially $\beta_2$ADR with evidence both for and against involvement. The preponderant evidence suggests that there is a real, although modest and not universally penetrant, role in the risk of higher BP and HT. Two linkage studies of the human Ch5q region[61] and of genome-wide linkage[62] that showed a modest hit (P = 0.0076) are weakly suggestive of linkage to HT around 5q32-34 (see primary HT section). Study has also suggested a role for $\beta_1$ADR variations in determining resting HR[63] and for specific variations in $\alpha_{2C}$ and $\beta_1$ADR in cardiac hypertrophy failure.[64]

The role of variation in the $\alpha_{1A}$, $\alpha_{1D}$, and $\alpha_{2A}$ in HT in general and additionally of $\alpha_{2B}$ in salt-sensitive HT and of $\beta_2$ in HT during exercise, or specifically when there is SNS overactivity, are strongly suggested from knockout mouse studies but have not yet been seriously addressed in the clinic. There is the potential to develop $\alpha$ADR antagonists, with a different selectivity to that of prazosin, which may be clinically useful. The findings of knockout mouse studies definitively conclude that variation in single genes especially in the $\alpha$-adrenergic limbs of the SNS can cause long-term changes in BP and, thus, may influence the risk of HT in humans. The more precise mechanisms through which this long-term effect develops and the strength of parallels in human pathophysiology will be the subject of future work, although the renal pressure natriuresis mechanism is likely to be affected. It seems probable that the human $\alpha$-adrenergic SNS will merit more careful consideration for roles relating to long-term BP control than has been appreciated. How $\beta$-blockers have their widely useful BP-lowering effect in humans remains unclear. The answer is likely to be of considerable value.

### The Endothelin System

By comparison, the ET system is a more recent discovery, although it has been known for more than a decade to be a powerful vasoconstrictor system resulting from three related homologous peptides ET-1, ET-2, and ET-3, which are activated by endothelin-converting enzymes (ECEs, especially ECE1). ET-1 is particularly important in vasoconstrictor responses, acting as the preferential ligand at ET-A receptors *in vitro* and in short-term experiments *in vivo*, although its role in long-term BP control is more complex and is still being elaborated. Some opposing vasodilatory and natriuretic actions of ETs occur on binding the ET-B receptor, to which all three ETs bind with similar affinity. Knockout experiments have revealed developmental roles for this system, and homozygous null mice having severe developmental problems not directly related to the ET system role in BP control (see the sections on candidate gene and primary HT). The finding that ET-1 +/− mice have mild HT is puzzling because these mice have a reduction in the production of ET-1, a peptide that mediates very powerful short-term vasoconstriction especially via ET-A receptors. The HT has not been fully explained. One explanation is that mild ET-1 +/− developmental respiratory difficulties raise BP as a long-term consequence of hypoxic SNS activation.[45] An alternative view suggests that the HT in ET-1 +/− is a consequence of somewhat altered ET-A/ET-B activation balance, perhaps because less renal ET-B binding and less vasodilation and natriuresis cause HT. This view is supported by the finding that ET-B +/− mice have raised BP and prolonged half-life of labeled plasma ET-1 (compared with normal and ET-A +/− mice). HT in ET B +/− was restored to normal by antagonists selective for ET-A (BQ-123) but not for ET-B (BQ-788). This indicates that the expression level of ET-B can alter long-term BP. Thus, ET-B level and the supply of ET-1 ligand are important. However, a key question is where such BP regulatory effects are based.

Tissue-specific knockouts of ET-1 and ET-B support the importance of expression level and binding of renal ET-B (±ET-A/ET-B balance). Thus, ET-1 CD −/− mice are hypertensive with impaired water and possibly Na$^+$ excretion.[36] Because ET-B CD −/− mice have been generated, the important issues of the role of ET-B in control of BP and renal function can be addressed, with some insight into renal epithelial versus renal vascular actions. Certainly ET-B seems to exert a natriuretic action in CD (possibly signaling via src), antagonizing the pathway promoting Na$^+$ reabsorption via ENaC. It has been recognized that renal medullary hypoxia somewhat upregulates ET-1 production locally in CD, whereas *in vivo* in humans renal ET-B mediates a net vasodilation.[65] ET-A is a net renal vasoconstrictor that seems to assume a greater effect when there is less stimulation of AngII receptors (e.g., during AT1 blocker treatment[66]). Thus, the renal ET system can alter long-term BP, and renal ET-A/ET-B stimulation balance would seem important. Renal hypoxia and angiotensin levels can modulate intrarenal ET-1 production and ET-A mediated vasoconstriction, respectively.

Some further evidence from ET3 −/− and ET-A −/− mice indicate that these components of the ET system may play limited (ET-A) or no role (ET-3) in normal BP control (at least in early life).[67] Thus, the other ETs (especially ET-1) and ET-B are important in the effects that the ET system has on longer term BP. The position in human HT is likely to become clearer because ET receptor blocking agents have now become clinically available for treating HT, initially with agents blocking both ET-A and ET-B such as bosentan.[65] Selective ET-A blockers (which may mimic ET-1 +/− lowering of BP) and inhibitors of ECE have also been developed.[68] There are other therapeutic roles in addition to systemic HT for such new agents[68]; they now show promise in pulmonary HT[69] and perhaps in situations in which local vasoconstriction relief would be beneficial[70] and in renal disease. Thus, the ET system is implicated in the long-term control of BP. However, the role of genetic variation in the component genes in human primary HT has only been relatively superficially assessed so far.

### The Nitric Oxide Signaling Pathways

The NO signaling pathways are able to alter blood flow and short- and long-term BP. NO is generated by NOS; this enzyme activity oxidizes the amino-acid L-arginine to citrulline.[71] Three different NOS enzymes have been identified in mammalian cells—eNOS, nNOS, and iNOS. Normally, in the absence of inflammation, iNOS is regarded as having only a minor role in normal human cardiovascular regulation. In inflammatory and infectious disease, iNOS may cause vasodilation and lower BP, which in severe acute disease may contribute to septic shock. In contrast eNOS and nNOS are constitutively expressed and contribute to regulation of vascular tone and BP. The neuronal form nNOS is expressed in several tissues, notably in specific sites within the CNS, in nonadrenergic noncholinergic neurons of the autonomic nervous system, and in the macula densa, which regulates TGF in nephrons. The endothelial form eNOS is expressed in endothelial cells of vasculature throughout the body. In addition, eNOS and nNOS contribute to expression in other sites including kidney, brain, and heart. NO is short lived so this system is operates at a local/paracrine or autocrine level. Nonetheless, its widespread presence in the vasculature and in other sites such as myocardium, renal epithelia, and CNS, which influence circulatory and renal function, make it clear that these locally acting phenomena do drive changes capable of regulating systemic BP. The most widely studied effect is the role of NO as endothelium-dependent relaxing factor (EDRF),[71] an important normal counterbalance to vasoconstrictor influence along with vasodilator arachidonic acid derived metabolites (e.g., prostacyclin[72] and EETs[73]) and endothelium-dependent hyperpolarizing factor (EDHF).[74-76] NO made in endothelial cells diffuses to adjacent VSM cells and activates soluble guanylate cyclase then generating cGMP, which, before degradation by phosphodiesterases, causes activation of a series of G-kinases to bring about VSM relaxation and vasodilation. NO generation by eNOS is a powerful contributor to vasodilatory regulation of vascular tone and flow and is widely impaired in HT. Such impairment contributes to insulin resistance often when there is coexisting dyslipidemia. The fact that mice deficient in eNOS (−/−) develop all these features,[77] (i.e., HT, insulin resistance, and dyslipidemia) indicates that primary defects in this pathway may contribute to the cause of these conditions rather than be a consequence of them. Several drug classes acting on the NO system also affect long-term BP. Thus, NOS inhibition by L-NAME lowers the NO levels and produces HT that, with continued treatment, is persistent. NO donor agents such as sodium nitroprusside raise the "NO tone" and lower BP, as do soluble guanylate cyclase activators. Specific phosphodiesterase inhibitors (e.g., sildenafil [Viagra]) produce beneficial localized vasodilation by potentiating the effect of NO (increasing the half-life of cGMP elevation). If coadministered with nitrate NO donors, more generalized changes and marked falls in BP result. Thus, there is powerful evidence this NO pathway may regulate systemic BP and local blood flow. NOS effects outside vascular endothelial cells may play an important part in the effects of the NO pathway on longer term BP. Thus, in the kidney NO promotes natriuresis at least in the TAL, partly via cGMP, to reduce Na$^+$ reabsorption[78] (a signaling pathway also used by ANP) and also in nonguanylate cyclase actions of NO through alteration on arachidonic acid metabolites, 20HETE ±EETs, which also have natriuretic effects.[73] NO also plays some role in elevation of renin in response to hypotension, especially during baroreflex activation or with salt depletion[79] and in the regulation of TGF.[80] These seem to be indirect effects of nNOS in the macula densa causing cGMP generation in JG cells. However, it is a modulatory role and other mediators (acting through macula densa adenosine and vasodilator prostaglandin release and effecting changes in JG cell intracellular Ca$^{2+}$ and cAMP) are emerging as the primary regulators.[79,80] Both eNOS and nNOS are expressed in the CNS, and there is emerging evidence that CNS nNOS is part of a pathway tonically restraining sympathetic (especially α) adrenergic outflow from the brainstem and hypothalamus. Alteration in CNS NO signaling can limit central sympathetic outflow overactivity and, thus, have influence on the risks of HT.[81]

NOS is also expressed in the heart where it has a negative inotropic influence. One pathway coupled to cardiac NO release is via $\beta_3$ADR coupling to inhibitory $G_i$-signaling and increasing NO release. Both $\beta_3$ADR $-/-$ and eNOS $-/-$ mice seem to lose at least part of this negative inotropic feedback on the heart, which restrains responses to adrenergic overactivity indicating that this probably beneficial negative feedback mechanism within the heart involves eNOS and at least partly is activated by $\beta_3$ADR. The role of NOS in cardiac function is a very complex field, and although this negative inotropic influence has the potential to alter CO, and the $\Delta CO \leftrightarrow \Delta TPR$ autoregulation in sympathetic overactivity, the long-term effect on BP is not known. In the absence of heart disease, the key roles of the NO pathway in long-term BP control are likely to lie in regulating vessel tone, through actions within the kidney and through effects on sympathetic outflow and overactivity. In the absence of inflammation, the eNOS branch of the NO pathways seems most implicated in such actions and capable of affecting long-term BP. Mice lacking eNOS $-/-$ had an increase in MAP of 20 to 30 mm Hg,[34] whereas mice overexpressing eNOS had a mean reduction of 18 mm Hg.

Thus far, human association and linkage studies of the NOS system to BP and HT have concentrated on the eNOS gene (see candidate genes section). However, variations in other genes in this pathway have not been assessed. Clearly the NO pathways can become dysregulated through processes causing endothelial damage, dysfunction, NOS downregulation, or inhibition. AngII brings about impaired endothelium-dependent vasodilation, and this may occur in HT with elevated AngII through the inactivation of NO by superoxide formed by NADPH oxidase.[82,83] NADPH oxidase can be induced by AngII, inflammatory cytokines, and by vessel wall shear stress and thus by worsening HT itself.[83] ACE inhibitors, by reversing all these stimuli, reduce NO inhibition (and elevate bradykinin, which promotes NO pathways) and assist in restoring endothelium-dependent vasodilation.[82] It is also possible that HT will be promoted by reduced NO pathway activity, through depletion of the natural antioxidant defenses in vasculature (e.g., glutathione) or the accumulation of circulating inhibitors of NOS such as methylated arginines (e.g., asymmetric dimethyl arginine [ADMA]) in renal failure.[84] These inhibitors appear to be increased in atherosclerosis and diabetes, secondary to their reduced hydrolysis by dimethylarginine dimethylaminohydrolase (DDAH) in the damaged endothelium or through its inhibition by hyperglycemia,[85] respectively. Compounding this are findings that eNOS deficiency causes insulin resistance and HT[77] and that an intact NO system helps protect against the hypertensive effects of chronic hyperglycemia. Thus, the hypertensive effects of L-NAME (on NO formation) together with hyperglycemia (from glucose infusion) are much more than the sum of these two treatments sepa-

rately.[86] Clearly, inhibition of the NO pathway and eNOS in particular may be particularly involved in HT when there is coexisting diabetes, atherosclerosis, renal impairment, or high AngII levels.

### The Dopaminergic System

The cardiovascular roles of the dopaminergic system are still incompletely understood, but there are now thought to be five separate dopaminergic receptors DRD 1 to 5 (DRD1 and DRD5 are sometimes called DRD1A and DRD1B, respectively). An older pharmacologic classification into D1-like (DRD1 and 5) and D2-like (DRD2, 3, and 4) receptors was based on D1-like stimulating adenyl cyclase (and coupling through stimulatory $G_s$ and/or $G_q$) and D2-like inhibiting adenyl cyclase (perhaps then coupling through inhibitory $G_i$). This classification is near obsolete, and although older literature uses these terms there must be caution in pooling D2 to 4 as D2-like. Dopamine acting on the kidney promotes natriuresis; in the lowest dose, this seems to relate to inhibition of $Na^+$ reabsorption particularly in PT, whereas at a slightly higher dose (or with higher doses of D1-agonists) there is also a further antinatriuretic effect from renal vasodilation. These effects were thought to be D1-like and certainly DRD1 mediates a proportion, but how much other receptor classes contribute requires clarification. Certainly it seems that DRD3 plays some role in natriuresis and diuresis, and DRD2 and DRD5 are now also implicated in long-term BP control. Although some dopamine may be filtered at the glomerulus, the supply of ligand L-DOPA, which is selectively taken up in PTs, converted to dopamine by dopa-decarboxylase, and re-exported, contributes to the supply of ligand binding the receptors[87] on the apical membranes of the tubules (e.g., DRD1 in PT). Outside the CNS D1-like receptors were described in VSM, JG apparatus, and renal tubules, whereas D2-like were described on glomeruli, postganglionic sympathetic nerve terminals, adrenal zona glomerulosa cells, and renal tubules. DRD1, 2, 3, and 5 have been identified in kidney. The concentration of D1-like receptors was highest in PT, and DRD1 is abundant in this site also. D1-like activity in PT activating adenyl cyclase leads to inhibition of $Na^+$ transport both apically at NHE3 (including via PKA and NHE3 phosphorylation[88]) and basolaterally at $Na^+$-$K^+$-ATPase[89] (including via PKC and 20-HETE). DRD1 is involved, but it is not yet clear if other receptors are too. There was controversy about the requirement for both D1-like and D2-like stimulation for inhibition of $Na^+$-$K^+$-ATPase,[87] and DRD3 at least seems likely to be involved in natriuretic actions. Other dopamine natriuretic effects are described on the TAL and CD $Na^+$-$K^+$-ATPase, but the PT effect is thought to be the most important, especially in the short term. Dopamine also exerts a vasodilatory effect on renal arterioles, and in the JG cells this seems most consistent with a cAMP elevation and, thus, a D2-like action. Aldosterone production is known to be under inhibitory tone from dopaminergic neurons (D2-like), but the role of this system in dysregulation of aldosterone in HT is not clear. Presynaptic D2-like actions on adrenergic nerve terminals also bring about more general vasodilation that is dependent on the extent of sympathetic vasoconstrictor tone.[87] Dopamine pathways are abundant in several regions of the CNS, but the best understood role of these relate to noncardiovascular functions.

Despite the very incomplete level of understanding of the peripherally acting dopaminergic system, the evidence for a role in BP control and a possible role in HT has considerable support. Thus, dopamine and some agonists (e.g., dopexamine or the D1-selective fenoldopam[90]) at DRDs lower BP, reduce renal vascular resistance, and promote natriuresis in humans and animals. Patients with malignant catecholamine-secreting tumours such as neuroblastomas that secrete appreciable quantities of dopamine have hypotension that can be severe or paroxysmal. Recently all five of the DRDs have been separately knocked out in mice.[91,92] At least four of these develop HT; DRD1[91] and DRD3[92] are particularly important because the heterozygote mice also have HT, demonstrating that both of these receptors are required to maintain normotension. The DRD1 knockout mice have HT with reduction in renal tubular cAMP stimulation and inhibition of Na[+] transport in renal tubules; this confirms that this receptor plays an important part in the proximal tubular natriuretic effect of dopamine.[91] The DRD3 knockout mice have HT with elevated renin and impaired natriuresis to acute volume expansion. Previous work in Dahl rats with selective DRD3-agonist and antagonist treatment concluded that DRD3 receptor deficiency could play an important role in salt-sensitive HT. The mechanism of HT in DRD2 −/− mice seems to relate to increased vasoconstriction via α-adrenergic receptors; increased stimulation of ET-B receptors was also found.[93] DRD5 knockout mice were recently reported to have HT by 3 months of age and show no compensatory changes in the expression level of the other DRDs. The mice have increased sympathetic outflow, and it was thought that the DRD5 knockout altered a pathway in the CNS, probably in the medulla that promoted the hyperadrenergic state.[94]

In humans, deficiency of synthesis and/or secretion of dopamine (often as reduced urinary dopamine metabolite measurements) has been reported in various forms of HT[87] including primary HT and in cases in which there is a significant family history. This finding is not always associated but seems more common in older and salt-sensitive HT patients. A subject with a family history of HT was reported to have a defect in dopa-decarboxylase (which would generate renal dopamine).[95] Other studies on low-renin primary hypertensives showed defects in renal tubular L-DOPA uptake and conversion to dopamine.[96] Isolation and culture of proximal tubular cells from subjects with primary HT had marked impairment of D1-agonist stimulated adenyl cyclase compared with normotensives suggesting a defect in receptor coupling selective for the dopamine pathway because there were no similar impairments of parathyroid hormone receptor signaling. A similar D1-like desensitization is present in obese (hypertensive) but not lean Zucker rats and has been attributed to hyperinsulinemia and insulin resistance, which the PPARγ agonist rosiglitazone reduces restoring the renal tubular D1-like sensitivity. In

human hypertensives further investigation identified a single base mutation in GRK4 (type 4 G-protein receptor kinase) changing the amino acid A142V. This increases phosphorylation of D1 receptors at a serine residue, causing their uncoupling from their signal transduction (by binding of uncoupling proteins called arrestins). This is a mechanism with parallels for many G-protein-coupled receptors. Moreover, transgenic mice with this GRK4$_{A142V}$ have HT with impaired diuretic and natriuretic capacity but not the acute hypotensive effects of D1-agonist stimulation.[97] These findings provide a mechanism for the D1 receptor coupling defect in the kidney that the same group had previously reported. Whether insulin resistance, hyperinsulinemia, or obesity affect D1-mediated natriuretic responses in humans remains to be studied.

The role of dopaminergic pathways in HT has been the subject of considerable interest in the past but the link with urinary dopamine and primary HT was not always found, and there have been problems developing clinically useful oral drugs that were effective and selective. Fenoldopam is a relatively D1-selective agonist licensed in some countries for use (intravenously) in patients with severe or accelerated HT; in recent reports it is viewed to be as effective as sodium nitroprusside.[90] Recent advances suggest opportunities for novel antihypertensive drugs acting on the dopaminergic system, and there has been considerable interest over this issue,[98] especially with the elucidation of DRD1-5. A full complement of at least two (DRD1[91] and DRD3[92]) are required for normal BP, and two others DRD2[93] (and DRD5[94]) and the related gene GRK4[97] can all cause HT if abnormal. Unless there are very major species differences, activity of at least some of these genes can play a role in HT in humans. There has been very little study of the genes of the dopaminergic system for linkage or association to primary HT and similarly little in the way of selective DRD blockers and agonists are available for clinical studies to further clarify the role of this system in human HT.

### Arachidonic Acid Metabolite Pathways

These metabolite pathways fall into three major branches shown in Figure 31-4: (1) COX metabolites[72] including prostacyclin (PGI$_2$, an important vasodilator), thromboxanes (e.g., TXA$_2$, a vasoconstrictor), and prostaglandins (e.g., the vasodilator PGE$_2$ and the vasoconstrictors PGF$_2$α and PGH$_2$); (2) the lipoxygenase (LOX) metabolites[72] including 12-HPETE and 12-HETE, which mediate vasoconstrictor effects especially of AngII by increasing intracellular Ca$^{2+}$ in VSM and inhibit prostacyclin synthase (thus reducing vasodilator stimuli); and (3) the CYP450 metabolites,[73] 20-hydroxyeicosatetraenoic acid (20-HETE), and epoxyeicosatrienoic acids (EETs). The former is made by CYP 4a enzymes with ω-hydroxylase activity in VSM causing vasoconstriction and in PT and TAL epithelial cells promoting natriuresis. The latter are EDHFs[73,75] (vasodilators acting via K$^+$ channels to relax VSM). The network of largely locally made and acting factors present a complex picture that a number of excellent reviews[72,73] cover in detail.

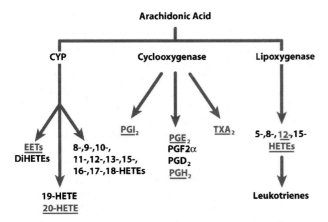

**FIGURE 31-4.** Branches and important products of arachidonic acid metabolism. The three major branches cyclo-oxygenase, lipoxygenase, and CYP generate classes of PGs, TXs, PI, HETEs, EETs, and dihydroxy-eicosatrienoic acids (DiHETEs). Those underlined have some involvement in processes affecting BP.

$PGI_2$ is an important vasodilator made by prostacyclin synthase in vasculature, regulating vessel tone, inhibiting noradrenaline release from nerve terminals, facilitating renal $Na^+$ and water excretion (especially in TAL), and also having antithrombotic effects. $PGI_2$ receptor knockout mice have normal BP.[99] However, a family has been identified with an inactivating prostacyclin synthase mutation (in intron 9 causing skipping of exon 9) in which all carriers of the mutation have HT with reduced $PGI_2$ urinary metabolites.[100] It is reported that renovascular $PGI_2$ metabolites seem higher in primary HT patients with high-renin HT than in low-renin HT, reflecting less $PGI_2$ production or more metabolism. AngII promotes $TXA_2/PGH_2$ (both act at the same receptor) vasoconstrictor signaling and inhibits $PGI_2$ signaling by upregulating 12-HPETE and 12-HETE, which inhibit prostacyclin synthase.[72] Animal and clinical studies with $TXA_2/PGH_2$ agonists and antagonists (ifetroban) show that these mediators raise BP and that this is dependent on peripheral (rather than CNS) $PGH_2$ receptors, an intact autonomic nervous system, and a substantial α-adrenergic contribution.[101] Although $TXA_2/PGH_2$ signaling plays some role in the sustained HT throughout Goldblatt 2-kidney-1-clip HT (modeling renovascular and renal end-organ damage HT),[102] these mediators seem to play no role in other rodent HT models including the SHR and SHR-SP taking saline. Knockout of the $TXA_2/PGH_2$ receptor (TP) does not cause HT in mice,[99] which have a bleeding tendency as the main finding; this is shared by some rare families with TP mutations.[103] Thus, the real importance of $TXA_2/PGH_2$ in long-term BP control is in doubt.

$PGE_2$ is an important prostaglandin that has largely vasodilator, natriuretic, and diuretic actions. It also influences the JG apparatus through release from the macula densa in response to low NaCl and promotes the elevation of renin and vasodilation. The natriuretic actions occur in several nephron segments and involve inhibition of transepithelial $Na^+$ transport including inhibition of $Na^+$-$K^+$-ATPase. There are four receptors for $PGE_2$, EP1

to 4. Within the kidney EP1 is expressed predominantly in CD and in some medullary renal vessels.[104] EP1 stimulates increased intracellular $Ca^{2+}$ and promotes diuresis and natriuresis.[104] Male (not female) EP1 −/− mice are hypotensive, with seemingly appropriately elevated renin.[105] EP2 immunohistochemistry and mRNA localization studies indicate that there is some EP2 expression in renal vessels in the medulla but only limited renal epithelial expression.[104] EP2 stimulates cAMP, and an EP2 agonist butaprost induces a hypotensive response.[106] EP2 −/− mice have salt-sensitive HT,[107] although at baseline, BP is normal or low (probably depending on the standard salt diet and strain background). In kidney, EP3 also has a largely medullary expression with strong expression in TAL, CD, and some renal vessels possibly including some expression in afferent arterioles.[104] EP3 mainly signals through Gi-proteins reducing cAMP, but a splicing variant (also seen in humans) has variant signaling via intracellular $Ca^{2+}$.[104] EP3 appears responsible for antagonizing renal concentrating actions of AVP in TAL and CD and causing diuresis and natriuresis.[104] In EP3 −/− mice, the urine diluting ability is impaired and $PGE_2$ causes a greater hypotensive effect as if EP3 assisted in countering hypotension.[106] It is not yet clear whether the baseline or salt-loaded BP of EP3 −/mice is normal.

EP4 is the main $PGE_2$ receptor expressed in renal cortex and is expressed in renal vessels and glomerulus including the afferent arteriole and JG cells (although there was some controversy about the latter). EP4 stimulates cAMP, and this promotes renin release and afferent arteriole vasodilation. It is known that low tubular fluid NaCl concentration passing the macula densa promotes production of vasodilator PGs, in particular $PGE_2$, and this can then cause elevation of renin and afferent arteriole dilation as TGF.[79,80,104] Hence, EP4 seems to be the likely receptor mediating these actions, whereas reports of an EP3 afferent arteriole vasoconstrictor action[108] may indicate a counterbalance to macula densa. EP4 −/− mice (like the other cAMP-coupled receptor) have salt-sensitive HT, inappropriately low renin, and at baseline slightly low BP (especially males) depending on the salt diet and strain background (one strain background had patent ductus arteriosus in EP4 −/−, closure of which is augmented by EP4 signaling).[99,106] Thus, three if not all four of the EP receptors cause long-term BP abnormalities if defective; EP2 and EP4 result in inappropriately low or dysregulated renin and salt-sensitive HT, and EP1 causes low BP. Together these receptors allow appropriate JG upregulation of renin and TGF to maintain GFR in low salt intake, whereas the medullary $PGE_2$ responses facilitate salt and water excretion in high salt intake. It seems likely that defects in these receptor pathways will affect BP in humans. The EP2 and EP4 −/− phenotype is similar to the acquired condition hyporeninemic hypoaldosteronism in which there is abnormal renin shut off and salt-sensitive HT and associated JG abnormalities and high-dose NSAID treatment (which inhibits cyclo-oxygenase) are predisposing factors. Overviews of the effect of NSAIDs on BP show an overall modest rise averaging approximately 5 mm Hg that affects between 1% to 10% of subjects.[109] However, it is clear that the rate of salt sensitivity would be expected to be higher. As for other prostaglandins, $PGD_2$ receptors seem to be barely expressed in kidney, and the $PGF_2\alpha$ receptor is expressed in DCT. However, the function of the $PGF_2\alpha$ receptor is not clear, and knockout of the corresponding receptors seem to have no effect on BP.[106]

The lipoxygenase pathway (Fig. 31-4) is less well understood, but 12-HPETE and 12-HETE certainly promote AngII vasoconstriction and inhibit prostacyclin synthesis.[72] This applies to potentiated vasoconstriction in large vessels and arterioles including efferent arterioles. Moreover, in patients with primary HT, 12-HETE levels and their urinary metabolites are increased above that of normotensives. The 20-HETE is an important product of the cytochrome P450 metabolism of arachidonic acid (Fig. 31-4), produced by isoforms of the CYP4 class of enzymes (principally specific isoforms within the CYP4A and 4F subclasses; details are still emerging[73]). This mediator is produced in VSM and potentiates the degree of vasoconstriction by reducing the open probability of $Ca^{2+}$-activated $K^+$-channels in vessel reflex responses to hypoxia and stretch (the myogenic reflex, for pressure-flow autoregulation). It is made in afferent arterioles potentiating vasoconstriction. Thus, inhibitors of 20-HETE synthesis block *in vivo* renal and cerebral blood flow autoregulation and interfere with normal TGF and vasoconstriction to excess $pO_2$ *in vivo*.[73] Production of 20-HETE is stimulated by vasoconstrictors, notably AngII (which also involves the AT 2 receptor), noradrenaline, ET-1, and vasopressin, whereas it is antagonized by NO and heme oxygenase generated carbon monoxide. Interestingly, these latter effects are cGMP independent and due to NO and carbon monoxide binding to the heme group in the CYP4A/F enzymes inhibiting 20HETE formation.[73] There are also some reports of a slower action of NO inducing 20-HETE synthesizing enzymes; the significance of this is currently unclear. Agonists at PPARα receptors (fibrates e.g., clofibrate) certainly increase the formation of 20-HETE by the induction of CYP4A/F enzymes. 20-HETE is made in renal epithelial cells where it promotes natriuresis and diuresis, especially in the PT and TAL.[73] In human primary HT, impaired 20-HETE responses seem to correlate with the presence of salt-sensitive HT indicating that 20-HETE normally participates in matching natriuresis to $Na^+$ load.[110] In PT, 20-HETE is involved in the D1-like natriuretic actions of dopamine inhibiting $Na^+$-$K^+$-ATPase through a PKC pathway.[87] EETs act as EDHFs: vasodilators that hyperpolarize VSM cells by activating $K^+$ channels.[73] EETs are also produced in renal epithelia. EETs are formed by several CYP subclasses especially isoforms of the CYP2B/C/J subclasses and CYP1A2.[73] The production of EETs and 20-HETE is altered in experimental and genetic models of HT, diabetes, and renal impairment. Given the powerful actions of these mediators, it is likely that they contribute to the associated changes in renal function and vascular tone. However, this field is still rapidly evolving, and it is not yet clear what roles may be played by LOX and CYP metabolites of arachidonic acid in HT. The genes involved in these or in prostaglandin action have not been carefully assessed for linkage and association to primary HT.

## The Natriuretic Peptide System

The pathways and other details of the NPS are dealt with in the candidate genes sections that follow. This system has the potential to make an important difference to long-term BP because there are actions at several physiologic targets that impact on the BP level. Thus, natriuresis is promoted through actions on the CD and also at the PT and afferent arteriole that increase the filtered load. Actions to antagonize renin and vasopressin will also facilitate reduction in TPR and diuresis. Thus, a powerful system (in theory) may be triggered in response to hypervolemia to cause a lowering of BP. It is now recognized that an excess of circulating ANP typically characterizes volume-expanded HT.[111] Brain natriuretic peptide (BNP), which despite its name originates largely in the heart ventricles, is also recognized as part of this NPS, and it too is typically high in hypervolemic HT, especially when the ventricles are under a particularly heavy load or are becoming hypertrophic.[112] Because the NPS is highly upregulated despite persistence of volume overload, either tissue resistance has developed or the system is overwhelmed by the power of the volume-pressure overload pathophysiology. Discovery of local degradation of ANP and BNP by proteolytic enzymes especially neutral endopeptidases (NEPs) and its sequestration and clearance by the NPRC receptor[113] explains local resistance because there may be little intact ANP and BNP left to bind to the functional receptor(s) NPRA (or NPRB for the third C-type natriuretic peptide; CNP was recently also proposed as an EDHF[76]). Neither inhibitors of NEP nor reduced clearance by NPRC markedly reestablish tissue sensitivity to the natriuretic peptide receptor system providing only weak long-term benefits. Transgenic mice overexpressing ANP have low BP, ANP −/− and +/− mice have salt-sensitive HT, and NPRA −/− and +/− have marked HT[39,99] (see later in candidate genes section). Such studies indicate that the NPS can cause long-term abnormalities in BP. Mice also develop resistance to the effects of strong activation of the NPS, in situations such as heart failure, indicating that the striking effect of knockout studies on BP are not merely due to major species differences in the extent to which resistance to the effect of circulating ANP and BNP develops. Thus, it seems that, in otherwise healthy individuals, changes in the NPS may have the potential to powerfully influence long-term BP especially in a salt-sensitive manner. Assessment for linkage and association of genes in this system have been mainly focused on the gene encoding ANP (NPPA) and largely find no association with HT. Other components await assessment. Elucidating the basis of ANP/BNP tissue resistance will be key in fully understanding this system. In addition to local proteolytic degradation and clearance receptor action, other explanations have included poor blood supply to the renal medullary sites of the natriuretic actions of ANP and induction of cGMP phosphodiesterase, which will clear the ANP/BNP cGMP second messenger quickly in target cells.[114]

## Kallikrein-Kinin System

In humans the plasma and tissue kallikrein-kinin systems (KKSs) generate bradykinin and kallidin peptides, respectively. KKS effects are implicated in inflammatory conditions, water and $Na^+$ excretion, and BP homeostasis and possibly cardioprotective effects relating to ischemic preconditioning. The levels of kinin peptides are higher in the tissues than in the blood where bradykinin levels exceed kallidin, whereas in urine kallidin exceeds bradykinin peptides.[115] ACE inhibitors increase levels of both bradykinin and kallidin, and in heart failure circulating kallidin especially is suppressed.[115] Kinins participate in the features of inflammation; they are vasodilators (and also promote vascular permeability, neutrophil chemotaxis, and pain) and promote natriuresis and diuresis. Plasma kallikrein forms bradykinin (BK) a nine amino acid peptide from (high molecular weight) kininogen, whereas tissue kallikrein forms kallidin (Lys0-BK, KBK) from kininogens (high and low molecular weight). Kinins act via two receptors, B1 and B2. B2 normally predominates, whereas B1 receptors, are upregulated with tissue injury. BK and KBK are more potent at B2 receptors, whereas their kininase I (carboxypeptidase) metabolites BK(1-8) and KBK(1-8) are more potent at B1.[116] ACE and NEP produce inactive BK(1-7) and KBK(1-7). Kallikrein is localized in arteries and arterioles especially in the endothelium. Kinins binding B2 receptors trigger generation of NO and cGMP and this causes vasodilation. In the nephron specifically TAL, this antagonizes vasopressin action and promotes diuresis and natriuresis. Although there is considerable evidence that kinins may influence BP, it is important to note that in humans with complete kininogen deficiency (William's trait) there are reported to be no abnormalities of BP and indeed normal health,[117] with only a laboratory clotting abnormality relating to the alternative clotting pathway of which kininogen is a trigger. Moreover, the beneficial effects of ACE inhibitors (which antagonize the RAS signaling by reducing AngII generation and promote the kinin system by reducing kinin breakdown) on lowering BP in many respects mimic selective blockade of AT1 receptors of the RAS; thus, there is some doubt regarding whether kinins contribute significantly to the effects of ACE inhibition on BP. The relative weakness of the NEP inhibitor (which limits breakdown of kinins and natriuretic factors) and icatibant (a B2 antagonist) effects on BP compared with ACE inhibitors does not lend any support to an important role for kinins in BP regulation. Thus, the evidence from clinical observations for an important effect of kinins on BP in humans is lacking. In contrast, kinin B2 receptor −/− mice develop salt-sensitive HT[118] (B1 −/− mice develop altered inflammatory responses but have no change in baseline BP). Transgenic mice overexpressing the B2 receptor or tissue kallikrein are hypotensive.[45] In addition, there are long-standing reports of reduced urinary kallikrein (and thus assumed lower renal kinin activation) in patients with primary HT. Thus, the animal studies support a significant role for the kinin system in long-term BP control and the risks of salt-sensitive HT, but the clinical findings are weak and largely circumstantial. So far candidate genes in this pathway have received little attention in linkage and association studies relating to human primary HT.

## Where in the Body Do Changes Initiating and Sustaining Hypertension Act?

### Kidney

Unless there is a defect in the renal pressure-natriuresis mechanism it is hard to see how long-term HT can persist, simply because this mechanism will return BP to normal. The pressure-natriuresis response is based in the kidney but integrates a number of stimuli deriving from extrarenal sources such as the SNS, aldosterone, AngII, ANP, and others. In addition, the bulk of renin production originates in the kidney, and other elements of the RAS are represented intrarenally, although most ACE and essentially all angiotensinogen synthesis is extrarenal. The role of the kidney was addressed in cross-transplantation experiments involving several rodent models of HT, for example, the Dahl[119], Milan,[120] and spontaneously hypertensive (SHR[121] and SHRSP[122]) rat models. In all these studies HT followed the kidney from prehypertensive donor to normal recipient, whereas a kidney from a normal donor provided the prehypertensive strain recipient with protection from developing what was otherwise inevitable later BP rise. Necessarily less direct and rigorous findings for human transplant recipients also suggest that the HT followed the kidney. Thus, HT develops more often in those receiving a kidney from a hypertensive donor[123,124] and in cadaveric donors having evidence of end-organ damage from HT (subarachnoid hemorrhage, more cardiac hypertrophy) than those without such findings.[125] In patients for whom essential HT was the likely cause of renal failure, there is long-term remission from HT after renal transplantation but not following removal of their native kidneys,[126] indicating that the native kidney had a defect in pressure natriuresis. This and other evidence indicates that the key mechanism of pressure natriuresis is intrinsic to the kidney, rather than dependent on extrarenal factors.

Human studies have also shown that abnormal renal $Na^+$ handling predates the development of essential HT in children with two hypertensive parents and that BP "tracks" with age from childhood. This and similar findings in animal models indicate that abnormalities in renal $Na^+$ handling are present at the prehypertensive stage in essential HT and occur in childhood so that the BP would be expected to track higher from this stage. The work of Lifton et al.[28] and others has contributed to these ideas indicating that multiple inherited $Na^+$ handling defects cause long-term alterations in BP and are due to defects intrinsic to the kidney rather than extrarenal signaling. In conclusion, impairment in pressure natriuresis is of central importance in the development of sustained HT.

In human secondary HT also, the renal pressure-natriuresis relationship has been shown to be abnormally shifted, such that on removal of the primary cause (renal artery stenosis or primary aldosterone excess) the pressure natriuresis relationship returned to normal in conjunction with restoration of normotension.[127] Similarly, some renal pathologies can be associated with HT and on transplantation the recipient may only develop recurrent HT when the pathology recurs in the transplant (e.g., IgA nephropathy, DM renal disease, amyloidosis). Here the chain of causation of the primary disease appears to begin outside but then later passes within the kidney to establish HT.

### Adrenal

The adrenal gland is the site of synthesis of aldosterone, cortisol, deoxycorticosterone, adrenaline, and noradrenaline. When overproduced, all of these often cause sustained HT, which can be severe. These abnormalities are discussed in later sections; those relating to aldosterone are also shown in Figure 33-4. Although there is some controversy regarding the prevalence of mineralocorticoid excess as a cause of HT, the contribution of all adrenal overproduction represents a small minority of total HT. Adrenocortical failure, however, has a BP lowering not restricted to a minority. If such patients are following a low-salt diet or taking diuretics, then life-threatening hypotension is likely to develop. The role of aldosterone deficiency is clear from the previous discussion because $FR_{Na}$ will fall, leading to a reduction in ECF volume and BP, unless dietary salt intake is high enough to keep up with losses. Patients with inherited aldosterone synthase deficiency (having isolated loss of aldosterone, cortisol is approximately normal) are salt wasting and hyperkalemic and have reduced BP responding to mineralocorticoid replacement like the more common primary adrenal deficiency. Losses will be less in those with coexisting renal failure in whom aldosterone loss may have less impact on BP than a significant change in salt diet will, but they will develop hyperkalemia. However, most HT patients with normal renal function, unless taking a high-salt diet, will have a diminution in HT, and, thus, aldosterone seems to be a permissive or amplifying factor for HT in general.

Cortisol deficiency occurs without any major aldosterone loss when there is ACTH deficiency. Although these patients are not uniformly hypotensive as patients with aldosterone loss are, they are prone to reduced vascular tone and relative refractoriness to effects of vasoconstrictors and have less synthesis of angiotensinogen[128]; however, they tend to have increased production of the vasodilator $PI_2$.[128] Finally, in acute illness, impaired repression of iNOS may lead to NO overproduction, causing marked drops in BP or collapse without glucocorticoid to limit its expression. Thus, it is hard to discount a role for glucocorticoids in the lower BP usually seen if adrenal cortical failure develops.

In summary, adrenal corticosteroids especially aldosterone may be effectively required to sustain significant HT in most patients, although this will be diminished in those on a high-salt diet and with renal impairment causing $Na^+$ retention. Thus, the adrenal probably plays at least a permissive role in most HT as distinct from the direct role played in adrenal causes of secondary HT.

### Heart, Sympathetic Nervous System, and Central Nervous System

No evidence appears to suggest a definite major etiologic role for the heart in initiating and sustaining long-term HT. For the nervous system, matters are less clear, suggesting a role in amplifying the severity of HT (by the SNS not downregulating) and may also support a primary etiologic role in some small subsets of hypertensives, especially with intracranial pathology and/or labile BP. The baroreceptor dampens swings in BP, but the long-term average BP remains unchanged. Thus, in animal studies in which the reflex is denervated there is initial HT from unsuppressed vasomotor center vasoconstriction, but BP then falls back to preexisting average levels after about 2 days. Similarly, increased peripheral resistance in established HT reduces with sympathectomy but over the course of weeks returns to previous levels. Despite this evidence, clinical studies report that many young hypertensives (and even those at a point before the development of established essential HT) have a hyperdynamic circulation and evidence consistent with elevated activity of the SNS. Moreover, such overactivity may increase renin angiotensin activation and hypertrophic changes of $\Delta CO \leftrightarrow \Delta TPR$.[129] Other clinical studies suggest that the baroreceptors reset at an inappropriately high rate in HT,[130] and it is hard to discount the fact that β- and α-blockers do have useful BP-lowering effects in human HT, which are not just short-lived, and that clinical experience indicated that surgical sympathectomy had some long-lasting benefit at least for those with severe HT.[131] Thus, there seems to be support for a role of the SNS in amplifying HT, especially in young patients, in those susceptible to the effects of stress, and in those with coexisting obesity.[132]

Extra-adrenal pheochromocytomas and paragangliomas cause HT through catecholamine excess. Lesions of the brainstem nucleus tractus solitarius can cause labile HT in experimental animals. Brainstem pathology,[18] raised intracranial pressure[19] or impaired medullary blood supply[17,18] can cause increased activation of the SNS via the CNS ischemic response reflex. Thus, another subset of human HT is driven by SNS overactivation that results from overactivation of a CNS reflex. Whether vertebrobasilar atherosclerosis in the elderly could cause HT in a larger group of HT patients[20] remains to be resolved.

The chemoreceptor and CNS ischemic response reflexes may play a role in the pathophysiology of HT when there are coexisting respiratory abnormalities, such as in obstructive sleep apnea (OSA)[133,134] in which the intermittent nature of the hypoxic and hypercapnic stimuli make acquiescence of the reflexes by resetting appear less likely. In OSA these hypoxia and hypercapnic reflexes, ongoing inspiratory effort against the obstructed airway (generating marked negative intrathoracic pressure and increased venous return), and intermittent arousals from sleep all play a role in the associated sympathetic activation. Normally the SNS activation from these reflexes is somewhat inhibited on inspiration by a counterbalancing reflex triggered by pulmonary stretch. However, this moderating pulmonary stretch effect is lacking and consequently the hypoxia and hypercapnia response is amplified by coincident apnea in OSA.[133] There is SNS overactivity in OSA with SNS activity not reducing (as is usual) overnight, and periodic upregulations in SNS activity peak at the point of arousal at the end of apneas. Moreover, OSA patients also have continuing daytime sleepiness and sympathetic activation during the day as well. OSA patients have increased vasoconstriction, and the prevalence of HT is raised in OSA (although obesity can be a confounder here). BP is typically increased both day and night (when there can be peaks of HT and associated SNS activation). Animal studies show that hypoxia with apnea results in vasoconstriction, which is greatly diminished with denervation of the carotid body or hypoxia alone. The frequent coexistence of obesity and mild polycythemia makes it hard to precisely quantify the proportionate contribution of SNS activation from hypoxia and hypercapnia, although it seems clear from most outcome studies that therapy that reduces the hypoxic and hypercapnic drive for OSA also have proven benefit in lowering BP[133,134] as has been shown for continuous positive airway pressure therapy (CPAP) and for surgical treatments of tracheostomy or uvulopalatopharyngoplasty. Studies with CPAP in particular confirm a fall in SNS activity with reduced plasma noradrenaline and urinary noradrenaline metabolites.[135]

## Vasculature

Altered compliance, especially of the large arteries with age and disease is a etiologic factor in ISH, especially in the elderly. This is recognized as an important risk factor for cardiovascular disease complications[136] and for renal impairment.[136] Genetic contributors to these risks acting through reduced compliance and higher systolic pressure are not understood, but alterations in structural proteins of large arteries seem to be involved. Thus, deficient or defective fibrillin-1[137] can lead to aneurysms not only in Marfan's syndrome[137] but also in other patients.[138] Fibrillin-1 genotype has now been associated in humans with increases in arterial stiffness and systolic pressure and greater coronary artery and aortic aneurysm disease risks independent of other risk factors.[138,139] Arterial disease lying between the aortic outflow and glomeruli causes HT, disconnecting the renal pressure-natriuresis system (and renin regulation) from exposure to actual systemic arterial pressure. Generalized rarefaction of the peripheral arterial tree would increase TPR, and there is some evidence that this is present early in the course of essential HT[140] and in young normotensives at increased risk of HT who have two parents with essential HT.[141] This suggests that there is a predisposition from early life to increased TPR, which could be inherited or derived from intrauterine fetal programming effects on vessel growth.[142] Importantly, the vasculature is intimately linked to the end-organ effects and the risk of tissue damage from HT. In other respects the extrarenal vasculature seems to play an amplifying role on HT initiated by other causes. By responding to the elevation in BP, vasoconstrictor and mitogenic stimulation (with a hypertrophic response) and impaired endothelium-dependent vasodilation TPR is elevated

and risk of vascular damage is increased. This engenders a vicious cycle of elevation in BP, impairment of vasodilation, hypertrophy, and permanent vessel damage. In cases of secondary HT, removal of the cause at an early stage and normalization of BP often results in restoration of endothelium-dependent vasodilation and regression of hypertrophic changes. In hypertensive patients with renal failure who start dialysis, assessment of BP can be difficult, but in careful studies aimed at dialyzing down to a consistent normal ECV it appears that a substantial proportion continue to have drops in BP for more than 4 weeks before the BP at the same body weight (and ECV) stabilizes. This has been interpreted as a progressive regression of peripheral vascular hypertrophy. Finally, vessels supplying muscle beds normally dilate on exercise and in response to elevations of insulin. In insulin resistance this response is impaired and may be a key factor in the degree of insulin resistance by limiting access of muscle tissue to glucose, insulin, and free fatty acids and by fostering greater hyperinsulinemia with attendant greater hypertensive effects.

## Other Tissues

Other tissues may play a role in HTL: (1) the immune system, which can cause inflammatory changes in the kidney (e.g., glomerulonephritis) and vasculature and (2) adipose tissue, which is a source of many vasoactive substances (thus, the potential load of these may increase markedly in obesity).[143] In one recent mouse model[144] the glucocorticoid regenerating enzyme 11β-hydroxysteroid dehydrogenase type 1 was overexpressed in adipose tissue on the basis that the centripetal abdominal obesity of both Cushing's syndrome and the metabolic syndrome (HT, obesity, dyslipidemia, and insulin resistance) suggested an important interaction of adipose tissue and glucocorticoid excess. Indeed, the mice had all the features of the metabolic syndrome including HT in association with renal abnormalities and elevated renin substrate (angiotensinogen) that derived from adipose tissue.[144] The RAS is present and active in fat but had previously been the subject of relatively little research.[145]

## Sites Considered Especially Important

The kidneys are of central importance with impairment of pressure natriuresis seeming to be a required part of the pathway to sustained HT. The larger vasculature plays an important role in SBP and pulse pressure. The peripheral vascular constitutes the site of TPR and is often labeled as damaged to explain the failure of BP to normalize after removal of a secondary cause. The vessels afferent to and within the kidney play an indisputable role in certain forms of HT. Vascular (end-organ) damage is also a key amplifier of HT. The adrenal and SNS probably play a more permissive role in the development of HT except in those cases in which overproduction of catecholamines or adrenal steroids is the primary drive to elevate BP.

# OVERVIEW OF CAUSES OF HYPERTENSION

## Primary and Secondary Hypertension

Primary or essential HT is HT in which no secondary cause for the HT is identified. The percentage that is primary HT is, thus, determined by what is included within secondary causes of HT (e.g., whether to include obesity or alcohol-related HT) and how carefully such secondary causes are looked for (thus affecting the rates of detection of secondary causes such as renal artery stenosis and pheochromocytoma). The definition of secondary HT is also important. An arbitrary line is often drawn beyond which a possible secondary cause for the HT is attributed (e.g., use of an aldosterone-to-renin ratio for mineralocorticoid excess). If a definitive treatment is available to remove such causes (e.g., surgery to remove an aldosterone-producing adenoma), then its use will help verify that the HT was indeed secondary to the cause. However, if there is unlikely to be such definitive curative treatment, then it becomes less clear if the condition is secondary or primary HT. Thus, if a considerably lower ratio of aldosterone-to-renin is used to define mineralocorticoid HT, it becomes much less likely that a curable aldosterone-producing tumor or even bilateral adrenal hyperplasia will be found and the spectrum of causes begins to merge with low-renin essential HT. Although the exact position of the dividing line can, thus, be difficult and is a source of some controversy in the case of mineralocorticoid excess,[146-148] the problem is to some extent present for most[149] causes of secondary HT because they merge, in less marked cases, into primary HT (e.g., by the percentage stenosis in renal artery stenosis and by the degree of elevation of catecholamine metabolites in pheochromocytoma). Probably slightly more secondary HT is detected and regarded as secondary with modern methods. However, because such cases typically are not among the mildest HT, it seems that, when the definition of HT in international guidelines now includes milder elevations in BP, this may somewhat dilute the percentage prevalence of secondary HT. Thus, secondary causes of HT probably still contributes approximately 5% of HT ($\geq$140/90 mm Hg). Traditionally, secondary HT includes coarctation, renovascular HT, renal HT, mineralocorticoid excess, pheochromocytoma and other adrenal causes (such as Cushing's syndrome), other endocrine causes (e.g., acromegaly), polycythemia and hyperviscosity, HT related to drug therapy, and OSA. HT with prominent association with obesity, diabetes, or alcohol has traditionally been classed as behavioral and lifestyle amplifiers (e.g., high-salt intake) of primary HT unless a more classical secondary cause is present (e.g., Cushing's syndrome). HT in pregnancy and malignant HT are separate entities. A number of rare syndromes have HT as a frequent feature (e.g., Bardet-Biedl syndrome) and it seems appropriate to consider them as rare forms of secondary HT. The remainder of HT is regarded as a polygenic, complex, quantitative trait, and, although it may have a normal frequency distribution, it is quite an assumption that primary HT is one entity best regarded without subdivision. The response to this concern has been to look for param-

eters with some etiologic credibility (e.g., directly linked to one of the major BP control or regulatory mechanisms discussed previously) and categorize primary HT into somewhat arbitrary subdivisions. Thus, there is low-, normal-, and high-renin HT; renin angiotensin modulators or nonmodulators; salt-sensitive and salt-resistant; and perhaps obese and nonobese or responders and nonresponders to the major classes of anti-HT treatment. It is important to subdivide primary HT, but the means and intermediate phenotypes to do so have yet to be defined.

## Evidence for a Genetic Component

Genetic component evidence comes from a range of studies including twin, adoption, and migration studies that estimate the extent to which HT clusters in families (e.g., monozygotic twins share ~75% of their variation in BP, dizygotic share ~50%), the degree to which individuals manifest differences in BP not explained by their shared environment, and how such differences survive major changes in environment. Distilling the clues from such studies down to a single percentage of BP variation that is genetic has yielded figures from 20% to 50% in the majority,[150-152] with occasional higher estimates from twin studies.[150] One of the more useful contexts in which to view this information is related to other common polygenic disorders and the extent to which the disorder clusters in a family. This is often expressed as the ratio ($\lambda$s) of the risk that the disorder will recur in another sibling of an affected person divided by the risk in the general population (Fig. 31-5). The analysis shown in Figure 31-5 shows that HT has a $\lambda$s = 3.5 and thus has a similar order of genetic contribution as ischemic heart disease ($\lambda$s = 2 to 3) and some forms of epilepsy ($\lambda$s = 4 to 5) and somewhat less than neural tube defects and psoriasis (both $\lambda$s = 15 to 20). Type 1 DM has a stronger genetic contribution ($\lambda$s $\approx$ 30) than mendelian conditions such as cystic fibrosis ($\lambda$s = 500) do. Because not all genetic factors are of equal strength and severe and mild mutations at the same genetic locus may well reveal themselves to very different extents, the percentage genetic contribution given as a range (such as 20% to 50%) seems less unsatisfactory. Similarly, it is sensible to have results from several different populations with different age and racial mixes before beginning to rely on estimates of strength of a genetic association with HT.

Table 31-3 lists different classes of genetic contributions to a phenotype, which in varying degrees make contributions to HT in a population. When a syndrome such as chromosome disorders or lesser cytogenetic abnormalities results in multiple pathologies, often in childhood or even in infancy, the extent to which BP is affected has understandably not been a focus of attention. However, when the burden of pathology is not so severe and the syndrome is relatively common the association of HT is clearer, and useful clues about the location of genes affecting BP or the origin of features predisposing to HT often emerge. Thus, Turner's syndrome (45 XO) is a common chromosome disorder with a substantially increased risk of HT and a greatly increased risk of coarctation of the aorta. Analysis of this and other disorders affecting the sex chromosomes indi-

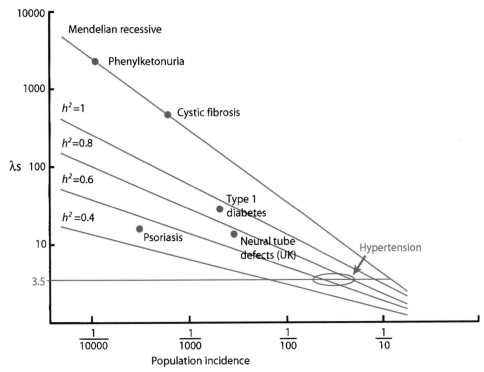

**FIGURE 31-5.** The extent to which disorders cluster in families. The risk of recurrence of disorders in a sibling of an affected individual (sibling incidence) divided by the average population incidence is designated $\lambda_s$. This index of familial clustering is plotted against population incidence for a range of disorders from mendelian single-gene disorders such as cystic fibrosis to polygenic diseases with a range of $\lambda_s$ values. The population incidence for HT reflects that found in youth rather than in old age. $h^2$, heritability. (*Modified from Cavalli-Sforza LL, Bodmer WF: The Genetics of Human Populations. WH Freeman and Co, New York, 1971.*)

cates that chromosomal regions predispose to coarctation and may involve imprinting effects. Williams' syndrome (Williams-Beuren syndrome)[153,154] is due to a cytogenetic abnormality (a deletion on chromosome 7q) and involves HT, supravalvular aortic, stenosis and hypercalcemia. Point mutations in the elastin gene on Ch 7q11.2 may cause isolated supravalvular aortic stenosis.

■ ■ ■

## TABLE 31-3   CLASSES OF GENETIC AND OTHER PHENOTYPE-MODIFYING FACTORS

**Class of Genetic Contribution**

Chromosome disorders
Lesser cytogenetic abnormalities
Single gene mutations
   Coding region
   Promoter
   Intronic
   Gene conversion
Polygenic and complex traits

**Other Phenotype Modifying Factors**

Incomplete penetrance
   Imprinting
   Gene-gene interactions
   permissive interacting genotypes
   somatic second hit in key tissue
   Gene-environment interactions
   Permissive environment
   Triggering environmental exposure
Susceptibility to end-organ damage

It seems that Williams' syndrome is a contiguous gene syndrome encompassing elastin gene involvement, which accounts for supravalvular aortic stenosis, and involvement and deletion of proximal genes, which cause hypercalcemia and HT. Thus, it seems that a gene capable of altering long-term BP is present on Ch 7q close to the elastin gene and its mutation or deletion can raise BP. Whether this effect requires hypercalcemia or aortic abnormalities requires further clarification. Close study of other cytogenetic syndromes may point to certain loci as probable sites of genes capable of altering long-term BP if abnormal or deleted. A number of mendelian single-gene disorders affect BP (lowering or raising it and causing HT). These involve both autosomal recessive and dominant disorders and mutations increasing, decreasing, or abolishing the activity of the gene product.[28] Some genes (e.g., MR or subunits of ENaC) mutated differently can either cause raised or lowered BP. All kinds of mutations have been involved in the causation of altered BP by such single-gene disorders including complete deletion of genes; partial deletions, microdeletions, and microinsertions; nonsense and missense point mutations; point mutations affecting splicing; and mutations that appear to leave the coding region unaffected but affect intronic sequence (e.g., WNK1 mutations causing the hypertensive Gordon's syndrome[155]). The details of the mutation can be very important; thus, as mentioned different mutations in the same gene can raise or lower BP (e.g., MR and β or γENaC), and in many cases the degree to which a mutation inactivates or activates the gene product appears to show some correlation with its effect on BP. However, for other genes the situation appears different. Thus, the spectrum of disease occurring in von Hippel Lindau (VHL) is affected by the nature of the mutation. Only 10% of mutations cause pheochromocytomas (and so HT), which are often a major feature in this group of patients; 96% of these mutations are missense (i.e., relatively mild in their effect compared with the nonsense premature stop codon). Deletion mutations are also often found and do not appear to cause pheochromocytomas or HT. The basis of this association of missense mutations with pheochromocytomas remains unresolved. Finally, in another mendelian disorder causing HT, glucocorticoid remediable aldosteronism (GRA) gene conversion mutations produce a unique chimeric gene from the recombination of the 5′half of one gene (CYP11B1) with a highly homologous region of the flanking gene (CYP11B2) just adjacent and 3′ on the same chromosome resulting in fusion with the 3′ half of this flanking gene to give a functional enzyme overproducing aldosterone in response to the ACTH responsive promoter of the "wrong" gene.[28]

Incomplete penetrance is an important factor to consider because this may modify or mask the otherwise simple mendelian inheritance of a condition and make such simple contributions to the disease phenotype easily missed. There are many reasons for incomplete penetrance; a special case is one in which imprinting of the genetic locus can modify inheritance so that only one allele is expressed and so that the disease may only be inherited from either mother or father. In one of the disorders causing pheochromocytomas and paragangliomas (see later) a region of Ch 11q is maternally imprinted so that causative mutations are only manifest if inheritance is from the father. Moreover, the imprinting is not present in all tissues; both alleles are expressed in lymphocytes but only one in tissues in which the pheochromocytomas or paragangliomas form. Interaction with other genes is another cause of incomplete penetrance. Thus, for a physiologic process such as $Na^+$ reabsorption a defect in one gene or pathway may be to some degree compensated by a related pathway or gene. If there is genetic variation within these compensatory genes or pathways, there will be a corresponding modification of the effects of the original mutation on phenotype. Thus, in kindreds in which a disease gene segregates (e.g., chimeric gene for GRA) those inheriting the gene may vary considerably in phenotype (BP and plasma $K^+$); when this cannot be attributed to variation in known key environmental factors (e.g., salt intake), the effects of interacting genes are thought to be a major reason for variation. Another reason for incomplete penetrance is that the disease mutation greatly predisposes to the disease (e.g., HT) but another hit is required to fully develop it. This hit can be a somatic mutation in a key tissue especially if that tissue also proliferates. Thus, in familial conditions that cause pheochromocytomas (e.g., VHL) there is loss or mutation of one copy of a key gene (usually a tumor suppressor), that is, heterozygosity, but for development of a pheochromocytoma loss of the remaining wild-type copy of the gene is required. This second hit occurs with a somatic mutation within the tissue itself, which can be shown to have lost heterozygosity, thus enabling pheochromocytoma formation and HT. Occasionally such a second hit can be at the locus of an interacting gene; this seems to be the case for two loci on Ch 11q at 11q13 and the SDHD gene on 11q25-26 where one gene is mutated and the other lost in somatic mutations. Thus, the enabling hit can generate pheochromocytomas or paragangliomas and cause HT. This special case represents a digenic disease. Just as incomplete penetrance can derive from interacting genes or requirement of enabling genetic hit, so can it be due to interactions with the environment (e.g., salt or calorie intake in diet), drug treatment (e.g., estrogen-containing contraceptive pill), alcohol consumption, or exposure to an infection or other antigen triggering an episode of glomerulonephritis. Thus, not all individuals are equally at risk for HT on receiving a high-salt or high-calorie diet (with attendant weight gain) or estrogens or on exposure to infections or antigens (with attendant renal and/or vascular damage). This can be viewed as incomplete penetrance or an inherited susceptibility or vulnerability that is only fully manifested if both genetic and environmental factors are present to interact.

Primary or essential HT is regarded as such a trait along with other common diseases and disorders prevalent in the West including diabetes (especially type II), atherosclerosis, dyslipidemia, and obesity. In the metabolic syndrome there is often coincidence of more than one and sometimes all of these factors; thus, etiologic factors are to some extent overlapping. Major insights into the cause of any of these conditions warrants consideration of an etiologic role in primary HT. Negative results should also be informative in excluding aspects of this overlap as important candidates in all cases. Thus, patients with most types of maturity-onset diabetes of the young (MODY) and Pima Indians with a high incidence of type 2 diabetes and obesity are not coincidentally affected by greatly increased risk of HT. Primary HT in some groups (e.g., African Americans or others of Afro-Caribbean background) is more often salt sensitive and associated with a high incidence of hypertensive nephrosclerosis. In some normotensive families predisposed to seemingly identical nephrosclerosis, genetic factors have been elucidated; thus, the cause of nephrosclerosis in these ethnic groups, previously assumed to be largely a HT complication, has been defined.

There is little fundamental information on which to base predictions about primary HT, but genetic modeling suggests that the near normal distribution of BP in large populations implicates genetic contributions from at least four genes with moderate effect rather than a smaller number with large effect. If there were such a very low number of genes (e.g., less than four), one would not expect to find good, homogeneous BP correlations among relatives across the BP range (i.e., parents with high BP tend to have children with high BP with approximately the same frequency as parents with average or low BP have children with average or low BP, respectively). Although a very small number of genes could have their effect very heavily modified by factors affecting penetrance (as outlined previously), it is generally assumed that such extreme masking of effects is unlikely without interacting genes being involved, thus again raising the number of genes that contribute to a higher number. Theoretical models fit increasingly well with the findings of the heritability of primary HT as the number of simple genetic contributors in a population rises above four. It is possible to model the features of primary HT within a population with a large number of genes each with small effect or with a smaller number (e.g., 10 to 20 genes) segregating in a mendelian fashion with high penetrance. If one introduces incomplete penetrance and major gene-gene interactions, the number of genes required to fit well can be lower. This has been an exciting realization. If it is hypothesized that the number of important genes in which variation contributes to BP variation in a population is not too numerous (say falling in the 4 to 20 or polygene range), then theory predicts that the identification of their loci is within reach. Based on such models of polygenetic contributions to primary HT, calculations have been made on the size of linkage studies required to detect the chromosomal loci of the more important hypothesized polygenes that have an effect on BP. This has led to genome-wide linkage studies to test these hypotheses and to identify such major gene loci using informative genetic markers (which vary person-to-person within the population) distributed across the genome by studying small but informative family groups (especially sib-pairs). Some of the first such "genome scan" linkage studies were in type 1 diabetes; they showed a spectacular major hit on human chromosome 6, near the HLA locus, now refined to a locus with a LOD score of 65 that contributes more than 50% of the genetic contribution to the risk of type 1 diabetes in many populations.[156] However, enough similar scans have now been carried out looking for loci of genes of major effect to know that no such *genes of huge effect* seem to be involved in adult BP variation in primary HT. As discussed later some loci have been identified but are relatively weak, and individual results, thus, require replication in other populations to verify that they are real effects. Parallels with loci identified on genome scans of rodent polygenic HT have reinforced the candidacy of some of the loci found on human genome scans because the corresponding syntenic region in the rodent studies also indicated a locus involved in the risk of HT was present—in particular this has strengthened the candidate loci for HT on human chromosomes 17[157] and appears to do so for other sites as well.

Association studies have also been widely used to identify genes of major effect in primary HT in humans. These studies look at how variations of a polymorphic locus adjacent to or within a candidate gene (especially related to a pathway regulating BP such as the RAS) segregate with HT or BP level within a population sample. As will be seen later, a number of candidates have been considered, and fewer were tested repeatedly in different populations with a good mix of ages and ethnic backgrounds. Thus, such results are currently inconclusive, although there is evidence that variations in the angiotensinogen gene, which alter its circulating level, seem to indicate a genuine albeit weak effect on BP and the risk of primary HT in a range of human populations.

Not only is primary HT caused by a genetic contribution deriving from multiple genes but it is also a complex trait in which incomplete penetrance and gene-gene interactions are certain to be at work. Moreover, there is an important and substantial, although elusive, contribution from the environment.

## Environment

There is evidence for substantial effects of environment on BP. The exact components of the environment responsible are very much less clear. Comparing societies around the world it is evident that the average BP varies widely. In primitive peoples such as Pacific Islanders, nomadic groups from Africa, and native Indians of the Amazon basin the BP is usually strikingly lower than in the West. Moreover, there is a great reduction or absence of the trend for adult BP to rise with age that is so prominent in the West.[158] Migration studies between environments of native populations with such striking differences in BP have shown that migrants coming into a more urbanized or Westernized society rapidly manifest changes in BP reflecting features prevalent in the new environment. For example Poulter et al.[159] studied migrants in East Africa from native small village communities to inner city locations with the attendant more urbanized environment and lifestyle and found that BP rose substantially within 1 month and began to show trends, detectable by 2 years, for BP to also rise with age.

The factors responsible for the change in BP in such studies and others addressing environmental effects on BP are not clear but are often attributed to changes in (1) diet: increased calories, from complex to simple carbohydrates, from vegetable protein and fats to more animal protein and more saturated fats, from low $Na^+$ and high $K^+$ (and magnesium) to high $Na^+$ and low $K^+$ (and magnesium); (2) reduction in exercise; (3) increase in body weight; (4) changes in the nature of stresses; and (5) other features such as higher smoking and alcohol use. There is every reason to expect that these features are the basis of some of the variation in BP not only between societies but also within a society and so may underpin differences observed between socioeconomic classes. Proving and estimating the contribution of individual environmental factors to BP has been difficult, but the contributions of salt intake, social stress, and especially obesity now seem reasonably well established even if the scale of the demonstrated effect appears weak. The Intersalt study across 52 populations confirmed an association of BP with $Na^+$ intake and $Na^+/K^+$ ratio of dietary intake. Although the effect was weak it was more convincing when change in BP with age was correlated with salt intake (24-hour urinary $Na^+$).[160] The strength of this effect and the extent to which estimates of the size of the effect made in cross-cultural studies can be viewed as relevant to estimate the effect within a culture have been sources of considerable controversy. However, more than 100 trials exploring the effect of dietary $Na^+$ on BP have been carried out; the prevailing evidence indicates that there is an average reduction of some 5/2 mm Hg in BP in HT patients when $Na^+$ intake is lowered to approximately 100 mmol/day. The effect was weaker for normotensive subjects and stronger if $Na^+$ intake was reduced further to 65mmol/day or less.[161] Maintaining a reasonably high $K^+$ intake has weaker BP-lowering effects probably of the order of lowering by 3/2 mm Hg.[161] Another dietary factor relates to higher calorie intake, weight gain, and adiposity. A number of studies have shown a strong effect of weight gain on BP; thus, in the Framingham study it was estimated that 60% to 70% of HT was attributable to adiposity with some 5 mm Hg increase in SBP for every 5-kg weight gain.[162] At long-term follow-up of up to more than 40 years, the risk of developing HT was largely explained by weight gain (i.e., BMI > 25) (relative risk 1.46 for men, and 1.75 for women).[163] Similarly the Nurses Health Study of 80,000 women found that 5-kg and 10-kg weight gains from weight at age 18 caused an increased relative risk of HT of 1.6 and 2.2, respectively.[164] Comparable rises have been found in other studies; the effect of weight gain on BP again is greater in women. Current lifestyle advice reflects the evidence for environmental and lifestyle impact on BP and the risk of HT. Six recommendations emerge in current guidance: (1) engage in moderate physical activity; (2) maintain normal body weight; (3) limit alcohol consumption; (4) reduce $Na^+$ intake; (5) maintain adequate intake of $K^+$; and (6) consume a diet rich in fruits, vegetables, and low-fat dairy products and reduced in saturated and total fat.[161] Studies on selected populations have also supported other factors such as social stress relating to long-term BP. For instance, one of the more radical of such comparisons demonstrated lower BP and lack of rise in BP with age in Italian women living as nuns within a secluded order compared with those continuing to live in "open society" nearby.[165] Further detailed consideration of individual putative environmental factors on HT is beyond the scope of this chapter.

Finally, the correlation of BP between relatives sharing 50% of genetic variation are not equal; correlation of BP for dizygotic twins is approximately 50%, between non-twin siblings approximately 25%, and between parents and offspring less still.[166,167] These differences have been ascribed to a greater shared environment of dizygotic twins versus other siblings versus parents and children and, thus, to the relative importance of the early environment. As studies have shown, indices of social deprivation in the adult are more closely correlated with adult cardiovascular disease (including HT) than indices of previous deprivation as a child. It is possible that the greater shared environment of twins and siblings relates to their shared intrauterine environment because they shared the same pregnancy or different pregnancies from the same mother (see fetal programming) or to other shared elements of their environment not attributable to social deprivation influences.

Finally, it is often the case that on migration of a population or on change of the prevailing environment that the population mean changes but in general individuals within the population retain a similar ranking within the stratification of the population by BP. If a family or ethnic group shifts its ranking within the stratification and with respect to the mean of the population, it suggests that they possess genes specifically interacting with the environmental change. Hence, people of Afro-Caribbean origin migrating to Western lifestyles often show disproportionate rise in BP, often attributed to greater salt sensitivity.

## Gender

BP differences exist between the sexes but are not large in comparison with those for example typically occurring between age groups. Typically BP is not significantly different between boys and girls in childhood, but from puberty the BP rise becomes steeper for boys leaving them on average with approximately 10/5 mm Hg higher BP at age 18. Beyond this age there is a tendency for both sexes to have increased BP with age in the West, and this rise is very similar initially in adulthood but by the 40s women have BP rising slightly more steeply. Thus, BP of women catches up and surpasses that of men by around age 60.[2] By this stage DBP is no longer rising and begins to fall slightly while SBP continues rising. Women have higher basal levels of endothelial NO release premenopausally[168] and tend to put on weight more than men after age 50[169]; these factors could explain part of the sex differences in BP levels. White coat HT is commoner in women. Women are at less risk for end-organ damage and complications of HT than men across the full range of BP. It is unclear if part of this effect relates to the higher proportion of women with white coat HT. Nonetheless, because HT is very common in the elderly and because women live longer than men the proportion of deaths in women related to complications of HT is greater

## Age

In most Westernized countries HT is very prevalent in the elderly because there is an upward trend in BP with age.[2,9] Thus, more than 50% have SBP greater than 140 mm Hg by age 65. SBP continues to rise unless there is concurrent debilitating illness. In contrast from the mid-50s DBP rise flattens and then falls slowly. Thus, the common pattern of HT in the elderly is ISH, which involves raised pulse pressure. In the elderly, baroreflex sensitivity is reduced, with increased BP variability and greater postural changes in BP. HT tends to be less responsive to β-blockers than in young hypertensives, often viewed as a reflection of altered β-adrenergic sensitivity in the elderly.[170] The relative risk of cardiovascular events is greater in the elderly at any given BP[9] because of concomitant rise in cardiovascular risk factors including age. In a large study of those older than 65 years for every 10 mm Hg rise in pulse pressure there was a 12% elevation in risk of coronary heart disease and a 6% rise in total mortality.[171] In the elderly there are some changes from the normal at younger ages: TPR is increased slightly, CO is usually normal or slightly reduced, plasma noradrenaline is increased but with diminished HR, and β-adrenergic responsiveness and RAS activity are lower (reduced renin and angiotensin and often lower aldosterone and vasopressin). Although there is a decline in renal function in the elderly, in health this is modest, and GFR is only about 20% lower. Increase in stiffness (reduced compliance) of large arteries is the major factor behind the increase in SBP and pulse pressure in ISH so common in the elderly. Pulse wave velocity has been used as an index of aortic stiffness and is powerfully linked to CVS risk in the elderly. In an assessment of almost 2000 hypertensive patients of 50 ±13 years followed for mean of approximately 9.5 years, pulse wave velocity (although not pulse pressure) was significantly and independently associated with all-cause and cardiovascular mortality with univariate odds ratios for relative risks of 2.14 and 2.67, respectively (both P < 0.0001).[172] This provides direct evidence that aortic stiffness is an independent predictor of mortality in essential HT especially in older patients. Factors appearing to affect large artery stiffness include physical inactivity, high salt intake, increased arterial wall collagen deposition, and reduced NO synthesis. Measures that offer some prospect for reduction in stiffness include aerobic exercise training,[173] decreased Na$^+$ intake,[174] ACE inhibitor[175] and nitrate[176] administration but probably not β-blocker treatment.[170] This suggests that the loss of arterial compliance with age in Westernized societies may not be totally due to irreversible structural changes.

## Fetal Programming

The observation that BP in adulthood shows a strong inverse relation to birth weight have been of great interest. This effect was not due to prematurity but rather to babies born small for dates that showed some evidence of slightly reduced growth *in utero*. A large number of studies focusing on different age ranges from 3 to older than 65 years and totaling thousands of subjects support this "early life origins" hypothesis. Together they represent evidence of a powerful inverse relationship of birth weight to adult BP (Fig. 31-6) such that there is a consistent average reduction in SBP in those of older than 50 years of 3 to 5 mm Hg/kg increase in birth weight, although some conclude a smaller effect. This may explain the observations that the concordance of BP is much higher between dizygotic twins (~50%) than non-twin siblings; even though both would have 50% genetic similarity, the difference may stem from the very early environment that they shared closely, which includes especially time *in utero* but also infancy. There is a long and extensive literature of work in several animal species that showed that events acting *in utero*, for limited periods, have lifelong effects on physiology and vulnerability to disease. This phenomenon is termed *fetal programming*.[177,178] Such studies have shown that altered glucocorticoid exposure *in utero* reduces birth weight and programs HT permanently in the adult offspring. Undernutrition in pregnancy may also alter intrauterine glucocorticoid effects and predisposes to low birth weight and subsequent HT in the offspring. This and other studies show that the early life environment can bring about these permanent effects. It remains unclear whether events such as stress to the

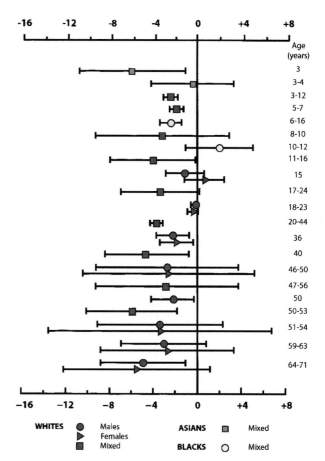

**FIGURE 31-6.** The association of low birth weight with subsequent lifelong elevation in BP in humans—fetal programming of HT. More than 20 studies at differing follow-up ages (shown on right) showing the mean ±95% confidence interval of the regression coefficient (X-axis) of SBP (in mm Hg) on birth weight (in kg) and current size (weight as children, BMI as adult). All except a couple of studies across pubertal ages reveal evidence that those of lower birth weight have higher average BP lifelong. *(Redrawn from Law CM, Shiell AW: Is blood pressure inversely related to birthweight? J Hypertens 1996; 14:935-941, with permission.)*

mother or fetus (changing fetal glucocorticoid exposure) during gestation or altered nutrition may be mediators of these effects. There may be effects from "catch up" growth of the low birth weight infant or from some contribution of maternal genes such as those that may impair insulin-mediated fetal growth and potentially then predispose to insulin resistance in adult life.[179] However, the fact that changes in the uterine environment have been shown to be capable of programming low birth weight and lifelong HT shows that events acting *in utero* can be sufficient, without the need to invoke a second independent induction of gene expression as an adult.[177,178,180]

One of the most compelling theories as to how low birth weight may link to adult HT is by an associated reduction in late gestational renal growth and impairment of the development of the full complement of nephrons—oligonephropathy.[180] There is support for this from animal[180] and human studies.[180-182] This change would affect the pressure-natriuresis mechanism that plays such a major role in long-term BP control.

Reduced nephron number will reduce the whole kidney ultrafiltration coefficient ($K_F$) and so leave a vulnerability to salt sensitivity and glomerular hyperfiltration in remaining nephrons, especially if renal damage of another kind further reduced nephron number. Raised glucocorticoids in later gestation tend to accelerate tissues from a proliferative to a more differentiated state. Doses used in late gestation for avoiding fetal respiratory distress should not be excessive because there is evidence that the lung would then downregulate its growth excessively leading to a degree of lung hypoplasia. Similarly glucocorticoids accelerate the urinary-concentrating abilities of the kidney, but excess glucocorticoid exposure *in utero* may inhibit generation of the full complement of nephrons *in utero*. In animal models, glucocorticoid exposure in late gestation is sufficient to program HT,[183] and nephron number is affected proportionately with body weight. Growth-retarding diets also reduce birth weight and nephron number in conjunction.[184] It is clear, however, that once nephron number is reduced it is not possible to catch up back to normal in the way that infant body growth may allow body weight to catch up to normal levels.[181] Thus, although much remains unknown about the mechanism of fetal programming of HT and the early life origins phenomenon, it seems that the hormonal environment and nutrition during gestation and their effect on growth and the kidney in particular are key factors in bringing about the observed lifelong predisposition to HT that accompanies low birth weight in humans.

## Amplification

Once a pathologic process has begun to raise BP there are ways in which a "vicious circle" can follow, and the damage that the pathology causes can promote more damage. For example, if glomeruli are damaged, the remaining glomeruli have to bear a greater load and

damage from hyperfiltration may ensue. Then, the reduced filtration in the damaged glomerulus leads to lower $Na^+$ load at the macula densa and elevated renin and so AngII. These processes tend to elevate BP and promote further renal decline. The vicious circle may be broken with the use of ACE inhibitor treatment. Once BP is significantly elevated those vulnerable to end-organ pathology may develop progressive renal damage that raises BP and causes further renal cumulative peripheral vasculature damage raising TPR and BP further. These processes of cumulative pathology and end-organ damage amplify the extent and risks associated with raised BP. It is clear that there is variation in the extent to which individuals are susceptible to such amplification.

## Summary Model

Figure 31-7 shows a model of how the development of HT can be viewed as a product of a predisposition, which in large part is in place in early life. This is in accord with the observation that BP "tracks" from childhood (i.e., individuals as they get older broadly retain their ranking within the population as stratified by BP). This predisposition is acted on by many environmental factors; some are very environmental and others foster the development of comorbid conditions such as obesity. Throughout there is an interaction of the environmental effects with the individual's vulnerability to them through genotype and any prehypertensive pathology already acquired. Aging brings predicable changes that seem inevitably in the West to foster a greatly increased rate of HT, but perhaps these may be substantially preventable and at least partly reversible. Finally, once HT is well established end-organ damage is a potent amplifier of HT and of risk of major cardiovascular complications. Again it appears that there may be ways to interrupt this vicious circle not only by lowering BP but also by spe-

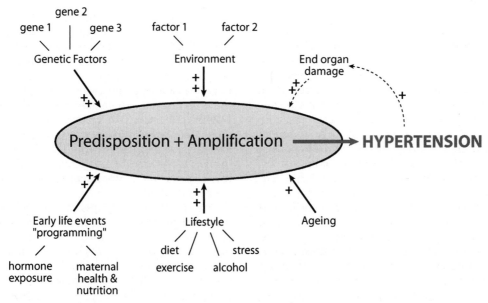

**FIGURE 31-7.** Overview of factors contributing to the development of HT.

cific approaches such as renin angiotensin blockade to preserve renal function and possible use of mineralocorticoid antagonists in situations in which fibrotic damage to the heart is accelerating.

## INDIVIDUAL GENES AND MOLECULES IMPLICATED IN PRIMARY AND ESSENTIAL HYPERENSION

In this and following sections the genes and molecules that are implicated in HT are discussed in some detail in the separate contexts of human primary (essential) HT, several forms of secondary HT, and also briefly in contexts in which HT is prominent in the presence of comorbid obesity and/or insulin resistance. This section deals with most human HT (85% to 95%) in which there is primary HT (HT is not known to be secondary to an identified cause).

Identifying the genetic variations that cause the sizable genetic contribution to human primary HT would transform the understanding of this condition and with time would facilitate identification of interacting environmental factors and the development of better and more individually appropriate treatment. Considerable progress has been made over the last 10 years in elucidating many of the genetic causes of some forms of human secondary HT[28] (Fig. 31-3 and see further discussion). However, attempting to identify the genetic factors involved in human primary HT, which is commoner, is a formidable undertaking because this is a polygenic complex trait, and although the methodology and theory[185] and enabling technologies to tackle such difficulties are firmly based and improving,[186,187] they are still in evolution.[188,189] In particular, assumptions have to be made about the type of candidate genes to scrutinize most carefully and in a more general sense about the rough number of genes that contribute to the major part of the polygenic variation and how best to choose a study population to maximize the chances that the study applied has sufficient power to detect at least the bigger of these single gene contributions.[185,189]

To address the issue of which genetic variations are involved in causing human primary HT two broad types of genetic study have been used: (1) a *candidate gene approach* and (2) a *genome wide "positional" approach*. The candidate gene approach assesses whether a gene thought to be a good candidate in contributing to causing human primary HT does have evidence of genetic variation, which is demonstrated to either show significant *linkage* to primary HT in family studies or show a significant *association* to primary HT in a population. Association studies simply assess whether the genetic variant is present significantly more commonly in those with raised BP than in others. Linkage studies require collection of hypertensive families, but then in addition to assessing the association of the genetic variation with HT such studies can also assess whether within families the segregation of HT and the candidate gene are unconnected and random or linked (i.e., segregate together more than by chance). Such linkage indicates effectively that the candidate gene and a genetic factor contributing

to HT share a locus on the same chromosome. Linkage studies give estimates of how likely linkage is as a LOD score (from the "Logarithm of ODds ratio"); a LOD score of zero is unlinked and in simple single gene studies a LOD score of 3 proves linkage. If linkage is suggested, an estimate of the size of the locus around the site of the gene marker used can be made in terms of genetic distance in centimorgans (cM) (1 cM is the chromosomal distance over which meiotic recombination occurs at a 1% frequency). The positional approach is not based around a candidate gene but rather uses large batteries of polymorphic genetic markers spaced throughout the genome in linkage analysis on collections of simple, but informative, families (e.g., sib-pairs concordant or discordant for HT). This allows genome-wide linkage analysis, often termed a genome scan, that aims to identify markers on any chromosome linked to HT. In practice if such linkage is seen, a series of raised LOD scores spanning adjacent markers is found and described in terms of the maximum LOD score. In such genome scans, hundreds and now thousands of markers are used. Because of the large number of points assessed for linkage, LOD score of 3.3 or greater indicate significant linkage (P $\leq$ 2.2 $\times$ $10^{-5}$),[190] and LOD scores down to 1.9[190] or 1.74 indicate, in contemporary genome scans,[191] "suggestive" linkage. These important statistical matters are referred to in greater detail again in the section relating to genome-wide linkage studies. A number of such genome scans have been carried out to identify loci (QTLs) linked to HT. This approach has been used in studies of human HT and in animal models to identify QTLs for high BP, analyzing large breeding crosses of HT strains of rats[192] and more recently of mice.[193-195] Primary HT is a condition in which it is expected that there will be gene-gene interactions, and although genome scans can find several QTLs or suggestive QTLs, the data set usually is not reanalyzed to see how each may interact with others to explain the variation in BP. The methods to allow reanalysis are now in part available, and it seems that some QTLs are indeed interacting significantly.[194] This requires that this analysis is standard so that the true significance of each putative QTL on BP can be determined. Similarly, some studies have incorporated attempts to see interactions with known environmental factors affecting BP (e.g., effect of variation of salt intake).[193] Finally, because the human genome sequence is now known, very large numbers of single nucleotide polymorphisms (SNPs) are cataloged, and chip-based technology for automation of genotyping at such SNPs is now established, it is feasible to genome scan at high enough density to contemplate genome-wide association studies[188,196] on populations or affected family members versus population controls.[189] These very powerful methods will raise the chances of pinpointing genetic factors involved in human primary HT, which to date have proved difficult. Studies examining candidate genes and genome wide linkage are considered later.

## Candidate Gene Studies

There are many genes that could affect BP if mutated. In humans determining those that actually do alter long-term BP can be assisted if there are rare individuals or families in whom this actually occurs because of severe mutations. Usually evidence is gathered by targeting and manipulating such credible candidate genes in rodents, especially mice, to clarify their function *in vivo*. Although mouse physiology is of course not a perfect mirror image of that in human, there are great physiologic similarities in many aspects. Intelligent scrutiny and follow-up of the results of such work can quickly sort out the unforeseen insights into human physiology from those in which the mouse model reveals a difference not reflected in humans. In addition, there may be selective pharmacologic agents acting on established and putative BP control pathways that allow clarification, if the genes acted on by such drugs do appear to have effects on long-term BP. In the absence of such *in vivo* evidence it can remain uncertain whether change in a particular gene, especially if not dramatically changed in function, would alter long-term BP because of other compensatory pathways. Finally, in actual genetic changes involved in complex diseases one has to anticipate that the genetic changes behind polygenic disease may in some cases be different from the spectrum of mutations causing single-gene disorders. In particular, mutations completely disabling a gene might not be so common, whereas those that alter the regulation of genes or even of several genes may be more common. Thus, in other polygenic diseases some of the polygenes and the responsible genetic changes have been found.[186] In type 2 diabetes, Horikawa et al.[187] hunted down a gene in which variation was responsible for an important QTL of moderate effect that caused type 2 diabetes in several populations. The causative mutation was in a gene previously unsuspected to have any relation to diabetes (Calpain 10), but just as important was the fact that the mutation was within an intron, thus certainly not affecting the coding sequence and not obviously in a position where either splicing or regulation of the gene would be altered. It seems likely that, as more polygene culprits are isolated, ideas about what a good candidate in polygenic HT will refine. Understandably at present a diverse range of genes have been investigated as candidate genes in human primary HT (Table 31-4), and more have no doubt been examined with negative results not reported in the literature. To date most candidates that have been supported by positive findings have only been examined in a very preliminary way, at times only by one study, and of those examined in multiple studies very few have a series of positive reports about their link to primary HT. In the past, some groups at the forefront of such research assessed several candidate genes over a number of years in broadly the same collection of families or populations, reporting results serially as they were completed.[197-202] There may now be some benefit in attempting when possible to reanalyze such data to detect and adjust for interactions between such genes, especially when there is an obvious physiologic link between their encoded products. In many ways although a great deal of such research has been carried out, the result is a series of candidates with interesting preliminary positive studies, and only angiotensinogen and perhaps the $\beta_2$-adrenergic recep-

■ ■ ■

### TABLE 31-4 CANDIDATE GENES INVESTIGATED IN PRIMARY HYPERTENSION

| Multiple Studies | Et-2 |
|---|---|
| Angiotensinogen | IGF1 |
| ACE | IRS1 |
| AT1 | Neutral endopeptidase |
| ADR-β2 | PG EP2 R |
| ADR-β3 | NKCC2 |
| GNß3 | NHE3 |
| Adducin | TGFβ1 |
| ENOS | SGK1 |
| ANP | TSC |
| Aldosterone synthase | NKCC2 |
| (CYP11B2) | NHE3 |
| ENaCα, β and γ | AVP V1R |
| | ADR-α1B |
| **Others** | ADR-α1C |
| Renin | ADLA |
| 11β-HSD2 | PNMT |
| NOS2A | Angiotensinase C |
| GNAS1 | NPR3 (NPRC) |
| TNFRSF1B | GUCyβ2 (soluble guanylate |
| ERβ (ER2) | cyclase) |
| Catalase | ENaCd |
| Glycogen synthase (GYS1) | COMT |
| APoA1 (PSF) | AHO2 |
| GR | Calpastatin |
| Et-1 | Kallikrein |
| Prostacyclin synthase | ADR-β1 |
| Glucagon receptor | GPRK2L (GRK4γ) |
| Leptin | Sah |
| Adenosine $A_{2A}R$ | NOS3 |
| NPRA (ANP-R) | CD36 |
| Bradykinin B2-R | PPAR? |
| DRD-1 | |

tor have received firm enough support to take them more seriously.

### Components of the Renin Angiotensin System

Studies have been carried out to look for association of variations in the genes of most components of the RAS with human primary HT. From these, angiotensinogen has emerged as the best candidate with good support for a modest role in the risk of primary HT. On the whole studies of other genes encoding components of the RAS have not supported them as a candidate gene in which genetic variation is of importance in human primary HT. Thus, angiotensinogen is discussed in some detail and briefer reference are made to other component genes.

### Angiotensinogen (AGT)

A large number of studies and three meta-analyses have shown that variation in the AGT gene is significantly associated with human primary HT. This has especially been the case for a coding polymorphism changing methionine 235 to threonine M235T; other variations such as upstream in the AGT promoter region, especially G-6A, have been much less examined. Several conclusions seem to emerge from what is still a rather contentious and somewhat sprawling literature. First, there appears to be a difference between ethnic groups. Thus, in those with African ancestry, the M235T genotype is commoner, and limited studies appear to show little association of M235T with BP.[203] In contrast, in those with Oriental ancestry or in whites there are a number of studies that have shown a significantly positive association of 235T with HT.

Three meta-analyses have concluded in such populations that there is a genuine although modest association (OR ±95% confidence interval) for HT with 235T of 1.2 to 1.31 (1.11 to 1.42).[204-206] The results merit careful consideration in assessing the AGT gene as a candidate gene in primary HT. Overall for more than 30 studies the TT and TM genotypes had an OR = 1.3 (P < 0.001) and 1.11 (P < 0.05) compared with MM, and these effects were more clearly seen in whites.[206] The genetic contribution to primary HT is being studied here, and it is preferable to compare families in which primary HT clusters or at least to compare HT individuals with a positive family history. Indeed meta-analysis based on those with a positive family history shows an OR = 1.42 (1.29 to 1.60),[204] whereas there is OR = 1.08 for those without a positive family history.[204] Ideally, such familial HT studies should have controls with a known negative family history for HT although this has not been a point for which care has been taken.[203,204,206] Finally, even those studies that individually failed to show an association of M235T with HT usually reported a nonsignificant excess of 235T in HT subjects giving even those negative studies a borderline association with HT: OR = 1.09 (1.02 to 1.167) on meta-analysis.[203,204] Although not proven beyond all doubts it seems fair to conclude that there is indeed a genuine association of the M235T AGT polymorphism with primary HT broadly in those of white and Oriental ancestry, but the effect is modest (OR ~1.2 to 1.31) and, thus, is seen more easily in families rather than wholly across unrelated individuals.

Such an association as M235T with HT has two interpretations.[185] First, M235T actually causes this effect. Second, M235T is not the real cause; another locus sufficiently close by it cosegregates with M235T very reliably (i.e., the two are in strong linkage disequilibrium). It has recently become much more clearly understood that the physical distance (in kb of DNA) over which linkage disequilibrium extends is nonuniform along chromosomes[188,196] because the probability of meiotic crossing over and recombination is similarly nonuniform. Thus, in theory it is possible that a functional genetic factor in linkage disequilibrium with M235T could be tens of kb away and outside the AGT gene. Until these new concepts are fully developed and an accepted "haplotype map" of the genome[188,196] emerges it has seemed speculative to search beyond the AGT gene, and those exploring the M235T association with HT have only seriously examined variant loci elsewhere in the AGT gene. Other variants in the AGT gene have been found, and some such as the G(-6)A variant in the AGT promoter seem often associated in a seldom varying G(-6)A, M235T haplotype. These studies are far from conclusive in identifying any of the AGT variants as the functional basis for the association of AGT with HT. Nevertheless, one can assume that local linkage disequilibrium does not extend widely around the AGT gene, and, thus, variations in AGT

must be the cause of the tendency to raised BP. The next question is, How?

Early studies from Jeunemaitre et al. who first reported the association of AGT with primary HT went on to report that the 235T haplotype was associated with a slightly higher circulating AGT level (by 15%).[207] In subsequent studies this has been confirmed with the AGT levels averaging 11% and 7% higher in the TT and TM genotypes compared with the MM genotype.[206] In one sense the level of activity of the RAS is limited by AGT in that in humans the AGT levels are often close to the Km for renin.[208] However, the RAS is dynamic and usually a rise in AGT levels, which can be four- to fivefold in some situations (e.g., pregnancy) through feedback, leads to a reduction of renin. Therefore, AngII levels are seen as independent of AGT levels unless a defect in feedback or "modulation" of renin levels is postulated (i.e., in "nonmodulators").[37,209] A higher AGT level will usually translate to a higher average AngII tone. Several studies do indeed show association of AGT polymorphisms (including M235T and often associated promoter variants; e.g., −6A present in the same haplotype) are linked to nonmodulation of the renin angiotensin responses at the tissue level in kidney (in modulating renal blood flow and natriuresis)[210] and adrenal (in modulating aldosterone).[209,210] Although AGT, which circulates is substantially derived from liver, there is extensive extrahepatic AGT production including in large arteries, kidney, adipose tissue, heart, and brain.[211] Because plasma AGT levels are close to the $K_m$ for renin, local tissue AGT production could easily raise the local AngII levels substantially if tissue ACE is present too. It has been estimated that 85% of angiotensin is formed in tissues rather than plasma.[212] Because M235T and −6A are associated with higher plasma AGT, a similar or greater increase in local tissue AGT (leading to persistently higher tissue AngII levels) has been seen as the link to nonmodulation of pressure-natriuretic and aldosterone responses, which constitute the nonmodulator intermediate phenotype associated with normal- or high-renin primary HT.[37,209] Similarly, higher AGT levels may be pathophysiologically involved in some forms of secondary HT (e.g., to the estrogen-containing oral contraceptive pill[213] and in preeclampsia).[214] AGT levels normally rise with estrogen,[215] and the lack of normal modulation has been invoked and an association with AGT polymorphisms similarly reported.[213,214] Thus, although the effect of AGT gene variation is not great and varies to some extent across ethnic groups, there seems to be a real effect and at least a possible explanation for a mechanism producing long-term BP change.

### Other Components

Studies assessing several other genes in the RAS for association with primary HT are very largely negative for renin and AT1R and independent of renal disease; BMI and other genotypes are also largely negative for ACE. At present, preliminary studies on other components do not allow a good basis for assessment. From the diverse literature that has grown up about the phenotypic consequences of the insertion/deletion (I/D) ACE gene polymorphism it seems that the DD genotype is associated with a somewhat increased risk of MI and an adverse rate of progression of renal pathologies, but objectively support is weak for an independent effect promoting HT and such an effect on BP is excluded unless small or of low penetrance.

## Renin

For renin, several linkage and association studies have been largely conclusively negative[197] with a few exceptions finding rather weak association in some different ethnic groups (Chinese[216] and Afro-Caribbeans[217]). Overall this seemed to leave little doubt that variation in the renin gene is not a generally important determinant of BP in primary HT. Hard to reconcile are positive studies associating polymorphisms of intron 1 (Bgl II) and especially intron 9 (Mbo I) with primary HT in populations in the United Arab Emerites (UAE) and United States.[218,219] Renin int1(−)int9(+) and int1(+)int9(+) haplotypes significantly associated with primary HT (OR = 3.35, corrected $P < 10^{-7}$) and stroke (OR = 4.31, $P < 10^{-7}$) are independent of classical risk factors relating to lipid, lipoproteins, and apolipoproteins levels in the U.S. cohort.[219] The int9(+) polymorphism was reported not associated with HT[220] but was associated with a positive family history of primary HT.[220] One possible reconciliation of these findings suggests late-onset HT, which may fit with an associated increased stroke risk.[219] Unless either key features of these UAE or U.S. populations or the functional QTL behind the int1int9(+) association is identified, the penetrance of a renin gene effect with lack of such findings in several other such studies is difficult to reconcile and to use to suggest the candidacy of the renin gene as one of the polygenes in primary HT.

## ACE

A large literature has developed on the phenotypic consequences of the 279bp insertion/deletion polymorphism in exon 16 of the ACE gene, the most prominent and by far most studied of more than 70 ACE gene molecular variants. More than 20 studies of diverse populations[221-223] show no linkage or association of this polymorphism with primary HT, and a comprehensive meta-analysis in 1997 of some 23 studies concurred in this conclusion.[224] It made no difference if there was exclusion of studies using the less robust early I/D PCR methods[224] that were later shown to falsely underrepresent D. A minority of studies report an association with primary HT of the D allele and DD genotype, whereas a few studies reported an association of the I allele with HT (sometimes salt-sensitive HT[225]). The I/D polymorphism is associated with approximately 50% of total variation in serum ACE level with the D allele accompanied by higher levels.[226] This allele is also associated with increase in MI and renal disease progression risk. The actual intronic I/D polymorphism may be functionally neutral and in linkage disequilibrium with a nearby QTL, proposed to be in the 3′ region of the ACE gene, although the adjacent growth hormone gene is an alternative possibility meriting some consideration. It

remains unclear, if this minority of studies finding an association of the D allele with HT represents a real subgroup. Some have suggested that their frequency varies by ethnic group invoking the possibility that linkage of the D allele to a putative real functional hypertensive QTL is broken across change in ethnic background. A higher proportion of studies appear to show association of DD with HT in subjects of Chinese[227-229] and possible also African ancestry.[230-232] Certainly a report of a recent meta-analysis of 18 relatively small Chinese studies totaling more than 3000 genotyped subjects concludes that for people with Han Chinese ancestral background there appears to be some support for a DD genotype effect with an OR = 1.37 (1.15 to 1.63, $P < 0.01$) versus ID or II. In terms of DD genotype frequencies, the overall differences between hypertensives and controls (23% vs. 19%, respectively) was relatively slender.[228] Otherwise the pattern of positive studies appears less clearly to segregate with ethnic background with a minority of positive studies on a range of other backgrounds such as whites from Europe, the United States, and Australia; Japanese; and those from the Indian subcontinent. Alternative explanations for such positive studies include coexisting higher risks of renal disease and its progression; gene-gene interaction effects that have been reported with variants of adducin and aldosterone synthase (CYP11B2) in some,[233,234] but not other studies[222]; and interaction with the reduced propensity of BP reduction on attaining physical fitness[235] may make the D allele effect somewhat less penetrant in an unfit more Westernized environment than in some other cultures. Finally poorly matched case and control BMI seems likely to be an important confounder because the DD genotype has been reported to interact with the effect of weight change on BP.[236] Whatever the reason it is hard to exclude a low-penetrance, small effect of the DD genotype (especially in those of Chinese[228] and possibly African ancestry[230-232]) with likely higher penetrance if there is a higher prevalence of obesity and renal damage. Overall, most studies indicate that the association of ACE genotype with primary HT is considerably weaker than for AGT and that an effect independent of coexisting renal abnormalities, BMI, or gene interactions may be restricted to certain ancestral genetic backgrounds or may not exist at all.

## Angiotensin II Type I Receptor (AT1R)

AT1R mediates the BP-elevating effects of AngII on the kidney and vessels and promotes aldosterone release. In contrast the less well understood AT2R and AT4R seem to act in some ways antagonistically, somewhat lowering BP, promoting natriuresis, and possibly antagonizing proliferation. AT1R is also the target blocked by the relatively new class of antihypertensives, the angiotensin receptor blockers such as losartan and irbesartan. AT1R represents a good candidate gene and more than 15 polymorphisms have been identified. Some, especially a 3′ SNP A1166C, have been used to look for linkage and association of AT1R with BP. One of the first studies examined AT1R polymorphisms in 60 HT subjects with a familial susceptibility to HT and found an increase only in the 1166C allele (P < 0.01) in hypertensives.[198] This was followed with a study for linkage in 267 sib-pairs from 138 pedigrees that showed no linkage of BP with a highly polymorphic marker for AT1R and that concluded that overall findings in these European subjects were compatible with "a common variant of AT1R imparting a small effect on BP."[198] Subsequently over two thirds of studies, a number of studies from Europe, China, Japan, and India, have not found a simple excess of the 1166C or CC genotype among hypertensives[237-240]; however, other studies from Australia,[241] China,[242] and Finland[243] did. Two studies that failed to find 1166C association with HT rather reported a weak association that BP was lower with 1166C than 1166A.[237,239] Overall these studies on the AT1R A1166C polymorphism appear to show no definite effect on the risk of HT. Only a very limited number of studies have been conducted with other polymorphic markers.

Finally two of the studies that failed to find general associations of HT with 1166C did find it significantly linked to SBP in subgroups that were hypercholestrolemic[240] or overweight and/or elderly[238] and to DBP if overweight.[238] Benetos et al.[244] reported that the 1166C allele is a strong independent determinant of aortic stiffness (and, thus, will promote elevated SBP), and this group has subsequently confirmed this finding in a study of 441 untreated HT subjects and showed the cosegregation of a second −153G AT1R SNP allele that further increases aortic stiffness in those older than 55 years.[245] Thus, the role of AT1R gene variations in arterial stiffness and systolic HT especially in the elderly may warrant further, hopefully large and conclusive studies.

## Sympathetic Nervous System Candidate Genes

The SNS is involved in the regulation of important cardiovascular responses and other fundamental aspects of physiology including energy metabolism. Thus, body-wide variation in SNS activity or responsiveness may alter cardiovascular function including BP in a context in which accompanying alteration in SNS responses of another kind (e.g., energy metabolism) will be probable and will depend on the specific aspect of the SNS affected. Although the roles of the SNS reflexes such as the baroreceptor and chemoreceptor reflexes are principally directed at relatively short-term control of BP, there seems little doubt that abnormal SNS overactivity accompanies early phases of HT in at least some subjects who later develop primary HT and that it continues to accompany HT associated with obesity. The general utility of $\alpha$-blockers and especially $\beta$-blockers in achieving some BP reduction in most primary HT and the potency of the hypertensive drive secondary to catecholamine excess in pheochromocytomas all represent evidence that indicate that inherited abnormalities in the SNS could, in theory at least, play key roles in long-term BP control and the risk of HT. Of the many potential candidate genes including catecholamine synthetic and degrading enzymes, reuptake mechanisms, and $\alpha$- and $\beta$-adrenergic receptors there has been a somewhat narrow focus on the undeniably important candidate genes encoding the $\beta$-adrenergic receptors.

## Adrenergic Receptors

The ADRs mediate the actions of the SNS and collectively have important physiologic influence on the circulation and other fundamental processes including energy metabolism. There are currently nine recognized ADRs that fall into three $\alpha_1$ ($\alpha_{1A}$, $\alpha_{1B}$, and $\alpha_{1D}$ on human Ch 8p21, Ch 5q32-4, and Ch 20p13, respectively), three $\alpha_2$ ($\alpha_{2A}$, $\alpha_{2B}$, and $\alpha_{2C}$ on human Ch 10, Ch 2, and Ch4p16), and three $\beta$ ($\beta_1$, $\beta_2$, and $\beta_3$, on human Ch 10q24-26, Ch 5q32-34 and Ch 8p12-11) receptor subtypes. It will be some time until the full roles of each receptor are appreciated. For $\alpha$ ADRs in particular, the lack of selective, clinically usable pharmacologic agents necessitates that the understanding of some important aspects of individual ADR subtype function must be gathered from largely nonclinical sources, including prototype-selective pharmacologic agents and mice with selective gene targeting. It seems that $\alpha_{1A}$ plays a key role in the basal level of vascular tone;[246] $\alpha_{1B}$ is the predominant $\alpha_1$ ADR in liver, heart, and at least larger vasculature (e.g., aorta), thus mediating the majority of the BP response to conventional $\alpha_1$-agonists.[50,246] The major portion of classic $\alpha_2$-agonist effects including arterial contraction seem to be mediated via the $\alpha_{2A}$ subtype, whereas $\alpha_{2C}$ may have a key role in regulating basal vascular, especially venous, tone.[246] Studies on transgenic mice indicate that both $\alpha_{2A}$ and $\alpha_{2C}$ are required for normal modulation of SNS neurotransmitter release; $\alpha_{2A}$ is required at high frequencies of firing and $\alpha_{2C}$ is required with lower firing frequencies (typically having more influence on venous tone).[54] Mice without normal $\alpha_{2A}$ or $\alpha_{2C}$ have elevated plasma noradrenaline and develop cardiac hypertrophy and reduced left-ventricular contractility.[54] $\beta_1$ ADR-mediated responses also affect cardiac contractility and HR.

In humans, coding polymorphisms in $\alpha_{2C}$ (causing deletion of amino acids 322 to 325 [del$_{322-325}$] that have decreased function) seem to have effects that impair left-ventricular function with an associated increased odds ratio of 5.65 for heart failure reported in Blacks homozygous for $\alpha_{2C\ del322-325}$.[247] Moreover, subjects who also carried a $\beta_1$ ADR variant (R389) that increased $\beta_1$ signal transduction had an associated higher risk of heart failure (OR 10.11).[247] This synergism most likely follows from $\alpha_{2C\ del322-325}$ mediated increased noradrenaline release to which $\beta_{1R389}$ already signals more strongly. The $\alpha_{2B}$ ADR subtype may play a role in regulating BMR. A human $\alpha_{2B}$ deletion variant ($\alpha_{2B\ del301-303}$ having reduced agonist-mediated desensitization) has been reported to be associated with a reduced BMR (by 5% to 6%, P < 0.01), hence suggesting a role of $\alpha_{2B}$ in body weight regulation.[248] It seems that $\beta_1$ and possibly also $\alpha_{2C}$ ADRs may also be involved in determining resting HR, which is a central factor in setting CO (and thus altering hemodynamics that affect BP); in addition, resting HR has been shown to be an important independent long-term predictor of cardiovascular mortality.[249] It has been estimated that the heritability of resting HR is approximately 40%, and it has been found linked to loci on human Ch 10, near the $\beta_1$ ADR gene and on Ch 4p where the $\alpha_{2C}$ ADR is, thus, a candidate gene.[250] Polymorphisms of $\beta_1$ ADR have been identified with variation in the encoding amino acids at S49G and R389G (as already mentioned previously); the former were significantly associated in one study with HR progressively by genotype such that HR: S/S > S/G > G/G, whereas polymorphisms of $\beta_{1R389G}$ and of $\beta_2$ and $\beta_3$ ADRs showed no correlation with HR.[63] It is hard to believe that a genetic effect likely to influence lifelong HR does not have the potential to affect BP, especially if interacting with factors that limit the ability of $\Delta CO \rightarrow \Delta TPR$ autoregulation, which may be factors influencing long-term vessel tone or circulatory filling via renal $Na^+$ reabsorption. The $\beta_2$ ADR has been the subject of considerable study, with several polymorphisms identified that affect the promoter 5'UTR or coding region including R16G and Q27E. $\beta_{2\,16G}$ appears to enhance agonist-mediated receptor downregulation, whereas possibly $\beta_{2\,27E}$ is resistant to such downregulation. Less studied in HT is another coding region polymorphism T164I with $\beta_{2\,164I}$ that has reduced agonist responsiveness. Such $\beta_2$ ADR polymorphisms have the potential to affect the $\beta/\alpha$ stimulation balance involved in adrenergic responses of major physiologic importance including those of the circulation and metabolism and in asthma. They have also been the subject of association studies relating to HT (see later) and obesity (see the section on obesity-related HT). Finally, the $\beta_3$ ADR plays a role in SNS responses in thermogenesis, especially in brown fat, and is seen as having a wider role in body weight homeostasis. The $\beta_{3\,W64R}$ polymorphism has been the subject of much investigation relating to body weight (see obesity-related HT) and to a lesser degree to HT (see later).

Most studies assessing linkage or association of adrenergic receptors genes with BP or risk of primary HT have assessed the $\beta_2$ ADR. Some assessment has been done with $\beta_3$, and very limited studies have been done on several others. Overall, the $\beta_2$ ADR results are frustratingly inconclusive but may well indicate a very modest real effect on the risk of HT, whereas results for other receptors appear negative and/or are too preliminary for the true position to be clear. Studies of the $\alpha_{1A}$[251] and $\alpha_{2B}$[252] genes have revealed no association with HT or BP. Some association with HT of RFLPs (using DRA I) in the $\alpha_{2A}$ gene ($\alpha2$ on Ch 10) is reported, both in a largely black (P = 0.008)[253] and in a white study population (P = 0.03).[254] Some association with variation in renal $Na^+$ excretion and baroreceptor sensitivity is also reported. Three other studies were negative; no association of $\alpha_{2A}$ RFLPs (using Bsu36I) with HT or BP or salt sensitivity was found. One study examined the $\beta_1$ ADR R389G and S49G polymorphisms and found that 389R was significantly (P = 0.0005) associated with HT (OR 1.9: 95% CI 1.3 to 2.7); there was significant association of the 389R/389R genotype with higher DBP and HR, but no positive associations for S49R.[255] As mentioned previously, another study found that $\beta_{1\,S49R}$ was significantly linked to resting HR.[63]

Two studies showed significant linkage of microsatellite markers very close to the $\beta_2$ ADR gene locus to HT[256,257]; only one found association of $\beta_2$ ADR polymorphisms with HT.[256] Another study failed to find such linkage. Studies allowing assessment of association of variation in the $\beta_2$ ADR gene with HT have involved over 12,000 subjects, often genotyping at the R16G and/or

E27Q polymorphism although occasionally at others or in early studies using RFLPs. Of more than 20 studies, most (slightly below two thirds) reported significant associations with BP or HT, for example[254,256,258-261]; however, this leaves a substantial minority of studies that found no association with HT,[257,262] and numbers in positive and negative studies are overall similar. None of the positive studies reported a very large effect on BP or on the risk of HT, with two of the larger studies finding odds ratios for HT risk of 1.35 (95% CI 1.08 to 1.7) for an association with $\beta_{2\,R16G}$[261] and 1.8 (95% CI 1.08 to 3) for an association with $\beta_{2\,Q27E}$ in a study that also demonstrated an excess of $\beta_{2\,R16G}$ in HT subjects.[260] Although some of the negative reports seem robust (e.g., Herrmann et al.[262] comprising two studies genotyping > 3000 subjects for four $\beta_2$ ADR polymorphisms), they must be weighed against the fact that even the component studies of Herrmann et al.'s report[262] was only powered to reliably detect an effect on HT risk of 1.6-fold or higher. Thus, they could easily fail to detect effects of the order of 1.35-fold as was found in some of the larger positive studies.[261] Although some of the positive association studies had findings that were only weakly supportive (e.g., only finding an association with DBP or SBP), others found highly significant associations (P < 0.00002),[258] combined positive linkage and association studies,[258] and some involved sizable study populations.[260,261] Overall these studies suggest that there may well be a minor effect of variations in or close to the $\beta_2$ ADR gene on the risk of HT. The coding $\beta_2$ ADR polymorphisms R16G and possibly also Q27E appear to have effects on receptor function that might be expected to be related to their association with BP or HT risk. The $\beta_{2\,R16G}$ allele associated with HT was 16G in some studies[256,258,260,261] and 16R in others, for example.[259] This appears to weaken the case for this being a functional polymorphism but is compatible with $\beta_{2\,R16G}$ being a marker for a haplotype linked to a functional locus near this site in $\beta_2$ ADR. The conflict between the positive and negative studies is probably most easily explained by an effect that is not actually due to a single tested polymorphism alone but rather to the aggregate of a whole $\beta_2$ ADR haplotype (haplotypes having so far been seldom studied) that incorporates the effect of promoter and coding polymorphisms (including R16G, Q27E, and T164I). However, one study examining haplotypes found no association with BP.[262] Finally, another possibility, perhaps less probable, is that the functional QTL affecting BP is further away outside the $\beta_2$ ADR gene.[257] Larger single studies may be required to resolve the uncertainty, but it seems likely that a $\beta_2$ ADR effect on HT risk really is modest; one positive study estimates that it accounts for approximately 1% of variation in SBP or DBP.

Studies on $\beta_3$ ADR relating to BP and HT largely relate to the $\beta_{3\,W64R}$ polymorphism studied in populations with coexisting insulin resistance, DM, and/or obesity. Most studies find no association with BP or HT risk,[263] although most of these are small.[263] A few positive studies[264,265] report largely weak effects in population subgroups and thus may reflect effects not typical or applicable to general primary HT. Overall, the evidence that $\beta_3$ ADR has an important effect on HT risk is not convincing; the effect on BP independent of effects of BMI or insulin resistance is even less convincing.

### Endothelin System

The ET system involves actions via two G-protein coupled receptors ET-A (Ch 4q31) and ET-B (Ch 13q22) mediated by three peptide ligands ET-1, ET-2, and ET-3.[266,267] These are the active 21 amino acid products of three corresponding genes on Ch 6p24.1, 1p34, and 20q13, respectively, that encode the preproendothelins that, on proteolytic splitting, yield big ETs (37 to 41 amino acids, low biologic activity). Each is finally cleaved to the corresponding fully active ET by ECE activities (especially ECE1 [Ch 1p36.1], but also ECE2 [Ch3q28] and other as yet unattributed ECE activities). ET-1 is predominantly secreted by vascular endothelial cells and remains the most potent vasoconstrictor of human vessels known. The vast majority of this action is mediated via the ET-A receptor in VSM cells, which preferentially binds ET-1. In contrast, ET-B binds ET1-3 equally, is prominent in endothelium, and often mediates vasodilation via NO release. ET-1 is continuously released from endothelial cells by a low-level constitutive pathway that contributes to basal vascular tone. In addition, regulated release occurs via an endothelial cell-specific vesicle (Weibel-Palade body) pathway triggered by external stimuli. ET-1 circulating concentrations are comparatively low, and local paracrine action is normally important. ET-2 has been less studied and is less abundant but is present in human cardiovascular tissues and potentially appears to be as potent a vasoconstrictor as ET-1 is. In some hypertensive rat models (e.g., Dahl rat) the ET-2 gene locus has been strongly linked to SBP. Substantial expression of ET-3 is present in human tissues including heart (but not endothelial cells), and mature ET-3 is detectable in plasma. ET-3 selectively binds ET-B receptors and is not usually seen as primarily a vasoconstrictor. Research especially relating to developmental actions indicates that effects of ET-3 and ET-B deficiency are almost identical (see later). ET-1 is highly expressed in lung and kidney (especially medulla) and plays a role in the special regulation of vascular tone in these sites along with other processes including airway tone, acid-base balance, and natriuresis.[267] In these organs, ET-B is also highly expressed, playing a role in nonvascular cells in some of these processes (e.g., natriuretic action in renal medullary CD via inhibition of ENaC conductance) and also playing an ET-B ET "clearance receptor" role. In some vascular beds, ET-B is located on VSM, not coupled to vasodilation in endothelium, and may mediate net vasoconstriction. Thus, ET-1 actions on vascular tone are dependent on several local factors: the balance of ET-A/ET-B and coupling of ET-B receptors and their stimulation by ET, both locally secreted and from local ECE conversion of circulating big ET. Local factors that impair endothelium-dependent NO release will perturb this balance to favor ET-A vasoconstriction.[268] Accordingly, the paracrine nature of ET actions is important,[267] although systemic changes in circulating ET levels poten-

tially have widespread effects if local receptor occupancy is changed and no compensatory mechanisms diminish the effects. ETs also have inotropic, chemotactic, and mitogenic effects that may play a role in tissue responses (e.g., in heart and kidney) to chronically elevated ET levels.

There are also other important noncardiovascular actions of ETs[267] during development, including actions on maturation of neural crest lineages (affecting e.g., melanocytes and autonomic nerves especially intrinsic to the gut) and pharyngeal arch structures affecting the heart, great vessels, neck, and face.[267] Accordingly, with lifelong severe defects in the ET system (in knockout mice or where identified in humans) there is prominent maldevelopment of neural crest structures for ET-B −/− or ET-3 −/− mice and patients with gut atony and Hirschsprung's disease.[267] For ET-A −/− (largely the same for ET-1 −/−) a variety of cardiac, great vessel, and facial defects occur that are fatal before or just after birth.[269] It seems likely in humans, too, that severe inactivating mutations of the ET system will have associated features akin to those affecting corresponding knockout mice. A patient with a mutation in ECE1(R742C, close to the active site) has been reported; the mutation reduced activity to less than 5% of normal and affected both ET-A and ET-B signaling.[270] The patient had labile BP, episodic HT, and defects relating to the branchial arch (craniofacial abnormalities and cardiac defects—ductus arteriosus and small atrial and ventricular septal defects) and neural crest (skip-lesion bowel aganglionosis of the Hirschsprung's type and autonomic lability of BP and temperature control) similar to the severe ET-A and ET-B signaling defects seen in knockout mice.[270] Thus, severe loss-of-function defects are complicated by severe problems not directly relating to the ET system's role in BP control. However, less severe defects as in ET-1 +/− mice escape such obvious developmental abnormalities; ET-1 +/− mice are mildly hypertensive.[271] There is still some uncertainty as to whether this reflects the effects of a structural developmental deficiency and hypoxic sympathetic activation[45] or more simply that the lower ET-1 levels cause an altered ET-A/ET-B activation balance perhaps with less renal ET-B vasodilation and less natriuresis causing HT. This view is supported by the findings that ET-B +/− mice have raised BP and half-life of labeled plasma ET-1 (compared with normal and ET-A +/− mice) and evidence of lack of BP regulatory roles of ET-3 and ET-A.[67] Thus, it seems that ET-B level and the supply of ET-1 ligand are important in influencing long-term BP, but a key question is where such BP regulatory effects are based. Tissue-specific knockouts of ET-1 and ET-B have been developed to answer such questions. ET-1 CD −/− mice are hypertensive with impaired water and possibly Na+ excretion.[36] ET-B CD −/− mice have now been generated, and this will allow the key issues of the role of ET-B in control of BP and renal function to be addressed with some insight into renal epithelial versus renal vascular actions. It is also known that renal medullary hypoxia upregulates ET-1 production locally in CD; that in humans in vivo renal ET-B mediates a net vasodilation[65]; and that ET-A, a net renal vasoconstrictor, assumes a greater effect when there is less stimulation of AngII receptors (e.g., during AT1 blocker treatment[66]). Thus, the renal ET system can alter long-term BP, and renal ET-A/ET-B stimulation balance would seem important. In addition, renal hypoxia and angiotensin levels can modulate intrarenal ET-1 production and ET-A mediated vasoconstriction, respectively. Transgenic ET-1 mice having two- to fourfold ET-1 elevation in the circulation and tissues (at least in the heart, kidney, and aorta) have normal BP[272] as do similar transgenic ET-2 rats with 2- to 2.5-fold elevations in ET-2.[273] These overexpressing animals gradually developed renal glomerulosclerosis[272,273] and other renal[272,274] and cardiac pathologies,[273] and in aged ET-1 overexpressing transgenic mice, when renal pathology was well established, the animals exhibited salt-sensitive HT.[274] Findings from these ET overexpression models indicate that effective compensation mechanisms maintaining normotension involved enhanced ET-B responses with NO-mediated vasodilation.[273] In separate work it is known that there is an increase in the ratio of intrarenal ET-1/NO in rodent kidney with aging, independent of BP, which may relatively impair vasodilator responses.[268]

A relatively small number of studies have looked for association with BP or HT of variation in genes of the ET system. These studies have found no overall association of HT with ET-1 gene polymorphisms causing a Taq1 RFLP at K198N[275]; SNPs elsewhere do not cause coding changes.[276] However, two of these studies did find weak associations with DBP overall[276] or selectively in overweight subjects only.[275] Significant association of ET-1$_{K198N}$ and SBP in pregnancy (not preeclampsia) has also been reported[277] Other studies found no association between ET-1 polymorphisms and risk of end-stage renal failure or pulse-wave velocity and aortic stiffness. Similarly for ET-2, although two studies found no significant associations across the total study population, they both found weak associations with DBP overall or only when compared within the HT group[276] or between the extreme quartiles of BP. Finally, studies on ET-A[276,278] or ET-B[278] found no overall association with HT, SBP, or DBP, although one ET-A study reported a weak association with pulse pressure.[278] Thus, although there have been some positive findings, no study to date has shown an overall strongly significant association of any ET system component gene to HT.

### Nitric Oxide Pathway

There are several ways in which the level and action of NO influences BP, and the three types of NOS enzymes play different roles in regulation of BP. The eNOS (NOS3: Ch 7q36) acts as an endothelial-dependent vasodilator. Neuronal NOS (NOS1: 12q24), in the macula densa, acts as an important component of autoregulation of renal Na$^+$ handling via TGF. Third, iNOS (NOS2A: 17q11 at ~26MB in the Ch 17 sequence), which affects BP in the short and medium term when it is strongly induced, affects renal medullary blood flow regulation. Incidentally, evidence suggests that the putative nearby NOS2B (17p11 at ~18.6MB) and NOS2C (17q11 ~0.1MB centromeric of NOS2A) genomic sequences exist and may by homology complicate some genetic analysis; however, they are at least partially accounted for by an unprocessed NOS pseudogene that cannot make any functional enzyme.[279] Thus, it is assumed that iNOS derives only from the NOS2A gene.

One study reported linkage in human primary HT to the iNOS locus on Ch 17[280] followed by a positive association study of HT with a NOS2A promoter polymorphism.[280] Another study has failed to find such an association between variants in the NOS2A promoter and HT or BP. However, eNOS has been the most assessed of the NOS enzymes as a candidate gene in primary HT. Multiple polymorphisms have been identified, in microsatellites flanking and more recently others within the eNOS gene on Ch 7q36 that involves the promoter (especially T-786C), several introns, including a variable tandem repeat VNTR in intron 4 (A and B alleles), and a widely used SNP in exon 7 (C894T, encoding a missense change Glu298Asp: E298D). More than 20 studies have assessed association (or linkage) of variation at these markers, especially E290D and intron 4 A/B, with BP or HT. The weight of evidence is against an important, widely penetrant contribution to primary HT. Thus, although several studies found association of BP or HT with the E298D polymorphism[281-285] (one with lower BP),[283] in other studies HT was associated with the 298D[284,285] allele in some or with the 298E allele in others.[281,282] This may mean that a real functional QTL was variably linked to the 298D or E alleles in different populations, but no evidence of more robust linkage elsewhere in the eNOS locus is established. Only some relatively weak associations with the intron 4A allele have been identified.[286] Moreover, most studies (more than 15) on eNOS find no association with HT or BP at the E298 locus, intron 4, or other polymorphic sites. Several of these negative studies are really rather robust (e.g., Tsujita et al.[287] genotyping more than 4000 subjects at two markers and Bonnardeaux et al.[199] finding no evidence of linkage to the eNOS locus in sib-pairs and then no association with HT using two biallelic markers for the gene). It is not easy to reconcile the studies with positive findings[284,285] with the large number of negative studies. There is some support for the idea that genetic variation in eNOS may be associated with the circulatory tolerance of hypervolemia[288] or may interact with insulin resistance.[283] Whether this extends to eNOS activity (which is more critical in influencing BP in volume-expanded insulin-resistant state) is as yet unclear; however, in pregnancy, eNOS gene variation associated with the risk of HT has been positive in most studies,[289-293] although not universally.[294]

### Guanine Nucleotide Binding Protein β3 Subunit (GNβ3)

The ubiquitously expressed third form of the G-protein β subunit (distinct from the 36-kd β1 and 35-kd β2 subunits) is localized to human Ch 12p13, and like other β subunits it associates with α and γ subunits to form heterotrimeric G-proteins. GNβ3 became a candidate as a gene contributing to the risk of primary HT following investigation by Siffert et al.[295] regarding the basis of enhanced pertussis-toxin-sensitive G-protein signal transduction in lymphoblasts and fibroblasts of selected patients with primary HT. This led to the identification of a C825T exon 10 polymorphism in which the 825T allele[295] and associated haplotype triggers a deletion of nucleotides 498 to 620 of exon 9 giving a shorter (GNβ3$_S$) subunit that appears to be responsible for the enhanced signal transduction. Other subsequent studies have suggested that 825T effects may be tissue specific; hence, in adipocytes the allele promoter lowers G-protein-mediated signal transduction and is associated with resistance to lipolytic stimuli. In early studies, Siffert et al.[295] reported evidence that 825T is linked to essential HT, associated with low renin, increased BMI, and obesity[296] especially developing in interaction with lifestyle and environmental effects such as low level of physical activity, high calorie diet, or the maternal weight gain during pregnancy.[297]

Now more than 20 studies have reported on the association of 825T to one or more of these factors. Overall, the number of positive and negative studies are close to evenly split, suggesting genuine variability, but taken in aggregate evidence does not support a large, widely penetrant independent effect of variation in the GNβ3 gene on BP. Thus, although there have been a number of studies reporting that 825T is significantly associated with higher BP or HT,[295,298,299] the degree of attributed effect on BP has never been very large and in some of the studies the significance of the association is borderline and/or applies predominantly to SBP,[298] DBP,[299] or men or women.[299] A similar number of studies reported no such independent association with HT or BP.[296,300-302] Some were robustly negative,[300-302] and one study reported an 825T association with reduced SBP[303] (rather than HT). Some subsequent studies have found that 825T associated with LVH, and others have not. In addition, findings are against a role in risk of MI or progression of nephropathy, except perhaps in post-transplant kidneys particularly with concurrent HT.[304] A report that GNβ3$_{825T}$ predicted a significantly greater response to thiazide diuretics in SBP and DBP (P < 0.0001)[305] has now to be reconciled with one showing no significant association of GNβ3$_{825T}$ with the salt sensitivity of BP.[306] Although a study on extremely obese children and adolescents[307] and another on adults showed no association of obesity or BMI with 825T, several others reported some[308] often firm[296,303,309,310] positive association with body weight and obesity, including a survey of many ethnic groups[296] and extending to evidence of 825T allele associated insulin resistance[309] or even amplification of the risk of developing diabetes.[296,309]

Because GNβ3 is not central to a well-understood BP control pathway (unlike e.g., angiotensinogen) it is harder to judge how best to further appraise this candidate gene if, as seems the case, there is genuine variability in findings that test the association with BP and BMI, which could be due to a modest effect that is not universally penetrant. The ethnic background of the study populations does not suggest a basis for this variability. Coincident end-organ damage promotion by GNβ3 genotype is not currently supported by findings. It is an attractive idea, given the previously discussed findings, that GNβ3$_{825T}$ may promote higher BP within an insulin-resistant, obese background in which sympathetic overactivity does not achieve the normal lipolytic weight-lowering effect resulting from the 825T allele or TT genotype. Siffert et al.[296] reported that, in some ethnic groups, an association of GNβ3 genotype and BP appears most likely via an effect on BMI without any body weight independent effect on BP. Studies of the association of variation in GNβ3 on BP in a large population with or without insulin resistance and/or obesity may help clarify these matters. However, currently it appears that a role for GNβ3 in body weight is a possibility, whereas an effect independent of BMI on BP would only be predicted as minor and, thus, not always manifested across a variable population genetic background.

### Adducin

Adducin 1 or α adducin (Ch 4p16.3) is a ubiquitous protein that forms heterodimers and tetramers with β or γ adducins and plays a role in normal cytoskeletal function. α Adducin became a candidate gene for both animal and human BP control and for the risk of HT from work on the Milan hypertensive rat (MHS). The MHS strain develops a genetic form of renal HT. When compared with its normotensive control strain (MNS), it shows higher GFR, lower renin, and increased renal Na$^+$ reabsorption most clearly in the prehypertensive and early hypertensive phases. These features tend to diminish and disappear when HT fully develops in MNS rats.[121] The Milan rat has been used as a model of human primary HT with the recognition of particular similarities to its low-renin subset. Bianchi et al. showed that one point mutation in each of α, β, and γ adducin was associated with BP level in the MHS; this explained up to 50% of the BP variance in this strain. More recently, a genome-wide linkage study has confirmed that that the most important of these changes is at the α adducin gene locus.[311] Studies have shown that the F316Y locus affects adducin interactions with the actin-spectrin cytoskeleton and importantly 316Y increases the surface expression and transport of Na$^+$-K$^+$-ATPase in renal epithelial cells.[312] Thus, α adducin was a credible candidate gene in primary human HT. In 1997 the Milan group reported significant linkage of primary human HT to the α adducin locus on 4p16.3. In a coreported association study on almost 800 French and Italian subjects the G460W polymorphism was found strongly associated with primary HT (P = 0.0003), and 460W was associated with higher BP.[313] Moreover, a subset assessed for Na$^+$ sensitivity showed that possession of the 460W allele conferred greater BP sensitivity to changes in Na$^+$ balance both acutely and after 2 months of thiazide diuretic treatment (P = 0.002). The authors suggested that the G660W polymorphism may help "identify patients who will benefit from diuretic treatment or maneuvers to reduce total body sodium."[313] Subsequent studies showed that recombinant human adducin stimulates Na$^+$-K$^+$-ATPase by altering the pump's apparent affinities for substrates and by accelerating the pump cycle. The apparent affinities for mutant human (and rat) adducins are higher than the corresponding wild-type proteins.[314] Another Italian study showed that 460W was associated with lower plasma renin and fractional excretion of Na$^+$ and a more salt-sensitive pressure-natriuresis relationship.[315]

Thus, this initial work indicated that variation in the α adducin gene may importantly influence BP in humans and now more than 30 studies have assessed the role of this gene and the 460W allele in primary HT in a wide range of ethnic backgrounds. The prevalence of the 460W allele has varied: 8% in native South Africans and North Canadian Indians, 13% to 27% in whites, 42% to 48% in Chinese, and 54% to 60% in Japanese. The tide of evidence has been against a general role for α adducin gene variation in influencing BP and the risk of primary HT. Although some studies[316-320] did report further support for an association in primary HT, this was only in a subset of their reported patients (e.g., in a weak association of G460W with HT in subjects from Milan but not Sardinia,[318] in a white study population but not the coreported Black study population,[319] and for SBP in Dutch hyperlipidemic patients but not for BP across the whole HT and control population[320]). Many more (>20) studies,[321-323] simply failed to find an association of 466W with BP or HT across Japanese; Chinese; Americans of Oriental or African ancestry; whites from Europe, North America, or Australia; or other ethnic groups. Two studies reported that adducin 460W was associated with lower BP. A few studies have re-examined linkage; two found linkage to the region of 4p close to adducin[321,322] but failed to confirm that linkage was due to adducin in follow-up association studies. Chinese studies found no linkage.[324,325] Incidentally, α adducin is not the sole candidate HT gene in this region. GPRK2L has also been suggested (G-protein coupled receptor kinase 2, also 4p16.3; also known as type 4 G-protein receptor kinase (GRK4), see dopaminergic system discussed previously). Several studies support the association of adducin 460W with low renin[313,315,318,326,327] and salt sensitivity,[313,318,326] (although not all do so[323]). A recent study in another form of low-renin HT (primary aldosteronism) has shown a significant interaction of 466W as a strong independent determinant of BP that along with alleles at the bradykinin B(2)R receptor locus account for 11% to 13% of the variability of both SBP and DBP.[328] Other studies have suggested that the 460W allele plays a role in determining long-term BP and the risk of HT within the low-renin subgroup of primary HT,[327] especially if there is also a family history of HT[326] or homozygosity for adducin.[329] Preliminary reports also suggest that 460W might be an adverse factor in the risk of progression of renal disease of diverse causes.[330]

It seems reasonable to conclude from this evidence that adducin has not been shown to have a significant effect on BP or the risk of HT in primary HT as a whole, whereas the 460W allele may well have an effect promoting HT that is penetrant in those with other factors predisposing them to low-renin and/or salt-sensitive HT, including a family history of low-renin HT,[326,327] mild aldosterone excess,[328] or renal abnormalities.[330] This may reflect the role of adducin in the MHS rat and may, thus, support the conclusion of Cusi et al.[313] mentioned previously (adducin G460W may be of assistance in identifying patients who will benefit particularly from diuretic treatment).[318]

## Natriuretic Peptides and Their Receptors

The natriuretic peptides ANP (Ch 1p36.2) and BNP (1p36.2) act mainly as cardiac hormones released from the atria and ventricles, respectively. CNP (C-type, 2q24-qter) is more broadly expressed, especially in CNS. These and the receptors to which the natriuretic peptides bind in mediating natriuretic actions (type A natriuretic peptide receptor NPRA, or NPR1, 1q21-22), vasoactive/dilator actions[331] (NPRB or NPR2, 9p21-12), and NPRC (or NPR3, 5p14-12), which appears not to signal intracellularly on binding natriuretic peptides but to act as a nonsignaling clearance receptor mechanism that modulate free natriuretic peptide availability, are all also potential candidate genes contributing to the causation of human primary HT. The natriuretic peptides are produced as larger precursors that are cleaved to release the active peptides. Corin, a serine protease (4p13-12) that is abundant in atrial myocytes, appears to be a pro-ANP converting enzyme that releases ANP and is expressed at lower levels in other tissues (e.g., kidney and bone). Studies in a number of gene-targeted and transgenic mice give valuable insight into how the NPS affects the circulation and other tissues and have confirmed the role of the NPS long-term BP control.[39,99] Thus, ANP −/− mice have HT that is salt sensitive, and ANP +/− develop HT on a raised salt intake. NPRA −/− and +/− mice have HT, which is clearer in +/− mice when on a high-salt diet.[39] Conversely, mice with three and four copies of NPRA have raised NPRA levels (twice normal for four-copy mice) and have lower BP (lowest also on a high-salt diet).[39] NPRA −/− mice also develop cardiac hypertrophy, which is disproportionate for the level of BP, and myocardial interstitial fibrosis resembling that seen in some human hypertensive heart disease. NPRC −/− mice are volume deplete and hypotensive, have reduced ability to concentrate urine, and have prolonged half-life of ANP—all consistent with NPRC locally modulating natriuretic peptide effects on cardiovascular and renal function. In addition, NPRC −/− mice have bone overgrowth skeletal deformities consistent with modulation of BNP and CNP effects locally on bone (see later). NPRC has been shown to downregulate with weight loss[332] and hypoxia and in kidney with high-salt diet.[333] This response is likely to contribute to moderation of BP. NPRC normally downregulates with weight loss.[332] Mice overexpressing BNP also have skeletal overgrowth (ANP overexpression causes no such bony phenotype), whereas BNP knockout mice have fibrotic lesions in the ventricles of the heart indicating that BNP has antifibrotic actions but not supporting BNP as important in long-term BP regulation.[334] CNP binds all three NPRs and is the peptide with highest affinity for NPRB. CNP knockout mice have achondroplasia-like dwarfism, but it remains unclear if CNP has significant effects on BP.

Lack of correlation of circulating ANP levels with long-term BP in clinical studies and lack of long-term BP-lowering benefits of peptidase inhibitor drugs (which reduce ANP degradation in humans) has raised doubt regarding the role of circulating levels of natriuretic peptides (especially ANP) as independent determinants of long-term BP in humans. This does not preclude key roles in BP control for local peptide levels (modulated by proteases and NPRC) and natriuretic peptide receptor expression levels (especially NPRA and NPRC). Several studies have examined the association of a range of different ANP gene variants with HT and BP. Other component genes of the NPS (including NPRA, NPRB, NPRC, and CNP) have been investigated for a link to HT to a limited degree.

Although there have been multiple studies investigating the association of variants in the ANP precursor gene (NPPA), this literature is somewhat unusual because several different polymorphisms have been investigated. Overall, evidence is against an important association of NPPA locus variation and primary HT. Single studies reported rather weak association of HT to NPPA polymorphisms (e.g., in intron 2[335]) or found weak linkage of a microsatellite marker close to NPPA (D151612) with young onset primary HT.[336] However, more than twice as many studies have found no association with a wide range of polymorphisms throughout the NPPA gene.[217] Although there are reports of NPPA variation ($-664$A, 1837A) associated with CVA in humans[337] as is the case in the SHR-SP rat strain, it will be important to see if this is confirmed in other human populations. A study of CNP precursor gene (NPPC) variants reported significant association of HT with a 3′UTR G2628A polymorphism and not three other polymorphisms.[338]

The receptor genes NPRA and NPRC are candidates deserving serious consideration, but findings are only preliminary. Studies on NPPA in Japan identified a 5′ 8 bp insertion/deletion polymorphism in which the rare deletion allele reduced NPRA transcription to less than 30% and was strongly associated with HT and LVH, although the numbers carrying the deletion allele were small.[339] Other studies showed no overall association with HT of NPRA variations at a 5′UTR TC/GA repeat and an exon3 M341I missense polymorphism, although in the latter case the 341I/341I homozygous genotype was found only in the HT group. Recently the NPRA gene has been completely sequenced in multiple individuals identifying 10 polymorphisms, and it has been shown that these noncoding polymorphisms have functional effects affecting NPRA gene expression by at least twofold.[340] By analogy with the transgenic mice carrying one to four NPRA gene copies causing twofold changes in NPRA expression (and accompanying effects on long-term BP)[39] it seems that these human polymorphisms are likely to influence BP and its response to salt intake and are likely to be the subject of further, hopefully large and conclusive studies. One study of the NPRC receptor reports that although overall the C-55A polymorphism showed no association with HT, there was a significant association in obese subjects (BMI > 30) of the common −55C allele with higher BP and lower ANP levels.[341] This is particularly interesting given that NPRC normally downregulates with weight loss.[332] Finally, in NPRB, an intron 2 GT repeat has been reported to be associated with HT,[342] whereas intron 18 insertion deletion polymorphisms were not.

Overall, evidence is against variation in the ANP precursor gene NPPA playing an important role in human primary HT, and results on the other NPS genes are too preliminary to judge although those on NPRC and especially NPRA are of considerable interest given the roles revealed for these genes in gene-targeted mice. Studies in subgroups of salt-sensitive and volume-dependent HT (perhaps when LVH is also prevalent) may reveal effects that are lost in a more heterogenous population.

### Genes Mediating Aldosterone Action and Renal Sodium Chloride Reabsorption

Several single-gene disorders affecting long-term BP in humans involve genes that are involved in renal Na⁺ reabsorption especially in the aldosterone-ENaC pathway (Fig. 31-3). Conn's syndrome and idiopathic adrenal hyperplasia are common causes of primary mineralocorticoid excess, the causes of which encompass common forms appearing sporadically and rarer familial forms[28] (notably familial hyperaldosteronism type II: recently linked to Ch 7p22[343]). Such idiopathic primary adrenal hyperplasia effectively merges in a continuum of aldosterone-to-renin ratios into low-renin primary HT. In secondary mineralocorticoid HT, across pedigrees of those affected by the same mutations, the degree of hypokalemia and alkalosis (consequent to the mineralocorticoid excess) varies and often neither feature is present despite HT. For example, hypokalemia is absent in many patients with primary mineralocorticoid excess and in the majority of those having glucocorticoid remediable aldosteronism (GRA).[344,345] Accordingly, milder mutations than those causing HT in primary mineralocorticoid and apparent mineralocorticoid excess are very credible candidates in contributing to commoner primary HT. All the genes in the aldosterone-ENaC pathway (Fig. 31-3) and others cross talking to this aldosterone pathway or in related pathways upregulating renal Na⁺ retention are potential candidate genes to contribute to the causation of primary HT or at least to its low-renin subset. Association studies on several such genes have been carried out especially on aldosterone synthase (CYP11B2), 11β-HSD2, and the subunits ENaC, which collectively assemble to form the limiting Na⁺ conductance in CD.

### Aldosterone Synthase

Aldosterone synthase (CYP11B2, Ch 8q21) is required to make aldosterone, which plays a key role in Na⁺ and ECF balance. Inactivating mutations of aldosterone synthase cause lower BP, salt wasting, and hyperkalemia in a very rare autosomal recessive syndrome.[346] Excessive aldosterone synthesis is the basis of primary aldosterone excess—a common cause of secondary HT with classically suppressed renin and hypokalemic alkalosis, which has several causes (Fig. 31-3). One such cause is a rare autosomal dominant mutations causing GRA, which involves gene conversion resulting in a chimeric gene, that joins the 3′ end of aldosterone synthase (CYP11B2) to the promoter and 5′ end of the adjacent highly homologous gene 11β-hydroxylase (CYP11B1). This functional chimeric gene synthesizes excess aldosterone, driving HT that is remediable by glucocorticoid treatment through suppression of ACTH and thereby the chimeric gene promoter and its aldosterone production.

Overall, studies on aldosterone synthase are not conclusive but appear against genetic variation in this gene playing an important role in human primary HT as a whole. Polymorphisms in the aldosterone synthase promoter, intron 2, exon 3 (missense K173R), and exon 7 (V386A) have been identified. Studies focused especially on the −377C/T polymorphism in the aldosterone synthase promoter (C-344T) at the regulatory site bound by the transcription factor steroidogenic factor 1 (SF-1). There was limited support for an overall association of variation at C-344T with BP or primary HT as a whole from several studies in European and Oriental populations. Although some studies found primary HT associated with −344C[347] or alternatively −344T[348] most (six studies), including some particularly large populations,[349] found no such association. However, when studies looked selectively at low-renin primary HT,[350,351] an association with variation in aldosterone synthase was found between HT and the −344T allele.[350,351] Studies found that the −377T allele was significantly associated with increased baroreflex sensitivity especially in the young[352] and with amplification of effects of Y chromosome loci on BP.[353] Further investigations found no association of aldosterone synthase alleles with salt sensitivity of BP[354,355] and are conflicting for associations with plasma aldosterone or aortic stiffness (some report increases with −377C, others with −377T, and others with no effect). One interesting study demonstrated that −377T was associated with both HT and higher aldosterone excretion rate.[348]

Overall, studies looking at variation in the aldosterone synthase gene (largely based on polymorphisms in the 5′ part of the gene) are against this gene having an important widely penetrant effect on BP in human primary HT as a whole. There remains the possibility of an effect in a subgroup especially in those having low-renin HT.[350,351] It would be of interest to know if the originally overall negative studies revealed association with BP if reanalyzed to look at low-renin subgroups. Finally, an association of aldosterone synthase haplotypes with BP in idiopathic hyperaldosteronism (IHA) appeared to support a role of aldosterone synthase variation in idiopathic low-renin HT; however, a subsequent report from the same group reported no association of −377T/C with BP in primary hyperaldosteronism including IHA.[328]

## 11β-HSD2

Studies on 11β-HSD2 gene (Ch 16q22) variation used a flanking microsatellite CA repeat D16S496 (usually ≥10 alleles) or an exon 3 SNP G534A (not affecting the coded amino acid 178E, but altering the presence of an Alu I cut site). The variant 534 A allele is not very common in reported populations usually averaging below 15%[356,357] in European studies and reported too rarely to be usable in a Japanese study.[358] Thus, other biallelic polymorphisms may assist wider study. The evidence using these 11β-HSD2 polymorphisms is limited but against an important widely penetrant effect of 11β-HSD2 gene variation on the risk of primary HT, although there is

some support for an effect on salt sensitivity and, thus, for higher BP on a high-salt diet.[359] Thus, there is some evidence of association of HT with 11β-HSD2 variation at D16S496[360] (in blacks with end-stage renal failure, a classically salt-sensitive HT group) and at G534A (but not D16S496) in a Swedish population.[357] However, other such studies are negative[200,356] as is one linkage study.[324] Two studies suggest that 11β-HSD2 variation affects salt sensitivity[354,359]; one also reported evidence from urinary steroid metabolites indicating that increased salt sensitivity was associated with increased 11β-HSD2 activity.

## ENaC Subunits

The amiloride-sensitive (epithelial) Na+ channel (ENaC) is composed of three different subunits α (CH 12p13.3), β, and γ (adjacent on 16p13). All subunits have two transmembrane domains between which there is a cysteine-rich extracellular loop and beyond which there are intracellular N- and C-terminal tails. No Na+ conductance has been generated with the β and γ subunits alone, and although a weak Na+ conductance is present with αENaC alone (possibly resulting from "$\alpha_4$ channels") this represents only approximately 1% of the conductance in channels having all three subunits (probably as $\alpha_2\beta\gamma$ heterotetramers). In humans, a δENaC (1p36) subunit exists and can substitute for α in active Na+ channels, but its expression is clearest in CNS, pancreas, and gonads.[361] In sites known to express classical ENaC conductance (e.g., distal nephron), δENaC is absent or at trivial levels, and apart from humans the presence of δENaC expression remains in some doubt. Thus, full ENaC function is regarded as requiring αβ and γ expression and αENaC has been regarded as essential for ENaC Na+ conductance in classical sites such as distal nephron. The nephron segment where ENaC exerts its major effects on BP is under renewed scrutiny with the provocative findings that mice homozygous null for αENaC in CD appear to have no clear defect in electrolyte handling or BP control even on low-Na+ diets.[33] Inactivating mutations in αβ or γ ENaC subunits can cause lower BP (in the salt-wasting condition autosomal recessive pseudohypoaldosteronism), whereas activating mutations affecting a short PY motif in a near C-terminal segment of β or γ ENaC increase ENaC surface half-life and conductance causing HT in Liddle's syndrome (see Fig. 31-3 and the section on mineralocorticoid HT). Recently a Liddle's-like phenotype was reported for a differently cited (N530S in the extracellular loop) γENaC subunit mutation that increased ENaC conductance and proposed to cause HT by increasing ENaC open probability.[362] Thus, the level of ENaC expression functioning at the cell surface seems key in long-term BP control. There has been interest in ENaC subunit mutations (especially in β and γ) producing subunits driving higher ENaC conductance. Attention has turned recently to whether promoter sequence variations in the ENaC subunits may contribute to essential HT. Some recent large studies carried out in Japan on ENaC subunit promoter variations provided interesting positive findings[363,364] in what had otherwise been an overall negative body of evidence against an important, widely penetrant role for ENaC subunit gene variation contributing to human primary HT. Another finding has been of considerable ethnic diversity in genetic variants in ENaC subunits, perhaps especially for βENaC with mutations found in peoples of African and Oriental ancestry that are rare or absent in other racial backgrounds. Many of these variations affect the amino acid sequence of subunits (especially βENaC), although some *in vitro* evidence suggests modest effects on conductance.[201] This may indicate that there is some environmental selection pressure of relatively recent effect and that the environmental factors that seem perhaps most likely to interact with ENaC variation are the climate and salt and water availability and intake. This diversity potentially makes the genetic "noise" in a study population of mixed ancestry higher, perhaps especially in the study of βENaC.

There have been several linkage studies that examined ENaC subunit loci. The first such study examined the common βγ locus on Ch 16p13 in an Australian population and found a linkage to SBP ($P \leq 0.001$) but not to DBP; the mean difference in SBP between sibs concordant at this locus was 7.1 mm Hg but was 14 mm Hg when nonconcordant.[365] Subsequent studies on Caribbean (on the βγ locus)[366] and Chinese populations (on α,β and γ loci[325] and γ[324]) have found no significant linkage to HT or BP. An early association study in a population of Afro-Caribbean origin in London found that the T594M polymorphism in the C-terminal βENaC exon was significantly commoner ($P = 0.029$) in those with HT (8.6%) than those with normal BP (2.1%), giving an odds ratio for HT in βENaC$_{T594M}$ carriers of 4.17 (95% CI 1.12 to 18.25). The association persisted, accounting for other factors including gender and BMI.[367] Among untreated hypertensives, plasma renin was significantly lower in βENaC$_{T594M}$ carriers.[367] Another study on a mixed white and African-American population from the United States reported a significant association of the αENaC$_{T663A}$ variation with lower BP and normotension in both whites ($P = 0.034$) and blacks ($P = 0.018$).[368] Expression of αENaC$_{T663A}$ in *Xenopus* oocytes showed no change in basal Na$^+$ current consistent with this polymorphism being in linkage disequilibrium with alleles at nearby functional loci.[368] A recent large study from Japan examined four promoter, three exonic and one intronic polymorphisms in αENaC; several associations were identified, especially the A(2139)G promoter variation associated with BP in preliminary studies and a finding in the whole study population (>3800 subjects) that HT was increased in αENaC$_{213G}$ (GA or GG genotypes, OR 1.31, $P = 0.015$) that was stronger in those older than 60 years (OR 1.7, $P = 0.0035$). Moreover, 2139G carriers had significantly greater proteinuria. MDCK kidney cell transient expression showed 2139G promoter activity to be higher than 2139A,[363] consistent with the αENaC$_{2139G}$ variant increasing αENaC expression and higher ENaC conductance that predisposes to HT. In a similar study examining γENaC on more than 4000 Japanese subjects, the same group identified four promoter and confirmed the presence of three exonic (two in exon 3, one in exon 13) polymorphisms.[364] The promoter polymorphisms were in tight linkage disequilibrium, and the G(−173)A and an exon 3 polymorphism were studied in the whole

study population. SBP and pulse pressure were significantly associated with γENaC$_{G(-173)A}$ (both $P = 0.005$); the AA genotype had 11 mm Hg and 8 mm Hg lower SBP and pulse pressure, respectively, and a higher prevalence of hypotension ($P < 0.02$).[364] Moreover, transient transfection in MDCK cells indicated that γENaC −173A had lower promoter activity than −173G, consistent with a −173A promoter effect of reduced γENaC subunit abundance and with the homozygous (AA) genotype having a limiting effect on ENaC conductance and BP.[364] These two studies from Osaka are of considerable interest and will stimulate further study of variations affecting the expression level of ENaC subunits. In addition, the rigorous approach with several polymorphisms and a large study population representative of the Japanese population as a whole are important because the γENaC promoter findings[364] suggest a recessive effect of γENaC$_{-173A}$. Because this allele was not common (8% to 9%), the prevalence of the AA genotype was low (0.7%) and a small study would not have detected the effect. The γENaC$_{-173G}$ allele has now been found significantly associated ($P = 0.019$) with HT in the overweight subgroup (BMI > 25) but not across the whole of an Australian white study population.[369] These association studies of γENaC[364,369] could be seen as consistent with the linkage of SBP to the βγENaC locus in a different Australian population mentioned previously.[365]

Despite these positive findings most studies (more than two thirds) have found no association of βγENaC genetic variation with HT or BP, including some particularly rigorous studies.[201,202] Studies on αENaC have been less common. One study in Japanese subjects[358] could not confirm the association of αENaC$_{T663A}$ with HT reported in African and whites in the United States,[368] although in this Japanese study αENaC$_{T663A}$ did show a borderline association ($P = 0.02$) with aldosterone-to-renin ratio.[358] Several studies have failed to find an association of BP or HT with variants of βENaC or γEna, including studies on white, Afro-Caribbean, and Japanese study populations. Two French studies are especially rigorous in looking at 400 to 600 subjects of mixed ethnic background, identifying several βENaC[201] (including T594M) and several γENaC[202] exonic polymorphisms, and finding none associated with HT or BP[201,202] and only small nonsignificant differences in ENaC conductance when those causing amino acid changes were expressed in *Xenopus* oocytes.[201,202]

### Other Genes Related to the Aldosterone-ENaC Pathway

Other genes in this pathway have received less attention; a few studies found no linkage or association of variation in the mineralocorticoid receptor (MR: Ch 4q31.1) with HT or BP.[324,354,358] However, a recent study looking at sgk1 (serum and glucocorticoid kinase: Ch 6q23), which is an aldosterone upregulated gene participating in the upregulation of ENaC conductance in distal nephron, found the sgk1 locus linked to DBP ($P < 0.0002$) and suggestive linkage to SBP ($P < 0.04$) using four microsatellite markers and two SNPs.[370] Analysis using the SNPs also confirmed significant association with both SNPs to BP.[370] It is likely that other studies on other genes involved in or crosstalking with the aldosterone-ENaC pathway such as channel activating protease 1 (CAP1, PRSS8: Ch 16p11.2) and NEDD4-2 (NEDD4L: Ch 18q21)[371] will be carried out.

### Other Genes Relating Directly to Renal Sodium and Chloride Reabsorption

Other genes involved in reabsorbing $Na^+$ in the kidney in response to diuretics and affecting sodium-lithium countertransport (an intermediate phenotype associated with essential HT) have been the subject of limited study. The target of thiazide diuretics, the thiazide sensitive cotransporter (TSC) (the major apical $Na^+$ transporter in DCT, Ch 16q13) was found not to be associated with HT or BP.[372] Some association of polymorphic alleles of NKCC2 (the target of loop diuretics and the major apical $Na^+$ transporter in the nephron TAL, ATP1A1: Ch 15q15.2) and $\alpha_1 Na^+$-$K^+$-ATPase (the major isoform of the $Na^+$ pump catalytic subunit in most tissues, including kidney, Ch 1p11.2) with HT and BP was reported in the same Sardinian hypertensive study population.[373] In other populations, $\alpha_1 Na^+$-$K^+$-ATPase showed no linkage to HT,[324] whereas for the $\alpha_2$ subunit of $Na^+$-$K^+$-ATPase (ATP1A2: Ch 1q22) one study reported no association with primary HT, a second found suggestive linkages (P = 0.01 to 0.013) for resting SBP and exercise DBP,[374] and a third found an $\alpha_2 Na^+$-$K^+$-ATPase RFLP significantly associated with HT (OR 7.7, 95% CI 1.9 to 31.4) but in a lead-exposed population in which the relevance to general primary HT remains less clear. Finally, polymorphisms in the main accessory subunit ($\beta_1$) of $Na^+$-$K^+$-ATPase (ATP1B1: Ch 1q23.2) in most tissues including in kidney have been associated with a rise in SBP on exercise in one study,[374] but another found no association with HT. $Na^+$-$H^+$ exchangers (NHEs) play important roles in cell volume regulation (especially NHE1: Ch 1p35.3) and in transepithelial $Na^+$ transport in kidney [several isoforms including NHE3 (Ch 5p15.33), the main apical $Na^+$ transporter in PT]. Studies showing no linkage of NHE1,[375,376] NHE2,[376] NHE3,[324,376] or NHE5[324,376] have been reported, whereas NHE5 was linked to the risk of end-stage renal failure in one of these studies.[376] Finally, WNK1 (Ch 12p13) and WNK4 (Ch 17q21.2) are two kinase genes in which recently identified mutations cause another monogenic form of HT affecting renal sodium chloride reabsorption (Gordon's syndrome or pseudohypoaldosteronism type II).[155] These are likely to be examined for association with BP and primary HT, especially because Gordon's syndrome responds well to thiazide diuretic treatment, which is also a useful treatment in a large proportion of human primary HT. Moreover, the WNK4 gene falls within a locus on human Ch 17q that has been identified as linked to human primary HT. The syntenic regions in the rat and mouse genomes are similarly linked to HT and BP in those species (see the section on genome scan). A third locus on Ch 1q31-42 for Gordon's syndrome has been identified, but the gene mutated at that site is not yet identified.[155]

### Other Genes

There is a long list of other genes that may be worth assessing to see if genetic variation in them results in variation in BP or in the risk of HT. Some such candidates are listed in Table 31-4, and some of particular interest will be mentioned briefly. If the proposed genome-wide association studies do become fully feasible in a robust form, it seems likely that the more weakly supported of such candidate genes will only continue to be the subject of investigation for association with primary HT if nearby markers show significant association with HT or BP. Thus, it may become obsolete to conduct single-gene association studies for more speculative candidate genes and conditions such as HT.

Bradykinin; dopamine; and arachidonic acid, prostaglandin, and prostacyclin are all mediators with proposed roles in regulating vascular tone, natriuresis, and BP. Polymorphisms in the bradykinin B2 receptor (B(2)R: Ch 14q32) at −58T/C have been linked to higher BP in primary aldosteronism (−58T allele)[328] and in primary HT (to −58C allele).[377] The A48G polymorphism of the type 1 dopamine receptor (D1 receptor, DRD1: Ch 5q35.1) has been associated with BP (especially DBP) in primary HT with 48G increased in HT (P < 0.01) and frequencies of AA, AG, and GG differing significantly between Japanese HT and normotensives (OR 2.1, CI 1.19 to 3.66).[378] Other studies show no association of variation in the D3 receptor (S9G in DRD3: Ch 3q13.3) with HT or BP or aldosterone levels in primary HT,[379] whereas a Taq1 polymorphism in the D2 dopamine receptor (DRD2: Ch 11q23) was weakly associated with BP in normoglycemic subjects.[380] A repeat polymorphism (VNTR: three to seven copies of a 9-bp repeat, R3 to R7) in the promoter of prostacyclin (prostaglandin $I_2$) synthase (Ch 20q13) was found to influence promoter activity in human endothelial cells; in a study of more than 4900 Japanese subjects it was associated with pulse pressure (P = 0.0005) and SBP (P = 0.013) with an increased risk of HT (OR 1.94, CI 1.19 to 1.32) in the R3/R4 genotype (1.6% of the population).[381] A different mutation in intron 9 affecting splicing of exon 9 and causing a premature stop in exon 10 is reported to cause familial HT with reduced urinary $PI_2$ metabolites.[382] However, two smaller studies from Japan have now failed to find an association with primary HT and the prostacyclin synthase promoter VNTR or another 5' SNP. Tyrosine hydroxylase (TH: Ch 11p15.5) is the rate-limiting enzyme in dopamine and catecholamine synthesis. The TH gene contains an internal short tandem repeat (STR) marker $(TCAT)_n$. Alleles at this STR have been found significantly linked to primary HT (P < 0.001),[383] but a small affected sib-pair study failed to show an association.[383] Another polymorphism (V81M) in linkage disequilibrium with the $(TCAT)_n$ STR was not associated with BP in two other studies, although there was an association with LV mass.

Some genes affecting the risk of obesity and insulin resistance (see corresponding sections) have been examined in a few studies for association with primary HT. Thiazolidinedione drugs and other ligands at PPARγ (Ch 3p25) increase CD36 expression and can lower BP (and reduce dyslipidemia and insulin resistance). In rare families, dominant negative mutations in PPARγ produce not only severe insulin resistance but also early-onset HT.[384] Some studies have found weakly significant associations of the PPARγ 12A allele with BP in obese diabetics,[385] nondiabetic controls,[385] and subjects with familial clustering of DM.[386] However, several other studies on similar populations found no association with HT or BP. One attempt to reconcile these differences showed that the PPARγ$_{12A}$ effect on BP is a recessive effect and because the 12A/12A genotype is rare the detection of the effect is variable[386] (in ethnic backgrounds studied the risk was only 1% to 2%). Although not conclusive, evidence is in favor of PPARγ$_{12A}$ associating with better glucose tolerance,[385,387] and, thus, the alternative, common, 12P allele is associated with worse glucose tolerance.[388] This predicts that 12A/12A predisposes to HT but against insulin resistance, in contrast to the rare families with dominant negative PPARγ mutations in which both insulin resistance and HT coexist.[384] Currently, PPARγ does not seem a strong candidate for importantly contributing to the risk of primary HT. CD36 (Ch 7q11.2) is a medium-long chain fatty acid translocase involved in absorption of free fatty acids into cells. CD36 deficiency is important in dyslipidemia and increased insulin resistance in hypertensive rats[389] (SHR) and seems likely to be similarly involved in humans in whom CD36 deficiency is common in peoples of African and Asian ancestry.[390] Early reports indicated that CD36-deficient human subjects were indeed dyslipidemic and insulin resistant and appeared to have BP higher than age-matched controls.[390] Moreover, CD36 has been reported to protect against dyslipidemic impairment of endothelium-dependent relaxation. However, several findings have now substantially weakened the concept that CD36 deficiency contributed to HT. First, in rats it was found that CD36 is not mutated in the related hypertensive and somewhat insulin-resistant stroke-prone SHR strain (SHR-SP).[391] Second, restoration of CD36 expression in the SHR rescues dyslipidemia and ameliorates insulin resistance but does not correct HT.[392] Third, short chain fatty acid treatment (which bypasses the CD36 deficiency as it transports longer chain fatty acids) also has no effect on BP in the SHR but ameliorates insulin resistance, which suggests a different mechanism for the HT. Fourth, study on a Japanese population examined the CD36 P90S substitution polymorphism (known to cause CD36 deficiency) and found that this polymorphism was associated with high plasma free fatty acids but not with any effect on BP or insulin resistance.[393] Thus, CD36 now appears to be a weaker candidate in human HT, although actual assessment has only been very preliminary. Studies of variants of the glucocorticoid receptor (GR: Ch 5q31) gene have found no overall significant linkage or association with BP or HT, although very weak, gender-specific subgroup associations with HT were identified in one of these studies.[394] Although one study in African Americans found no evidence for linkage of the leptin gene (Ch 7q31.3) to HT, another study found that a repeat polymorphism 3′ to the leptin gene is significantly associated with HT independent of BMI.[395] Studies have also reported linkage of the leptin receptor gene (Ch 1p31) to DBP[396] and association of its exon 6

Q223R polymorphism in men to BP on weight gain[397] and HT and BP in type II diabetes.[398]

### Conclusions from Association Studies in Human Primary HT (Table 31-5)

Conclusions emerging from this extensive body of work are shown in Table 31-5. The table also highlights difficulties with the study form often used and some potential ways to improve them so that future studies may yield a more conclusive picture. Although no candidate gene is implicated as having a major or even a moderately wide penetrant effect on the risk of human primary HT, it seems that genetic variation at the angiotensinogen locus may contribute to the risk of primary HT to a milder or less penetrant degree. Contributions of other genes are less clear and although, for example, it seems possible that the β$_2$-adrenergic receptor may also contribute, current studies have suggested interaction with genetic background and other factors (e.g., body weight) and have left the status of such putative weaker effects on BP unresolved. Now that these realities are known it should be possible to design more informative strategies for candidate gene studies (Table 31-5).

## The Positional Approach and Genome-Wide Linkage Studies

### Overview

The positional approach when applied to human primary HT (or other polygenic complex disorders) does not center around an identified candidate gene but rather seeks to identify the position of loci at which segregation of genetic variants is linked: risk of HT, variation in BP, or other quantitative traits that are seen as intermediate phenotypes for primary HT. These loci are referred to as QTLs, and the general approach is a linkage study, based on families that are of small or minimal size (e.g., affected sib-pairs). The most basic application tests for significant linkage of genetic variation at a single point in the genome with the risk of HT or variation in BP. Although segregation at a single specific point (one marker) can be assessed using pointwise significance levels (P < 0.05), many more studies use several markers, thus assessing an interval spanning several closely spaced points. Guidance has preferred stricter significance criteria even though the overall locus interval is very small compared with the whole genome (e.g., multiple markers across a 20cM interval needing a P < 0.01 threshold for significance).[190] The previous sections refer to instances in which linkage has been assessed at the chromosomal loci around important candidate genes, with positive linkage reported for genes such as angiotensinogen (Ch 1q42-43), β and γ ENaC subunits (both at 16p12), serum and glucocorticoid kinase (sgk1, 6q23), adducin (4p16.3), β$_2$-adrenergic receptor (β$_2$ ADR, 5q31-32), the ACE gene (on 17q23), and others. It is very important to appreciate that other linkage studies on these gene loci have been negative, and because there is a great deal more to the candidacy of such genes the reader is referred to the sections

■ ■ ■

## TABLE 31-5   LESSONS EMERGING FROM ASSOCIATION STUDIES IN HUMAN PRIMARY HYPERTENSION

### Realities Emerging about the Genetic Contribution to Primary HT

**Primary HT seems truly polygenic,** and currently there is no evidence of variation at a single gene having major or even moderate widely penetrant effect on BP. There could be genes of mild or incompletely penetrant moderate effect

**Effect of genes on BP influenced by interactions** with
Lifestyle and environment especially as affecting body weight, insulin resistance, and end-organ damage
Ancestral genetic background
Other single-gene variations especially within the same BP control pathway or influencing the same intermediate phenotype

**Across ancestral backgrounds the allele frequencies at a single locus and the haplotypes flanking them may completely change.** Thus, there may be drawbacks in too diverse a population mix of ancestral genetic backgrounds (high genetic "noise")

*Allele frequencies:* thus, if such a simple allelic marker is used in some backgrounds, it may barely show variation (no signal) or encounter diverse novel background-specific alleles (high noise) (e.g., some polymorphisms at the βENaC locus)

*Flanking haplotypes* may completely change—this may leave the same allele linked to functional variations raising BP in one genetic background but not in others (signal unreliable)

### Problems Affecting Past Studies

**Many studies did not have sufficient power** (see previous) being too small or otherwise suboptimally designed to reliably detect smaller genetic influences on BP or risk of HT

**Publication bias** of insufficiently powered positive studies may mislead because their outcome may reflect chance noise

**Often assessment of population BP was suboptimal**

**Inadequate assessment of gene-gene interactions.** Too often several genes are serially assessed and reported within the same population without their interaction being considered

### Potential Improvements

**Analysis for gene-gene interaction** effects on BP should be applied when multiple genes have been assessed in a population

**There should be more robust assessment of BP:**
**24-Hour ambulatory BP** in addition to single assessments
**Aim to increase penetrance or early detection** of primary HT (e.g., by salt loading or by changes in BP on exertion)
**Care in BP level used for those on antihypertensive treatment**
**Assess and limit other confounders** (e.g., variations in salt intake, BMI, glucose tolerance)

**Increase the signal-to-noise ratio** in detecting genetic effects on BP. All have advantages some have at least theoretical drawbacks:
**Larger well-conducted studies** more reliably detect smaller effects
**Younger hypertensive population** should have less secondary amplifying factors contributing to their BP (less noise) but may have less variation in BP levels (signal)
**Using intermediate phenotypes** to study a more homogeneous subset of primary HT (less noise) (e.g., phenotyping by renin level, response to different antihypertensives, BMI, salt sensitivity, etc.)

**Using less diverse populations** and within that large numbers of small informative families (e.g., sib-pairs and parents discordant for BP) will reduce noise

---

on the corresponding genes to put these studies in context. Some studies (e.g., some assessing loci near adducin[321,322] and β2 ADR[257]) reported strong linkage over a candidate locus and negative association with polymorphisms within the actual candidate gene. One constructive interpretation is that the functional QTL linked to BP is nearby, either elsewhere within the gene or possibly involving an adjacent gene. Overall, however, such approaches remain fundamentally candidate-centered rather than positional.

Two larger chromosomal regions of special interest (on 5q and 17q) have been assessed for linkage to HT and BP. The near-telomeric portion of human chromosome 5q is particularly rich in HT candidate genes including the adrenergic receptors β$_2$ADR (5q32-33.1, at 148 Mb along the Ch5 genomic sequence) and α$_1$B ADR (5q33.3-34, at 160 Mb) and the dopamine receptor DRD1 (5q35.1 at 175 Mb). Two studies have assessed regional linkage across the 5q31.1-35.3/ter interval spanning more than 50 Mb (>55 cM). Both studies reported significant linkage to BP and HT across the region. In one study the maximum linkage fell at a marker now localized in the human genome at approximately 144.9 Mb[257] and accordingly three polymorphisms of the nearby β$_2$ ADR gene were screened but showed no significant asso-

ciation with HT or BP. In the other study[61] maximum linkage fell across a two-marker interval now localized at 163.4-171.9 Mb; this was followed up by the same group who found a hit on Ch 5q34 for linkage to BP on a genome scan, maximum at a marker now localized at 167.5 Mb. Although the latter was the point with the third highest significance, this was at P = 0.0076,[62] which falls short of the threshold for taking seriously as an isolated finding (see later). However, the aggregate of all three of these independent studies seems to amount to suggestive (not significant) evidence of a QTL for HT in the region of Ch 5q32-34/35.1 (144.9-167.5 Mb). The genetic variation responsible for this possible QTL remains unknown.

A region of human chromosome 17q became of interest in human HT because it is homologous (syntenic) to a region of rat Ch10 harboring an important QTL for BP that was identified in the early 1990s.[399] In addition, the ACE gene (17q23 at 64.1 Mb) is encoded nearby as is WNK4 (17q21-22 at 43.2 Mb), one of the genes mutated in some cases of the autosomal dominant hypertensive condition Gordon's syndrome.[155] In an elegant study reported in 1997, Julier et al.[400] carried out regional linkage studies across a portion of Ch 17q in affected sib-pairs from Europe and identified significant linkage (P < 0.0001) of primary HT to a 5-cM region now known to fall over 17q21 at 38.8-43.4 Mb, which is sufficiently remote from the ACE gene to exclude it as a likely cause of this effect. A subsequent study in the United States with five markers spanning 12 cM crossing this interval found maximum linkage at a marker located at 17q21.1 (41.2 Mb) at a much greater significance level ($P < 0.0005$) than the threshold in replicating a hit across such a regional interval ($P < 0.01$, as indicated in the example quoted previously[190]). Although a smaller study in Afro-Caribbeans failed to show linkage to BP in this region, a more recent genome scan showed a hit, significant at the genome level (maximum LOD = 4.7, see later) spanning this locus.[401] This QTL on 17q21 was, thus, the first for human primary HT identified, and, although WNK4 represents a theoretically strong candidate now known to lie nearby, the cause of the QTL is not established.

### Genome Scan Studies Available and Their Analysis

Advances in mapping and methodology enabled genome-wide linkage analyses, or genome scans, that aim to identify sites anywhere in the genome linked to HT and use large batteries of polymorphic markers, typically 350 to 450 evenly dispersed at 10-cM intervals across the genome (autosomes and X at least). Such scans for HT and BP QTLs began in 1998 and now more than 20 have been reported. Moreover, there have already been a larger number of such scans carried out to detect QTLs for HT and BP in hypertensive strains of rat[192] and more recently in mice, too.[193-195] Findings from studies that are more directly relevant to human primary HT are laid out in Table 31-6[400-430] including hits found in the human scans (and two regional Ch 17q studies[400,402]). The locus in the human genome is shown with any corresponding syntenic mouse or rat QTLs. The primary criteria for including hits is their maximum LOD score greater than 1.74, pointwise $P < 0.0023$ indicative of at least suggestive linkage ($P < 1$) at the genome-wide level using the kind of genome scan marker density used in these scans.[191] The locus of the peak of the linkage hits are given (i.e., corresponding to the marker, or pair of markers, having the highest LOD score). Hits are also grouped into clusters using the conservative criteria of overlap of their peak ±7.5 Mb intervals (or additionally when peak LOD score > 3.3, and the original report indicates extension at LOD > 1.74 over other peak loci of members in the cluster). The human genome scans largely were for loci linked to SBP and DBP or HT, although one study examined basal BP supine and then also on standing.[403] Two studies examined BP basally and then the change brought about by a phase of standardized exercise endurance training; one focused on resting BP[404] and the other on exercise BP.[405] A study based on the Framingham Heart Study cohort used a derived index of long-term SBP and DBP phenotype.[401] Kotchen et al.[407] examined BP and also used anthropomorphic measurements including BMI and indirect measures of body fluid compartments (using impedance plethysmography[406]) to derive indices of HT-related intermediate phenotypes, comorbidities of ECF and volume overload, and adiposity and assessed these HT-associated traits for linkage. The

study populations are familial and derive from diverse origins: whites,[62,401-405,408-413] African,[62,402-405,407,409-413] and Mexican/Hispanic Americans,[414,415] Australian,[416] Canadian,[409] Nigerian,[417] European,[400,418-422] Icelandic,[423] Chinese,[424-426] or those of Chinese or Japanese ancestry.[427] Some populations are relatively isolated including those from Finland,[419] Iceland,[423] Sardinia,[421] rural China,[425,426] and Amish communities in the United States.[408] Subjects had especially young onset HT in one study,[419] whereas in two others there were more subjects with dyslipidemia[421] and obesity[409] and HT. Most studies used marker densities giving 10-cM coverage of the genome (350 to 450 markers), whereas one used more than 900 markers giving 3 to 4cM coverage.[423] Although most studies concentrated on analyzing one population throughout, one genome scan chose the especially rigorous approach of a three-stage process, each progressively narrowing in on a Ch 2 locus but using a different population of sib pairs (from a total of more than 1600) for each stage.[424]

### Significant and Suggestive Linkage: QTLs and Weaker Hits

Although there is some controversy about the thresholds to define genome-wide levels of significance, few would argue that if the criteria outlined by Lander and Kruglyak[190] are met for a pointwise significance level of $P < 2 \times 10^{-5}$ (LOD score ≥3.3 to ≥3.6, depending on study design) then there is *significant linkage* because genome-wide significance is established at the $P < 0.05$ level. In addition to such significant linkage hits it is useful to be aware of hits of lesser significance and as proposed by Lander and Kruglyak[190] the term *suggestive linkage* referring to a genome-wide probability in the range $0.05 \leq P < 1$ is a useful category for this purpose. Rao and Province[191] calculate that for typical genome scans with approximately 400 markers distributed every 10 cM or so the lower threshold for suggestive linkage hits (i.e., $P < 1$) corresponds to LOD score of 1.74 or higher and pointwise probability of $P < 0.0023$. Lander and Kruglyak[190] originally proposed a higher threshold for suggestive linkage (pointwise $P < 7 \times 10^{-4}$, LOD > 1.9 to 2.2 depending on study design); however, this was based on an infinitely dense pointwise map simulation of a genome scan and investigators do not routinely go on to finely linkage map over such weak suggestive linkage hits. Thus, the standard of Rao and Province[191] is preferred here for suggestive linkage. In contrast, investigators do tend to finely map over their most significant hits and so the $P < 2 \times 10^{-5}$ standard of Lander and Kruglyak[190] for significant linkage is best for distinguishing significant QTLs.

Accordingly we used these standards in compiling Table 31-6 in which the listed linkage hits have LOD score of 1.74, whereas column 2 only designates hits as QTLs if they have significant linkage (LOD score ≥3.3 to ≥3.6); the rest have suggestive linkage. Two genome scans, one reported at a relatively early stage[418] and one recently,[411] found no hits with LOD greater than 1.74. In essence, the QTLs are likely to be reliable, because in all the human genome scans to date one would expect only approximately 1 such $P < 2 \times 10^{-5}$ hit by chance and

**TABLE 31-6  GENOME SCAN HITS RELEVANT TO HT**

| Genome Scan Hits Relevant to HT Hit No | QTL[A] | Ch | Human Genome Scan Hits Relevant to BP and HT — Hit Clusters | Individual Hits — Cytogenetic Locus | MB | s/d§ | LOD¶ | Ref | Syntenic Mouse BP QTLs — Syntenic Human locus Cytogenetic | MB | Site of Mouse QTL Ch-marker/cM | Ref. | Syntenic Rat BP QTLs — Syntenic Human Locus Cytogenetic | Width, cM |
|---|---|---|---|---|---|---|---|---|---|---|---|---|---|---|
| 1 | 1 | 1 | | 1p36.32 | 3.5 | s | 2.48 | 414 | | | | | 1p35-p31 | 75.1 |
| 2 | | | | 1p34.1-32.3 | 45.9-56.8 | s | 2.7* | 416 | | | | | | |
| 3 | | | | 1p22.3 | 81.9-83.1 | s | 1.75 | 409 | | | | | | |
| 4 | | | | 1p11.2-11.1 | 115.8-119.4 | s | 1.77 | 409 | | | | | 1p13-q22 | 46.2 |
| 5 | | | 1q23.1-24.2 | 1q23.1 | 157.1 | d | 1.78 | 419 | 1q23.2-25.2 | 163.8-181.7 | 1/D1kMit14 | 193 | 1q21-q32 | 62.0 |
| 6 | | | | 1q23.1 | 158.5 | d | 2.96 | 412 | | | | | | |
| 7 | | | | 1q24.1 | 171.1 | d | 2.8 | 410 | | | | | | |
| 8 | 9[A] | | | 1q24.1-(24.2) | 172.2 | bmi | 3.7 | 407 | | | | | | |
| 9 | | 2 | | 2p25.1 | 11.3-11.5 | ht | 1.99 | 420 | | | | | | |
| 10 | | | | 2p22.1 | 41.7 | ht | 2.08 | 413 | | | | | | |
| 11 | | | | 2p13.2 | 68.4 | s | 1.88 | 404 | | | | | | |
| 12 | | | 2p11.2-q12.1 | 2p11.2-11.1 | 85.4 | d | 1.92 | 417 | | | | | | |
| 13 | | | | 2p11.2-11.1 | 85.4 | s | 2.22 | 409 | | | | | | |
| 14 | 1 | | | 2p11.2-q12.1 | 85.4-106 | d | 3.92 | 415 | Close to 2q13 | 107-108 | 10/D10Mit123/117 | 195 | 2q11-q14 | 10.3 |
| 15 | | | | 2q11.2 | 101.0 | s | 2.26 | 409 | | | | | | |
| 16 | | | | 2q24.1 | 154.8 | ht | 2.24 | 424 | 2q21.3-24.3 | 136.4-165.5 | 2/D2Mit149/92 | 195 | | |
| 17 | | | | 2q24.1 | 156.5 | ht | 1.76 | 428 | | | | | | |
| 18 | | | 2q31.3-32.3 | 2q31.3 | 178.3 | d | 2.96 | 419 | 2q24.3-32.1 | 165.5-186.6 | 2/D2Mit92/274 | 195 | | |
| 19 | 7 | | | 2q32.3 | 194.3 | d | 3.36 | 408 | | | | | | |
| 20 | | 3 | 3p26.3-25.3 | 3p26.3 | 1 | s | 1.84 | 404 | | | | | | |
| 21 | | | | 3p26.3 | 2-2.3 | s | 2.03 | 426 | | | | | | |
| 22 | | | | 3p26.1-25.3 | 6.9 | d | 2.28 | 417 | | | | | | |
| 23 | 10[A] | | | 3p21.31/(32) | 43.8 | ecv | 3.94 | 407 | | | | | 3p21.3-p11 | 98.4 |
| 24 | 2 | | | 3q24/25.1 | 149.4-154 | d | 4.04 | 419 | | | | | 3q21-q26.3 | 56.9 |
| 25 | | | | 3q28 | 187.5 | s | 1.8 | 404 | | | | | | |
| 26 | 3 | 4 | | 4p16.1-15.3 | 6.6-20.3 | s | 4.6 | 421 | | | | | | |
| 27 | | | | 4q23-26 | 104-120.4 | s | 2.25* | 416 | | | | | 4q25-q28 | 38.5 |
| 28 | 5 | 5 | 5p15.2-12 | 5p15.2-12 | 12.4-42.1 | s | 1.9 | 401 | 5p15.31-q11.2 | 9.1-45 | 15/D15Mit175/152 | 99,194 | 5p14-q11 | 35.6 |
| 29 | | | | 5p13.3 | 32.2 | s | 2.8 | 409 | | | | | | |
| 30 | | | | 5p13.2 | 34.8 | ecv | 4.49 | 407 | | | | | | |
| 31 | 11[A] | | | 5p13.1 | 67.8 | ht | 1.85 | 428 | | | | | | |
| 32 | | | | 5q15 | 96.8 | d | 1.83 | 417 | | | | | | |
| 33 | | 6 | 6p22.1 | 6p22.1 | 24.2 | s‡c | 1.9c | 403 | 6p21.31-22.1 | 20-24.2 | 13/D13Mit198 | 195 | | |
| 34 | | | | 6p12.1 | 55.2 | ecv | 2.79 | 407 | | | | | | |
| 35 | 8 | | 6q14.1-16.1 | 6q14.1 | 75.8 | s | 3.30 | 410 | 6q14.3-16.1 | 87.1-97 | 4/18±6cM | 429 | | |
| 36 | | | | 6q14.1-16.1 | 75.8-94.1 | d | 2.5 | 421 | | | | | | |
| 37 | | | | 6q16.1 | 92.6 | ecv | 2.52 | 407 | | | | | | |
| 38 | | | | 6q23.2-24.1 | 137.1-144.4 | s | 3.1** | 62 | 6q16.2-24.3 | 100.4-152 | 10/D10Mit123/117 | 195 | | |
| 39 | | | | 6q27 | 169.8 | ht | 3.21 | 428 | | | | | | |
| 40 | | 7 | 7q11.21-23 | 7q11.21 | 65.9 | d | 1.99 | 417 | 7q11.21-23 | 65-74.5 | 5/D5Mit31 | 193 | | |
| 41 | | | | 7q11.23 | 77.8 | ecv | 3.16 | 407 | | | | | | |
| 42 | | | 7q21.3-22.1 | 7q21.3-22.1 | 94.6 | d | 2.07 | 417 | Close to QTL below and another (~90.9MB): mouse Ch5/9±9cM | | | 429 | 7q21-35 | 60.1 |
| 43 | | | | 7q22.1 | 99.7 | s | 2.51 | 414 | 7q22.1 | 98.1-100.7 | 5/D5Mit31 | 193 | | |

| # | Ch | Hit cluster | Cytoband | Position (cM) | s/d | LOD | Ref | Synteny note | Interval (cM) | Rat QTL | Ref | Human chr | LOD |
|---|---|---|---|---|---|---|---|---|---|---|---|---|---|
| 44 | | ⎡7q31.32-32.2 | 7q31.32 | 119.9 | s | 2.00 | 410 | | | | | | |
| 45 | | | 7q32.2 | 127.7 | s | 2.26 | 409 | | | | | | |
| 46 | | ⎣ | 7q35/(36.1) | 145.7 | s | 2.6 | 410 | | | | | | |
| 47 | 8 | | 8p21.2 | 22.8 | d | 1.8 | 421 | Close QTL 8p21.1 and p22(−17.8 and 28.8-MB): mouse Ch8/D8Mit64/205 | | | 195 | 8p23-p12 | 5.8 |
| 48 | | | 8q12.3 | 67 | s | 2.24 | 409 | | | | | | |
| 49 | 12^A | ⎡8q24.21-24.3 | 8q24.21 | 127.6 | bmi | 3.43 | 407 | | | | | | |
| 50 | | | 8q24.3 | 144.4 | d | 1.92 | 415 | | | | | | |
| 51 | 9 | ⎣ | 8q24.3 | 144.4 | Δs | 2.36 | 405 | | | | | | |
| 52 | | | 9q34.13 | 127.1 | ht | 2.24 | 428 | | | | | | |
| 53 | 10 | | 10p14 | 11.5 | ht | 2.5 | 427 | | | | | | |
| 54 | | | 10q21.1 | 56.5 | d | 2.29 | 417 | 10q11.22-22.1 | 54-75 | 10/D10Mit123/117 | 195 | 10q11.2-q23.3 | 32.6 |
| 55 | | | 10q23.33 | 95.2 | s | 1.84 | 405 | | | | | | |
| 56 | 11 | | 11q13.1 | 60.0 | s | 2.07 | 426 | 11q12.2-13.1 | 58.1-60.1 | 2/D2Mit92/274 | 195 | 11q14.1-14.3 | 10.4 |
| 57 | | | 11q13.4 | 81.5 | s | 1.98 | 404 | 11q13.4-14.3 | 81.5-91.9 | 7/42cM (Bpq7) | 194 | | |
| 58 | 12 | | 12q21.31 | 83 | s | 2.4 | 410 | | | | | | |
| 59 | | 12q21.31-21.32 | 12q21.32 | 91.3 | d | 2.35 | 404 | | | | | | |
| 60 | 15 | ⎡15q26.1-26.3 | 15q26.1 | 86.3-86.9 | s | 1.7** | 409 | Close to 15q 25.1-25.3/26.1 | 76.3-84.1 | 7/42cM(Bpq7) | 194 | | |
| 61 | | | 15q26.2 | 89.9 | s | 2.4 | 410 | | | | | | |
| 62 | 4 | ⎣ | 15q26.2/26.3 | 93.5 | d | 3.77 | 425 | | | | | | |
| 63 | 16 | | 16p12.2 | 25.7 | s | 2.25* | 416 | | | | | 16p11-12.2 | 14.6 |
| 64 | | | 16q11.2 | 51.2 | s | 2.74 | 426 | | | | | | |
| 65^B | 17 | | 17p13.1 | 12.0 | s | 2.16 | 426 | | | | | | |
| 66^B | 5 | ⎡17q11.2-23.2, | 17q11.2-23.2 | 34.6-58.8 | s | 4.7 | 401 | | | | | 17p11-q21 | 74.4 |
| 67 | | core = 17q21 | 17q21.1 | 41.2 | ht | 2.71^B | 402 | | | | | 17q23.1 | 6 |
| 68 | | ⎣ | 17q21.1-21.31 | 38.8-43.4 | ht | 3***^B | 400 | | | | | | |
| 69 | | | 17q21.33 | 53.9 | d | 2.1 | 401 | | | | | | |
| 70 | | | 17q25.1 | 72.2 | s | 2.2 | 401 | | | | | | |
| 71 | 18 | | 18p11.31 | 3.05 | d | 2.1 | 401 | | | | | | |
| 72 | | ⎡18q21.2-22.1 | 18q21.2 | 54.8 | s‡ | 2.6 | 403 | | | | | 18q21-23 | 52.4 |
| 73 | 6 | | 18q21.31-22.1 | 57-61.4 | ht | 4.6 | 423 | | | | | | |
| 74 | | ⎣ | 18q22.3-23 | 74.5 | s | 2.09 | 415 | | | | | | |
| 75 | 19 | ⎡19p13.3-12 | 19p13.3 | 3.1 | s | 2.4 | 421 | 19p13.3 | 0.7-4.1 | 10/D10Mit123/117 | 195 | | |
| 76 | | | 19p13.3 | 3.2 | s | 2.1 | 409 | | | | | | |
| 77 | | | 19p13.11 | 16.1 | s | 2.39 | 417 | Close to 19p13.12 | 15.4-15.6 | | | | |
| 78 | | | 19p12 | 22.0 | s | 2.14 | 404 | | | | | | |
| 79 | | ⎣ | 19q13.33 | 51.3 | s | 2.65 | 417 | | | | | | |
| 80 | 21 | | 21q22.13 | 35.8 | s | 2.82 | 415 | | | | | | |
| 81 | 22 | | 22q12.2 | 30.2 | d | 2.07 | 419 | 22q12.2 | 29.5-30.2 | 10/D10Mit123/117 | 195 | | |
| 82 | X | ⎡Xp11.4 | Xp11.4 | 39.4 | s | 2.4* | 416 | | | | | | |
| 83 | | ⎣ | Xp11.4 | 41.2 | s | 2.41 | 419 | | | | | | |

^AQuantitative trait loci (QTLs) 1 to 6 show linkage to BP or HT with LOD ≥ 3.6, clearly meeting criteria for genome-wide significant linkage;[190] QTL7 and 8 are borderline significant LOD ≥ 3.3 to 3.6, and QTL 9 to 12 are significantly linked to HT-associated intermediate phenotypes. Ch, chromosome; MB, locus in megabases from chromosome short-arm telomere. §s/d column = nature of QTL, including QTL analysis based on −d, DBP; s, SBP; ht, HT status; s‡, post-standing SBP (†post-standing DBP also linked (lod 1.7) to hit 33 locus[403]); Δs, change in SBP after endurance training minus baseline; bmi and ecv are body mass index and extracellular fluid volume/total body water (or total body water level itself) and were used in one genome scan as indices to assess HT-associated intermediate phenotypes of obesity or circulatory volume expansion respectively. ¶ LOD score of QTL column, when followed by *, **, *** LOD score is derived from different statistical expressions of linkage used in the original reports, specifically: *this study[416] reported findings as nonparametric Z-score statistics of Z = 3.5, 3.2, 3.2, and 3.3 for the Ch 1, 4, 16, and X loci; ‡this study[62] used the t statistic of Risch and Zhang[430] and associated P values were P = 0.00009 and P = 0.0033 for the Ch 6 and 15 loci; and ***having linkage significance at the P < 0.0001 level.[400] ‡Rat QTL information,[192] width refers to the width in centimorgans (cM) of the QTL interval on the syntenic human chromosome. The square brackets indicate which hits are included within each hit cluster (hit cluster column).

there have been 12. In contrast, the suggestive linkage hits are not independently reliable and require other support to be taken seriously. Thus, with all the human genome scans to date one would expect of the order of approximately 20 (perhaps 10 to 30) such $P < 0.0023$ suggestive hits by chance and there are more than 70 in Table 31-6; thus, a third to a half are likely to be artifactual noise. What can separate the real linkage signal in this suggestive hit group from the noise? Three factors are key: first, as the LOD score (Table 31-6, column 8) of the hit rises, especially approaching 3.3, it becomes increasingly unlikely to be artifact; second, if other hits are present at the same genome site from independent studies (i.e., the presence of a cluster of hits) (Table 31-6 column 4), it is unlikely to be artifact; and third if the syntenic region of genomes in other species contains an important QTL for BP (right half Table 31-6), artifact is unlikely. We have included the two regional linkage studies[400,402] on 17q referred to previously (hits 67, 68). Finally, we have also included 1 hit (hit 60) with LOD score ≈ 1.7 that seems unlikely to be artefact and is part of a cluster; the exact LOD score is complicated by the non-LOD statistical analysis used in this early study but is very close to the (LOD > 1.74) threshold for suggestive linkage. Finally, hit 33 for SBP coincides with a hit at the same locus in the same study for DBP having LOD score of 1.7.[403]

### Syntenic Analysis

The syntenic analysis makes use of the completed human and mouse genome project data and comparative mapping tools[431] wherever possible anchoring marker locations to the physical location on the genomes in Mb (megabases from chromosome short-arm telomere) in preference to cytogenetic banding position or location on the Marshfield human genetic map. Accordingly, the MB positions in Table 31-6 rather than the accompanying cytogenetic banding is preferred for finer comparison between the location of human linkage hits and the human syntenic position of mouse BP QTLs. In constructing the synteny analysis for the mouse in Table 31-6 a relatively conservative mouse QTL span width ±7.5-Mb flanking markers delimiting peak LOD score point or interval of the QTL has been used. A considerably wider interval would include regions and complexity with increasingly diminishing chances of a real cross-species QTL involvement. The complexity of the syntenic relationship between human and mouse (and rat) genomes is strikingly nonuniform, and this can be viewed as having three levels of complexity: (1) simple—in some regions large proportions of human chromosomes translate seemingly undisturbed to a syntenic rodent counterpart, notably most of human Ch 17p, 20p+q with mouse Ch 11 and 2, respectively, and similarly a 50-Mb region of human Ch 1q flanking the human linkage hit cluster centered on QTL9 (hit 8) with mouse Ch 1; (2) shredded—in many regions although large proportions of human chromosomes translate to a single syntenic rodent counterpart, the syntenic region is shredded and the various shreds (which can be as small as a fraction of a Mb but usually is much larger) are

altered in their order and orientation. This happens notably for the human Ch 17q with mouse Ch 11 and between X chromosomes and similar portions of human 7q (65-91Mb, 96-104Mb) and mouse Ch 5 flanking human linkage hit clusters at 7q11 and 7q21-22 (hits 40-41 and 42-43, respectively); and (3) complex—in many regions an interval from a human chromosome is shredded, and synteny of the shreds falls across more than one rodent chromosome, and, preferably, each shred is considered separately. This is a notable feature in the synteny of human Ch 2q where the centromeric half 93-130 Mb has synteny shredding across seven different mouse chromosomes and for human Ch 19p (0-23 Mb) across five mouse chromosomes, and in inverse the interval of mouse Ch 10, where the strongest BP QTL to date has been located,[99,195] shreds across seven human chromosomes and remarkably five of these syntenic loci contain or closely flank human linkage hits for BP (Ch 2q, QTL1 (hit14); Ch 6q, hit 38; Ch 10q, hit 54; Ch 19p, hits 75-76 ± also hits 77-78; and Ch 22q, hit 81). The evolutionary process that generated such syntenic complexity are intriguing. Although such matters lie well outside the scope of this chapter, this shredding of synteny has two very relevant consequences. First, if a real QTL were to fall within a relatively small syntenic shred, then the limited extent of the shred interval would dramatically assist in locating the gene or genetic element responsible for the effect on BP in both species. Second, if a real QTL falls close to a shred boundary, its functioning may differ between species. If this involved an important gene, one would assume that function would survive intact and that any difference may be reflected in aspects of its regulation. Thus, as a syntenic shred gets smaller there are both pros and cons in pursuing it as a potential locus in harboring genetic elements altering BP across species. The large body of work relating to genome scans for BP and HT in hypertensive rat strains will come into sharper focus after completion and full annotation of the rat genome. At this point it is appropriate to pool overlapping significant QTLs into larger rat BP QTL clusters and to derive a syntenic location for the major syntenic regions of these rat QTL clusters on the human genome in terms of cytogenetic location and the width of these syntenic intervals in cM[192] as in Table 31-6. These syntenic loci for rat QTL clusters are predominantly wide and when coincident with those from mouse or human linkage hits the rat-derived region is usually overarching, not delimiting. An exception occurs where the human hit cluster centered around hit 14 (QTL1) on Ch 2 spans an interval across which the syntenic rodent chromosome changes, and, thus, the rat BP QTL cluster that exists on one of these rodent chromosomes only partly overlaps this human hit cluster interval.

### Findings

Although some aspects of the information in Table 33-6 can be interpreted in diverse ways, some very important points emerge. First, no single human genome locus shows up as a hit in the majority or even a substantial minority of what is now a number of genome scans for BP and HT. This simply means that the genetic contribution to human primary HT shows no widely pene-trant dominant locus (i.e., no gene of huge effect) in contrast to type 1 diabetes in which most scans pick up the Ch 6 HLA locus that recently was estimated to have a linkage LOD score of 65 and to contribute more than 50% of the genetic contribution to the risk of type 1 dia-betes in many populations.[156] This conclusion is echoed by a meta-analysis (analyzing > 6000 relatives) of four recent genome scans carried out in the United States, which encompassed samples within four familial popu-lation networks and found no significant or even sug-gestive linkage hits spanning all ethnic backgrounds.[432] Second, as mentioned previously in essence the QTLs (Table 31-6, column 2) are likely to be reliable because in all the human genome scans to date one would expect only approximately 1 (perhaps 0 to 2) such $P < 2 \times 10^{-5}$ hit(s) by chance and there have been 12. There are several explanations for differences among studies. The most important one is that genome scans are not powered to detect real but reasonably small QTLs with more than 80% reliability. Other explanations include the age and racial mix of the population and aspects of the exact trait being assessed (HT risk; SBP/DBP; and those studies examining effect of postural change, exer-cise training, and HT-associated intermediate pheno-types). Third, of the 12 QTLs identified, 9 form part of a linkage hit cluster, and all but 2 (QTL 7 and 12) of these 9 clusters meet the conservative criteria that clustered hits have an overlap of their peak ±7.5 Mb loci. QTL 2, 3, and 10 clearly stood in isolation at the time of this writing. Similarly nine of the QTLs overlapped regions syntenic to mouse or rat BP and HT QTLs and QTLs 9 and 11 (and possibly the 2q portion of the QTL1 inter-val) were sites where significant linkage to BP and HT appeared to extend syntenically across all three species. QTL4 was close to overlap with the syntenic region to a mouse BP QTL but for QTL3 and 12 there was no over-lap. The extent of this clustering of other linkage hits and syntenic overlap around the site of these human QTLs was greater than that expected by chance, repre-senting independent confirmations that they are likely sites of real genetic influence on BP. QTL3, however, had no support on either count; QTL10 has not yet been linked to human HT or BP (only indirectly via HT-asso-ciated fluid-volume phenotype). In contrast, support was particularly strong for QTL1, 5, 8, 9, and 11. Fourth, some other linkage hit clusters (beyond those around QTLs) are apparent on Ch 2q24.1, 3p26, 7q11, 7q21, 7q31, 12p21, and 19p13-12, and, although these are not in themselves independently significant, the strength of some are suggestive (e.g., 19p13-12 has four linkage hits all within 20 Mb and overlap with a mouse QTL; 3p26 at the tip of Ch 3 has three hits within 6 Mb; the 7q11 clus-ter has a hit almost reaching significance [LOD = 3.1]; and all three 7q clusters have overlapping rodent syn-teny [7q21 for mouse and rat] and may not all be inde-pendent). Clearly these suggestive hit clusters are not as strong candidates as the QTLs, but it is highly likely that at least one of these regions harbors a real BP locus. If larger populations were added to the original studies or the original populations of the studies in the clusters pooled and genotyped with the same marker sets, this

would likely reveal which suggestive hit clusters achieve significance. Fifth, although identification of BP QTLs in human is recent and the genetic elements responsible are not known, considerable effort is under-way to identify some of the more important rodent BP QTLs, including some with synteny to those linked to BP in humans. Clearly if these efforts were successful, it would greatly increase the importance of the syntenic hit. For example, this might transform the view of linkage hits 54 and 57, which overlap syntenic regions for QTLs in both mouse and rat but remain weak candi-dates (having LOD scores less than 2.3 and occurring in isolation outside clusters). Finally, from Table 31-6 clusters of hits typically combine those for SBP and DBP. Two possible exceptions are QTL 7 that has two very strong hits both for DBP and the suggestive hit cluster on Ch 19p13-12 that has four hits all for SBP.

## Conclusions from Genome Scans

The previous analysis suggests that human primary HT has no widely penetrant genes of huge or even major effect dominating the genetic contribution to this disor-der; instead, there are multiple polygenes of modest effect. Human genome scans appear to have amassed suf-ficient evidence to identify up to 12 QTLs for HT/BP/HT-associated phenotypes of modest effect. Independent confirmation of these loci in more than one human genome scan and their overlap with regions syntenic to BP QTLs in mice, rats, or both (see Table 31-6) have pro-duced evidence highlighting certain loci (Table 31-7) for a role in BP and HT for humans, which is strongest over-all for QTL1 (Ch 2p11-q12), QTL5 (17q11-23 especially 17q21), QTL8 (6q14-16 especially 6q14), QTL9 (1q23-24), and QTL11 (5p15-12 especially 5p13); evidence is moderately strong for QTLs 4, 6, 7, and 12 and support-ive but weaker for QTL2 and 3 because, although both these loci were linked to human BP with significant LOD scores in their original reports, they have not been linked to it subsequently (although QTL2 overlaps a region syn-tenic to a BP QTL in rats). The final QTL (QTL10) has not been directly linked to human BP or HT originally or subsequently; the original linkage was to potentially related body fluid volume phenotypes. Thus, the status of this QTL in relation to human BP remains unsubstan-tiated, despite overlapping with a syntenic QTL for HT in rats. Likewise, a number of linkage hits falling short of significance individually have, by their repetitive occur-rence in tightly colocalized clusters especially on Ch19p13-12, 3p26 and regions of 7q11-31, raised the possibility of linkage to BP at these sites. These hits are reinforced and suggestive of linkage to human BP but require a more conclusive study to establish this at a genome-wide significant level. Overlap of the 19p and 7q sites with those syntenic to rodent QTLs for HT seems to corroborate their candidacy further.

## The Y Chromosome and Mitochondrial DNA

For several reasons genome-wide assessments have not included coverage of some areas of the genome, particu-larly for the Y chromosome and mitochondrial genome.

■ ■ ■

**TABLE 31-7** CONCLUSIONS ON LOCI SHOWING SIGNIFICANT LINKAGE (QTLS) OR MULTIPLE INSTANCES OF SUGGESTIVE LINKAGE (HIT CLUSTERS) TO BLOOD PRESSURE IN HUMANS

| Evidence | Good Evidence | | | Moderate Evidence | | Quite Weak, Unconfirmed | | Speculative, Suggestive Only | |
|---|---|---|---|---|---|---|---|---|---|
| QTL/ Cluster | Name | Locus | | Name | Locus | Name | Locus | Name | Locus |
| | | Interval | Core | | | | | | |
| | QTL1, | 2p11-q12 | | QTL4, | 15q26 | QTL2, | 3q24/25 | QTL10 | 3p21.31/(32) |
| | QTL5, | 17q11-23 | 17q21 | QTL6, | 18q21-22 | QTL3 | 3p16-15 | | |
| | QTL8, | 6q14-16 | 6q14 | QTL7, | 2q32 | | | Hit | 2q24.1 |
| | QTL9, | 1q24 | | QTL12 | 8q24 | | | Clusters | 3p26.3-25.3 |
| | QTL11. | 5p15-12 | 5p13 | | | | | | 7q11.21-23 |
| | | | | | | | | | 7q21.3-22.1 |
| | | | | | | | | | 7q31.32-32.2 |
| | | | | | | | | | 12q21.31-21.32 |
| | | | | | | | | | 19p13.3-12 |
| | | | | | | | | | Xp11.4 |

Inheritance patterns at such loci have their own unique aspects, and although this may complicate some aspects of analysis there are reasons not to neglect these portions of the genome that play special roles in male and maternally inherited effects.

In most assessments, between puberty and age 50 to 60 men have higher BP. One explanation relates to genetic effects on the Y chromosome. In rodent models, especially the SHR, reports of inherited male-accentuated HT have suggested an effect of Y chromosome loci.[433,434] Assessments of the importance of Y chromosome effects on BP were initially conflicting, but more recent work in rats has shown that Y chromosome loci can have important effects on SBP, DBP, and the risk of HT. The size of the effect reported varies and has often been larger for SBP, whereas the effect of salt loading has been somewhat variable. The most dramatic effects have been reported in the SHRSP strain in which SHRSP Y chromosome ancestry conferred significantly higher BP, with mean increments in BP over control WKY strain Y chromosome ancestry of 19.8 mm Hg (21 mm Hg on salt loading) for SBP and 14.6 mm Hg (15.8 mm Hg on salt loading) for DBP.[434] Others found more modest effects with less straightforward effects of salt loading. More recently, use of consomic strains (having control strain autosomes and the hypertensive strain Y chromosome and vice versa) that allowed effects of the SHR and SHRSP Y chromosome and autosomes to be separately assessed have confirmed that the Y chromosome does carry genetic variation (having effect on SBP and DBP in the SHR[435] and especially SHRSP[436] strains) and that these effects positively interact with other loci carried on the hypertensive strain autosomes. In such strains there is evidence that the Y chromosome affects plasma lipids,[435] the stress response, basal Na+ intake, noradrenaline content and turnover in heart and kidney, and urinary electrolyte responses including K+ excretion level and Na+/K+ ratios.[437]

In human HT subjects, one study from Japan found no association of a Y chromosome insertion polymorphism with HT.[438] However, two studies on white populations found significant association of a HindIII biallelic marker on the nonrecombinant region of Y with DBP in

Australian subjects[439] and with higher mean SBP (3.1 to 5 mm Hg) and DBP (1.4 to 2.6 mm Hg) in subjects from Scotland or Poland.[353] In the latter study, polymorphisms of the aldosterone synthase gene were also genotyped and a potential interaction with the Y chromosome locus was suggested because the combined Y(HindIII(+))/aldosterone synthase (−344T/−344T) genotype was significantly associated with HT (P = 0.023) with an odds ratio of 3.92 (CI 1.21 to 12.65). This possible interaction is interesting in view of the reports in animal models of Y chromosome loci affecting urinary K+ and Na+/K+ ratios[437] and salt sensitivity. A high-resolution scan of the Y chromosome in a suitably large human cohort for linkage with HT and effect on BP with and without salt loading would be of interest.

Mitochondrial DNA variations have recently been found to be significantly associated with HT in blacks with end-stage renal failure. Two nucleotide changes in the ND3 gene (at A10398G and A10086G) and a third in the CO1 gene (causing a HaeIII RFLP) are significantly associated with HT even after adjustment for the multiple comparisons made (P = 0.0038).[440] It is also known that mutations and variations of the mitochondrial genome can affect the risks of renal impairment (especially from focal segmental glomerulosclerosis[441]) and diabetes and its complications, which of course can all secondarily affect the risk of HT.

Markers of the Y chromosome and mitochondrial DNA should be included in genome scans. Analysis for appropriate inheritance patterns should be incorporated to allow detection of effects on BP and HT risk.

## SECONDARY HYPERTENSION AND SINGLE-GENE DISORDERS WITH PROMINENT HYPERTENSION

### Coarctation

In coarctation, localized aortic vessel narrowing, which reduces pressure and flow distally, can be (1) postductal (~95% cases), that is, between the origin of the ductus arteriosus and left subclavian artery; (2) preductal (~5%

cases, the majority presenting with serious problems in infancy), causing a larger diffuse narrowing upstream of the ductus arteriosus, which remains patent; or (3) elsewhere in the aorta (rare < 1%), which may be affected by less aortic-specific causes of stenoses in large arteries (e.g., fibromuscular dysplasia [FMD] or Takayasu's arteritis). In early childhood and especially in infancy, coarctation is a major cause of marked HT (up to 30% to 50%[442,443]), is commonly preductal, and is complicated by patent ductus arteriosus (PDA) and heart failure in particular. Later in childhood and early adolescence a second rise in incidence (of postductal cases) presents with HT. As many as 20% of cases present from later adolescence[442] into adulthood, although this becomes rare after 30 years of age. Fifty percent to 75% of all cases are associated with a bicuspid aortic valve. Preductal cases have associated PDA and less commonly patent septal defects and/or other features of a hypoplastic left heart,[442] whereas postductal and later presenting cases have such features much less often. Extracardiac associations include short stature, circle of Willis aneurysms, platelet abnormalities, and other clusters of features that are characteristic of a number of syndromes. Coarctation has a limited number of very strong syndromic associations with (1) Turner's syndrome (occurring in 1/2500 live female births and including 45X and 45X/46XY mosaicism), (2) other sex chromosome disorders with Turner's-like features (e.g., 46XYp[−444]), (3) Kabuki syndrome[445] (OMIM #147920) (most described in Japan, incidence of 1/32000 infants, and a significant minority having demonstrable Yp or X chromosome abnormalities), (4) Noonan's syndrome[446] (OMIM #163950) a largely autosomal dominant disorder (resulting from mutations of a nonreceptor tyrosine phosphatase SHP2 on Ch12q24.1) with some phenotypic overlap with Turner's syndrome. The incidence of congenital heart disease (CHD) (1/125 live births in the general population) and coarctation (6% to 7% CHD) is greatly increased in these syndromes; Turner's syndrome has 23% to 50% CHD rate, with 30% to 70% being clinically important coarctation largely post-truncal. In Kabuki syndrome, CHD occurs in 30% to 58%[445,447] of which coarctation makes up 20% to 25%.[445,447] CHD occurs in 50% to 70% of patients with Noonan's syndrome; coarctation is less prominent (8% to 9%)[446] than pulmonary stenosis (40% to 50%+).[446]

Coarctation and other CHD, with which it is most commonly associated (e.g., septal defects, PDA), can occur with hypoplastic left heart syndrome. This is linked to a region on 11q23-24[448] along with a platelet disorder (Paris-Trousseau type [PTT][449] and related abnormalities). Families with 11q23 deletion have PTT in association with isolated coarctation,[449] suggesting that genes linked to these CHD defects (including coarctation) map close to the locus 11q23-24 that causes this platelet disorder.[449] Interestingly, familial aortic aneurysm has now also been linked to 11q23.2-q24.1. Wilson et al.[450] reported a family that has a 22q11 deletion; three siblings have aortic arch abnormalities and two of these cases are coarctation. This implicates 22q11 as a potential locus for coarctation. There are other isolated families whose genetic analysis suggests mendelian inheritance involv-

ing coarctation; for example, in one family, familial coarctation involved four members in three generations. Currently no other studies reporting significant linkage in such families have been reported. Finally, a study has shown that the embryonic methylenetetrahydrofolate reductase (MTHFR, 1p36.3) 677T genotype has been significantly associated with the development of some forms of CHD; it is present in 9.2% of controls and 38% to 67% of those with coarctation[451] and other aortic and hypoplastic left heart abnormalities or pulmonary stenosis.

It has been proposed that compression of the aortic arch during development by distension of the thoracic lymph ducts[452] and cystic hygromas may be a mechanism of formation of coarctation especially in Turner's syndrome. Lymphedema is a characteristic feature of Turner's syndrome, and webbing of the neck is associated with increased frequency of coarctation[453] (e.g., in 25% with neck webbing and only 3% with normal neck).[452] Moreover, prevertebral cystic hygromas have been found in stillborn Turner's fetuses in association with generalized subcutaneous edema and coarctation. In Noonan's syndrome, lymphedema, neck webbing, and prenatal cystic hygromas are common; however, the spectrum of CHD is different, and it is unclear if particular lymphatic abnormalities associate with coarctation in Noonan's syndrome.

Thus, there seems to be an association of coarctation with sex chromosome abnormalities. Such cardiac abnormalities are rarer in those who are Turner-mosaics (45X:46XY). In Turner's syndrome the X chromosome is of maternal origin in two thirds and paternal in one third of cases; some studies found that maternal X is associated with both CHD and neck webbing but not with renal manifestations.[454] This suggests that a region of the maternal X subject to imprinting increases the risk of both lymphatic congestion and aortic and coarctation abnormalities but that this locus is "recessive" to paternal X (where the same locus would be imprinted differently) or Y, especially Yp (resulting from a second interacting gene). It will be of interest to know if coarctation with lymphatic abnormalities is seen in Kabuki's syndrome especially when associated with Yp or X (including ring X) chromosome abnormalities.

Thus, although the overall cause of coarctation is not clear, a proportion of coarctation is associated with syndromes, especially Turner's syndrome, and very rare familial occurrences. For the remainder of nonsyndromic, nonfamilial cases preductal or postductal coarctation is most likely to have resulted from environmental causes acting during development. The nature of such environmental triggers remains obscure apart from reports of a very small number of cases of gestational use of certain drugs including phenytoin and sodium valproate. There is no analysis of whether such environmental cases have any associated intrathoracic or mediastinal abnormalities related to lymphatic dysfunction. Clarifying the loci and identifying the genes contributing to the high rate of the syndromic coarctations will help identify populations susceptible to coarctation and enable the hunt for environmental factors that alter the penetrance of this feature of the syndromes. Factors relating to lymphatic abnormalities, thoracic and mediastinal developmental changes, or folate metabolism would be of particular interest.

## Renal Artery Stenosis

Renal artery stenosis of sufficient severity can promote HT by activating nonsuppressible renin release from the JG cells of downstream afferent arterioles. This in turn leads to higher AngII and aldosterone driving up BP via vasoconstriction and proximal nephron $Na^+$ reabsorption (AngII) and distal nephron $Na^+$ reabsorption (aldosterone). The rise in BP drives pressure natriuresis in the contralateral kidney and feeds back to downregulate renin (especially directly and via renal sympathetic innervation), suppressing it fully in the contralateral kidney but only partly in the "stenosis" kidney. This moderates BP rise, but this remains significant if the renal artery stenosis is severe, thus mimicking the situation in Goldblatt 2-kidney-1-clip (2K-1C) HT.[455,456] Moreover, the arterial stenosis causes renal ischemia and concomitant persisting nonsuppressible activation of the RAS, which can exacerbate the ischemic effects via AngII constriction of the efferent arteriole and limitation of peritubular blood flow and via profibrogenic actions of AngII in the renal interstitium. If the resulting HT is untreated, damaging changes occur in the nonstenosed kidney causing it to contribute to longer term maintenance of the HT. Finally, if the renal artery of the second kidney is also affected by stenotic changes, this exacerbates matters by limiting pressure-natriuresis, resulting in a higher volume state and increasing risks of bilateral renal ischemia and fibrotic interstitial damage depleting renal reserve further, thus mimicking Goldblatt HT with all renal arteries stenoses (i.e., Goldblatt −2K-2C or 1K-1C HT).[455,456]

The prevalence of significant renal artery stenosis is probably around 1% of HT generally. It is commoner in whites than in Afro-Caribbeans. In childhood, renal artery stenosis is not common, although as a proportionate cause of HT its prevalence is higher (<6%) than in adult HT. In the West, atherosclerosis is the commonest cause largely in older patients (>50 years), whereas FMD predominates from childhood to younger adulthood, especially in women aged 20 to 50, giving relative frequencies overall for adults of 2 to 3:1 for atherosclerosis-to-FMD depending on the age and gender mix.[457] In non-Western regions, especially in Asia, Takayasu's arteritis (a chronic inflammatory arteritis of the aorta and/or its large branches) is also a significant contributing cause in younger adults and adolescents (female > male, ratio varying geographically) and children, becoming the commonest cause in this younger age-group.[443] A high frequency of HLA B52 or B39 or their subhaplotypes have been found in Takayasu's arteritis, especially A24-B52-DR2 in Japanese, Indian, and Korean patients. Hence, the causation also varies with the region and ethnic mix of the population.

Atherosclerotic renal artery stenosis normally affects the proximal one third of the artery; 8% to 17% of stenoses progress to occlusion in 3 to 4 years.[458] Renal artery stenosis in FMD predominantly affects the distal two thirds with alternating stenoses and dilations corresponding to a "string of beads" appearance on angiography in most adult cases (~75%) and dysplastic and fibrotic changes in multiple vessel layers on histology, predominantly in the media. In this form of FMD, progression to occlusion is rare[459] and appears usually limited to renal arteries. However, FMD encompasses a wider spectrum and can be less benign with occlusive complications increasing the risk of associated accelerated phase HT, strokes, and MI in young patients. Less benign outcomes are associated with alternative radiographic appearances (single and multiple tight stenoses with no intervening dilation), alternative histologic appearances (predominantly intimal or periarterial fibroplasia), or involvement of multiple arterial beds. (FMD especially affects renal and carotid but also vertebral, iliac, subclavian and can involve visceral, cerebral or coronary arteries[459]).

The cause of FMD remains obscure, and it is possible that the spectrum of symptoms are different facets or stages of a single condition that seems best described as a (usually) low-grade noninflammatory arterial disease.[459] There are certainly indications of a subset with a familial basis when this has been investigated. Thus, radiologic screening of relatives of patients with angiographically demonstrated FMD revealed one or more first-degree relatives affected in 10% of cases (likely to be an underestimate of the familial prevalence[460]). Familial cases more often have bilateral renal artery stenosis. Rushton[461] analyzed 20 families with at least one documented FMD case and found that in 60% of families there were between 1 and 11 other family members with a clinical history strongly suggestive of FMD (e.g., strokes, MI, or other peripheral vascular symptoms or events at a young age), although investigations confirming these cases were not carried out. Both studies suggest an autosomal dominant inheritance with incomplete penetrance and an observed female preponderance (84%[460] and 60%[459]). One study that examined elastin gene polymorphisms reported no evidence of linkage to this locus in French families with FMD. Nonetheless, there is evidence of elastin defects associated with FMD. In explaining nongenetic occurrence for FMD, others have hypothesized mural ischemia (resulting from paucity of vasa vasorum), vessel wall traction/stress, effects of female hormones. and postinfectious (rubella) or inflammatory causes.[459]

FMD causing renal artery stenosis occurs in von Recklinghausen neurofibromatosis (NF1, caused by autosomal dominant mutations in neurofibromin 1, Ch 17q11.2) and is one of the causes of HT in this condition[462] especially in children, although approximately 30% of such cases occur in adults. One series found a 20% incidence of NF1 amongst 25 childhood cases of FMD. It has been hypothesized that NF1 associated Swann cell proliferation relates to the intimal ± medial dysplasia usually found. There are reports of FMD in three other autosomal dominant conditions involving mutations in vascular collagen (collagen type III, alpha-1 chain, Ch 2q31; Ehlers Danlos type IV, OMIM #130050), elastin (Ch 7q12, familial supravalvular aortic stenosis [SVAS] OMIM #185500), or the milder autosomal dominant form of cutis laxa (OMIM #123700). Further cases that involved FMD with renal artery stenosis and HT[154] are reported in Williams-Beuyrens syndrome (OMIM #194050), an autosomal dominant contiguous gene syndrome involving deletions within 7q11.23 that involves the elastin gene and usually has supravalvular aortic stenosis. These conditions raise the possibility that defects in structural proteins in such arteries are behind many more FMD cases. *In vitro* studies show that deficiencies and disruption in elastin increases the risk of vessel wall proliferation (by arterial smooth muscle cells) and segmental occlusive vessel disease by multilayer thickening of the tunica media and then formation of hyperplastic intimal lesions.[153] Elastin deficiency and disruption can, thus, lead to such FMD pathologies in familial SVAS, WBS, and cutis laxa. It is of interest that cutis laxa can be acquired on an autoimmune basis[463] and that *in vitro* TGFβ (a cytokine involved in the regulation of wound healing) can reverse the pathologic elastin deficiency in fibroblasts from congenital cutis laxa families by stabilizing its mRNA.[464] This suggests that susceptibility resulting from abnormal healing responses in arterial media would be a route whereby such FMD pathology may be acquired.

## Renal (Parenchymal) Disease

Given the central role of the kidney in long-term BP control it is not surprising that in a wide range of renal disease there is an associated rise in BP particularly when there is (1) widespread decrease in arterial pressure reaching the glomerular afferent arterioles, resulting from upstream afferent vascular resistance ($R_A$, triggering renin release in the supplied nephrons); or (2) a significant reduction in whole-kidney ultrafiltration coefficient ($K_F = k_fN$) either by deterioration in glomerular filtration per nephron (reducing single nephron ultrafiltration coefficients [$k_f$]) and filtration fraction across a substantial number of glomeruli and/or by reductions in nephron number (N, often then causing hyperfiltration with increased filtration fraction in the remaining nephrons); or (3) an inappropriate increase in the fractional reabsorption of $Na^+$ ($FR_{Na}$). All such pathologies lead to impairment of the maintenance of normal long-term BP control, and their relative contribution affects the extent to which there will likely be attendant raised renin, to maintain GFR, and the threat of ischemic nephropathy, glomerular HT and hyperfiltration (especially damaging in a shrinking nephron population), and salt sensitivity. The range of renal pathologies encompasses intrinsic renal vascular diseases, glomerulonephritis, renal cystic diseases, chronic pyelonephritis, reflux nephropathy, other tubulointerstitial diseases, and systemic diseases with renal involvement such as amyloid and diabetic nephropathy. Causes are equally diverse encompassing mendelian disorders, syndromic conditions, and disorders of complex cause (e.g., diabetic renal disease and focal segmental glomerulosclerosis [FSGS]) in which genetic factors in causation and susceptibility are currently being sought and identified (e.g., in FSGS[465,466] and IgA nephropathy).[467] Coverage of this topic in detail is beyond the scope of this chapter; thus, the reader is referred to general nephrology texts on specific renal diseases.[468]

Consideration of an important series of mendelian tubular disorders affecting $FR_{Na}$ and altering BP by salt retention (e.g., Liddle's syndrome) or salt loss causing hypotension (e.g., Bartter's syndrome) are mentioned in sections on mineralocorticoid excess/salt retention and renal pressure natriuresis.

### Vulnerability to Renal Damage

When renal pathology and coexisting HT worsen, it is of interest to know whether the HT causes the renal decline or the renal decline causes the HT. Where investigated there is major individual variability in the susceptibility to common forms of hypertensive renal injury such as worsening diabetic nephropathy. Some of these differences segregate strongly across ethnic and racial groups but have a substantial individually determined genetic basis predetermining the individual vulnerability to such injury. Thus, renal pathologies such as FSGN, often thought of as a "final common pathway" of renal injury from HT, and other conditions (e.g., diabetes) causing renal glomerular damage can develop as an inherited condition,[465,466] in which other causes of renal injury are absent and HT is not at all prominent. Such separation of the renal pathology from HT affords opportunities to identify causative genes and elucidate the interrelationships of such pathologies with HT. Other genetic factors related to the response to nephron loss (e.g., cyclin-dependent kinase inhibitor 1A [CDKN1A or p21, Ch 6p21.2]) have also been identified. Thus, p21 $-/-$ mice seem resistant to the usual spiraling renal decline following partial renal ablation.[469] Such studies shows some promise in elucidating genetic factors relating to the risk of spiraling renal decline and HT subsequent to renal damage. This could also be relevant to the lifetime risk of renal decline when there is reduced nephron number at birth,[180,184] which may occur in association with low birth weight related to fetal programing and may predispose to later HT.[180,182,184]

## Mineralocorticoid Excess and Salt Retention

The aldosterone-ENaC pathway regulating $Na^+$ reabsorption in the late distal tubule and CD is a primary BP control mechanism (Fig. 31-2) and has a very clear and powerful effect on long-term BP in humans. Primary abnormalities that alter pathway activity at any point cause BP disorders (Fig. 31-3); those that elevate pathway activity cause HT (with salt retention and predisposition to hypokalemic alkalosis), whereas those that reduce pathway activity cause secondary hypotension (with salt wasting and predisposition to hyperkalemic acidosis). Mineralocorticoid HT is always a form of low-renin HT. The excess mineralocorticoid drive is the primary abnormality in contrast to secondary aldosterone excess driven by high-renin states (e.g., rare renin-secreting tumors and to a variable degree in renal artery stenosis). Mineralocorticoid HT is thus a subset of low-renin HT, and it is the indices of primary aldosterone-ENaC overactivity that define this mineralocorticoid HT subset.

The disorders that may produce mineralocorticoid HT are shown in Table 31-8. All these disorders have

**TABLE 31-8** CONDITIONS THAT MAY PRODUCE HYPERTENSION SECONDARY TO MINERALOCORTICOID PATHWAY OVERACTIVITY

| A | Class of Abnormality | | Specific Condition | Steroid-Driving Effects | Rarity |
|---|---|---|---|---|---|
| 1a | Primary aldosteronism | | Adrenocortical (Conn's) adenoma, (AngII insensitive) | Aldosterone | Common |
| 1b | | | (AngII sensitive) | Aldosterone | Unusual |
| 2a | | | Idiopathic adrenocortical hyperplasia, bilateral, | Aldosterone | Common |
| 2b | | | unilateral | Aldosterone | Unusual |
| 3 | | Inherited (dominant) | Glucocorticoid-remediable aldosteronism (GRA, FH I) | Aldosterone | Unusual |
| 4 | | Inherited (?dominant) | Familial hyperaldosteronism type II (FH II) | Aldosterone | Unusual |
| 5 | | | Adrenocortical carcinoma | Aldosterone ±others | Rare |
| 6 | | | Extra-adrenal tumor | Aldosterone ±others | Very rare |
| 7 | Congenital adrenal hyperplasia | Inherited (recessive) | 11β-Hydroxylase deficiency | DOC? | Rare |
| 8 | | Inherited (recessive) | 17α-Hydroxylase deficiency | DOC + metabolites | Very rare |
| 9 | Primary DOC excess | | DOC-secreting tumor | DOC | Very rare |
| 10 | Mineralocorticoid spillover of severe circulating glucocorticoid excess | Ectopic ACTH syndrome | Paraneoplastic syndrome | Cortisol± corticosterone | Unusual |
| 11 | | Inherited (recessive) | Glucocorticoid resistance: GR mutation | ±Aldosterone | Very rare |

| B | Class of Abnormality | | Specific Condition | Steroid-Driving Effects | Rarity |
|---|---|---|---|---|---|
| 1 | Defective 11β-HSD2 activity | Inherited (recessive) | Syndrome of apparent mineralocorticoid excess (SAME) | Normal levels of cortisol ±corticosterone | Very rare |
| 2 | | Acquired, temporary | 11β-HSD2 inhibition: habitual licorice intake, carbenoxolone | | Unusual |
| 3 | Abnormal MR | Inherited (dominant) | MR S810L mutation | Normal progesterone ±cortisone levels | Very rare |
| 4 | Activating βγENaC mutations | Inherited (dominant) | Liddle's syndrome (PPXY motif + some loop mutations) | None | Very rare |

Most mineralocorticoid hypertension is due to Conn's tumors or idiopathic bilateral adrenal hyperplasia (Table 31-8A, 1a and 2a, respectively). Table 31-8A shows conditions in which the mineralocorticoid overactivity is *systemically driven* by circulating excess of a steroid with mineralocorticoid activity. Table 31-8B shows conditions in which the mineralocorticoid pathway overactivity and hypertension are *intrinsically driven* by alterations in pathway components in association with normal or low circulating steroid levels.

excessive mineralocorticoid signaling either *systemically driven* (Table 31-8, part A) by excess of a circulating steroid, usually aldosterone but alternatively others (e.g., deoxycorticosterone [DOC] in 11β hydroxylase deficiency; see steroid synthesis pathway shown in Fig. 31-8) or *intrinsically driven* (Table 31-8, part B) by molecular abnormalities within the pathway resulting in Na+ retention and HT feeding back to suppress circulating aldosterone. Thus, when mineralocorticoid HT is systemically driven, aldosterone or another steroid with mineralocorticoid activity is elevated, whereas in intrinsically driven mineralocorticoid HT there is no circulating mineralocorticoid excess. The names of these syndromes reflect this fact so that 11β-HSD2 deficiency is known as the syndrome of apparent mineralocorticoid excess (SAME), whereas activating mutations of ENaC cause Liddle's syndrome, a condition also known as pseudo(hyper)aldosteronism.

In the past, the presence of some degree of hypokalemic alkalosis was viewed as important in the diagnosis of min-

eralocorticoid HT, but today mineralocorticoid HT is seen as the commonest form of secondary HT.[146,470] There is no clear boundary between mineralocorticoid HT and low-renin essential HT. Thus, the point in the continuous spectrum of aldosterone-to-renin or urinary steroid ratios and spironolactone or amiloride responsiveness at which the line delimiting mineralocorticoid HT is drawn is controversial.[147,148,471] The role of the genes in the aldosterone-ENaC pathway in human primary HT is considered in sections on primary HT candidate genes. Some forms of low-renin HT involve overactivity of other renal salt reabsorption pathways in addition to that mediated by ENaC. The role that these play in long-term BP control is currently less certain and is discussed along with disorders affecting such other pathways (e.g., Gordon's, Gitelman's, and Bartter's syndromes; see the section on renal pressure natriuresis and Table 31-1). This section deals with HT seen as secondary to mineralocorticoid excess with some mention of the corresponding secondary hypotensive disorders (Fig. 31-3).

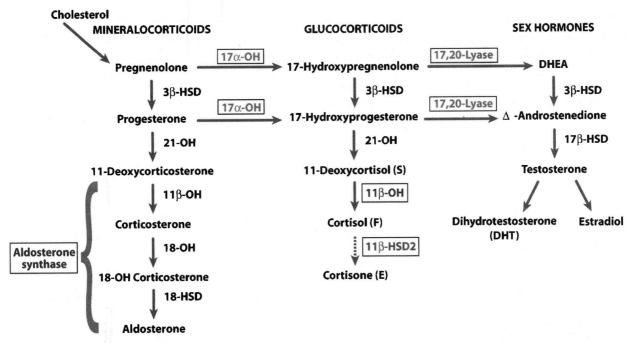

**FIGURE 31-8.** Steroid hormone synthetic pathways. Cholesterol metabolism gives rise to mineralocorticoids (aldosterone and DOC), gluco-corticoids (cortisol and corticosterone), and sex steroids through the sequential metabolic activity of steroid hydroxylases (OHs) and hydroxy-steroid dehydrogenases (HSDs). Congenital adrenal hyperplasia from impaired 17α-hydroxylase (17α-OH) or the final enzyme making cortisol 11β-hydroxylase (11β-OH) usually leads to raised mineralocorticoids and HT. In converting DOC to aldosterone the aldosterone synthase enzyme incorporates three steps, and these intermediates can give rise to useful marker 18-hydroxylated steroid such as 18OH cortisol especially when there is abnormal mineralocorticoid overproduction. The enzyme 11β-HSD2 is present in a range of tissues and inactivates physiologic glucocorti-coids.

## Primary Aldosteronism

This is the commonest form of mineralocorticoid excess. The primary abnormality, inappropriately high circulat-ing aldosterone levels that do not suppress normally, sys-temically drives Na$^+$ retention causing mineralocorticoid HT. Prevalence estimates for primary aldosteronism when hypokalemia was included in the diagnostic crite-ria varied from 0.05% to 2% of HT,[146,470] whereas with modern criteria that dispense with the need for hypokalemia this is the commonest form of secondary HT, with prevalence estimates ranging from 5% to 10% of those with HT[146,470] (higher in a referral center for resist-ant HT). Although the absolute numbers of subjects with HT considered to have primary aldosteronism has risen, it is not clear if this percentage really would apply across the large numbers with mild HT included by mod-ern guideline definitions of HT.[2,3,6] Primary aldostero-nism has mixed causes (Table 31-8) commonly (in >95% cases) resulting from either (1) an adrenocortical aldos-terone-producing adenoma (APA, or Conn's tumor that is almost always >90% AngII insensitive) or (2) idiopathic adrenal hyperplasia (IAH), often exhibiting multinodular characteristics and mostly bilateral. Rarely, it is due to autosomal dominant familial hyperaldosteronism (FH types I and II; FH I is GRA) or even more rarely from malignant tumors (adrenal carcinoma or extra-adrenal tumors). Distinguishing between these conditions is important because their management differs; surgery is usually best for tumors, and medical treatment differs between the common IAH (usually involving MR-blockade; e.g., spironolactone or eplerenone ± ENaC-blockade

with amiloride) and GRA, in which glucocorticoids also play a role. Much has been written about how to best distinguish the conditions giving rise to mineralocorti-coid HT in general and primary aldosteronism in partic-ular. This is relevant to considering these conditions, their discrimination from primary HT, and their causes. Thus, some brief comments are made on discriminating these conditions, but for detailed consideration of these matters other sources[147,470,472,473] should be consulted.

In primary mineralocorticoid HT, renin is suppressed. When this is due to primary aldosteronism, the aldosterone is inappropriately elevated in the face of (1) Na$^+$ retention and HT and (2) a serum K$^+$ that is not raised (but normal or low). The higher the BP and the lower the K$^+$ the clearer it is that aldosterone is inappropriately high and by inference not normally suppressible. For less clear-cut abnormalities with less resistant HT one can use the aldos-terone-to-renin ratio as a guide for when to screen further. The lack of standardized use of the aldosterone-to-renin ratio is currently a problem[148] to which there is no con-sensus solution, but some have begun to move toward standardizations (sample in morning, upright, K$^+$ replete, etc.[472]) and use of a ratio above approximately 900 as a threshold to prompt further screening (ratio of 700 to 900[472,473] with aldosterone in pmol/L and plasma renin activity in ng/mL/hour [25 to 32.5 ng/dL per mg/mL/hour]). Of course there should be more caution if the aldosterone is in the normal range because a high ratio may be more a reflection of low renin (or worse the renin assay quality) than aldosterone excess. Renin is more often proportionately low in the elderly and those on β-blockers.

Because more than 95% of primary aldosteronism is due to two common causes, Conn's tumors and IAH (Table 31-8, 1 and 2), distinguishing these is normally important, and there are several approaches. One useful approach exploits the fact that hyperplasia is more closely related to the normal aldosterone-producing zone of adrenal (zona glomerulosa, retaining some aldosterone response to AngII) than most Conn's tumors, which show some features of the cortisol-producing zone (zona fasciculata, being more responsive to ACTH). Moreover, Conn's tumors often possess enzymes to make both cortisol and aldosterone in the same cells (which does not normally happen). A useful marker of this mixed synthetic activity is overproduction of a "hybrid" steroid normally only seen at low levels—18 hydroxy cortisol (18OHF). ACTH is higher at 8 to 9 am than at noon, and AngII normally increases changing from supine (lying down for >30 minutes) to erect posture. A useful postural test allows the relative effects of AngII and ACTH on aldosterone to be compared. Classically in Conn's tumors or GRA 8 to 9 am supine aldosterone is greater than noon erect aldosterone (i.e., ACTH predominates), whereas the opposite (AngII predominant) is true in normal subjects and in IAH.[474] Performed carefully, this is certainly one of the best discriminators, which had an overall 85% predictive accuracy in a number of studies involving more than 200 surgically proven Conn's tumors.[475] In addition, 18OHF levels are highest in GRA[473,476] and higher in Conn's tumor patients than in IAH or in normal subjects.[476] Molecular tests are now readily available to amplify the hybrid gene in GRA. Aldosterone also exhibits a more complete glucocorticoid suppression in GRA. On imaging (CT or MRI scan of adrenals) both GRA and IAH usually show bilateral adrenal enlargement, whereas classically a unilateral lesion occurs in Conn's tumor. Imaging has improved but small tumors and incidental adrenal lumps can still be notoriously misleading. Thus, before surgery for a presumed Conn's tumor, it is often prudent to clarify by adrenal venous sampling that there is a unilateral source (the other adrenal being suppressed) and with spironolactone treatment to show that the HT is likely to respond to its removal. Although occasionally (≤10% to 15%) a Conn's adenoma is AngII responsive (aldosterone rising on standing, which may indicate a different cause) or IAH is unilateral, such cases are unusual and may similarly require assessment for a unilateral source and BP responsive to spironolactone. Thus, in distinguishing the causes of primary aldosteronism this approach is generally useful[477] and inherently suggests that different causes are at work in Conn's tumors and in IAH.

To date, no useful cytogenetic abnormalities, gene polymorphism associations, or candidate gene expression studies have revealed the pathologic processes responsible. Occasional cases of aldosterone-producing adrenocortical adenomas have been reported in multiple endocrine neoplasia type 1 (MEN 1) and Bechwith-Wiedmann syndrome. However, such tumors are rare in MEN 1, and loss of heterozygosity at the MEN 1 gene locus is probably not uncommon in later adrenal tumor progression and may not indicate an important etiologic link. Work on a familial form of Cushing's syndrome with adrenal nodular hyperplasia (Carney complex, with associated pigmentation and myxomas) has made progress in identifying a causative gene (protein kinase A regulatory subunit 1-alpha, PRKAR1A Ch 17q23-q24) relating to protein kinase A signaling.[478] Thus, a clear molecular pathway for the different types of hyperplasia giving rise to primary aldosteronism may soon be elucidated. Other factors apart from AngII, K+, and ACTH are known to influence adrenal release of aldosterone and/or related growth of the adrenal cortex. These include non-ACTH POMC peptides, vasopressin, dopamine (inhibition of aldosterone release via D2-like receptors), ANP, catecholamines, somatostatin, and other factors.[479] As yet attempts to define a change in receptor number or response to such mediators have not given consistent insight into the cause of Conn's tumors or IHA.

### Familial Hyperaldosteronism Type I (Glucocorticoid Remediable Aldosteronism, FH I) and Type II (FH II)

Among the large numbers of apparently sporadic cases of primary aldosteronism familial cases represent a minority (<approximately 5%, depending on the presence of large kindreds in the catchment area). GRA (or FH I) is an autosomal dominant disorder, resulting from a gene-conversion mutation that joins the 3′ end of aldosterone synthase gene (CYP11B2) to the promoter and 5′ end of the adjacent gene, 11β-hydroxylase (CYP11B1), see also Figure 31-8. (Both genes lie on Ch 8q21 and are highly [>90%] homologous.[28]) This functional chimeric gene synthesizes excess aldosterone, which drives HT, and is remediable by glucocorticoid treatment through suppression of ACTH action on the chimeric gene promoter. There is a marked overproduction of the unusual steroid marker 18OHF well above that usually seen in cases with Conn's adenoma. Reports have indicated that the homologous breakpoints allowing the chimeric recombination varied in site between different pedigrees but were always located somewhere between intron 2 and intron 4 of the CYP11B genes. *In vitro* studies have shown that, if the fusion was further 3′ into the CYP11B2 gene at intron 5, the chimeric gene lacks aldosterone synthase activity, indicating that residues crucial for this activity are present in CYP11B2 exon 5. Two changes to CYP11B1 (S288G in exon 5 and V320A in exon 6) are sufficient to convert this to an enzyme with aldosterone synthase activity, confirming that exon 5 (and 6) are crucial in defining the activity of these enzymes.[480]

In GRA pedigrees, HT shows incomplete penetrance, but it is nonetheless often marked at a young age even in childhood.[345,481] There is an increased risk of CVA especially from intracranial aneurysm and hemorrhage.[345,481,482] (This can be viewed as an additional feature of the disorder in at least some pedigrees.) Overall, HT in GRA appears more severe in males[482] and possibly when maternally inherited (and thus entailing aldosterone excess exposure *in utero*). Hypokalemia is typically absent in the majority of those having GRA.[344,345] It is important to appreciate that suppression of the hypothalamic-pituitary-adrenal axis does not always normalize BP in GRA and may reflect coexisting primary HT, effects of prior HT end-organ damage, or the observed phenomenon of autonomous aldosterone production in long-standing GRA. Thus, treatment of HT in GRA requires only partial suppression of ACTH.[482] Any residual HT does not require marked suppression of ACTH but requires alternative treatment such as reduced salt intake, MR-blockade (e.g., spironolactone/eplerenone), and/or ENaC-blockade (amiloride 5 to 30 mg/day).[472]

FH II is a different familial disorder with hyperaldosteronism that is not suppressible with glucocorticoid. It appears to have autosomal dominant inheritance but is otherwise biochemically and morphologically indistinguishable from apparently sporadic primary aldosteronism, and families with aldosterone-producing adenomas, IHA, or both within the pedigrees have been described. FH II has taken on a more defined nature recently, with reports of large kindreds and linkage to a locus on Ch 7p22.[343]

### Congenital Adrenal Hyperplasia from Deficiency of 11β-Hydroxylase or 17α-Hydroxylase Enzymes

HT is a common accompaniment in the 11β-hydroxylase and 17α-hydroxylase forms of congential adrenal hyperplasia. In 11β-hydroxylase (CYP11B1) deficiency, the glucocorticoids cortisol and corticosterone are not efficiently produced from 11-deoxycortisol and 11-deoxycorticosterone (DOC), respectively (Fig. 31-8). The reduced glucocorticoid feedback raises ACTH, which drives overproduction of adrenal glucocorticoid precursors and adrenal androgens. This results in masculinization, hirsutism, and amenorrhea in females; accelerated skeletal growth and maturation in both sexes; and precocious puberty in males. Affected homozygotes for this autosomal recessive condition occur at the overall rate of approximately 1/100,000 live births (up to 1/5000 in Jews from Morocco). Heterozygotes and those homozygous for the mild nonclassical form of the disorder are characteristically normotensive.[483] However, approximately two thirds of patients with severe classic 11β-hydroxylase deficiency have HT, often with onset in the first few years of life.[483] A minority have other signs of mineralocorticoid excess (hypokalemia, muscle weakness), which correlate poorly with BP. Glucocorticoid treatment of the condition reduces ACTH drive and HT, which like GRA may need additional treatment with spironolactone/amiloride. The cause of HT in 11β-hydroxylase deficiency is not very well understood. Renin and aldosterone levels are usually suppressed. Despite assumptions that the HT is driven by elevated DOC levels, these correlate poorly with BP.[483] Although DOC metabolites (e.g., 18-hydroxy DOC or 19-nor) may be more potent mineralocorticoids, these have not been shown to be elevated in 11β-hydroxylase deficiency, and, because they may require 11β-hydroxylase for their synthesis, scope for their overproduction is questionable[483] (although 19nor-DOC can result from extra-adrenal conversion[484]). Despite this uncertainty, the HT is assumed to be due to inappropriate elevation of a non-aldosterone mineralocorticoid (DOC ± metabolites) that is suppressed, along with the HT, by glucocorticoid treatment.

In the rare autosomal recessive disorder of 17α-hydroxylase deficiency there is blocked cortisol, adrenal androgen, and sex steroid production, whereas production of corticosterone and DOC and its 18OH and 19-nor metabolites is unimpaired (see Fig. 31-8) and driven to high levels by elevated ACTH, until corticosterone (a glucocorticoid normally circulating at approximately 10% of cortisol levels) levels allow some feedback inhibition of the ACTH drive.[485] The elevated DOC and its metabolites (thought to derive from 18OHase actions of CYP11B1) are seen as the basis for the HT (± hypokalemic tendency) that affects most patients.[485] This can present in infancy and be severe but typically develops or at least comes to attention at or after pubertal age when the consequences of the concomitant sex-steroid deficiency (pubertal failure, both sexes phenotypically female) bring unrecognized cases to medical attention. Treatment includes judicious replacement of sex steroids and is otherwise similar to the treatment in 11β-hydroxylase deficiency with the use of glucocorticoids to reduce ACTH drive and HT. In addition, there may be a benefit from supplementary eplerenone/amiloride treatment.[485] In affected kindreds a prenatal diagnosis allows minimization of the adverse consequences that can attend a late diagnosis.

### 11β-Hydroxysteroid Dehydrogenase Type 2 Deficiency(11β-HSD2): Syndrome of Apparent Mineralocorticoid Excess (SAME)

The important enzyme 11β-hydroxysteroid dehydrogenase type 2 (11β-HSD2) inactivates physiologic glucocorticoids (cortisol and corticosterone) leaving aldosterone unmetabolized[486,487] (Fig. 31-3). In mineralocorticoid target tissues such as the distal nephron there is abundant 11β-HSD2 expression,[486,488] which acts as a barrier allowing selective access by aldosterone to MR while eradicating the 100- to 1000-fold circulating excess of glucocorticoids. Because MR has equal affinity for aldosterone and these vastly more abundant glucocorticoids it is only because of this 11β-HSD2 prereceptor metabolism that normal mineralocorticoid regulation of renal Na+ reabsorption occurs.[489,490] In SAME, inactivating 11β-HSD2 mutations allow glucocorticoids to flood past to rossly overactivate the MR-ENaC pathway causing mineralocorticoid HT with Na+ retention and hypokalemia.[487] Renin, aldosterone, and other mineralocorticoids are also suppressed because the normal glucocorticoid levels that gain illicit access to distal nephron MR produce these features of apparent mineralocorticoid excess. A similar milder syndrome occurs in subjects taking carbenoxolone or excessive licorice, because both carbenoxolone and a related licorice-derivative, glycyrrhetic acid, strongly inhibit 11β-HSD2.[489,490] SAME is a rare autosomal recessive syndrome with severe HT, which usually presents in childhood or infancy and causes considerable morbidity if untreated. There are reports of CVAs at young ages and often marked hypokalemia (with some reports of consequent rhabdomyolysis).[487] The impaired cortisol inactivation is reflected in an elevated plasma half-life of cortisol (from normal of ~80 minutes to 120 to >190 minutes in SAME patients). The diagnosis of impaired 11β-HSD2 activity is most often made on urinary steroid metabolite ratios; reflecting its action, an elevated tetrahydrocortisol WD + allotetrahydrocortisol/tetrahydrocortisone (THF+alloTHF/THE) or perhaps a urinary free cortisol/ free cortisone ratio (E/F) are used.[487] 11β-HSD2 −/− knockout mice share the features of SAME in humans with increased mortality, marked HT, and hypokalemic tendency.[491] In humans, the severity of the 11β-HSD2 defect correlates well with the age of presentation and biochemical abnormalities in SAME patients but not with mean BP, SBP, or DBP.[487] Recently, a rare case in which a patient with SAME developed renal failure and had a renal transplant was reported. The transplantation resolved the features of SAME and corrected the underlying disorder,[492] thus confirming the pathophysiology of the condition in humans.

### Activating Mutations of MR and ENaC (Liddle's Syndrome)

Recently, a unique family with an activating mutation of MR (S810L) was reported to result in an autosomal dominant form of mineralocorticoid HT; the mutant showed 25% of maximal constitutive activation in the absence of ligand and remarkably an altered spectrum of activating steroids that is now known to include progesterone, cortisone, and spironolactone.[493] The strong $MR_{S810L}$ activation by progesterone led to the presentation of very severe HT in late pregnancy[493] (when progesterone concentrations are highest), although it seems that the HT in men and nonpregnant women may at least partly relate to chronic MR activation via binding of cortisone (a steroid not causing significant activation of normal wild-type MR).[494]

Liddle's syndrome is a rare autosomal dominant condition resulting from mutations that activate ENaC conductance, causing excess $Na^+$ reabsorption, HT, and a tendency to hypokalemia. The responsible activating mutations affect a short PPXY amino acid motif in a near C-terminal segment of the β or γENaC subunits and increase ENaC surface half-life and conductance, causing HT[28,495] (see Fig. 31-3). Recently, a Liddle's-like phenotype was reported for a differently cited γENaC subunit mutation (N530S in the extracellular loop) that increased ENaC conductance and that was proposed to cause HT by increasing ENaC open probability.[362] Gene-targeted mice carrying a βENaC Liddle's mutation develop salt-sensitive mineralocorticoid HT with hypokalemia,[495] although the relatively low expression level of the Liddle's β-ENaC subunit in these mice (probably for technical reasons relating to the gene targeting) resulted in the mice having a mild phenotype. The PPXY motif in ENaC subunits is now known to be the site of protein-protein interaction between the ENaC subunits and a ubiquitin ligase NEDD4-2 that participates in regulating the retrieval of ENaC from the apical membrane and in regulating the channel half-life.[371] One can see that mutations in NEDD4-2 could potentially alter BP, and, thus, there is active interest in identifying further genes regulating ENaC and its surface expression. Another such gene is

sgk1, a kinase that is upregulated by aldosterone in renal CD[30]; when knocked out in mice it causes low BP[31] and is related to surface expression of EnaC.[371] Treatment of these activating mutation causes of mineralocorticoid HT involves use of amiloride, salt restriction, and $K^+$ supplementation.

### Other Causes of Mineralocorticoid-Like HT or Conversely Mineralocorticoid Insufficiency/Salt Wasting and Lower BP

Rarely, adrenocortical tumors that make DOC rather than aldosterone as the principal steroid occur. This has been reported for adrenocortical adenoma, hyperplasia, and carcinoma. HT occurs in 80% or more of those with Cushing's syndrome because of glucocorticoid excess, and this is especially likely to exhibit mineralocorticoid HT-related features (hypokalemia, volume expansion, $Na^+$ retention, alkalosis, etc.) in ectopic ACTH syndrome.[496] This relates in part to the higher average glucocorticoid levels attending such cases of Cushing's syndrome, which overwhelm the 11βHSD2 barrier in cortisol inactivation overload.[496] An additional contribution to their mineralocorticoid nature from cosecretion of other mineralocorticoids seems likely from these more malignant tumors. Cushing's syndrome has other features that contribute to HT such as upregulation of angiotensinogen, increased insulin resistance, and greater risks of obesity. In more slowly developing, pituitary-dependent Cushing's syndrome, these factors and comorbid obesity are typically more prominent and the HT bears less mineralocorticoid excess features than in typical ectopic ACTH cases without marked obesity. Familial or sporadic glucocorticoid resistance is characterized by elevated cortisol with or without minimal stigmata of Cushing's syndrome, and many such patients present with HT, with or without hypokalemic alkalosis.[497] The elevated cortisol and resistance of ACTH to feedback lead to elevated ACTH levels, which drive the increase of other salt-retaining steroids (e.g., DOC) probably acting together with high cortisol levels, through MR. Mutations have been identified (both in familial and sporadic cases) in the ligand-binding domain of GR, including cases with autosomal dominant inheritance resulting from $GR\alpha_{1559N}$ (causing retention of GR in the cytoplasm) or $GR\alpha_{1747M}$ (disturbing normal coactivator/corepressor interactions at the GR AF2 region).[497] Treatment of glucocorticoid resistance usually involves dexamethasone ± some MR blockade treatment to reduce ACTH and limit mineralocorticoid HT.

As shown in Figure 31-3 many of the causes producing mineralocorticoid HT have corresponding opposites in which there is mineralocorticoid insufficiency and salt wasting and lower BP. Thus, inactivating mutations of aldosterone synthase (CYP11B2) cause lower BP, salt wasting, and hyperkalemia in a very rare autosomal recessive syndrome.[346] Severe mutations in congenital adrenal hyperplasia affecting the mineralocorticoid branch of adrenal steroid synthesis also cause such salt wasting; the commonest such disorder is severe 21-hydroxylase deficiency. Similarly, pseudohypoaldosteronism type I (PHA I) resulting from inactivating mutations in MR or ENaC (any of the three subunits) all cause similar salt-wasting low BP and tendency to hyperkalemic acidosis, but aldosterone is raised in these mineralocorticoid-resistant states (hence, the term pseudohypoaldosteronism). The PHA I syndrome resulting from inactivating MR mutations is autosomal dominant. Symptoms are most severe in the early postnatal months, after which the condition becomes milder[498] indicating that MR is important at this early stage when the other renal salt-conserving mechanisms (especially in PT) are immature. MR has been knocked out in mice, and, although MR +/− are well, MR −/− mice develop PHA I with salt wasting and hypotension and die[499] unless given a forced high-salt intake, which permits survival to adulthood, when they display increased $Na^+$ loss and tendency to hyperkalemia[500] that is exacerbated by a low-salt diet. The renal ENaC activity is greatly reduced in MR −/− mice, but there is only minor if any downregulation of ENaC subunit mRNAs[499] confirming that other mineralocorticoid regulated genes are key in the normal activation of ENaC to permit normal regulation of $Na^+$ absorption and BP. In these mice, glucocorticoids can induce a similar but weaker induction (25% to 50% of that for MR +/+ mice) of ENaC and ENaC-mediated current in kidney and colon,[500] but it is clear that elevation of glucocorticoid levels alone is insufficient to allow survival of the MR −/− mice. In some dominant PHA I cases no MR mutations have been found.[498] Inactivating mutations of any of the subunits of ENaC cause autosomal recessive PHA I in humans[501] with more severe salt wasting and hypotension than in the dominant cases. Again knockout of the corresponding genes in mice produces PHA I[495] (although ENaCα −/− mice also suffer a more severe lung abnormality not seen in the severe form in humans). Hence, it is clear that reduced activity of the aldosterone-ENaC pathway at any stage causes reduced BP and salt wasting in both humans and animals.

## Pheochromocytoma and Paraganglioma

The SNS originates from neural crest, giving rise to neuroblasts, sympathetic ganglion progenitors, and chromaffin tissue. Tumors of all these lineages may produce hypertensive catecholamines (especially noradrenaline), although amounts are usually modest in neuroblastoma and ganglioblastoma (tumors rarely seen outside childhood). There may be coproduction of hypotensive catecholamines (especially dopamine), especially in neuroblastoma. Accordingly, significant HT is much less consistently a feature of these tumors than in it is in pheochromocytomas. Pheochromocytoma is the major type of catecholamine-producing tumor. Surgical removal is usually curative, whereas undiagnosed it eventually has a high morbidity and mortality. Pheochromocytomas can arise at any age from chromaffin tissue of the adrenal medulla (85% of cases) or less commonly extra-adrenally and proximate to SNS ganglia (paragangliomas). They produce excess noradrenaline and/or adrenaline. They cause HT and/or paroxysmal features such as rapid rises in BP, headache, tachycardia, palpitations, and anxiety. One large study found that 60% to 65% of patients with pheochromocytoma had sustained HT, half with superimposed paroxysmal features, and an additional 25% had HT only during paroxysms.

Normally in the SNS, active catecholamines are stored in vesicles and their release is regulated centrally such as during "flight or fight responses" to stressful or threatening situations or by reflexes such as the baroreflex that regulates BP across postural changes. In pheochromocytoma, active catecholamine production and release is not dependent on normal controls and usually shows a net increase, which is partly constitutive and exhibits inappropriate episodic discharges (which can cause dramatic spikes in circulating catecholamines). Increase in tumor catecholamine synthetic enzymes without increase, indeed a decrease, in catecholamine degradation and vesicle numbers produces a constitutive spillover of the active catecholamines in excess of vesicle capacity into the circulation. Tumor discharge of catecholamines may be inappropriately triggered by stimuli such as direct pressure, pharmacologic treatments, and so forth. Moreover, concomitant dysregulation of SNS reflexes may contribute to overall elevated noradrenaline release, but because of a lack of normal postural reflex modulation, postural hypotension is a common symptom. Elevated circulating noradrenaline predominates and via α-adrenergic receptor pathways leads to long-term HT with elevation in SBP and DBP; TPR is increased and plasma volume reduced if elevated BP is sustained.

Tumors with elevated adrenaline are usually well differentiated, hyperplastic, and adrenal or rarely infra-aortic or para-aortic (at the site of the organ of Zuckerkandl, a mass of SNS tissue that normally regresses after birth). With corelease of adrenaline, β-adrenergic effects of tachycardia, palpitations, apprehension, sweating and widening of pulse pressure become more prominent, especially in paroxysmal symptoms that follow discharge from adrenal pheochromocytomas. Rarely, dopamine is coreleased, suggesting a less differentiated or frankly malignant tumor, which may cause episodic hypotension through its natriuretic and other hypotensive properties.

Most estimates attribute 0.1% to 1% of HT to pheochromocytoma. Autosomal dominant inheritance is seen in 10% to 20% of cases, either as an isolated pathology or with other features indicating multiple endocrine neoplasia type 2 (MEN 2), VHL, less commonly NF1, or very rarely in other syndromes with neurocutaneous associations (e.g., tuberose sclerosis, ataxia telangiectasia, or Sturge-Weber syndrome). The elucidation of the genes causing these conditions allows insight into causation of pheochromocytoma and allows assessments of the extent to which these genes are mutated in cases of isolated familial or apparently sporadic pheochromocytomas. Early studies suggest that 8% to 23% of apparently sporadic pheochromocytomas may harbor MEN 2 or VHL mutations and that in some VHL families (with missense VHL mutations) pheochromocytomas may be the only feature.[502] In all these syndromes the mutated genes are tumor suppressors, typically those that affected inheritance of one mutated copy and the loss of the other copy through a subsequent somatic mutation (indicated by loss of heterozygosity [LoH]) giving rise to the hyperplasias and tumors of the syndromes. Thus, in neurofibromatosis, pheochromocytomas almost invariably show LoH for NF1, whereas ret gene LoH has been noted in pheochromocytomas in MEN 2. One study on pheochromocytomas in VHL found 45% LoH in the VHL gene, and one third of the others had hypermethylation of the wild-type VHL allele, attenuating expression and effectively causing LoH. Moreover, loss of additional tumor suppressor genes appears common in pheochromocytomas (e.g., NF1 expression is reduced or absent in 25% to 50% of familial non-NF1 pheochromocytomas, including VHL and MEN 2). High rates of loss of the p53 tumor suppressor gene is reported in multiple and malignant pheochromocytomas. Several cytogenetic abnormalities associate with pheochromocytomas in particular (1) in sporadic pheochromocytomas LoH at Ch 1p (42% to 71%), 3p (16% to 24%, VHL is at 3p26), 17p (24%), 21q (53%), or 22q (31%) are all often found[503,504]; (2) in pheochromocytomas in NF1, LOH at 14q32-ter is common (40%) and may occur in other pheochromocytomas; (3) pheochromocytomas in VHL have LOH at Ch11 loci; and (4) MEN 2 have loci at 1p, 3p, 6, or 22q.[503,504] It is hoped that identification of tumor suppressor genes at these loci will lead to a better understanding of the underlying processes, pathogenesis, and phenotypic behavior of pheochromocytomas. The latter Ch 11 finding is of interest because two maternally imprinted loci are now identified on 11q, mutation of which predisposes to nonchromaffin paragangliomas (which may nonetheless be associated with catecholamine secretion and HT).

Most pheochromocytomas appear sporadically but at least 20% to 25% have an inherited basis, and the proportion is much higher if they are multiple, affect the adrenals bilaterally, or arise in unusual extra-adrenal sites.[502] The syndromes most commonly responsible are all autosomal dominant, and, thus, the chances of other affected family members is high. With appropriate genetic testing and screening other syndromic pathologies may be detected early. As the understanding of the molecular basis of these syndromes advances it will also elucidate the basis of more general pheochromocytoma and associated HT. Syndromes with which pheochromocytoma is associated include MEN 2 (both MEN 2a and MEN 2b); VHL with missense mutations and paraganglioma-pheochromocytoma syndromes[502]; less commonly NF1; and rarely other neuroectodermal syndromes of tuberous sclerosis, ataxia telangiectasia, and Sturge-Weber syndrome (all autosomal dominant). Association of pheochromocytoma in the Carney triad (extra-adrenal pheochromocytoma [or paraganglioma], gastric leiomyosarcoma, and pulmonary chondroma) appears to be sporadic and to affect young women.[505] Importantly, one recent study of 217 apparently nonfamilial, nonsyndromic pheochromocytomas found that 66 (24.5%) had germline mutations for VHL (11%), MEN 2 (5%), or paraganglioma-pheochromocytoma syndromes (SDHB [4%], SDHD [4-5%], see later).

## MEN 2

MEN 2 is an autosomal dominant syndrome in which 50% of patients have pheochromocytomas and virtually 100% develop medullary carcinoma of the thyroid. It is subtyped on the basis of other features: hyperparathyroidism or cutaneous amyloid in MEN 2a or marfanoid habitus and intestinal/mucosal ganglionoma/neuroma in MEN 2b in which medullary carcinoma of the thyroid is prone to early spread. MEN 2 is due to mutation in the Ret proto-oncogene with the site of the mutation determining the 2A/2B phenotype on human chromosome 10q11. This gene consists of 21 exons and encodes a 150 to 170 kd transmembrane protein with alternatively spliced and glycosylated forms. Ret is a receptor tyrosine kinase, which is one subunit of a receptor monomer to which glial-derived neurotrophic factor (GDNF) binds. The other ret-associated subunit forming the receptor monomer is an extracellular membrane anchored protein called GFRα-1 (GDNF receptor α-1). Other possible ligands at the ret-GRF are the peptides neuturin, persephin, and artemin.[506] GDNF binds two ret-GFRα-1 monomers and the resulting receptor dimer has intracellular tyrosine kinase activity, which is important in signal transduction relating to Ras and GTP hydrolysis. Such signaling via ret has been shown to have a number of effects, including changes in cell-cell interactions, growth, and differentiation. Both subtypes of MEN 2 are caused by mutations of ret but in different regions with MEN 2a having mutations of the cysteine residues of the extracellular ligand binding domain, whereas in MEN 2b the intracellular tyrosine kinase active site is mutated. Pheochromocytomas in MEN 2 are usually adrenal (extra-adrenal is rare), are often bilateral, often are associated with adrenal medullary nodular hyperplasia, and most often, secrete a high proportion of adrenaline and exhibit paroxysms. Malignancy is rare but reported.[502] The high adrenaline ratio (which can be useful in screening in MEN 2) is in keeping with palpitations and anxiety attacks that often predate problematic HT, by which time a larger tumor and unequivocally elevated urinary metabolites of adrenaline ± noradrenaline are common. The increased proportion of adrenaline indicates a likely role of ret in regulation of the enzyme para-N-methyl transferase (PNMT) converting noradrenaline into adrenaline. Ret mutations producing MEN 2a account for approximately 90% of germline mutations described in MEN 2 families, especially in codon 634; the MEN 2b cases (<10% of MEN 2) predominantly have mutations at codon 918. Analysis of DNA from sporadic pheochromocytomas indicates an 8% prevalence of ret mutations[502] and a proportionately higher representation of MEN 2b mutations than in the MEN 2b family germline mutations.

## Von Hippel Lindau

VHL is an autosomal dominant syndrome, is estimated as present in 1 in approximately 40,000 live births, and is especially associated with CNS hemangioblastomas and retinal angiomas and less consistently with renal and pancreatic cysts and occasionally with tumors. Pheochromocytoma is a feature in 10% to 20% of cases, but it occurs with very different frequencies across kindreds. In contrast within a kindred the prevalence rate of pheochromocytomas is consistent, either very unlikely or very common; some families have a 90% prevalence of pheochromocytomas, which may be the dominant or only manifestation. The gene mutated in VHL is on chromosome 3p25-26 and is relatively small, consisting of three exons and encoding a 283 amino acid protein. The gene functions as a tumor suppressor and has roles in signaling hypoxic effects on gene expression and angiogenesis. More than 300 germline mutations causing VHL have been reported across all three exons, but only approximately 10% of these in kindreds with pheochromocytomas and most missense mutations are in this subset (especially at codon 238). The other features of VHL seem to dominate, and pheochromocytoma is rare when there are other more drastic mutations (deletions, frameshifts, and nonsense mutations).

The VHL protein binds to transcription factors (elongin b, elongin c, Cullin2, and rbx-1; all bind a region often mutated in VHL), which inhibit transcription that is upregulated in hypoxia. Loss of VHL is associated with upregulation of hypoxia-induced pathways, including inappropriate accumulation of VEGF or other factors that promote angiogenesis in keeping with the hypervascular pathology of VHL. Pheochromocytomas in VHL have primarily an elevation in noradrenaline and may be multiple. They are more commonly extra-adrenal or malignant than those in MEN 2 are. Screening sporadic pheochromocytoma patients has revealed 8% to 20% prevalence of germline VHL mutations.[502] Because VHL is usually seen as a condition with high penetrance, these reports, if replicated, have considerable implications for family members. In addition, VHL must be considered in patients who have what is assumed to be sporadic pheochromocytomas.

### Neurofibromatosis Type 1 (NF1)

NF1 is an autosomal dominant condition in which the tumor suppressor gene neurofibromin on chromosome 17q12 is mutated, giving rise to a number of features, in particular the formation of neurofibromas along the course of peripheral nerves and café au lait spots—both of which are seen on the skin. Pheochromocytomas arise in approximately 1% of cases of NF1; however, among those with HT the prevalence may be higher than 50%.[507] Pheochromocytomas in NF1 usually make both noradrenaline and adrenaline, are most commonly adrenal, and rarely occur outside the abdomen. Mice rarely develop pheochromocytomas, but those heterozygous for NF1 knockout (NF1 +/−) have a strongly increased prevalence of pheochromocytomas. NF1 expression is reduced or absent in 25% to 50% of cases of familial pheochromocytomas (including MEN 2 and VHL).

### Mitochondrial Complex 2 Subunits: Paraganglioma-Pheochromocytoma Syndromes

Paraganglioma is a term used to indicate extra-adrenal paraganglia-related tumors and may be used to refer to extra-adrenal pheochromocytomas or other nonchromaffin paragangliomas such as those more vascular tumors arising from tiny anatomically dispersed paraganglia located at the base of the skull and temporal bone (glomus jugulare tumors) or most commonly related to the carotid bifurcation and its associated chemoreceptors (carotid body tumors, chemodectomas).[508,509] It has recently been found that germline mutations in three of the four subunits (succinate dehydrogenase—ubiquinone oxoreductase complex subunits B, C, or D [SDHB, SDHC, and SDHD]) comprising complex II of the mitochondrial respiratory chain are responsible for cases of familial nonchromaffin paragangliomas and associated pheochromocytomas (especially extra-adrenal[509,510]). Mutations in two of the subunits (SDHB and SDHD) are common, whereas reports of cases involving the third subunit (SDHC) remain extremely rare. In addition to familial cases, germline mutations in the three SDH complex II subunits have been found in approximately 20% of unselected patients with apparently sporadic paraganglioma, and approximately 8% of patients with apparently sporadic pheochromocytomas have germline mutations in SDHB or SDHD.[502]

In familial cases, inheritance is consistent with an autosomal dominant pattern for subunits SDHB on chromosome 1p36.1-p35 and SDHC on 1q21 but shows parental restricted dominant inheritance consistent with maternal imprinting for the third subunit (SDHD on 11q23) and also for an as yet unidentified gene at a similarly maternally imprinted positioned locus more proximally on 11q (localized to 11q13.1, LOD score 7.6) that also is involved in causation of paraganglioma. The two loci on 11q are of particular interest because the imprinting is not body wide; thus, there is restricted paternal only (monoallelic) expression in paraganglioma and carotid body cells, whereas both maternal and paternal alleles (biallelic) are expressed in several other tissues examined (lymphocytes, brain, kidney).[511] Such tissue-restricted imprinting is found in other syndromes such as brain-limited imprinting of the UBE3A gene in Angleman's syndrome. Moreover, it is proposed the two 11q loci are tumor suppressor genes, and loss of both is required for tumor formation (paraganglioma or pheochromocytomas). Thus, the maternal copy of each is lost by imprinting, the paternal copy of one is mutated in the germline mutations found, and it is predicted that the final hit to allow tumor formation will, thus, be a somatic mutation and loss at the complementary 11q locus within the tumors. Limited studies suggest that this may be the case but do not conclusively prove that the two loci on 11q represent a true digenic disorder (comparable to one digenic form of retinitis pigmentosa in which a mutation in each of two genes, RDS and ROM1, was causative).

The discovery that pheochromocytomas are caused by defects in the three genes (SDHB, SDHC, and SDHD) and the associated 11q13 gene is a recent finding. The role of these genes in causation of pheochromocytomas is under assessment. Already it is clear that SDHB and SDHD mutations cause adrenal and extra-adrenal pheochromocytomas with or without apparent associated nonchromaffin paragangliomas. As yet cases arising from mutations of SDHC or the 11q13 locus are too rare to be sure about the spectrum of disease resulting.

The parallels are striking between the effects of mutations in these SDH subunits and in effects of VHL gene mutations. Both cause a syndrome with pheochromocytomas in association with highly vascular tumors, especially of the head and neck. Both genes are involved in pathways affected by hypoxia. Mitochondrial complex enzymes have been involved in oxygen sensing in the carotid body (chemoreceptors), and such vascular paragangliomas are mirrored by hypertrophy (and increased tumor incidence) at the same sites occurring in some chronic hypoxic states (e.g., associated with respiratory insufficiency or high altitude).[512,513] Of course the fact that the chemoreceptor reflex is one of the fundamental mechanisms that can be involved in regulation of BP (Fig. 31-2) makes the pathway in which the SDHB, SDHC, and SDHD subunits participate of considerable interest because alterations in this pathway could have a bearing on HT more generally if it rendered the chemoreceptor reflex constitutively overactive.

## Obstructive Sleep Apnea (OSA)

OSA is a condition that appears surprisingly common[134,514] and particularly affects those with upper body obesity especially with increased neck circumference. During sleep the upper airway tone allows the airway to collapse at the end of expiration, thus obstructing inspiration. There follows an apneic period of ongoing inspiratory effort against the obstructed airway (resembling a Müller maneuver: inspiration against a closed glottis) during which negative intrathoracic pressure increases enhancing venous return, and some hypoxia and hypercapnia develop. Eventually the apnea is terminated by arousal from sleep and re-establishment of increased tone and movement in the upper airway allowing inspiration. Consequently, sleep is often disturbed, and there is accompanying daytime sleepiness (again with obstructive apnea). Intermittent hypoxia and hypercapnia are associated with increased SNS activation with raised TPR and HT. The mechanisms that produce the high rate of systemic HT in OSA (which is close to 50%[514]) appear to relate to both OSA effects and the usual comorbid obesity. Certainly the rate of HT is higher in OSA (~50%) than in comparable obese subjects without OSA (~20%).[514] Overall, treatment studies of OSA show a concomitant reduction in HT[133,134] with the use of CPAP, surgical treatments of tracheostomy or uvulopalatopharyngoplasty, or even postural therapy, whereas weight reduction has perhaps an even greater benefit in lowering BP.[515] A degree of secondary polycythemia may develop in OSA but is rarely more than minor and is unlikely to contribute substantially to HT. Finally, reduction in growth hormone levels is reported to often accompany OSA and is linked to the development of upper body obesity and insulin resistance, whereas treatment of OSA restored GH levels to normal. This may, thus, represent a link between OSA and the development of accompanying obesity. The way in which OSA hypoxia, hypercapnia, and apnea are linked to 24-hour SNS activation is discussed in the section on the role of the SNS is CNS in HT. The mechanisms of obesity-driven HT are also discussed separately. It seems that a tendency to OSA and coincident weight gain are powerful coamplifiers, largely through the increase in SNS activation

and TPR to raise BP. In OSA, swings in BP, $pO_2$, and vasoconstriction may predispose to subtle changes in the kidney, as do mechanisms of renal interstitial deposits,[149] and predisposition to glomerular hyperfiltration[516] that are proposed in obesity. However, no studies describing renal function changes as HT develops in OSA or responds to its treatment are available. Finally, a number of conditions predispose to OSA, especially those causing upper body obesity such as the common metabolic syndrome and other uncommon conditions with upper airway laxity or structural changes (e.g., Hallermann-Streiff syndrome) including conditions such as achondroplasia, an autosomal dominant disorder caused by mutations in the FGF-R3 gene on chromosome 4p16.3 causing nonsymmetrical dwarfism and increased OSA. No genetic factors directly associated with commoner nonsyndromic OSA have been identified.

## OTHER COMPLEX TRAITS WHERE MARKED HT IS COMMONLY ASSOCIATED

### Obesity

It has been appreciated for many years that the genetic contribution to obesity is substantial and estimated at 50% to 70%. It is now clear that the causes of obesity encompass common obesity, another complex polygenic trait, and rare single-gene disorders, such as deficiencies in the signaling pathway of leptin and syndromes in which obesity is one of often many striking features (e.g., Prader Willi or Bardet Biedl syndromes). The metabolic syndrome appears most likely a product of Western environment and lifestyle (high calorie intake, relative physical inactivity, etc.). In this environment common genetic factors confer vulnerability to comorbidities from obesity, insulin resistance, HT, and dyslipidemia, which commonly cross-amplify one another such that their coincidence is the rule. Nonetheless, the underlying susceptibility to each of these comorbid features varies such that among the spectrum there are communities or kindreds in which one or more of the features such as insulin resistance or HT is totally absent although the others are strikingly present. Approaches to study the causation to identify genes involved in the metabolic syndrome as a whole are underway, as are efforts to do the same when each comorbid feature is proportionately prominent or occurs in isolation. One useful explanation of why HT and obesity are so common in the West sees the root causes in ancestral selection pressure for a "thrifty genotype." Thus, in ancestral times, genes promoting appetite and reducing BMR are likely to have conferred a survival advantage especially in times of famine and illness, whereas diet-induced thermogenesis may have been disadvantageous in very hot climates. These survival traits will predispose to obesity in a Westernized environment. A similar survival advantage is likely from genes allowing efficient conservation of salt (and, thus, ECF volume because primitive diets are low in salt). In very hot and dry climates this may even have extended to an advantage in suppression of normal natriuretic responses or in the propensity to develop mild salt-retaining nephropathy after adult maturity when obligatory water and salt loss would normally rise somewhat from related renal changes. These survival traits will predispose to HT and obesity in a Westernized environment. However, this implies coincidence of separately segregating polygenes rather than a common genetic basis. The overlap in the genes of primary causation of obesity and HT may be small. A gene conferring a survival advantage during both famine and drought in a hot climate would be especially powerfully selected for. However, such a gene could as likely affect appetite (in bringing in more salt with the calories) and have some point of overlap such as insulin action between metabolism and salt and water balance. Detailed discussion of such theories is beyond the scope of this chapter, but whatever the accuracy of these predictions it seems inevitable that the fundamental causes of primary HT have some overlap with those of common obesity. However, the genetic extent of this is not known, will not be constant across ethnic background and kindreds, and may be rather small.

Once obesity is established, HT is secondarily promoted, and weight gain further amplifies hypertensive susceptibility. Again the basis of this is not well understood. Landsberg[517] and others believe that weight gain initiates a cycle of sympathetic overactivity. Insulin resistance and related endothelial dysfunction promote increased CO and vasoconstriction, which impairs vasodilation and natriuresis and generates a volume expanded, initially raised CO. Later, normalized CO, raised TPR hypertensive state, coexisting insulin resistance, and hyperinsulinemia result. This fits the findings in some forms of obesity-associated HT.[517] The variable extent of coexisting insulin resistance has led Hall to propose that an obesity-related renal change is the key pathophysiologic link to secondarily associated HT. Obesity-related nephropathy impairing normal pressure natriuresis is involved more directly than contributions from insulin resistance.[149] Others, notably Ahima and Flier,[143] believe that the growing fat mass, especially visceral fat, is a potent factory of mediators including angiotensinogen that exaggerate insulin resistance, which could promote HT.[518] In Edinburgh, a mouse model of the metabolic syndrome has been generated,[144] in which features of the metabolic syndrome (central obesity, insulin resistance, and HT) that are shared by glucocorticoid excess states (e.g., glucocorticoid treatment side effects, Cushing's syndrome) were reproduced. Glucocorticoid metabolism was selectively altered in fat without systemic glucocorticoid excess but with elevated leptin, angiotensinogen, and HT. These provocative findings show that adipose tissue may indeed be an active player rather than have passive consequence in the metabolic syndrome and obesity-associated HT. Moreover, altered adipose tissue steroid metabolism and adipose tissue derived mediators affecting BP warrant investigation in the link between visceral obesity and HT. Systemic glucocorticoid excess in humans causes increased leptin release from adipose tissue and central resistance to its effects promote increased apetite.[519] In common obesity, too, there is resistance to the appetite-reducing effects of leptin, and

now it appears that leptin has peripheral effects, including stimulation of the SNS and catecholamine release from the adrenal. Thus, the continued production of leptin may have a role in sympathetic overactivity. Although these and other findings, which indicate that leptin increases central SNS outflow and renal sympathetic tone,[145] may appear to implicate leptin signaling in BP control, the pathways involved are unclear. Although elevated leptin is reported in some studies of HT,[145] other studies looking at the correlation of leptin with HT reported no association.[520] It is also reported that variations in the leptin receptor are strongly correlated with the rise in BP on weight gain,[397] which may have a bearing on the tendency to weight gain and HT in times of stress.[519]

The identification of genes involved in obesity is an emerging field; several rare causes have been identified in humans relatively recently that are largely mirrored phenotypically by equivalent gene defects in mice. Thus, very rare autosomal recessive causes of obesity have been found to include (1) leptin deficiency[521] with early-onset marked obesity showed responsive to leptin (equivalent in ob/ob mouse, which was how leptin was identified); (2) leptin receptor deficiency[522] with early-onset marked obesity and inappropriately high leptin resulting from leptin resistance (equivalent in db/db mice); (3) deficiency of prohormone convertase-1 (PC1) in a patient who had marked childhood-onset obesity but appropriate leptin for body mass and deficient processing (resulting from PC-1 loss) of proinsulin to insulin, POMC to ACTH, and α-MSH and β-MSH[523] (similar to fat/fat mouse in which the next enzyme in the PC1 pathway carboxypeptidase E is defective); and (4) POMC deficiency, which leads to marked obesity beginning around 4 months of age, deficient ACTH leading to adrenal insufficiency, and deficiency of MSH and its actions in the CNS at MC4 (melanocortin type 4) receptors, which are thought to cause the obesity and peripherally at MC1R cause red hair and pale skin.[524] Importantly, mutations in MC4R have been shown to cause a usually autosomal dominant occasionally recessive[525] form of marked obesity (usually BMI > 40) that also has early onset and appears free from other disorders, although those affected tend to be tall and have high bone mineral density as well. This disorder is much commoner, contributing to 3% to 5% of nonsyndromic obesity, although a recent study from Italy found a prevalence lower than 1%. A pathway has, thus, emerged whereby leptin released from adipose tissue binds to leptin receptor in the CNS, stimulates POMC neurons (in the hypothalamus), and upregulates α-MSH and has several other described neuropeptide modulatory actions[526] including an influence on the thyroid hormone axis (at the level of TRH and TSH and in the SNS).[145] MSH acts on MC4R and to some degree on other MCRs. Work on transgenic mice indicates that MC3R and MC4R play a role in normal body weight homeostasis, through distinct and complementary mechanisms. MC4R regulates food intake and possibly energy expenditure, whereas MC3R influences weight gain and food intake and the partitioning of fuel stores into fat.[527] Although there is much to clarify, especially regarding how fully this pattern may apply in normal human physiology, it is hard to deny, given the inherited disorders described previously and the equivalent conditions in mice, that the pathway from leptin-receptor-POMC-α-MSH-MC4R regulates weight in humans because interruption at any point causes marked obesity. The extent to which this pathway relates to the BP elevations accompanying weight gain remains to be clarified.

In common obesity apart from the 4% to 5% or less that is now attributable to MC4R mutations, the basis of the substantial genetic contribution to common nonsyndromic obesity and obesity-related HT remains unclear. As with primary HT the candidate and genome scan approaches have been used to further understanding of the underlying polygenic factors. A wide and diverse range of candidate genes have been subjected to analysis in one or two association studies, but a much smaller number have received substantial attention, especially relating to the leptin pathway and β-adrenergic pathways (which is proposed to play a role in BMR and thermogenesis). Unfortunately, there are no clearly undisputed candidates. A meta-analysis recently indicated that there is no overall association of obesity or BMI to the leptin receptor in studies based on more than 3000 subjects.[528] Three meta-analyses have assessed evidence on the $\beta_3$-adrenergic receptor, a good candidate gene involved in regulation of BMR and thermogenesis in brown fat, although the very limited role of brown fat in humans makes the theoretical basis of the candidacy of this gene less strong. Frustratingly, in 1998 two separate meta-analyses studies on more than 7000 genotyped individuals[529,530] evaluated whether the W64R coding variation in this gene is linked to BMI or obesity and came to opposite conclusions. In 2001, a further meta-analysis from another group looked at the then more than 6700 individuals who were genotyped for the W64R variant in 35 studies on Japanese subjects and who had a relatively high prevalence of the variant. The conclusion was that a small increment in BMI of 0.26 kg/m (95% CI 0.18 to 0.42, P < 0.01) was present for those who were heterozygous for the variant compared with those who were not. Although there have been several studies on two coding region variants of the $\beta_2$ adrenergic receptor, the initial strong effects reported[531] for the Q27E variant were not uniformly found. The finding that the 27Q (rather than the 27E) allele was associated with obesity was also reported. A number of genome scans have been carried out, with linked loci reported particularly on Ch 10p12 (on several occasions[532]); Ch 2p21 (close to the POMC gene); Ch 3p24-27 (close to the PPARγ gene); and on more than one occasion on Ch 7p15, Ch7q22, 17p11, and Ch 22. To date there have been no major genome scans that focused solely on obesity-linked HT, and none of the QTLs for obesity have isolated the causative mutation.

## Insulin Resistance and Diabetes Mellitus

The focus of this section is on insulin resistance. Both type 1 and type 2 (maturity onset) DM are associated with an increased risk of HT. The increased risk is less for type 1 DM (10% to 30%), which is primarily a state of reduced insulin action with little contribution from insulin resistance. HT in type 1 DM is particularly closely associated with coexisting diabetic nephropathy. In type 2 diabetes, HT is commoner (30% to 50%, more than 80% having BP > 140/90 mm Hg in some studies), insulin resistance and often hyperinsulinemia are prominent, and HT occurs in those with and without renal disease. As a whole in HT in type 2 DM there is typically volume expansion, glomerular hyperfiltration, a tendency to proteinuria, and 24-hour ambulatory BP measurements more often show a "nondipping" pattern. This latter finding has several possible explanations but may reflect a combination of the tendency to impaired natriuresis and autonomic disturbance. Thus, in DM the association of HT with insulin resistance largely relates to type 2 DM, and it is HT in the context of insulin resistance that is considered here. HT secondary to renal parenchymal disease is considered elsewhere. Type 2 DM is a polygenic complex trait with usual onset in adulthood, typically at 40 to 60+ years but also younger if there is coexisting obesity. The penetrance of type 2 DM is possibly mainly in the 20% to 40% range, and affected individuals are typically overweight or obese and have features of the metabolic syndrome: diabetes, insulin resistance, HT, and hypertriglyceridemia. As in HT, attempts have been made to define the genes involved in type 2 DM using candidate gene and positional and genome scan approaches. Some of the main candidates relate directly to the insulin signaling pathway and are of central importance to insulin resistance; these are discussed in the following. A number of genome scans seeking to identify genes for type 2 DM have been carried out, and, although there are no genes of huge effect (e.g., HLA locus in type I DM), some loci have been reported. Importantly, one such locus, NIDDM1, seems to have the greatest effect on NIDDM risk in Mexican Americans, Finns, and Germans, although not in all populations. The causative genetic variation has been identified and turns out to be in a gene previously unsuspected to have any connection with diabetes—calpain 10 (Ch 2q37.3; a protease destined to be much investigated although the mutation involved an intron[187]). Other loci have not yet had the gene responsible identified, including loci on Ch 12q24.2 (NIDDM2[533]) and 20q12-13.1. In addition to the polygenic majority of type 2 DM, there are a number of extremely rare single-gene disorders that cause type 2 DM, including several related MODY syndromes, type A insulin resistance syndromes,[534] and lipodystrophies.[535-537] MODY syndromes have a younger onset younger than 25 years, and the syndromes are not characterized by obesity nor features, in addition to diabetes, of the metabolic syndrome. Type A insulin resistance syndromes involve mutations in the insulin signaling pathway at receptor or postreceptor levels, and features usually include marked insulin resistance and acanthosis nigricans. Familial lipodystrophies are characterized by insulin resistance and deficiency of adipose tissue, which can be partial[535] or complete (also known as Berardinelli-Seip congenital lipodystrophy) for which two causative genes have recently been identified BSCL2[537] and AGPAT2.[536] The latter is an enzyme in the normal synthesis of adipose tissue lipids. Lacking normal adipose tissue complement, patients with lipodystrophy have deficiency of the normal storage site for lipids but have an increased appetite (low leptin) with dyslipidemia, impaired glucose tolerance or diabetes, and marked insulin resistance. This section concentrates on insulin resistance and its relation with HT.

The association of insulin resistance with HT extends beyond the context of DM. Thus, in some surveys of HT the rate of coincident insulin resistance is surprisingly high (e.g., overall >30% in a white population by middle age).[538] The proportion of those that are insulin resistant who have HT varies markedly with the degree of obesity and the genetic background of the population. Thus, in whites a relatively high percentage of those with marked insulin resistance have HT, in contrast in other racial groups (e.g., Mexican Americans[539]) there is marked insulin resistance without a higher rate of HT. Although insulin resistance is much commoner when there is abdominal obesity, the association of HT with increased insulin resistance persists in nonobese populations at a lower coincidence level (halving to 15% in the study referred to previously[538]). It is argued that this nonobese group will have a higher rate of "subtle" obesity with increased visceral fat and higher body fat content without being overweight and so the proportion with truly nonobese, normal body fat content insulin

resistance and HT may be lower still. At least in whites, a pathophysiologic connection between insulin resistance and HT appears probable and is probably amplified by obesity.

The insulin sensitive pathway is increasingly understood at the molecular level[540] (see Fig. 31-9) with insulin binding to the insulin receptor (IR) activating its intracellular tyrosine kinase, which then phosphorylates several intracellular substrates including insulin receptor substrates 1 to 4 (IRS1 to IRS4), the proto-oncogene Cbl isoforms of Shc, and others (Gab-1, p60[doK], APS). The phosphotyrosine activations of these substrates act as docking sites for SH2 proteins, facilitating major branches of insulin signaling including (1) binding to IRSs of the p85 subunit of the key enzyme PI(3)kinase, which causes kinase cascades affecting intermediary metabolism; (2) binding to phosphorylated Cbl of CrkII to seed formation of a multiprotein complex in lipid rafts of the plasma membrane facilitating glucose transport; and (3) binding to IRSs or Shc of GRb2 and SHP2 that, respectively, recruit a RAS containing protein complex and activate it to trigger MAP kinase cascades largely responsible for many insulin-mediated effects on tissue growth and differentiation. Insulin-mediated glucose transport involves the membrane protein complex and the PI(3)kinase cascades in triggering three downstream kinases (PKB(Akt) and two atypical protein kinase C isoforms (aPKCs)—PKCλ and PKCζ.[540] Interestingly, in muscle it is now clear that an alternative pathway of activating glucose transport, which is independent of insulin but

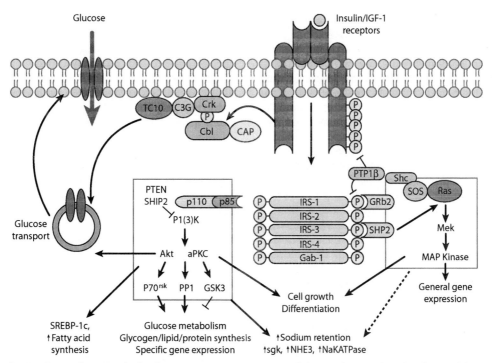

FIGURE 31-9. Insulin signaling pathway. Insulin binding its receptor triggers intracellular signaling via phosphorylation of the insulin receptor substrates (IRSs) to activate PI(3)kinase, MAP kinase, and a third Cbl/CAP pathway occurs. Many processes are influenced but especially glucose transport, fatty acid synthesis especially via the transcription factor SREBP-1c, cell growth, and importantly effects on smooth muscle (vessel) tone and sodium reabsorption (in the nephron). In insulin resistance there may be selective blockade of signaling with branches or tissues remaining sensitive, whereas others are resistant. Hyperinsulinemia may accompany resistance and overdrive the still-sensitive signaling.

cross talks distally to the branch pathways and via Glut 4, is active, and this seems one of the major explanations for the surprising finding of near normal basal and exercise-augmented glucose uptake into muscle in muscle-specific IR −/− mice.[541,542] PI(3)kinase cascades regulate several other key anabolic intermediary metabolism activities including gluconeogenesis and fatty acid synthesis via regulation of the expression of the key transcription factor SREBP-1c.[543] Interestingly, PI(3)kinase cascades also include activation of sgk1, a kinase that in the distal nephron participates in the aldosterone pathway that activates $Na^+$ retention via ENaC (Fig. 31-3) and possibly also participates in activation of $Na^+$ retention via NKCC2 in the loop of Henle.[544] A feature typical of insulin resistance accompanying HT is that the branches are not all equally resistant. Thus, despite elevated circulating insulin levels, there are typically defects in intermediary metabolism of glucose and lipids. Resistance in branches in muscle, fat, and liver is commonly accompanied by insulin-mediated hypertrophic changes (relating to overstimulation of the less resistant branch signaling [IRSs or Shc of GRb2 and SHP2] at sites of diabetic tissue damage including in kidney) that facilitate HT and overactive renal $Na^+$ retention, because of reduced branch insulin resistance in renal epithelia and augmented sgk1 activity promoting distal nephron $Na^+$ retention.[544] Overactive renal $Na^+$ retention also seems to involve activation of $Na^+$- $K^+$-ATPase probably in PT and distal nephron,[545] which may involve both tyrosine phosphorylation of the $\alpha 1 Na^+$-$K^+$-ATPase subunit in PT and other mechanisms (e.g., desensitization of dopaminergic inhibition of $Na^+$-$K^+$-ATPase[546]), and upregulation of NHE3,[547] which appears to require the permissive effect of glucocorticoids.

It is clear from knockout studies in mice that severe mutations in key mediators of insulin signaling (e.g., IRS-1 or IRS-2) cause severe insulin resistance and some growth and trophic abnormalities;[540] more severe IR −/− causes fatal ketoacidosis after birth in mice. Severe mutations in insulin signaling also give rise to insulin-resistant states in humans (e.g., leprechaunism [IR mutations in both alleles impairing function]) and type A syndrome of insulin resistance.[534] Of wider relevance is the finding that IR +/− mice have a low rate of diabetes (up to 5%), whereas IRS-1 +/− (and IRS-2 +/−) mice are "normal," with normal insulin sensitivity and glucose tolerance when lean,[548] but the compound heterozygotes IR (+/−)/IRS-1(+/−), and IR(+/−)/IRS-1(+/−)/IRS-2(+/−) have a DM rate of 17% and 40% mimicking polygenic type 2 DM.[549] This indicates that such relatively mild single hits such as IRS-1 +/− on the insulin signaling pathway may only be penetrant and cause significant insulin resistance if a coincident second hit affecting the pathway occurred. Moreover, when lean IRS-1 +/− mice become obese their insulin sensitivity changes from normal to profound insulin resistance compared with similarly obese IRS-1 +/+.[548] Thus, double heterozygote mice show that a second hit can be inherited or acquired as obesity. Recent work suggests specific points at which obesity-mediated insulin resistance impairs insulin signaling. One such point appears to involve PKC and IkappaB kinaseβ (IκkB) signaling.[550] This is blocked by high-dose salicylate treatment (which blocks IκkB).[550] This suggests that selective IκkB inhibitors would be useful insulin-sensitizing agents.

Other phenomena can contribute toward an acquired hit making a latent tendency to insulin resistance and diabetes manifest. Insulin resistance is more prominent during pregnancy and at times of chronic stress and with infection and inflammation, glucocorticoid treatment (or endogenous Cushing's syndrome), aging, physical inactivity, dyslipidemia, and acromegaly and also results from the predisposition to features of the metabolic syndrome that accompany early life events causing low birth weight (see fetal programming). Some of the mechanisms by which such conditions exacerbate insulin resistance are briefly mentioned. First, impairment of endothelial-dependent relaxation (EDR) reduces blood flow and is regulation by insulin and intermediary metabolites. Such reduced blood flow reduces insulin delivery to tissues and somewhat limits postprandial plasma glucose and fatty acid influx to sites of their uptake, especially muscle. Normally insulin directly stimulates EDR vasodilation via IRSs and Akt stimulation of eNOS and NO production. This insulin action is, thus, attenuated in insulin resistance and also with aging, dyslipidemia, and obesity. Physical inactivity limits exercise-mediated vasodilation and insulin-independent glucose and fatty acid uptake in muscle.[542,551] Second, TNFα is a cytokine that increases with aging (and typically has greater increases in inflammatory states) and that exacerbates insulin resistance (less established in human studies). This action is antagonized by thiazolidinedione drugs acting at PPARγ.[551] Third, glucocorticoids and growth hormone are hormones with actions that antagonize aspects of insulin action; cortisol is elevated during Cushing's syndrome but also in stressful and inflammatory states. Moreover, the key enzyme 11β-HSD1, which generates active glucocorticoid locally in tissues, is abundant in liver and active in visceral fat where it appears capable of amplifying predispositions to all the features of the metabolic syndrome including insulin resistance and HT, as illustrated by the metabolic syndrome phenotype of the adipose tissue 11βHSD1 overexpressing mouse[144] (see obesity section). Insulin resistance causes problems with inadequate uptake of glucose and with nonesterified fatty acids (NEFAs), which originate in visceral adipose tissue and exacerbate insulin resistance in skeletal muscle (reducing glucose uptake) and in liver (affecting VLDL and glucose output and probably reducing uptake).[551,552] Tissue-specific knockouts of the insulin receptor in mice have revealed unexpected consequences of communication between insulin-sensitive processes and organs. Thus, the IR knockout in muscle produces a mild phenotype in muscle but features of the metabolic syndrome elsewhere, especially with elevation of abdominal fat mass and dyslipidemia.[541] The liver-specific IR knockout shows marked glucose intolerance with resistance to the glucose-lowering effect of insulin thus driving hyperinsulinemia that importantly then appears to cause a further increase in insulin resistance in the liver via downregulation of the insulin signaling cascade.[553] Other hyperinsulinemic states appear to trigger a similar vicious cycle exaggerating hepatic insulin resistance. Thus, one can see that, if several mild genetic variations (e.g., single IRS-1 mutations) in the insulin signaling or cross talking pathways segregated commonly in a population, then carriers of with no metabolic abnormalities might easily develop such abnormalities as they get older, become less physically active, and develop abdominal obesity. A superimposed stressful episode or infection could then trigger the development of hyperglycemia and hyperinsulinemia, and a vicious cycle that worsens hepatic resistance persists beyond the infection. This scenario bears some resemblance to the pattern of presentation of some cases of polygenic type 2 DM and mirrors for DM the general scheme shown in Figure 31-9 for HT.

HT is associated with insulin resistance but exactly where the causal balance lies between these two conditions is usually hard to discern. That HT can follow from insulin resistance is clearer in mice with knockouts within insulin signaling pathways (e.g., IRS-1 −/−[554] or GLUT-4 +/− mice[555]) or when insulin resistance is more severe. There are several possible mechanisms that can be invoked to explain such HT. There may be coincident obesity (see previous section). In insulin resistance there is impaired EDR, as explained previously; eNOS −/− mice seem relevant here because they have both mild HT (10 to 15 mm Hg elevation) and insulin resistance.[77] The basis of the HT in eNOS −/− mice is not clear,[556] but there is normal renal blood flow, increased renal vascular resistance, and reduction in renal renin. There may be an increase in transepithelial electrolyte transport in the TAL because eNOS normally represses chloride transport.

NEFA overproduction has also been seen as a possible basis for HT in insulin-resistant states. Thus, infusions with lipids (intralipid) raise BP and TPR in animal and clinical studies.[551,552] Infusion of oleic acid into the portal vein (mimicking NEFA from abdominal fat) raises BP; this appears to be mediated by an $\alpha_1$-adrenergic pathway because $\alpha_1$-blockers abolish this effect, whereas ACE inhibition does not.[557,558] More widely appreciated are the mechanisms of sympathetic overactivity and renal Na$^+$ retention that are equally relevant in obesity. The latter may relate to overactivity of distal nephron tubular absorption,[544] or in more severe insulin resistance, it may follow from renal hyperfiltration that begins with PT overabsorption[559] or other dyslipidemic nephropathy.[149]

The genes CD36 and PPARγ have been of interest in insulin-resistant states and their causation. CD36 is a medium-long chain fatty acid translocase via which free fatty acids are absorbed into cells. CD36 deficiency is important in dyslipidemia and increased insulin resistance in hypertensive rats[389] (SHR) and seems likely to be similarly involved in humans. CD36 deficiency is common in peoples of African and Asian ancestry.[390] Iidinedione drugs and other ligands at PPARγ increase CD36 expression and can lower BP (and reduce dyslipidemia and insulin resistance). These genes are discussed further in the section on other candidate genes for primary HT. Initial enthusiasm on the key role of these genes in BP elevation has diminished because associations with BP seem weaker than was initially thought.

## REFERENCES

1. Beevers G, Lip GY, O'Brien E: ABC of hypertension: Blood pressure measurement. Part II. Conventional sphygmomanometry: Technique of auscultatory blood pressure measurement. [see comments.] [review] [13 refs]. BMJ 2001;22:1043-1047.
2. Chobanian AV, Bakris GL, Black HR, et al: The Seventh Report of the Joint National Committee on Prevention, Detection, Evaluation and Treatment of High Blood Pressure: The JNC 7 Report. JAMA 2003;289:2560-2573.
3. Ramsay LE, Williams B, Johnston GD, et al: British Hypertension Society guidelines for hypertension management 1999: Summary. BMJ 1999;319:630-635.
4. Flack JM, Neaton J, Grimm R Jr, et al: Blood pressure and mortality among men with prior myocardial infarction: Multiple Risk Factor Intervention Trial Research Group. Circulation 1995;92: 2437-2445.
5. O'Brien E, Staessen JA: Critical appraisal of the JNC VI, WHO/ISH and BHS guidelines for essential hypertension. Expert Opin Pharmacother 2000;1:675-682.
6. 1999 World Health Organization-International Society of Hypertension Guidelines for the Management of Hypertension. Guidelines Subcommittee. J Hypertens 1999;17:151-183.
7. Update on the 1987 Task Force Report on High Blood Pressure in Children and Adolescents: A working group report from the National High Blood Pressure Education Program. National High Blood Pressure Education Program Working Group on Hypertension Control in Children and Adolescents. Pediatrics 1996;98:649-658.
8. Report of the National High Blood Pressure Education Program Working Group on High Blood Pressure in Pregnancy. Am J Obstet Gynecol 2000;183:S1-S22.
9. National High Blood Pressure Education Program Working Group Report on Hypertension in the Elderly: National High Blood Pressure Education Program Working Group. Hypertension 1994;23:275-285.
10. Devereux RB, Case DB, Alderman MH, et al: Possible role of increased blood viscosity in the hemodynamics of systemic hypertension. Am J Cardiol 2000;85:1265-1268.
11. Fowkes FG, Lowe GD, Rumley A, et al: The relationship between blood viscosity and blood pressure in a random sample of the population aged 55 to 74 years. Eur Heart J 1993;14:597-601.
12. Resch KL, Ernst E, Matrai A, Paulsen HF: Fibrinogen and viscosity as risk factors for subsequent cardiovascular events in stroke survivors. Ann Intern Med 1992;117:371-375.
13. Wannamethee G, Perry IJ, Shaper AG: Haematocrit, hypertension and risk of stroke. J Intern Med 1994;235:163-168.
14. Nakanishi N, Yoshida H, Okamoto M, et al: Hematocrit and risk for hypertension in middle-aged Japanese male office workers. Ind Health 2001;39:17-20.
15. Guyton AC, Coleman TG, Cowley AV Jr, et al: Arterial pressure regulation: Overriding dominance of the kidneys in long-term regulation and in hypertension. Am J Med 1972; 52:584-594.
16. Hall JE, Guyton AC, Brands MW: Pressure-volume regulation in hypertension. Kidney Int Suppl 1996;55:S35-S41.
17. Morise T, Horita M, Kitagawa I, et al: The potent role of increased sympathetic tone in pathogenesis of essential hypertension with neurovascular compression. J Hum Hypertens 2000; 14:807-811.
18. Jannetta PJ, Segal R, Wolfson SK Jr: Neurogenic hypertension: Etiology and surgical treatment. I. Observations in 53 patients. Ann Surg 1985;201:391-398.
19. Plets C: Arterial hypertension in neurosurgical emergencies. Am J Cardiol 1989;63:40C-42C.
20. Dickenson CJ: Neurogenic Hypertension: A Synthesis and Review. London, Chapman & Hall, 1991.
21. Schnermann J: Sodium transport deficiency and sodium balance in gene-targeted mice. Acta Physiol Scand 2001;173:59-66.
22. Goyal S, Vanden Heuvel G, Aronson P: Renal expression of novel Na+-H+ exchanger isoform NHE8. Am J Physiol Renal Physiol 2003; 284:F467-473.
23. Cruz DN, Simon DB, Nelson-Williams C, et al: Mutations in the Na-Cl cotransporter reduce blood pressure in humans. Hypertension 2001;37:1458-1464.

24. Simon DB, Lifton RP: Mutations in Na(K)Cl transporters in Gitelman's and Bartter's syndromes. Curr Opin Cell Biol 1998;10:450-454.

25. Birkenhager R, Otto E, Schurmann MJ, et al: Mutation of BSND causes Bartter syndrome with sensorineural deafness and kidney failure. Nat Genet 2001;29:310-314.

26. Estevez R, Boettger T, Stein V, et al: Barttin is a Cl⁻ channel beta-subunit crucial for renal Cl⁻ reabsorption and inner ear K⁺ secretion. Nature 2001;414:558-561.

27. Lorenz JN, Baird NR, Judd LM, et al: Impaired renal NaCl absorption in mice lacking the ROMK potassium channel: A model for type II Bartter's syndrome. J Biol Chem 2002;277:37871-37880.

28. Lifton RP, Gharavi AG, Geller DS: Molecular mechanisms of human hypertension. Cell 2001;104:545-556.

29. Chen SY, Bhargava A, Mastroberardino L, et al: Epithelial sodium channel regulated by aldosterone-induced protein sgk. Proc Natl Acad Sci USA 1999;96:2514-2519.

30. Hou J, Speirs HJ, Seckl JR, Brown RW: Sgk1 gene expression in kidney and its regulation by aldosterone: Spatio-temporal heterogeneity and quantitative analysis. J Am Soc Nephrol 2002;13:1190-1198.

31. Wulff P, Vallon V, Huang DY, et al: Impaired renal Na(+) retention in the sgk1-knockout mouse[comment]. J Clin Invest 2002;110:1263-1268.

32. Wang J, Barbry P, Maiyar AC, et al: SGK integrates insulin and mineralocorticoid regulation of epithelial sodium transport. Am J Physiol Renal Fluid Electrolyte Physiol 2001;280:F303-F313.

33. Rubera I, Loffing J, Palmer L, et al: Collecting duct-specific gene inactivation of alpha-ENaC in the mouse kidney does not impair sodium and potassium balance. J Clin Invest 2003; 112:554-565.

34. Huang PL, Huang Z, Mashimo H, et al: Hypertension in mice lacking the gene for endothelial nitric oxide synthase. Nature 1995;377:239-242.

35. Lopez MJ, Wong SK, Kishimoto I, et al: Salt-resistant hypertension in mice lacking the guanylyl cyclase-A receptor for atrial natriuretic peptide. Nature 1995;378:65-68.

36. Ahn DW, Stricklett PK, Nelson RD, et al: Collecting duct-specific knockout of endothelin-1 in mice causes hypertension and impaired fluid excretion [abstract]. J Am Soc Nephrol 2002;13:SU-FC257.

37. Williams GH, Dluhy RG, Lifton RP, et al: Non-modulation as an intermediate phenotype in essential hypertension. Hypertension 1992;20:788-796.

38. Fisher ND, Hurwitz S, Jeunemaitre X, et al: Adrenal response to angiotensin II in black hypertension: Lack of sexual dimorphism. Hypertension 2001;38:373-378.

39. Smithies O, Kim HS, Takahashi N, Edgell MH: Importance of quantitative genetic variations in the etiology of hypertension. Kidney Int 2000;58:2265-2280.

40. Yanai K, Saito T, Kakinuma Y, et al: Renin-dependent cardiovascular functions and renin-independent blood-brain barrier functions revealed by renin-deficient mice. J Biol Chem 2000;275:5-8.

41. Sharp MG, Kantachuvesiri S, Mullins JJ: Genotype and cardiovascular phenotype: Lessons from genetically manipulated animals and diseased humans. Curr Opin Nephrol Hypertens 1997;6:51-57.

42. Mullins JJ, Peters J, Ganten D: Fulminant hypertension in transgenic rats harbouring the mouse Ren-2 gene. Nature 1990;344:541-544.

43. Kantachuvesiri S, Fleming S, Peters J, et al: Controlled hypertension, a transgenic toggle switch reveals differential mechanisms underlying vascular disease. J Biol Chem 2001;276:36727-36733.

44. Pinto YM, Paul M, Ganten D: Lessons from rat models of hypertension: From Goldblatt to genetic engineering. Cardiovasc Res 1998;39:77-88.

45. Bader M, Bohnemeier H, Zollmann FS, et al: Transgenic animals in cardiovascular disease research. Exp Physiol 2000;85:713-731.

46. Civantos CB, Aleixandre DA: Alpha-adrenoceptor subtypes. Pharmacol Res 2001;44:195-208.

47. Tanoue A, Koshimizu TA, Tsujimoto G: Transgenic studies of alpha(1)-adrenergic receptor subtype function. Life Sci 2002;71:2207-2215.

48. Rohrer DK: Physiological consequences of beta-adrenergic receptor disruption. J Mol Med 1998;76:764-772.

49. Jarajapu YP, Johnston F, Berry C, et al: Functional characterization of alpha1-adrenoceptor subtypes in human subcutaneous resistance arteries. J Pharmacol Exp Ther 2001;299:729-734.

50. Cavalli A, Lattion AL, Hummler E, et al: Decreased blood pressure response in mice deficient of the alpha1b-adrenergic receptor. Proc Natl Acad Sci USA 1997;94:11589-11594.

51. Rokosh DG, Simpson PC: Knockout of the alpha 1A/C-adrenergic receptor subtype: The alpha 1A/C is expressed in resistance arteries and is required to maintain arterial blood pressure. Proc Natl Acad Sci USA 2002;99:9474-9479.

52. Tanoue A, Nasa Y, Koshimizu T, et al: The alpha(1D)-adrenergic receptor directly regulates arterial blood pressure via vasoconstriction. J Clin Invest 2002;109:765-775.

53. Rudner XL, Berkowitz DE, Booth JV, et al: Subtype specific regulation of human vascular {alpha}1-adrenergic receptors by vessel bed and age. Circulation 1999;100:2336-2343.

54. Hein L, Altman JD, Kobilka BK: Two functionally distinct alpha2-adrenergic receptors regulate sympathetic neurotransmission. Nature 1999;402:181-184.

55. Makaritsis KP, Johns C, Gavras I, Gavras H: Role of alpha(2)-adrenergic receptor subtypes in the acute hypertensive response to hypertonic saline infusion in anephric mice. Hypertension 2000;35:609-613.

56. Makaritsis KP, Handy DE, Johns C, et al: Role of the alpha2B-adrenergic receptor in the development of salt-induced hypertension. Hypertension 1999;33:14-17.

57. Rohrer DK, Chruscinski A, Schauble EH, et al: Cardiovascular and metabolic alterations in mice lacking both beta1- and beta2-adrenergic receptors. J Biol Chem 1999;274:16701-16708.

58. Chruscinski A, Brede ME, Meinel L, et al: Differential distribution of beta-adrenergic receptor subtypes in blood vessels of knockout mice lacking beta(1)- or beta(2)-adrenergic receptors. Mol Pharmacol 2001;60:955-962.

59. Chruscinski AJ, Rohrer DK, Schauble E, et al: Targeted disruption of the beta2 adrenergic receptor gene. J Biol Chem 1999;274:16694-16700.

60. Bachman ES, Dhillon H, Zhang CY, et al: Beta AR signaling required for diet-induced thermogenesis and obesity resistance. Science 2002;297:843-845.

61. Krushkal J, Xiong M, Ferrell R, et al: Linkage and association of adrenergic and dopamine receptor genes in the distal portion of the long arm of chromosome 5 with systolic blood pressure variation. Hum Mol Genet 1998;7:1379-1383.

62. Krushkal J, Ferrell R, Mockrin SC, et al: Genome-wide linkage analyses of systolic blood pressure using highly discordant siblings. Circulation 1999;99:1407-1410.

63. Ranade K, Jorgenson E, Sheu WH, et al: A polymorphism in the beta1 adrenergic receptor is associated with resting heart rate. Am J Hum Genet 2002;70:935-942.

64. Small KM, Liggett SB: Identification and functional characterization of alpha(2)-adrenoceptor polymorphisms. Trends Pharmacol Sci 2001;22:471-477.

65. Davenport AP, Maguire JJ: Of mice and men: Advances in endothelin research and first antagonist gains FDA approval. Trends Pharmacol Sci 2002;23:155-157.

66. Montanari A, Carra N, Perinotto P, et al: Renal hemodynamic control by endothelin and nitric oxide under angiotensin II blockade in man. Hypertension 2002;39:715-720.

67. Kuwaki T, Ishii T, Ju K, et al: Blood pressure of endothelin-3 null (−/−) knockout mice and endothelin A receptor null (−/−) knockout mice under anaesthesia. Clin Sci (Lond) 2002;103(Suppl)48:48S-52S.

68. Doggrell SA: The therapeutic potential of endothelin-1 receptor antagonists and endothelin-converting enzyme inhibitors on the cardiovascular system. Expert Opin Investig Drugs 2002;11:1537-1552.

69. Rubin LJ, Badesch DB, Barst RJ, et al: Bosentan therapy for pulmonary arterial hypertension [erratum N Engl J Med 2002;18:1258]. N Engl J Med 2002;346:896-903.

70. Krejci V, Hiltebrand LB, Erni D, Sigurdsson GH: Endothelin receptor antagonist bosentan improves microcirculatory blood flow in splanchnic organs in septic shock. Crit Care Med 2003;31:203-210.

71. Moncada S, Higgs A: The L-arginine-nitric oxide pathway. N Engl J Med 1993;329:2002-2012.

72. Nasjletti A: Arthur C. Corcoran Memorial Lecture: The role of eicosanoids in angiotensin-dependent hypertension. Hypertension 1998;31:194-200.

73. Roman RJ: P-450 metabolites of arachidonic acid in the control of cardiovascular function. Physiol Rev 2002;82:131-185.

74. Busse R, Edwards G, Feletou M, et al: EDHF: Bringing the concepts together. Trends Pharmacol Sci 2002;23:374-380.

75. Archer SL, Gragasin FS, Wu X, et al: Endothelium-derived hyperpolarizing factor in human internal mammary artery Is 11,12-epoxyeicosatrienoic acid and causes relaxation by activating smooth muscle BKCa channels. Circulation 2003;107:769-776.

76. Chauhan SD, Nilsson H, Ahluwalia A, Hobbs AJ: Release of C-type natriuretic peptide accounts for the biological activity of endothelium-derived hyperpolarizing factor. PNAS 2003;100:1426-1431.

77. Duplain H, Burcelin R, Sartori C, et al: Insulin resistance, hyperlipidemia, and hypertension in mice lacking endothelial nitric oxide synthase. Circulation 2001;104:342-345.

78. Bailly C: Transducing pathways involved in the control of NaCl reabsorption in the thick ascending limb of Henle's loop. Kidney Int Suppl 1998;65:S29-S35.

79. Bader M, Ganten D: Regulation of renin: New evidence from cultured cells and genetically modified mice. J Mol Med 2000;78:130-139.

80. Schnermann J, Levine DZ: Paracrine factors in tubuloglomerular feedback: Adenosine, atp, and nitric oxide. Annu Rev Physiol 2003;65:501-529.

81. Patel KP, Li YF, Hirooka Y: Role of nitric oxide in central sympathetic outflow [review] [74 refs]. Exp Biol Med 2001;226:814-824.

82. Hanna IR, Taniyama Y, Szocs K, et al: NAD(P)H oxidase-derived reactive oxygen species as mediators of angiotensin II signaling. Antioxid Redox Signal 2002;4:899-914.

83. Griendling KK, Sorescu D, Ushio-Fukai M: NAD(P)H oxidase: Role in cardiovascular biology and disease. Circ Res 2000;86:494-501.

84. Vallance P, Leone A, Calver A, et al: Accumulation of an endogenous inhibitor of nitric oxide synthesis in chronic renal failure. Lancet 1992;339:572-575.

85. Lin KY, Ito A, Asagami T, et al: Impaired nitric oxide synthase pathway in diabetes mellitus: Role of asymmetric dimethylarginine and dimethylarginine dimethylaminohydrolase. Circulation 2002;106:987-992.

86. Claxton CR, Brands MW: Nitric oxide opposes glucose-induced hypertension by suppressing sympathetic activity. Hypertension 2003;41:274-278.

87. Hussain T, Lokhandwala MF: Renal dopamine receptors and hypertension. Exp Biol Med 2003;228:134-142.

88. Beheray S, Kansra V, Hussain T, Lokhandwala MF: Diminished natriuretic response to dopamine in old rats is due to an impaired D1-like receptor-signaling pathway. Kidney Int 2000;58:712-720.

89. Chibalin AV, Ogimoto G, Pedemonte CH, et al: Dopamine-induced endocytosis of Na+, K+-ATPase is initiated by phosphorylation of Ser-18 in the rat alpha subunit and Is responsible for the decreased activity in epithelial cells. J Biol Chem 1999;274:1920-1927.

90. Murphy MB, Murray C, Shorten GD: Fenoldopam: A selective peripheral dopamine-receptor agonist for the treatment of severe hypertension. N Engl J Med 2001;345:1548-1557.

91. Albrecht FE, Drago J, Felder RA, et al: Role of the D1A dopamine receptor in the pathogenesis of genetic hypertension. J Clin Invest 1996;97:2283-2288.

92. Asico LD, Ladines C, Fuchs S, et al: Disruption of the dopamine D3 receptor gene produces renin-dependent hypertension. J Clin Invest 1998;102:493-498.

93. Li XX, Bek M, Asico LD, et al: Adrenergic and endothelin B receptor-dependent hypertension in dopamine receptor type-2 knockout mice. Hypertension 2001;38:303-308.

94. Hollon TR, Bek MJ, Lachowicz JE, et al: Mice lacking D5 dopamine receptors have increased sympathetic tone and are hypertensive. J Neurosci 2002;22:10801-10810.

95. Kuchel O, Shigetomi S: Defective dopamine generation from dihydroxyphenylalanine in stable essential hypertensive patients. Hypertension 1992;19:634-638.

96. Iimura O, Shimamoto K: Salt and hypertension: Water-sodium handling in essential hypertension. Ann NY Acad Sci 1993;676:105-121.

97. elder RA, Sanada H, Xu J, et al: G protein-coupled receptor kinase 4 gene variants in human essential hypertension. Proc Natl Acad Sci USA 2002;99:3872-3877.

98. Velasco M, Contreras F, Cabezas GA, et al: Dopaminergic receptors: A new antihypertensive mechanism. J Hypertens 2002;20(Suppl):8.

99. Sugiyama F, Yagami K, Paigen B: Mouse models of blood pressure regulation and hypertension. Curr Hypertens Rep 2001;3:41-48.

100. Nakayama T, Soma M, Watanabe Y, et al: Splicing mutation of the prostacyclin synthase gene in a family associated with hypertension. Biochem Biophys Res Commun 2002;297:1135-1139.

101. Gao H, Welch WJ, DiBona GF, Wilcox CS: Sympathetic nervous system and hypertension during prolonged TxA2/PGH2 receptor activation in rats. Am J Physiol 1997;273:H734-H739.

102. Wilcox CS, Cardozo J, Welch WJ: AT1 and TxA2/PGH2 receptors maintain hypertension throughout 2K,1C Goldblatt hypertension in the rat. Am J Physiol 1996;271:R891-R896.

103. Hirata T, Kakizuka A, Ushikubi F, et al: Arg60 to Leu mutation of the human thromboxane A2 receptor in a dominantly inherited bleeding disorder. J Clin Invest 1994;94:1662-1667.

104. Breyer MD, Breyer RM: G protein-coupled prostanoid receptors and the kidney [review] [195 refs.] Annu Rev Physiol 2001;63:579-605.

105. Stock JL, Shinjo K, Burkhardt J, et al: The prostaglandin E2 EP1 receptor mediates pain perception and regulates blood pressure. J Clin Invest 2001;107:325-331.

106. Kobayashi T, Narumiya S: Function of prostanoid receptors: Studies on knockout mice. Prostaglandins Other Lipid Mediators 2002;68-69:557-573.

107. Kennedy CR, Zhang Y, Brandon S, et al: Salt-sensitive hypertension and reduced fertility in mice lacking the prostaglandin EP2 receptor. Nat Med 1999;5:217-220, 1999.

108. Tang L, Loutzenhiser K, Loutzenhiser R: Biphasic actions of prostaglandin E(2) on the renal afferent arteriole: Role of EP(3) and EP(4) receptors. Circ Res 2000;86:663-670.

109. Frishman WH: Effects of nonsteroidal anti-inflammatory drug therapy on blood pressure and peripheral edema. Am J Cardiol 2002;89:18D-25D.

110. Laffer CL, Laniado-Schwartzman M, Wang MH, et al: Differential regulation of natriuresis by 20-hydroxyeicosatetraenoic acid in human salt-sensitive versus salt-resistant hypertension. Circulation 2003;107:574-578.

111. Sagnella GA, Markandu ND, Buckley MG, et al: Atrial natriuretic peptides in essential hypertension: Basal plasma levels and relationship to sodium balance. Can J Physiol Pharmacol 1991;69:1592-1600.

112. Takeda T, Kohno M: Brain natriuretic peptide in hypertension. Hypertens Res 1995;18:259-266.

113. Hollister AS, Inagami T: Atrial natriuretic factor and hypertension: A review and metaanalysis. Am J Hypertens 1991;4:850-865.

114. Lee EY, Humphreys MH: Phosphodiesterase activity as a mediator of renal resistance to ANP in pathological salt retention. Am J Physiol 1996;271:F3-6.

115. Campbell DJ: The kallikrein-kinin system in humans. Clin Exp Pharmacol Physiol 2001;28:1060-1065.

116. Regoli D, Rhaleb NE, Drapeau G, Dion S: Kinin receptor subtypes. J Cardiovasc Pharmacol 1990;15(Suppl 6):S30-S38.

117. Cheung PP, Kunapuli SP, Scott CF, et al: Genetic basis of total kininogen deficiency in Williams' trait. J Biol Chem 1993;268:23361-23365.

118. Alfie ME, Yang XP, Hess F, Carretero OA: Salt-sensitive hypertension in bradykinin B2 receptor knockout mice. Biochem Biophys Res Commun 1996;224:625-630.

119. Dahl LK, Heine M: Primary role of renal homografts in setting chronic blood pressure levels in rats. Circ Res 1975;36:692-696.

120. Cusi D, Bianchi G: Renal mechanisms of genetic hypertension: From the molecular level to the intact organism. Kidney Int 1996;49:1754-1759.

121. Bianchi G, Fox U, Di Francesco GF, et al: Blood pressure changes produced by kidney cross-transplantation between spontaneously hypertensive rats and normotensive rats. Clin Sci Mol Med 1974;47:435-448.

122. Rettig R: Does the kidney play a role in the aetiology of primary hypertension? Evidence from renal transplantation studies in rats and humans. J Hum Hypertens 1993;7:177-180.

123. Guidi E, Menghetti D, Milani S, et al: Hypertension may be transplanted with the kidney in humans: A long-term historical prospective follow-up of recipients grafted with kidneys coming from donors with or without hypertension in their families. J Am Soc Nephrol 1996;7:1131-1138.

124. Merino GE, Kjellstrand CM, Simmons RL, Najarian JS: Late hypertension in renal transplant recipients: Possible role of the donor in late primary hypertension. Proc Clin Dial Transplant Forum 1976;6:145-152.

125. Strandgaard S, Hansen U: Hypertension in renal allograft recipients may be conveyed by cadaveric kidneys from donors with subarachnoid haemorrhage. BMJ Clin Res Ed 1986;292:1041-1044.

126. Curtis JJ, Luke RG, Dustan HP, et al: Remission of essential hypertension after renal transplantation. N Engl J Med 1983;309:1009-1015.

127. Saito F, Kimura G: Antihypertensive mechanism of diuretics based on pressure-natriuresis relationship. Hypertension 1996;27:914-918.

128. Stockigt JR, Hewett MJ, Topliss DJ, et al: Renin and renin substrate in primary adrenal insufficiency: Contrasting effects of glucocorticoid and mineralocorticoid deficiency. Am J Med 1979;66:915-922.

129. Brook RD, Julius S: Autonomic imbalance, hypertension, and cardiovascular risk. Am J Hypertens 2000;13:112S-122S.

130. Izzo JL Jr, Taylor AA: The sympathetic nervous system and baroreflexes in hypertension and hypotension. Curr Hypertens Rep 1999;1:254-263.

131. Thorpe JJ, Welch WJ, Poindexter CA: Bilateral thoracolumbar sympathectomy for hypertension. Am J Med 1950;9:500-515.

132. Grassi G, Seravalle G, Dell'Oro R, et al: Adrenergic and reflex abnormalities in obesity-related hypertension. Hypertension 2000;36:538-542.

133. Narkiewicz K, Somers VK: The sympathetic nervous system and obstructive sleep apnea: Implications for hypertension. J Hypertens 1997;15:1613-1619.

134. Malhotra A, White DP: Obstructive sleep apnoea. Lancet 2002;360:237-245.

135. Hedner J, Darpo B, Ejnell H, et al: Reduction in sympathetic activity after long-term CPAP treatment in sleep apnoea: Cardiovascular implications. Eur Respir J 1995;8:222-229.

136. Gasowski J, Fagard RH, Staessen JA, et al: Pulsatile blood pressure component as predictor of mortality in hypertension: A meta-analysis of clinical trial control groups. J Hypertens 2002;20:145-151.

137. Pereira L, Lee SY, Gayraud B, et al: Pathogenetic sequence for aneurysm revealed in mice underexpressing fibrillin-1. Proc Natl Acad Sci USA 1999;96:3819-3823.

138. Powell JT, MacSweeney ST, Greenhalgh RM, et al: Interaction between fibrillin genotype and blood pressure and the development of aneurysmal disease. Ann NY Acad Sci 1996;800:198-207.

139. Medley TL, Cole TJ, Gatzka CD, et al: Fibrillin-1 genotype is associated with aortic stiffness and disease severity in patients with coronary artery disease. Circulation 2002;105:810-815.

140. Antonios TF, Singer DR, Markandu ND, et al: Rarefaction of skin capillaries in borderline essential hypertension suggests an early structural abnormality. Hypertension 1999;34:655-658.

141. Noon JP, Walker BR, Webb DJ, et al: Impaired microvascular dilatation and capillary rarefaction in young adults with a predisposition to high blood pressure. J Clin Invest 1997;99:1873-1879.

142. Boudier HA: Arteriolar and capillary remodelling in hypertension. Drugs 1999;58(Spec No 1):37-40.

143. Ahima RS, Flier JS: Adipose tissue as an endocrine organ. Trends Endocrinol Metab 2000;11:327-332.

144. Masuzaki H, Paterson J, Shinyama H, et al: A transgenic model of visceral obesity and the metabolic syndrome. Science 2001;294:2166-2170.

145. Engeli S, Sharma AM: Emerging concepts in the pathophysiology and treatment of obesity-associated hypertension. Curr Opin Cardiol 2002;17:355-359.

146. Stowasser M: Primary aldosteronism: Rare bird or common cause of secondary hypertension? Curr Hypertens Rep 2001;3:230-239.

147. Padfield PL: Primary aldosteronism, a common entity? The myth persists. J Hum Hypertens 2002;16:159-162.

148. Montori VM, Young WF Jr: Use of plasma aldosterone concentration-to-plasma renin activity ratio as a screening test for primary aldosteronism. A systematic review of the literature. Endocrinol Metab Clin North Am 2002;31:619-632.

149. Hall JE, Crook ED, Jones DW, et al: Mechanisms of obesity-associated cardiovascular and renal disease [review] [79 refs]. Am J Med Sci 2002;324:127-137.

150. Williams RR, Hunt SC, Hasstedt SJ, et al: Are there interactions and relations between genetic and environmental factors predisposing to high blood pressure? Hypertension 1991;18(Suppl):37.

151. Mitchell BD, Kammerer CM, Blangero J, et al: Genetic and environmental contributions to cardiovascular risk factors in Mexican Americans: The San Antonio Family Heart Study. Circulation 1996;94:2159-2170.

152. Cui J, Hopper JL, Harrap SB: Genes and family environment explain correlations between blood pressure and body mass index. Hypertension 2002;40:7-12.

153. Urban Z, Riazi S, Seidl TL, et al: Connection between elastin haploinsufficiency and increased cell proliferation in patients with supravalvular aortic stenosis and Williams-Beuren syndrome. Am J Hum Genet 2002;71:30-44.

154. Rose C, Wessel A, Pankau R, et al: Anomalies of the abdominal aorta in Williams-Beuren syndrome: Another cause of arterial hypertension. Eur J Pediatr 2001;160:655-658.

155. Wilson FH, Disse-Nicodeme S, Choate KA, et al: Human hypertension caused by mutations in WNK kinases. Science 2001;293:1107-1112.

156. Cox NJ, Wapelhorst B, Morrison VA, et al: Seven regions of the genome show evidence of linkage to type 1 diabetes in a consensus analysis of 767 multiplex families. Am J Hum Genet 2001;69:820-830.

157. Zimdahl H, Kreitler T, Gosele C, et al: Conserved synteny in rat and mouse for a blood pressure QTL on human chromosome 17. Hypertension 2002;39:1050-1052.

158. Truswell AS, Kennelly BM, Hansen JD, Lee RB: Blood pressures of Kung bushmen in Northern Botswana. Am Heart J 1972;84:5-12.

159. Poulter NR, Khaw KT, Hopwood BE, et al: The Kenyan Luo migration study: Observations on the initiation of a rise in blood pressure. BMJ 1990;300:967-972.

160. Elliott P, Stamler J, Nichols R, et al: Intersalt revisited: further analyses of 24 hour sodium excretion and blood pressure within and across populations: Intersalt Cooperative Research Group. [erratum in BMJ 1997;315:458.] BMJ 1996;312:1249-1253.

161. Whelton PK, He J, Appel LJ, et al: Primary prevention of hypertension: Clinical and public health advisory from The National High Blood Pressure Education Program. JAMA 2002;288:1882-1888.

162. Kannel WB, Garrison RJ, Dannenberg AL: Secular blood pressure trends in normotensive persons: The Framingham study. Am Heart J 1993;125:1154-1158.

163. Wilson PW, D'Agostino RB, Sullivan L, et al: Overweight and obesity as determinants of cardiovascular risk: The Framingham experience. Arch Intern Med 2002;162:1867-1872.

164. Huang Z, Willett WC, Manson JE, et al: Body weight, weight change, and risk for hypertension in women. Ann Intern Med 1998;128:81-88.

165. Timio M, Lippi G, Venanzi S, et al: Blood pressure trend and cardiovascular events in nuns in a secluded order: A 30-year follow-up study. Blood Pressure 1997;6:81-87.

166. Mongeau JG: Heredity and blood pressure in humans: An overview [review] [30 refs]. Pediatr Nephrol 1987;1:69-75.

167. Mongeau JG, Biron P, Sing CF: The influence of genetics and household environment upon the variability of normal blood pressure: The Montreal Adoption Survey. Clin Exp Hypertens A Theory Pract 1986;8:653-660.

168. Forte P, Kneale BJ, Milne E, et al: Evidence for a difference in nitric oxide biosynthesis between healthy women and men. Hypertension 1998;32:730-734.

169. Kuch B, Muscholl M, Luchner A, et al: Gender specific differences in left-ventricular adaptation to obesity and hypertension. J Hum Hypertens 1998;12:685-691.

170. Messerli FH, Grossman E, Goldbourt U: Are beta-blockers efficacious as first-line therapy for hypertension in the elderly? A systematic review. JAMA 1998;279:1903-1907.

171. Vaccarino V, Berger AK, Abramson J, et al: Pulse pressure and risk of cardiovascular events in the systolic hypertension in the elderly program. Am J Cardiol 2001;88:980-986.

172. Laurent S, Boutouyrie P, Asmar R, et al: Aortic stiffness is an independent predictor of all-cause and cardiovascular mortality in hypertensive patients. Hypertension 2001;37:1236-1241.

173. Seals DR, Stevenson ET, Jones PP, et al: Lack of age-associated elevations in 24-h systolic and pulse pressures in women who exercise regularly. Am J Physiol 1999;277:H947-H955.

174. Avolio AP, Clyde KM, Beard TC, et al: Improved arterial distensibility in normotensive subjects on a low salt diet. Arteriosclerosis 1986;6:166-169.

175. Benetos A, Cambien F, Gautier S et al.: Influence of the angiotensin II type 1 receptor gene polymorphism on the effects of perindopril and nitrendipine on arterial stiffness in hypertensive individuals. Hypertension 1996;28:1081-1084.

176. Wilkinson IB, Qasem A, McEniery CM, et al: Nitric oxide regulates local arterial distensibility in vivo. Circulation 2002;105:213-217.

177. Langley-Evans SC: Fetal programming of cardiovascular function through exposure to maternal undernutrition. Proc Nutr Soc 2001;60:505-513.

178. Seckl JR, Cleasby M, Nyirenda MJ: Glucocorticoids, 11beta-hydroxysteroid dehydrogenase, and fetal programming [review] [74 refs]. Kidney Int 2000;57:1412-1417.

179. Hattersley AT, Tooke JE: The fetal insulin hypothesis: An alternative explanation of the association of low birthweight with diabetes and vascular disease. Lancet 1999;353:1789-1792.

180. Mackenzie HS, Brenner BM: Fewer nephrons at birth: A missing link in the etiology of essential hypertension? Am J Kidney Dis 1995;26:91-98.

181. Manalich R, Reyes L, Herrera M, et al: Relationship between weight at birth and the number and size of renal glomeruli in humans: A histomorphometric study. Kidney Int 2000;58:770-773.

182. Keller G, Zimmer G, Mall G, et al: Nephron number in patients with primary hypertension [comment]. N Engl J Med 2003;348:101-108.

183. Levitt NS, Lindsay RS, Holmes MC, Seckl JR: Dexamethasone in the last week of pregnancy attenuates hippocampal glucocorticoid receptor gene expression and elevates blood pressure in the adult offspring in the rat. Neuroendocrinology 1996;64:412-418.

184. Marchand MC, Langley-Evans SC: Intrauterine programming of nephron number: The fetal flaw revisited. J Nephrol 2001;14:327-331.

185. Lander ES, Schork NJ: Genetic dissection of complex traits. [erratum appears in Science 1994;266:353.]. Science 1994;265:2037-2048.

186. Korstanje R, Paigen B: From QTL to gene: The harvest begins. Nat Genet 2002;31:235-236.

187. Horikawa Y, Oda N, Cox NJ, et al: Genetic variation in the gene encoding calpain-10 is associated with type 2 diabetes mellitus. [erratum in Nat Genet 2000;26:502]. Nat Genet 2000;26:163-175.

188. Gabriel SB, Schaffner SF, Nguyen H, et al: The structure of haplotype blocks in the human genome. Science 2002;296:2225-2229.

189. Tabor HK, Risch NJ, Myers RM: Opinion: Candidate-gene approaches for studying complex genetic traits: Practical considerations. Nat Rev Genet 2002;3:391-397.

190. Lander E, Kruglyak L: Genetic dissection of complex traits: Guidelines for interpreting and reporting linkage results. Nat Genet 1995;11:241-247.

191. Rao DC, Province MA: The future of path analysis, segregation analysis, and combined models for genetic dissection of complex traits. Hum Hered 2000;50:34-42.

192. Stoll M, Kwitek-Black AE, Cowley AW Jr, et al: New target regions for human hypertension via comparative genomics. Genome Res 2000;10:473-482.

193. Sugiyama F, Churchill GA, Higgins DC, et al: Concordance of murine quantitative trait loci for salt-induced hypertension with rat and human loci. Genomics 2001;71:70-77.

194. Sugiyama F, Churchill GA, Li R, et al: QTL associated with blood pressure, heart rate, and heart weight in CBA/CaJ and BALB/cJ mice. Physiol Genomics 2002;10:5-12.

195. Wright FA, O'Connor DT, Roberts E, et al: Genome scan for blood pressure loci in mice. Hypertension 1999;34:625-630.

196. Judson R, Salisbury B, Schneider J, et al: How many SNPs does a genome-wide haplotype map require? Pharmacogenomics 2002;3:379-391.

197. Jeunemaitre X, Rigat B, Charru A, et al: Sib pair linkage analysis of renin gene haplotypes in human essential hypertension. Hum Genet 1992;88:301-306.

198. Bonnardeaux A, Davies E, Jeunemaitre X, et al: Angiotensin II type 1 receptor gene polymorphisms in human essential hypertension. Hypertension 1994;24:63-69.

199. Bonnardeaux A, Nadaud S, Charru A, et al: Lack of evidence for linkage of the endothelial cell nitric oxide synthase gene to essential hypertension. Circulation 1995;91:96-102.

200. Brand E, Kato N, Chatelain N, et al.: Structural analysis and evaluation of the 11beta-hydroxysteroid dehydrogenase type 2 (11beta-HSD2) gene in human essential hypertension. J Hypertens 1998;16:1627-1633.

201. Persu A, Barbry P, Bassilana F, et al: Genetic analysis of the beta subunit of the epithelial Na$^+$ channel in essential hypertension. Hypertension 1998;32:129-137.

202. Persu A, Coscoy S, Houot AM, et al: Polymorphisms of the gamma subunit of the epithelial Na$^+$ channel in essential hypertension. J Hypertens 1999;17:639-645.

203. Catanzaro DF: Angiotensinogen: Physiology, molecular biology and relevance to hypertension. In Oparil S, Weber MA (eds): Hypertension: A Companion to Brenner and Rector's The Kidney. Philadephia, WB Saunders Philadelphia, 2000, pp 77-89.

204. Kunz R, Kreutz R, Beige J, et al: Association between the angiotensinogen 235T-variant and essential hypertension in whites: A systematic review and methodological appraisal. Hypertension 1997;30:1331-1337.

205. Kato N, Sugiyama T, Morita H, et al: Angiotensinogen gene and essential hypertension in the Japanese: Extensive association study and meta-analysis on six reported studies. J Hypertens 1999;17:757-763.

206. Staessen JA, Kuznetsova T, Wang JG, et al: M235T angiotensinogen gene polymorphism and cardiovascular renal risk. J Hypertens 1999;17:9-17.

207. Jeunemaitre X, Soubrier F, Kotelevtsev YV, et al: Molecular basis of human hypertension: Role of angiotensinogen. Cell 1992;71:169-180.

208. Newton MA, Sealey JE, Ledingham JG, Laragh JH: High blood pressure and oral contraceptives: Changes in plasma renin and renin substrate and in aldosterone excretion. Am J Obstet Gynecol 1968;101:1037-1045.

209. Williams GH, Fisher ND, Hunt SC, et al: Effects of gender and genotype on the phenotypic expression of nonmodulating essential hypertension. Kidney Int 2000;57:1404-1407.

210. Hopkins PN, Hunt SC, Jeunemaitre X, et al: Angiotensinogen genotype affects renal and adrenal responses to angiotensin II in essential hypertension. Circulation 2002;105:1921-1927.

211. Stock P, Liefeldt L, Paul M, Ganten D: Local renin-angiotensin systems in cardiovascular tissues: Localization and functional role. Cardiology 1995;86(Suppl):8.

212. Campbell DJ: The site of angiotensin production. J Hypertens 1985;3:199-207.

213. Mulatero P, Rabbia F, di Cella SM, et al: Angiotensin-converting enzyme and angiotensinogen gene polymorphisms are nonrandomly distributed in oral contraceptive-induced hypertension. J Hypertens 2001;19:713-719.

214. Kobashi G, Shido K, Hata A, et al: Multivariate analysis of genetic and acquired factors; T235 variant of the angiotensinogen gene is a potent independent risk factor for preeclampsia. Semin Thromb Hemost 2001;27:143-147, 2001.

215. Azizi M, Hallouin MC, Jeunemaitre X, et al: Influence of the M235T polymorphism of human angiotensinogen (AGT) on plasma AGT and renin concentrations after ethinylestradiol administration. J Clin Endocrinol Metab 2000;85:4331-4337.

216. Chiang FT, Hsu KL, Tseng CD, et al: Association of the renin gene polymorphism with essential hypertension in a Chinese population. Clin Genet 1997;51:370-374.

217. Barley J, Carter ND, Cruickshank JK, et al: Renin and atrial natriuretic peptide restriction fragment length polymorphisms: Association with ethnicity and blood pressure. J Hypertens 1991;9:993-996.

218. Frossard PM, Lestringant GG, Malloy MJ, Kane JP: Human renin gene BglI dimorphism associated with hypertension in two independent populations. Clin Genet 1999;56:428-433.

219. Frossard PM, Malloy MJ, Lestringant GG, Kane JP: Haplotypes of the human renin gene associated with essential hypertension and stroke. J Hum Hypertens 2001;15:49-55.

220. Okura T, Kitami Y, Hiwada K: Restriction fragment length polymorphisms of the human renin gene: Association study with a family history of essential hypertension. J Hum Hypertens 1993;7:457-461.

221. Zaman MM, Yoshiike N, Date C, et al: Angiotensin converting enzyme genetic polymorphism is not associated with hypertension in a cross-sectional sample of a Japanese population: The Shibata Study. J Hypertens 2001;19:47-53.

222. Clark CJ, Davies E, Anderson NH, et al: Alpha-adducin and angiotensin I-converting enzyme polymorphisms in essential hypertension. Hypertension 2000;36:990-994.

223. Schmidt S, van Hooft IM, Grobbee DE, et al: Polymorphism of the angiotensin I converting enzyme gene is apparently not related to high blood pressure: Dutch Hypertension and Offspring Study. J Hypertens 1993;11:345-348.

224. Staessen JA, Wang JG, Ginocchio G, et al: The deletion/insertion polymorphism of the angiotensin converting enzyme gene and cardiovascular-renal risk. J Hypertens 1997;15:1579-1592.

225. Giner V, Poch E, Bragulat E, et al: Renin-angiotensin system genetic polymorphisms and salt sensitivity in essential hypertension. Hypertension 2000;35:512-517.

226. Rigat B, Hubert C, Alhenc-Gelas F, et al: An insertion/deletion polymorphism in the angiotensin I-converting enzyme gene accounting for half the variance of serum enzyme levels. J Clin Invest 1990;86:1343-1346.

227. Jeng JR, Harn HJ, Jeng CY, et al: Angiotensin I converting enzyme gene polymorphism in Chinese patients with hypertension. Am J Hypertens 1997;10:558-561.

228. Qu H, Lu Y, Lin S: [Meta-analysis on the association of ACE/ID polymorphism and essential hypertension in Chinese population (English abstract)]. Zhonghua Yu Fang Yi Xue Za Zhi 2001;35:408-411.

229. Liu Y, Qiu C, Zhou W, et al: Gene polymorphisms of the renin-angiotensin system in essential hypertension. Chin Med J (Engl) 1999;112:115-120.

230. Zhu X, Yan D, Cooper RS, et al: Linkage disequilibrium and haplotype diversity in the genes of the renin-angiotensin system: Findings from the family blood pressure program. Genome Res 2003;13:173-181.

231. Barley J, Blackwood A, Miller M, et al: Angiotensin converting enzyme gene I/D polymorphism, blood pressure and the renin-angiotensin system in Caucasian and Afro-Caribbean peoples. J Hum Hypertens 1996;10:31-35.

232. Duru K, Farrow S, Wang JM, et al: Frequency of a deletion polymorphism in the gene for angiotensin converting enzyme is increased in African-Americans with hypertension. Am J Hypertens 1994;7:759-762.

233. Barlassina C, Schork NJ, Manunta P, et al: Synergistic effect of alpha-adducin and ACE genes causes blood pressure changes with body sodium and volume expansion. Kidney Int 2000;57:1083-1090.

234. Staessen JA, Wang JG, Brand E, et al: Effects of three candidate genes on prevalence and incidence of hypertension in a Caucasian population. J Hypertens 2001;19:1349-1358.

235. Zhang B, Sakai T, Miura S, et al: Association of angiotensin-converting-enzyme gene polymorphism with the depressor response to mild exercise therapy in patients with mild to moderate essential hypertension. Clin Genet 2002;62:328-333.

236. Kostis JB, Wilson AC, Hooper WC, et al: Association of angiotensin-converting enzyme DD genotype with blood pressure sensitivity to weight loss. Am Heart J 2002;144:625-629.

237. Castellano M, Muiesan ML, Beschi M, et al: Angiotensin II type 1 receptor A/C1166 polymorphism: Relationships with blood pressure and cardiovascular structure. Hypertension 1996;28:1076-1080.

238. Szombathy T, Szalai C, Katalin B, et al: Association of angiotensin II type 1 receptor polymorphism with resistant essential hypertension. Clin Chim Acta 1998;269:91-100.

239. Liu Y, Zhuoma C, Shan G, et al: A1166C polymorphism of the angiotensin II type 1 receptor gene and essential hypertension in Han, Tibetan and Yi populations. Hypertens Res 2002;25:515-521.

240. Morisawa T, Kishimoto Y, Kitano M, et al: Influence of angiotensin II type 1 receptor polymorphism on hypertension in patients with hypercholesterolemia. Clin Chim Acta 2001;304:91-97.

241. Wang WY, Zee RY, Morris BJ: Association of angiotensin II type 1 receptor gene polymorphism with essential hypertension. Clin Genet 1997;51:31-34.

242. Jiang Z, Zhao W, Yu F, Xu G: Association of angiotensin II type 1 receptor gene polymorphism with essential hypertension. Chin Med J (Engl) 2001;114:1249-1251.

243. Kainulainen K, Perola M, Terwilliger J, et al: Evidence for involvement of the type 1 angiotensin II receptor locus in essential hypertension. Hypertension 1999;33:844-849.

244. Benetos A, Gautier S, Ricard S, et al: Influence of angiotensin-converting enzyme and angiotensin II type 1 receptor gene polymorphisms on aortic stiffness in normotensive and hypertensive patients. Circulation 1996;94:698-703.

245. Lajemi M, Labat C, Gautier S, et al: Angiotensin II type 1 receptor-153A/G and 1166A/C gene polymorphisms and increase in aortic stiffness with age in hypertensive subjects. J Hypertens 2001;19:407-413.

246. Civantos CB, Aleixandre dA: Alpha-adrenoceptor subtypes. Pharmacol Res 2001;44:195-208.

247. Small KM, Wagoner LE, Levin AM, et al: Synergistic polymorphisms of beta1- and alpha2C-adrenergic receptors and the risk of congestive heart failure. N Engl J Med 2002;347:1135-1142.

248. Heinonen P, Koulu M, Pesonen U, et al: Identification of a three-amino acid deletion in the alpha2B-adrenergic receptor that is associated with reduced basal metabolic rate in obese subjects. J Clin Endocrinol Metab 1999;84:2429-2433.

249. Kannel WB, Kannel C, Paffenbarger RS Jr, Cupples LA: Heart rate and cardiovascular mortality: The Framingham study. Am Heart J 1987;113:1489-1494.

250. Wilk JB, Myers RH, Zhang Y, et al: Evidence for a gene influencing heart rate on chromosome 4 among hypertensives. Hum Genet 2002;111:207-213.

251. Xie HG, Kim RB, Stein CM, et al: Alpha1A-adrenergic receptor polymorphism: Association with ethnicity but not essential hypertension. Pharmacogenetics 1999;9:651-656.

252. Baldwin CT, Schwartz F, Baima J, et al: Identification of a polymorphic glutamic acid stretch in the alpha2B-adrenergic receptor and lack of linkage with essential hypertension. Am J Hypertens 1999;12:853-857.

253. Lockette W, Ghosh S, Farrow S, et al: Alpha 2-adrenergic receptor gene polymorphism and hypertension in blacks. Am J Hypertens 1995;8:390-394.

254. Svetkey LP, Timmons PZ, Emovon O, et al: Association of hypertension with beta2- and alpha2c10-adrenergic receptor genotype. Hypertension 1996;27:1210-1215.

255. Bengtsson K, Melander O, Orho-Melander M, et al: Polymorphism in the beta(1)-adrenergic receptor gene and hypertension. Circulation 2001;104:187-190.

256. Busjahn A, Li GH, Faulhaber HD, et al: Beta-2 adrenergic receptor gene variations, blood pressure, and heart size in normal twins. Hypertension 2000;35:555-560.

257. Tomaszewski M, Brain NJ, Charchar FJ, et al: Essential hypertension and beta2-adrenergic receptor gene: Linkage and association analysis. Hypertension 2002;40:286-291.

258. Kotanko P, Binder A, Tasker J, et al: Essential hypertension in African Caribbeans associates with a variant of the beta2-adrenoceptor. Hypertension 1997;30:773-776.

259. Timmermann B, Mo R, Luft FC, et al: Beta-2 adrenoceptor genetic variation is associated with genetic predisposition to essential hypertension: The Bergen Blood Pressure Study. Kidney Int 1998;53:1455-1460.

260. Bray MS, Krushkal J, Li L, et al: Positional genomic analysis identifies the beta(2)-adrenergic receptor gene as a susceptibility locus for human hypertension. Circulation 2000;101:2877-2882.

261. Ranade K, Shue WH, Hung YJ, et al: The glycine allele of a glycine/arginine polymorphism in the beta2-adrenergic receptor gene is associated with essential hypertension in a population of Chinese origin. Am J Hypertens 2001;14:1196-1200.

262. Herrmann SM, Nicaud V, Tiret L, et al: Polymorphisms of the beta2 -adrenoceptor (ADRB2) gene and essential hypertension: The ECTIM and PEGASE studies. J Hypertens 2002;20:229-235.

263. Ghosh S, Langefeld CD, Ally D, et al: The W64R variant of the beta3-adrenergic receptor is not associated with type II diabetes or obesity in a large Finnish sample. Diabetologia 1999;42: 238-244.

264. Strazzullo P, Iacone R, Siani A, et al: Relationship of the Trp64Arg polymorphism of the beta3-adrenoceptor gene to central adiposity and high blood pressure: Interaction with age: Cross-sectional and longitudinal findings of the Olivetti Prospective Heart Study. J Hypertens 2001;19:399-406.

265. Ringel J, Kreutz R, Distler A, Sharma AM: The Trp64Arg polymorphism of the beta3-adrenergic receptor gene is associated with hypertension in men with type 2 diabetes mellitus. Am J Hypertens 2000;13:1027-1031.

266. Haynes WG, Webb DJ: Endothelin as a regulator of cardiovascular function in health and disease. J Hypertens 1998;16:1081-1098.

267. Kedzierski RM, Yanagisawa M: Endothelin system: The double-edged sword in health and disease. Annu Rev Pharmacol Toxicol 2001;41:851-876.

268. Barton M, Lattmann T, d'Uscio LV, et al: Inverse regulation of endothelin-1 and nitric oxide metabolites in tissue with aging: Implications for the age-dependent increase of cardiorenal disease. J Cardiovasc Pharmacol 2000;36:S153-S156.

269. Clouthier DE, Hosoda K, Richardson JA, et al: Cranial and cardiac neural crest defects in endothelin-A receptor-deficient mice. Development 1998;125:813-824.

270. Hofstra RM, Valdenaire O, Arch E, et al: A loss-of-function mutation in the endothelin-converting enzyme 1 (ECE-1) associated with Hirschsprung disease, cardiac defects, and autonomic dysfunction. Am J Hum Genet 1999;64:304-308.

271. Kurihara Y, Kurihara H, Suzuki H, et al: Elevated blood pressure and craniofacial abnormalities in mice deficient in endothelin-1. Nature 1994;368:703-710.

272. Hocher B, Thone-Reineke C, Rohmeiss P, et al: Endothelin-1 transgenic mice develop glomerulosclerosis, interstitial fibrosis, and renal cysts but not hypertension. J Clin Invest 1997;99: 1380-1389.

273. Liefeldt L, Schonfelder G, Bocker W, et al: Transgenic rats expressing the human ET-2 gene: A model for the study of endothelin actions in vivo. J Mol Med 1999;77:565-574.

274. Shindo T, Kurihara H, Maemura K, et al: Renal damage and salt-dependent hypertension in aged transgenic mice overexpressing endothelin-1. J Mol Med 2002;80:105-116.

275. Asai T, Ohkubo T, Katsuya T, et al: Endothelin-1 gene variant associates with blood pressure in obese Japanese subjects: The Ohasama Study. Hypertension 2001;38:1321-1324.

276. Brown MJ, Sharma P, Stevens PA: Association between diastolic blood pressure and variants of the endothelin-1 and endothelin-2 genes. J Cardiovasc Pharmacol 2000;35(Suppl):43.

277. Barden AE, Herbison CE, Beilin LJ, et al: Association between the endothelin-1 gene Lys198Asn polymorphism blood pressure and plasma endothelin-1 levels in normal and pre-eclamptic pregnancy. J Hypertens 2001;19:1775-1782.

278. Nicaud V, Poirier O, Behague I, et al: Polymorphisms of the endothelin-A and -B receptor genes in relation to blood pressure and myocardial infarction: The Etude Cas-Temoins sur l'Infarctus du Myocarde (ECTIM) Study. Am J Hypertens 1999; 12:304-310.

279. Korneev S, O'Shea M: Evolution of nitric oxide synthase regulatory genes by DNA inversion. Mol Biol Evol 2002;19:1228-1233.

280. Rutherford S, Johnson MP, Curtain RP, Griffiths LR: Chromosome 17 and the inducible nitric oxide synthase gene in human essential hypertension. Hum Genet 2001;109:408-415.

281. Lacolley P, Gautier S, Poirier O, et al: Nitric oxide synthase gene polymorphisms, blood pressure and aortic stiffness in normotensive and hypertensive subjects. J Hypertens 1998;16: 31-35.

282. Shoji M, Tsutaya S, Saito R, et al: Positive association of endothelial nitric oxide synthase gene polymorphism with hypertension in northern Japan. Life Sci 2000;66:2557-2562.

283. Chen W, Srinivasan SR, Elkasabany A, et al: Combined effects of endothelial nitric oxide synthase gene polymorphism (G894T) and insulin resistance status on blood pressure and familial risk of hypertension in young adults: The Bogalusa Heart Study. Am J Hypertens 2001;14:1046-1052.

284. Miyamoto Y, Saito Y, Kajiyama N, et al: Endothelial nitric oxide synthase gene is positively associated with essential hypertension. Hypertension 1998;32:3-8.

285. Jachymova M, Horky K, Bultas J, et al: Association of the Glu298Asp polymorphism in the endothelial nitric oxide synthase gene with essential hypertension resistant to conventional therapy. Biochem Biophys Res Commun 2001;284:426-430.

286. Uwabo J, Soma M, Nakayama T, Kanmatsuse K: Association of a variable number of tandem repeats in the endothelial constitutive nitric oxide synthase gene with essential hypertension in Japanese. Am J Hypertens 1998;11:125-128.

287. Tsujita Y, Baba S, Yamauchi R, et al: Association analyses between genetic polymorphisms of endothelial nitric oxide synthase gene and hypertension in Japanese: The Suita Study. J Hypertens 2001;19:1941-1948.

288. Yokoyama K, Tsukada T, Nakayama M, et al: An intron 4 gene polymorphism in endothelial cell nitric oxide synthase might modulate volume-dependent hypertension in patients on hemodialysis. Nephron 2000;85:232-237.

289. Bashford MT, Hefler LA, Vertrees TW, et al: Angiotensinogen and endothelial nitric oxide synthase gene polymorphisms among Hispanic patients with preeclampsia. Am J Obstet Gynecol 2001;184:1345-1350.

290. Kobashi G, Yamada H, Ohta K, et al: Endothelial nitric oxide synthase gene (NOS3) variant and hypertension in pregnancy. Am J Med Genet 2001;103:241-244.

291. Arngrimsson R, Hayward C, Nadaud S, et al: Evidence for a familial pregnancy-induced hypertension locus in the eNOS-gene region. Am J Hum Genet 1997;61:354-362.

292. Yoshimura T, Yoshimura M, Tabata A, et al: Association of the missense Glu298Asp variant of the endothelial nitric oxide synthase gene with severe preeclampsia. J Soc Gynecol Invest 2000; 7:238-241.

293. Tempfer CB, Dorman K, Deter RL, et al: An endothelial nitric oxide synthase gene polymorphism is associated with preeclampsia. Hypertens Pregnancy 2001;20:107-118.

294. Lade JA, Moses EK, Guo G, et al: The eNOS gene: A candidate for the preeclampsia susceptibility locus? Hypertens Pregnancy 1999;18:81-93.

295. Siffert W, Rosskopf D, Siffert G, et al: Association of a human G-protein beta3 subunit variant with hypertension. Nat Genet 1998; 18:45-48.

296. Siffert W, Forster P, Jockel KH, et al: Worldwide ethnic distribution of the G protein beta3 subunit 825T allele and its association with obesity in Caucasian, Chinese, and Black African individuals. J Am Soc Nephrol 1999;10:1921-1930.

297. Siffert W: G protein beta 3 subunit 825T allele, hypertension, obesity, and diabetic nephropathy. Nephrol Dial Transplant 2000; 15:1298-1306.

298. Poch E, Gonzalez-Nunez D, Compte M, de La SA: G-protein beta3-subunit gene variant, blood pressure and erythrocyte sodium/lithium countertransport in essential hypertension. Br J Biomed Sci 2002;59:101-104.

299. Dai SP, Shi JP, Ding Q, et al: [Polymorphism analysis of 825C/T of the G-protein beta 3 subunit in high risk population of hypertension in the northeast China]. [Japanese, English Abstract]. I Chuan Hsueh Pao Acta Genetica Sinica 2002;29:294-298.

300. Brand E, Herrmann SM, Nicaud V, et al: The 825C/T polymorphism of the G-protein subunit beta3 is not related to hypertension. Hypertension 1999;33:1175-1178.

301. Ishikawa K, Imai Y, Katsuya T, et al: Human G-protein beta3 subunit variant is associated with serum potassium and total cholesterol levels but not with blood pressure. Am J Hypertens 2000;13: 140-145.

302. Snapir A, Heinonen P, Tuomainen TP, et al: G-protein beta3 subunit C825T polymorphism: No association with risk for hypertension and obesity. J Hypertens 2001;19:2149-2155.

303. Hegele RA, Harris SB, Hanley AJ, et al: G protein beta3 subunit gene variant and blood pressure variation in Canadian Oji-Cree. Hypertension 1998;32:688-692.

304. Beige J, Kreutz R, Tscherkaschina I, et al: Matrix analysis for the dissection of interactions of G-Protein beta3 subunit

C825T genotype, allograft function, and posttransplant hypertension in kidney transplantation. Am J Kidney Dis 2002;40: 1319-1324.

305. Turner ST, Schwartz GL, Chapman AB, Boerwinkle E: C825T polymorphism of the G protein beta(3)-subunit and antihypertensive response to a thiazide diuretic. Hypertension 2001;37: 739-743.

306. Gonzalez-Nunez D, Giner V, Bragulat E, et al: [Absence of an association between the C825T polymorphism of the G-protein beta 3 subunit and salt-sensitivity in essential arterial hypertension]. [Spanish, English abstract]. Nefrologia 2001;21:355-361.

307. Hinney A, Geller F, Neupert T, et al: No evidence for involvement of alleles of the 825-C/T polymorphism of the G-protein subunit beta 3 in body weight regulation. Exp Clin Endocrinol Diabetes 2001;109:402-405.

308. Benjafield AV, Lin RC, Dalziel B, et al: G-protein beta3 subunit gene splice variant in obesity and overweight. Int J Obes 2001;25: 777-780.

309. Poch E, Giner V, Gonzalez-Nunez D, et al: Association of the G protein beta3 subunit T allele with insulin resistance in essential hypertension. Clin Exp Hypertens (NY) 2002;24:345-353.

310. Siffert W, Naber C, Walla M, Ritz E: G protein beta3 subunit 825T allele and its potential association with obesity in hypertensive individuals. J Hypertens 1999;17:1095-1098.

311. Zagato L, Modica R, Florio M, et al: Genetic mapping of blood pressure quantitative trait loci in Milan hypertensive rats. Hypertension 2000;36:734-739.

312. Tripodi G, Valtorta F, Torielli L, et al: Hypertension-associated point mutations in the adducin alpha and beta subunits affect actin cytoskeleton and ion transport. J Clin Invest 1996;97:2815-2822.

313. Cusi D, Barlassina C, Azzani T, et al: Polymorphisms of alpha-adducin and salt sensitivity in patients with essential hypertension [erratum in Lancet 1997;350:524]. Lancet 1997;349: 1353-1357.

314. Ferrandi M, Salardi S, Tripodi G, et al: Evidence for an interaction between adducin and Na(+)-K(+)-ATPase: Relation to genetic hypertension. Am J Physiol 1999;277:H1338-H1349

315. Manunta P, Cusi D, Barlassina C, et al: Alpha-adducin polymorphisms and renal sodium handling in essential hypertensive patients. Kidney Int 1998;53:1471-1478.

316. Barlassina C, Norton GR, Samani NJ, et al: Alpha-adducin polymorphism in hypertensives of South African ancestry. Am J Hypertens 2000;13:719-723

317. Tamaki S, Iwai N, Tsujita Y, et al: Polymorphism of alpha-adducin in Japanese patients with essential hypertension. Hypertens Res Clin Exp 1998;21:29-32.

318. Glorioso N, Manunta P, Filigheddu F, et al: The role of alpha-adducin polymorphism in blood pressure and sodium handling regulation may not be excluded by a negative association study. Hypertension 1999;34:649-654.

319. Province MA, Arnett DK, Hunt SC, et al: Association between the alpha-adducin gene and hypertension in the HyperGEN Study. Am J Hypertens 2000;13:710-718.

320. Beeks E, Janssen RG, Kroon AA, et al: Association between the alpha-adducin Gly460Trp polymorphism and systolic blood pressure in familial combined hyperlipidemia. Am J Hypertens 2001;14:1185-1190.

321. Allayee H, de Bruin TW, Michelle DK, et al: Genome scan for blood pressure in Dutch dyslipidemic families reveals linkage to a locus on chromosome 4p. Hypertension 2001;38:773-778.

322. Busjahn A, Aydin A, von Treuenfels N, et al: Linkage but lack of association for blood pressure and the alpha-adducin locus in normotensive twins. J Hypertens 1999;17:1437-1441.

323. Wang WY, Adams DJ, Glenn CL, Morris BJ: The Gly460Trp variant of alpha-adducin is not associated with hypertension in white Anglo-Australians. Am J Hypertens 1999;12:632-636.

324. Chu SL, Zhu DL, Xiong MM, et al: Linkage analysis of twelve candidate gene loci regulating water and sodium metabolism and membrane ion transport in essential hypertension. Hypertens Res Clin Exp 2002;25:635-639.

325. Niu T, Xu X, Cordell HJ, et al: Linkage analysis of candidate genes and gene-gene interactions in chinese hypertensive sib pairs. Hypertension 1999;33:1332-1337.

326. Fisher ND, Hurwitz S, Jeunemaitre X, et al: Familial aggregation of low-renin hypertension. Hypertension 2002;39:914-918.

327. Sugimoto K, Hozawa A, Katsuya T, et al: Alpha-adducin Gly460Trp polymorphism is associated with low renin hypertension in younger subjects in the Ohasama study. J Hypertens 2002;20: 1779-1784.

328. Mulatero P, Williams TA, Milan A, et al: Blood pressure in patients with primary aldosteronism is influenced by bradykinin B(2) receptor and alpha-adducin gene polymorphisms. J Clin Endocrinol Metab 2002;87:3337-3343.

329. Grant FD, Romero JR, Jeunemaitre X, et al: Low-renin hypertension, altered sodium homeostasis, and an alpha-adducin polymorphism. Hypertension 2002;39:191-196.

330. Nicod J, Frey BM, Frey FJ, Ferrari P: Role of the alpha-adducin genotype on renal disease progression. Kidney Int 2002;61: 1270-1275.

331. Drewett JG, Fendly BM, Garbers DL, Lowe DG: Natriuretic peptide receptor-B (guanylyl cyclase-B) mediates C-type natriuretic peptide relaxation of precontracted rat aorta. J Biol Chem 1995;270:4668-4674.

332. Dessi-Fulgheri P, Sarzani R, Rappelli A: The natriuretic peptide system in obesity-related hypertension: New pathophysiological aspects. J Nephrol 1998;11:296-299.

333. Sun JZ, Chen SJ, Majid-Hasan E, Oparil S, Chen YF: Dietary salt supplementation selectively downregulates NPR-C receptor expression in kidney independently of ANP. Am J Physiol Renal Physiol 2002;282:F220-F227.

334. Tamura N, Ogawa Y, Chusho H, et al: Cardiac fibrosis in mice lacking brain natriuretic peptide. Proc Natl Acad Sci USA 2000;97:4239-4244.

335. Nkeh B, Tiago A, Candy GP, et al: Association between an atrial natriuretic peptide gene polymorphism and normal blood pressure in subjects of African ancestry. Cardiovasc J South Africa 2002;13:97-101.

336. Pan WH, Chen JW, Fann C, et al: Linkage analysis with candidate genes: The Taiwan young-onset hypertension genetic study. Hum Genet 2000;107:210-215.

337. Rubattu S, Ridker P, Stampfer MJ, et al: The gene encoding atrial natriuretic peptide and the risk of human stroke. Circulation 1999;100:1722-1726.

338. Ono K, Mannami T, Baba S, et al: A single-nucleotide polymorphism in C-type natriuretic peptide gene may be associated with hypertension. Hypertens Res Clin Exp 2002;25:727-730.

339. Nakayama T, Soma M, Takahashi Y, et al: Functional deletion mutation of the 5′-flanking region of type A human natriuretic peptide receptor gene and its association with essential hypertension and left ventricular hypertrophy in the Japanese. Circ Res 2000;86: 841-845.

340. Knowles JW, Erickson LM, Guy VK, et al: Common variations in noncoding regions of the human natriuretic peptide receptor A gene have quantitative effects. Hum Genet 2003;112:62-70.

341. Sarzani R, Dessi-Fulgheri P, Salvi F, et al: A novel promoter variant of the natriuretic peptide clearance receptor gene is associated with lower atrial natriuretic peptide and higher blood pressure in obese hypertensives. J Hypertens 1999;17: 1301-1305.

342. Rehemudula D, Nakayama T, Soma M, et al: Structure of the type B human natriuretic peptide receptor gene and association of a novel microsatellite polymorphism with essential hypertension. Circ Res 1999;84:605-610.

343. Lafferty AR, Torpy DJ, Stowasser M, et al: A novel genetic locus for low renin hypertension: Familial hyperaldosteronism type II maps to chromosome 7 (7p22). J Med Genet 2000;37:831-835.

344. Litchfield WR, Coolidge C, Silva P, et al: Impaired potassium-stimulated aldosterone production: A possible explanation for normokalemic glucocorticoid-remediable aldosteronism. J Clin Endocrinol Metab 1997;82:1507-1510.

345. Jamieson A, Slutsker L, Inglis G, et al: Clinical, biochemical and genetic features of five extended kindred's with glucocorticoid-suppressible hyperaldosteronism. Endocr Res 1995;21: 463-469.

346. Pascoe L, Curnow KM, Slutsker L, et al: Mutations in the human CYP11B2 (aldosterone synthase) gene causing corticosterone

methyloxidase II deficiency. Proc Natl Acad Sci USA 1992;89: 4996-5000.

347. Tsukada K, Ishimitsu T, Teranishi M, et al: Positive association of CYP11B2 gene polymorphism with genetic predisposition to essential hypertension. J Hum Hypertens 2002;16:789-793.

348. Davies E, Holloway CD, Ingram MC, et al: Aldosterone excretion rate and blood pressure in essential hypertension are related to polymorphic differences in the aldosterone synthase gene CYP11B2. Hypertension 1999;33:703-707.

349. Tsujita Y, Iwai N, Katsuya T, et al: Lack of association between genetic polymorphism of CYP11B2 and hypertension in Japanese: The Suita Study. Hypertens Res Clin Exp 2001;24: 105-109.

350. Komiya I, Yamada T, Takara M, et al: Lys(173)Arg and −344T/C variants of CYP11B2 in Japanese patients with low-renin hypertension. Hypertension 2000;35:699-703.

351. Rossi E, Regolisti G, Perazzoli F, et al: −344C/T polymorphism of CYP11B2 gene in Italian patients with idiopathic low renin hypertension. Am J Hypertens 2001;14:934-941.

352. Ylitalo A, Airaksinen KE, Hautanen A, et al: Baroreflex sensitivity and variants of the renin angiotensin system genes. J Am Coll Cardiol 2000;35:194-200.

353. Charchar FJ, Tomaszewski M, Padmanabhan S, et al: The Y chromosome effect on blood pressure in two European populations. Hypertension 2002;39:353-356.

354. Poch E, Gonzalez D, Giner V, et al: Molecular basis of salt sensitivity in human hypertension. Evaluation of renin-angiotensin-aldosterone system gene polymorphisms. Hypertension 2001;38: 1204-1209.

355. Brand E, Schorr U, Ringel J, et al: Aldosterone synthase gene (CYP11B2) C-344T polymorphism in Caucasians from the Berlin Salt-Sensitivity Trial (BeSST). J Hypertens 1999;17:1563-1567.

356. Smolenicka Z, Bach E, Schaer A, et al: A new polymorphic restriction site in the human 11 beta-hydroxysteroid dehydrogenase type 2 gene. J Clin Endocrinol Metab 1998;83:1814-1817.

357. Melander O, Orho-Melander M, Bengtsson K, et al: Association between a variant in the 11 beta-hydroxysteroid dehydrogenase type 2 gene and primary hypertension. J Hum Hypertens 2000; 14:819-823.

358. Sugiyama T, Kato N, Ishinaga Y, et al: Evaluation of selected polymorphisms of the Mendelian hypertensive disease genes in the Japanese population. Hypertens Res Clin Exp 2001;24: 515-521.

359. Lovati E, Ferrari P, Dick B, et al: Molecular basis of human salt sensitivity: The role of the 11beta-hydroxysteroid dehydrogenase type 2. J Clin Endocrinol Metab 1999;84:3745-3749.

360. Watson B, Jr., Bergman SM, Myracle A, et al: Genetic association of 11 beta-hydroxysteroid dehydrogenase type 2 (HSD11B2) flanking microsatellites with essential hypertension in blacks. Hypertension 1996;28:478-482.

361. Waldmann R, Champigny G, Bassilana F, et al: Molecular cloning and functional expression of a novel amiloride-sensitive Na⁺ channel. J Biol Chem 1995;270:27411-27414.

362. Hiltunen TP, Hannila-Handelberg T, Petajaniemi N, et al: Liddle's syndrome associated with a point mutation in the extracellular domain of the epithelial sodium channel gamma subunit. J Hypertens 2002;20:2383-2390.

363. Iwai N, Baba S, Mannami T, et al: Association of a sodium channel alpha subunit promoter variant with blood pressure. J Am Soc Nephrol 2002;13:80-85.

364. Iwai N, Baba S, Mannami T, et al: Association of sodium channel gamma-subunit promoter variant with blood pressure. Hypertension 2001;38:86-89.

365. Wong ZY, Stebbing M, Ellis JA, et al: Genetic linkage of beta and gamma subunits of epithelial sodium channel to systolic blood pressure. Lancet 1999;353:1222-1225.

366. Munroe PB, Strautnieks SS, Farrall M, et al: Absence of linkage of the epithelial sodium channel to hypertension in black Caribbeans. Am J Hypertens 1998;11:942-945.

367. Baker EH, Dong YB, Sagnella GA, et al: Association of hypertension with T594M mutation in beta subunit of epithelial sodium channels in black people resident in London. Lancet 1998;351: 1388-1392.

368. Ambrosius WT, Bloem LJ, Zhou L, et al: Genetic variants in the epithelial sodium channel in relation to aldosterone and potassium excretion and risk for hypertension. Hypertension 1999;34:631-637.

369. Morris B, Benjafield A, Ishikawa K, Iawi N: Polymorphism (−173G>A) in promoter of human epithelial sodium channel gamma subunit gene (SCNN1G) and association analysis in essential hypertension. Hum Mutat 2001;17(2):157.

370. Busjahn A, Aydin A, Uhlmann R, et al: Serum- and glucocorticoid-regulated kinase (SGK1) gene and blood pressure. Hypertension 2002;40:256-260.

371. Debonneville C, Flores SY, Kamynina, E et al: Phosphorylation of Nedd4-2 by Sgk1 regulates epithelial Na(+) channel cell surface expression. EMBO J 2001;20:7052-7059.

372. Song Y, Herrera VL, Filigheddu F, et al: Non-association of the thiazide-sensitive Na,Cl-cotransporter gene with polygenic hypertension in both rats and humans. J Hypertens 2001;19: 1547-1551.

373. Glorioso N, Filigheddu F, Troffa C, et al: Interaction of alpha(1)-Na,K-ATPase and Na,K,2Cl-cotransporter genes in human essential hypertension. Hypertension 2001;38:204-209.

374. Rankinen T, Perusse L, Deriaz O, et al: Linkage of the Na,K-ATPase alpha 2 and beta 1 genes with resting and exercise heart rate and blood pressure: Cross-sectional and longitudinal observations from the Quebec Family Study. J Hypertens 1999;17:339-349.

375. Lifton RP, Hunt SC, Williams RR, et al: Exclusion of the Na(+)-H+ antiporter as a candidate gene in human essential hypertension. Hypertension 1991;17:8-14.

376. Yu H, Freedman BI, Rich SS, Bowden DW: Human Na⁺/H⁺ exchanger genes: Identification of polymorphisms by radiation hybrid mapping and analysis of linkage in end-stage renal disease. Hypertension 2000;35:135-143.

377. Mukae S, Aoki S, Itoh S, et al: Bradykinin B(2) receptor gene polymorphism is associated with angiotensin-converting enzyme inhibitor-related cough. Hypertension 2000;36:127-131.

378. Sato M, Soma M, Nakayama T, Kanmatsuse K: Dopamine D1 receptor gene polymorphism is associated with essential hypertension. Hypertension 2000;36:183-186.

379. Soma M, Nakayama K, Rahmutula D, et al: Ser9Gly polymorphism in the dopamine D3 receptor gene is not associated with essential hypertension in the Japanese. Med Sci Monitor 2002;8: CR1-CR4.

380. Thomas GN, Critchley JA, Tomlinson B, et al: Relationships between the taqI polymorphism of the dopamine D2 receptor and blood pressure in hyperglycaemic and normoglycaemic Chinese subjects. Clin Endocrinol 2001;55:605-611.

381. Iwai N, Katsuya T, Ishikawa K, et al: Human prostacyclin synthase gene and hypertension: The Suita Study. Circulation 1999;100: 2231-2236.

382. Nakayama T, Soma M, Watanabe Y, et al: Splicing mutation of the prostacyclin synthase gene in a family associated with hypertension. Biochem Biophys Res Commun 2002;297:1135-1139.

383. Sharma P, Hingorani A, Jia H, et al: Positive association of tyrosine hydroxylase microsatellite marker to essential hypertension. Hypertension 1998;32:676-682.

384. Barroso I, Gurnell M, Crowley VE, et al: Dominant negative mutations in human PPARgamma associated with severe insulin resistance, diabetes mellitus and hypertension [see comments]. Nature 1999;402:880-883.

385. Douglas JA, Erdos MR, Watanabe RM, et al: The peroxisome proliferator-activated receptor-gamma2 Pro12A1a variant: Association with type 2 diabetes and trait differences. Diabetes 2001;50: 886-890.

386. Hasstedt SJ, Ren QF, Teng K, Elbein SC: Effect of the peroxisome proliferator-activated receptor-gamma 2 pro(12)ala variant on obesity, glucose homeostasis, and blood pressure in members of familial type 2 diabetic kindreds. J Clin Endocrinol Metab 2001;86:536-541.

387. Chuang LM, Hsiung CA, Chen YD, et al: Sibling-based association study of the PPARgamma2 Pro12Ala polymorphism and metabolic variables in Chinese and Japanese hypertension families: A SAPPHIRe study. Stanford Asian-Pacific Program in Hypertension and Insulin Resistance. J Mol Med 2001;79:656-664.

388. Altshuler D, Hirschhorn JN, Klannemark M, et al: The common PPARgamma Pro12Ala polymorphism is associated with decreased risk of type 2 diabetes. Nat Genet 2000;26:76-80.

389. Aitman TJ, Glazier AM, Wallace CA, et al: Identification of Cd36 (Fat) as an insulin-resistance gene causing defective fatty acid and glucose metabolism in hypertensive rats. Nat Genet 1999;21:76-83.

390. Miyaoka K, Kuwasako T, Hirano K, et al: CD36 deficiency associated with insulin resistance. Lancet 2001;357:686-687.

391. Collison M, Glazier AM, Graham D, et al: Cd36 and molecular mechanisms of insulin resistance in the stroke-prone spontaneously hypertensive rat. Diabetes 2000;49:2222-2226.

392. Pravenec M, Landa V, Zidek V, et al: Transgenic rescue of defective Cd36 ameliorates insulin resistance in spontaneously hypertensive rats. Nat Genet 2001;27:156-158.

393. Kajihara S, Hisatomi A, Ogawa Y, et al: Association of the Pro90Ser CD36 mutation with elevated free fatty acid concentrations but not with insulin resistance syndrome in Japanese. Clin Chim Acta 2001;314:125-130.

394. Lin RC, Wang WY, Morris BJ: Association and linkage analyses of glucocorticoid receptor gene markers in essential hypertension. Hypertension 1999;34:1186-1192.

395. Shintani M, Ikegami H, Fujisawa T, et al: Leptin gene polymorphism is associated with hypertension independent of obesity. J Clin Endocrinol Metab 2002;87:2909-2912.

396. Bray MS, Boerwinkle E, Hanis CL: Linkage analysis of candidate obesity genes among the Mexican-American population of Starr County, Texas. Genet Epidemiol 1999;16:397-411.

397. Rosmond R, Chagnon YC, Holm G, et al: Hypertension in obesity and the leptin receptor gene locus. J Clin Endocrinol Metab 2000;85:3126-3131.

398. Zheng Y, Xiang K, Zhang R, et al: [Association of Gln223Arg variant in leptin receptor gene with metabolic abnormalities and hypertension in type II diabetes mellitus in Shanghai "Han" population]. Chung-Hua Nei Ko Tsa Chih Chin J Intern Med 1999;38(3):174-177.

399. Jacob HJ, Lindpaintner K, Lincoln SE, et al: Genetic mapping of a gene causing hypertension in the stroke-prone spontaneously hypertensive rat. Cell 1991;67:213-224.

400. Julier C, Delepine M, Keavney B, et al: Genetic susceptibility for human familial essential hypertension in a region of homology with blood pressure linkage on rat chromosome 10. Hum Mol Genet 1997;6:2077-2085.

401. Levy D, DeStefano AL, Larson MG, et al: Evidence for a gene influencing blood pressure on chromosome 17. Genome scan linkage results for longitudinal blood pressure phenotypes in subjects from the framingham heart study. [see comments]. Hypertension 2000;36:477-483.

402. Baima J, Nicolaou M, Schwartz F, et al: Evidence for linkage between essential hypertension and a putative locus on human chromosome 17. Hypertension 1999;34:4-7.

403. Pankow JS, Rose KM, Oberman A, et al: Possible locus on chromosome 18q influencing postural systolic blood pressure changes. Hypertension 2000;36:471-476.

404. Rice T, Rankinen T, Chagnon YC, et al: Genomewide linkage scan of resting blood pressure: HERITAGE Family Study. Health, Risk Factors, Exercise Training, and Genetics. Hypertension 2002;39:1037-1043.

405. Rankinen T, An P, Rice T, et al: Genomic scan for exercise blood pressure in the Health, Risk Factors, Exercise Training and Genetics (HERITAGE) Family Study. Hypertension 2001;38:30-37.

406. Foster KR, Lukaski HC: Whole-body impedance–what does it measure? Am J Clin Nutr 1996;64:388S-396S.

407. Kotchen TA, Broeckel U, Grim CE, et al: Identification of hypertension-related QTLs in African American sib pairs. Hypertension 2002;40:634-639.

408. Hsueh WC, Mitchell BD, Schneider JL, et al: QTL influencing blood pressure maps to the region of PPH1 on chromosome 2q31-34 in Old Order Amish. Circulation 2000;101:2810-2816.

409. Rice T, Rankinen T, Province MA, et al: Genome-wide linkage analysis of systolic and diastolic blood pressure: The Quebec Family Study. Circulation 2000;102:1956-1963.

410. Hunt SC, Ellison RC, Atwood LD, et al: Genome scans for blood pressure and hypertension: The National Heart, Lung, and Blood Institute Family Heart Study. Hypertension 2002;40:1-6.

411. Kardia SLR, Rozek LS, Krushkal J, et al: Genome-wide linkage analyses for hypertension genes in two ethnically and geographically diverse populations. Am J Hypertens 2003;16:154-157.

412. Thiel BA, Chakravarti A, Cooper RS, et al: A genome-wide linkage analysis investigating the determinants of blood pressure in whites and African Americans. Am J Hypertens 2003;16:151-153.

413. Rao DC, Province MA, Leppert MF, et al: A genome-wide affected sibpair linkage analysis of hypertension: The HyperGEN network. Am J Hypertens 2003;16:148-150.

414. Cheng LS, Davis RC, Raffel LJ, et al: Coincident linkage of fasting plasma insulin and blood pressure to chromosome 7q in hypertensive hispanic families. Circulation 2001;104:1255-1260.

415. Atwood LD, Samollow PB, Hixson JE, et al: Genome-wide linkage analysis of blood pressure in Mexican Americans. Genet Epidemiol Suppl 2001;20:373-382.

416. Harrap SB, Wong ZY, Stebbing M, et al: Blood pressure QTLs identified by genome-wide linkage analysis and dependence on associated phenotypes. Physiol Genomics 2002;8:99-105.

417. Cooper RS, Luke A, Zhu X, et al: Genome scan among Nigerians linking blood pressure to chromosomes 2, 3, and 19. Hypertension 2002;40:629-633.

418. Sharma P, Fatibene J, Ferraro F, et al: A genome-wide search for susceptibility loci to human essential hypertension. Hypertension 2000;35:1291-1296.

419. Perola M, Kainulainen K, Pajukanta P, et al: Genome-wide scan of predisposing loci for increased diastolic blood pressure in Finnish siblings. J Hypertens 2000;18:1579-1585.

420. Angius A, Petretto E, Maestrale GB, et al: A new essential hypertension susceptibility locus on chromosome 2p24-p25, detected by genomewide search. Am J Hum Genet 2002;71:893-905.

421. Allayee H, de Bruin TW, Michelle DK, et al: Genome scan for blood pressure in Dutch dyslipidemic families reveals linkage to a locus on chromosome 4p. Hypertension 2001;38:773-778.

422. Caulfield M, Lavender P, Newell-Price J, et al: Linkage of the angiotensinogen gene locus to human essential hypertension in African Caribbeans. J Clin Invest 1995;96:687-692.

423. Kristjansson K, Manolescu A, Kristinsson A, et al: Linkage of essential hypertension to chromosome 18q. Hypertension 2002;39:1044-1049.

424. Zhu DL, Wang HY, Xiong MM, et al: Linkage of hypertension to chromosome 2q14-q23 in Chinese families. J Hypertens Suppl 2001;19:55-61.

425. Xu X, Yang J, Rogus J, et al: Mapping of a blood pressure quantitative trait locus to chromosome 15q in a Chinese population. Hum Mol Genet 1999;8:2551-2555.

426. Xu X, Rogus JJ, Terwedow HA, et al: An extreme-sib-pair genome scan for genes regulating blood pressure. Am J Hum Genet 1999;64:1694-1701.

427. Ranade K, Hinds D, Hsiung CA et al: A genome scan for hypertension susceptibility loci in populations of Chinese and Japanese origins. Am J Hypertens 2003;16:158-162.

428. Caulfield M, Munroe P, Pembroke J, et al: Genom-wide mapping of human loci for essential hypertension. Lancet 2003;361:2118-2123.

429. Paigen B: The genetics of blood pressure variation in mice. Program of the 2002 annual meeting of the American Society of Nephrology. J Am Soc Nephrol 13(9):62P and http://pga.jax.org/hypertension_qtl.html, 2002.

430. Risch N, Zhang H: Extreme discordant sib pairs for mapping quantitative trait loci in humans. Science 1995;268:1584-1589.

431. Human genome NCBI NT release build 31, mouse genome MGSC v3 NT release build 29; NCBI homology map using NCBI genome assembly vs mouse genome database (MGD) map and Ensembl Syntenyview Ensembl Human Genome browser v9.30a.1 vs Ensembl MGSC Mouse Genome browser v9.3a.1. NCBI (www.ncbi.nlm.nih.gov), Ensembl (www.ensembl.org) 2003.

432. Province MA, Kardia SLR, Ranade K, et al: A meta-analysis of genome-wide linkage scans for hypertension: The National Heart, Lung and Blood Institute Family Blood Pressure Program. Am J Hypertens 2003;16:144-147.

433. Ely DL, Turner ME: Hypertension in the spontaneously hypertensive rat is linked to the Y chromosome. Hypertension 1990;16:277-281.

434. Davidson AO, Schork N, Jaques BC, et al: Blood pressure in genetically hypertensive rats. Influence of the Y chromosome. Hypertension 1995;26:452-459.

435. Kren V, Qi N, Krenova D, et al: Y-chromosome transfer induces changes in blood pressure and blood lipids in SHR. Hypertension 2001;37:1147-1152.

436. Negrin CD, McBride MW, Carswell HV, et al: Reciprocal consomic strains to evaluate Y chromosome effects. Hypertension 2001;37:391-397.

437. Dumas P, Kren V, Krenova D, et al: Identification and chromosomal localization of ecogenetic components of electrolyte excretion. J Hypertens 2002;20:209-217.

438. Shoji M, Tsutaya S, Shimada J, et al: Lack of association between Y chromosome Alu insertion polymorphism and hypertension. Hypertens Res 2002;25:1-3.

439. Ellis JA, Stebbing M, Harrap SB: Association of the human Y chromosome with high blood pressure in the general population. Hypertension 2000;36:731-733.

440. Watson B, Jr., Khan MA, Desmond RA, Bergman S: Mitochondrial DNA mutations in black Americans with hypertension-associated end-stage renal disease. Am J Kidney Dis 2001;38:529-536.

441. Doleris LM, Hill GS, Chedin P, et al: Focal segmental glomerulosclerosis associated with mitochondrial cytopathy. Kidney Int 2000;58:1851-1858.

442. Uhari M, Koskimies O: A survey of 164 Finnish children and adolescents with hypertension. Acta Paediatri Scand 1979;68:193-198.

443. Hari P, Bagga A, Srivastava RN: Sustained hypertension in children. Indian Pediatr 2000;37:268-274.

444. Blagowidow N, Page DC, Huff D, Mennuti MT: Ullrich-Turner syndrome in an XY female fetus with deletion of the sex-determining portion of the Y chromosome. Am J Med Genet 1989;34:159-162.

445. Digilio MC, Marino B, Toscano A, et al: Congenital heart defects in Kabuki syndrome. Am J Med Genet 2001;100:269-274.

446. Marino B, Digilio MC, Toscano A, et al: Congenital heart diseases in children with Noonan syndrome: An expanded cardiac spectrum with high prevalence of atrioventricular canal. J Pediatr 1999; 135:703-706.

447. Hughes HE, Davies SJ: Coarctation of the aorta in Kabuki syndrome. Arch Dis Child 1994;70:512-514.

448. Phillips HM, Renforth GL, Spalluto C, et al: Narrowing the critical region within 11q24-qter for hypoplastic left heart and identification of a candidate gene, JAM3, expressed during cardiogenesis. Genomics 2002;79:475-478.

449. Krishnamurti L, Neglia JP, Nagarajan R, et al: Paris-Trousseau syndrome platelets in a child with Jacobsen's syndrome. Am J Hematol 2001;66:295-299.

450. Wilson DI, Cross IE, Goodship JA, et al: DiGeorge syndrome with isolated aortic coarctation and isolated ventricular septal defect in three sibs with a 22q11 deletion of maternal origin. Br Heart J 1991;66:308-312.

451. Junker R, Kotthoff S, Vielhaber H, et al: Infant methylenetetrahydrofolate reductase 677TT genotype is a risk factor for congenital heart disease. Cardiovasc Res 2001;51:251-254.

452. Clark EB: Neck web and congenital heart defects: A pathogenic association in 45 X-O Turner syndrome? Teratology 1984;29: 355-361.

453. Berdahl LD, Wenstrom KD, Hanson JW: Web neck anomaly and its association with congenital heart disease. Am J Med Genet 1995;56:304-307.

454. Chu CE, Donaldson MD, Kelnar CJ, et al: Possible role of imprinting in the Turner phenotype. J Med Genet 1994;31:840-842.

455. Thurston H: Experimental models of hypertension: Goldblatt, coarctation and Page experimental models of renovascular hypertension. In Swales JD (ed): Textbook of Hypertension. Oxford, Blackwell Scientific Publications 1994, 477-493.

456. Brunner HR, Kirshman JD, Sealey JE, Laragh JH: Hypertension of renal origin: Evidence for two different mechanisms. Science 1971;174:1344-1346.

457. Bookstein JJ, Abrams HL, Buenger RE et al: Radiologic aspects of renovascular hypertension. II. The role of urography in unilateral renovascular disease. JAMA 1972;220:1225-1230.

458. Schreiber MJ, Pohl MA, Novick AC: The natural history of atherosclerotic and fibrous renal artery disease. Urol Clin North Am 1984;11:383-392.

459. Luscher TF, Lie JT, Stanson AW, et al: Arterial fibromuscular dysplasia. Mayo Clin Proc 1987;62:931-952.

460. Grimbert P, Fiquer-Kempf B, Coudol P, et al: [Genetic study of renal artery fibromuscular dysplasia] [French, English abstract]. Arch Maladies Coeur Vaisseaux 1998;91:1069-1071.

461. Rushton AR: The genetics of fibromuscular dysplasia. Arch Intern Med 1980;140:233-236.

462. Stanley JC, Fry WJ: Pediatric renal artery occlusive disease and renovascular hypertension. Etiology, diagnosis, and operative treatment. Arch Surg 1981;116:669-676.

463. Tsuji T, Imajo Y, Sawabe M, et al: Acquired cutis laxa concomitant with nephrotic syndrome. Arch Dermatol 1987;123:1211-1216.

464. Zhang MC, He L, Giro M, et al: Cutis laxa arising from frameshift mutations in exon 30 of the elastin gene (ELN). J Biol Chem 1999;274:981-986.

465. Boute N, Gribouval O, Roselli S, et al: NPHS2, encoding the glomerular protein podocin, is mutated in autosomal recessive steroid-resistant nephrotic syndrome. [erratum appears in Nat Genet 2000;25:125]. Nat Genet 2000;24:349-354.

466. Kaplan JM, Kim SH, North KN, et al: Mutations in ACTN4, encoding alpha-actinin-4, cause familial focal segmental glomerulosclerosis. Nat Genet 2000;24:251-256.

467. Gharavi AG, Yan Y, Scolari F, et al: IgA nephropathy, the most common cause of glomerulonephritis, is linked to 6q22-23. Nat Genet 2000;26:354-357.

468. Brenner BM, Rector FC: Brenner and Rector's the Kidney, 6th ed. Philadelphia, WB Saunders, 2000.

469. Megyesi J, Price PM, Tamayo E, Safirstein RL: The lack of a functional p21WAF1/CIP1 gene ameliorates progression to chronic renal failure. PNAS 1999;96:10830-10835.

470. Young WF Jr: Primary aldosteronism: Management issues Ann NY Acad Sci 2002;970:61-76.

471. Lim PO, Jung RT, MacDonald TM: Raised aldosterone to renin ratio predicts antihypertensive efficacy of spironolactone: A prospective cohort follow-up study. Br J Clin Pharmacol 1999;48: 756-760.

472. Dluhy RG, Lawrence JE, Williams GH: Endocrine hypertension. In Larsen PR, Wilson JD, Melmed S, et al. (eds): Williams Textbook of Endocrinology, 10th ed. Philadelphia, WB Saunders, 2003, pp 552-585.

473. Connell JMC, Fraser R: Primary aldosteronism. In Wass JAH, Shalet SM (eds): Oxford Textbook of Endocrinology and Diabetes. Oxford, Oxford University Press, 2002, 791-799.

474. Ganguly A, Melada GA, Luetscher JA, Dowdy AJ: Control of plasma aldosterone in primary aldosteronism: Distinction between adenoma and hyperplasia. J Clin Endocrinol Metab 1973;37:765-775.

475. Young WF Jr, Klee GG: Primary aldosteronism: Diagnostic evaluation. Endocrinol Metab Clin North Am 1988;17:367-395.

476. Ulick S, Blumenfeld JD, Atlas SA, et al: The unique steroidogenesis of the aldosteronoma in the differential diagnosis of primary aldosteronism. J Clin Endocrinol Metab 1993;76:873-878.

477. Phillips JL, Walther MM, Pezzullo JC, et al: Predictive value of preoperative tests in discriminating bilateral adrenal hyperplasia from an aldosterone-producing adrenal adenoma. J Clin Endocrinol Metab 2000;85:4526-4533.

478. Kirschner LS, Carney JA, Pack SD, et al: Mutations of the gene encoding the protein kinase A type I-alpha regulatory subunit in patients with the Carney complex. Nat Genet 2000;26:89-92.

479. Quinn SJ, Williams GH: Regulation of aldosterone secretion. Annu Rev Physiol 1988;50:409-426.

480. Curnow KM, Mulatero P, Emeric-Blanchouin N, et al: The amino acid substitutions Ser288Gly and Val320Ala convert the cortisol producing enzyme, CYP11B1, into an aldosterone producing enzyme. Nat Struct Biol 1997;4:32-35.

481. Dluhy RG, Anderson B, Harlin B, et al: Glucocorticoid-remediable aldosteronism is associated with severe hypertension in early childhood. J Pediatr 2001;138:715-720.

482. Stowasser M, Gordon RD: Familial hyperaldosteronism. J Steroid Biochem Mol Biol 2001;78:215-229, 2001.

483. White PC: Steroid 11 beta-hydroxylase deficiency and related disorders. Endocrinol Metab Clin North Am 2001;30:61-79.

484. Melby JC, Dale SL, Holbrook M, Griffing GT: 19-Norcorticosteroids in experimental and human hypertension. Clin Exp Hypertens A 1982;4:1851-1867.

485. Auchus RJ: The genetics, pathophysiology, and management of human deficiencies of P450c17. Endocrinol Metab Clin North Am 2001;30:101–119.

486. Brown RW, Chapman KE, Kotelevtsev Y, et al: Cloning and production of antisera to human placental 11 beta-hydroxysteroid dehydrogenase type 2. Biochem J 1996;313:1007–1017.

487. White PC: 11beta-hydroxysteroid dehydrogenase and its role in the syndrome of apparent mineralocorticoid excess. Am J Med Sci 2001;322:308–315.

488. Albiston AL, Obeyesekere VR, Smith RE, Krozowski ZS: Cloning and tissue distribution of the human 11 beta-hydroxysteroid dehydrogenase type 2 enzyme. Mol Cell Endocrinol 1994;105:R11–R17.

489. Funder JW, Pearce PT, Smith R, Smith AI: Mineralocorticoid action: Target tissue specificity is enzyme, not receptor, mediated. Science 1988;242:583–585.

490. Stewart PM, Wallace AM, Valentino R, et al: Mineralocorticoid activity of liquorice: 11-beta-hydroxysteroid dehydrogenase deficiency comes of age. Lancet 1987;2:821–824.

491. Kotelevtsev Y, Brown RW, Fleming S, et al: Hypertension in mice lacking 11beta-hydroxysteroid dehydrogenase type 2. J Clin Invest 1999;103:683–689.

492. Palermo M, Cossu M, Shackleton CH: Cure of apparent mineralocorticoid excess by kidney transplantation. N Engl J Med 1998;339:1787–1788.

493. Geller DS, Farhi A, Pinkerton N, et al: Activating mineralocorticoid receptor mutation in hypertension exacerbated by pregnancy. Science 2000;289:119–123.

494. Rafestin-Oblin ME, Souque A, Bocchi B, et al: The severe form of hypertension caused by the activating S810L mutation in the mineralocorticoid receptor is cortisone related. Endocrinology 2003;144:528–533.

495. Rossier BC, Pradervand S, Schild L, Hummler E: Epithelial sodium channel and the control of sodium balance: Interaction between genetic and environmental factors. Annu Rev Physiol 2002;64:877–897.

496. Torpy DJ, Mullen N, Ilias I, Nieman LK: Association of hypertension and hypokalemia with Cushing's syndrome caused by ectopic ACTH secretion: A series of 58 cases. Ann NY Acad Sci 2002;970:134–144.

497. Kino T, Vottero A, Charmandari E, Chrousos GP: Familial/sporadic glucocorticoid resistance syndrome and hypertension. Ann NY Acad Sci 2002;970:101–111.

498. Geller DS, Rodriguez-Soriano J, Vallo BA, et al: Mutations in the mineralocorticoid receptor gene cause autosomal dominant pseudohypoaldosteronism type I. Nat Genet 1998;19:279–281.

499. Berger S, Bleich M, Schmid W, et al: Mineralocorticoid receptor knockout mice: Lessons on Na+ metabolism [review] [23 refs]. Kidney Int 2000;57:1295–1298.

500. Schulz-Baldes A, Berger S, Grahammer F, et al: Induction of the epithelial Na+ channel via glucocorticoids in mineralocorticoid receptor knockout mice. Pflugers Arch Eur J Physiol 2001;443:297–305.

501. Chang SS, Grunder S, Hanukoglu, A et al: Mutations in subunits of the epithelial sodium channel cause salt wasting with hyperkalaemic acidosis, pseudohypoaldosteronism type 1. Nat Genet 1996;12:248–253.

502. Neumann HP, Hoegerle S, Manz T, et al: How many pathways to pheochromocytoma? Semin Nephrol 2002;22:89–99.

503. Mulligan LM, Gardner E, Smith BA, et al: Genetic events in tumour initiation and progression in multiple endocrine neoplasia type 2. Genes Chromosomes Cancer 1993;6:166–177.

504. Khosla S, Patel VM, Hay ID, et al: Loss of heterozygosity suggests multiple genetic alterations in pheochromocytomas and medullary thyroid carcinomas. J Clin Invest 1991;87:1691–1699.

505. Carney JA, Stratakis CA: Familial paraganglioma and gastric stromal sarcoma: A new syndrome distinct from the Carney triad. Am J Med Genet 2002;108:132–139.

506. Mason I: The RET receptor tyrosine kinase: Activation, signalling and significance in neural development and disease. Pharmaceut Acta Helvet 2000;74:261–264.

507. Kalff V, Shapiro B, Lloyd R, et al: The spectrum of pheochromocytoma in hypertensive patients with neurofibromatosis. Arch Intern Med 1982;142:2092–2098.

508. Strauchen JA: Germ-line mutations in nonsyndromic pheochromocytoma. N Engl J Med 2002;347:854–855.

509. Maher ER, Eng C: The pressure rises: Update on the genetics of phaeochromocytoma. Hum Mol Genet 2002;11:2347–2354.

510. Benn DE, Croxson MS, Tucker K et al: Novel succinate dehydrogenase subunit B (SDHB) mutations in familial phaeochromocytomas and paragangliomas, but an absence of somatic SDHB mutations in sporadic phaeochromocytomas. Oncogene 2003;22:1358–1364.

511. Baysal BE, Ferrell RE, Willett-Brozick JE, et al: Mutations in SDHD, a mitochondrial complex II gene, in hereditary paraganglioma. Science 2000;287:848–851.

512. Rodriguez-Cuevas S, Lopez-Garza J, Labastida-Almendaro S: Carotid body tumors in inhabitants of altitudes higher than 2000 meters above sea level. Head Neck 1998;20:374–378.

513. de la Monte SM, Hutchins GM, Moore GW: Peripheral neuroblastic tumors and congenital heart disease: Possible role of hypoxic states in tumor induction. Am J Pediatr Hematol Oncol 1985;7:109–116.

514. Hla KM, Young TB, Bidwell T, et al: Sleep apnea and hypertension. A population-based study. Ann Intern Med 1994;120:382–388.

515. Rauscher H, Formanek D, Popp W, Zwick H: Nasal CPAP and weight loss in hypertensive patients with obstructive sleep apnoea. Thorax 1993;48:529–533.

516. Kimura G, Frem GJ, Brenner BM: Renal mechanisms of salt sensitivity in hypertension. Curr Opin Nephrol Hypertens 1994;3:1–12.

517. Landsberg L: Insulin-mediated sympathetic stimulation: Role in the pathogenesis of obesity-related hypertension (or, how insulin affects blood pressure, and why). J Hypertens 2001;19:523–528.

518. Frederich RC Jr, Kahn BB, Peach MJ, Flier JS: Tissue-specific nutritional regulation of angiotensinogen in adipose tissue. Hypertension 1992;19:339–344.

519. Bjorntorp P: Do stress reactions cause abdominal obesity and comorbidities? Obes Rev 2001;2:73–86.

520. Sudi KM, Gallistl S, Weinhandl G, et al: No evidence for leptin as an independent associate of blood pressure in childhood and juvenile obesity. J Pediatr Endocrinol Metab 2000;13:513–521.

521. Montague CT, Farooqi IS, Whitehead JP, et al: Congenital leptin deficiency is associated with severe early-onset obesity in humans. Nature 1997;387:903–908.

522. Clement K, Vaisse C, Lahlou N, et al: A mutation in the human leptin receptor gene causes obesity and pituitary dysfunction. Nature 1998;392:398–401.

523. Jackson RS, Creemers JW, Ohagi S, et al: Obesity and impaired prohormone processing associated with mutations in the human prohormone convertase 1 gene. Nat Genet 1997;16:303–306.

524. Krude H, Biebermann H, Luck W, et al: Severe early-onset obesity, adrenal insufficiency and red hair pigmentation caused by POMC mutations in humans. Nat Genet 1998;19:155–157.

525. Farooqi IS, Yeo GS, Keogh JM, et al: Dominant and recessive inheritance of morbid obesity associated with melanocortin 4 receptor deficiency. J Clin Invest 2000;106:271–279.

526. Jequier E: Leptin signaling, adiposity, and energy balance. Ann NY Acad Sci 2002;967:379–388.

527. Cummings DE, Schwartz MW: Melanocortins and body weight: A tale of two receptors. Nat Genet 2000;26:8–9.

528. Heo M, Leibel RL, Boyer BB, et al: Pooling analysis of genetic data: The association of leptin receptor (LEPR) polymorphisms with variables related to human adiposity. Genetics 2001;159: 1163–1178.

529. Allison DB, Heo M, Faith MS, Pietrobelli A: Meta-analysis of the association of the Trp64Arg polymorphism in the beta3 adrenergic receptor with body mass index. Int J Obes Relat Metab Disord 1998;22:559–566.

530. Fujisawa T, Ikegami H, Kawaguchi Y, Ogihara T: Meta-analysis of the association of Trp64Arg polymorphism of beta 3-adrenergic receptor gene with body mass index. J Clin Endocrinol Metab 1998;83:2441–2444.

531. Arner P, Hoffstedt J: Adrenoceptor genes in human obesity. J Intern Med 1999;245:667–672.

532. Hager J, Dina C, Francke S, et al: A genome-wide scan for human obesity genes reveals a major susceptibility locus on chromosome 10. Nat Genet 1998;20:304–308.

533. Bektas A, Suprenant ME, Wogan LT, et al: Evidence of a novel type 2 diabetes locus 50 cM centromeric to NIDDM2 on chromosome 12q. Diabetes 1999;48:2246–2251.

534. Taylor SI, Arioglu E: Syndromes associated with insulin resistance and acanthosis nigricans [review] [76 refs]. J Basic Clin Physiol Pharmacol 1998;9:419–439.

535. Cao H, Hegele RA: Nuclear lamin A/C R482Q mutation in Canadian kindreds with Dunnigan-type familial partial lipodystrophy. Hum Mol Genet 2000;9:109–112.

536. Agarwal AK, Arioglu E, De Almeida S, et al: AGPAT2 is mutated in congenital generalized lipodystrophy linked to chromosome 9q34. Nat Genet 2002;31:21–23.

537. Magre J, Delepine M, Khallouf E, et al: Identification of the gene altered in Berardinelli-Seip congenital lipodystrophy on chromosome 11q13. Nat Genet 2001;28:365–370.

538. Lind L, Berne C, Lithell H: Prevalence of insulin resistance in essential hypertension. J Hypertens 1995;13:1457–1462.

539. Haffner SM, D'Agostino R, Saad MF, et al: Increased insulin resistance and insulin secretion in nondiabetic African-Americans and Hispanics compared with non-Hispanic whites. The Insulin Resistance Atherosclerosis Study. Diabetes 1996;45:742–748.

540. Saltiel AR, Kahn CR: Insulin signalling and the regulation of glucose and lipid metabolism. Nature 2001;414:799–806.

541. Bruning JC, Michael MD, Winnay JN, et al: A muscle-specific insulin receptor knockout exhibits features of the metabolic syndrome of NIDDM without altering glucose tolerance. Mol Cell 1998;2:559–569.

542. Wojtaszewski JF, Higaki Y, Hirshman MF, et al: Exercise modulates postreceptor insulin signaling and glucose transport in muscle-specific insulin receptor knockout mice. J Clin Invest 1999;104:1257–1264.

543. Shimomura I, Bashmakov Y, Ikemoto S, et al: Insulin selectively increases SREBP-1c mRNA in the livers of rats with streptozotocin-induced diabetes. Proc Natl Acad Sci USA 1999;96:13656–13661.

544. Lang F, Klingel K, Wagner CA, et al: Deranged transcriptional regulation of cell-volume-sensitive kinase hSGK in diabetic nephropathy. Proc Natl Acad Sci USA 2000;97:8157–8162.

545. Feraille E, Doucet A: Sodium-potassium-adenosinetriphosphatase-dependent sodium transport in the kidney: Hormonal control. Physiol Rev 2001;81:345–418.

546. Tsuchida H, Imai G, Shima Y, et al: Mechanism of sodium load-induced hypertension in non-insulin dependent diabetes mellitus model rats: Defective dopaminergic system to inhibit Na-K-ATPase activity in renal epithelial cells. Hypertens Res 2001;24:127–135.

547. Klisic J, Hu MC, Nief V, et al: Insulin activates Na$^+$/H$^+$ exchanger 3: Biphasic response and glucocorticoid dependence. Am J Physiol Renal Physiol 2002;283:F532–F539.

548. Shirakami A, Toyonaga T, Tsuruzoe K, et al: Heterozygous knockout of the IRS-1 gene in mice enhances obesity-linked insulin resistance: A possible model for the development of type 2 diabetes. J Endocrinol 2002;174:309–319.

549. Kido Y, Burks DJ, Withers D, et al: Tissue-specific insulin resistance in mice with mutations in the insulin receptor, IRS-1, and IRS-2. J Clin Invest 2000;105:199–205.

550. Yuan M, Konstantopoulos N, Lee J, et al: Reversal of obesity- and diet-induced insulin resistance with salicylates or targeted disruption of Ikkbeta.[erratum appears in Science 2002;295:277]. Science 2001;293:1673–1677.

551. Corry DB, Tuck ML: Selective aspects of the insulin resistance syndrome. Curr Opin Nephrol Hypertens 2001;10:507–514.

552. Steinberg HO, Paradisi G, Hook G, et al: Free fatty acid elevation impairs insulin-mediated vasodilation and nitric oxide production. Diabetes 2000;49:1231–1238.

553. Kitamura T, Kahn CR, Accili D: Insulin receptor knockout mice. Annu Rev Physiol 2003;65:313–332.

554. Abe H, Yamada N, Kamata K, et al: Hypertension, hypertriglyceridemia, and impaired endothelium-dependent vascular relaxation in mice lacking insulin receptor substrate-1. J Clin Invest 1998;101:1784–1788.

555. Stenbit AE, Tsao TS, Li J, et al: GLUT4 heterozygous knockout mice develop muscle insulin resistance and diabetes. Nat Med 1997;3:1096–1101.

556. Ortiz PA, Garvin JL: Cardiovascular and renal control in NOS-deficient mouse models. Am J Physiol Regul Integr Comp Physiol 2003;284:R628–R638.

557. Egan BM, Hennes MMI, Stepniakowski KT, et al: Obesity hypertension is related more to insulin's fatty acid than glucose action. Hypertension 1996;27:723–728.

558. Grekin RJ, Dumont CJ, Vollmer AP, et al: Mechanisms in the pressor effects of hepatic portal venous fatty acid infusion. Am J Physiol 1997;273:R324–R330.

559. Vallon V, Blantz RC, Thomson S: Glomerular hyperfiltration and the salt paradox in early type 1 diabetes mellitus: A tubulo-centric view. J Am Soc Nephrol 2003;14:530–537.

■ ■ ■ c h a p t e r **3 2**

# Molecular Biology of Transplantation and Xenotransplantation

*Patrick Hildbrand*
*Daniel R. Salomon*

In recent years there has been remarkable progress in the understanding of the molecular mechanisms of transplantation immunology. Transplantation immunology has also moved into the mainstream of cell biology by considering the fundamental mechanisms and consequences of cell adhesion, migration, cell death and apoptosis, intracellular signaling, and the genetic regulation of cell differentiation and tissue development. At the bedside, clinical trials in transplantation have been undertaken using a new generation of therapeutic molecules. In parallel, groundbreaking work is moving forward to induce transplantation tolerance and make xenotransplantation successful. Thus, the design and conduct of future clinical trials will require researchers and physicians who have an understanding of both immunity and cell biology at the molecular level.

In this chapter we review the molecular basis of the immune response to alloantigen in transplantation and xenotransplantation and describe present and possible future therapeutic approaches to overcome graft rejection. In many areas the molecular details are too complex for the scope of this review. Moreover, many aspects of the basic mechanisms are still unknown and disputed so that some connections made in this chapter between the molecular basis and clinical events are speculative. Thus, the aim is to create a set of unifying concepts that can transcend the details and yet be reconsidered in the constant flux of progress.

## ANTIGEN-ANTIBODY COMPLEXES AND ACTIVATION OF THE COMPLEMENT SYSTEM

A primary immunologic barrier in transplantation is the presence of circulating, antigraft antibodies. These antibodies can be present prior to transplantation or develop as part of the immune response after transplantation. The attempt to transplant an organ into a patient with preformed antibodies results in a destructive activation of the immune system, either hyperacute or accelerated acute rejection. In allotransplantation (i.e., human-to-human organ transplants) these antibodies are directed against donor-specific major histocompatibility complex (MHC or HLA) antigens called alloantigens. In xenotransplantation (i.e., animal donor to human transplants) these antibodies reflect what is called natural immunity and represent exposure to antigens present in the environment such as intestinal bacterial and parasitic flora. In either case, preexisting antigraft antibodies can lead to graft rejection via activation of the complement system or by antibody-dependent cell-mediated cytotoxicity (ADCC).

Several mechanisms can account for the presence of preexisting antibodies specific for alloantigens. Patients receiving multiple blood transfusions can develop antibodies to MHC molecules expressed by allogeneic leukocytes that contaminate the transfused blood. During pregnancy, a woman can be exposed to paternal alloantigens expressed in fetal blood components, particularly at the time of delivery. A third type of exposure to alloantigens occurs in patients that have had a previous transplant, a situation that is common in kidney transplantation but less common in heart transplants. Finally, it is important to acknowledge that circulating anti-blood group antibodies (e.g., against both major and minor blood group antigens) are another powerful barrier to successful transplants and that these antibodies are really a type of natural immunity as described later.

The good news is that the development of sensitive assays for detecting preexisting antibodies in patients before transplantation, called crossmatching, has allowed physicians to minimize the risks of hyperacute and accelerated acute rejection mediated by these preformed antibodies. It is also true that many heart transplants are performed without full crossmatching because of time considerations. Fortunately, the impact of preexisting antialloantigen antibodies on heart transplants appears to be less devastating than on kidney transplants. On the other hand, the immune response to the transplant can also lead to the development of antidonor antibodies after transplantation. These new alloantibodies can cause an antibody-mediated graft injury that results in either acute or chronic rejection.

In the context of immune mechanisms, the downstream events of antibody-mediated activation of complement and coagulation cascades and recruitment of inflammatory cells are similar for preexisting antidonor antibodies and antibodies formed after transplant. The key point is that preexisting antidonor antibodies are present in high titer very early in the transplant process when they can mediate a very rapid form of immune injury. In contrast, antibodies formed after transplant occur more gradually and after the patient is fully immunosuppressed so that their impact is modified significantly.

## Natural Antibodies in Xenotransplantation

A *discordant* xenograft is one that comes from a distantly related species (i.e., pig to human), whereas a *concordant* xenograft refers to an organ from a more closely related species (i.e., nonhuman primate to human). Thus, in a concordant xenograft, hyperacute reaction is normally not seen, although an antibody-mediated immune response often develops within days or weeks. This latter response can be called an accelerated or delayed acute rejection depending on the timing. In contrast, the use of a discordant donor results in a very fast and catastrophically destructive reaction toward the graft, called hyperacute rejection, that can lead to vascular thrombosis and complete graft loss in minutes to hours.

Why have recent events in xenotransplantation focused on the pig as the donor? The availability, breeding potential, experience in animal health care, size of organs, cost of maintaining a breeding colony, and ethical concerns raised by the alternative idea of large herds of captive nonhuman primates explain why the pig is the frontrunner of potential xenograft donors. However, the choice of a discordant donor species presents the very major barrier of hyperacute rejection mediated by circulating natural antibodies.

Natural antibodies are mostly of the IgM class, directed to a specific sugar moiety expressed by pig endothelial cells called galactose (alpha 1-3) galactose (Gal$\alpha$1-3Gal). At a molecular level, this antigen is structurally related to the human major blood group antigens (i.e., ABO). Contrary to the pig, humans, apes, and Old World monkeys do not express the enzyme, alpha 1-3 galactosyltransferase that is required to synthesize Gal$\alpha$1-3Gal. Therefore, humans do not express this antigen and have naturally occurring antibodies specific for these sugars. Moreover, these antibodies are produced by continuous antigenic stimulation from environmental exposure to bacteria, viruses, and other parasitic organisms such as normal gastrointestinal flora. Their biologic function is to represent an immune barrier to invasion and infection.

The importance of the Gal$\alpha$1-3Gal sugar structure as a target of xenoreactive antibodies was first indicated *in vitro*; removing anti-Gal antibodies could prevent the lysis of pig cells by human serum. Treatment of endothelial cells by $\alpha$-galactosidase also inhibited antibody binding, and, as predicted, anti-Gal antibodies contained in human serum lysed a monkey cell line transfected with cDNA for the 1,3-galactosyltransferase enzyme. *In vivo* experiments showed that baboons (that have anti-Gal antibodies) hyperacutely reject the organs of New World monkeys, which express the Gal$\alpha$1-3Gal sugars. In addition, several reports document that the specific depletion of anti-Gal from monkeys or baboons prevents hyperacute rejection of porcine xenografts. Knockout mice that do not express the Gal$\alpha$1-3Gal sugars develop natural anti-Gal antibodies and will reject organs from otherwise identical donor mice. Finally, several groups have created transgenic pigs with human complement regulatory proteins (CRPs) expressed on the endothelium. Hyperacute rejection of these pig organs in nonhuman primates was either prevented or significantly reduced.

The finding that specific depletion of anti-Gal antibodies prevents lysis of porcine cells *in vitro* and hyperacute rejection *in vivo* is not meant to imply that the anti-Gal antibodies are the only antibody barrier to successful xenotransplantation. Anti-pig but non-Gal antibodies also appear in significant amounts in xenograft recipients. These antibodies are directed against a large number of porcine proteins although their significance in mediating graft injury is uncertain at this point. The recent creation of 1,3-galactosyltransferase knockout pigs will eventually allow the direct determination of the roles that these non-gal anti-pig antibodies will play in xenotransplantation immunity.[1]

## Mechanisms of Complement Activation in Transplantation

The activation of the complement system is the main effecter mechanism in hyperacute and accelerated acute graft rejection. The proteins and glycoproteins of the complement system circulate in the blood in functionally inactive forms. Activation of the complement system involves a sequential enzyme cascade in which the resulting product of one step becomes the enzymatic catalyst of the next step. Another characteristic feature is that the activated components have a short half-life and are inactivated rapidly. Thus, this is a very dynamic system, which is fitting for a system involved in nearly instantaneous and destructive reactions.

The first part of complement activation results in the accumulation of the C5b component. This can occur via three pathways: (1) the classical pathway, (2) the alternative pathway, and (3) a lectin pathway.[2] The final common pathway for all three is the formation of the membrane-attack complex (C5b-9; MAC), which leads to cell lysis (Fig. 32-1).

For some xenotransplants, such as the guinea pig to rat model, the fixation of complement is primarily due to the alternative pathway (antibody independent). However, two lines of evidence support the predominance of the classical pathway (antibody dependent) in pig organs transplanted into primates. First, depletion of xenoreactive antibodies prevents hyperacute rejection. Second, pig organs transplanted into newborn baboons that have an intact complement system, but only low

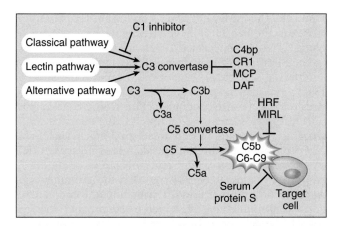

**FIGURE 32-1.** Illustration of the complement cascade and its regulation. Three pathways result in the accumulation of the C5b component. Ultimately the cascade leads to the formation of the MAC (C5b,C6-C9) that inserts into the cell membrane causing lysis of the cell. In addition, there is a series of complement regulatory proteins that act at the different steps along the cascade.

level of xenoreactive antibodies, do not have hyperacute rejection. Certainly the activation of the complement cascade in human-to-human allotransplantation is predominantly antibody-dependent (classical pathway) and mediated by antidonor antibodies. As already noted, these antidonor antibodies may be present before transplantation because of presensitization of the patient by blood transfusions, previous transplants, or pregnancy. However, the immune response posttransplantation can also produce antidonor antibodies, typically T helper cell-dependent, and these have been shown to play a role in both acute and chronic rejection. Thus, for example, an increased amount of IgG anti-donor antibody in endomyocardial biopsies is associated with an increased incidence of rejection and chronic graft dysfunction.[3,4]

The formation of soluble antibody-antigen complexes or the binding of antibody on a cell surface initiates the activation of the complement cascade via the classical pathway. The binding of the antibody to its antigen leads to a conformational change of its Fc-portion exposing a binding side for the C1 component of complement. The C1 protein is actually a complex, C1qr2s2, consisting of C1q, C1r, and C1s. The C1q component binds the Fc-CH2 domain of the antibody. The C1 complex must bind via C1q to at least two Fc-sites for a stable C1-antibody interaction. Pentameric IgM provides at least three binding sides for C1q, which explains why IgM is more effective in activating the complement cascade then IgG with its single C1q binding site.

The enzymatically active form of C1q converts the C1r molecule to its active form, which in turn converts C1s. C4 and C2 are then cleaved to two molecules each (C4a, C4b, C2a, and C2b) by the active C1s. The C4b fragment binds to the cell surface near the C1 complex and forms a complex with the C2a fragment. This complex is called C3 convertase (C4aC2b), and it converts the C3 proenzyme to the active form C3b. The formation of the C3b component is a major amplification step in the complement cascade. One C3 convertase complex can activate 200 C3b molecules. This tremendous amplification

is one reason for the elaborate natural regulation of this step of the cascade and why it is a natural target for xenotransplantation therapies (see later). C3b can then bind to C3 convertase to form C5 convertase (C4aC2bC3b), or it can diffuse away and coat immune complexes to function as an opsonin (mediating activated cell uptake by macrophages). The terminal sequence of the complement system is a sequential interaction of the C5b, C6, C7, C8, and C9 to create the membrane attack complex (MAC). This complex displaces the phospholipid membrane bilayer and forms a channel that enables ions and molecules to pass through it freely. The result is death and lysis of the cell.

## COMPLEMENT REGULATION IN TRANSPLANTATION

If one approaches the complexity of complement activation as a system design problem, then it is not surprising that there is an elaborate regulation system in place. One mechanism is that labile components are formed that undergo spontaneous inactivation once they diffuse away from the cell. For example, C3b undergoes spontaneous hydrolysis once it has diffused away from C3 convertase. This mechanism limits binding to adjacent cells.

In addition, there is a series of CRPs that act at the following steps:

*C1 complex.* C1 inhibitor is a soluble serine protease inhibitor that disrupts the C1 complex by causing C1r2s2 to dissociate from C1q.

*C3 convertase.* The soluble C4-binding protein (C4bp) can interfere with C3 convertase by preventing its assembly via binding the C4b component, leading to cleavage by a soluble protein (factor I). Two endothelial cell membrane proteins called complement receptor 1 (CR1; CD35) and the membrane cofactor protein (MCP; CD46) can block the formation of C3 convertase and mediate the disassociation of the assembled complex. The cell membrane-bound protein decay-acceleration factor (DAF; CD55) interferes only with the already assembled complex.

The key point for xenotransplantation is that pig endothelium does not express cell-associated regulator molecules (i.e., MIRL, DAF) capable of regulating human complement components. This reflects the species specificity of complement regulation. Thus, transgenic expression of human DAF on pig endothelium was the strategy used to construct the first pigs for xenotransplantation.[5] Pigs are now being produced that are transgenic for human CD46 and for multiple CRPs.

*MAC.* Serum protein S binds to C5b67 inducing a hydrophobic transition and blocking the ability of the complex to insert into the cell membrane. The homologous restriction factor (HRF) and the membrane inhibitor of reactive lysis (MIRL, CD59) protect the cells from nonspecific complement-mediated lysis by binding to C8 and preventing assembly of the MAC.

In conclusion, the complexity of complement activation is matched by the complexity of its regulation. In human-to-human transplantation, the formation of antidonor antibodies through either presensitization or posttransplant immunity can lead to a range of destructive rejections from hyperacute to chronic. In the clinical setting, the identification of patients with preformed antidonor antibodies by crossmatching is very useful although in many heart transplants there is not sufficient time for prospective crossmatches. However, once antibodies are formed, the reality is that the current immunosuppressive strategies are ineffective in preventing their assault on the transplant. The hope of developing new anticomplement activation drugs is only fulfilled thus far with a first generation of modestly active inhibitors. In parallel, newer immunosuppressive drugs and biologicals are being tested for their ability to inhibit B cell activation and the T cell/B cell signaling required for creating antidonor antibodies post transplantation. For xenotransplantation, the rules are very similar except that the preformed antibodies are primarily the natural IgM antibodies, and any human patient considered will be presensitized. The advantage for xenotransplantation is that genetic engineering of the pig has allowed a number of strategies to circumvent the natural antibody barrier including the recent development of the galactosidase knockout pigs.[1]

## INDIRECT AND DIRECT ANTIGEN PRESENTATION

The initial step in T cell-mediated immune responses is the recognition of antigen. There are two mechanisms of antigen presentation, direct and indirect. The relative contribution of each mechanism is a matter of great interest and importance.

Intracellular (endogenous) and extracellular (exogenous) antigens present different challenges to the immune system. In the intracellular pathway, endogenous proteins are degraded in the cytoplasm by the proteasome complex. A portion of the resulting peptides is transported from the cytoplasm into the lumen of the endoplasmic reticulum by a transmembrane ATP-binding transporter called transporter associated with antigen processing (TAP).[6] MHC Class I molecules associated with the TAP complex bind the peptides and the MHC-antigen complex is transported through the Golgi complex to the cell surface membrane where it can be recognized by CD8+ cytotoxic T cells.

In contrast, exogenous antigens (e.g., foreign proteins or bacteria) are taken up by the cells by endocytosis, phagocytosis, or both. Hydrolytic enzymes and the acidic condition of the lysosomes, intracellular organelles involved in the traffic of cellular and extracellular materials, degrade the exogenous antigens into peptides. Class II MHC molecules synthesized in the endoplasmic reticulum move through the Golgi complex into the lysosomal compartment with a special protein called Class II-associated invariant chain peptide (CLIP) that protects the antigen-binding groove. Proteolytic digestion of CLIP in the lysosome allows the antigenic peptides access to

bind and the resulting MHC Class II-antigen complex moves to the cell surface membrane, where it is accessible to CD4+ helper T cells.

The MHC is also called the HLA complex in humans. It represents a set of genes located on chromosome 6. There is an enormous diversity between MHC molecules within a species. Diversity results from inherited genetic polymorphisms creating multiple alleles for each MHC locus in a species. In contrast, antibodies and T-cell receptors generate diversity for antigen binding through an ongoing process of gene rearrangement during development. By generating many clones, the combinatorial diversity of antibodies and T cells for antigen recognition can be selected and shaped to respond to changes and challenges throughout the life of the organism. In the context of transplantation, a foreign donor tissue is defined by the immune system as "nonself" based on recognition of predominantly the MHC molecules of the organ donor.

The structure of each MHC molecule creates a groove that binds only certain peptides efficiently. The structural diversity of the MHC dictates that theoretically every MHC molecule has a different groove and can present a different set of peptides or antigens. Thus, each human has inherited a set of MHC molecules that determine a repertoire of antigenic peptide presentation. This correlation between MHC structure and the presentation of specific peptides helps explain how certain diseases such as diabetes mellitus and ankylosing spondylitis can be linked to specific MHC molecules. It also explains the higher incidence of autoimmune disease in certain families. The hypothesis is that the inheritance of certain MHC combinations favors the presentation of peptides that trigger the autoimmune response. There is also another inheritable connection between antigen presentation and the MHC. A number of the genes involved in antigen/peptide processing are located in the same chromosomal region as the MHC genes. These antigen-peptide processing genes encode structural and transport proteins in the proteolysosomes. Therefore, inherited differences in antigen-processing genes are linked to MHC alleles and may also regulate which antigenic peptides are selected for presentation in the groove of the MHC molecules. If this thinking about the genetics and structure of MHC molecules is extended to transplantation, it provides a genetics theory for the clinical experience that some patients never reject their grafts, whereas others reject their grafts no matter how intense the immunosuppression.

### Indirect Antigen Presentation

Indirect antigen presentation involves host antigen-presenting cells (APCs) that process and present exogenous antigens to T cells. Different cells can function as APCs (dendritic cells, macrophages, B cells, and endothelial and epithelial cells). The requirements for an APC are (1) the expression of MHC molecules, (2) the ability to process and present antigenic peptides, and (3) the expression of necessary costimulatory molecules that are discussed later. The term *indirect* is used to denote a mechanism whereby transplant antigens are taken away from donor cells and presented in the context of "self" MHC molecules as antigenic peptides. In other words, the patient's T cells encounter the transplant antigens on the surface of the patient's own APCs and the patient's own MHC molecules. This mechanism requires that the patient's APCs traffic to the transplant to get the donor antigens or donor cells derived from the transplant must traffic to lymphoid tissues (Fig. 32-2).

In what compartment does indirect antigen recognition occur? One can distinguish at least three compartments: (1) peripheral (spleen, lymph nodes), (2) central (thymus), and (3) local (within the transplant). Donor cells could traffic out of a transplant and interact with the patient's APC in the peripheral compartment. This type of donor antigen exposure is one basis of the "passenger leukocytes" theory discussed later in the context of tolerance. Alternatively, the patient's APCs can obtain donor antigen by binding soluble antigenic proteins released into the circulation by a local inflammatory response or donor cell injury and death resulting from an inflammatory injury or ischemia in the transplanted heart. Released antigens can be encountered in the peripheral, central, and local compartments. This mechanism could be involved in the setting of acute vascular rejection or could be the consequence of ischemic injury caused before or during organ procurement. The implication of this important step is considered further in the adhesion molecule paradigm. Of course, the patient's APCs could traffic to the heart transplant and physically encounter donor antigens on the vascular surface or within the tissue. Interestingly, the central compartment in the thymus appears to be able to recruit activated APCs after antigen engagement. The results of thymic antigen presentation may be either immune enhancement or paradoxically suppression of the immune response.

How can the current understanding of indirect antigen presentation suggest a strategy to create tolerance or donor-specific immune unresponsiveness? A central approach would involve manipulating the process of antigen recognition in the thymus. In this context, one should note that T cell development in the thymus has two objectives: (1) elimination of T-cell clones that recognize self-antigen and (2) selection of T-cell clones that efficiently recognize foreign antigens (nonself).

Every individual inherits a given set of MHC molecules whose antigen-presenting grooves are designed to present a finite set of potential immunogenic peptides. The same MHC molecules present self-MHC in the thymus and foreign antigenic peptides in the periphery. Thus, there is a common structural motif inherited for each individual, which directs the types of self and foreign peptides that can be presented. During the last decade, the gene and protein sequences of most MHC molecules have been described. Therefore, the structure of their antigen groove can be predicted. Thus, the next challenge is to understand the rules for antigen selection and presentation in the context of groove structure.

Once these secrets are discovered, it may be possible to choose a set of peptides for a specific set of MHC molecules and take the next step toward rational tolerance induction. Hypothetically, if the peptides presented in the thymus can be manipulated, the outcome of T cell selection could be selectively manipulated. Thus, if the MHC of the recipient and the donor is known, the patient could be given peptides chosen to fool developing T cells into thinking that the donor transplanted antigens are self. Alternatively, a similar strategy could be used to selectively inhibit antigen presentation in the peripheral lymphoid system or locally in the transplant. This could be accomplished either by using immunogenic peptides matched to donor MHC sequences to tie up or inhibit free T cell receptors or by using peptides that bind to patient's own MHC molecules with high affinity so that they can compete with or even displace the foreign donor MHC peptides before an immune response can be triggered.

Unfortunately, the initial attempts in the early 1990s to put these strategies into practice for immune manipulation and vaccine construction were not successful. As a result, the area was largely abandoned. However, basic scientists are continuing to make significant progress in integrating the results of protein sequence and crystal structure to understand the physical rules of protein-protein interactions and folding. Therefore, at some point, more powerful bioinformatics tools and methods to create and screen large libraries of stable peptides or small molecule peptide analogs will present another opportunity to test this possible strategy for immune manipulation and/or tolerance.

## Direct Antigen Presentation

Direct antigen presentation involves the recognition of antigens directly on the surface of transplanted donor cells. In other words, there is no antigen processing or

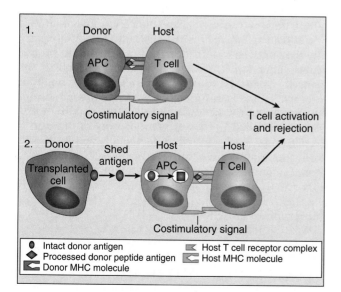

**FIGURE 32-2.** Two mechanisms of antigen presentation. I. Direct antigen presentation in which host T cells respond directly to donor antigenic peptides presented by donor-MHC molecules. II. Indirect antigen presentation in which processing of a donor antigen by a host APC leads to presentation of antigenic peptides in the context of self-MHC molecules.

presentation by self-MHC molecules. Instead, host T cells directly recognize the donor MHC molecules as foreign or nonself antigens. It is uncertain whether this interaction involves recognition of fixed structural epitopes on donor MHC molecules or the donor-derived peptides contained in the MHC's binding grooves (Fig. 32-2).

Direct recognition assumes that the patient's T-cell antigen receptor (TCR) is flexible enough to recognize the donor's self-antigenic peptides in the groove of the donor's allogeneic MHC molecules. The immune system has evolved the T-cell receptor to deal with self and foreign or nonself antigens presented by its own body's cells, not to deal with transplanted cells and foreign MHCs. Thus, the major portions of the structure of the TCR that mediate MHC molecule binding are similar between various individuals. The big differences are in the small, highly variable regions of the TCR that interact with antigenic peptides and a few key amino acids flanking the peptide groove on the presenting MHC molecule. These conclusions regarding structure and function are directly supported by the recent elucidation of the x-ray crystallographic structure of TCR, demonstrating its orientation to the MHC molecule and the peptide-binding groove.[7]

Direct recognition also implies that the donor's self-peptides are a component of the antigen. This is a fascinating molecular insight into the unique nature of the transplant immune response. For example, before organ harvesting a heart cell in the donor would have a specific set of self-derived peptides in the groove of its MHC molecules. Because of thymic selection, these self-peptides do not induce an immune response by the donor's T cells. However, immediately after transplantation, this same heart cell is suddenly the target for the patient's T cells. Another interesting feature of this interaction with donor MHC molecules on target cells is the implication that the population of peptides carried in the groove of one target cell is distinct from those in the groove of another. In other words, MHC molecules are usually loaded with peptides derived from endogenous proteins and, thus, it is reasonable to hypothesize that the peptides from an endothelial cell will be different than those from an epithelial cell. This might explain why a patient can have vascular rejection and little cellular rejection or vice versa.

Another key question is whether the self-peptides in the groove of donor's heart cells are different than the self-peptides that were in the groove of recipient's heart cells. If every MHC molecule tends to present a different set of peptides based on the structure of its binding groove, then the transplanted heart cells should present a different set of self peptides than recipient's heart cells. If so, the patient's T cells should recognize the allogeneic target cell and its self-peptide-MHC complex as nonself. There is a counter argument. Many of the peptides eluted from MHC molecules are derived from intracellular proteins.[8,9] Therefore, at least simplistically, two structurally identical heart cells, one from the patient and the other from the donor, could have many of the same self-peptides if these peptides are derived from mitochondrial proteins or intracytoplasmic enzymes characteristic of heart cells. However, the reality of genet-

ics is that there are many different alleles for enzymes in the population. Thus, these allelic differences may actually serve to describe individuals for the transplantation immune response as effectively as MHC molecule differences. Such non-MHC determined differences might be one explanation for the fact that transplantation across racial barriers despite good MHC matching is still associated with higher rejection rates and poor long-term graft survival. It would also explain why the effect of MHC matching on rejection and long-term graft survival is not as great as would be expected if the only difference recognized was simply MHC structure.

The next important molecular insight is that direct antigen recognition may not be as efficient as indirect antigen recognition. The definition of efficient in the context of antigen presentation and immunity is important to consider for transplantation. The arguments develop as follows. The job of the thymus is to select only those T cells with receptors that have the best match for efficient nonself peptide recognition. *Efficient* in this context means that mature immune responses to foreign or altered self antigens will be productive and controlled to achieve rapid clearance of any challenge, yet protect the organism from the risk of an autoimmune backlash. In other words, the system uses efficiency to balance the immune response. The structure of a TCR determines its avidity or antigen-binding capability. During early T cell development in the thymus, the immature T cells rearrange the germline sequence of two chains of antigen receptor to create millions of combinations. In the next step, called thymic selection, all of these T cell receptor combinations are sorted and tested for recognition of self-peptides presented by self-MHC molecules. Self–MHC-peptide complexes are presented by thymic epithelial cells in the cortex and by bone marrow-derived dendritic cells in the medulla.

The objective of thymic selection is to kill any T cells whose antigen receptors have either too low an affinity or too high an affinity for self-MHC. If TCR affinity is too low, then antigen recognition is too inefficient to protect against infection. On the other hand, if affinity is too high, it would be difficult to regulate the immune response, possibly resulting in overreactions or autoimmunity. More than 90% of all T cells produced in the thymus die there. Thus, the T-cell receptors of circulating T cells have been carefully selected to work optimally with the body's own MHC molecules. Therefore, in transplantation, direct antigen recognition of nonself or donor MHC-peptide molecules should not be as efficient as antigen recognition via the indirect pathway based on interactions with self-MHC.

## THE ROLE OF COSTIMULATORY MOLECULES IN T CELL ACTIVATION

A remarkable feature of the immune response is that the recognition of antigen is not sufficient to trigger the full activation of the T cell. In other words, the TCR may determine the exquisite antigen specificity of a T cell clone, but it cannot produce T cell activation without the

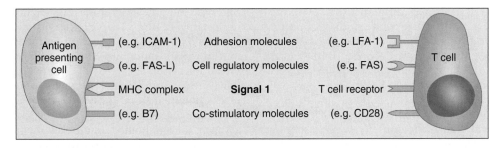

**FIGURE 32-3.** Activation of T cells. Recognition of antigen (Signal 1) is not sufficient to trigger the full activation of the T cell. Engagement of one or more costimulatory molecules flanking the T-cell receptor is necessary (Signal 2).

participation of additional signaling mechanisms. Thus, additional costimulatory signals must be delivered in collaboration with successful antigen engagement (Fig. 32-3).

Experiments in the late 1980s demonstrated that T cell clones failed to proliferate in the absence of costimulatory signals and were subsequently unresponsive to further stimulation.[10-16] This T cell anergy (unresponsive to further stimulation) was dramatic and relevant to clinical strategies for inducing transplantation tolerance or as therapy for autoimmune disease. Therefore, these results stimulated a search for additional costimulatory signals that in the following years identified multiple candidates (Table 32-1).

One costimulatory pathway for T cell activation is the CD28/B7 pathway. This pathway remains one of the most potent and well-characterized costimulatory interactions. The effectiveness of costimulatory blockade for transplantation was first demonstrated in the early 1990s using CTLA-4Ig, an engineered fusion protein that binds the two ligands of CD28, B7-1 (CD80), and B7-2 (CD86), with high affinity.[17,18] This antagonist inhibited islet xenograft rejection and induced long-lasting immune tolerance.[19] In addition, short-term treatment with CTLA-4Ig at the time of graft implantation induced long-term acceptance of cardiac allografts in rats.[20] However, the complexity of costimulatory regulation of

T cells has become apparent in recent years with a growing number of pathways. Thus, the relative importance of various costimulation pathways is dependent on tissue expression, the order in which the pathways are engaged, the state of activation of the T cells, the repertoire of different T cell subsets, and the nature of inflammatory responses.

To understand the concept of costimulation in the context of T cell activation, three phenomena must be explained:

First, the physical strength of the bond between the TCR and the MHC molecule presenting an antigenic peptide is too weak to stabilize the binding of the T cell to the APC surface. This finding led to the original discovery that the CD4 and CD8 molecules of the T cell bind to the MHC molecules of the APC to create a bridge that stabilizes the T cell-APC interaction. Another feature of costimulatory molecules is that the expression and/or signaling activity of these ligands is also regulated by inflammatory cytokines such as a growing number of interleukins, TNF, and the IFNs. This explains why the cytokine-activated "professional" APCs (i.e., dendritic cells and some macrophages) are much more efficient in activating T cells than naïve or resting dendritic cells or macrophages. This cytokine activation seems to be even more important for the function of "amateur" APCs like endothelial cells or B cells because their costimulatory properties for T cells are almost entirely dependent on cytokine activation.

Second, although stable cell-cell adhesion is a critical step in T cell activation, it is also not sufficient. These adhesion molecules trigger the activation of a complex series of cytoplasmic signaling pathways. Intracellular signals linked to cell surface adhesion events are required for full expression of the T cell activation program. The signaling role of adhesion molecules is a major discovery and promises a whole new set of potential drug targets for immunosuppression.

Third, costimulatory signals balance the immune response. For example, the blockade of the CD28/CD86 pathway can affect the cytokine balance to protect or to exacerbate disease depending on the nature of disease pathogenesis and the ability of the reactive T cells to expand in the absence of adequate costimulation. It is known that the CD28/CD86 pathway regulates the Th1/Th2 differentiation toward a Th1

■ ▦ ■

## TABLE 32-1   COSTIMULATORY MOLECULES IN T-CELL ACTIVATION

| Receptor | Ligand |
| --- | --- |
| CD4 | MHC class II |
| CD8 | MHC class II |
| LFA-1 (CD11a) | ICAM-1 (CD54) |
| LFA-1 (CD11a) | ICAM-2 (CD102, ICAM-3 (CD50) |
| CD2 | LFA-3 (CD58) |
| CD28, CTLA4 | B7-1 (CD80) |
| CD28, CTLA4 | B7-2 (CD86) |
| VLA4 (α4β1) | VCAM-1 (CD106) |
| L-Selectin (CD62L) | MadCam-1 |
| P-Selectin (CD62P) | Sialyl-LewisX |
| (α4β7) | MadCam-1, VCAM-1 |
| PECAM-1 (CD31) | CD31 |
| CD31 | (αvβ3) |
| CD45 | Glycolipids |
| CD40 | CD40 ligand (CD154) |
| CD44 | Hyaluronate PLNad |

phenotype. Th1 produce inflammatory cytokines such as IFN-$\gamma$ and TNF-$\alpha$ that mediate immune responses in transplantation. In contrast Th2 cells produce cytokines such as IL-4, IL-5, and IL-10 that are important for the humoral immune response and critical for downmodulating the Th1 response.

The concept of costimulation has several direct applications to clinical transplantation. If a T cell requires costimulatory signals in addition to the engagement of antigen by the TCR, it follows that one level of regulating the immune response is to control the setting in which the T cell encounters antigen. As described previously if a T cell encounters an APC (signal 1) with no costimulatory ligands (signal 2), the T cell will become anergic (unresponsive) to further antigen exposure.[14] The precise basis of how a T cell survives but is anergic to further activation remains unclear but the advantages of purposefully creating anergy after a transplant are evident.

The exposure of APCs to inflammatory cytokines increases the expression of costimulatory ligands and minimizes the possibility that any T cell will encounter antigen without an abundance of "second signal" present. This is exactly what the immune system is designed to do. Thus, when rejection or infection is present, the efficiency of antigen presentation and T cell activation is substantially enhanced. This also occurs in the immediate postsurgical period, when wound healing demands a rich milieu of inflammatory cytokines. The primary biologic function of the immune system is to protect the host in states of trauma, and an increase in antigen-presenting efficiency in such situations is very useful. However, this may explain why rejection is most common in the first months after transplantation and why stable transplant patients with active viral infections may suddenly have acute rejection. A brain-dead donor is often stressed by serious trauma, hypothermia, brain injury, hemodynamic instability, or subclinical bacteremia resulting from multiple intravenous lines before organ retrieval. Thus, the association of increased rejection posttransplant with compromised donors or complications during organ procurement is due to cytokine-induced increases in costimulatory ligand expression in the graft. Thus, it is extremely important for clinical transplant teams to optimize the medical condition of the donors pretransplant.

APCs such as dendritic cells normally express higher levels of Class II MHC and costimulatory ligands and are often called professional APCs. In a transplantation setting these professionals are involved in indirect antigen recognition. Next in APC efficiency are macrophages, particularly activated macrophages. Finally, at the bottom of the APC ladder are B cells, endothelial cells, and potentially even epithelial cells. For example, in heart transplantation the endothelial cells of the donor heart are presumably responsible for the earliest direct antigen presentation.

Considering the implications of indirect and direct antigen presentation in the context of costimulatory molecule expression, it seems reasonable that T cell interactions with the different classes of APCs triggers different immune responses. For example, the relative importance of host versus donor costimulatory molecule expression in allograft rejection has been examined in a murine heart model. Vascularized heart allografts survived long-term in B7-1/B7-2 deficient recipients in which the professional APCs are affected. However, hearts obtained from either wild-type or B7-1/B7-2 deficient animals were rejected with the same kinetics after allograft transplantation. In other words, the lack of these costimulatory molecules on the transplanted heart had no influence on rejection. These findings suggest that this particular costimulatory pathway plays its role in indirect antigen recognition.[21,22] In contrast, a recent study in a mouse xenograft model demonstrated that immunization of mice with peptides derived from pig B7 (CD86) led to the induction of an anti-pig CD86 antibody response that blocked subsequent xenograft rejection. These results suggest that the direct pathway may be involved in donor xenograft recognition.[23]

Another point to consider is that a strict application of the two signal hypothesis to direct antigen recognition involving nonprofessional APCs predicts that T cell anergy, not activation, should result. This is because direct antigen presentation by a donor endothelial cell, for example, involves a very low level of costimulatory ligands (second signals). One explanation for why T cell anergy is not the case in clinical transplantation may be the expression of inflammatory cytokines in the transplanted organ; in this circumstance the ability of nonprofessional APCs such as endothelial and epithelial cells to present antigen may be greatly enhanced by increased expression of costimulatory molecules. A better understanding of these mechanisms of antigen presentation could lead to strategies for reducing the risk of rejection starting with approaches to better management of the donor patient before organ harvest.

The CD28 and CTLA-4 molecules on T cells and their APC ligands B7-1 and B7-2 are differentially expressed and dependent on activation. One theory is that APC activation through CTLA-4 may favor T cell anergy or at least provide a negative signal that blocks IL-2 production and T-cell proliferation.[24] Because both CTLA-4 and CD28 are expressed on fully activated lymphocytes, it supports the concept that these two receptors may regulate the results of signaling each other. However, blocking the CD28 pathway appears to produce T cell anergy but not transplantation tolerance.[25,26]

Another costimulatory pathway is the CD40/CD40 ligand interaction (CD40L or CD154). Blocking their interaction by using anti-CD40L mAbs in experimental rodent and primate transplant models demonstrated a strategy to prevent graft rejection. In rodents, this treatment prevented acute cardiac allograft rejection,[27,28] and more importantly it prolonged graft survival of kidneys and islets in nonhuman primates after discontinuation of therapy.[29-31] Moreover, the combination of CD40/CD40L and CD28/B7 blockade has synergistic effects in preventing both acute and chronic rejection.[27,29]

CD40/CD40L or CD28/B7 blockade during transplantation inhibits alloreactive T cell proliferation and may induce an increase in cell death by apoptosis.[28,32,33] In contrast, engagement of CTLA-4 suppresses IFN-$\gamma$ and

IL-2 production that would reduce the risk of rejection but may also inhibit the induction of tolerance to allografts.[32-36] There is evidence that the routinely used calcineurin inhibitors (i.e., cyclosporine and FK506) may also inhibit tolerance induction and antagonize the therapeutic effects of costimulation blockade. These lines of evidence illustrate the paradoxical concept that intact T cell receptor signaling is required for both rejection and tolerance induction to allografts.

In summary, clinical investigators will play a major part in advancing the understanding of T cell activation. Several strategies to selectively inhibit the delivery of costimulatory signals in transplantation have been created. Molecular engineering has been used to create soluble fusion proteins of costimulatory ligands or their receptors. These can be delivered intravenously, and they effectively block or compete with endogenous receptor-ligand binding. A second approach has been to create humanized monoclonal antibodies against these molecules. Humanized antibodies have the advantage over mouse monoclonals in that they can remain functional in the circulation for up to 6 weeks, allowing for the real possibility of blocking these signals in a clinical situation. A third approach has been to create novel peptide analogs or small molecular weight inhibitors of costimulatory signaling. Clinical trials with these new agents will offer a number of unique opportunities for immunologists to study the different effects of signal blockade. Overall, this complex pathway of T-cell stimulation is likely to yield potent immunosuppressive strategies. On the other hand, so much is unknown about the primary logic of this system that the current designs and rationales for clinical trials must still be considered complex experiments.

## INTERCELLULAR AND INTRACELLULAR SIGNALS

Once the T cell recognizes its target, the next step in T cell activation occurs in the cytoplasm. The model of cytoplasmic signaling is as complex as the T cell subsets, cytokines, and surface receptors determining the course of the immune response outside of the cell. It is beyond the scope of this chapter to describe the intracellular signaling pathway in great detail; however, a few unifying concepts are introduced.

Intracellular enzymes called tyrosine kinases deliver many primary signals by phosphorylation of defined tyrosine groups on target molecules. It is useful to group these as "receptor-associated" when they are an integral part of cell surface receptors or their complexes and "nonreceptor-associated" when they normally are present in the cytoplasm and are recruited to sites of activation. The target molecules for these kinases can be other enzymes that result in phosphorylation or dephosphorylation of other molecules or proteins without enzymatic activity called adapter proteins that are signaling intermediates. The level of phosphorylation is balanced by phosphatases (e.g., tyrosine and serine-threonine phosphatases). Interestingly, the phosphatases not only regulate the phosphorylation level, but also are important molecules in the delivery of signals independent of the protein kinases.

Adapter proteins express a variety of modular binding domains (e.g., SH2 and SH3) or tyrosine-based signaling motifs, which enable them to mediate constitutive or inducible protein-protein or protein-lipid interactions. The main function of adapter proteins is to coordinate receptor-mediated signals at a cell surface membrane or intracellular level. They couple signal transduction receptor complexes to intracellular effecter systems by organizing the dynamic assembly of signaling scaffolds. For example, it is now known that T cell activation involves the creation of a supramolecular activation complex (SMAC) that includes the T cell receptor for antigen complex, CD4 or CD8, CD45, and a set of integrin adhesion molecules such as leukocyte function antigen 1 (LFA-1) and other costimulatory molecules.[37] A major research objective for this area is to understand the molecular basis and regulation of assembling these signaling complexes at the cell surface in response to activation of receptors there.

The intracellular calcineurin complex is a serine-threonine kinase and is the target of both cyclosporine and FK506 when either drug is bound to its carrier protein. There is a family of small molecular weight GTP-binding proteins (e.g., Ras and Rho) that are activated by GTP and subsequently catalyze phosphorylation of various substrates such as mitogen-activated protein kinase (MAPK) and mitogen-activated protein kinase kinase (MAPKK), which have been directly linked to activation of nuclear-binding proteins, specific gene transcription factors, cell cycle activation, and control of programmed cell death (apoptosis). Also important in cell signaling networks is PKC, which is activated downstream of membrane phosphoinositide cleavage by phosphoinositol lipase $C\gamma$ (PLC $\gamma$) and formation of diacylglycerol (DG). Another critical signal network is initiated by phosphoinositol 3 kinase (PI3K) that interacts downstream with a series of different adaptor molecules and members of the GTPase family such as Rac and Cdc42 (Fig. 32-4).

There are at least four basic cellular roles for intracellular signaling relevant to immune-mediated rejection:

*Cell activation.* Cell activation has already been discussed in the context of antigen recognition and costimulatory molecules, the first and second signals.

*Coordination and support of cell functions.* For example, intracellular signals regulate the expression of costimulatory ligands (e.g., ICAM-1) and the production of various cytokines, which, in turn, determine the consequences of cell activation and cell survival (e.g., apoptosis). Intracellular signals also regulate gene transcription for the synthesis of effecter molecules, such as granzymes and perforin required for killing by cytotoxic T cells.

*Cell cycle control.* The control of cell division is a complex and regulated process that proceeds from DNA synthesis to the physical separation of duplicated chromosomes into two new cells, which is amplified by costimulatory signals and cytokines (growth factors) such as IL-2, INF-$\gamma$, TNF, and IL-4.

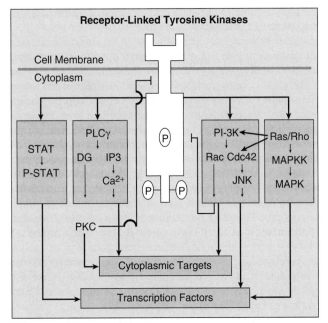

**FIGURE 32-4.** Pathways activated by receptor-linked tyrosine kinases: The boxes represent four distinct signaling pathways that are activated by receptor–linked tyrosine kinases. Also shown are stimulatory and inhibitory or regulatory signals of the different pathways. The different pathways can modulate cytoplasmic events and/or transcriptional factors required for specific gene activation in the nucleus.

*Cell traffic adhesion and migration.* Immunity depends on the ability of cells to traffic to sites of inflammation, migrate into tissue, bind to the surface of target cells, release specific enzymes involved in cell killing, or provide costimulatory and/or cytokine support for other inflammatory cells migrating into the site.

Some aspects of intracellular signaling that are related to the immune response are understood in some detail. For example, the TCR-CD3 complex is directly involved in the generation of cytoplasmic signals for T cells. Several cytoplasmic tyrosine kinases such as Ssrc, Zap 70, and Fyn can bind to the cytoplasmic tails of the CD3 complex proteins and are activated when the TCR engages its antigen on the exterior surface of the cell. In addition, the close physical location of costimulatory CD4 or CD8 molecules creates a bridge between the kinases bound to the cytoplasmic tails of the CD3 complex and receptor-associated kinases such as Lck, which are bound to the cytoplasmic tails of CD4 or CD8 molecules. As a functional unit, this is what has been called the SMAC (see previous discussion). Also in close proximity are various adhesion molecules (e.g., integrins such as LFA-1), which stabilize T cell adhesion to the APC. An example of an adhesion-specific kinase is focal adhesion kinase (FAK), which rapidly localizes at the cytoplasmic side of clustered integrin molecules binding a cellular ligand [i.e., intercellular adhesion molecule-1 (ICAM-1) the ligand of LFA-1] or an extracellular matrix protein (i.e., fibronectin). Activation of nearby cytokine or growth factor receptors also links membrane-bound G-proteins and calcium channels with subsequent acti-

vation of PKC and generation of DG and phosphoinositol intermediaries of cell activation.

Another major discovery is that the cell surface membrane is organized into functional units, literally floating lipid rafts. These rafts effectively partition sets of cell membrane-associated signaling molecules and cell receptors into movable groups.[38-40] Although in a resting cell the localization and movement of these rafts in the membrane is probably random, when cells are stimulated by external phenomenon, the rafts carrying their complement of receptors appear to move and localize to key cellular sites. For example, two transmembrane proteins linker for activation of T cells (LAT) and phosphoprotein associated with glycosphingolipid-enriched microdomains (PAG) have been shown to reside in a class of membrane rafts termed glycolipid-enriched membrane domains (GEMs) or detergent-resistant membrane domains (DRMs). Within these floating "icebergs" in the lipid bilayer of cell membranes, LAT and PAG have relatively long intracellular sequences that serve as binding sites for a number of important signaling proteins such as Src and Csk kinases and PLCγ. Conceptually, part of antigen engagement by the TCR complex involves the recruitment of GEMs to the same site on the cell membrane to serve as a platform for amplification of downstream signaling cascades. In this regard studies have shown that exclusion of LAT from the GEMs impairs signaling via the TCR.[41,42] Thus, these insights provide another whole set of drug targets to small molecule screening for new immunosuppressive agents.

Ultimately, cellular functions described in the context of transplantation involve the transcription of specific genes. Gene transcription mediates the synthesis of cytokines, cell surface receptors, intracellular signaling molecules, and a variety of enzymes involved in processes as diverse as cell replication, antibody production, and cytotoxic T cell killing. The connection between cell signaling and gene transcription is made via nuclear transcription factors. These proteins can bind directly to specific sequences of genes, called enhancer or promoter elements, which are required for transcription of the genes typically located immediately downstream of the factor binding sites.

In a resting cell the transcription factors are often complexed in the cytoplasm with inhibitor molecules that prevent their translocation into the nucleus. Either phosphorylation or dephosphorylation results in the loss of the inhibitory complex, allowing the transcription factor to translocate into the nucleus, bind the promoter elements, and initiate gene transcription. The transcription of a gene is not solely dependent on one transcription factor. Different transcription factors can influence each other and the right mix leads to the transcription of a gene. Thus, a critical function of the intracellular signaling pathways is to regulate the activation of a complex mix of cytoplasmic transcription factors.

It would make sense that specific transcription factors are associated with specific signal pathways. The best support for this hypothesis is the association of the cytokine receptors for IL-2 and IL-4 with the JANUS family kinases (JAK kinases) and members of the STAT family of transcription factors.[43] It appears that both the IL-2 and IL-4 receptors share a common γ chain and can trigger the same JAK kinases after receptor engagement. If so, how can the cell know whether it has bound IL-2 or IL-4? The answer appears to be that it is the association of two different STAT transcription factors with the unique αβ chains of each receptor that determines the specificity of the cell response that follows.[44,45]

What remains a mystery is how all these individual-signaling pathways are regulated to mediate specific cell function. Nonetheless, understanding of this complex system will reveal a whole new set of drug targets for more specific immunosuppression and tolerance induction. One feature of this endeavor is that cell signaling is a fundamental property of all cells not only of lymphocytes. Thus, cell signaling has moved transplant immunology into the mainstream of cell biology. Once the basic principles of these intracellular cell signal cascades are understood, then their specific application in the immune response can be studied and the right targets for transplantation can be identified.

## CELL DEATH

At the center of the immune response is the clonal expansion of activated T and B cells. However, an uncontrolled proliferation could lead to a malignant state or autoimmune disease. Therefore, the immune system has a number of ways to eliminate activated lymphocytes. A challenge to the field at this time is to sort out the molecular mechanisms of cell death associated with necrosis and programmed cell death (apoptosis).

In simple terms, cell death associated with ischemia or tissue destruction during rejection is due largely to necrosis. However, a remarkable discovery was that cells also possess several highly regulated receptor- and enzyme-mediated death pathways that have been termed collectively apoptosis. Although it seemed for some time that these two mechanisms of cell death would be exclusive, it now appears increasingly difficult to sort these out definitively in biologic systems and pathologic states such as rejection.

Cell death can be initiated by receptor-mediated activation of nuclear DNA degradation or induced by mitochondria. The classic cell death receptor is Fas (CD95 or APO-1), a member of the TNF receptor (TNFR) family. Ligation of Fas by Fas ligand (FasL) results in the recruitment of the Fas-adaptor protein FADD. FADD contains two death effecter domains (DEDs), which activate Caspase-8 and Caspase-10.

Caspases are cytoplasmic proenzymes or zymogens that, when cleaved at specific sequences comprised of four amino acids located amino-terminal to an aspartic acid, are activated as enzymes. The preferred tetrapeptide recognition motif differs significantly among Caspases and explains their diversity as a family. Activated Caspase-8/10 promotes cleavage of several downstream Caspases including Caspase-3, Caspase-6, and Caspase-7. These smaller Caspases, also called "effecter Caspases," can degrade cytoskeletal proteins (e.g., foldrin and gelsolin) or lead to activation of DNA degradation enzymes.

Another important part of the intracellular death machinery is the Bcl-2 family of cytoplasmic and mitochondrial membrane binding proteins including Bcl-2, Bid, Bcl-$x_L$, and BAD.[46] For example, Caspase-8 can cleave and activate Bid. Activated Bid complexes with and inhibits the function of Bcl-2, which is located in the outer mitochondrial membrane, to initiate a mitochondrial death sequence. In addition to mitochondrial dysfunction this pathway involves activation of Caspase-9 by a cytoplasmic complex of cytochrome c released from the mitochondria and the protein Apaf-1.[47] In turn, activated Caspase-9 can activate Caspase-3, Caspase-6, and Caspase-7 with the same consequences as already described for Caspase-8/10 downstream of FAS. Thus, in the case of the TNFR family receptors such as FAS, cell death can be triggered by at least two interacting pathways—receptor-induced and mitochondrial.

In a recent review[48] the mitochondria are compared with nuclear reactors. They provide cells with energy through oxidative phosphorylation and glycolysis but can be disastrous to the cell on their meltdown. The inner membrane of the mitochondria is the primary place of energy production. Certain Bcl-2 family members (e.g., Bcl-2, Bcl-$x_L$) are located in the outer membrane and support the maintenance of the intramitochondrial $H^+$ concentration. As already described for Caspase-8 cleavage of Bid, a number of cytoplasmic molecules can be cleaved and activated to complex with members of the Bcl-2 family and inhibit their function. As an end result, the integrity of the mitochondrial outer membrane is compromised allowing the release of several critical mediators of apoptosis into the cytoplasm. The classic member of these mitochondrial-derived mediators is cytochrome c that complexes with Apaf-1 in the cytoplasm. The cytochrome c/Apaf-1 complex recruits and activates Caspase-9 to create what has been called an "apoptosome." The apoptosome mediates the downstream activation of Caspase-3. In the final mechanism of the pathway, endonucleases are activated that mediate the degradation of chromosomal DNA in the cell nucleus resulting in cell death (Fig. 32-5).

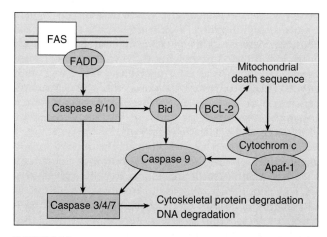

**FIGURE 32-5.** Apoptosis and cell death. Cell death can be initiated by receptor-mediated or mitochondrial-mediated death pathways that lead to activation of enzymes of the Caspase family that cause nuclear DNA degradation.

## Five Applications of Cell Death Directly Relevant to Transplantation

First, the adult T cell repertoire is created in the thymus during T cell development by positive and negative selection. Several members of the TNFR family have been reported to contribute to negative selection, although a precise understanding remains to be resolved. In addition, several molecules positively influence the survival of developing thymocytes including glucocorticoids, cytokines, extracellular matrix, and nitric oxide. Therefore, a better understanding of cell death mechanisms in T cell selection could suggest new strategies to eliminate donor-reactive T cell clones after transplantation to produce tolerance.

Second, it is clear that costimulatory signals for T cell activation can play a role in protecting cells from apoptosis. For example, cells activated by low levels of antigen may undergo apoptosis that can be prevented by engagement of an integrin adhesion molecule with its ligand fibronectin.[49] Alternatively, T cells activated without costimulation may become anergic. There must be a rationale for whether a cell becomes anergic or undergoes apoptosis when sufficient second signal is not delivered with antigen recognition. Recent evidence suggests that only certain kinds of costimulatory signals can produce anergy. This suggests that the immune response regulates its pace and outcome via the interplay of signal pathways that can mediate at least three conflicting outcomes: costimulation leading to cell activation, incomplete activation leading to anergy, and cell death by apoptosis.

Third, manipulating the Fas-FasL pathway has been suggested directly as a strategy for preventing rejection in transplantation. It has been known for some time that the testes is an immune-privileged site capable of supporting both allogeneic and xenogeneic transplants in several models (i.e., islet transplants). FasL is highly expressed by rodent Sertoli cells, although not on their human counterparts. Transplantation of Sertoli cells from strains of mice with a genetic loss of FasL resulted in rapid rejection as compared with transplantation of FasL-expressing Sertoli cells from control animals.[50] The theory is that the FasL on the Sertoli cell surface triggers apoptosis of infiltrating T cells in the early stages of the immune response. This mechanism of targeting cells for death is supported by the fact that cytotoxic T cells use expression of FasL as one mechanism for killing their targets. Thus, it has been proposed that the purposeful expression of FasL on transplanted cells via gene therapy might form the basis for a novel strategy to accomplish successful cell transplantation.

Fourth, apoptosis plays a role in the induction and maintenance of tolerance (see the section on tolerance).

Fifth, not only T cells are subject to cell death; epithelial and endothelial cells are also subject to apoptosis and necrosis. Various physical insults associated with transplantation such as rejection, complement activation, ischemia, heat, pressure, superoxides, and exogenous toxins can trigger the apoptosis pathways leading to cell death. One theory is that there is a working relationship between pathologic cell death (necrosis) and physiologic cell death (apoptosis).[51] For example, a mild insult might injure some cells but the majority could still recover. In contrast, a more severe insult, crossing some kind of cellular threshold, would trigger apoptosis. Therefore, strategies to protect cells from triggering apoptosis could be used to limit the final extent of ischemic reperfusion injury or rejection-induced tissue injury. If one also looks at the progressive ischemia, vascular injury, and interstitial fibrosis that characterizes chronic transplant rejection, it is tempting to speculate that long-term protection of stressed or injured cells might slow or prevent chronic rejection.

## ADHESION MOLECULES AND THE PHYSICS OF THE IMMUNE RESPONSE

So far adhesion molecules have been defined in the context of stabilizing T-cell interactions with APCs during antigen presentation and delivery of costimulatory signals. In this regard CD4, CD8, the TCR, and even HLA are adhesion molecules. However, *adhesion* for the cell biologist has a different sense and defines the mechanisms by which cells adhere to extracellular matrix proteins or adjacent cells. In this context, cell adhesion determines the fetal development of the organism, maintains the adult structure and function of the body's tissues, and heals the body when injured. Therefore, to relate adhesion to transplantation, the role of at least three different families of adhesion molecules must be considered: the integrins, selectins, and sialic acid-binding Ig-like lectins (SIgLecs).

A broader view of adhesion in transplantation immunology explains several basic mechanisms of how a successful immune response works. First, it explains how leukocytes and APCs can traffic to a site of acute inflammation, accumulate, and mediate an immune response. Second, it explains how local epithelial, endothelial, and stromal cells use adhesion molecules to move into sites of damage to repair tissue injury and restore organ structure and function after acute inflammation subsides. Third, it explains how the structure of transplanted tissues or cells is affected by the events surrounding a transplant including how transplants are revascularized. We briefly describe examples of these three aspects of adhesion biology.

The process of inflammatory cell extravasation from the vascular space to the tissue space can be divided into three sequential steps: rolling, adhesion, and transendothelial migration. The best established model for the first step is the loose attachment of cells to the endothelium by low-affinity selectin-carbohydrate interactions.[52] Cytokines and other immunoregulatory mediators act on the graft endothelium, leading to increased expression of adhesion molecules of the selectin family. Endothelial-selectin (E-selectin) binds to adhesion molecules on circulating inflammatory cells. Leukocyte-selectin (L-selectin) expressed on circulating T cells and macrophages interacts with the highly glycosylated CD34 molecules on the endothelium. These initial cell-cell interactions oppose the sheer force of the circulating blood, albeit incompletely, and the circulating cell soon detaches again. This process is repeated, so that the cell tumbles end over end along the endothelium, also referred to as rolling. As the cells are slowed, a second set of interactions between integrins and immunoglobulin superfamily adhesion molecules are recruited to stabilize the adhesion of the cell to the endothelium (i.e., VLA-4/VCAM-1, LFA-1/ICAM-1, ICAM-2, ICAM-3). In contrast to selectins, integrins mediate the firm attachment of cells with high enough bond strength to oppose the sheer force generated by the blood flow. This stops the selectin-mediated rolling on the endothelial surface. Integrins also mediate the third phase of the extravasation process, cell migration, which requires a regulated mix of both adhesion and cell locomotion. The resulting transendothelial migration of the flow-arrested inflammatory cells into the tissue involves the direct migration of the cells through interendothelial cell junctions (Fig. 32-6).

One key element of cell extravasation is that both integrins and selectins can be activated to enhance binding efficiency. For example, a number of inflammatory cytokines mediate integrin and selectin activation. These cytokines also stimulate the expression of the cellular ligands for these receptors. Thus, IL-1 and TNF-α are potent stimulators of endothelial VCAM-1 expression, which is a target ligand for two leukocyte integrins, VLA-4 (α4β1) and α4β7. Furthermore, certain integrins are also capable of delivering costimulatory signals required for T cell activation (i.e., LFA-1 binding to ICAM-1). In contrast, there is no evidence that any of the selectins are costimulatory. A second key element is that the strength of the blood flow, expressed in physics as shear stress, is an important factor. The physical complex of any adhesion molecule with its ligand has a tensile strength that must be measured under flow conditions.[53] Therefore, it is logical to propose that adhesion in the high shear stress of an arteriole will involve receptor-ligand interactions fundamentally different than those required for adhesion in the low shear conditions of the postcapillary venules.

This hypothesis can be applied to transplantation as follows. The pathology of rejection demonstrates that early accumulation of inflammatory cells after trans-plantation and during initiation of classical acute transplant rejection begins in the postcapillary venules (low shear stress). The interstitial rejection infiltrate that results is characterized by the accumulation of activated lymphocytes, cytokine release, and cell-mediated cytotoxicity. Thus, this process would seem to involve efficient T cell adhesion and a prompt migration into the underlying tissue. In contrast, acute vascular rejection including xenotransplant rejection typically starts on the arteriolar side of the capillary bed (high shear stress) and is initially dominated by leukocytes followed only later by activated T cells. Hypothetically, leukocytes may initiate local injury and ischemia and release cytokines that increase endothelial ligand expression levels. Increased adhesion receptor activity and higher ligand concentrations enhance the ability of the T cells to arrest their forward motion on an endothelial surface in the high sheer stress environment of the artery.

Adhesion molecule pathways are promising potential targets for manipulating the immune response. If cells cannot get to the transplant, then antigen recognition will clearly be limited, particularly the direct route of antigen recognition. Moreover, even if the first wave of T cells are activated, interfering with their traffic to the transplant or their migration into the interstitium could be used to suppress rejection. Blocking adhesion molecules might even induce tolerance or T cell anergy if any of the adhesion receptor-ligand combinations previously described are critical costimulatory signals for T cell activation.

However, these same adhesion molecules, by definition, are also required for a wide variety of normal cellular mechanisms. Although it is beyond the scope of this chapter, it is important to mention the critical role that adhesion molecules play in creating the three-dimensional structure of all tissues during development. Perhaps even more critical to consider in the context of transplantation is the role adhesion molecules play in the maintenance of tissue structure in the adult organism. To the extent that tissue structure determines tissue function, it is reasonable to stress the close relationship between successful transplantation and the ability to protect the normal structure of the

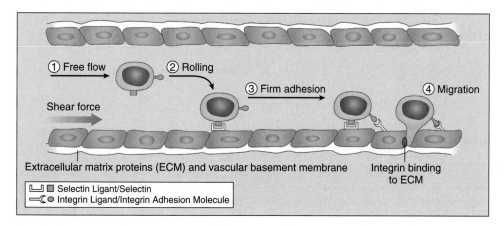

**FIGURE 32-6.** The physics of the immune response. Different adhesion molecules regulate four distinct stages in the process of taking a lymphocyte: flowing in the bloodstream, rolling along the endothelium, firm adhesion at sites of inflammation or tissue injury, and migration of lymphocytes across the endothelial wall and into the tissues during rejection.

transplanted tissue. Moreover, when tissue injury occurs by any mechanism after a transplant, it is the adhesion molecule system that plays a major part in determining the repair and restoration of the transplanted tissue to normal function. All of these considerations put a special emphasis on carefully testing these new reagents intended to manipulate adhesion molecules in transplantation.

## TOLERANCE

Although it is has been possible to induce immune tolerance by several means in a number of animal models for over two decades, a successful clinical strategy for tolerance induction in a human patient still remains one of the ultimate goals for clinical transplantation. Before going further, it is important to clarify the definitions of tolerance. The classical definition for immunologists has been a complete lack of an immune response to a donor antigen set. This can be obtained by deleting the T cells that can recognize the antigens or by creating super regulatory cells that effectively suppress any kind of donor antigen-specific immunity. In clinical transplantation, physicians have come to view tolerance in more pragmatic terms. To a transplant clinician, the ultimate objective would be long-term transplant survival and function without immunosuppression. Although this could be achieved by classical tolerance induction, it could also be accomplished by a more limited adaptation of the immune system to just the specific graft. In other words, this would not require the true tests of tolerance: loss of donor antigen immune

responses represented by no response to new transplants from the same or a matched donor including skin grafts, hematopoietic cells, or other cells and organs. Another situation producing long-term survival of a transplant without classic tolerance would be adaptation of the graft to the host immune system so that the exposed endothelial surfaces might express little or no donor MHC or no costimulatory molecules to trigger the first steps in immune recognition.

Induction of tolerance can be divided into an initial induction phase, in which the acute rejection of the graft is inhibited, and a subsequent maintenance phase, which is required to sustain long-term graft survival. In animal models, the initial induction of tolerance may be easily broken. For example, treatment with IL-2 can reverse the acceptance of a graft induced by costimulatory blockade.[54] This may explain why patients with early acute rejections have significantly reduced long-term graft survival. However, it may be one argument for the use of immunosuppression early posttransplant during the induction phase of tolerance. In contrast, stable tolerance cannot be broken by IL-2,[55] and this is accompanied by the presence of circulating regulatory T cells that are able to transfer donor antigen-specific tolerance to naive recipients, often called "adoptive tolerance"[55] (Fig. 32-7). These kinds of experiments in animal models of tolerance suggest that immunologic tolerance results from early mechanisms that facilitate graft acceptance and from long-term mechanisms of immunologic regulation that oppose or counter-regulate T-cell-mediated activation and responses. Therefore, the mechanisms that induce tolerance are probably distinct from those that maintain it, a balance that must be

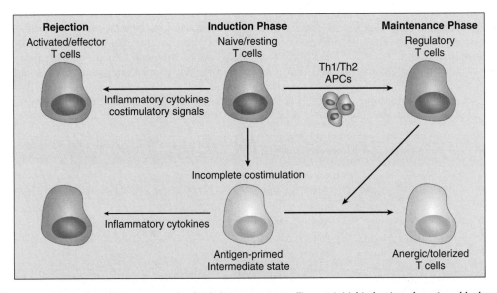

**FIGURE 32-7.** The successful creation of tolerance can be divided into two stages. First, an initial induction phase (e.g., blockage of T cell activation such as by costimulation signal blockade and deviation of helper T cell cytokine production) in which the acute rejection of the graft is inhibited. Second, a tolerance maintenance phase, which is required to sustain long-term graft survival (e.g., regulatory T cells and T cell anergy). The concept of an intermediate T cell that is antigen-primed but still able to "choose" between activation and rejection or tolerance-inducing T cell anergy is shown indicating the complexity of the immune response that has made single strategy approaches to creating transplantation tolerance difficult. It is important for the reader to note that in tolerance strategies involving bone marrow transplantation that the mechanisms are probably very different than what is shown in this figure. In the purest form of bone marrow-induced tolerance, the circulating T cells should not recognize the transplant as foreign so that the very first signal of the immune response, T-cell receptor activation, does not occur.

considered in the ongoing clinical trials testing new strategies to produce tolerance. A good example of this problem was the excitement that originally followed the results that blockade of the costimulatory molecule CD40 ligand protected kidney and islet transplants in nonhuman primates.[29-31] Although this was a remarkable experimental result and a powerful proof of concept for costimulatory blockade, the initial conclusion that this was the tolerance breakthrough for the field was shattered a year later when it was clear that the organs rejected when immunosuppression was stopped.

Tolerance created by clonal deletion of antigen-reactive T cells is most likely to occur in the thymus (central tolerance). The thymus is where natural clonal deletion of autoreactive T cells occurs, a process required to prevent autoimmune disease. However, there are still T cells that are not eliminated and can react to self-antigen in the periphery. Thus, mechanisms do exist in the periphery to regulate or delete these autoreactive T cells. In the case of transplantation, a high frequency of alloantigen-reactive T cells exists, representing up to 5% of the circulating T cells. Similar to clonal deletion in the thymus, the apoptotic deletion of alloreactive T cells is allied with tolerance induction. However, the high levels of alloreactive T cells in the circulation effectively "raises the bar" for strategies to use this approach for clinical tolerance.

One mechanism to control the "pool size" of alloreactive T cells involves apoptosis.[56] The theory is that if a large number of alloreactive T-cell clones are activated posttransplant, the corresponding immunoregulatory cells will not be sufficient to control the alloreactive T cells resulting in acute or chronic rejection. Thus, strategies to induce apoptosis of activated T cells posttransplant, such as costimulatory molecule blockade or signaling through apoptosis receptors such as the TNF family, could adjust this balance in favor of long-term graft survival.

A key point is that deletional control of alloreactive T cell clones requires their activation and initial expansion. This is dependent on a number of proinflammatory cytokines such as IL-2. The irony is that the most effective clinical immunosuppressive drugs, the calcineurin inhibitors cyclosporine and FK506, rapamycin, and steroids all interfere with this early and critical production of cytokines or their immediate effects on T cell activation. Thus, although immunosuppression is very effective in preventing rejection, it may also dramatically reduce the efficiency of any purposeful manipulations of activation-induced deletional or regulatory pathways intended to induce tolerance.[28]

A nondeletional immunoregulatory concept is that of immune deviation of T helper cells (Th), or the Th1/Th2 hypothesis. Currently, the evidence is that one class of Th is Th1 cells that produce primarily Il-2, INF-$\gamma$, and TNF-$\alpha$. A second class, called Th-2 cells, produce primarily IL-4, IL-5, IL-6, IL-10, and IL-13.[38,39] Experiments in the mouse indicate that the Th1 pathway mediates development of cell-mediated immunity, whereas the Th2 pathway favors humoral immune mechanisms and may also mediate a feedback suppression of the Th1 pathway. Based on this observation, it was suggested that transplant rejection represents a primary Th1 response, whereas transplant tolerance is favored by a Th2 response. It was hypothesized that any strategy to induce tolerance should be characterized by an immune deviation from a primary Th1 response to a Th2 response.

Several studies followed that documented relative increases in Th2 cytokine gene transcripts and Th2 cells in tolerant animals, favoring this immune deviation theory for tolerance. Nevertheless, despite the logical attraction of this simple binary Th1 versus Th2 paradigm for transplantation, there is increasing evidence that the immune response to transplantation in humans is more complex.[39,57] For example, a simple application of the paradigm would predict the following result. In separating the peripheral T cell population of two groups of patients, one with acute rejection and another that never had a rejection, a distinct Th1 predominance in the rejecting patients and Th2 predominance in the nonrejecting group should be found. However, this has not been reported. It could be countered that the T helper cells in the peripheral blood may not be representative of the immune response to the transplant. This would require analysis of the T cells in the graft. Therefore, a number of investigators studied Th1 versus Th2 cytokine message levels in biopsy specimens from stable and rejecting patients but with no better results. It could still be argued that most cells in the biopsy are kidney epithelium and interstitial stroma such that the sensitivity of even PCR-based cytokine assays are not sufficient to identify the deviation.

Nonetheless, messages for both Th1 and Th2 cytokines are detectable by PCR in rejecting transplant biopsy specimens. Immunosuppressed patients often demonstrate a preponderance of Th2 cytokines such as Il-4 and IL-10 in the periphery or the biopsies. This apparent paradox is actually not surprising based on the potent suppression of proinflammatory Th1 cytokine gene transcription by immunosuppressive drugs. Thus, the theory of immune deviation predicts that the use of immunosuppression effectively blocks the cytokines responsible for Th1 development and, thus, favor immune deviation to the Th2 phenotype. This is supported in mouse and rat transplant model studies in which a short course of cyclosporine at the time of transplantation can produce long-term tolerance. Unfortunately, whatever immunosuppression is doing to Th1/Th2 profiles in human patients, the fact that no one would think of using only a week of immunosuppression and that chronic rejection is still the primary problem in transplantation suggests that tolerance is not being produced. These contrasting observations in murine and human transplantation may eventually be explained by critical differences in the logic of the Th1/Th2 paradigm in higher mammals. This exemplifies another ongoing controversy regarding the true utility of small animal rodent models for preclinical development of new transplantation strategies.

It is also important to acknowledge the possible connection between the theory of immune deviation and the concept of apoptosis. First, apoptosis of APCs could alter the net presentation of costimulatory ligands, which might influence the balance of costimulation-mediated T cell activation. The extent to which certain costimulatory signals or the net amount of costimulation may favor Th1 or Th2 development could determine the nature of cytokines present in a given environment. In turn, the amount and kind of cytokines in a local site will also determine the efficiency of antigen presentation. Second, as indicated previously, immunosuppression inhibits the IL-2-dependent deletion of reactive T cells by apoptosis. So one could imagine the situation following early induction therapy posttransplant: as immunosuppression levels are tapered the alloreactive T cell pool remains too large; thus, even a successful deviation of the immune response to the regulatory Th2 cells will fail to control rejection. Thus, although the field continues to focus on specific pathways to induce stable tolerance, we propose that success might eventually require integrating several strategies to deal with the early posttransplantation induction period very differently than the long-term maintenance phase.

One of the most promising strategies to induce transplantation tolerance is bone marrow stem cell transfer. The pioneering work of Sir Peter Medawar and colleagues in the late 1940s provided the first insight into the feasibility of bone marrow stem cell transfer for which the Nobel Prize was eventually awarded. Building on observations made with calves sharing a placenta during development, a hypothesis was made that sharing of cells between donors at an early point in the development of the immune system resulted in a perfect tolerance induction.[58,59] For example, when newborn mice were immunized with allogeneic spleen cells, the animals grew up to accept transplants from the allogeneic donors with absolutely no immune response—classic tolerance.

Over the last several decades it was recognized that a similar situation to neonatal tolerance could be reprised in adults by fully ablating the bone marrow compartment and rescuing with a hematopoietic stem cell transplant along with some allogeneic donor cells. With an understanding of immune repertoire development based on thymic T cell selection, it was realized that ablation of the adult immune system required a re-education of the newly developing T cells in the thymus following the successful stem cell transplant. If donor alloantigen was presented in the thymus during this reeducation presumably by donor-derived APCs, then the new T cell clones that recognized these alloantigens would be deleted in the thymus as autoreactive. The resulting "hole" in the adult immune repertoire is specific for the donor antigens and allows transplantation without immune recognition despite the fact that all other immune responses are normal.

As proof of this concept, a number of patients have been transplanted with bone marrow from fully HLA-matched siblings for hematologic malignancies and later received kidney transplants from the same donors with complete tolerance.[60,61] One should note that these siblings are fully HLA-matched but not HLA-identical twins because in the latter situation there would be no

immune response regardless of the induction and transplant. Thus, in the field of bone marrow transplantation, fully HLA-matched siblings that are not identical twins are called allogeneic donors, and there is a 50% or greater incidence of acute or chronic graft versus host disease in this setting. The obvious limitations of a bone marrow transplant approach are that a fully ablative bone marrow transplant is a very severe regimen for organ transplantation and that most patients do not have the required HLA-matched donor.

The obvious question was whether a nonmyeloablative regimen engineered to establish a mixed hematopoietic chimerism with donor and patient would also be effective. If so, how mixed would this chimerism need to be—a few detectable donor cells or equal portions with the recipient? A clue that dramatically influenced the field was a series of observations made on successful liver transplant patients that, after 10 to 20 years, had stopped all their immunosuppressive medications.[62-64] Barely detectable levels of donor cells, called microchimerism, were observed to roughly correlate with patients who did not reject after stopping immunosuppression. The hypothesis was that small numbers of donor-derived APCs, called passenger leukocytes by some,[65-67] were carried over in the transplanted organ and were sufficient to create some level of functional tolerance in the long term. A number of reports in kidney, heart, and lung transplant patients seemed to suggest the same correlations, and a series of rodent transplant models were used to confirm that protocols to create mixed chimerism did produce long-term allograft survival and functional tolerance.[68]

The next logical clinical step was to infuse allogeneic donor cells obtained from bone marrow aspirations at the time of organ harvest. In these studies, bone marrow was obtained from cadaveric organ donors for kidney transplants and the patients were given relatively standard immunosuppression rather than any kind of myeloablative protocol.[69] Unfortunately, the results were only modestly better than standard transplantation protocols, and the perfect correlations between rejections, long-term graft function, and survival with the levels of donor chimerism detectable were not observed. Although several studies representing various protocol refinements are still underway, it now appears that a more aggressive regimen of myeloablation and donor hematopoietic stem cell transplantation will be necessary if the quality of the results are to improve sufficiently to allow real tolerance induction as measured by reduction or even elimination of long-term immunosuppression.

Therefore, a series of new clinical trials has been initiated in which various levels of myeloablation, some fully ablative and others nonmyeloablative, combined with allogeneic donor-derived stem cells are being combined for kidney transplant recipients.[61,70] If one accepts the proof that fully ablative induction and HLA-matched stem cell transplantation leads to functional tolerance induction, it is reasonably likely that refinement of these regimens as currently underway will produce strategies suitable for clinical organ transplantation in some portion of patients. The big question is whether successful tolerance induction can be done with hematopoietic stem cell transplants in such a way that a relatively low-risk, low-toxicity regimen can be implemented for all patients. This is far from clear at this point but would obviously change the whole field if accomplished.

## CONCLUSIONS

The whole field of transplantation has changed dramatically in the last decade. The key has been the integration of this clinical specialty into the mainstreams of cell biology, genomics, chemistry, and molecular medicine. Nonetheless, its future will still be written by the successful interchanges between basic and clinical scientists. It will require from both groups an even greater appreciation of the complexity of the immune system and the complexity of the mechanisms that maintain the health of functioning tissues. As attractive as binary mechanisms and single-agent therapies are to everyone, the reality is much more likely to require a highly integrated, multifactorial approach.

## REFERENCES

1. Dai Y, Vaught TD, Boone J, et al: Targeted disruption of the alpha1,3-galactosyltransferase gene in cloned pigs. Nat Biotechnol 2002; 20:251-255.
2. Fujita T: Evolution of the lectin-complement pathway and its role in innate immunity. Nat Rev Immunol 2002;2:346-353.
3. Hammond EH, Ensley RD, Yowell RL, et al: Vascular rejection of human cardiac allografts and the role of humoral immunity in chronic allograft rejection. Transplant Proc 1991;23(2 Suppl 2): 26-30.
4. Ratkovec RM, Hammond EH, O'Connell JB, et al: Outcome of cardiac transplant recipients with a positive donor-specific cross-match–preliminary results with plasmapheresis. Transplantation 1992;54:651-655.
5. McCurry KR, Kooyman DL, Alvarado CG, et al: Human complement regulatory proteins protect swine-to-primate cardiac xenografts from humoral injury. Nat Med 1995;1:423-427.
6. Lankat-Buttgereit B, Tampe R: The transporter associated with antigen processing TAP: Structure and function. FEBS Lett 1999;464:108-112.
7. Garcia KC, Degano M, Stanfield RL, et al: An alphabeta T cell receptor structure at 2.5 A and its orientation in the TCR-MHC complex. Science 1996;274:209-219.
8. Chicz RM, Urban RG: Analysis of MHC-presented peptides: Applications in autoimmunity and vaccine development. Immunol Today 1994;15:155-160.
9. Sayegh MH, Perico N, Gallon L, et al: Mechanisms of acquired thymic unresponsiveness to renal allografts: Thymic recognition of immunodominant allo-MHC peptides induces peripheral T cell anergy. Transplantation 1994;58:125-132.
10. Jenkins MK, Pardoll DM, Mizuguchi J, et al: T-cell unresponsiveness in vivo and in vitro: Fine specificity of induction and molecular characterization of the unresponsive state." Immunol Rev 1987; 95:113-135.
11. Jenkins MK, Pardoll DM, Mizuguchi J, et al: (1987). Molecular events in the induction of a nonresponsive state in interleukin 2-producing helper T-lymphocyte clones. Proc Natl Acad Sci USA 1987;84:5409-5413.
12. Jenkins MK, Ashwell JD, Schwartz RH: Allogeneic non-T spleen cells restore the responsiveness of normal T cell clones stimulated with antigen and chemically modified antigen-presenting cells. J Immunol 1988;140:3324-3330.
13. Schwartz RH, Mueller DL, Jenkins MK, et al: T-cell clonal anergy. Cold Spring Harbor Symp Quant Biol 1989;54(Pt 2):605-610.
14. Schwartz RH: A cell culture model for T lymphocyte clonal anergy. Science 1990;248:1349-1356.
15. Jenkins MK, Mueller D, Schwartz RH, et al: Induction and maintenance of anergy in mature T cells. Adv Exp Med Biol 1991;292: 167-176.
16. Schwartz RH: T cell clonal anergy. Curr Opin Immunol 1997; 9:351-357.
17. Linsley PS, Wallace PM, Johnson J, et al: Immunosuppression in vivo by a soluble form of the CTLA-4 T cell activation molecule. Science 1992;257:792-795.
18. Gudmundsdottir H, Turka LA: T cell costimulatory blockade: New therapies for transplant rejection. J Am Soc Nephrol 1999;10: 1356-1365.
19. Lenschow DJ, Zeng Y, Thistlethwaite JR, et al: Long-term survival of xenogeneic pancreatic islet grafts induced by CTLA4Ig. Science 1992;257:789-792.
20. Turka LA, Linsley PS, Lin H, et al: T-cell activation by the CD28 ligand and B7 is required for cardiac allograft rejection in vivo. Proc Natl Acad Sci USA 1992;89:11102-11105.
21. Mandelbrot DA, Furukawa Y, McAdam AJ et al: Expression of B7 molecules in recipient, not donor, mice determines the survival of cardiac allografts. J Immunol 1999;163:3753-3757.
22. Szot GL, Zhou P, Sharpe AH, et al: Absence of host B7 expression is sufficient for long-term murine vascularized heart allograft survival. Transplantation 2000;69:904-909.
23. Rogers NJ, Mirenda V, Jackson I, et al: Costimulatory blockade by the induction of an endogenous xenospecific antibody response. Nat Immunol 2000;1:163-168.
24. Schwartz LM, Osborne BA: Programmed cell death, apoptosis and killer genes. Immunol Today 1993;14:582-590.
25. Allison JP, Krummel MF: The Yin and Yang of T cell costimulation. Science 1995;270:932-933.
26. Waterhouse P, Penninger JM, Timms E, et al: Lymphoproliferative disorders with early lethality in mice deficient in Ctla-4. Science 1995;270:985-988.
27. Larsen CP, Alexander DZ, Hollenbaugh D, et al: CD40-gp39 interactions play a critical role during allograft rejection: Suppression of allograft rejection by blockade of the CD40-gp39 pathway. Transplantation 1996;61:4-9.
28. Li Y, Li XC, Zheng XX, et al: Blocking both signal 1 and signal 2 of T-cell activation prevents apoptosis of alloreactive T cells and induction of peripheral allograft tolerance. Nat Med 1999;5: 1298-1302.
29. Kirk AD, Harlan DM, Armstrong NN, et al: CTLA4-Ig and anti-CD40 ligand prevent renal allograft rejection in primates. Proc Natl Acad Sci USA 1997;94:8789-8794.
30. Kenyon NS, Chatzipetrou M, Masetti M, et al: Long-term survival and function of intrahepatic islet allografts in rhesus monkeys treated with humanized anti-CD154. Proc Natl Acad Sci USA 1999; 96:8132-8137.
31. Kenyon NS, Fernandez LA, Lehmann R, et al: Long-term survival and function of intrahepatic islet allografts in baboons treated with humanized anti-CD154. Diabetes 1999;48:1473-1481.
32. Dai Z, Konieczny BT, Lakkis FG: The dual role of IL-2 in the generation and maintenance of CD8+ memory T cells. J Immunol 2000;165:3031-3036.
33. Iwakoshi NN, Mordes JP, Markees TG, et al: Treatment of allograft recipients with donor-specific transfusion and anti-CD154 antibody leads to deletion of alloreactive CD8+ T cells and prolonged graft survival in a CTLA4-dependent manner. J Immunol 2000;164: 512-521.
34. Judge TA, Tang A, Spain LM, et al: The in vivo mechanism of action of CTLA4Ig. J Immunol 1996;156:2294-2299.
35. Dai Z, Konieczny BT, Baddoura FK, et al: Impaired alloantigen-mediated T cell apoptosis and failure to induce long-term allograft survival in IL-2-deficient mice. J Immunol 1998;161:1659-1663.
36. Konieczny BT, Dai Z, Elwood ET, et al: IFN-gamma is critical for long-term allograft survival induced by blocking the CD28 and CD40 ligand T cell costimulation pathways. J Immunol 1998;160: 2059-2064.
37. Monks CR, Freiberg BA, Kupfer H, et al: Three-dimensional segregation of supramolecular activation clusters in T cells. Nature 1998; 395:82-86.

38. Seder RA: Acquisition of lymphokine-producing phenotype by CD4+ T cells. J Allergy Clin Immunol 1994;94:1195–1202.

39. Kelso A: Th1 and Th2 subsets: Paradigms lost? Immunol Today 1995;16:374–379.

40. Harder T, Simons K: Caveolae, DIGs, and the dynamics of sphingolipid-cholesterol microdomains. Curr Opin Cell Biol 1997;9:534–542.

41. Zhang W, Trible RP, Samelson LE: LAT palmitoylation: its essential role in membrane microdomain targeting and tyrosine phosphorylation during T cell activation. Immunity 1998;9:239–246.

42. Lin J, Weiss A, Finco TS: Localization of LAT in glycolipid-enriched microdomains is required for T cell activation. J Biol Chem 1999;274:28861–28864.

43. Taniguchi T: Cytokine signaling through nonreceptor protein tyrosine kinases. Science 1995;268:251–255.

44. Darnell JE Jr: The JAK-STAT pathway: Summary of initial studies and recent advances. Recent Prog Horm Res 1996;51:391–403; discussion 403–404.

45. Ihle JN: Janus kinases in cytokine signalling. Philos Trans R Soc Lond B Biol Sci 196;351:159–66.

46. Chao DT, Korsmeyer SJ: BCL-2 family: regulators of cell death. Annu Rev Immunol 1998;16:395–419.

47. Budihardjo I, Oliver H, Lutter M, et al: Biochemical pathways of caspase activation during apoptosis. Annu Rev Cell Dev Biol 1999;15:269–290.

48. Budd RC: Activation-induced cell death. Curr Opin Immunol 2001;13:356–362.

49. Zhang Z, Vuori K, Reed JC, et al: The alpha 5 beta 1 integrin supports survival of cells on fibronectin and up-regulates Bcl-2 expression. Proc Natl Acad Sci USA 1995;92:6161–6165.

50. Bellgrau D, Gold D, Selawry H, et al: A role for CD95 ligand in preventing graft rejection. Nature 1995;377:630–632.

51. Vaux DL, Strasser A: The molecular biology of apoptosis. Proc Natl Acad Sci USA 1996;93:2239–2244.

52. Rossiter H, Alon R, Kupper TS: Selectins, T-cell rolling and inflammation. Mol Med Today 1997;3:214–222.

53. Alon R, Hammer DA, Springer TA: Lifetime of the P-selectin-carbohydrate bond and its response to tensile force in hydrodynamic flow. Nature 1995;374:539–542.

54. Sayegh MH, Turka LA: The role of T-cell costimulatory activation pathways in transplant rejection. N Engl J Med 1998;338:1813–1821.

55. Tran HM, Nickerson PW, Restifo AC, et al: Distinct mechanisms for the induction and maintenance of allograft tolerance with CTLA4-Fc treatment. J Immunol 1997;159:2232–2239.

56. Wells AD, Li XC, Li Y, et al: Requirement for T-cell apoptosis in the induction of peripheral transplantation tolerance. Nat Med 1999;5:1303–1307.

57. Thompson CB: Distinct roles for the costimulatory ligands B7-1 and B7-2 in T helper cell differentiation? Cell 1995;81:979–982.

58. Owen R: Immunogenetic consequences of vascular anastomoses between bovine twins. Science 1945;102:400–401.

59. Billingham R, Brent L, Medawar, PB: Actively acquired tolerance of foreign cells. Nature 1953;172:603.

60. Sayegh MH, Fine NA, Smith JL, et al: Immunologic tolerance to renal allografts after bone marrow transplants from the same donors. Ann Intern Med 1991;114:954–955.

61. Dey B, Sykes M, Spitzer TR: Outcomes of recipients of both bone marrow and solid organ transplants. A review. Medicine (Baltimore) 1998;77:355–369.

62. Starzl TE, Demetris AJ, Murase N, et al: Donor cell chimerism permitted by immunosuppressive drugs: A new view of organ transplantation. Immunol Today 1993;14:326–332.

63. Starzl TE, Zinkernagel RM: Antigen localization and migration in immunity and tolerance. N Engl J Med 1998;339(26): 1905–1913.

64. Starzl TE, Zinkernagel RM: Transplantation tolerance from a historical perspective. Nat Rev Immunol 2001;1:233–239.

65. Batchelor JR, Phillips BE, Grennan D: Suppressor cells and their role in the survival of immunologically enhanced rat kidney allografts. Transplantation 1984;37:43–46.

66. Braun MY, McCormack A, Webb G, et al: Evidence for clonal anergy as a mechanism responsible for the maintenance of transplantation tolerance. Eur J Immunol 1993;23:1462–1468.

67. Hornick PI, Mason PD, Yacoub MH, et al: Assessment of the contribution that direct allorecognition makes to the progression of chronic cardiac transplant rejection in humans. Circulation 1998;97:1257–1263.

68. Sachs DH, Sykes M, Greenstein JL, et al: Tolerance and xenograft survival. Nat Med 1995;1:969.

69. Mathew JM, Garcia-Morales R, Fuller L, et al: Donor bone marrow-derived chimeric cells present in renal transplant recipients infused with donor marrow. I. Potent regulators of recipient anti-donor immune responses. Transplantation 2000;70:1675–1682.

70. Fuchimoto Y, Huang CA, Yamada K, et al: Mixed chimerism and tolerance without whole body irradiation in a large animal model. J Clin Invest 2000;105:1779–1789.

# chapter 33

# Viral Infections of the Heart

*Kirk U. Knowlton*
*Hervé Duplain*

Viral infections have been implicated in a broad spectrum of cardiovascular diseases that include congenital heart disease, myocarditis, dilated cardiomyopathy, pericarditis, endocardial fibroelastosis, atherosclerosis, and cardiac allograft vasculopathy (Table 33-1). In some of these, a cause-effect relationship has been established. However, in many, associations have been repeatedly demonstrated, but the evidence for a clear cause-effect relationship is still incomplete. This chapter summarizes the evidence that virus infection can cause or contribute to a variety of cardiovascular diseases, and it addresses the molecular mechanisms that are important for viral infection, replication, and pathogenesis using the extensively studied enteroviral-mediated cardiomyopathy as a prototype.

## ESTABLISHING A CAUSE-EFFECT RELATIONSHIP BETWEEN VIRAL INFECTION AND DISEASE

In the late 19th century, Robert Koch, a country doctor in a small German village, identified the anthrax bacillus as the cause of anthrax and the tubercle bacillus as the cause of tuberculosis. Based on his experience he established guidelines known as Koch's postulates, criteria that are often used as the standard to establish that a particular infectious organism is the causative agent for a disease. The criteria are as follows:

1. The organism must be regularly found in the lesions of the disease.
2. The organism must be isolated in pure culture.
3. Inoculation of such a pure culture of organisms into a host should initiate the disease.
4. The organisms must be recovered once again from the lesions of the host.

It is generally agreed that when these criteria are met, there is strong evidence that a particular organism causes a disease; however, it is interesting that it was only when these rules broke down and failed to yield a causative agent that the concept of a virus was born.[1] Advances in viral isolation have allowed fulfillment of Koch's postulates for a number of viral diseases. However, as an understanding of the complexity of viral pathogenesis and the ability to detect evidence of viral infection has improved, there is a growing list of diseases that may be caused by viruses but do not fulfill all of Koch's postulates. Nevertheless, recognition of this difficulty does not preclude the need to maintain standards that are comparable to those established by Koch for determination that infection with a particular organism causes a given disease.

## DIAGNOSTIC VIROLOGY

A key characteristic of modern virology is the use of multiple strategies for the detection of viral infections. Although an extensive review of the diagnostic techniques used to identify a virus as a cause of a disease is beyond the scope of this chapter, they are discussed briefly.

### Viral Culture

Unlike bacteria, viruses require cellular proteins and machinery to replicate and are, therefore, usually grown in living cells, generally in culture but occasionally in mice. Culture of a virus from a specimen of interest allows further analysis of the virus and meets one of Koch's postulates. Unfortunately, there is a relatively limited range of viruses that can be easily grown in culture, and it is becoming evident that some viruses can exist as a persistent infection, in which case, they may have a pathogenic role in a disease, but for a variety of reasons are not easily identified by culture.

### Serology

Identification of antibodies directed against viral antigens was one of the first techniques used to identify viral infection. Antibody titers may be negative at the onset of the disease but become positive several weeks following infection. The initial antibody response is usually characterized by an increase in IgM antibody, an indication of a more acute infection, followed by increases in specific IgG antibodies that may persist for the life of the individual. This is used as a measure of immunity and/or previous infection with a particular virus.

The advantage of serology is that it is a very sensitive assay that can be performed on a patient's serum. The disadvantages include the fact that the antibody titer is often negative during the acute phase of the infection when therapy might be most beneficial, and, if positive, it is difficult to determine if the elevated titer indicates that the virus that it recognizes is the cause of the dis-

**TABLE 33-1** CARDIOVASCULAR DISEASES ASSOCIATED WITH VIRAL INFECTION

| Disease | Virus(es) Implicated |
| --- | --- |
| Congenital rubella syndrome | Rubella virus |
| Myocarditis, dilated cardiomyopathy, and pericarditis | |
| | Enteroviruses, adenovirus, echovirus, influenza, cytomegalovirus, hepatitis C, varicella, poliomyelitis, mumps, rabies, rubella, herpes, and others |
| Endocardial fibroelastosis | Mumps virus |
| Cardiac allograft vasculopathy | Cytomegalovirus |
| Increased cardiac transplant rejection | Cytomegalovirus, adenovirus, coxsackievirus, parvovirus, others. |
| Atherosclerosis | Cytomegalovirus, herpes virus, others |

ease or only representative of a previous infection with that virus.

## Viral Nucleic Acid Detection

### In Situ Hybridization

*In situ* hybridization was one of the earliest methods used to detect viral nucleic acid sequences in the tissue of interest.[2] This is accomplished by direct binding of labeled nucleic acid probes that are complementary and specific to a given virus in a histologic section of the tissue of interest[3] (Fig. 33-1). The advantage of this strategy is its high degree of specificity. The corresponding disadvantage is the relatively low sensitivity of the assay that has been reported to require from $10^4$ to $10^5$ copies of the target sequence.

### Polymerase Chain Reaction (PCR)

A more sensitive strategy for detection of viral nucleic acids involves amplification of the nucleotide sequence of interest using PCR. This is performed by amplification of the DNA using small nucleotide probes that serve as primers for DNA amplification and bind specifically to the target viral DNA. Viral RNA can also be detected using reverse transcriptase (rt)-PCR. Newer techniques have been developed to increase sensitivity and to simplify the assay. One that is gaining widespread use is real-time PCR. This assay allows detection and quantitation of the amount of viral RNA or DNA in a given sample.

Advantages of PCR and rt-PCR include the high sensitivity of the assay and the relative ease with which the assay can be performed. The disadvantage is the correspondingly high probability of contamination with small amounts of DNA or RNA.

### Histology

Occasionally, viruses can be identified directly in histologic specimens, most commonly using electron microscopy to identify viral particles within the tissue of interest. Because the area examined with an electron microscope is very small, visualization is guided by indirect evidence of viral infection on light microscopy, such as the presence of inclusion bodies or virus-induced cytopathic effects. Histologic examination is enhanced when combined with immunohistochemistry or immunofluorescence using antiviral antibodies to detect viral proteins in the tissue (Fig. 33-1).

These assays and others, used either singly or in combination, are the major tools used to identify viral infection in cardiovascular disease.

## CARDIOVASCULAR DISEASES ASSOCIATED WITH VIRAL INFECTION

Infectious agents have recently been implicated in a number of noncardiac diseases in which there was

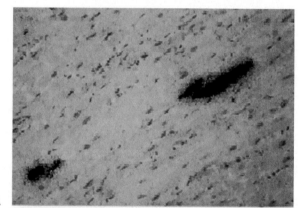

**FIGURE 33-1.** *A,* Detection of the coxsackievirus genome within the human myocardium using *in situ* hybridization between the viral RNA and a [35]S-labeled coxsackievirus specific probe.[3] (Magnification ×160), *B,* Detection of coxsackieviral protein within the myocardium from a coxsackievirus-infected mouse using a polyclonal anti-coxsackievirus antibody (magnification ×200). (*B, Courtesy H. Duplain, unpublished.*)

initially little suspicion of an infectious cause. These include cervical cancer caused by human papillomavirus,[4] Kaposi's sarcoma caused by human herpes virus-8,[5] Burkitt's lymphoma caused by Epstein-Barr virus,[6] peptic ulcer disease caused by *Helicobacter pylori*,[7] and others. These examples demonstrate that viral infection may contribute to diseases that are not typically thought to be secondary to infection. However, rigorous standards should be required before it becomes generally accepted that a virus can cause or contribute to a cardiovascular disease. Accordingly, this section reviews some of the cardiovascular diseases that have been most clearly associated with viral infection. We discuss the evidence that the virus may be causative and in some cases review the mechanisms by which the virus may contribute to the disease.

## Congenital Rubella Syndrome

Perhaps one of the most compelling examples of a viral infection causing cardiovascular disease is the congenital heart disease that is part of the congenital rubella syndrome. This is caused by maternal infection with rubella virus during the first trimester of pregnancy. The common cardiovascular manifestations of congenital rubella syndrome include a patent ductus arteriosus, atrial septal defects, and pulmonary valvular or pulmonary arterial stenosis.[8] Other common manifestations of congenital rubella syndrome include hearing loss, psychomotor retardation, cataracts or glaucoma, retinopathy, neonatal thrombocytopenic purpura, hepatosplenomegaly, and intrauterine growth retardation.[9]

Rubella infection was generally considered to cause only a mild disease until 1941 when an ophthalmologist, Norman Gregg, identified a large number of children with cataracts, many of whom also had serious congenital defects. He noted that this apparent epidemic followed a large rubella outbreak. He proposed that the syndrome was a consequence of maternal infection during pregnancy.[10] After some initial reluctance to the idea that rubella could cause this syndrome, it was ultimately accepted by the scientific community as a likely cause. The introduction of the rubella virus vaccine in 1969 has been remarkably successful at preventing both postnatal rubella and its teratogenic effects in the United States.[11,12] Unfortunately, rubella is still endemic in underdeveloped countries, but the precise incidence of both postnatal and congenital rubella syndrome is difficult to determine.[13]

Rubella virus is an enveloped, positive-strand RNA. In early gestation, the rubella virus can infect the placenta leading to placental hypoplasia and macroscopic placentitis.[14] The virus is then able to spread throughout the developing fetus infecting almost any organ.[15] This leads to a chronic, generally nonlytic infection. It has been demonstrated that infection of cultured cells from many different organs results in slowed growth of the cells and reduced survival, suggesting a direct viral-mediated cytopathic effect that may contribute to the observed congenital abnormalities. There is also evidence of immune activation directed against the rubella

virus that may also have a role in the congenital rubella syndrome.[16]

Since the original description of congenital rubella syndrome in 1946, evidence has accumulated to demonstrate that maternal infection with rubella during the first trimester of pregnancy can cause the congenital rubella syndrome. The virus has been consistently isolated from affected tissues. However, the most convincing argument that rubella is the cause of the disease is the markedly decreased incidence of congenital rubella since the introduction of the rubella vaccine in 1969.

## Viral-Mediated Cardiomyopathy and Myocarditis

Most of the viral mediated heart muscle diseases fit the broad classification of cardiomyopathy as defined by the World Health Organization, "diseases of the myocardium associated with cardiac dysfunction."[17] However, there is overlap between the definitions of dilated cardiomyopathy and inflammatory cardiomyopathy. Dilated cardiomyopathy is "...characterized by dilation and impaired contraction of the left ventricle or both ventricles. It may be idiopathic, familial/genetic, viral and/or immune, alcoholic/toxic..." The definition for inflammatory cardiomyopathy is "myocarditis in association with cardiac dysfunction." As molecular and histopathologic diagnostic tools improve, the classification of cardiomyopathies will likely evolve. However, the current limitations in terminology should be kept in mind as one reviews the literature that identifies the association of viral infection with cardiomyopathy.

### Evidence of Enteroviral Infection in Human Cardiomyopathy

Viral infection has been clearly associated with acute episodes of myocarditis that often present with cardiomyopathy and heart failure. Many different infectious agents have been attributed as the cause of viral myocarditis including enteroviruses such as the coxsackieviruses from groups A and B, adenovirus,[18] cytomegalovirus,[19] hepatitis C virus,[20] influenza virus, dengue virus, echovirus, encephalomyocarditis virus, Epstein-Barr virus, hepatitis A, herpes simplex virus, varicella-zoster virus, HIV, Junin virus, lymphocytic choriomeningitis, measles virus, mumps virus, parvovirus, poliovirus, rabies virus, respiratory syncytial, rubella, vaccinia virus, variola virus, and yellow fever virus.[21] Among the most commonly identified infectious causes are the group B coxsackieviruses (CVB), members of the enterovirus genera of the picornavirus family.

The association of acute myocarditis with coxsackievirus infection was identified as early as the mid-1950s.[22-24] Reports of isolation of coxsackievirus from the heart or pericardial fluid of patients with acute myocarditis date back to the mid-1960s[25] with numerous reports since then that have isolated virus from the heart or pericardial fluid or demonstrated the presence of viral proteins in diseased heart tissue.[26-31] According to World

Health Organization surveys from many different countries, 34.6 per 1000 of all CVB infections are associated with cardiovascular disease.[32]

In addition to the clear association between enteroviral infection and acute myocarditis, it has been shown that dilated cardiomyopathy can also be a sequela of viral myocarditis.[33] Attempts to isolate virus from the myocardium of patients with chronic forms of dilated cardiomyopathy have been unsuccessful. However, serologic evidence and the presence of enteroviral genomes in heart tissue of patients with dilated cardiomyopathy have been demonstrated using molecular biologic techniques such as slot blot,[34] *in situ* hybridization[2,35] and rt-PCR.[36-38] Recently, using a pan-enteroviral antibody, viral proteins were also shown to be present in the myocardium of a subset of patients with dilated cardiomyopathy.[39]

Identification of enteroviral RNA and protein in myocardial tissue establishes an association between enteroviral infection and dilated cardiomyopathy. Although results vary between studies, the most commonly reported enterovirus detection rates from published studies are in the 10% to 30% range; however, the reported incidence ranges from 0% to 75%.[38] It should be noted that many of these studies do not represent consecutive patients and they may not differentiate acute forms of the disease from chronic forms of dilated cardiomyopathy.

The studies described previously indicate that, in cases of acute myocarditis, Koch's first and second postulates can be met because the virus can be found in the diseased tissue and can be isolated in pure culture. It is also clear that in a subset of patients with dilated cardiomyopathy, the first postulate has been met, but the second is lacking. These reports establish associations between viral infection and heart disease, but, of themselves, do not establish a clear cause-effect relationship.

### Mouse Models of Myocarditis

Establishment of a cause-effect relationship between virus infection and cardiomyopathy is strengthened by animal models that allow validation of Koch's postulates three and four: "inoculation of such a pure culture of organisms into a host should initiate the disease, and the organisms must be recovered once again from the lesions of the host." In 1969, Wilson et al.[40] found that acute infection with CVB3 in weanling Swiss mice was followed by marked fibrosis, dystrophic mineralization in the heart, and microscopic myocardial hypertrophy, which persisted for at least 6 months. Subsequently, they observed the natural history of the mice that were infected with CVB3 and forced to swim. They found that the cardiomyopathy worsened after 15 months, a natural course resembling acute myocarditis that progresses to dilated cardiomyopathy in humans.[41] Coxsackieviral infection of mice has, subsequently, been used widely to study the acute effects of viral infection on the myocardium. Following inoculation with coxsackievirus, the virus can be consistently isolated from the heart. Therefore, the murine model of viral myocarditis fulfills the third and fourth of Koch's postulates for the acute phase of viral heart disease. However, it

has been more challenging to experimentally demonstrate a cause-effect relationship between viral infection and the pathogenesis of chronic dilated cardiomyopathy.

Insights into the mechanisms by which coxsackieviral infection and viral persistence could contribute to dilated cardiomyopathy were provided by Klingel et al.[42] in a murine model of CVB3-induced myocarditis. In their study, murine hearts were examined by *in situ* hybridization for the presence of CVB3 genomic RNA. The areas of the myocardium where viral RNA was detected were further analyzed for the extent of myocardial damage and inflammatory cell infiltration. In the first 3 days after infection, myocytes containing CVB3 RNA were randomly distributed throughout the myocardium, presumably indicating hematogenous infection during viremia. By day 6, infected myocytes were adjacent to foci of inflammatory cells. The greatest numbers of CVB3-infected myocardial cells were noted from days 6 to 9. This correlated with a significant increase in myocardial injury. From days 15 to 30 after inoculation, infectious virus could no longer be isolated from the myocardium, but CVB3 genomes could still be detected in myocardial cells. These positive cells were found primarily within foci of myocardial lesions characterized by fibrosis, myocardial necrosis, and mononuclear cell infiltrates. These observations demonstrate that the CVB genomes can persist in the myocardium of infected hearts. Furthermore, the association between the presence of viral RNA and areas with evidence of abnormal myocardial pathology suggests that persistence of the viral genome in CVB-infected mice may contribute to the pathogenesis of some cases of chronic myocarditis. Interestingly, although there was evidence of persistent viral infection in A.CA/SnJ, A.BY/SnJ, and SWR/J mice, DBA/1J mice, which were capable of terminating the inflammatory processes through elimination of the virus from the heart, showed no evidence of persistent viral RNA in the myocardium.[43]

To demonstrate that low-level expression of enteroviral genomes in the heart can cause cardiomyopathy, transgenic mice were generated that expressed replication-defective enteroviral genomes in myocardium driven by the cardiac-specific MLC-2v promoter.[44] This allowed for low-level expression of coxsackieviral genomes in the heart without formation of infectious virions, thus preventing a productive viral replication cycle. In addition, the MLC-2v promoter directs expression in the heart at day 8.5 of embryogenesis,[45] thus avoiding activation of a potent immune response against viral antigens. As hypothesized, heart muscle-specific expression of the CVB3 mutant led to the synthesis of viral plus- and minus-strand RNA without formation of infectious viral progeny. Histopathologic analysis of transgenic hearts revealed typical morphologic features of myocardial interstitial fibrosis, hypertrophy, and degeneration of myocytes, thus resembling dilated cardiomyopathy in humans. These findings in the CVB3 transgenic mice demonstrate that restricted replication of enteroviral genomes in the heart without formation of infectious virions can induce cardiomyopathy with characteristics that are typical of dilated cardiomyopathy in humans.[44]

## Pericarditis

The level of evidence for a relationship between viral infection and pericarditis is similar to that for acute viral myocarditis. This includes isolation of virus from the pericardial fluid in patients with acute pericarditis. Furthermore, in animal models of CVB myocarditis, there is also evidence of accompanying pericarditis.[46,47] Less is known about the pathogenesis of this disease process. It is likely that activation of the immune response has a significant role in the disease because treatments with antiinflammatory agents are effective.

## Endocardial Fibroelastosis

Endocardial fibroelastosis is defined as a fibrous and elastic thickening of the left-ventricular endocardial lining.[46,48] Although a number of heart diseases are associated with endocardial fibroelastosis, one of the interesting insights into this disease was made from analysis of autopsy samples from 29 children that had endocardial fibroelastosis and died between 1955 and 1992, before extensive mumps vaccination. Mumps RNA could be identified in 21 of the 29 (72%) patients using rt-PCR, whereas none of the 65 control samples from patients with other heart disease were positive for mumps RNA.[49] The association between endocardial fibroelastosis and mumps infection is further supported by a fall in incidence associated with widespread mumps vaccination.[50] However, little is known about potential mechanisms by which mumps virus could induce endocardial fibroelastosis.

## Atherosclerosis

The potential link between both viral and bacterial infections and the pathogenesis of atherosclerosis has been described by several groups.[51-54] A possible role for infectious diseases in atherosclerosis was suggested in the late 1970s, when it was shown that administration of an avian herpes virus could cause atherosclerotic lesions in the chicken that were similar to those observed in humans.[55] Since then, several sero-epidemiologic studies in humans have found a positive association between atherosclerotic heart disease and both viral and bacterial pathogens, such as cytomegalovirus (CMV), herpes simplex virus (HSV), *Chlamydia pneumoniae, H. pylori,* hepatitis A virus, and enteroviruses.[56-61]

Although more than 70 articles have been published that implicate *C. pneumoniae* in atherosclerosis, it is important to note that the majority of evidence is obtained from seroepidemiologic data. The presence of antibodies in the sera may be a reflection of a relatively acute infection and does not determine whether the infection is in the arterial wall or in an unrelated location. Furthermore, most of these pathogens are common and there is little known about factors that determine susceptibility to develop coronary artery disease. In addition, some large-scale prospective studies show only a weak link between bacterial pathogens and atherosclerosis.[62,63] Another study showed no increased risk with *C. pneumoniae, H. pylori,* or hepatitis A virus but did

report an increase risk in patients that were seropositive for CMV.[64]

The presence of *C. pneumoniae,* CMV, and HSV antigen has been demonstrated in endarterectomy tissues from patients with carotid atherosclerosis.[65] HSV, CMV, and Epstein-Barr virus nucleic acids were detected in the aorta of a higher percentage of patients with atherosclerosis when compared with nonatherosclerotic patients.[66] In addition, to evidence that infections are associated with atherosclerosis, an increased incidence of restenosis after coronary angioplasty has been reported in patients that have antibodies to CMV.[67]

An emerging concept relates to the role of multiple infections or "pathogen burden." Previous studies have tried to focus on the role of a single agent in the pathogenesis of atherosclerosis; however, more recent reports have highlighted the importance of the aggregate number of pathogens by which a single individual is infected. A cross-sectional study demonstrated that although individual pathogens (CMV, hepatitis A, HSV-1, HSV-2, and *C. pneumoniae*) are variably associated with the risk of coronary artery disease, it was the association of multiple pathogens that most significantly correlated with atherosclerosis.[68-70] Many of these studies indicate that risk is primarily attributable to seropositivity to viral rather than bacterial pathogens.[71] It has been proposed that a herpes burden (aggregate seropositivity to CMV, HSV-1, HSV-2, and Epstein-Barr virus) is a more efficient cardiovascular seropredictor[70] (Fig. 33-2). Increased pathogen burden has also been associated with endothelial dysfunction, measured as changes in coronary vascular resistance to acetylcholine.[72]

Despite the numerous studies that show an association between infection and atherosclerosis, little is known about the mechanisms by which infection can promote atherosclerosis. It has been shown that infections with CMV can lead to smooth muscle cell accumulation by inhibiting apoptosis and promoting smooth

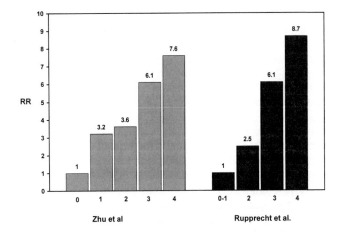

**FIGURE 33-2.** The risk of cardiovascular mortality and myocardial infarction increases with increased viral pathogen burden. Relative risk (RR) for death or myocardial infarction[69] or cardiovascular death[70] based on seropositivity for different viruses. The numbers along the X-axis represent the number of seropositive tests in a given individual. *(Adapted from Muhlestein JB, Anderson JL: Infectious serology and atherosclerosis: How burdensome is the risk? Circulation 2003;107:220-222.)*

muscle cell migration and proliferation.[52] CMV has been shown to inhibit the tumor suppressor gene *p53*, thereby stimulating the cells to divide.[73] Another mechanism by which CMV could lead to cellular proliferation is the stimulation of the production of growth factors.[74] Virus infection of smooth muscle cells also leads to increased lipid accumulation by decreasing the cholesterol esterase activity and increasing the uptake of oxidized LDL.[75,76] Herpes virus infection promotes the synthesis of tissue factor, increases the generation of thrombin on the endothelial cell surface, and increases platelet adherence, leading to a procoagulant phenotype of the endothelium.[77-79] Furthermore, patients, who are seropositive for CMV, have an impaired endothelium-mediated coronary vasodilator response.[52] Promotion of inflammation in the vessel wall is also thought to play a major role because viral infection can induce the production of reactive oxygen species and cytokines.[80-82] Recently, antigen mimicry between pathogen and host tissue epitopes, leading to the induction of autoimmunity, has been postulated in the pathogenesis of atherosclerosis.[83]

Because a significant percentage of patients with atherosclerosis lack conventional risk factors, it is likely that additional mechanisms play a major role in this disease. The presence of infectious agents has been established in atherosclerotic lesions and, from *in vitro* experiments, possible causal mechanisms have been identified. However, the precise role of viral or bacterial infection in human coronary artery disease has not yet been firmly established and further studies are warranted.

# Virus Infection and Transplant Pathology

## Cardiac Allograft Vasculopathy

Cardiac allograft vasculopathy is the most common cause of death and retransplantation following heart transplantation. Cardiac allograft vasculopathy has several characteristics that differentiate it from typical atherosclerosis. Most prominent of these is the concentric nature of the lesions associated with smooth muscle cell hyperplasia. Numerous studies have implicated viral infection in this process. Most of these studies have identified a seroepidemiologic association with CMV infection and allograft vasculopathy.[84-88] However, it has been difficult to identify virus within the arterial lesions in humans.

In an attempt to establish a cause-effect relationship between CMV and atherosclerosis, a post-hoc analysis of a randomized trial of ganciclovir, an anti-CMV agent, was demonstrated to have a protective effect against transplant vasculopathy but only in a subset of patients.[89] In line with the association between CMV and allograft vasculopathy in human, a rat model of heart transplantation shows an increase in arterial disease following CMV infection that can be inhibited by gancyclovir.[90]

Despite a significant body of evidence implicating CMV in posttransplant vasculopathy, there is persistent controversy about its role. To establish a clinically significant relationship between these two processes, it will be important to determine whether the vasculopathy can be decreased in a randomized, double-blind trial of ganciclovir treatment in patients undergoing cardiac transplantation.

## Viral Triggers to Cardiac Allograft Dysfunction

Because both viral infection and heart transplant rejection are associated with potent activation of the cellular immune response, it has been hypothesized that viral infection of the transplant recipient may contribute to cardiac transplant rejection. This argument is strengthened by evidence implicating viral infection in allograft disease of other organs such as the lung and liver.[91,92] PCR of endomyocardial biopsy specimens for a variety of viruses demonstrated that viral nucleic acids could be detected in 21 out of 40 pediatric heart transplant recipients with findings consistent with acute unexplained rejection.[93]

In a larger study that analyzed 553 consecutive biopsies from 149 pediatric heart transplant recipients, viral genomic sequences were identified by PCR in 48 samples from 34 (23%) patients. Adenovirus was found in 30 samples, enterovirus in 9 samples, parvovirus in 5 samples, cytomegalovirus in 2 samples, HSV in 1 sample, and Epstein-Barr virus in 1 sample. In 85% of the PCR- or rt-PCR-positive patients, an adverse event occurred within 3 months of obtaining the positive specimen, whereas adverse events occurred in only 34% of PCR- or rt-PCR-negative patients within 3 months.[94] A potential limitation of this study in regard to establishing a cause-effect relationship between viral infection and rejection is that it is conceivable that patients that have evidence for rejection may be more susceptible to viral infection. However, in some patients the biopsy specimen was positive for a viral genome but negative for rejection and only biopsies obtained at a later time point showed evidence of rejection. In addition, it is not clear if the association between viral infection and rejection occurs in adult cardiac transplant recipients. To date, there are no studies that demonstrate whether treatment for viral infection or immunization against potential viral pathogens would significantly decrease the incidence of rejection and adverse events.

# Cardiovascular Disease in HIV infection

Cardiovascular involvement in AIDS was underappreciated in the early course of the epidemic, but it is now recognized as a frequent complication of HIV infection. In retrospective analysis and autopsy series, cardiac involvement is varied from 25% to 75% of the cases.[95] The clinical cardiovascular manifestations of HIV include myocarditis, dilated cardiomyopathy, pericarditis, infective endocarditis, cardiac malignancies, vasculitis, accelerated atherosclerosis, and arrhythmias. A number of coincident etiologic factors have been postulated to contribute to these abnormalities. They include HIV, coxsackievirus, CMV, toxoplasma, Ebstein-Barr virus, bacterial infection, nutritional deficiencies, and drug toxicity.

Global ventricular hypokinesia was found in roughly 15% of randomly selected HIV positive patients.[96]

Myocarditis, characterized by lymphocytic infiltration, is present in 40% to 52% of patients who died of AIDS, and opportunistic infections were found in the heart in less than 20% of these cases (*Toxoplasma gondii, Cryptococcus neoformans,* HSV-2, *Mycobacterium tuberculosis, and Mycobacterium avium intracellulare*).[97]

Although it is clear that HIV infection is associated with ventricular dysfunction, the mechanisms by which HIV infection causes this are not clear. The HIV genome has been detected in cardiac tissue of some,[98,99] but not all,[100] AIDS patients. In addition, because of the complex nature of the AIDS pathologies (immunodeficiency, opportunistic infections, drug toxicity, terminal nature of the disease), it is difficult to determine whether HIV infection of the myocardium is the cause of the ventricular dysfunction in humans. In a transgenic mouse model with cardiac restricted overexpression of the HIV-Tat protein, cardiac abnormalities were found, including left-ventricular hypertrophy, reactivation of the fetal gene program, and morphologic mitochondrial abnormalities. This implies that expression of an HIV protein in the heart can have a pathogenic role in HIV-mediated heart disease[101] but does not exclude other contributing factors.[95,102]

## MECHANISMS OF VIRAL HEART DISEASE

To illustrate mechanisms that are important for viral-mediated heart disease, the following sections focus primarily on the well-studied coxsackievirus myocarditis model for two main reasons. First, enteroviruses, such as coxsackievirus, are among the most commonly implicated viruses in human myocarditis and viral-mediated cardiomyopathy. Second, a well-characterized murine model is available that allows delineation of the mechanisms by which a virus can cause heart disease.

## Mechanisms of Enteroviral Infection and Replication

Coxsackievirus is a member of the picornavirus family and is part of the enterovirus genus. It is a small virus (24 to 30 nm in diameter) consisting of a 7.4-kb positive-strand RNA genome encapsidated by 60 copies of each of four structural proteins—VP1, VP2, VP3, and VP4—forming the icosahedral shell structure of CVB3[103] (Fig. 33-3).

### Viral Receptors

To infect a target cell, the virus must attach to a viral receptor or receptor complex. In 1997, a common receptor for coxsackie and adenovirus, the coxsackie adenovirus receptor (CAR), was identified.[104] CAR mediates cell attachment and entry into the cell. In the case of coxsackievirus, CAR collaborates with a coreceptor, decay accelerating factor (DAF also known as CD55) (Fig. 33-3). DAF facilitates the binding of the virus onto the receptor-coreceptor complex, whereas CAR is thought to be responsible for the internalization of the virus. DAF has been shown to cause CVB attachment to

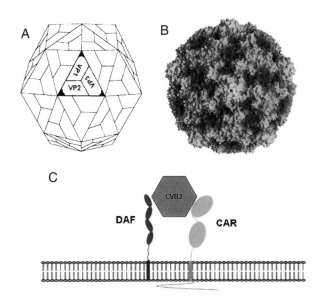

**FIGURE 33-3.** *A*, Schematic of the coxsackievirus capsid packaging arrangement of VP1, VP2, and VP3; VP4 lies buried. *B*, 3.5-Angstrom resolution structure of CVB3. *C*, Interaction of coxsackievirus with the CAR and the DAF. DAF facilitates the binding of the virus onto the receptor-coreceptor complex, whereas CAR is thought to be responsible for internalization of the virus into the cell. (*A, From Rueckert R: Picornaviridae: The viruses and their replication. In Fields B, Knipe D, Howley P (eds): Fields Virology. Philadelphia, Lippincott-Raven, 1996, pp 609–654; B, from Muckelbauer JK, Kremer M, Minor I, et al: The structure of coxsackievirus B3 at 3.5 A resolution. Structure 1995;3:653–667.)*

the surface but is insufficient to mediate entry of the virus into the cell.[105]

### Replication in the Host Cell

On entry into the host cell the single positive-strand RNA is released from the capsid, and viral protein synthesis is initiated by host cell translational mechanisms using the positive-strand viral RNA as template. The viral genome is translated as a single monocistronic polypeptide containing VP0, VP3, VP1, 2A, 2B, 2C, 3A, 3B, 3C, and 3D. This polypeptide is then cleaved at specific proteolytic cleavage sites during translation by the viral proteases protease 2A and 3C. The cleavage of VP0 into VP4 and VP2 occurs through an autocatalytic process. A 22 amino acid peptide (VPg) is covalently bound to the 5′-end of the viral RNA. The VPg peptide is uridylylated by the 3D polymerase and serves as a primer for the synthesis of the negative- and positive-strand RNA.[106] The viral protein 3D is an RNA-dependent RNA polymerase that initially synthesizes negative-strand RNA using the positive-strand RNA as template. From the negative-strand RNA, additional positive stands are formed that provide additional templates for translation or for incorporation into newly formed virus particles[107] (Fig. 33-4).

### Viral Protease Cleavage of Host Proteins

In addition to cleavage of the viral polypeptide, enteroviral proteases can cleave host cell proteins at highly

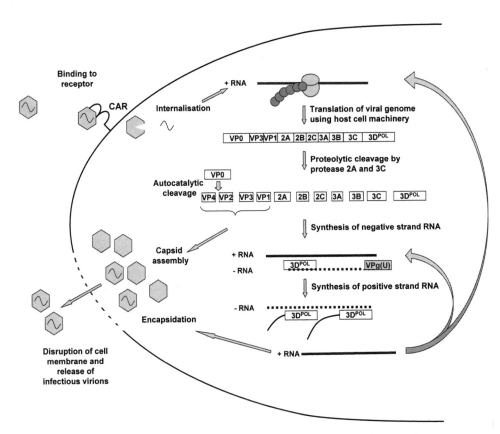

**FIGURE 33-4.** Schematic of coxsackievirus infection and replication cycle (see text for details).

specific proteolytic sites. Protease 2A has been shown to cleave host proteins involved in translation, such as eukaryotic initiation factors 4G (eIF4G)-1[108] and eIF4G-2[109] and the polyadenylate binding protein (PABP).[110] In addition, it was discovered that protease 2A could cleave the cytoskeletal proteins dystrophin[111] (Fig. 33-5) and cytokeratin-8,[112] a process that facilitates release of virus from the cell.[113] Protease 3C can cleave the TATA-binding protein,[114] and has been associated with the cleavage of the poly(A)-binding protein[115] and the poly(ADP-ribose) polymerase (PARP), a nuclear protein involved in DNA repair.[116]

The factors eIF4G-1 and eIF4G-2 are part of the translation initiation complex that is required for efficient translation of host cell, capped mRNA, which includes the majority of eukaryotic mRNA. Picornaviruses, however, possess an internal ribosomal entry site (IRES) that can bind the translation initiation complex in the presence of a cleaved eIF4G. The IRES is an RNA sequence in the 5' untranslated region of the viral genome. Its secondary structure enables cap-independent initiation of translation that occurs in the absence of full-length eIF4G. Enteroviral-mediated cleavage of eIF4G, therefore, results in inhibition of host cell, cap-dependent translation in favor of viral, IRES-mediated protein synthesis (Fig. 33-5).

### Coxackievirus-Induced Cellular Signaling

In addition to the cleavage of host proteins by viral proteases, additional signaling mechanisms have been demonstrated to occur with coxsackieviral infection. On entry and during its replication cycle, CVB activates ERK1/2, members of the mitogen-activated protein kinase (MAPK) family.[117,118] Activation of ERK1/2 is a well-documented cell-protective response in hypertrophy[119] and ischemia-reperfusion injury.[120] In Hela cells, it was demonstrated that the viral stimulation of ERK1/2 involves the activation of Ras, Raf-1, and MEK1 and is associated with cleavage of the p21$^{ras}$ GTPase-activating protein (RasGAP),[121] leading to further activation of Ras (positive feedback loop).[122] However, in cardiomyocytes, the exact mechanism by which coxsackievirus infection activates ERK1/2 is not clear (Fig. 33-6). This appears to be important for replication of coxsackievirus, because inhibition of ERK activation results in decreased viral titers and viral protein synthesis, decreased cleavage of host proteins by viral proteases, and attenuation of host cell death.[117,122] Phosphorylation of other proteins have been shown to occur in CVB infected cells, but the significance is not known.[123]

Another signaling mechanism that is an important determinant of CVB pathogenicity is the sarcoma family kinase, p56$^{lck}$. Mice deficient in p56$^{lck}$ are resistant to CVB-induced acute myocarditis and are protected against CVB-mediated cardiomyopathy. This effect is specific for CVB, because infection with another myocarditic picornavirus, encephalomyocarditis virus, resulted in increased heart disease in p56$^{lck}$-deficient mice. T cells appear to play a central role in this interaction between p56$^{lck}$ and CVB, because reintroduction of T-cells expressing p5b$^{lck}$ in knockout animals was suf-

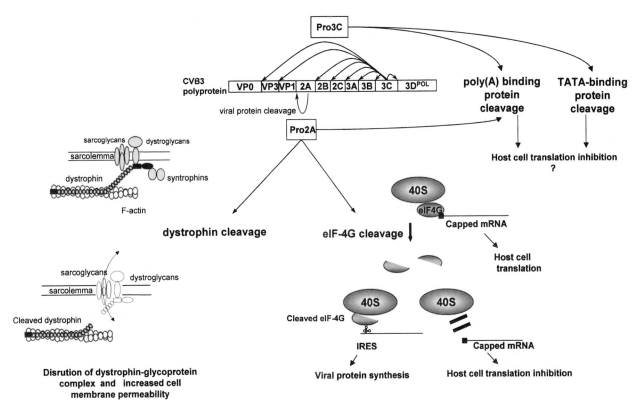

**FIGURE 33-5.** Viral protease cleavage of host proteins. Protease 2A cleaves the cytoskeletal protein dystrophin, leading to disruption of the dystrophin-glycoprotein complex and increased membrane permeability, a process that facilitates release of virus from the cell. Proteases 2A and 3C also can cleave proteins involved in translation, such as eIF4G and PABP, leading to inhibition of host cell translation synthesis in favor of viral protein synthesis. Protease 3C can also cleave the TBP decreasing transcription of host cell RNA.

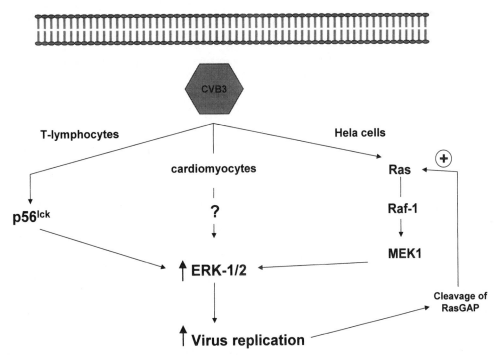

**FIGURE 33-6.** A proposed model of ERK1/2 activation after coxsackievirus infection. In the T cell, ERK1/2 activation is mediated by the sarcoma family kinase, p56^lck. In Hela cells, stimulation of ERK1/2 is a multistep process that involves activation of Ras, Ras-1, and MEK1. Activation of ERK1/2 leads to RasGAP cleavage, which in turn leads to further activation of ERK1/2. The mechanisms of activation in cardiomyocytes have not yet been fully explained.

ficient to restore CVB susceptibility to the same level as in the wild-type mice. Expression of p56[lck] is required for efficient CVB replication in Jurkat T cells, and it was, therefore, postulated that T cells represent a reservoir for viral replication during CVB infection.[124] In addition, it has been shown that p56[lck] is required in T cells for the activation of ERK1/2.[117]

### Release of Virus from the Cell

After the viral replication cycle and incorporation of the genome into the capsid, infectious virions disrupt the cell membrane to exit the cell and infect adjacent cells. As previously mentioned, coxsackieviral protease 2A cleaves the cytoskeletal protein dystrophin. Dystrophin is a 427-kd protein that links cytoskeletal actin to plasma membrane glycoproteins and is known to mechanically stabilize the cell membrane.[125] Cleavage of dystrophin results in disruption of the dystrophin-glycoprotein complex, in turn leading to an increase in cell membrane permeability facilitating release of virus from the infected myocyte.[111,113] Therefore, protease 2A mediated dystrophin cleavage facilitates release of infectious particles from the cardiomyocyte. Interestingly, viral protease mediated cleavage of cytoskeletal proteins is a phenomenon that is conserved among many viruses. For example, adenovirus can cleave the cytoskeletal protein cytokeratin.[18,46]

## HOST DEFENSE

Host defense mechanisms can be divided into two categories: innate and adaptive. Both have been reviewed elsewhere[126]; therefore, only examples of the processes are discussed here. Although more effective, the onset of the adaptive immune response is slow (several days). Meanwhile, to prevent extensive damage by a pathogenic agent, the rapid, albeit nonantigen-specific, innate immune response is activated. It includes the activation of natural killer cells and the production of cytokines.

### Innate Immune Mechanisms

#### Natural Killer Cells

After coxsackievirus infection, NK cells are activated roughly 2 days postinoculation. Depletion of NK cells leads to increased viral replication in the heart, demonstrating the importance of this cell type in the innate host defense.[127] Although the mechanisms of target recognition by NK cells is not totally understood, they are able to identify infected cells and destroy them through perforin-mediated mechanisms.[128]

#### Double-Stranded RNA

Production of double-stranded RNA (dsRNA) is a part of the coxsackievirus replication cycle. It has been shown that dsRNA is able to directly stimulate a dsRNA-activated

protein kinase (PKR). A major substrate of PKR is the $\alpha$ subunit of the eukaryotic translation initiation factor 2 (eIF-2$\alpha$). Phosphorylation of eIF-2$\alpha$ greatly reduces the rate of initiation of translation and inhibits viral translation. Production of dsRNA also activates NF-$\kappa$B in turn, leading to the production of several proinflammatory cytokines including IFN-$\alpha$ and IFN-$\beta$, IL-1, IL-2, IL-6, and TNF-$\alpha$.[129]

### Nitric Oxide

NO is a reactive molecule produced by the nitric oxide synthesis (NOS) during the oxidation of the amino acid substrate L-arginine to L-citrulline. NO has been shown to play a major role in cardiovascular and metabolic homeostasis and acts as a neurotransmitter and as a cytotoxic effector molecule of the immune system. Three distinct NOS isoforms have been identified: nNOS (NOS1), iNOS (NOS2), and eNOS (NOS3). Both eNOS and nNOS are constitutively active, their activity is calcium and calmodulin dependent, and they have been shown to be expressed in the heart. The inducible form iNOS was first isolated from macrophages but has been shown to be expressed in many other cell types including cardiomyocytes.[130] It is transcriptionally regulated by several cytokines such as IL-1$\beta$, TNF-$\alpha$, and IFN-$\gamma$. Because these cytokines play a role in antiviral response, it was postulated that iNOS or more broadly NO could play a major role in the host defense against coxsackievirus infection. In a cell culture model, an NO-donor inhibited coxsackievirus replication and viral protein synthesis.[131] *In vivo*, coxsackievirus infection in mice resulted in induction of iNOS in the heart. Pharmacologic inhibition of NOS increased the mortality and cardiac virus replication in these animals.[132] In addition, mice deficient in iNOS are more susceptible to coxsackieviral-mediated myocarditis[133] and pancreatitis.[134] The mechanisms by which NO can specifically inhibit coxsackievirus pathogenic effects may be related to protease inhibition. It was shown that NO can inhibit the catalytic activity of proteases 2A and 3C through S-nitrosylation of the catalytic cysteine.[135,136]

### Apoptosis

Apoptosis may be used by the host to defend against invading microbes, as a way of getting rid of infected cells. Viruses can trigger apoptosis through cytotoxic T cells, viral-mediated disruption of cellular metabolism and cell cycle regulation, and induction of proinflammatory cytokines such as TNF.[137] However, several viruses (adenovirus, cowpox, gamma herpes virus, poxvirus) have developed strategies to avoid apoptosis. Infection of cells with mutant viruses lacking the genes conferring antiapoptotic properties often results in premature programmed cell death and altered yields of progeny virus, indicating that antiapoptotic proteins are necessary for efficient virus replication.[138,139] NF-$\kappa$B is a transcription factor central to immune and inflammatory responses and to viral replication.[129,140] Activation of NF-$\kappa$B also inhibits some forms of apoptosis. Coxsackievirus, through dsRNA and/or cell stimulation by proinflammatory cytokines such as TNF-α, enables rapid nuclear translocation of NF-κB. Mice with targeted disruption of the NF-κB1 subunit, p50 (p50 −/− mice), although more susceptible to certain bacterial pathogens, are resistant to a myocarditic picornavirus, the murine encephalomyocarditis virus (EMCV).[141] This was initially attributed to elevated IFN-β levels in the mice. However, subsequent experiments performed in p50 −/− mice also lacking the IFN type 1 receptor showed that increased apoptosis rather than increased type I IFN signaling was responsible for the viral resistance in these p50 −/− mice.[142] Therefore, viral activation of NF-κB may be a double-edged sword—it leads to production of proinflammatory cytokines, resulting in activation of the innate immune system; however, it also promotes survival, enhancing virus replication before death of the infected cells.

### Cytokines

Cytokines are an important component of the host defense against viruses. On coxsackievirus infection, several proinflammatory cytokines have been shown to be induced in cultured cardiomyocytes (IL-1α, IL-1β, IL-6, IL-7, TNF-α),[143] cardiac fibroblasts (IL-6 and IL-8),[144] or in murine models of coxsackievirus myocarditis (IL-1α, IL-1β, IL-2, IL-5, IL-6, IL-7, IL-10, IL-12, TNF-α, TNF-β, IFN-β, and IFN-γ.[143] Production of these cytokines either by infected cardiomyocytes or by activated leukocytes leads to activation and modulation of the immune response.

IFNs are cytokines that play a central role in host defense against invasive viruses. It has been shown that administration of IFN-α or IFN-β can inhibit viral myocarditis in the early stages of infection,[145] but whole-animal knockouts of the IFN-α/β or IFN-γ receptor had no effect or only a modest effect, respectively, on the extent of viral replication in the heart during the early stages of infection.[146] However, extracardiac IFN signaling pathways appear to play a major role in the pathogenesis of coxsackievirus infection as evidenced by increased virus replication and cytopathic effects in the liver of IFN-α/β receptor knockout mice leading to increased mortality in these animals.[146] In addition, mice with pancreatic-restricted forced expression of IFN-γ are resistant to coxsackievirus infection.[147]

Elucidation of IFN-signaling mechanisms led to the discovery of the Janus kinase (JAK) and the signal transducers and activators of transcription (STAT) signaling pathway that is required for expression of IFN-responsive genes. These include the suppressors of cytokine signaling (SOCS) that negatively regulate activation of the JAK-STAT pathway. JAK-STAT signaling is the converging pathway of several cytokines including IFNs, IL-6, cardiotrophin-1 (CT-1), and leukemia inhibitory factor (LIF). Coxsackievirus infection activates the cardiac JAK-STAT signaling pathway in the heart, as evidenced by STAT1 and STAT3 phosphorylation and induction of IFN-responsive genes. In addition to activation of JAK-STAT signaling, CVB3 infection of the murine heart leads to induction of the suppressor of cytokine signaling (SOCS) 1 and SOCS3. The SOCS molecules act as a negative feedback loop for JAK-STAT signaling by inhibiting JAK. The importance of this signaling pathway in coxsack-

ieviral myocarditis is highlighted by the increased virus replication and virus-mediated cytopathic effects in transgenic mice that express a cardiac restricted SOCS1 transgene inhibiting the JAK-STAT signaling in the hearts of the infected animals. In line with these observations, adenoassociated virus-mediated expression of a dominant negative SOCS1 molecule inhibited coxsackievirus-induced myocardial damage in the heart[148] (Fig. 33-7).

IL-1 might also play a role in the host defense against coxsackievirus because it has been shown that IL-1 infusion augmented the virus-mediated cardiac pathogenic effects.[144,149] In addition, cardiac injection of a plasmid encoding the IL-1 receptor antagonist resulted in improved survival rates, decreased myocardial inflammation, and decreased viral proliferation in the heart of infected mice.[150]

## Adaptive Immunity

Focal infiltration with inflammatory cells associated with areas of necrotic myocytes is a histopathologic hallmark of coxsackievirus myocarditis in humans and in mice.[144,151,152] These inflammatory cells consist of macrophages, T helper lymphocytes, NK cells, and CD8+ cells.[153] The cellular infiltrate has been implicated as a protective mechanism against viral infection and as a mediator of the myocardial damage that is associated with viral infection. The importance of the role of T lymphocytes in coxsackievirus infection has been highlighted in experiments using T-lymphocyte-deficient mice or mice with severe combined immunodeficiency (SCID). When challenged with coxsackievirus, T cell-deficient mice developed more extensive myocardial lesions and virus replication increased.[154,155] The precise T cell response appears to be dependent on which inbred strain is infected.[156,157] However, two different T lymphocyte populations could be identified during coxsackievirus infection of the heart. One reacts against viral infected cells *in vitro*,[152,158] whereas another reacts against uninfected syngeneic host cells in culture[159] (see later).

As previously mentioned, antibodies are formed during coxsackievirus infection. In mice, it was shown that the humoral response was strongly gender dependant.[160] In female mice the onset of the antibody production, of IgG1 subtype, was quicker and associated with Th2 cell response, whereas in male mice the response involved mostly IgG2a antibodies, which were predominantly produced in association with the Th1 cell response.[161] Additional studies in mice have shown that although the humoral response can play a protective role in coxsackievirus myocarditis,[162,163] it is insufficient to totally prevent myocardial lesions and to clear the virus.[164] For further details, this topic has been extensively studied and reviewed elsewhere.[126,127,165,166]

## Autoimmunity

Heart-reactive autoantibodies are found in a significant percentage of patients with myocarditis but are rare in patients with ischemic heart disease. These antibodies have been shown to be directed against cardiac myosin;

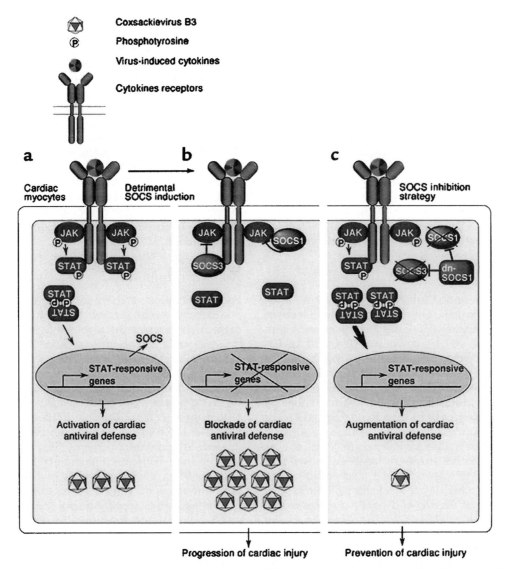

**FIGURE 33-7.** JAK-STAT antiviral defense in the cardiomyocyte and SOCS inhibition to limit early virus-induced cardiac injury. *A,* Virus infection of the heart stimulates cytokine-receptor signaling through the JAK-STAT pathway. Activation of the JAK-STAT pathway induces antiviral target gene transcription stimulating the innate viral defense in the cardiomyocyte. *B,* Although activation of the JAK-STAT pathway has an important role in antiviral defense, phosphorylated STAT also induces SOCS expression that attenuates the innate antiviral defense by inhibiting JAK signaling. As in SOCS1-transgenic mice, increased expression of SOCS in cardiomyocytes results in robust virus replication and cardiac injury. *C,* The strategies aimed at inhibition of SOCS potentiate the innate antiviral actions of cytokines that use the JAK-STAT pathway, resulting in the prevention of virus-mediated myocardial injury. P, phosphorylated.

β$_1$-adrenergic receptor; adenine nucleotide translocator; branched chain keto acid dihydrogenase; and other sarcolemmal, connective tissue, and extracellular matrix proteins.[127] Cross reactivity between these antibodies and coxsackievirus epitopes suggest that antigen mimicry is responsible for the initiation of the autoimmune response.[167] To determine the role of autoantibodies in the pathogenesis of viral myocarditis, monoclonal anticoxsackieviral antibodies, which were found to also react against the cardiac isoform of myosin, were injected into mice. Although they cannot induce cardiac lesions in healthy mice, these monoclonal antibodies exacerbated cardiac injury during coxsackievirus infection.[168] Similarly, autoreactive T cell clones appear to play a role in the pathogenesis of coxsackievirus myocarditis, because it was demonstrated that transfer of lympho-

cytes from an infected to a uninfected mouse can cause myocarditis and pancreatitis.[169] Similarly, transfer of lymphocytes obtained from a patient suffering from myocarditis into severe combined immunodeficiency mice can induce myocarditis in these animals.[170] In line with this concept, cardiac myosin alone or adenine nucleotide translocator (ANT) can induce myocarditis when injected into susceptible strains of mice.[171,172]

## SUSCEPTIBILITY TO VIRUS INFECTION

Infection with coxsackievirus can lead to an illness that ranges from a mild flulike disease to fatal myocarditis. From that observation a crucial question arises: what factors predispose one individual to severe coxsackieviral-mediated disease, whereas others have only mild symptoms without apparent cardiac pathology?

## Nutritional Deficiency

Keshan disease was originally identified as an endemic cardiomyopathy of unknown origin in China. It was observed exclusively in rural areas, where nutritional selenium deficiency was present. Further studies showed that an infectious agent caused Keshan disease, which was then identified as coxsackievirus.[173] The selenium deficiency was thought to contribute to the increased susceptibility to coxsackievirus because the disease could be prevented by selenium supplementation.[174] The importance of adequate selenium intake was confirmed in various murine models of coxsackievirus infection. Mice fed with a selenium-deficient diet were more susceptible to coxsackievirus myocarditis.[175] Interestingly, however, selenium deficiency affected the cardiovirulence of coxsackievirus causing the viral genome to mutate. Virus recovered from the heart of selenium-deficient mice that were infected with the benign CVB3/0 were able to elicit myocarditis in selenium-fed mice, whereas virus recovered from selenium-fed mice were not able to cause myocarditis.[176] Vitamin E deficiency had the same potentiating effects on the infection of mice with coxsackievirus as selenium deficiency did.[175]

## Immune System

The immune system seems to be an important determinant of the host susceptibility to coxsackievirus. For example, in SCID mice that lack both T and B cells, CVB3 infection induces severe disease.[155] Further studies using genetic manipulations (CD4, CD8, T-cell receptor, major histocompatibility genes) showed that the individual components of the immune system can differentially modulate the severity of the myocarditis and the survival in coxsackievirus-infected animals.[177,178]

## Dystrophin

Dystrophin is a subsarcolemmal rod-shaped protein that stabilizes the sarcolemma by attaching the actin cytoskeleton to the extracellular matrix through the dystrophin-associated glycoprotein complex.[125] This connection protects muscle cells from contraction-induced damage.[179] Enteroviruses are typically released from the cell by disruption of the cell membrane or by cell lysis.[107] In line with these concepts, it was shown in mice that dystrophin deficiency predisposed to coxsackievirus-induced cardiac cytopathic effects and led to increased virus-replication in the hearts of dystrophin-deficient animals.[113] In addition, cell culture experiments showed that dystrophin expression was protective against coxsackievirus-mediated cellular damage.[113] The markedly increased susceptibility of dystrophin-deficient mice to viral infection of the heart suggests that one of the mechanisms for increased cardiomyopathy in Duchenne's muscular dystrophy is through increased susceptibility to virus infection of the heart.

## DETERMINANTS OF CARDIOTROPISM

Although it is not entirely clear why myocarditic viruses infect the heart, there are several parameters that are likely to contribute. These range from myocyte selective expression of viral receptors to differences in the immune response in the heart versus other organs.

The CAR has been shown to be a major receptor for two of the most commonly identified viruses that cause cardiomyopathy, coxsackievirus, and adenovirus.[104] Interestingly, the level of CAR expression is higher in the heart than in other organs in humans and mice.[180] It is, therefore, likely that this pattern of expression is one of the factors that contributes to the ability of these viruses to enter cardiomyocytes.

Although entry into a cell is required for organ-specific infection, the host immune response can also have a significant role. IFN stimulation can be one of the most potent antiviral mechanisms in some cells. Disruption of IFN signaling has a profound effect on mortality in mice infected with a number of different pathogens[181,182] including coxsackievirus.[146] However, careful analysis of coxsackievirus-infected mice that lack the IFN-α/β (type I) receptor demonstrates that, in the absence of type I IFN signaling, the tropism of the virus changes dramatically from a primarily cardiotropic virus to a hepatotropic virus with a marked increase in viral RNA in the liver. This indicates that, although coxsackievirus can infect both the heart and the liver, the normal type I IFN signaling in the liver markedly inhibits viral replication in that organ. On the other hand, type I INF signaling appeared to have little effect on the early phase of viral replication in the heart, suggesting that type I IFN signaling may have little impact in the wild-type, infected cardiomyocyte. This demonstrates that, although viral receptors undoubtedly have a major role in determining viral tropism, other mechanisms such as viral defense mechanisms can also have a significant role.[146]

## SUMMARY

The body of evidence is growing that implicates infectious pathogens in diseases that were not previously recognized to be related to an infectious cause. Gradually, a role for viral pathogens in cardiovascular diseases is becoming apparent. Although it is important to maintain strict scientific criteria to define the cause-effect relationship between viral infection and disease, it is equally important that investigators keep an open and inquisitive attitude toward the potential interactions between the genetic makeup of the host and environmental influences to better understand the role of infectious etiologies in the pathogenesis of heart diseases.

## REFERENCES

1. Levine AJ: The origins of virology. In Fields B, Knipe D, Howley P (eds): Fields Virology. Philadelphia, Lippincott-Raven, 1996, pp 1–14.

2. Kandolf R, Ameis D, Kirschner P, et al: In situ detection of enteroviral genomes in myocardial cells by nucleic acid hybridization: An approach to the diagnosis of viral heart disease. Proc Natl Acad Sci USA 1987;84:6272-6276.

3. Kandolf R, Sauter M, Aepinus C, et al: Mechanisms and consequences of enterovirus persistence in cardiac myocytes and cells of the immune system. Virus Res 1999;62:149-158.

4. Munoz N, Bosch FX: The causal link between HPV and cervical cancer and its implications for prevention of cervical cancer. Bull Pan Am Health Organ 1996;30:362-377.

5. Chang Y, Cesarman E, Pessin MS, et al: Identification of herpesvirus-like DNA sequences in AIDS-associated Kaposi's sarcoma. Science 1994;266:1865-1869.

6. Epstein MA, Achong BG, Barr YM: Virus particles in cultured lymphoblasts from Burkitt's lymphoma. Lancet 1964;1:702-703.

7. Suerbaum S, Michetti P: Helicobacter pylori infection. N Engl J Med 2002;347:1175-1186.

8. Venables AW: The syndrome of pulmonary stenosis complicating maternal rubella. Br Heart J xxxx;27:491965.

9. Webster WS: Teratogen update: Congenital rubella. Teratology 1998;58:13-23.

10. Gregg N: Congenital cataract following German measles in the mother. Trans Ophthalmol Soc Aust 1941;3:35-46.

11. Schluter WW, Reef SE, Redd SC, Dykewicz CA: Changing epidemiology of congenital rubella syndrome in the United States. J Infect Dis 1998;178:636-641.

12. Cochi SL, Edmonds LE, Dyer K, et al: Congenital rubella syndrome in the United States, 1970-1985: On the verge of elimination. Am J Epidemiol 1989;129:349-361.

13. Cutts FT, Robertson SE, Diaz-Ortega JL, Samuel R: Control of rubella and congenital rubella syndrome (CRS) in developing countries. 1. Burden of disease from CRS. Bull World Health Organ 1997;75:55-68.

14. Garcia AG, Marques RL, Lobato YY, et al: Placental pathology in congenital rubella. Placenta 1985;6:281-295.

15. Bellanti JA, Artenstein MS, Olson LC, et al: Congenital rubella: Clinicopathologic, virologic, and immunologic studies. Am J Dis Child 1965;110:464-472.

16. Singer DB, Rudolph AJ, Rosenberg HS, et al: Pathology of the congenital rubella syndrome. J Pediatr 1967;71:665-675.

17. Report of the 1995 World Health Organization/International Society and Federation of Cardiology Task Force on the Definition and Classification of Cardiomyopathies. Circulation 1996;93:841-842.

18. Towbin JA, Griffin LD, Martin AB, et al: Intrauterine adenoviral myocarditis presenting as nonimmune hydrops fetalis: Diagnosis by polymerase chain reaction. Pediatr Infect Dis J 1994;13:144-150.

19. Maisch B, Schonian U, Crombach M, et al: Cytomegalovirus associated inflammatory heart muscle disease. Scand J Infect Dis Suppl 1993;88:135-148.

20. Matsumori A, Yutani C, Ikeda Y, et al: Hepatitis C virus from the hearts of patients with myocarditis and cardiomyopathy. Lab Invest 2000;80:1137-1142.

21. Feldman AM, McNamara D: Myocarditis. N Engl J Med 2000;343:1388-1398.

22. Fechner RE, Smith MG, Middelkamp JN: Coxsackie B virus infection of the newborn. Am J Pathol 1963;42:493-505.

23. Kibrik S, Bernirschke K: Severe disease (encephalomyocarditis) occurring in the newborn period and due to infection with coxsackie virus, group B. Pediatrics 1958;22:857-874.

24. Dalldorf G: The coxsackie viruses. Annu Rev Microbiol 1955;9:277-296.

25. Sun NC, Smith VM: Hepatitis associated with myocarditis: Unusual manifestation of infection with Coxsackie virus group B, type 3. N Engl J Med 1966;274:190-193.

26. Grist NR, Bell EJ: Coxsackie viruses and the heart. Am Heart J 1969;77:295-300.

27. Lerner AM, Wilson FM: Virus myocardiopathy. Prog Med Virol 1973;15:63-91.

28. Sainani GS, Dekate MP, Rao CP: Heart disease caused by coxsackie virus B infection. Br Heart J 1975;37:819-823.

29. Li Y, Bourlet T, Andreoletti L, et al: Enteroviral capsid protein VP1 is present in myocardial tissues from some patients with myocarditis or dilated cardiomyopathy. Circulation 2000;101:231-234.

30. Sutinen S, Kalliomaki JL, Pohjonen R, Vastamaki R: Fatal generalized coxsackie B3 virus infection in an adolescent with successful isolation of the virus from pericardial fluid. Ann Clin Res 1971;3:241-246.

31. Burch GE, Sun SC, Chu KC, et al: Interstitial and coxsackievirus B myocarditis in infants and children: A comparative histologic and immunofluorescent study of 50 autopsied hearts. JAMA 1968;203:1-8.

32. Gerzen P, Granath A, Holmgren B, Zetterquist S: Acute myocarditis: A follow-up study. Br Heart J 1972;34:575-583.

33. Martino TA, Liu P, Sole MJ: Viral infection and the pathogenesis of dilated cardiomyopathy. Circ Res 1994;74:182-188.

34. Bowles NE, Richardson PJ, Olsen EG, Archard LC: Detection of Coxsackie-B-virus-specific RNA sequences in myocardial biopsy samples from patients with myocarditis and dilated cardiomyopathy. Lancet 1986;1:1120-1123.

35. Kandolf R, Klingel K, Zell R, et al: Molecular pathogenesis of enterovirus-induced myocarditis: Virus persistence and chronic inflammation. Intervirology 1993;35:140-151.

36. Martino TA, Liu P, Sole MJ: Viral infection and the pathogenesis of dilated cardiomyopathy. Circ Res 1994;74:182-188.

37. Martino TA, Liu P, Martin P, Sole MJ: Enteroviral myocarditis and dilated cardiomyopathy: A review of clinical and experimental studies. In Rotbart HA (ed): Human Enterovirus Infections. Washington DC, American Society for Microbiology, 1995, pp 291-351.

38. Baboonian C, Davies MJ, Booth JC, McKenna WJ: Coxsackie B viruses and human heart disease. Curr Top Microbiol Immunol 1997;223:31-52.

39. Li Y, Bourlet T, Andreoletti L, et al: Enteroviral capsid protein VP1 is present in myocardial tissues from some patients with myocarditis or dilated cardiomyopathy. Circulation 2000;101:231-234.

40. Wilson FM, Miranda QR, Chason JL, Lerner AM: Residual pathologic changes following murine coxsackie A and B myocarditis. Am J Pathol 1969;55:253-265.

41. Reyes MP, Ho KL, Smith F, Lerner AM: A mouse model of dilated-type cardiomyopathy due to coxsackievirus B3. J Infect Dis 1981;144:232-236.

42. Klingel K, Hohenadl C, Canu A, et al: Ongoing enterovirus-induced myocarditis is associated with persistent heart muscle infection: Quantitative analysis of virus replication, tissue damage, and inflammation. Proc Natl Acad Sci 1992;89:314-318.

43. Klingel K, Kandolf R: The role of enterovirus replication in the development of acute and chronic heart muscle disease in different immunocompetent mouse strains. Scand J Infect Dis Suppl 1993;88:79-85.

44. Wessely R, Klingel K, Santana LF, et al: Transgenic expression of replication-restricted enteroviral genomes in heart muscle induces defective excitation-contraction coupling and dilated cardiomyopathy. J Clin Invest 1998;102:1444-1453.

45. O'Brien TX, Lee KJ, Chien KR: Positional specification of ventricular myosin light chain 2 expression in the primitive murine heart tube. Proc Natl Acad Sci USA 1993;90:5157-5161.

46. Chen PH, Ornelles DA, Shenk T: The adenovirus L3 23-kilodalton proteinase cleaves the amino-terminal head domain from cytokeratin 18 and disrupts the cytokeratin network of HeLa cells. J Virol 1993;67:3507-3514.

47. Chow LH, Gauntt CJ, McManus BM: Differential effects of myocarditic variants of Coxsackievirus B3 in inbred mice: A pathologic characterization of heart tissue damage. Lab Invest 1991;64:55-64.

48. Moller JH, Lucas RV, Adams P, et al: Endocardial fibroelastosis: A clinical and anatomic study of 47 patients with emphasis on its relationship to mitral insufficiency. Circulation 1964;30:759-782.

49. Ni J, Bowles NE, Kim YH, et al: Viral infection of the myocardium in endocardial fibroelastosis: Molecular evidence for the role of mumps virus as an etiologic agent. Circulation 1997;95:133-139.

50. Colan S, Newburger J: Acquired heart disease in children. In Braunwald E (ed): Heart Disease: A Textbook of Cardiovascular Medicine. Philadelphia, WB Saunders, 2001, pp 1622-1642.

51. Danesh J, Collins R, Peto R: Chronic infections and coronary heart disease: Is there a link? Lancet 1997;350:430-436.

52. Epstein SE, Zhou YF, Zhu J: Infection and atherosclerosis: Emerging mechanistic paradigms. Circulation 1999;100:e20-e28.

53. Libby P, Egan D, Skarlatos S: Roles of infectious agents in atherosclerosis and restenosis: An assessment of the evidence and need for future research. Circulation 1997;96:4095–4103.

54. Mattila KJ, Valtonen VV, Nieminen MS, Asikainen S: Role of infection as a risk factor for atherosclerosis, myocardial infarction, and stroke. Clin Infect Dis 1998;26:719–734.

55. Minick CR, Fabricant CG, Fabricant J, Litrenta MM: Atheroarteriosclerosis induced by infection with a herpesvirus. Am J Pathol 1979;96:673–706.

56. Adam E, Melnick JL, Probstfield JL, et al: High levels of cytomegalovirus antibody in patients requiring vascular surgery for atherosclerosis. Lancet 1987;2:291–293.

57. Saikku P, Leinonen M, Mattila K, et al: Serological evidence of an association of a novel Chlamydia, TWAR, with chronic coronary heart disease and acute myocardial infarction. Lancet 1988;2:983–986.

58. Sorlie PD, Nieto FJ, Adam E, et al: A prospective study of cytomegalovirus, herpes simplex virus 1, and coronary heart disease: The atherosclerosis risk in communities (ARIC) study. Arch Intern Med 2000;160:2027–2032.

59. Siscovick DS, Schwartz SM, Corey L, et al: Chlamydia pneumoniae, herpes simplex virus type 1, and cytomegalovirus and incident myocardial infarction and coronary heart disease death in older adults: The Cardiovascular Health Study. Circulation 2000;102:2335–2340.

60. Mendall MA, Goggin PM, Molineaux N, et al: Relation of Helicobacter pylori infection and coronary heart disease. Br Heart J 1994;71:437–439.

61. Roivainen M, Alfthan G, Jousilahti P, et al: Enterovirus infections as a possible risk factor for myocardial infarction. Circulation 1998;98:2534–2537.

62. Danesh J, Whincup P, Walker M, et al: Chlamydia pneumoniae IgG titres and coronary heart disease: Prospective study and meta-analysis. BMJ 2000;321:208–213.

63. Danesh J, Wong Y, Ward M, Muir J: Chronic infection with Helicobacter pylori, Chlamydia pneumoniae, or cytomegalovirus: Population based study of coronary heart disease. Heart 1999;81:245–247.

64. Smieja M, Gnarpe J, Lonn E, et al. for the Heart Outcomes Prevention Evaluation (HOPE) Study Investigators: Multiple infections and subsequent cardiovascular events in the Heart Outcomes Prevention Evaluation (HOPE) study. Circulation 2003;107:251–257.

65. Chiu B, Viira E, Tucker W, Fong IW: Chlamydia pneumoniae, cytomegalovirus, and herpes simplex virus in atherosclerosis of the carotid artery. Circulation 1997;96:2144–2148.

66. Shi Y, Tokunaga O: Herpesvirus (HSV-1, EBV and CMV) infections in atherosclerotic compared with non-atherosclerotic aortic tissue. Pathol Int 2002;52:31–39.

67. Zhou YF, Leon MB, Waclawiw MA, et al: Association between prior cytomegalovirus infection and the risk of restenosis after coronary atherectomy. N Engl J Med 1996;335:624–630.

68. Zhu J, Quyyumi AA, Norman JE, et al: Effects of total pathogen burden on coronary artery disease risk and C-reactive protein levels. Am J Cardiol 2000;85:140–146.

69. Zhu J, Nieto FJ, Horne BD, et al: Prospective study of pathogen burden and risk of myocardial infarction or death. Circulation 2001;103:45–51.

70. Rupprecht HJ, Blankenberg S, Bickel C, et al: Impact of viral and bacterial infectious burden on long-term prognosis in patients with coronary artery disease. Circulation 2001;104:25–31.

71. Muhlestein JB, Anderson JL: Infectious serology and atherosclerosis: How burdensome is the risk? Circulation 2003;107:220–222.

72. Prasad A, Zhu J, Halcox JP, et al: Predisposition to atherosclerosis by infections: Role of endothelial dysfunction. Circulation 2002;106:184–190.

73. Speir E, Modali R, Huang ES, et al: Potential role of human cytomegalovirus and p53 interaction in coronary restenosis. Science 1994;265:391–394.

74. Lemstrom KB, Aho PT, Bruggeman CA, Hayry PJ: Cytomegalovirus infection enhances mRNA expression of platelet-derived growth factor-BB and transforming growth factor-beta 1 in rat aortic allografts: Possible mechanism for cytomegalovirus-enhanced graft arteriosclerosis. Arterioscler Thromb 1994;14:2043–2052.

75. Hajjar DP, Pomerantz KB, Falcone DJ, et al: Herpes simplex virus infection in human arterial cells: Implications in arteriosclerosis. J Clin Invest 1987;80:1317–1321.

76. Zhou YF, Guetta E, Yu ZX, et al: Human cytomegalovirus increases modified low density lipoprotein uptake and scavenger receptor mRNA expression in vascular smooth muscle cells. J Clin Invest 1996;98:2129–2138.

77. Visser MR, Tracy PB, Vercellotti GM, et al: Enhanced thrombin generation and platelet binding on herpes simplex virus-infected endothelium. Proc Natl Acad Sci USA 1988;85:8227–8230.

78. Key NS, Vercellotti GM, Winkelmann JC, et al: Infection of vascular endothelial cells with herpes simplex virus enhances tissue factor activity and reduces thrombomodulin expression. Proc Natl Acad Sci USA 1990;87:7095–7099.

79. Etingin OR, Silverstein RL, Friedman HM, Hajjar DP: Viral activation of the coagulation cascade: Molecular interactions at the surface of infected endothelial cells. Cell 1990;61:657–662.

80. Billstrom Schroeder M, Worthen GS: Viral regulation of RANTES expression during human cytomegalovirus infection of endothelial cells. J Virol 2001;75:3383–3390.

81. Visseren FL, Verkerk MS, Bouter KP, et al: Interleukin-6 production by endothelial cells after infection with influenza virus and cytomegalovirus. J Lab Clin Med 1999;134:623–630.

82. Speir E, Yu ZX, Ferrans VJ, et al: Aspirin attenuates cytomegalovirus infectivity and gene expression mediated by cyclooxygenase-2 in coronary artery smooth muscle cells. Circ Res 1998;83:210–216.

83. Epstein SE, Zhu J, Burnett MS, et al: Infection and atherosclerosis: Potential roles of pathogen burden and molecular mimicry. Arterioscler Thromb Vasc Biol 2000;20:1417–1420.

84. McDonald K, Rector TS, Braulin EA, et al: Association of coronary artery disease in cardiac transplant recipients with cytomegalovirus infection. Am J Cardiol 1989;64:359–362.

85. Everett JP, Hershberger RE, Norman DJ, et al: Prolonged cytomegalovirus infection with viremia is associated with development of cardiac allograft vasculopathy. J Heart Lung Transplant 1992;11:S133–S137.

86. Koskinen PK, Nieminen MS, Krogerus LA, et al: Cytomegalovirus infection and accelerated cardiac allograft vasculopathy in human cardiac allografts. J Heart Lung Transplant 1993;12:724–729.

87. Loebe M, Schuler S, Zais O, et al: Role of cytomegalovirus infection in the development of coronary artery disease in the transplanted heart. J Heart Transplant 1990;9:707–711.

88. Grattan MT, Moreno-Cabral CE, Starnes VA, et al: Cytomegalovirus infection is associated with cardiac allograft rejection and atherosclerosis. JAMA 1989;261:3561–3566.

89. Valantine HA, Gao SZ, Menon SG, et al: Impact of prophylactic immediate posttransplant ganciclovir on development of transplant atherosclerosis: A post hoc analysis of a randomized, placebo-controlled study. Circulation 1999;100:61–66.

90. Lemstrom K, Sihvola R, Bruggeman C, et al: Cytomegalovirus infection-enhanced cardiac allograft vasculopathy is abolished by DHPG prophylaxis in the rat. Circulation 1997;95:2614–2616.

91. Heng D, Sharples LD, McNeil K, et al: Bronchiolitis obliterans syndrome: Incidence, natural history, prognosis, and risk factors. J Heart Lung Transplant 1998;17:1255–1263.

92. Lautenschlager I, Hockerstedt K, Linnavuori K, Taskinen E: Human herpesvirus-6 infection after liver transplantation. Clin Infect Dis 1998;26:702–707.

93. Schowengerdt KO, Ni J, Denfield SW, et al: Diagnosis, surveillance, and epidemiologic evaluation of viral infections in pediatric cardiac transplant recipients with the use of the polymerase chain reaction. J Heart Lung Transplant 1996;15:111–123.

94. Shirali GS, Ni J, Chinnock RE, et al: Association of viral genome with graft loss in children after cardiac transplantation. N Engl J Med 2001;344:1498–1503.

95. D'Amati G, di Gioia CR, Gallo P: Pathological findings of HIV-associated cardiovascular disease. Ann NY Acad Sci 2001;946:23–45.

96. Herskowitz A, Vlahov D, Willoughby S, et al: Prevalence and incidence of left ventricular dysfunction in patients with

human immunodeficiency virus infection. Am J Cardiol 1993; 71:955-958.

97. Rerkpattanapipat P, Wongpraparut N, Jacobs LE, Kotler MN: Cardiac manifestations of acquired immunodeficiency syndrome. Arch Intern Med 2000;160:602-608.

98. Grody WW, Cheng L, Lewis W: Infection of the heart by the human immunodeficiency virus. Am J Cardiol 1990;66:203-206.

99. Herskowitz A, Wu TC, Willoughby SB, et al: Myocarditis and cardiotropic viral infection associated with severe left ventricular dysfunction in late-stage infection with human immunodeficiency virus. J Am Coll Cardiol 1994;24:1025-1032.

100. Bowles NE, Kearney DL, Ni J, et al: The detection of viral genomes by polymerase chain reaction in the myocardium of pediatric patients with advanced HIV disease. J Am Coll Cardiol 1999;34:857-865.

101. Raidel SM, Haase C, Jansen NR, et al: Targeted myocardial transgenic expression of HIV Tat causes cardiomyopathy and mitochondrial damage. Am J Physiol Heart Circ Physiol 2002;282: H1672-H1678.

102. Barbaro G, Lipshultz SE: Pathogenesis of HIV-associated cardiomyopathy. Ann NY Acad Sci 2001;946:57-81.

103. Muckelbauer JK, Kremer M, Minor I, et al: The structure of coxsackievirus B3 at 3.5 A resolution. Structure 1995;3:653-667.

104. Bergelson JM, Cunningham JA, Droguett G, et al: Isolation of a common receptor for coxsackie B viruses and adenoviruses 2 and 5. Science 1997;275:1320-1323.

105. Shafren DR, Bates RC, Agrez MV, et al: Coxsackieviruses B1, B3, and B5 use decay accelerating factor as a receptor for cell attachment. J Virol 1995;69:3873-3877.

106. Paul AV, van Boom JH, Filippov D, Wimmer E: Protein-primed RNA synthesis by purified poliovirus RNA polymerase. Nature 1998;393:280-284.

107. Rueckert R: Picornaviridae: The viruses and their replication. In Fields B, Knipe D, Howley P (eds): Fields Virology. Philadelphia, Lippincott-Raven, 1996, pp 609-654.

108. Lamphear BJ, Yan R, Yang F, et al: Mapping the cleavage site in protein synthesis initiation factor eIF-4 gamma of the 2A proteases from human coxsackievirus and rhinovirus. J Biol Chem 1993;268:19200-19203.

109. Gradi A, Imataka H, Svitkin YV, et al: A novel functional human eukaryotic translation initiation factor 4G. Mol Cell Biol 1998;18:334-342.

110. Kerekatte V, Keiper BD, Badorff C, et al: Cleavage of Poly(A)-binding protein by coxsackievirus 2A protease in vitro and in vivo: Another mechanism for host protein synthesis shutoff? J Virol 1999;73:709-717.

111. Badorff C, Lee GH, Lamphear BJ, et al: Enteroviral protease 2A cleaves dystrophin: Evidence of cytoskeletal disruption in an acquired cardiomyopathy. Nat Med 1999;5:320-326.

112. Seipelt J, Liebig HD, Sommergruber W, et al: 2A proteinase of human rhinovirus cleaves cytokeratin 8 in infected HeLa cells. J Biol Chem 2000;275:20084-20089.

113. Xiong D, Lee GH, Badorff C, et al: Dystrophin deficiency markedly increases enterovirus-induced cardiomyopathy: A genetic predisposition to viral heart disease. Nat Med 2002;8:872-877.

114. Clark ME, Lieberman PM, Berk AJ, Dasgupta A: Direct cleavage of human TATA-binding protein by poliovirus protease 3C in vivo and in vitro. Mol Cell Biol 1993;13:1232-1237.

115. Kuyumcu-Martinez NM, Joachims M, Lloyd RE: Efficient cleavage of ribosome-associated poly(A)-binding protein by enterovirus 3C protease. J Virol 2002;76:2062-2074.

116. Barco A, Feduchi E, Carrasco L: Poliovirus protease 3Cpro kills cells by apoptosis. Virology 2000;266:352-360.

117. Opavsky MA, Martino T, Rabinovitch M, et al: Enhanced ERK-1/2 activation in mice susceptible to coxsackievirus-induced myocarditis. J Clin Invest 2002;109:1561-1569.

118. Blenis J: Signal transduction via the MAP kinases: Proceed at your own RSK. Proc Natl Acad Sci 1993;90:5889-5892.

119. Ruwhof C, van der Laarse A: Mechanical stress-induced cardiac hypertrophy: Mechanisms and signal transduction pathways. Cardiovasc Res 2000;47:23-37.

120. Bogoyevitch MA, Gillespie-Brown J, Ketterman AJ, et al: Stimulation of the stress-activated mitogen-activated protein kinase subfamilies in perfused heart: p38/RK mitogen-activated protein kinases and c-Jun N-terminal kinases are activated by ischemia/reperfusion. Circ Res 1996;79:162-173.

121. Huber M, Watson KA, Selinka HC, et al: Cleavage of RasGAP and phosphorylation of mitogen-activated protein kinase in the course of coxsackievirus B3 replication. J Virol 1999;73: 3587-3594.

122. Luo H, Yanagawa B, Zhang J, et al: Coxsackievirus B3 replication is reduced by inhibition of the extracellular signal-regulated kinase (ERK) signaling pathway. J Virol 2002;76:3365-3373.

123. Huber M, Selinka HC, Kandolf R: Tyrosine phosphorylation events during coxsackievirus B3 replication. J Virol 1997;71: 595-600.

124. Liu P, Aitken K, Kong YY, et al: The tyrosine kinase p56lck is essential in coxsackievirus B3-mediated heart disease. Nat Med 2000;6:429-434.

125. Durbeej M, Campbell KP: Muscular dystrophies involving the dystrophin-glycoprotein complex: An overview of current mouse models. Curr Opin Genet Dev 2002;12:349-361.

126. Huber SA, Gauntt CJ, Sakkinen P: Enteroviruses and myocarditis: Viral pathogenesis through replication, cytokine induction, and immunopathogenicity. Adv Virus Res 1998;51:35-80.

127. Gauntt CJ: Introduction and historical perspective on experimental myocarditis. In Cooper LT (ed): Myocarditis: From Bench to Bedside. Totowa, NJ, Humana Press, 2002, pp 1-22.

128. Barber GN: Host defense, viruses and apoptosis. Cell Death Differ 2001;8:113-126.

129. Iordanov MS, Wong J, Bell JC, Magun BE: Activation of NF-{kappa}B by double-stranded RNA (dsRNA) in the absence of protein kinase R and RNase L demonstrates the existence of two separate dsRNA-triggered antiviral programs. Mol Cell Biol 2001; 21:61-72.

130. Bloch W, Addicks K, Hescheler J, Fleischmann BK: Nitric oxide synthase expression and function in embryonic and adult cardiomyocytes. Microsc Res Tech 2001;55:259-269.

131. Zaragoza C, Ocampo CJ, Saura M, et al: Nitric oxide inhibition of coxsackievirus replication in vitro. J Clin Invest 1997;100: 1760-1767.

132. Lowenstein CJ, Hill SL, Lafond-Walker A, et al: Nitric oxide inhibits viral replication in murine myocarditis. J Clin Invest 1996; 97:1837-1843.

133. Zaragoza C, Ocampo C, Saura M, et al: The role of inducible nitric oxide synthase in the host response to Coxsackievirus myocarditis. Proc Natl Acad Sci USA 1998;95:2469-2474.

134. Flodstrom M, Horwitz MS, Maday A, et al: A critical role for inducible nitric oxide synthase in host survival following coxsackievirus B4 infection. Virology 2001;281:205-215.

135. Badorff C, Fichtlscherer B, Rhoads RE, et al: Nitric oxide inhibits dystrophin proteolysis by coxsackieviral protease 2A through S-nitrosylation: A protective mechanism against enteroviral cardiomyopathy. Circulation 2000;102:2276-2281.

136. Saura M, Zaragoza C, McMillan A, et al: An antiviral mechanism of nitric oxide: Inhibition of a viral protease. Immunity 1999;10: 21-28.

137. Shen Y, Shenk TE: Viruses and apoptosis. Curr Opin Genet Dev 1995;5:105-111.

138. Brooks MA, Ali AN, Turner PC, Moyer RW: A rabbitpox virus serpin gene controls host range by inhibiting apoptosis in restrictive cells. J Virol 1995;69:7688-7698.

139. Pilder S, Logan J, Shenk T: Deletion of the gene encoding the adenovirus 5 early region 1b 21,000-molecular-weight polypeptide leads to degradation of viral and host cell DNA. J Virol 1984;52:664-671.

140. Baeuerle PA, Henkel T: Function and activation of NF-kappa B in the immune system. Annu Rev Immunol 1994;12:141-179.

141. Sha WC, Liou HC, Tuomanen EI, Baltimore D: Targeted disruption of the p50 subunit of NF-kappa B leads to multifocal defects in immune responses. Cell 1995;80:321-330.

142. Schwarz EM, Badorff C, Hiura TS, et al: NF-kappaB-mediated inhibition of apoptosis is required for encephalomyocarditis virus virulence: A mechanism of resistance in p50 knockout mice. J Virol 1998;72:5654-5660.

143. Seko Y, Takahashi N, Yagita H, et al: Expression of cytokine mRNAs in murine hearts with acute myocarditis caused by coxsackievirus b3. J Pathol 1997;183:105-108.

144. Henke A, Zell R, Ehrlich G, Stelzner A: Expression of immunoregulatory cytokines by recombinant coxsackievirus B3 variants confers protection against virus-caused myocarditis. J Virol 2001;75:8187-8194.

145. Lutton CW, Gauntt CJ: Ameliorating effect of IFN-beta and anti-IFN-beta on coxsackievirus B3-induced myocarditis in mice. J Interferon Res 1985;5:137-146.

146. Wessely R, Klingel K, Knowlton KU, Kandolf R: Cardioselective infection with coxsackievirus B3 requires intact type I interferon signaling: Implications for mortality and early viral replication. Circulation 2001;103:756-761.

147. Horwitz MS, La Cava A, Fine C, et al: Pancreatic expression of interferon-gamma protects mice from lethal coxsackievirus B3 infection and subsequent myocarditis. Nat Med 2000;6:693-697.

148. Yasukawa H, Yajima T, Duplain H, et al: The suppressor of cytokine signaling-1 (SOCS1) is a novel therapeutic target for enterovirus-induced cardiac injury. J Clin Invest 2003;111:469-478.

149. Huber SA, Polgar J, Schultheiss P, Schwimmbeck P: Augmentation of pathogenesis of coxsackievirus B3 infections in mice by exogenous administration of interleukin-1 and interleukin-2. J Virol 1994;68:195-206.

150. Lim BK, Choe SC, Shin JO, et al: Local expression of interleukin-1 receptor antagonist by plasmid DNA improves mortality and decreases myocardial inflammation in experimental coxsackieviral myocarditis. Circulation 2002;105:1278-1281.

151. McManus BM, Gauntt CJ, Cassling RS: Immunopathologic basis of myocardial injury. Cardiovasc Clin 1988;18:163-184.

152. Leslie K, Blay R, Haisch C, et al: Clinical and experimental aspects of viral myocarditis. Clin Microbiol Rev 1989;2:191-203.

153. Godeny EK, Gauntt CJ: In situ immune autoradiographic identification of cells in heart tissues of mice with coxsackievirus B3-induced myocarditis. Am J Pathol 1987;129:267-276.

154. Schwimmbeck PL, Huber SA, Schultheiss HP: Roles of T cells in coxsackievirus B-induced disease. Curr Top Microbiol Immunol 1997;223:283-303.

155. Chow LH, Beisel KW, McManus BM: Enteroviral infection of mice with severe combined immunodeficiency. Evidence for direct viral pathogenesis of myocardial injury. Lab Invest 1992;66:24-31.

156. Huber SA, Lodge PA: Coxsackievirus B-3 myocarditis. Identification of different pathogenic mechanisms in DBA/2 and Balb/c mice. Am J Pathol 1986;122:284-291.

157. Huber SA: Coxsackievirus-induced myocarditis is dependent on distinct immunopathogenic responses in different strains of mice. Lab Invest 1997;76:691-701.

158. Huber SA, Weller A, Herzum M, et al: Immunopathogenic mechanisms in experimental picornavirus-induced autoimmunity. Pathol Immunopathol Res 1988;7:279-291.

159. Guthrie M, Lodge PA, Huber SA: Cardiac injury in myocarditis induced by coxsackievirus group B, type 3 in Balb/c mice is mediated by Lyt 2 + cytolytic lymphocytes. Cell Immunol 1984;88:558-567.

160. Wong CY, Woodruff JJ, Woodruff JF: Generation of cytotoxic T lymphocytes during coxsackievirus B-3 infection. III. Role of sex. J Immunol 1977;119:591-597.

161. Huber SA, Pfaeffle B: Differential Th1 and Th2 cell responses in male and female BALB/c mice infected with coxsackievirus group B type 3. J Virol 1994;68:5126-5132.

162. Cho CT, Feng KK, McCarthy VP, Lenahan MF: Role of antiviral antibodies in resistance against coxsackievirus B3 infection: Interaction between preexisting antibodies and an interferon inducer. Infect Immun 1982;37:720-727.

163. Takada H, Kishimoto C, Hiraoka Y: Therapy with immunoglobulin suppresses myocarditis in a murine coxsackievirus B3 model. Antiviral and anti-inflammatory effects. Circulation 1995;92:1604-1611.

164. Sato S, Tsutsumi R, Burke A, et al: Persistence of replicating coxsackievirus B3 in the athymic murine heart is associated with development of myocarditic lesions. J Gen Virol 1994;75:2911-2924.

165. Fairweather D, Kaya Z, Shellam GR, et al: From infection to autoimmunity. J Autoimmun 2001;16:175-186.

166. Maisch B, Ristic AD, Hufnagel G, Pankuweit S: Pathophysiology of viral myocarditis: The role of humoral immune response. Cardiovasc Pathol 2002;11:112-122.

167. Huber SA: Cellular autoimmunity in myocarditis. In Cooper LT (ed): Myocarditis: From Bench to Bedside. Totowa, NJ, Humana Press, 2002, pp 55-76.

168. Gauntt CJ, Arizpe HM, Higdon AL, et al: Molecular mimicry, anti-coxsackievirus B3 neutralizing monoclonal antibodies, and myocarditis. J Immunol 1995;154:2983-2995.

169. Blay R, Simpson K, Leslie K, Huber S: Coxsackievirus-induced disease. CD4+ cells initiate both myocarditis and pancreatitis in DBA/2 mice. Am J Pathol 1989;135:899-907.

170. Schwimmbeck PL, Badorff C, Schultheiss HP, Strauer BE: Transfer of human myocarditis into severe combined immunodeficiency mice. Circ Res 1994;75:156-164.

171. Liao L, Sindhwani R, Leinwand L, et al: Cardiac alpha-myosin heavy chains differ in their induction of myocarditis: Identification of pathogenic epitopes. J Clin Invest 1993;92:2877-2882.

172. Smith SC, Allen PM: Myosin-induced acute myocarditis is a T cell-mediated disease. J Immunol 1991;147:2141-2147.

173. Li Y, Peng T, Yang Y, et al: High prevalence of enteroviral genomic sequences in myocardium from cases of endemic cardiomyopathy (Keshan disease) in China. Heart 2000;83:696-701.

174. Cheng YY, Qian PC: The effect of selenium-fortified table salt in the prevention of Keshan disease on a population of 1.05 million. Biomed Environ Sci 1990;3:422-428.

175. Beck MA: Increased virulence of coxsackievirus B3 in mice due to vitamin E or selenium deficiency. J Nutr 1997;127:966S-970S.

176. Beck MA, Shi Q, Morris VC, Levander OA: Rapid genomic evolution of a non-virulent coxsackievirus B3 in selenium-deficient mice results in selection of identical virulent isolates. Nat Med 1995;1:433-436.

177. Opavsky MA, Penninger J, Aitken K, et al: Susceptibility to myocarditis is dependent on the response of {alpha}{beta} T lymphocytes to coxsackieviral infection. Circ Res 1999;85:551-558.

178. Huber SA, Stone JE, Wagner DH Jr, et al: Gamma delta + T cells regulate major histocompatibility complex class II (IA and IE)-dependent susceptibility to coxsackievirus B3-induced autoimmune myocarditis. J Virol 1999;73:5630-5636.

179. Petrof BJ, Shrager JB, Stedman HH, et al: Dystrophin protects the sarcolemma from stresses developed during muscle contraction. Proc Natl Acad Sci 1993;90:3710-3714.

180. Tomko RP, Xu R, Philipson L: HCAR and MCAR: The human and mouse cellular receptors for subgroup C adenoviruses and group B coxsackieviruses. Proc Natl Acad Sci 1997;94:3352-3356.

181. Fiette L, Aubert C, Muller U, et al: Theiler's virus infection of 129Sv mice that lack the interferon alpha/beta or interferon gamma receptors. J Exp Med 1995;181:2069-2076.

182. Huang S, Hendriks W, Althage A, et al: Immune response in mice that lack the interferon-gamma receptor. Science 1993;259:1742-1745.

Page numbers in italics refer to illustrations; page numbers followed by t refer to tables.